Advanced Therapy of
INFLAMMATORY BOWEL DISEASE

Advanced Therapy of

INFLAMMATORY BOWEL DISEASE

Theodore M. Bayless, MD

Stephen B. Hanauer, MD

2001

B.C. Decker Inc.

Hamilton • London

B.C. Decker Inc.
20 Hughson Street South
P.O. Box 620, L.C.D. 1
Hamilton, Ontario L8N 3K7
Tel: 905-522-7017/1-800-568-7281
Fax: 905-522-7839
E-mail: info@bcdecker.com
Website: www.bcdecker.com

01 02 03 04 / BP / 6 5 4 3 2

ISBN 1-55009-122-0
Printed in Canada

Sales and Distribution

United States
B.C. Decker Inc.
P.O. Box 785
Lewiston, NY 14092-0785
Tel: 905-522-7017 / 1-800-568-7281
Fax: 905-522-7839
E-mail: info@bcdecker.com
Website: www.bcdecker.com

Canada
B.C. Decker Inc.
20 Hughson Street South
P.O. Box 620, L.C.D. 1
Hamilton, Ontario L8N 3K7
Tel: 905-522-7017 / 1-800-568-7281
Fax: 905-522-7839
E-mail: info@bcdecker.com
Website: www.bcdecker.com

Foreign Rights
John Scott & Company
International Publishers' Agency
P.O. Box 878
Kimberton, PA 19442
Tel: 610-827-1640
Fax: 610-827-1671

U.K., Europe, Scandinavia, Middle East
Harcourt Publishers Limited
Customer Service Department
Foots Cray High Street
Sidcup, Kent
DA14 5HP, UK
Tel: 44 (0) 208 308 5760
Fax: 44 (0) 181 308 5702
E-mail: cservice@harcourt_brace.com

Australia, New Zealand
Harcourt Australia Pty. Limited
Customer Service Department
STM Division
Locked Bag 16
St. Peters, New South Wales, 2044
Australia
Tel: (02) 9517-8999
Fax: (02) 9517-2249
E-mail: stmp@harcourt.com.au
Website: www.harcourt.com.au

Japan
Igaku-Shoin Ltd.
Foreign Publications Department
3-24-17 Hongo
Bunkyo-ku, Tokyo, Japan 113-8719
Tel: 3 3817 5680
Fax: 3 3815 6776
E-mail: fd@igaku.shoin.co.jp

Singapore, Malaysia, Thailand, Philippines, Indonesia, Vietnam, Pacific Rim
Harcourt Asia Pte Limited
583 Orchard Road
#09/01, Forum
Singapore 238884
Tel: 65-737-3593
Fax: 65-753-2145

This book is dedicated to the late Mrs. Lyn Pancoe Meyerhoff who, along with her husband, Harvey M. Meyerhoff, conceived and established The Harvey M. and Lyn P. Meyerhoff Center at The Johns Hopkins Medical Institutions. Her vision was of a center devoted to excellence in patient care, patient education, patient support, and basic research. During her term as President of the National Foundation for Ileitis and Colitis, she had markedly increased the number of supporters of IBD research. Mrs. Meyerhoff had also organized a major NFIC basic science meeting on IBD at Princeton, New Jersey, which in turn led to many of the successful research projects subsequently funded by the NFIC. This book is intended to bring together current opinions on patient management in all of these scientific and personal support areas that are vital to excellence in IBD management. We will always be grateful to Mrs. Meyerhoff for her foresight and leadership.

PREFACE

This is the second edition of a book devoted to the details of medical, surgical, and supportive management of patients with Crohn's disease and ulcerative colitis. The first edition, entitled *Current Management of Inflammatory Bowel Disease*, appeared in 1989. Readers and reviewers appreciated the 90 well-written "consultations" from experts of note who were able to present their views on management, treatment, and prognosis both clearly and concisely. Those authors were asked to focus on a relatively narrow and specific topic, trying to avoid generalizations and platitudes. The editor added brief comments to many of the chapters to call attention to other views or other areas of potential interest. This format provided a particularly useful book.

The current edition, entitled *Advanced Therapy of Inflammatory Bowel Disease*, includes the original 90 topics with new authors, plus 48 topics new to the book. Stephen B. Hanauer, an experienced clinician who has participated in the design and conduct of many of the controlled trials that provide the evidence base for many of our therapeutic decisions, is the coeditor. We have assumed that many of the readers of this text will be experienced and competent digestive disease specialists who have already made the correct diagnosis and are now looking for another opinion regarding a new or controversial treatment modality. Just as each of us would be tempted to call the expert on anti-TNF-alpha or on unresponsive pouchitis or on adenomas in patients with IBD, we have persuaded the experts to write a brief chapter on her or his approach to that problem. The authors have been generous with their insights and recommendations.

In these past 10 years there have been many exciting developments in IBD management. New therapies have been developed and tested; concepts of remission induction and of maintenance have been widely accepted; surgical techniques have been developed and are now widely used; experience with the management of IBD in children and teenagers has expanded; concepts of surveillance for dysplasia have been expanded to Crohn's disease and to ileoanal pouches; management of complications has become more specialized; and awareness of the quality of life and supportive services are receiving more attention.

Certain topics, such as immunomodulators and anticytokine therapy are covered in more than one chapter. Clearly there are divergent opinions on a number of medical and surgical topics, and we have considered it worthwhile to hear from proponents on several sides of various issues. Most chapters end with a list of supplemental readings and references. This has been more useful than asking the author to document every opinion. We want to know what they do and this usually goes beyond the results of clinical trials and evidence-based medicine. As in many phases of medicine, there still are a lot of unanswered questions that we as clinicians face almost daily. There are more chapters on "humanistic" aspects of the management of chronic digestive diseases than one finds in most medical or surgical books. These reflect our interests in the natural history of IBD and in patient–physician interactions. We are keenly aware of the need for additional laboratory and clinical research to provide further understanding of the etiology, genetics, and pathogenesis of Crohn's disease and ulcerative colitis. The future will include even better care and hopefully a cure and prevention of these chronic and potentially devastating illnesses. Ensuing editions will chronicle those improvements in management of IBD.

We are grateful to our patients who have taught us the importance of many of the issues in this book; to the authors, who generously shared their views with us; to our colleagues at the Meyerhoff IBD Center at Johns Hopkins and at the Joseph B. Kirsner IBD Center at the University of Chicago, who have participated in the patient care and research that form many of our views of IBD management; to the members, officers, and staff of the Crohn's & Colitis Foundation of America (CCFA), who have helped us to appreciate the many-faceted needs of patients with IBD; and to our publisher Brian Decker of B.C. Decker Inc., and his editorial staff, notably Laurie Thomas and Jon Pressick. Thanks to Donna Rode, our administrative assistant in Baltimore who coordinated the entire effort. Our profound thanks to our wives, children, and grandchildren who gave up *their* time to permit this type of endeavor.

T. M. Bayless, MD
S.B. Hanauer, MD

CONTRIBUTORS

Kareem Abu-Elmagd, MD, PhD
Associate Professor of Surgery
University of Pittsburgh
    Medical Center
Pittsburgh, Pennsylvania

Grant J. Anhalt, MD
Professor of Dermatology and
    Pathology
Johns Hopkins Hospital
Baltimore, Maryland

Robert D. Baker, MD, PhD
Co-Director, Pediatric GI/Nutrition/
    Hepatology
Medical University of South Carolina
Charleston, South Carolina

Susan S. Baker, MD, PhD
Department of Pediatrics
Medical University of South Carolina
Charleston, South Carolina

Peter A. Banks, MD
Professor of Medicine
Harvard Medical School
Director, Clinical Gastroenterology
    Service
Brigham and Women's Hospital
Boston, Massachusetts

Theodore M. Bayless, MD
Professor of Medicine
Clinical Director
Meyerhoff Inflammatory Bowel
    Disease Center
Johns Hopkins Hospital
Baltimore, Maryland

James M. Becker, MD
James Utley Professor and Chairman
Boston University School of Medicine
Surgeon-in-Chief
Boston University Medical Center
Boston, Massachusetts

Charles N. Bernstein, MD, FRCPC
Associate Professor of Medicine
University of Manitoba
University of Manitoba Health
    Sciences Centre
Winnipeg, Manitoba

**Ingvar Bjarnason, MD, MSc,
    FRCPath, DSc**
Professor of Medicine
Guy's King's St Thomas' School
    of Medicine
Consulting Physician and
    Gastroenterologist
London, United Kingdom

Jason H. Bodzin, MD
Clinical Associate Professor of Surgery
Wayne State University School of
    Medicine
Detroit, Michigan
William Beaumont Hospital
Royal Oak, Michigan

Steven R. Brant, MD
Assistant Professor of Medicine
Johns Hopkins University School
    of Medicine
Director, Meyerhoff Genetics
    Laboratory
Johns Hopkins Hospital
Baltimore, Maryland

Teresa A. Brentnall, MD
Assistant Professor in
    Gastroenterology
University of Washington
University of Washington
    Medical Center
Seattle, Washington

Jean-Marc Brunetaud, MD, PhD
Professor of Medicine
Director, Centre des Lasers
Lille Medical School
Lille University Hospital
Lille, France

Alan L. Buchman, MD, MSPH
Division of Gastroenterology and
    Hepatology
Northwestern University
    Medical School
Northwestern Memorial Hospital
Lakeside Veterans Administration
    Medical Center
Chicago, Illinois

Robert Burakoff, MD
Gastroenterology Chief
Washington Hospital Center
Washington, District of Columbia

Massimo Campieri, MD
Professor of Internal Medicine
Department of Internal Medicine and
    Gastroenterology
University of Bologna
Bologna, Italy

Dina F. Caroline, MD
Professor of Radiology
Temple University School of Medicine
Section Head, Abdominal Radiography
Temple University Hospital
Philadelphia, Pennsylvania

H. Ballentine Carter, MD
Professor of Urology
Johns Hopkins Medical Institutions
Baltimore, Maryland

David Y. Chan, MD
Department of Surgery
Johns Hopkins Medical Institutions
Baltimore, Maryland

Judy H. Cho, MD
Assistant Professor of Medicine
University of Chicago
The Martin Boyer Laboratories
Gastroenterology Section
Department of Medicine
Chicago, Illinois

Robynne Chutkan, MD
Assistant Professor of Medicine
Division of Gastroenterology
Georgetown University Medical Center
Washington, District of Columbia

Maria I. Clavell, MD
Department of Pediatrics
Medical University of South Carolina
Children's Hospital Medical University
of South Carolina
Charleston, South Carolina

Harris R. Clearfield, MD
Professor of Medicine
Section Chief of Gastrointestinal
Division
MCP-Hahnemann University
Hahnemann University Hospital
Philadelphia, Pennsylvania

Ray E. Clouse, MD
Professor of Medicine and
of Psychiatry
Washington University
Physician
Barnes-Jewish Hospital
St. Louis, Minnesota

Dominique Cochelard
Senior Lecturer
Lille Medical School
Lille, France

**Stephen M. Collins, MBBG,
FRCP(UK), FRCPC**
Professor of Medicine
McMaster University
Chief of Gastroenterology
Hamilton Health Sciences Corporation
Hamilton, Ontario

Jean-Frédéric Colombel, MD
Professor, Lille University
Lille, France

Janice C. Colwell, RN, MS, CWOCN
Clinical Nurse Specialist in Wound,
Ostomy, and Skin Care
University of Chicago Hospitals
Chicago, Illinois

Antoine Cortot, MD
Professor, Lille University
Lille, France

Marcia Cruz-Correa, MD
Fellow, Gastroenterology
Johns Hopkins Hospital
Baltimore, Maryland

Carmen Cuffari, MD
Assistant Professor of Pediatrics
Johns Hopkins Hospital
Baltimore, Maryland

Henry Cymorek, MD
Fellow, Division of Gastroenterology
University of Connecticut
Health Center
Farmington, Connecticut

Geert D'Haens, MD, PhD
University of Leuven
Imelda General Hospital
University Hospital, Sasthuisberg
Bonheiden, Belgium

**Benedict M. Devereaux, MB, BS,
FRACP**
ERCP Fellow
Division of Gastroenterology
Indiana University Medical Center
Indianapolis, Indiana

Douglas A. Drossman, MD
Professor of Medicine and Psychiatry
Department of Medicine, Division
of Digestive Diseases
University of North Carolina at
Chapel Hill
Co-Director, UNC Center for
Functional Gastrointestinal and
Motility Disorders
Chapel Hill, North Carolina

David Edwin, PhD
Associate Professor
Department of Psychiatry and
Behavioral Sciences
Johns Hopkins University School of
Medicine
Division of Medical Psychology
Johns Hopkins Hospital
Baltimore, Maryland

Laurence J. Egan, MD
Assistant Professor of Medicine
Mayo Clinic
Rochester, Minnesota

Charles O. Elson, MD
Basil I Hirschowitz Chair
in Gastroenterology
University of Alabama
University Hospital
Birmingham, Alabama

**Paula Erwin-Toth, MSN, RN, ET,
CWOCN, CNS**
Director, R.B. Turnbull Jr School of
Enterostomal Therapy Nursing
Cleveland Clinic Foundation
Cleveland, Ohio

Maria Esteve, MD
Senior Research Fellow
University Hospital
Barcelona, Spain

Z. Myron Falchuk, MD
Associate Professor of Medicine
Harvard Medical School
Chief, Clinical Gastroenterology
Beth Israel Deaconess Medical Center
Boston, Massachusetts

James J. Farrell, MD
Harvard Medical School
Gastrointestinal Unit
Massachusetts General Hospital
Boston, Massachusetts

Richard J. Farrell, MD, MRCPI
Instructor in Medicine
Harvard Medical School
Staff Gastroenterologist
Beth Israel Deaconess Medical Center
Boston, Massachusetts

Forough Farrokhyar, PhD
McMaster University
Hamilton, Ontario, Canada

Victor W. Fazio, MB, MS, FRACS, FACS
Professor of Surgery
Ohio State University School
of Medicine
Cleveland Clinic Health Sciences
Center
Rupert Turnball Chairman
Department of Colrectal Surgery
Cleveland Clinic Foundation
Cleveland, Ohio

Brian G. Feagan, MD
Professor of Medicine, Epidemiology,
and Biostatistics
University of Western Ontario
London Health Sciences Centre
University Campus
London, Ontario

George D. Ferry, MD
Professor of Pediatrics
Baylor College of Medicine
Chief, Gastrointestinal and Nutrition
Clinic
Texas Children's Hospital
Houston, Texas

Rosemarie L. Fisher, MD
Professor of Medicine
Yale University School of Medicine
Yale–New Haven Hospital
New Haven, Connecticut

Eliot K. Fishman, MD
Professor of Radiology and Oncology
Department of Radiology
Johns Hopkins Medical Institutions
Baltimore, Maryland

Sandy L. Fogel, MD
Assistant Professor of Surgery
Johns Hopkins School of Medicine
Johns Hopkins Hospital
Baltimore, Maryland

Eric W. Fonkalsrud, MD
Professor and Chief of Pediatric
Surgery
University of California, Los Angeles
School of Medicine
Los Angeles, California

Sonia Friedman, MD
Instructor in Medicine
Harvard Medical School
Associate Physician in Medicine
Brigham and Women's Hospital
Boston, Massachusetts

Lawrence S. Friedman, MD
Associate Professor of Medicine
Harvard Medical School
Physician, Gastrointestinal Unit
Chief, Walter Bauer Firm
Massachusetts General Hospital
Boston, Massachusetts

Christoph Gasche, MD
Associate Professor of Medicine
University of Vienna
Vienna, Austria

Miguel A. Gassull, MD, PhD
Associate Professor of Medicine
Head of the Department of
Gastroenterology and Hepatology
University Hospital
Barcelona, Spain

Kevin T. Geraci, MD
Clinical Associate Professor
Case Western University
University Hospital of Cleveland
Cleveland, Ohio

Francis M. Giardiello, MD
Associate Professor
Johns Hopkins University School of
Medicine
Director, Gastroenterology Division
Johns Hopkins Hospital
Baltimore, Maryland

Geoffrey Gibson, MD
Department of Gastroenterology
Royal Adelaide Hospital
Adelaide, Australia

Allen L. Ginsberg, MD
Professor of Medicine
Director, Division of Gastroenterology
George Washington University School
of Medicine
Washington, District of Columbia

Seth N. Glick, MD
Department of Radiology
Temple University Hospital
Philadelphia, Pennsylvania

Ranjana Gokhale, MD
Assistant Professor
University of Chicago
University of Chicago Children's
Hospital
Chicago, Illinois

Julio A. Gonzalez, MD
Johns Hopkins University School
of Medicine
Johns Hopkins Hospital
Baltimore, Maryland

Gordon R. Greenberg, MD, FRCP(C)
Professor of Medicine
University of Toronto
Head, Division of Gastroenterology
Mount Sinai Hospital
Toronto, Ontario

Adrian J. Greenstein, MD
Professor of Surgery
Mount Sinai School of Medicine
Mount Sinai Hospital
New York, New York

Anne M. Griffiths, MD, FRCP(C)
Associate Professor of Pediatrics
University of Toronto
Director, Inflammatory Bowel Disease
Program
The Hospital for Sick Children
Toronto, Ontario

Matthew B. Grisham, PhD
Professor
Department of Molecular and Cellular
Physiology
Louisiana State University Health
Sciences Center
Shreveport, Louisiana

Stephen B. Hanauer, MD
Professor of Medicine and Clinical
Pharmacology
Director, Section of Gastroenterology
and Nutrition
University of Chicago
Chicago, Illinois

Mary Lawrence Harris, MD
Associate Professor of Medicine
Johns Hopkins Hospital
Baltimore, Maryland

David B. Hellmann, MD
Mary Betty Stevens Professor
    of Medicine
Johns Hopkins University School
    of Medicine
Co-Director, Johns Hopkins Vasculitis
    Center
Director, Medicine
Johns Hopkins-Bayview Hospital
Baltimore, Maryland

Robert J. Hilsden, MD, MSc, FRCPC
Department of Community Health
    Sciences
University of Calgary
Calgary, Alberta

Humphrey J.F. Hodgson, MD, FRCP
Professor of Medicine, University
    College
Chief, Hepatology and Gastro-
    enterology
Royal Free Hospital
London, United Kingdom

Peter A. Holt, MD
Associate Professor of Rheumatology
Good Samaritan Hospital
Baltimore, Maryland

Karen M. Horton, MD
Assistant Professor, Department of
    Radiology
Johns Hopkins Medical Institutions
Baltimore, Maryland

Tracy L. Hull, MD
Department of Colon and Rectal
    Surgery
Cleveland Clinic Foundation
Cleveland, Ohio

Sharon A. Hunt, BSN, RN
Blaine Franklin Newman
    Inflammatory Bowel Disease
    Nurse Advocate
Meyerhoff Inflammatory Bowel
    Disease Center
Johns Hopkins Hospital
Baltimore, Maryland

Roger D. Hurst, MD
Assistant Professor of Clinical Surgery
Department of Surgery
University of Chicago
University of Chicago Hospitals
Chicago, Illinois

Jeffrey S. Hyams, MD
Professor of Pediatrics
University of Connecticut School
    of Medicine
Pediatric Gastroenterologist
Connecticut Children's Medical Center
Hartford, Connecticut

Nuzhat Iqbal, MD
Gastroenterology Division
University of Alabama
Birmingham, Alabama

E. Jan Irvine, MD
Professor of Medicine
McMaster University
Staff Gastroenterologist
Hamilton Health Sciences Corporation
Hamilton, Ontario

Kim L. Isaacs, MD, PhD
Associate Professor of Medicine
University of North Carolina
Division of Digestive Diseases and
    Nutrition
University of North Carolina Hospitals
Chapel Hill, North Carolina

Douglas A. Jabs, MD, MBA
Professor of Ophthalmology
    and Medicine
Johns Hopkins University School
    of Medicine
Professor of Epidemiology
Johns Hopkins University School of
    Public Health and Hygiene
Johns Hopkins Hospital
Baltimore, Maryland

Stephen P. James, MD
Head of Gastroenterology
University of Maryland School
    of Medicine
University of Maryland Medical
    Center
Baltimore, Maryland

Gunnar Järnerot, MD, PhD, FRCP
Professor of Gastroenterology
Health University
Consultant Gastroenterologist
Örebro Medical Center Hospital
Örebro, Sweden

Anthony N. Kalloo, MD
Associate Professor of Medicine
Director of Endoscopy
Johns Hopkins Hospital
Baltimore, Maryland

Theodore J. Kalogeris, PhD
Assistant Professor
Departments of Surgery and
    Molecular and Cellular Physiology
Louisiana State University Health
    Sciences Center
Shreveport, Louisiana

Sunanda V. Kane, MD, MSPH
Inflammatory Bowel Disease Center
University of Chicago Hospitals
Chicago, Illinois

Marshall M. Kaplan, MD
Tufts University School of Medicine
New England Medical Center
Boston, Massachusetts

Loren C. Karp, MA
Researcher/Specialist
Cedars-Sinai Inflammatory Bowel
    Disease Center
Los Angeles, California

Jeffry A. Katz, MD
Assistant Professor of Medicine
Case Western Reserve University
Cleveland, Ohio

Seymour Katz, MD
Clinical Professor of Medicine
New York University School
    of Medicine
North Shore University Hospital -
    Long Island Jewish Health System
Great Neck, New York

Keith A. Kelly, MD
Professor of Surgery
Mayo Medical School
Mayo Clinic
Scottsdale, Arizona

Barbara S. Kirschner, MD
Professor of Pediatrics and Medicine
University of Chicago
Section of Pediatric Gastroenterology,
    Hepatology & Nutrition
University of Chicago Children's
    Hospital
Chicago, Illinois

Andrew S. Klein, MD
Associate Professor of Surgery
Chief, Division of Transplantation
Director, Comprehensive Transplant
    Center
Johns Hopkins University School
    of Medicine
Baltimore, Maryland

Gary I. Kleiner, MD, PhD
Mount Sinai Medical Center
New York, New York

Walter A. Koltun, MD
Associate Professor of Surgery
Pennsylvania State College
    of Medicine
Chief, Section of Colon and
    Rectal Surgery
Milton S. Hershey Medical Center
Hershey, Pennsylvania

Burton I. Korelitz, MD
Clinical Professor of Medicine
New York University Medical Center
Chief of Gastroenterology
Lenox Hill Hospital
New York, New York

Asher Kornbluth, MD
Associate Clinical Professor
    of Medicine
Mount Sinai School of Medicine
New York, New York

Richard A. Kozarek, MD
Clinical Professor of Medicine
University of Washington
Chief of Gastroenterology
Virginia Mason Medical Center
Seattle, Washington

Prasanna Kumaranayake, BSc, MD, FRCPC
University of Western Ontario
Department of Gastroenterology
London Health Sciences Centre
London, Ontario

Alex Ky, MD
Resident in Colorectal Surgery
Mount Sinai School of Medicine
New York, New York

Bret A. Lashner, MD
Director, Center for Inflammatory
    Bowel Disease
Cleveland Clinic Foundation
Cleveland, Ohio

Paul A. Latkany, MD
Assistant Professor, Department of
    Ophthalmology
Johns Hopkins University School
    of Medicine
Johns Hopkins Hospital
Baltimore, Maryland

Ian C. Lavery, MBBS, FRACS, FACS
Ohio State University
Cleveland Clinic
Cleveland, Ohio

Konstantinos N. Lazaridis, MD
Fellow in Gastroenterology
Division of Gastroenterology
    and Hepatology
Mayo Clinic
Rochester, Minnesota

Jeffrey H. Lee, MD
Assistant Professor
Yale University School of Medicine
New Haven Hospital
New Haven, Connecticut

Kenneth K. W. Lee, MD, FACS
Department of Surgery
University of Pittsburgh School
    of Medicine
University of Pittsburgh Medical
    Center
Pittsburgh, Pennsylvania

Linda A. Lee, MD
Assistant Professor
Johns Hopkins University School
    of Medicine
Johns Hopkins Hospital
Baltimore, Maryland

Scott D. Lee, MD
Senior Fellow, Gastroenterology
University of Washington
Seattle, Washington

Young-Mee Lee, MD
Tufts University School of Medicine
New England Medical Center
Boston, Massachusetts

Glen A. Lehman, MD
Professor of Medicine
Department of Gastroenterology
Indiana University Medical Center
Indianapolis, Indiana

Joel B. Levine, MD
Professor of Medicine
Division of Gastroenterology
University of Connecticut Health
    Center
Farmington, Connecticut

Gary R. Lichtenstein, MD
Associate Professor of Medicine
University of Pennsylvania School
    of Medicine
Director, Center for Inflammatory
    Bowel Diseases
Philadelphia, Pennsylvania

Keith D. Lindor, MD
Professor of Medicine
Consultant and Chair, Division of
    Gastroenterology and Hepatology
Mayo Clinic
Rochester, Minnesota

Ian C. Lindsey, MBBS, FRACS
Fellow, Colorectal Unit
John Radcliffe Hospital
Oxford, United Kingdom

Robert Löfberg, MD, PhD
Associate Professor of Medicine
Karolinska Institute
Head, Inflammatory Bowel
    Disease Unit
Huddinge University Hospital
Huddinge, Sweden

Richard P. MacDermott, MD
Professor of Medicine
Head, Division of Gastroenterology
Albany Medical College
Albany, New York

Peter W. Marcello, MD
Assistant Professor of Surgery
Tufts University School of Medicine
Staff Surgeon, Lahey Clinic
Burlington, Massachusetts

Jay Soloman Markowitz
Assistant Professor of Surgery
Johns Hopkins University
Baltimore, Maryland

Sharon Masel
Inflammatory Bowel Disease Center
University of Chicago
Chicago, Illinois

Lloyd Mayer, MD
Chairman, Immunobiology Center
Professor of Medicine,
    Immunobiology and Microbiology
Mount Sinai Medical Center
New York, New York

Marcovalerio Melis, MD
Research Associate
Department of Surgery
University of Chicago
University of Chicago Hospitals
Chicago, Illinois

Marjorie Merrick
Director of Research and Education
Crohn's & Colitis Foundation
    of America
New York, New York

Fabrizio Michelassi, MD
Professor and Vice Chairman
Chief, Section of General Surgery
University of Chicago
University of Chicago Hospitals
Chicago, Illinois

Pierre Michetti, MD
Harvard Medical School
Division of Gastroenterology
Beth Israel Deaconess Medical Center
Boston, Massachusetts

Jeffrey W. Milsom, MD
Professor of Surgery
Co-Director, Minimally Invasive
    Surgery Center
Mount Sinai School of Medicine
Mount Sinai Medical Center
New York, New York

Philip B. Miner Jr., MD
Clinical Professor, Oklahoma
    University School of Medicine
President and Medical Director
Oklahoma Foundation For Digestive
    Research
Oklahoma City, Oklahoma

Neil J. McC. Mortensen, MD, FRCS
Consultant Colorectal Surgeon,
    Colorectal Unit
John Radcliffe Hospital
Oxford, United Kingdom

Gabriele Moser, MD
Head, Psychosomatic Outpatient
    Clinic
Department of Gastroenterology
    and Hepatology
Vice-Rector
University of Vienna
Vienna, Austria

Douglas G. Moss, MD
Department of Obstetrics
Mount Sinai Hospital
Mount Sinai School of Medicine
New York, New York

Ulf Müller-Ladner, MD
Department of Internal Medicine
University of Regensburg
Regensburg, Germany

Sateesh Nair, MD
Fellow, Gastroenterology Division
Johns Hopkins Hospital
Baltimore, Maryland

Peter Nielsen
Former Mr. America and Mr. Universe
Fitness Consultant
Detroit, Michigan

Hossein C. Nousari, MD
Department of Dermatology
Johns Hopkins Hospital
Baltimore, Maryland

Patrick L. O'Kane, MD
Department of Radiology
Temple University Hospital
Philadelphia, Pennsylvania

Choon Jin Ooi, MD
Center for the Study of Inflammatory
    Bowel Diseases
Harvard Medical School
Gastrointestinal Unit
Massachusetts General Hospital
Boston, Massachusetts

**Timothy R. Orchard, MA, MD, DM,
MRCP**
Research Fellow
Gastroenterology Unit
Radcliffe Infirmary
Oxford, United Kingdom

John H. Pemberton, MD
Professor of Surgery
Mayo Medical School
Mayo Clinic
Rochester, Minnesota

Mark A. Peppercorn
Professor of Medicine, Harvard
    Medical School
Director of Center for Inflammatory
    Bowel Disease
Division of Gastroenterology
Beth Israel Deaconess Medical Center
Boston, Massachusetts

Robert E. Petras, MD
Chair, Department of Anatomic
    Pathology
Cleveland Clinic Foundation
Cleveland, Ohio

Sidney F. Phillips, MD
Professor of Medicine
Mayo Medical School
Karl F. and Marjory Hasselmann
    Professor of Research
Mayo Clinic
Rochester, Minnesota

Michael F. Picco, MD, PhD
Assistant Professor of Medicine
Mayo Medical School
Mayo Clinic
Jacksonville, Florida

Alan J. Pikarsky, MD
Clinical Fellow
Department of Colorectal Surgery
Cleveland Clinic
Fort Lauderdale, Florida

Daniel K. Podolsky, MD
Mallinckrodt Professor of Medicine
Harvard Medical School
Chief, Gastrointestinal Unit
Massachusetts General Hospital
Boston, Massachusetts

Kathleen L. Potter, RN, BSN, COCN
Department of Surgery
Johns Hopkins Hospital
Baltimore, Maryland

Cosimo Prantera, MD
Chief of the Division of
    Gastroenterology
Azienda Ospedialiera S.
    Camillo-Forianini
Rome, Italy

Daniel H. Present, MD
Clinical Professor
Mount Sinai School of Medicine
Attending Physician
Mount Sinai Hospital
New York, New York

Thomas T. Provost, MD
Department of Dermatology
Johns Hopkins Medical Institutions
Baltimore, Maryland

Ramona Rajapakse, MD
Gastroenterology Division
Lenox Hill Hospital
New York, New York

Feza H. Remzi, MD
Department of Colorectal Surgery
Cleveland Clinic Health Sciences
    Center
Cleveland, Ohio

John Rhodes
Professor of Medicine
Department of Gastroenterology
University Hospital of Wales
Cardiff, United Kingdom

Elena Ricart, MD
Research Fellow of the Inflammatory
    Bowel Disease Clinic
Mayo Clinic
Rochester, Minnesota

Arvey I. Rogers, MD, FACP
Professor of Medicine
University of Miami
University of Miami Hospital
    and Clinics
Miami, Florida

Richard P. Rood, MD, FACP
Assistant Clinical Professor
    of Medicine
Case Western Reserve University
School of Medicine
Cleveland, Ohio

William A. Rowe, MD
Section of Gastroenterology and
    Hepatology
Pennsylvania State University College
    of Medicine
Milton S. Hershey Medical Center
Hershey, Pennsylvania

Peter H. Rubin, MD
Clinical Associate Professor of Medicine
Mount Sinai School of Medicine
Attending Physician
Mount Sinai Hospital
New York, New York

Paul J. Rutgeerts, MD, PhD, FRCP
Professor of Medicine
Department of Medicine
University of Leuven
Leuven, Belgium

Murray Saltzman, DDS, DHL, DD
Rabbi Emeritus
Baltimore Hebrew Congregation
Baltimore, Maryland

William J. Sandborn, MD
Associate Professor of Medicine
Mayo Medical School
Head, Inflammatory Bowel Disease
    Clinic
Mayo Clinic
Rochester, Minnesota

R. Balfour Sartor, MD
Professor of Medicine, Microbiology,
    and Immunology
University of North Carolina School
    of Medicine
Director, Multidisciplinary Center for
    Inflammatory Bowel Disease
    Research and Therapy
Chapel Hill, North Carolina

Lawrence R. Schiller, MD
Department of Gastroenterology
University of Texas Southwestern
    Medical School
Baylor University Medical Center
Dallas, Texas

David J. Schoetz Jr, MD
Professor of Surgery
Tufts University School of Medicine
Chairman, Department of Colon
    and Rectal Surgery
Lahey Clinic
Burlington, Massachusetts

Jürgen Schölmerich, MD
Department of Internal Medicine
University of Regensburg
Regensburg, Germany

Maria Lia Scribano, MD
Gastroenterologist
Division of Gastroenterology
Azienda Ospedialiera S.
    Camillo-Forianini
Rome, Italy

David A. Schwartz, MD
Gastroenterology Section
Mayo Clinic
Rochester, Minnesota

Ernest G. Seidman, MD, FRCPC
Departments of Pediatrics and
    Nutrition
University of Montreal
Chief, Gastrointestinal & Nutrition
    Division
Ste Justine Hospital
Montreal, QC, Canada

Joseph Sellin, MD
Division of Gastroenterology and
    Hepatology,
University of Texas—Houston Health
    Sciences Center
Memorial Hermann Hospital
Houston, Texas

Harry S. Shabsin, PhD
Psychologist
Baltimore, Maryland

Stuart Sherman, MD
Department of Gastroenterology
Indiana University Medical Center
Indianapolis, Indiana

John W. Singleton, MD
Professor of Medicine
University of Colorado Health
 Sciences Center
University of Colorado Hospital
Denver, Colorado

Michael D. Sitrin, MD
Professor of Medicine
University of Chicago
Chicago, Illinois

Simon Smale, BMBS, MRCP
Department of Gastroenterology
Kings College Hospital
Denmark Hill
London, United Kingdom

Konrad H. Soergel, MD
Professor of Medicine
Medical College of Wisconsin
Division of Gastroenterology and
 Hepatology
Froedtert Memorial Lutheran Hospital
Milwaukee, Wisconsin

Peter S. Staats, MD
Assistant Professor
Anesthesiology and Critical Care
 Medicine
Johns Hopkins University School
 of Medicine
Johns Hopkins Hospital
Baltimore, Maryland

Scott A. Strong, MD
Department of Colorectal Surgery
Cleveland Clinic Foundation
Cleveland, Ohio

Christina M. Surawicz, MD
Professor of Medicine
University of Washington School of
 Medicine
Chief, Gastroenterology
Harborview Medical Center
Seattle, Washington

**Lloyd R. Sutherland, MDCM, MSc,
 FRCPC, FACP**
Professor, Head, Department of
 Community Health Sciences
University of Calgary
Foothills Hospital
Calgary, Alberta

Francisco A. Sylvester, MD
Assistant Professor of Pediatrics
University of Connecticut School
 of Medicine
Pediatric Gastroenterologist
Connecticut Children's Medical Center
Hartford, Connecticut

Mark A. Talamini, MD
Associate Professor of Surgery
Director of Minimally Invasive
 Surgery
Johns Hopkins Hospital
Baltimore, Maryland

Henkie Tan, MD, PhD
Fellow, Gastroenterology Division
Johns Hopkins University
Johns Hopkins Hospital
Baltimore, Maryland

Stephan R. Targan, MD
Professor of Medicine
University of California, Los Angeles
School of Medicine
Cedars-Sinai Medical Center
Los Angeles, California

Mark L. Teitelbaum, MD
Associate Professor of Psychiatry
 and Medicine
Johns Hopkins University School
 of Medicine
Attending Psychiatrist
Johns Hopkins Hospital
Baltimore, Maryland

Gareth Thomas, MD, BSc, MRCP
Department of Gastroenterology
University Hospital of Wales
Cardiff, United Kingdom

Paul J. Thuluvath, MD, FRCP
Associate Professor of Medicine
Johns Hopkins University
Johns Hopkins Hospital
Baltimore, Maryland

William J. Tremaine, MD
Associate Professor of Medicine
Director, Inflammatory Bowel
 Disease Clinic
Mayo Clinic
Rochester, Minnesota

Alethea Trinkaus, MPH
Crohn's & Colitis Foundation of
 America
New York, New York

Georgia B. Vogelsang
Professor of Oncology
Johns Hopkins University
Johns Hopkins Hospital
Baltimore, Maryland

H. Richard Waranch, PhD
Assistant Professor
Medical Psychology and Psychiatry
Johns Hopkins Medical Institutions
Baltimore, Maryland

Bryan F. Warren, MB, ChB, MRCPath
Consultant Gastrointestinal
 Histopathologist
John Radcliffe Hospital
Oxford, United Kingdom

Jerome D. Waye, MD, FACP
Clinical Professor of Medicine
Mount Sinai Medical Center
Chief, Gastrointestinal Endoscopy Unit
Mount Sinai Hospital
New York, New York

Steven D. Wexner, MD
Professor of Surgery
Ohio State University
Chairman and Chief of Staff
Department of Colorectal Surgery
Cleveland Clinic Florida
Fort Lauderdale, Florida

Christopher Willet, MD
Harvard Medical School
Massachusetts General Hospital
Boston, Massachusetts

C. Noel Williams, MRCS, LRCP, FRCP(C), FACP
Professor of Medicine
Dalhousie University
Staff Gastroenterologist
Queen Elizabeth II Health Sciences Centre
Halifax, Nova Scotia

Harland S. Winter, MD
Associate Professor of Pediatrics
Harvard Medical School
Director, Pediatric Inflammatory Bowel Disease Center
Massachusetts General Hospital
Boston, Massachusetts

Douglas C. Wolf, MD
Clinical Assistant Professor of Medicine
Emory University School of Medicine
Atlanta, Georgia

Jacqueline L. Wolf, MD
Associate Professor of Medicine
Harvard Medical School
Director, Inflammatory Bowel Disease Center
Brigham and Women's Hospital
Boston, Massachusetts

Bruce R. Yacyshyn, MD, FRCPC
Associate Professor
University of Alberta
University of Alberta Hospital
Edmonton, Alberta

Albert M. Yunich, MD
Professor of Medicine
Albany Medical College
Head, Division of Gastroenterology
Albany Medical Center
Albany, New York

Thomas A. Zizic, MD
Associate Professor of Rheumatology
Johns Hopkins Hospital
Baltimore, Maryland

TABLE OF CONTENTS

INTRODUCTION

1. Patient-Doctor Interactions   1
    Stephen B. Hanauer, MD

2. Pediatric Patient, Family, Doctor Interactions   5
    George D. Ferry, MD

3. Adherence Issues in Management of Inflammatory Bowel Disease   9
    Sunanda Kane, MD, MSPH

4. Managing Inflammatory Bowel Disease in the Managed Care Era   13
    Seymour Katz, MD

5. Medical-Surgical Collaboration in Patient Management   19
    Fabrizio Michelassi, MD, and Stephen B. Hanauer, MD

6. Consultations and the Patient with Inflammatory Bowel Disease   23
    Harris R. Clearfield, MD

DIAGNOSTIC METHODOLOGY

7. Measures of Disease Activity   25
    John W. Singleton, MD

8. Computer Database for Patients with Inflammatory Bowel Disease   29
    Jean-Frédéric Colombel, MD, Dominique Cochelard, PhD, Antoine Cortot, MD,
    and Jean-Marc Brunetaud, MD, PhD

9. Useful Biologic Markers as Activity Indices   35
    Jeffry A. Katz, MD

10. Imaging of Mucosal Inflammation   39
    Dina F. Caroline, MD, Seth N. Glick, MD, and Patrick L. O'Kane, MD

11. Crohn's Disease: Computed Tomographic Scanning in Clinical Decision Making   47
    Karen M. Horton, MD, and Elliot K. Fishman, MD

12. Transabdominal Bowel Sonography in Clinical Decision-making   55
    Christoph Gasche, MD

PROCTO-SIGMOIDITIS

13.   Mode of Action of Anti-inflammatory Agents   63
      Theodore Kalogeris, PhD, and Matthew B. Grisham, PhD

14.   Management of Distal Colitis   69
      Massimo Campieri, MD

15.   Topically Active Corticosteroids for Colitis   73
      Gordon R. Greenberg, MD, FRCP(C)

16.   Pseudo-intractability of Inflammatory Bowel Disease   77
      Arvey I. Rogers, MD, FACP

17.   Refractory Distal Colitis   81
      Philip B. Miner Jr., MD

18.   Coexistence of Inflammatory Bowel Disease and Irritable Bowel Syndrome   87
      Stephen M. Collins, MBBG, FRCP(UK), FRCPC

19.   Coexistent Irritable Bowel Syndrome and Inflammatory Bowel Disease   91
      Theodore M. Bayless, MD

20.   Infectious Agents as Aggravating Factors in Inflammatory Bowel Disease   95
      Scott D. Lee, MD, and Christina M. Surawicz, MD

21.   Use of Nicotine and Tobacco in Colitis   99
      Elena Ricart, MD, and William J. Sandborn, MD

22.   Immunomodulator Use in Patients with Distal Colitis   103
      Stephen P. James, MD

23.   Mucosal Protective and Repair Agents in the Treatment of Colitis   107
      John Rhodes and Gareth Thomas, MD, BSc, MRCP

ULCERATIVE COLITIS

24.   Therapeutic Expectations: Medical Management of Ulcerative Colitis   111
      Stephen B. Hanauer, MD

25.   Sequential and Combination Therapy of Ulcerative Colitis   115
      William J. Tremaine, MD

26.   Ulcerative Colitis: A Diverse Disease with Diverse Questions and Diverse Solutions   119
      Kevin T. Geraci, MD

27.   Aminosalicylates Therapy for Ulcerative Colitis   123
      Stephen B. Hanauer, MD

28.   Systemic Corticosteroids in Inflammatory Bowel Disease   127
      Humphrey J.F. Hodgson, MD, FRCP

29.   Steroid Unresponsiveness in Inflammatory Bowel Disease   133
      Miquel A. Gassull, MD, PhD, and Maria Esteve, MD

30. Immunomodulators in Ulcerative Colitis — 139
Asher Kornbluth, MD

31. Management of Severe Ulcerative Colitis — 143
Gunnar Järnerot, MD, PhD, FRCP

32. Use of Antibiotics and Other Anti-infectious Agents in Ulcerative Colitis — 149
Pierre Michetti, MD, and Mark A. Peppercorn, MD

33. Management of Ulcerative Colitis in Children — 153
Harland S. Winter, MD

34. Indeterminate Colitis — 157
Richard P. MacDermott, MD

35. Dietary Recommendations for Active and Inactive Ulcerative Colitis — 161
Geoffrey Gibson, MD

36. Novel Manipulations of Inflammatory Mediator Pathways — 165
Bruce R. Yacyshyn, MD, FRCPC

SURGERY FOR ULCERATIVE COLITIS

37. Therapeutic Expectations: Surgical Management of Ulcerative Colitis — 171
Keith A. Kelly, MD

38. Indications for Colectomy and Choice of Procedures — 175
James M. Becker, MD

39. Role of the Enterostomal Therapy Nurse — 179
Janice C. Colwell, RN, MS, CWOCN

40. Brooke Ileostomy — 185
Jason H. Bodzin, MD

41. Continent Ileostomy (Kock Pouch) — 191
Sandy L. Fogel, MD

42. Ileoanal Pouch Anastomosis — 197
Feza H. Remzi, MD, and Victor W. Fazio, MB, MS, FRACS, FACS

43. Long-Term Results with Ileoanal pouch — 203
John H. Pemberton, MD

44. Ileoanal Pouch: Evaluation of Excessive Bowel Movements — 209
Lawrence J. Egan, MD, and Sidney F. Phillips, MD

45. Ileoanal Pouch Surgery in Childhood — 215
Eric W. Fonkalsrud, MD

46. Chronic Pouchitis — 219
David A. Schwartz, MD, and William J. Sandborn, MD

47. Endoscopy in Evaluating Ileal Pouches — 225
Robynne Chutkan, MD, and Jerome D. Waye, MD, FACP

48. Role of the Pathologist in Evaluating Chronic Pouches   229
    Robert E. Petras, MD

49. Support for Patients Who Undergo Ostomy and Pouch Surgery   233
    Kathleen L. Potter, RN, BSN, COCN

50. Ileorectal Anastomosis   237
    Ian C. Lavery, MBBS, FRACS, FACS

51. Indeterminate Colitis: Surgical Approaches   241
    Ian Lindsey, MBBS, FRACS, Bryan F. Warren, MB, ChB, MRCPath,
    and Neil Mortensen, MD, FRCS

COMPLICATIONS OF INFLAMMATORY BOWEL DISEASE

52. Growth and Nutritional Problems in Pediatric Inflammatory Bowel Disease   245
    Ernest G. Seidman, MD, FRCPC

53. Dysplasia Surveillance Programs   251
    Teresa A. Brentnall, MD

54. Cancer Prevention Strategies in Inflammatory Bowel Disease   257
    Charles N. Bernstein, MD, FRCPC

55. Dysplasia Surveillance in Crohn's Disease   263
    Peter H. Rubin, MD

56. Extra-intestinal Manifestations   267
    Kim L. Isaacs, MD, PhD

57. Cutaneous Manifestations of Inflammatory Bowel Disease   271
    Hossein C. Nousari, MD, Thomas T. Provost, MD, and Grant J. Anhalt, MD

58. Ocular Manifestations of Inflammatory Bowel Disease   275
    Paul A. Latkany, MD, and Douglas A. Jabs, MD, MS

59. Arthritis Associated with Inflammatory Bowel Disease   279
    Timothy R. Orchard, MA, MD, DM, MRCP

60. Lessons from Treatment of Rheumatoid Arthritis   283
    Ulf Müller-Ladner, MD, and Jürgen Schölmerich, MD

61. Osteopenia and Osteoporosis: Prevention and Treatment   289
    Jeffrey H. Lee, MD, and Jacqueline L. Wolf, MD

62. Ischemic Necrosis of Bone   293
    Thomas M. Zizic, MD, and Peter A. Holt, MD

63. Sclerosing Cholangitis   299
    Young-Mee Lee, MD, and Marshall M. Kaplan, MD

64. Stricture Management in Primary Sclerosing Cholangitis   303
    Anthony N. Kalloo, MD, FACP

65. Liver Transplantation for Primary Sclerosing Cholangitis   305
    Paul J. Thuluvath, MD, FRCP, Henkie Tan, MD, PhD, Sateesh Nair, MD, and Andrew Klein, MD

66. **Cholangiocarcinoma in The Inflammatory Bowel Disease Patient**   311
Benedict M. Devereaux, MB, BS, FRACP, Stuart Sherman, MD, and Glen A. Lehman, MD

67. **Gallstone Management in Inflammatory Bowel Disease**   317
Konstantinos Lazaridis, MD, and Keith D. Lindor, MD

68. **Urologic Complications**   321
David Y. Chan, MD, and H. Ballentine Carter, MD

69. **Hematologic Problems in Inflammatory Bowel Disease**   325
Henry Cymorek, MD, and Joel B. Levine, MD

70. **Pancreatitis in Inflammatory Bowel Disease**   329
Sonia Friedman, MD, and Peter A. Banks, MD

CROHN'S DISEASE

71. **Crohn's Disease: Therapeutic Implications of Disease Subtypes**   333
Lloyd R. Sutherland, MDCM, MSc, FRCPC, FACP

72. **Therapeutic Expectations of Medical Management of Crohn's Disease**   337
Theodore M. Bayless, MD, and Michael F. Picco, MD, PhD

73. **Sequential and Combination Therapy for Small Bowel Disease**   343
Geert D'Haens, MD, PhD

74. **Oral 5-Aminosalicylic Acid Medications in Crohn's Disease**   347
Cosimo Prantera, MD, and Maria Lia Scribano, MD

75. **Clinical Questions in Crohn's Disease Not Answered by Controlled Trials**   353
Richard J. Farrell, MD, MRCPI, and Z. Myron Falchuk, MD

76. **Antibiotics as Therapeutic Agents in Crohn's Disease**   359
R. Balfour Sartor, MD

77. **Appropriate Use of Corticosteroids in Inflammatory Bowel Disease**   363
Francisco A. Sylvester, MD, and Jeffrey S. Hyams, MD

78. **Topically Active Steroid Preparations**   367
Robert Löfberg, MD, PhD

79. **Azathioprine and 6-Mercaptopurine Use in Crohn's Disease**   373
Ramona O. Rajapakse, MD, and Burton I. Korelitz, MD

80. **Azathioprine Metabolism in Inflammatory Bowel Disease: Correlation with Efficacy and Toxicity**   377
Carmen Cuffari, MD

81. **Methotrexate in Inflammatory Bowel Disease**   383
Brian Gordon Feagan, MD, and Prasanna Kumaranayake, MD

82. **Cyclosporine in Crohn's Disease**   387
Mary Lawrence Harris, MD

83. Anticytokine Therapy in Crohn's Disease 389
Loren C. Karp, MA, and Stephan R. Targan, MD

84. Perianal Fistula 395
Daniel H. Present, MD

85. Options in Managing Enteral Fistulae in Inflammatory Bowel Disease 401
Charles O. Elson, MD, and Nuzhat Iqbal, MD

86. Bowel Rest and Parenteral Nutrition 405
Rosemarie L. Fisher, MD

87. Enteral Nutrition and Dietary Management 409
Anne M. Griffiths, MD, FRCP(C)

88. Crohn's Disease in Children and Adolescents 415
Ranjana Gokhale, MD, and Barbara S. Kirschner, MD

89. Gastroduodenal Crohn's Disease 421
Robert Burakoff, MD

90. Crohn's Jejunoileitis 425
C. Noel Williams, MRCS, LRCP, FRCP(C), FACP

91. Medical Therapy of Crohn's Colitis 429
E. Jan Irvine, MD, MSc, FRCPC, and Forough Farrokhyar, PhD

92. Fistulizing and Perforating Crohn's Disease 435
Gary R. Lichtenstein, MD

SURGERY FOR CROHN'S DISEASE

93. Therapeutic Expectations: Surgical Management of Crohn's disease 439
Jeffrey W. Milsom, MD, and Alex Ky, MD

94. Indications and Procedures for Surgery of Small Bowel Crohn's Disease 443
Adrian J. Greenstein, MD, FACS, FRCS

95. Perioperative Nutrition Support 449
Michael D. Sitrin, MD

96. Laparoscopically Assisted Bowel Resection 453
Mark A. Talamini, MD

97. Surgery for Crohn's Disease: Strictureplasty 457
Scott A. Strong, MD

98. Gastroduodenal Crohn's Disease: Surgical Management 461
Peter W. Marcello, MD, and David J. Schoetz Jr, MD

99. Measures to Minimize Postoperative Recurrences of Crohn's Disease 465
Paul J. Rutgeerts, MD, PhD, FRCP

100. Diarrhea Following Small Bowel Resection 471
Lawrence R. Schiller, MD

101. Hyperoxaluria and Nephrolithiasis 475
William A. Rowe, MD, CNSP

102. Clinical Management of Short-Bowel Syndrome 479
Alan L. Buchman, MD, MSPH, and Joseph Sellin, MD

103. Intestinal Transplantation 485
Kenneth K.W. Lee, MD, FACS, and Kareem Abu-Elmagd, MD, PhD, FACS

104. Management of Postoperative Fistulae 491
Walter A. Koltun, MD

105. Surgery for Crohn's Colitis 495
Roger D. Hurst, MD, Marcovalerio Melis, MD, and Fabrizio Michelassi, MD

106. Perianal Disease 501
Alon J. Pikarsky, MD, and Steven D. Wexner, MD

107. Endoscopic Management of Small Bowel, Anastomotic, and Colonic Strictures in 509
Crohn's Disease
Richard A. Kozarek, MD

108. Rectovaginal Fistulae 515
Tracy L. Hull, MD, FACS

109. Fate of Excluded Bowel 519
Bret A. Lashner, MD

PATIENT SUPPORT SERVICES

110. Inflammatory Bowel Disease Genetics 523
Steven R. Brant, MD, and Judy H. Cho, MD

111. Managing Patients' Concerns 527
Gabriele Moser, MD, and Douglas A. Drossman, MD

112. Life-Style Issues and Inflammatory Bowel Disease 531
Richard P. Rood, MD, FACP

113. Inflammatory Bowel Disease Nurse Advocate 535
Sharon A. Hunt, BSN, RN

114. Crohn's & Colitis Foundation of America: Information and Support Services 539
Marjorie Merrick, Director of Research and Education

115. Pediatric Patient and Family Support 543
Maria I. Clavell, MD, Robert D. Baker, MD, PhD, and Susan S. Baker, MD, PhD

116. Nutritional Consultation and Guidance 547
Allen L. Ginsberg, MD

117. Questions Frequently Asked of a Support System 551
Alethea Trinkaus, MPH

118. Insurance and Disability Advocacy Issues in Inflammatory Bowel Disease 555
Douglas C. Wolf, MD

119. Sexual Adjustments and Body Image 561
Paula Erwin-Toth, MSN, RN, ET, CWOCN, CNS

120. Role of Clergy and the Patient with Chronic Disease 565
Rabbi Murray Saltzman, DDS, DHL, DD

BEHAVIORAL THERAPY

121. Appreciation of Psychosocial Factors 569
Ray E. Clouse, MD

122. Psychiatric Complications of Inflammatory Bowel Disease 573
Mark L. Teitelbaum, MD

123. Psychological Perspectives on the Care of Patients with Inflammatory Bowel Disease 577
David Edwin, PhD

124. Stress Management 583
H. Richard Waranch, PhD

125A. Behavioral Pain Management 587
Harry S. Shabsin, PhD

125B. Pain Management 593
Julio A. Gonzalez, MD, and Peter S. Staats, MD

126. Fitness Program 599
Peter Nielson

127. Alternative Patient Care Methods 603
Robert J. Hilsden, MD, MSc, FRCPC

SPECIAL SITUATIONS

128. Fertility and Pregnancy in Inflammatory Bowel Disease 607
Douglas G. Moss, MD

129. Pregnancy and Inflammatory Bowel Disease 613
Daniel H. Present, MD

130. Colitis in the Elderly 619
James J. Farrell, MD, and Lawrence S. Friedman, MD

131. Nonsteroidal Anti-inflammatory Drugs, Enterocolonic Ulceration, and Inflammatory Bowel Disease 625
Simon Smale, BMBS, MRCP, and Ingvar Bjarnason, MD, MSc, FRCPath, DSc

132. Collagenous and Lymphocytic Colitis 631
Marcia Cruz-Correa, MD, and Francis M. Giardiello, MD

133. Radiation Enterocolitis 635
Choon Jin Ooi, MD, Christopher G. Willet, MD, and Daniel K. Podolsky, MD

134. **Colitis and Enteritis in Immunocompromised Individuals**   639
Gary I. Kleiner, MD, PhD, and Lloyd Mayer, MD

135. **Lymphoma in Inflammatory Bowel Disease**   645
Sharon Masel, MD, and Stephen B. Hanauer, MD

136. **Gastrointestinal Complications in Stem Cell Transplantation**   649
Linda A. Lee, MD, and Georgia B. Vogelsang, MD

137. **Behçet's Disease**   655
David B. Hellman, MD

138. **Therapy of Ulcerative Jejunoileitis**   659
Konrad H. Soergel, MD

CHAPTER 1

PATIENT–DOCTOR INTERACTIONS

STEPHEN B. HANAUER, MD

When a physician presents the diagnosis of ulcerative colitis (UC) or Crohn's disease (CD) to a patient and family and explains that the disease does not have a known cause or medical cure, these often are the last words that are heard during the encounter. Yet, this decree sets the stage for all future interactions between the doctor and the patient and his or her family. The medical team must henceforth guide the patient through an uncommon, socially embarrassing, painful, and, at times, disfiguring illness. The physician and affiliated staff must be able to respond to unanswerable questions and provide compassion, sympathy, and ultimate optimism regarding the future for young, fearful, and denying patients and family members who often are unwilling to accept the uncertainty and vagaries of an idiopathic disease. The physician must begin a course of education and support coinciding with nutritional, life-style, pharmaceutical, and, potentially, surgical recommendations.

Education

Educating the patient and family regarding inflammatory bowel disease (IBD) can begin with referencing UC and CD among other inflammatory diseases. Comparison may be made to other familiar diseases of unknown etiology, such as arthritis, lupus, multiple sclerosis, or Alzheimer's disease, as well as common conditions such as coronary heart disease and cancer. Admittedly, although considerable understanding has been achieved regarding the diagnosis, treatment, and prognosis, infectious diseases are the only human ailments with known causation and cure. Nevertheless, despite a lack of understanding regarding the causation or medical cure, patients can be assured that they can live a normal life span, have a normal quality of life, develop or continue their career, and raise a family. Yes, there may be "speed bumps" along the way, but the major milestones are attainable.

With this introduction, the physician initiates education regarding the anatomy and function of the gastrointestinal (GI) tract and describes the location of disease and anticipated physiologic impact of the inflammation that translates into symptoms. An anatomic diagram is useful, because most lay individuals do not have significant knowledge of digestive tract components or function. Interpretation of symptoms is explained according to the

disease location, and treatment is discussed according to site of disease (eg, why topical mesalamine is useful for distal colitis, the pharmacology of sulfasalazine, the reasons for selecting a specific mesalamine delivery system). The physician explains why bleeding or diarrhea occurs and discusses normal defecation and why the loss of rectal compliance leads to urgency or, rarely, incontinence.

It is important from the outset that the patients recognize that IBD is a chronic disease requiring a two-phase medical approach: *induction* and then *maintenance of remission* for both UC and CD. Too often, patients seek second opinions simply because they have not had sufficient education regarding therapeutic expectations. Unless it is made clear to patients that continuation of maintenance therapy is necessary to prevent recurrence, it is human nature for patients to attempt self-tapering or discontinuation of maintenance drugs as long as they are feeling well. It must be emphasized that it is usually easier to prevent relapse than to treat active disease and that long-term compliance (adherence) helps to minimize long-term complications and exposure to therapies with more severe side effects. There is another chapter on compliance that provides additional strategies.

The educational process does not end with the first visit or series of visits. It is the beginning of a long-term series of discussions that evolve according to the patient's age and life experiences. Children have little interest in an illness. Teenagers, in particular, are primarily concerned with conforming to their peer group activities and life style. Teens need to develop an involvement in and control of their illness that will allow them to participate with their peers in school and social events. They need to learn that adherence, in contrast to denial, is the best means of sustaining normal peer activities. There are four chapters on dealing with teenage patients with IBD.

Young adults have different priorities and educational needs. They may be more inquisitive regarding medication side effects and impact on career, dating, or family. They may be more responsive to educational literature, books, or the Internet for background information and options. Significant others may assume educational responsibilities to support their mate. Physician encounters require sufficient time to allow for questions from family or a mate and responses to their personal

1

research into these diseases from lay literature or Internet chat rooms.

Older patients may expect their physicians to guide them without the need for explanations or provision of options that younger patients have come to expect. Inflammatory bowel disease in the older patient requires consideration of concurrent illness and impact on different components of quality of life. For example, surgical options for UC (ileostomy vs ileoanal anastomosis) have different implications for older patients with coexistent health problems but, otherwise, stable family lives. Older patients often have to deal with multiple medications, drug interactions, and costs of polypharmacy. Impact of the disease and therapies need to be explained in the context of age, morbidity, and risk of mortality.

Support

Psychosocial support for patients and their families begins with the initial physician–patient encounter. After education regarding the disease, prognosis, and therapy, it is important to allow time (over subsequent visits) for the patient or family to assimilate the new information and to express their questions and concerns. These differ according to the patient's age, social status, and level of education. Studies have demonstrated that patient concerns are different in UC and CD. Patients with UC are more concerned with the risk of ostomies and cancer, whereas patients with CD focus on pain, surgery, and loss of social function. Certainly, individuals need specific support, according to the disease complications, such as those facing resections and the risk of recurrence, colectomy and ileostomy, or a multistage pelvic pouch, or women with perianal or rectovaginal fistulae.

Although support begins with the physician, it extends to the ancillary staff from receptionist, office nurses, procedure room staff, dietitian, social worker, and ostomy nurse. Patients expect respect and maintenance of dignity despite embarrassing symptoms and physical signs, uncomfortable procedures and tests, and hospitalizations or surgeries with loss of control. These patients need explanations of procedures and tests, rationale for dietary or life-style changes, and patience from the medical staff when they appear hesitant, afraid, or contradictory. In many situations, the loss of autonomy unmasks regressive or contentious behavior. At times, medications, particularly steroids or narcotics, cause personality changes or complications. Staff should be able to comprehend the psychosocial or medicinal explanations for apparent counterproductive behavior and the phases of acceptance of a chronic illness, including denial, anger, bargaining, and so on.

Most patients do not require formal psychosocial support. They and their families need to understand that these are not psychosomatic illnesses or diseases caused by stress or parental neuroses. An explanation of how stress can impact on *symptoms* rather than *inflammation* helps to alleviate guilt that often affects parents of children with IBD. These diseases impact upon the entire family, and it is important for families to avoid focusing on the patient, alone, without appropriate energies distributed to siblings. Accounting should be made of the family dynamics (for any age patient) to anticipate isolation, anger, or resentment against the patient, spouse, sibling, or parent. Social workers can assist if family dynamics become dysfunctional or impair therapy. Rarely, formal psychiatric consultation may become necessary. The chapters on the roles of psychiatry, psychology, social work, and the clergy provide additional insights.

Life Style and Nutrition

Inflammatory bowel disease comes with a lot of "baggage." There is guilt and embarrassment on the part of the patient and family. The family must be informed that these are not psychosomatic diseases or caused in any way by the parents, siblings, or patient. Yet, it is counterintuitive that "stress" does not contribute to these diseases or that diet is not an important therapeutic (or contributing) factor.

Patients should be reassured that they will be able to maintain a normal life style, social relationships, and occupation. It is extremely rare that an individual will need to change his or her career intentions because of IBD. There has been a tremendous turnabout over the past 40 years; patients once expected to be hospitalized for months while undergoing special diets or psychotherapy. With the advent of newer therapies, patients with CD rarely require hospitalization (aside from the need for surgical resections) and patients with severe UC can be maneuvered through medical or surgical treatment within a maximum of 2 weeks.

Studies have demonstrated that the majority of patients are able to maintain their occupation and that the number of patients on disability benefits is not significantly different from the general population. Inflammatory bowel disease in either male or female patients does not rule out conception, and the percentage of healthy children delivered to parents with IBD is comparable to that among healthy cohorts of similar age.

Myths regarding dietary therapies range to both ends of the spectrum. Most people would like to believe that there is something in the diet that causes or contributes to IBD. On the other hand, it does not make sense to simply state that "diet does not matter." Families need to hear a further explanation and clarification that, although there is no known specific environmental or dietary factor that causes these diseases, dietary factors can contribute to the symptoms of disease rather than contributing to inflammation. Patients need dietary advice to minimize their symptoms and maintain their overall nutritional status. The chapters on dietary advice, alternative medicine, and nutritional issues are helpful in this regard.

Gastroenterologists as Primary Care Providers

Most patients with IBD are young and otherwise healthy. Because of the complexity of IBD presentations, complications, and therapies, the gastroenterologist often is the primary care provider. In any case, the gastroenterologist needs to be aware of other health issues and to remain cognizant of other health encounters or referrals. It is important that patients inform their physician of any other doctor recommendations or prescriptions, to avoid complications, such as the use of nonsteroidal anti-inflammatory drugs (NSAIDs) for rheumatologic, neurologic, or gynecologic complaints. The physician needs to know of antibiotic therapy in case of disease exacerbation or persisting diarrhea. Many extraintestinal complications, such as erythema nodosum, pyoderma gangrenosum, ocular inflammation, nephrolithiasis, or osteoporosis, are best comanaged with the input of the gastroenterologist.

A major expectation of patients is to have a single care giver managing their course and to provide advice and reassurance through the variety of coexistent illnesses, surgery, and postsurgical care. Patients should have access to their primary care giver, who needs to be experienced with the spectrum of IBD presentations, complications, and therapies. Usually, this is the gastroenterologist by choice or default.

For the patient and family confronted with a medically incurable disease of unknown cause and varied course, the doctor–patient relationship is of paramount importance to assure them of the best medical outcome and maintenance of quality of life.

Supplemental Reading

Akobeng AK, Miller AV, Firth D, et al. Quality of life of parents and siblings of children with inflammatory bowel disease. J Pediatr Gastroenterol Nutr 1999;28:S40–2.

Andersson P, Olaison G, Bodemar G, et al. Low symptomatic load in Crohn's disease with surgery and medicine as complementary treatments. Scand J Gastroenterol 1998;33:423–9.

Eaden JA, Abrams K, Mayberry JF. The Crohn's and Colitis Knowledge Score: a test for measuring patient knowledge in inflammatory bowel disease. Am J Gastroenterol 1999;94:3560–6.

Hilsden RJ, Scott CM, Verhoef MJ. Complementary medicine use by patients with inflammatory bowel disease (see comments). Am J Gastroenterol 1998;93:697–701.

Loudon CP, Corroll V, Butcher J, et al. The effects of physical exercise on patients with Crohn's disease. Am J Gastroenterol 1999;94:697–703.

Munkholm P, Langholz E, Davidsen M, Binder V. Disease activity courses in a regional cohort of Crohn's disease patients. Scand J Gastroenterol 1995;30:699–706.

Ramchandani D, Schindler B, Katz J. Evolving concepts of psychopathology in inflammatory bowel disease. Implications for treatment. Med Clin North Am 1994;78:1321–30.

Talal AH, Drossman DA. Psychosocial factors in inflammatory bowel disease. Gastroenterol Clin North Am 1995; 24:699–716.

CHAPTER 2

PEDIATRIC PATIENT, FAMILY, DOCTOR INTERACTIONS

GEORGE D. FERRY, MD

Caring for children with inflammatory bowel disease (IBD) often involves multiple family members (Figure 2–1) and requires an understanding of pediatric and adolescent behavior patterns, denial of symptoms, poor compliance, fear of tests, and special support needs (Table 2–1). In addition to one or both parents, grandparents, and, in many cases, stepfathers or stepmothers may be intimately involved as care givers. Dealing with this extended family is an important part of managing pediatric patients with IBD and is both rewarding and challenging. The rewards come from a better understanding of family dynamics, sharing in the family's care and concern, and helping each child and family member cope with the many problems associated with IBD. The challenge is to educate the extended family so as to maximize and coordinate care as the child moves from one home to another. Providing care to children whose parents are divorced is especially challenging, as communication between divorced parents and their respective families is often nonexistent. This leads to poor compliance with medication and inaccurate reporting of symptoms. Meeting and working with the extended family in the office setting gives an opportunity to answer questions and outline treatment objectives. Including each family member as part of the team will cut down on phone calls, avoid conflicting messages, and improve patient care and compliance.

While most patients come to the doctor because they need help, some adolescents are brought to the doctor unwillingly. Even in cases of moderate to severe IBD, adolescents often deny symptoms and do everything possible to avoid being different from their peers. Obtaining a history or doing an adequate physical examination is very difficult in this setting. Great patience and understanding is required from the physician and other members of the medical team. It takes a real interest and commitment to gain the trust of an angry or unhappy child or adolescent and it may require many visits to establish any kind of meaningful doctor-patient relationship.

History and Physical Examination

Since many pediatric patients arrive at the office *en masse* with one or both parents, siblings, grandparents, and or friends, one often must ask members of the family to stay

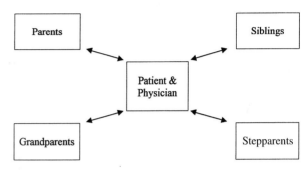

FIGURE 2–1. Physician/patient interaction—who is involved?

outside for some or all of the visit. At the same time, it may require input from all of the extended family to obtain the history, depending on who has the most contact with the patient. Children may not be good historians, but it is important to ask them about how they feel and about any specific complaints. Talking directly to a young patient helps gain their confidence, helps the doctor assess their level of understanding, and leads to better cooperation with the physical examination. Young children respond in a positive manner when physicians talk to them directly and many will be appreciative, grateful, and excited to see their physician in spite of the many uncomfortable procedures that we often prescribe and perform.

As children move into adolescence, it is important to see them separate from their parents. Whenever there is a battle going on in the examining room between a child and parent, separating them and getting individual histories is mandatory. Visiting alone with an adolescent helps develop rapport and it helps the adolescent to be comfortable in sharing fears and problems. In addition, talking alone often allows better discussion about compliance issues, parental interactions, depression, and issues of

TABLE 2–1. Critical Issues in Patient, Family, Doctor Interaction

Multiple care givers
Normal patterns of adolescent denial
Seeing adolescents away from parents — confidentiality
Normal independence and control issues
Compliance
Fear of tests and procedures
Education of the family
Value in teen support (for family and patient)

sexuality. Teenagers will talk about feelings and fears when the physician is a good listener and nonjudgmental. Confidentiality is critical in this setting, but at the same time the patient has to know up front that critical health and psychological issues will be shared with parents.

Talking with parents either alone or in the same room as the patient at the beginning of the visit gives the physician the opportunity to hear issues that can be discussed with the patient separately. Bringing the family together again at the end of a visit is reassuring to family members. This also gives the opportunity to educate all of the care givers in the progress or complications of IBD, any tests needed, and the treatment plan. It also gives parents an opportunity to ask questions and share any additional concerns.

Both boys and girls, from the earliest age through adolescence, are often quite embarrassed about examination of the rectum and perineum. This takes great sensitivity on the physician's part to help a child through this. With young children, a complete but simple explanation is important. For example, a child should know that a rectal examination can be uncomfortable, but not overly painful. Truthful explanations are the key. If a child or adolescent is totally resistant, it may be best to put off the examination until another time. A clash between the doctor, parent, and child rarely leads to a successful examination and can take up valuable time. On a different day, a child may react quite differently.

Independence and Control Issues

Due to worry and fear over a chronic disease, parents often tend to take more control over their children's lives, becoming restrictive in activities and diet and nagging about symptoms and medications. One of the most useful ways to confront this is to discuss it openly with the patient and parents, helping each to understand their needs and fears. Teens need to "not be different" from their peers and the need to develop independence is critical in understanding adolescent behavior. Chronic disease often strips them of this independence. A parent's fear of complications combined with the long-term outlook for a chronic illness leads him or her to become overprotective. The physician can play a critical and vital role in helping the patient and family cope better. It is very helpful to let teens know that you believe they can take responsibility, and offer tips on how they might take control over their disease (eg, defining their own solution for remembering their medications, calling the doctor's office themselves to report symptoms, etc.). Acknowledging the adolescent's need for independence and "fitting in" will improve compliance and reporting of symptoms and will establish excellent rapport with both the patient and the family.

At times there is a lack of connection between the severity of symptoms and functioning reported by parents and children. Many teenagers minimize and under-report symptoms. The family's input here is critical. Since there is no ideal marker for active inflammation, careful attention to days missed from school, avoidance of activities with friends, signs of depression, or loss of appetite may be the only clues to disease activity. At the same time, overprotective parents can push for more and more intervention when in fact the patient may be functioning reasonably well in spite of the chronic inflammatory bowel disease. This is especially difficult in a hospital setting where the parent is at the bedside all day long making all of the decisions for the patient. In this setting, it can be hard or impossible to evaluate the degree of illness, pain, and other symptoms. While there is no easy solution to developing coping skills in this setting, there are two resources of great value. One is involving a pediatric social worker with experience with IBD. A social worker can provide another voice of reason and give support to the family in helping them cope. A second resource is teen support. Either individually or in a group, peers can often do more to encourage and help with coping skills than the medical team. We have age-matched patients who are willing to come to the hospital to meet other teens and we have a video of teens talking about IBD, how they cope, what their fears and concerns are, and how they get beyond the fear and frustration. We use everything we can think of to encourage and help our patients and parents cope with IBD and function normally.

Parents and patients often ask for help with school-related problems. I am often asked to write absentee excuses for missing school because of IBD-related symptoms. In my experience, this has generally been legitimate and I have had very few children or adolescents abuse this. I am also asked to write excuses to avoid physical education. There is no question that cramps and diarrhea interfere with sports, but my goal with all patients is to help them live as normal lives as possible. Temporary excuses are clearly needed, but I try to stress getting back into routine school activities just as soon as possible. In some cases, home schooling becomes necessary to avoid failing and being held back a year in school. This is a very important decision and one that requires input from the family, the patient, the physician, and the school.

Preparing a Child for Tests and Procedures

Young children are often quite fearful of procedures, including blood drawing, radiography, and endoscopy. The major concerns are pain or discomfort and embarrassment. Providing a brief, realistic description of all tests is useful. Since conscious sedation or anesthesia avoids pain, it is important to reassure children that you will make any testing as easy as possible. At the same time, not all children want to know a lot about tests and the physician must be careful to evaluate each patient and family in terms of how much they want or need to know.

Saying too much can be a disadvantage and lead to extreme anxiety, making cooperation for tests or even conscious sedation impossible. While this is not common in adolescents, it is a big problem in children 5 to 12 years of age. A parent's insight into how their child reacts is critical in planning how and when tests should be performed.

Patient and Family Education

Family education about inflammatory bowel disease is the key to establishing rapport and getting good follow-up and compliance. It has always interested me that children frequently do not want to know anything about their disease and will totally disengage when you try to explain IBD. At the same time, they hear more than they let on. Even though they do not ask questions, as soon as they get home, they are often full of questions and the parents are faced with providing answers. Children rarely read materials given to parents, but they do browse the Internet and are especially attracted to chat pages or opportunities to find out from other teens what is really going on.

One of the best opportunities for young people to develop coping skills is summer or weekend camps with other children with IBD or similar diseases. Adolescents begin to talk with each other and share very intimate concerns and ideas and it helps them to feel less alone and less isolated. As part of this experience, we include our pediatric social workers. In addition to just being in camp, they lead discussion groups to help our patients adjust and cope with their chronic illness. The doctors are usually asked to stay out of these sessions.

The doctors and nurses who serve as counselors (and look after any emergency medical needs) benefit greatly from the camp experience. You see your patients in a different setting, have a wonderful opportunity to interact much more personally, and develop friendships that are life-long. This type of interaction makes the doctor, patient and family interaction very special and adds immeasurably to the enjoyment of caring for young people with IBD.

Supplemental Reading

Ferry G, Bartholomew L. Living with IBD. CCFA Publication. Updated 1999.

Ferry G. Quality of life in inflammatory bowel disease. J Pediatr Gastroenterol Nutr 1999;28:S15–18.

McCartney S, Ballinger A. Growth failure in inflammatory bowel disease. Nutrition 1999;15:169–71.

Polito JM II, Childs B, Mellits ED, et al. Crohn's disease: influence of age at diagnosis on site and clinical type of disease. Gastroenterology 1996:111:580–6.

CHAPTER 3

ADHERENCE ISSUES IN MANAGEMENT OF INFLAMMATORY BOWEL DISEASE

SUNANDA KANE, MD, MSPH

Ulcerative colitis (UC) and Crohn's disease (CD) are chronic, recurring conditions requiring life-long management. Most often, patients take their medicines when they are sick, but nonadherence is a common phenomenon with quiescent disease. Many clinicians incorrectly assume that their patients are adherent to prescribed therapeutic recommendations. Unfortunately, whereas literature on other chronic diseases, such as coronary artery disease, congestive heart failure, and diabetes, has tried to address the issue of medication noncompliance and determine its risk factors, the impact of medication adherence on specific inflammatory bowel disease (IBD) outcomes has not been fully explored. The published literature on the efficacy of IBD maintenance medications underestimates the extent of the problem, as patients often conceal their failure to take medications as directed once outside of controlled clinical trial environments. The degree of adherence that patients are able to achieve early in the course of disease may decrease markedly after 1 to 2 years. Particularly after remission has been established, patients may not believe (or understand) the importance of continuing maintenance therapy.

Once remission has been established, patients often enter a "honeymoon" phase of maintenance therapy. After a period of time, they may tire of taking their medications. Thus, during the transition from inductive to maintenance therapy, education regarding the importance of continued adherence to prevent relapse of disease or complications is paramount. Failure to comply with recommended maintenance regimens increases the risk of recurrent active disease, possible hospitalization, or steroid exposure and the consequences of prolonged steroid use. It is worth considering that nonadherence also is associated with the risk of extra-intestinal manifestations of IBD that parallel gastrointestinal disease activity, and nonadherence may be an important factor regarding long-term cancer risks. Furthermore, the issue of compliance is not limited to medicines but includes life-style modifications (smoking cessation, dietary restrictions) and other follow-up care (surveillance colonoscopies and monitoring blood tests for certain medications).

Patterns of Medication Nonadherence

Patterns of nonadherence include under- or overconsuming medication, taking doses at inappropriate intervals, or administering medication incorrectly (as in enema therapy). Although clinicians do not want to give the impression that missing doses is acceptable, this possibility should be discussed with patients. As a component of ongoing education, patients should learn what to do if they miss a dose, when it is permissible to skip a dose, or when to double a subsequent dose. Elderly patients require special attention, because they are at particular risk for inappropriate consumption secondary to dementia or complicated medication regimens. During discussion of these issues, exploring the reasons why doses are missed is also warranted. However, it is important to keep in mind that despite any instructions or dialogue, the patient may not ever fill the prescription. According to pharmacy studies, as many as 15 percent of patients never fill a prescription provided by their physician.

Inappropriate altering of dosing regimens is another pattern of nonadherent behavior that may be secondary to life style. Many patients find it difficult to take their medicines while at work, and younger patients feel inhibited or embarrassed about taking medicines at school. In this scenario, it may be possible to increase adherence by changing to a twice- or even once-daily regimen.

Incorrect administration of topical therapies arises from inadequate instruction from both physician and pharmacist. Rectal administration of medication can be embarrassing to discuss in an open manner, and patients, rather than admit to ignorance, attempt to self-administer enemas inappropriately, potentially rendering them ineffective.

Factors That Influence Adherence

Factors that influence long-term adherence include those related to the health care provider, the patient, and also the medication itself. In terms of the health care provider, important factors include (1) degree of knowledge regarding disease and its treatment, (2) commitment to patient education, and (3) provisions for monitoring and follow-up of patients.

For example, physicians caring for patients with IBD should be aware of the key literature that may help to convince patients that taking medications is important. There are two important studies correlating nonadherence with sulfasalazine therapy to the development of colorectal cancer. In a retrospective case control study, Pinczowski et al (1994) found that a minimum of 3 months of therapy with sulfasalazine had a protective effect against colon cancer. There was a 62 percent reduction in risk with any history of therapy in the 102 patients studied. The second study also was a retrospective study of 168 patients with at least a 10-year history of UC. The outcome measure of cancer risk was assessed based upon use of sulfasalazine. A patient was classified as noncompliant if there was clear evidence in the medical record of failure to take prescribed medications. The crude cancer rate was 3 percent in "compliant" patients and 31 percent in those "not compliant." Since the authors found rates of colectomy and cancer similar to those of previously published series, they concluded that adherence to medications was beneficial for reducing cancer risk.

Factors related to the patient include (1) degree of disease-specific education received from health care providers, (2) comprehension of instructions for proper medication use, (3) understanding of potential consequences of nonadherence, (4) extent of self-management skill and abilities, and (5) strength of a support system. Only by recognizing and addressing these issues can patients be expected to adhere to any medical regimen.

In terms of therapeutics, factors affecting adherence include (1) efficacy in maintaining remission and controlling symptoms, (2) safety profile (real as well as perceived), (3) convenience (ie, number of pills and dosing regimen), (4) formulation (pill size and mode of delivery), and, finally, (5) cost. Medicines such as sulfasalazine and 6-mercaptopurine have genetic polymorphisms in their metabolism, and assays have been developed to quantify particular metabolites and the potential to measure adherence. Early compliance studies were with sulfasalazine, a medication with both dose-related efficacy and side effects. Monitoring serum levels of the sulfapyridine metabolite revealed that 41 percent of patients with quiescent UC had subtherapeutic levels just 4 weeks after hospital discharge. Seemingly, lack of compliance was at least one factor. The authors suggested that estimations of serum sulfapyridine concentrations, as well as identification of the patient's acetylation phenotype, might be useful in decreasing the incidence of side effects and assessing compliance.

In addition, recent work with immunomodulators has shown a therapeutic benefit within target serum levels. Variability in levels can occur because of genetic aspects of metabolism or drug interactions. Once confirmed in prospective trials, use of therapeutic monitoring for 6-mercaptopurine metabolites or the thiopurine methyl-transferase enzyme activity may prove to be useful tools to measure compliance, optimize therapeutic outcomes, and minimize complications. At present, particularly in the pediatric population, gastroenterologists have used these assays to document a patient's nonadherence if or when drug levels are undetectable.

Apart from adherence to medical therapies, adherence to the recommendations regarding surveillance colonoscopy is of considerable importance. One of the most important methods available to reduce the risk of colorectal cancer in long-standing UC is via surveillance colonoscopies. Unfortunately, many patients do not adhere to the recommended intervals because of a variety of factors, including cost, inconvenience, and fear of the procedure (or its results) or need for colectomy. To encourage patients to adhere to surveillance schedules, clinicians must emphasize the value of the procedure in detecting precancerous changes and preventing the consequences of progression to colorectal cancer. The literature supports the relation between adherence with a surveillance program and a decreased risk of colorectal cancer. In a cohort of 121 patients with UC, for longer than 7 years, 7 patients developed cancer within the observation period. Two of these seven had not complied with recommendations for repeat colonoscopy or colectomy after dysplasia was found. Both patients had clinically quiescent disease and presented years later with tumor-related obstructive symptoms. The authors concluded that diminished compliance when a patient is asymptomatic increases the risk of cancer.[*]

Methods to Optimize Adherence

Optimizing adherence is most effective when open lines of communication characterize the relationship between physician and patient. Allowing the patient the time to voice his or her concerns and questions is the first step in effective education. Open-ended questions during a patient visit can be time consuming, but setting an appropriate tone so as not to overestimate the patient's level of education is paramount in establishing a good relationship between physician and patient. A recent study from the psychology literature featuring patients with IBD revealed that, when asked, their greatest concern was the uncertain nature of their disease. Patients also expressed a significant concern about the effect of medications on their disease. The chapter on an IBD nurse advocate position emphasizes the role of the nurse in getting and giving information on medications.

Physicians tend to overestimate patient comprehension in regard to instructions and education. A pool of

---

[*] Editor's Note: Patients with primary sclerosing cholangitis (PSC) commonly have relatively quiescent colitis that can go undiagnosed for years. Even if surveillance is closely pursued, 58 percent of our series of 35 patients had dysplasia or cancer by 28 years. (TMB)

TABLE 3–1. Health Communication Model for Optimizing Adherence

1. Provide explicit directions
2. Emphasize the importance of therapy
3. Supply written information combined with oral counseling
4. Clarify the purpose of the medication or intervention
5. Repeat important points
6. Give consistent advice

patients with IBD indicated that 62 percent of patients with UC and 78 percent of patients with CD felt ill-informed about their disease (Martin et al, 1992). Whereas 86 percent of respondents knew of the increased risk of cancer, only 44 percent know that it was possible to screen for dysplasia and possibly prevent invasive cancer. The Health Communication model for optimizing adherence contains six main strategies (Table 3–1).

Techniques to help patients remember to take their medications include linking medications with activities of daily living, such as brushing teeth or drinking a morning cup of coffee. Supplying the patient with a pill organizer box also can help to avoid missed or inconsistent dosing. Prescribing medications in 3-month versus 1-month allotments, when feasible, decreases the number of times the patient has to visit the pharmacy and increases long-term adherence. Another way to help patients is to simplify the regimen when possible. For example, oral mesalmine can be dosed bid, tid, or qid, depending upon patient preference and schedule. Providing the patient with a combination of written materials and pictures for review also is helpful. The Crohn's and Colitis Foundation of America has an award-winning Website (*www.cccfa.org*) that is another reliable source of information and should be offered to those with access to the Internet. This is discussed in a separate chapter.

Support Systems

The nature of a patient's support systems can be an important asset in terms of ensuring adherent behavior. There are data to suggest that single men have a higher risk for nonadherent behavior than those who are married. Having a family member or spouse accompany the patient to office visits allows for clarification of instructions and another source for behaviors outside the clinic setting.

Individualizing Therapy

The key to an adherent patient is to individualize therapy. The medications prescribed and recommendations made

have to be based on each individual's disease and therapeutic history, prior response and adherence to medications, and pharmacoeconomic issues. Physicians need to be flexible and should change a regimen, when possible, to accommodate individual patients and their unique situations. Successful management of IBD will come from employing a full range of treatment modalities as well as consideration of psychosocial and emotional aspects of the disease.

Physicians cannot do this alone. The integration of other health care term members, such as nurses, social workers, and pharmacists, is as important to the overall care of patients with IBD as are office visits. A team approach using the strengths, knowledge, and experience of each member will ultimately lead to the best medical care.

Establishing the prevalence and impact of nonadherence is important, since the magnitude and significance of this determines the degree to which potential benefits of intervention are unrealized. Small retrospective and prospective studies support the claim that patient compliance is associated with positive outcomes. However, larger, population-based prospective studies are needed to document true compliance rates, as well as the association of noncompliance with significant clinical outcomes.

References

Martin A, Leone L, Castagliuolo I, et al. What do patients want to know about their inflammatory bowel disease? Ital J Gastroenterol 1992;24:477–80.

Pinczowski D, Ekbom A, Baron J, et al. Risk factors for colorectal cancer in patients with ulcerative colitis: a case-control study. Gastroenterology 1994;107:117–20.

Supplemental Reading

Horwitz R, Horwitz SM. Adherence to treatment and health outcomes. Arch Intern Med 1993;153:1863–8.

Moody GA, Jayanthi V, Probert CS, et al. Long-term therapy with sulfasalazine protects against colorectal cancer in ulcerative colitis: a retrospective study of colorectal cancer risk and compliance with treatment in Leicestershire. Eur J Gastroenterol Hepatol 1996;8:1179–83.

Riley S, Mani V, Goodman MJ, Lucas S. Why do patients with ulcerative colitis relapse? Gut 1990;31:179–83.

van Hees PA, van Tongeren JH. Compliance to therapy in patients on a maintenance dose of sulfasalazine. J Clin Gastroenterol 1982;4:333–6.

Von Korff M, Gruman J, Schaefer J, et al. Collaborative management of chronic illness. Ann Intern Med 1997;127:1097–102.

MANAGING INFLAMMATORY BOWEL DISEASE IN THE MANAGED CARE ERA

SEYMOUR KATZ, MD

The published guidelines for therapy in inflammatory bowel disease have been written by Drs. Hanauer, Meyers, Sachar, and Kornbluth in as clear and unambiguous a manner as possible as disseminated by the American College of Gastroenterology in 1997.

What is not clear and certainly not unambiguous is the implementation of these guidelines by the clinician within the limitations set by managed care organizations (MCOs).

The clinician is besieged daily by restraints from utilizing diagnostic and therapeutic modalities for the IBD patient requiring lengthy and often unproductive pre-certification phone calls, written waivers, or outright rejection of what he/she perceives to be the correct care. Indeed, we will review the present vexing problems facing the clinician in this new "paradigm" of care, that is, the MCO, and attempt to offer some insight into recent legal and legislative inroads with MCO policy. We hope to provide the clinician with a user-friendly and "hands-on" approach to dealing with the problems and obstacles of operating in such a paradigm. This review is not meant to be encyclopedic in detail but instead as practical and pragmatic as possible.

Problems

A sampling of the daily difficulties facing the clinician include:

(1) The MCO's refusal to pay for a flexible sigmoidoscopy on the same day as an office visit for an established IBD patient even though the need for such an investigation is clear to the clinician. The consequences are profound for the patient and the clinician. The patient's family may need to take another day off from work or travel great distances, or the patient may become reluctant to be evaluated and consequently may "fall through the cracks." To prevent this from happening, any responsible physician will perform the procedure at his/her expense.

(2) The MCO may interfere with a physician's request for a CT scan in a Crohn's disease patient suspected of mass or abscess by either refusing outright or directing that patient be sent to an MCO contract laboratory that may be geographically inconvenient for the patient or have a delayed appointment schedule that may threaten the patient's health.

Again, the physician must intercede for the patient at personal loss of time and office reserves (and without remuneration.)

(3) An MCO pharmacy may not carry a specific medication (eg 5-ASA in place of sulfasalazine) or prohibit dispensing an established dose of 4.8 g of 5-ASA as recognized in clinical use, and, instead, limiting the prescription to 2.4 g as listed in the *Physician's Desk Reference*.

(4) MCOs may delay payment or simply refuse to pay for services rendered even when those services were pre-approved and "pre-certified." For example, an MCO was notified for their consent prior to anti-TNF infusion therapy in Crohn's disease. A pre-certification approval also was obtained and the infusion given at a cost of $2000 per patient. When billed for the procedure, the MCO refused payment, claiming they approved of its use, but did not say they would pay for the therapy.

What issues drive the MCOs to take such adversarial positions this late in the evolution of managed care and what progress has been made in affording the clinician and the patient some relief from this frustrating and counterproductive position?

It Is All a Matter of Money

The bewildering legal, financial, and ethical issues emerging from the financial constraints in the managed care arena of the late 1990s continue to confound physicians and patients.

Health care costs are on the rise, again with a twofold increase anticipated by the year 2007. A threefold increase in prescription drug expenditures with an 8 to 10% increase in HMO premiums and a 28.8 percent increase in indemnity premiums were noted in 1999.

Presumably, the rise in HMO premiums resulted from slowed utilization improvements, fewer savings from a

Editor's Note: This chapter and the attached letters represent the author's opinion and no specific legal advice is intended. The "changing paradigm" of health care for IBD is in flux and the reader is advised to keep current on this as well as all other medical topics.

shift to outpatient setting, tougher negotiations with hospitals and MDs, and losses from Medicare and Medicaid programs.

An Issue of Ethics

The resultant knee-jerk response is a further "squeeze" on health care providers regarding capitating risk or creating risk pools with incentives presumably for "quality and efficiency."

Of 766 California Primary Care Physicians (PCPs) surveyed, 35 percent were offered bonuses on performance, (eg, 75% felt "pressured" to see more patients/day, 57% were "pressured" to limit referrals). A median incentive was $10500 but 13 percent of PCPs received $40000.

Thus, ethical concerns exist with HMO incentives in the form of cash bonuses, which Dr. Jerome Kassirer, editor of *The New England Journal of Medicine*, stated may "create intolerable threat to physicians' integrity if strong enough to *shun* sick patients."

Medical Necessity Decisions

The physician is in a precarious position when tests, procedures, referral to specialists, or treatment programs are denied by health plans.

The ethical position, as stated by *AMA Code of Ethics* (Opinion E8:13), is clear: "Physicians are required to be advocates for *any* care they believe will materially benefit their patients."

The legal position is equally clear in that a physician has a legal duty to advocate on behalf of his/her patient when a health plan denies coverage. If a physician fails to do so, he/she can be held liable to the patient. (*Wichline vs. California* 1986).

Since the Employment Retirement Income Security Act (ERISA of 1974) that limits exposure and liability of an employer- or union-sponsored plan extends to an MCO, the physician remains the only source or target for a patient's suit. Compound this concern with the physician's fear of *deselection* "without cause" from a health plan when he/she assumes the role as patient advocate.

The good news is that the courts, state agencies, and legislatures are beginning to hold health plans accountable and *liable* for utilization review decisions that are contrary to the *documented advice* of attending physicians.

Good News: The judicial system

(1) In July 1997, a California arbitrator ruled that InterValley Health Plan, Inc. must pay $1.1 million to a kidney disease patient after the HMO repeatedly refused to authorize, and delayed authorization of, referrals, treatments, and tests authorized by the patient's primary care physician.

(2) In Murphy vs. Arizona Board of Medical Examiners (1997), the Arizona court of appeals ruled that a medical director of an insurance company can be disciplined by the state Board of Medical Examiners for a coverage decision. The medical director refused to approve coverage for gallbladder surgery, deciding that it was not medically necessary. The surgeon proceeded with the operation, which revealed a diseased liver. The insurer subsequently paid the medical bill.

(3) In Shea vs. Esensten (1997), the United States Court of Appeals for the Eighth Circuit held that an HMO's behind-the-scenes financial incentives to curb specialist referrals violated the HMO's fiduciary duty under ERISA.

(4) In 1995, an Oregon HMO settled for $1 million with a patient who alleged that she was denied timely surgery for a compressed nerve root on her head. The plaintiff's primary care physician appealed the denial and 7 months later, the HMO approved the surgery, but significant nerve damage occurred in the interim that could not be corrected by surgery.

(5) In Fox vs. Health Net (1994), a California jury awarded $89 million to the family of a patient denied a bone marrow transplant that was recommended by two treating physicians. The plaintiff's attorney showed that the Health Net executive who made the decision was compensated on the basis of how much money he saved the company.

(6) In Dunn vs. Praiss (1995), the New Jersey Supreme court held that the New Jersey HMO Act permits HMOs to be sued directly by a patient for medical malpractice and that a physician can assert a cross claim against an HMO in a malpractice claim for breach of contract based on the HMO's failure to coordinate care.

(7) In Johnson vs. Humana, Inc. (October 21, 1998), a Kentucky jury awarded $13.1 million damage (second largest award) against Humana for failure to cover care recommended by the enrollee's doctor for refusal to pay for hysterectomy for pre-invasive cervical cancer.

(8) In Shannon vs. Health America of Pennsylvania (October 5, 1998), the Pennsylvania appeals court held the HMO responsible for a medical decision by assigning the HMO the same standards of malpractice it holds for physicians and hospitals regarding the death of a premature infant.

(9) A new use of disability legislation was found in Zamora J, et al vs. Humana Health Plans of Texas, PacifiCare of Texas, HealthTexas Medical Group of San Antonio and PrimaryCare Net of Texas. Federal Judge Fred Biery ruled that disabled Medicare patients and their physicians have the right to sue Medicare HMOs under the Americans with Disabilities Act, Section 504. He further held that the medical HMO had in fact discriminated against the patient. This ruling may apply to commercial HMO members if the insurer offers Medicare as well.

(10) A striking example of some relief occurred in the NYS Supreme Court Appellate Division (First Dept. Nealy vs. U.S. Healthcare & Ralph Young, M.D. [6/18/98]), which ruled that a medical malpractice action against a general practitioner (G.P.) was *pre-empted under Federal ERISA status* after it was alleged that the MD failed to obtain the HMO's permission to refer the patient to an approved specialist.

In this case, the patient sought the advice and care of a cardiologist who cared for the patient during prior cardiac surgery but who did not participate in the new U.S. Healthcare plan, which the patient joined when he changed jobs. The GP completed the necessary forms and requests for such a consultation on behalf of the patient, which the HMO rejected on two occasions. U.S. Healthcare claimed it had its own qualified cardiologists on its roster. The GP explained the out-of-pocket expenses to the patient if he wished his original cardiologist to continue care. A visit was scheduled but the patient suffered a fatal heart attack before the visit. The patient's family sued the GP and U.S. Healthcare.

The resultant scenario began when U.S. Healthcare was removed by the federal court because of statutory pre-emption under ERISA. The GP requested similar dismissal under ERISA but the local court refused such dismissal, claiming the physician was subject to state law for malpractice and was not covered under ERISA.

The Appeals court disagreed: The lawsuit was not based on failure to properly diagnose and treat but failure to *urgently* obtain approval for referral to the cardiologist; the GP's records documented that such help was needed immediately and his involvement was as a "facilitator" for such referral.

If a malpractice trial were to occur, the court would have to focus on the MD's procedures for claims processing and denial of benefits, which is the area pre-empted from suit by ERISA.

The lessons to be learned are that the GP advised the patient and clearly documented the immediate need for cardiologist's referral *regardless of the uncertainty of coverage.*

Encouraging as these results may be, MDs are not absolved of liability to patients if bad results occur from a utilization review decision. The key to protection is a *well-documented* challenge to coverage and utilization review decisions. The process is dependent on *written* and *confirmed* documentation to the health plan regarding opposition to denial or decision and detailed reason for conflict with the MD's medical judgment.

Good News: State agencies have begun to penalize HMOs that deny care

(1) In June 1997, the Florida Agency for Health Care Administration fined PacifiCare $200000 after on-site review found deficiencies in 28 of 44 standards, including delayed referrals to specialists and delayed second opinions.

(2) Pursuant to a 1997 settlement with the Texas Department of Insurance, a health plan paid a $1 million fine for alleged quality-of-care violations, including denial of payment for emergency services after plan employees had instructed patients to use the services, and denial of emergency room payment when enrollees reasonably believed emergency care was needed.

(3) In 1996, the Oregon Department of Consumer and Business Services fined an HMO $420000 for improper denial of emergency room claims.

(4) In 1995, the California Department of Corporations fined an HMO $500000 for failing to provide a young cancer patient with a qualified specialist and retaliating against her parents for seeking services of a qualified specialist out-of-network.

Good News: Legislation is being enacted to hold health plans accountable for such denials, eg, Texas law

(1) In September 1998, Judge Vanessa Gilmore ruled for the first time that Texas' Health Care Liability Act is *not* pre-empted by federal law since it addresses quality of care and not federally protected benefits. Remember, ERISA had limited a state's right to regulate employee health and pension benefits and essentially protected HMOs from state legislation. Judge Gilmore's decision essentially upheld Texas law holding HMOs liable for denying medically necessary care but is now under appeal by United States Circuit Court of Appeals in New Orleans. Missouri is the only other state allowing such suits and Pennsylvania may follow.

(2) In a further decision, United States District Judge Gilmore upheld the liability portion of law challenged by Aetna but struck down a provision requiring binding *independent* reviews for denial of coverage. Latter decision now *stayed* permitting 240 cases to be evaluated with equal split regarding overturning or upholding HMO decisions.

(3) In Plocica vs. NYLCare of Texas (October 19, 1997), Plocica charged NYLCare of Texas with malpractice in ordering hospital discharge due to coverage denial of a patient leading to his suicide. The HMO had promised not to overrule this legislation.

Inappropriate Use of Clinical Guidelines

Many HMOs base their guidelines denying access or coverage based on the Milliman and Robertson six volumes of guidelines.

Yet:

(a) The scientific basis of these guidelines has never been established.

(b) As originally crafted, the top 10 percent of outcomes were based on *assumptions* of appropriate support services and gradual implementation with local MDs. However, these guidelines are now applied, often indiscriminately as an economy measure.

(c) The original Milliman and Robertson text disclaims its role as a substitute for professional medical judgment; yet the guidelines are often applied in a diagnostic manner that does *indeed* substitute for an MD's judgment, for example, 24-hour discharge after delivery originated in these guidelines in contradistinction to recommendations by the American College of Obstetrics and Gynecology.

Lessons and Suggestions

Remember, the physician is *not* relieved of liability even if the MCO denied coverage of a treatment or procedure.

If a patient is harmed because he/she failed to undergo the necessary test or treatment, the non-coverage by the MCO is *not* a defense if the patient was not informed of the medical necessity for such treatment. As an example, NYS requires, in case of MCO denial:

(1) The physician explains to the patient why such test/treatment is necessary and risks if such test/treatment is not obtained.

(2) The physician assists the patient in the appeals process with MCO.

(3) If still denied, the MD must inform the patient of medical necessity to undergo procedure notwithstanding non-coverage by the plan. (ie, patient must pay costs).

(4) Documentation of all of the above must be clear and unequivocal.

(5) Finally, the question of legal action to be sought by the patient against the MCO should be considered after all avenues of relief have been exhausted.

Indeed, 18 states have a formal dispute resolution process, but this is underutilized.

The factors to consider before embarking on this external appeal process include:

(1) Documentation that the HMO internal appeal systems has been exhausted.

(2) The patient be aware of application fees ($50 in NY; $25 in MA; CT and RI require the patient to pay 50% of costs appeal).

(3) Time limit for appeal from the adverse plan decision or internal appeal decision to filing date may be limited to 30 to 60 days. The independent review panel usually responds *within* 30 days and in 3 days in emergencies (effective 7/1/99 in New York State).

(4) The limitation of external appeals may apply only to experimental therapies in the terminally ill in certain states (CA and OH), but New York will permit appeals on such therapy or clinical trials.

(5) The low rate of appeal is used as a defense by HMOs to limit legislation permitting patients to sue plans. Yet, external reviews overturned HMO decisions in 32 to 65 percent of cases. The costs averaged $500/case (eg, Texas $460 to $650/case), and Medicare cases averaged $300/case. The appeals reviews are *binding* on Plans with Medicare patients in all states except PA and NJ. Therefore, patients should be encouraged to utilize the appeal process.

Alternative Strategies Re: Unionization

In an attempt to obtain some clout in dealing with HMOs, the AMA House of Delegates, on June 23, 1999, voted to endorse unionization for doctors but only those who are certified salaried employees or medical residents. This is an attempt to obtain some clout in bargaining with HMOs.

Existing unions such as the National Doctors Alliance (with 15,000 members) and the Doctors Council (with 2,500 members) are affiliates of larger structures such as the Physician Service Employees International Union, the American Federation of Teachers, and American Federation of State, County and Municipal Employees.

It must be emphasized that federal law does not permit private practitioners to unionize (ie, self-employed MDs) since this is interpreted as a violation of anti-trust law as conspiring to restrain trade. The Campbell bill (H.R. 1304, Health Care Quality Coalition Act of 1999) is an attempt to overcome this barrier.

The present climate of the Justice Department and Federal Trade Commission is still stacked against any exemption from anti-trust by practitioners. The fear is that such exemption would limit competition among health providers and lead to runaway (ie, higher) costs, copayments and insurance premiums.

A further setback occurred on a local level when the National Labor Relations Board (MRB) denied a request of 650 New Jersey physicians to unionize, refusing to consider their positions as "employees of an HMO."

The present situation is that HMOs are indeed dictating care via limiting treatment and diagnostic decisions. They are overwhelming MDs with regulatory paperwork, thus restricting time for patient care with the added loss of autonomy by the patient and their physicians.

What to Do When Payment Is Denied

Overall Strategy

(1) The physician's staff must verify authorization regarding the correct insurance carrier prior to initiating care. Failure to confirm the carrier for their specific responsibility or prior history of a different carrier's denial of care (eg, patient offers one insurance company when Medicare is actual carrier) will lead to immeasurable nuisance calls and expenditures of valuable resources.

(2) Document accuracy of claim for care even down to:
  (a) Typographical errors, blank spaces on requests, etc., that may have sidetracked action as well as administrative errors, that is, wrong department receiving claim.
  (b) Ask yourself: "Were all diagnoses recorded accurately and legibly? Did any diagnosis change during my care? Were these charges documented in a timely and exact manner?"
(3) Develop lines of communication with key personnel in each of the contracted health plans.
(4) Assign a physician *each day* to spend time reviewing denials. That MD may be distinctly more successful in overturning a denial via direct communication with a health plan medical director than the office or ancillary staff, for example, justifying a treatment or extended hospital stay. Dedicating a physician to this task will be worth the cost with money saved on denials. This is as important a task as time spent on consultations or office visits.
(5) Maintain active familiarity with Medicare and Medicaid regulations. Often the same physician battling denials will become skilled in understanding such regulations and their frequent revisions.
(6) Appeal all denials!
  (a) Begin by initiating a letter justifying claim that is in dispute,
  (b) then create "audit trail of appeals", that is:
    • Dates due and sent of insurer-requested records;
    • Name of insurer personnel contacted, date and time;
    • Confirmation of faxes, courier, or overnight mail;
    • Time and dates of appeals.
(7) Periodically, review and scrutinize your contract regarding: compliance and appeal process (should be done at initiation of contract). Pay attention to reimbursement guidelines or policies of denials.
(8) *Finally*, if insurer simply refuses to pay for a service that is covered under provider's contract:
  (a) Send a certified letter to insurer stating your position acknowledging that the payer is not compliant with terms of your contract.
  (b) If still unresolved, arrange a "face to face" session with the insurer's senior official.
  (c) Failing this and if you are convinced of the righteousness of your cause, then:
    • Notify employers and patients that their health plan is *not* providing proper payment for agreed-upon services.
    • Notify the medical society and other physicians having similar problems. If so, consider a joint communication to the carrier on the society's letterhead.

• Last, begin legal action (but remember to avoid adversarial actions if possible).

"Late Payment"

Serious financial burdens exist for MDs whose practices rely on plans with delinquent payment.
(1) Merging health plans claim delay due to system complexities.
(2) Oxford Health Plan (NY) claimed a new computer system was responsible for delay in payment, in some instances over a year.
  Note: Health plans enhance their financial structure by delaying cash payments to MDs. Oxford earned millions of dollars in interest with such delays, prompting the NYS Attorney General to force this MCO to institute interest cost to physicians and hospitals.
(3) Several states provide penalties to HMOs for delayed payment. California requires a 10 percent penalty if a claim is not paid in 30 days, but insurance commissioners vary considerably in enforcement of such laws. NYS and Florida are attempting to enact such laws.

Strategies for Recovery of Payments Due

(1) If there appears to be an unusual delay in reimbursements, the MD's office must ensure that "clean claims," that is, no missing or incorrect data, have been submitted. If you are convinced that your claims are correct, then:
  (a) Document the follow-up communications that are being ignored,
  (b) Provide documentation that such "clean claims" are being manipulated to allow payment delay, that is, redundant or unnecessary inquiries from MCO for data clearly stated on original claims.
(2) Alert the state/county medical society to determine if such delays are widespread, as well as the AMA advocacy resource center (ARC) and Division of Representation.
(3) Mobilize efforts with colleagues "in the same boat" to pressure MCOs for payment, particularly in states with late payment penalty legislation.
(4) Notify the plan, asking for explanations of delay and cite the relevant section of the state's insurance code that interest is due on the unpaid claim and that such documentation will be forwarded to the state's commissioner of insurance.
(5) Discuss this policy of dealing with delayed payment with legal counsel since health plans have the potential to terminate MDs without cause.

Conclusion

Principle 1: "Always, always do what you feel is best for the patient." As a physician, you will never be chastised for interceding on behalf of the patient and you will win more times than you expected.

Principle 2: Persevere! Many MCOs approach requests with initial denials irrespective of the merits of the case. An organized and sustained response will help immeasurably.

Principle 3: Enlist the support of the patients by communicating to the MCOs those services that are rightfully due them and that their physicians should be compensated accordingly.

Late Payment Letter

Dear Mr./Ms. _____ :

I am writing in regards to the attached claims that I have submitted to __(Health Plan)__ . These claims, which were submitted between __(Date)__ and __(Date)__ have not been paid, and I have not received any explanation for this delay in payment.

Please contact my office at the earliest possible convenience to explain the reason for the delay and to indicate when we will receive payment. Because I know that the issue of delayed payment is of increasing concern to many physicians, I intend to report this to the state insurance commissioner if the situation is not rectified.

Thank you for your prompt attention to this matter.

Sincerely,

(Physician Name)

Request for Explanation of Delay in Payment

Dear Mr./Ms. _____ :

Attached is correspondence I sent to __(Health Plan)__ on __(Date)__ regarding late payment of my claims. I have received no response from the plan.

As you may know, the physician community is increasingly concerned about chronic late payment of claims. This is a troubling trend that makes it extremely difficult to run a practice. I hope that your agency will take note of this trend and take steps to put an end to this practice.

Thank you for your consideration of this matter.

Sincerely,

(Physician Name)

Dear Mr./Ms. _____ :

This letter confirms our conversation today about the care of __(Patient's Name)__ . As a physician, I have an ethical and legal duty to advocate for any care that I believe will materially benefit my patients. As you recall,

I recommended __(Describe procedure, course of treatment, referral, etc.)__ , which I believe is medically necessary for the following reasons: __(State reasons)__ .

The Plan has made a decision to deny this care. I will inform my patient in writing of this decision, including his/her options: __(List options)__ . In addition, I will include this letter as part of his/her medical record.

If this is not accurate, please advise me promptly. Again, I restate my belief that this __(Procedure, test, course treatment)__ is medically necessary and that in my clinical judgment, Plan's denial of coverage is not in the best interest of the patient.

In the event that __(Patient's Name)__ , his/her family, or employer wish to hear your reasoning, I will refer them directly to you to avoid any misrepresentation.

Sincerely,

(Physician Name)

Process of Dealing with MCO Denial of Services/Care

The Physician:
(1) Must explain to the patient why such a test or treatment may be necessary and the risks if such a test or treatment is not obtained.
(2) Must assist the patient in the appeals process within the MCO.
(3) Must inform the patient of the medical necessity of undergoing the procedure notwithstanding noncoverage by the plan (ie, patient must pay costs).
(4) Must document all of the above to be clear and unequivocal.
(5) May assist in an external review mechanism for managed care denials in that state if available.
(6) Finally, the question of legal action to be sought by the patient against the MCO should be considered after all avenues of relief have been exhausted.

Supplemental Reading

American Medical Association Code of Ethics (Opinion E8:13).
Grumbach K, Osmond D, Vranizan K, et al. Primary care physicians' experience of financial incentives in managed-care systems. N Engl J Med 1998;339:1516–21.
Hanauer SB, Meyers S. Management of Crohn's disease in adults. Am J Gastroenterol 1997;92:559–66.
Kaiser Family Foundation. American Medical Association News 1998; Dec 7th edition.
Kassirer JP. Doctor discontent. N Engl J Med 1998;339:1543 (editorial).
Kornbluth A, Sachar DB. Ulcerative colitis practice guidelines in adults. Am J Gastroenterol 1997;92:204–11.
Milliman, Robertson. Healthease management guidelines.
Wichline v. California 1986.

CHAPTER 5

MEDICAL-SURGICAL COLLABORATION IN PATIENT MANAGEMENT

FABRIZIO MICHELASSI, MD, AND STEPHEN B. HANAUER, MD

Ulcerative colitis (UC) and Crohn's disease (CD) are chronic inflammatory bowel diseases (IBDs) whose clinical courses are represented by periods of medically or surgically induced clinical remissions interrupted by exacerbations. Throughout the course, both medical and surgical complications can occur. Therefore, continuity of therapy for IBD typically requires teamwork between medical and surgical counterparts to guide therapy and monitor for sequelae of the disease and of medical and surgical treatment. Since nearly one-quarter of patients with UC and over one-half of patients with CD ultimately require surgery, the team effort should define the appropriate indications, timing, and postoperative management for surgical and medical intervention.

The decision to proceed with surgery rarely is easy. The patient and gastroenterologist need to understand that a safe and expertly conducted surgical procedure can alleviate disease- and therapy-related symptoms and restore the patient's quality of life. Conversely, surgery does not cure CD and can have a detrimental impact upon the quality of life for patients with quiescent UC requiring colectomy owing to dysplasia or cancer. Therefore, the decision to proceed with surgery requires concurrence between the patient, gastroenterologist, and surgeon with collaboration from pathologists and radiologists. An active collaboration between gastroenterologist and surgeon is instrumental in obtaining excellent results in the treatment of patients affected by IBD.

Ulcerative Colitis

Preoperative decisions in UC are influenced by the expanding surgical options for proctocolectomy and ileostomy, subtotal colectomy, and ileorectal or ileoanal anastomosis. Many factors, including the patient's age, clinical status, disease duration and complications, life style, and surgical findings, determine the ultimate choice of surgical procedure. Whether surgery is elective or emergent, the medical-surgical team must collaborate to optimize the clinical status as well to educate the patient and family as to the short- and long-term physical, emotional, and life-style implications of surgery. The authors engage in individual and mutual discussions with the patient and offer general nursing support as well as specialized enterostomy nurse input whenever feasible.

Patients and family members have access to a videotape presentation of surgical techniques and alternatives that allow them to understand the implications of various surgical options and expectations.

Management of severe or fulminant colitis is a classic scenario necessitating cooperative medical and surgical teamwork. Patients with fulminant colitis or toxic megacolon admitted to a medical service should be followed from the onset by experienced surgeons. Physicians should initiate education regarding surgical options early and make certain that patients are prepared for surgery if the clinical condition deteriorates or fails to improve. Since surgical morbidity is increased in the setting of perforation or abscess, avoiding these complications must be balanced against the potential improvement with intensive medical therapy. Optimizing timing for an urgent or emergent colectomy requires continuous communication between the medical and surgical teams.

Whereas proctocolectomy and end-ileostomy usually are curative, patients still require preoperative and postoperative education to minimize complications related to diet or life style. Patients who undergo procedures to maintain continuity, such as ileorectal anastomoses, usually require continued medical therapy to the residual colon and long-term surveillance for dysplasia. Those who select restorative pelvic or Kock pouches also require dietary counseling and surveillance for dysplasia as well as potential collaborative management of recurrent pouch inflammation. Depending upon the time frame of complications, these strategies may be initiated at surgical or medical follow-up. Therefore, continued communication between medical and surgical teams is essential for the long-term management of colectomized patients.

Crohn's Disease

Since CD cannot be cured by medical or surgical therapy, and the majority of patients require surgical intervention at some time during their course, collaboration between gastroenterologists and surgeons occurs over a long term. As in UC, surgery may be elective or urgent. In either case, patient preparation and education are essential to optimize outcomes and minimize complications. In addition, there has been a change in attitude toward surgery for CD with the recognition that surgery can rapidly restore a patient's quality of life and with the advent of potential medical therapies that delay postoperative recurrence.

Hospitalization for medical therapy of CD is declining with the advent of newer medical alternatives. Therefore, most patients who require hospitalization for complications of CD (eg, obstruction, abscess) benefit from combined medical and surgical decision-making. Emergent surgery often can be deferred until resolution of an acute obstruction but may be necessary if the patient does not improve or deteriorates. Medical or surgical morbidity can be minimized by cooperative strategies to decompress proximal dilatation and to maintain or restore nutritional deficiencies.

With the availability of interventional radiographic techniques to drain abscesses, emergent surgical procedures often are converted to elective procedures. These approaches also require combined medical-surgical management to maintain the clinical status and nutrition support during staged management. With appropriate management and timing, complications from medical therapies (eg, steroids) and nutritional complications are minimized or avoided. The chapter on perioperative nutritional management provides useful information on the proper use of preoperative total parenteral nutrition (TPN) or elemental diet.

Similarly, evolving operative strategies using minimally invasive surgery, limited resections, or strictureplasty offer patients rapid return to baseline well-being without extensive hospital stay or postoperative morbidity. Therefore, surgical management is more rapidly transitioned to postoperative medical therapy to minimize complications, such as diarrhea secondary to fat or bile salt malabsorption, or metabolic bone disease.

Prior therapeutic nihilism regarding the potential to reduce postoperative recurrence has been replaced by new optimism regarding a variety of strategies to reduce clinical recurrence or repeated surgery. These potential approaches require consideration of the patient's clinical status, predicted risk of recurrence, motivation, and estimated adherence to prophylactic medical therapies. Preoperative discussions, concurrence, and support between medical and surgical counterparts are important to the development of individualized strategies.

University of Chicago Approach

Historic Perspective

At the University of Chicago, gastroenterologists and surgeons have collaborated in the treatment of patients with UC and CD for several decades. The collaboration has been reciprocal and based on the traditional clinical, educational, and academic components of a university practice. Through this continuous collaboration, mentors of the authors, Drs. Joseph B. Kirsner and George E. Block,

were able to decrease the morbidity and mortality associated with medical and surgical treatment of IBD; facilitate cross-fertilization and mutual education; allow for the education of medical students, residents, and fellows; and produce seminal publications. They taught by example how important for the patient and fruitful for the physician this collaboration can be. Under the authors' leadership, this collaboration has evolved into a regular bimonthly clinical and educational conference, a common IBD outpatient clinic, and interactive inpatient management.

Facilities

OUTPATIENT CLINIC

In 1989, a combined IBD outpatient clinic was initiated. In adjacent suites, patients were scheduled to see either the medical team or the surgical team, with easy access to either group. In addition, enterostomy therapists, dietitians, and social workers were available for immediate consultation. Patients were scheduled for endoscopic or radiographic procedures to be reviewed at the same outpatient visit, which significantly increased patient satisfaction and improved physician-to-physician communication. Both groups were able to discuss patients seen primarily by the gastroenterologist or surgeon whether for potential surgery or during routine postoperative visits. This proximity and availability allowed easy communication for patients and their family members and continuity of care as patients transitioned between medical therapy and surgery, or vice versa.

The model of a unified clinic started by the authors 10 years ago has now matured into an institutional model where several gastroenterologists and surgeons, all involved in the treatment of patients with IBD, work efficiently together.

INPATIENT FACILITIES

Over the past 15 years, the authors have tried, with varying degrees of success, to admit medical and surgical patients with IBD to a common hospital wing. In doing so, the same unified approach created in the outpatient facility is maintained for hospitalized patients. Patients admitted to this wing remain there for their medical and surgical treatment, being cared for by the same nurses knowledgeable in the medical as well as the postoperative treatment of IBD. Instead of being the only patients in the hospital or unit with an uncommon condition, patients and family members are reassured to be on a unit where the nursing, dietary, and social work staff are familiar with the unique needs and specialized care. In addition, in an era of managed care and limited hospital stay, the combined unit concept facilitates presurgical management of severely ill patients and the development of critical pathways to expedite both medical and surgical management.

Whether on the same or different floors, patients are visited daily by both the gastroenterologist and the surgeon during their preoperative and postoperative course.

Clinical Conference

In addition to the outpatient and inpatient services directly for patients, the medical and surgical IBD services meet twice a month to discuss routine and complicated cases in conjunction with pathologists and radiologists interested or involved in the care of the patients with IBD. The meeting also is open to medical and surgical residents and gastrointestinal fellows. Associated IBD nurses, research nurses, and data managers participate as well.

The conference has immense clinical and educational value, and it facilitates clinical research. All difficult cases are discussed in a multidisciplinary fashion and the contributions of the pathologist and radiologist are balanced against the clinical impressions of the gastroenterologist and surgeon to individualize the treatment for the patient being discussed. Using an advanced audiovisual system, endoscopic pictures, radiographs, and histopathologic slides are projected on a full screen, allowing everybody to visualize and appreciate the abnormalities being discussed. Difficult cases are presented before the anticipated endoscopic, radiologic, or histopathologic studies are performed to seek advice and counseling on the proper diagnostic sequence and to alert endoscopists, radiologists, and pathologists to the difficulty of the case and the expected diagnostic goals to be achieved. Integration of the endoscopic, radiologic, and pathologic findings with the description of the clinical course, physical examination, and other appropriate data makes for an extraordinary and highly valuable educational conference for students, residents, fellows, faculty members, and visiting physicians from other domestic and international centers. The conference also allows the opportunity to assign patients to the most appropriate research protocols with immediate notification of the data manager and research nurses.

Conclusions

Inflammatory bowel diseases are chronic illnesses that benefit from collaboration between medical and surgical counterparts to optimize short-term management and long-term outcomes and to elucidate patient and family expectations. These interactions occur over years, necessitating ongoing communication and concurrent management decisions between gastroenterologists, surgeons, and their mutual ancillary support.

Supplemental Reading

Cohen RD, Brodsky AL, Hanauer SB. A comparison of the quality of life in patients with severe ulcerative colitis after total colectomy versus medical treatment with intravenous cyclosporin. Inflamm Bowel Dis 1999;5:1–10.

Fleshner PR, Michelassi F, Rubin M, et al. Morbidity of subtotal colectomy in patients with severe ulcerative colitis unresponsive to cyclosporin. Dis Colon Rectum 1995;38:1241–5.

Hurst RD, Finco C, Rubin M, Michelassi F. Prospective analysis of perioperative morbidity in one hundred consecutive colectomies for ulcerative colitis. Surgery 1995;118:748–54; discussion 754–5.

Hurst RD, Michelassi F. Strictureplasty for Crohn's disease: techniques and long-term results. World J Surg 1998;22:359–63.

Hurst RD, Molinari M, Chung TP, et al. Prospective study of the features, indications, and surgical treatment in 513 consecutive patients affected by Crohn's disease. Surgery 1997;122:661–7; discussion 667–8.

Stein RB, Hanauer SB. Medical therapy for inflammatory bowel disease. Gastroenterol Clin North Am 1999;28:297–321.

CHAPTER 6

Consultations and the Patient with Inflammatory Bowel Disease

Harris R. Clearfield, MD

Effective medical care of the patient with inflammatory bowel disease (IBD) not only requires concern for the patient's medical and psychosocial problems but also necessitates an understanding of the gastroenterologist/referring physician interface. The chronic nature of these disorders should prompt managed care organizations to recognize the importance of promoting a coordinated approach. Most primary care physicians are uncomfortable with assuming significant responsibility for the overall supervision of IBD patients, yet they usually do not wish to be excluded from the decision-making process. The following are some personal views of the IBD consultative process, observations of the generalist/gastroenterologist interface as it relates to IBD, and several clinical suggestions regarding IBD patient management.

The Initial Consultation

The consultation process actually begins when the appointment is made. The receptionist must insist that the patient bring actual radiographs (as well as reports), plus all other pertinent records from the referring and previous physicians. The gastrointestinal radiographs should be personally reviewed and, if indicated, evaluated by a trusted radiologist with an interest in IBD. Some erroneous IBD diagnoses, based on inadequate barium studies, are continuously perpetuated if the original studies are not evaluated. The same confirmation approach should apply to other imaging studies and biopsies. It is frustrating for both the patient with IBD and the physician when the patient is sent to the consultant without such records. This problem is complicated further by a referral for only one visit in a managed care setting.

Parents and the Inflammatory Bowel Disease Consultation

Many IBD patients are teenagers who will be accompanied by one or both parents. The parents, understandably, will be concerned and protective. They often wish to play an active and perhaps dominant role in the interview session. It is important to carve out some personal one-on-one discussion time with these young patients to explore emotionally charged issues such as family dynamics, work or school stresses, social pressures, recreational drug and alcohol use, and the effect of the IBD on the patient's ability to function. I find that this works best during the physical examination when parents can be asked to wait in the consultation room. Chapter 2 on the pediatric patient presents additional ideas on this topic.

Information Seeking

Many patients with IBD are remarkably well informed about their disease, having obtained information from the Crohn's and Colitis Foundation of America (CCFA) or from the Internet. The latter source, unfortunately, may stimulate anxiety, particularly if emotionally charged issues are uncovered in chat rooms, or if MEDLINE information is obtained that cannot be reasonably interpreted by the patient. It is best to praise patients for their interest and explain why the Internet literature they have retrieved does not (or does) pertain to their particular problem. Casual dismissal of the patient's information-seeking efforts may evoke hostility. Patients should not be discouraged from Internet information retrieval but need to be counseled regarding the possibility of obtaining information (in chat rooms or from other sources) that may be inaccurate or misleading. The announcements of TNF-α inhibitor therapy (infliximab), for example, prompted many Internet-connected patients with ulcerative colitis or stable Crohn's disease, who were not candidates for treatment, to seek such therapy.

Hereditary Concerns

Although the familial incidence of IBD is 10 to 20 percent, patients rarely express concern as to the risks of their parents or siblings developing the disease. Their concern is usually directed toward the risk for their existing or future children. The lifetime risk for the children of patients with Crohn's disease is 2 to 17 percent, with the higher percentage occurring in those of Ashkenazi Jewish descent. The risk for offspring of patients with ulcerative colitis is approximately 3 percent. The chapter on genetic aspects of IBD contains additional answers to some patient questions.

Unprepped Proctoscopy or Sigmoidoscopy

If rectal disease is likely, an "unprepped" proctosigmoidoscopy using the rigid sigmoidoscope can be informative and avoids the excess mucus production and hypermia that can follow use of phosphosoda enemas. Information regarding rectal activity often can be obtained for therapeutic decisions. The unprepped rigid sigmoidoscopy can also provide some measure of the activity of ulcerative colitis and the response to therapy. The rigid open scope or an anoscope provides more information about hemorrhoids and anal fissure disease than does a flexible instrument.

Communications with the Referring Physician

Consultants often complain that referred patients frequently appear without adequate information, while the referring physicians are not pleased with the lack of contact from their consultants. Direct phone contact with the referring physician regarding the assessment of symptomatic patients is a useful approach.

Letters should be dictated the same day as the evaluation. It is helpful to keep a database of all referring physicians and determine whether they prefer to have their reports mailed, faxed, mailed and faxed, or e-mailed. The referral letter is also an opportunity to provide educational materials, such as a copy of therapy guidelines or a review of the efficacy of a new therapy such as infliximab.

Multiple Visits

Inflammatory bowel disease patients may require multiple visits to the consultant in order to discuss the findings of the laboratory and imaging studies, review the early response to therapy, and follow the clinical course so that medication adjustments can be made. There has been interest in the concept of "principal care," wherein the specialist assumes total responsibility for the patient's care. This entails other responsibilities, including checking cholesterol levels, immunizations, and appropriate mammographic and gynecologic screening. Other arrangements include "co-care," which permits unlimited consultant visits without the primary physician relinquishing control.

Imaging Studies

There can be differences in the quality of barium studies and I try, if possible, to schedule referred patients with radiologists who have demonstrated an interest and skill in performing these examinations. Unfortunately, some managed care patients are capitated to radiography departments that may lack expertise in the performance of barium small bowel radiographs or enteroclysis. Personally reviewing the films, perhaps by tele-radiography, can be helpful.

Surgical Referral

Gastroenterologists usually have strong feelings about the choice of a surgeon for various disorders but the referring physician also may want to influence that decision. Ideally, IBD surgery, whether it is complicated small bowel Crohn's disease with skip areas and fistulas or ulcerative colitis that requires a J-pouch, should be performed by experienced GI surgeons. If local surgeons have marginal experience with J-pouch procedures or other complicated IBD surgery, patients now have the option of independently inquiring about surgeons or hospital centers located through the Internet. If surgery is being considered, the referring physician should be apprised of this; otherwise, the patient may ask for his/her opinion without any available background information from the gastroenterologist.

Role of the Referring Physician

The referring physician needs to be part of the "team" care process. For example, immunosuppressive therapy will require hematologic monitoring and patients on steroid therapy will require DEXA scans and intermittent ophthalmologic examinations. Unexpected changes in a patient's status should prompt referral back to the consultant. Since the IBD management of a previous physician, either a primary physician or another gastroenterologist, may have been different from your approach, it is helpful to explain that legitimate differences in terms of dosage or sequencing of therapies exist among physicians.

There are other chapters devoted to emotional factors in the IBD patient and to the overlap of irritable bowel syndrome with IBD. The consultant may also have to address insurance and disability issues, which are also discussed in separate chapters.

Conclusion

The IBD consultation requires evaluation of the impact of IBD on the patient's ability to function as well as other clinical factors. The referring physician may either wish to delegate ongoing IBD care to the consultant or may intermittently refer the patient for reevaluation. In either case, close attention to letters after each visit and efforts to keep the referring physician involved in the management process are essential.

Supplemental Reading

Clearfield HR. Consultant strategies for the gastroenterologist. Am J Gastroenterol 1999;94:1453–56.

Emmanuel LL. The consultant and the patient-physician relationship. Arch Intern Med 1994;154:1785–90

Peeters M, Nevens H, Baert F, et al. Familial aggregation in Crohn's disease: increased age-adjusted risk and concordance in clinical characteristics. Gastroenterology 1996;111:597–603.

Roth MP, Petersen GM, McElree C, et al. Familial empiric risk estimates of inflammatory bowel disease in Ashkenazi Jews. Gastroenterology 1989;96:1016–20.

Travis SPL. Review article: insurance risks for patients with ulcerative colitis or Crohn's disease. Aliment Pharmacol Ther 1997;11:51–9.

CHAPTER 7

MEASURES OF DISEASE ACTIVITY

JOHN W. SINGLETON, MD

The notion that it might be useful to express activity of inflammatory bowel disease (IBD) quantitatively arose with the first controlled clinical trials in England in the 1950s. The three-level classification of severity of ulcerative colitis, published by Truelove and Witts in 1955 (Table 7–1), is still a useful tool. A plethora of quantitative and detailed indexes for expressing activity of both ulcerative colitis and Crohn's disease have followed, including indexes specially adapted for proctitis, perianal disease, and pediatric patients. Recently, the need for measurement of patients' subjective responses to inflammatory bowel disease has led to development of "quality of life" indexes. This chapter selects for review those instruments judged most useful for the quantitatively minded clinician.

General Indexes: Several definitional dilemmas have made indexes of IBD activity controversial from the start. First, "What is activity?" Is IBD activity "degree of inflammation" or is it "degree of illness?" The practicing clinician, and the patient, may be more interested in illness than inflammation. The interests of the clinical trial investigator might be just the opposite. Second, "How much weight should be given to the patient's, or the physician's, subjective assessment?" A major objection to the Crohn's Disease Activity Index (CDAI) was its heavy weighting of the patient's assessment of degree of illness. On the other hand, the Inflammatory Bowel Disease Questionnaire (IBDQ) was developed because of the perception that the CDAI and other indexes did not adequately measure the effect of IBD on patients' lives. Third,

TABLE 7–1. Truelove and Witts' Activity Categories for Ulcerative Colitis

Severe	Diarrhea >6 motions/day, with blood
	PM temperature >37°C
	Average pulse >90 beats/min
	Anemia with hemoglobin ≤75%
	ESR >30 mm/hr
Mild	Diarrhea <4 motions/day, non-bloody
	No fever
	No tachycardia
	Anemia "not severe"
	ESR <30 mm/hr
Moderately severe	Intermediate between mild and severe

TABLE 7–2. St Mark's Clinical Illness Score for Ulcerative Colitis

Item	Points	Range
General health	0–3	Good to unable to work
Abdominal pain	0–2	None to prolonged
Bowel frequency	0–2	<3 to >6 per day
Blood in stool	0–2	None to more than trace
Stool consistency	0–2	Formed to liquid
Anorexia	0–1	Absent to present
Nausea/vomiting	0–1	Absent to present
Abdominal tenderness	0–4	None to rebound
Extra-intestinal manifestations	0–3	None to severe (or >1)
Temperature	0–2	Normal to >38°C
Sigmoidoscopy	0–2	Nonhemorrhagic to spontaneous bleeding

"Is it desirable or possible to express IBD activity for every patient on a single numerical or ordinal scale?" An index like the CDAI forces its users to accept the choices made by the authors of the index. Despite all of these problems, several general indexes have proven useful.

Ulcerative Colitis

The localization of mucosal disease in the distal colon makes sigmoidoscopic observation an easy way to judge severity of bowel involvement in ulcerative colitis. Several classification schemes have been proposed; the most reproducible avoid characteristics, such as edema and color, for which interobserver variation is great, and include hemorrhage, ulceration, and friability where consensus is more easily obtained. However, severity of systemic illness may correlate poorly with severity of mucosal disease. To address this problem, Truelove and Witts proposed a classification (see Table 7–1) of severity of systemic disease. It continues to be the standard system for classifying systemic severity of ulcerative colitis. Although it has been used in several large controlled trials, it lacks sensitivity, having only three levels of severity. It is also not clear how to classify patients who exhibit only some of the criteria specified for each level. The St. Mark's Index (Table 7–2) is more specific and offers a continuous numeric scale while remaining easy to use. Lichtiger et al proposed an index of severity for patients

TABLE 7–3. Crohn's Disease Activity Index*

Item (daily sum per week)	Weight
Number of liquid or very soft stools	2
Abdominal pain score in 1 week, rating 0–3	5
General well-being (rating 1–4)	7
Sum of findings per week: Arthritis/arthralgia Mucocutaneous lesions (e.g., E. nodosum) Iritis/uveitis Anal disease (fissure, fistula, etc.) External fistula (enterocut./vessicle, etc.) Fever > 36.8°C	20
Antidiarrheal use (eg, diphenoxylate)	30
Abdominal mass (none = 0, equivocal = 2, definite = 5)	10
47 minus hematocrit (males) or 42 minus hematocrit (females)	6
100 x (1 – [body weight divided by standard weight])	1

*Adapted from Best et al.

hospitalized with ulcerative colitis and being considered for cyclosporine therapy. This index was not validated prior to the study. A pouchitis index (Sanborn et al) is used in some studies of that problem.

Crohn's Disease

Crohn's Disease Activity Index: The CDAI (Table 7–3) was derived by choosing from among a number of clinical and common laboratory measurements those that best predicted the physician's global assessment of the clinical status of a large group of Crohn's disease patients. It then was validated in another large group of patients. In the past 25 years, the CDAI has been used in over 50 controlled clinical trials, continuing to the present. It offers a standardized scale with which to compare patients and their responses over time and space, within clinical trials and everyday practice. It is sufficiently sensitive to changes in clinical status to allow recognition of therapeutic effect in a relatively small, economically feasible clinical trial. It requires determination of the hematocrit and that the patient keep a daily diary of stool number and subjective degree of illness for a week prior to the day the index is calculated; these requirements make assessments cumbersome at a single office visit.

The Harvey-Bradshaw, or Simple Index (Table 7–4), requires only data available at the time of the visit and correlates well (r = .80) with the CDAI. It also has been used in numerous controlled clinical trials. A Pediatric Crohn's Disease Activity Index includes data on symptoms (pain, diarrhea, well-being), laboratory assessment (hematocrit, ESR, albumin), physical examination (abdominal tenderness, perianal disease, extra-intestinal manifestations), and growth (weight gain/loss, growth channel, velocity). It has been used extensively in clinical trials and is recommended for use with children and adolescents. For survey research, Sandler and colleagues have modified the CDAI, including only elements that could

TABLE 7–4. Harvey-Bradshaw (Simple) Index*

Item	Scale
General well-being	0 = very well, 1 = slightly below par, 2 = poor, 3 = very poor, 4 = terrible
Abdominal pain	0 = none, 1 = mild, 2 = moderate, 3 = severe
Number of liquid stools per day	
Abdominal mass	0 = none, 1 = dubious, 2 = definite, 3 = definite and tender
Complications: arthritis, uveitis, erythema nodosum, apthous ulcers, pyoderma gangrenosum, anal fissure, new fistula, abscess	Score 1 per item

*Adapted from Harvey and Bradshaw.

be obtained by interview (stool frequency, abdominal pain, sense of well-being). The new index correlated very well with the CDAI from which it was derived (r = .87, p < .001).

Patient-specific Treatment Goals: Present et al devised a system of patient-specific treatment goals for their controlled trial of 6-mercaptopurine in Crohn's disease. Treatment success or failure was determined by whether or not improvement occurred in one or more of three clinical arenas: reduction of steroid dosage, healing of fistulas, and amelioration of other specific clinical signs and symptoms. Improvement or worsening in each goal item was judged at 3-month intervals on a scale of +3 for excellent improvement, through 0 for no change, to –3 for severe worsening. While this system avoids the "one size fits all" objection raised to numerical indexes, it introduces an arbitrary choice of goals as well as the subjective judgment of the clinician as to improvement or worsening. It has been used in several trials, often along with the CDAI or the Harvey-Bradshaw index.

Other general indexes: The Van Hees, or Dutch Index (Table 7–5), was developed specifically to avoid subjective elements. It correlates poorly with the CDAI but has been useful in several clinical trials. It is somewhat cumber-

TABLE 7–5. The Van Hees (Dutch) Index*

Regression Variable $x_{(1-9)}$	Index Item
1	Serum albumin (g/L)
2	ESR (mm after 1 hour)
3	Quetelet index[†]
4	Abdominal mass (grade 1–5)[#]
5	Sex (male = 1, female = 2)
6	Temperature (°C) daily average for week
7	Stool consistency (rating 1–3)[$]
8	Intestinal resection (no = 1, yes = 2)
9	Extra-intestinal lesions

* Adapted from Van Hees et al.

The Index score is obtained by inserting each dependent variable value (x_n) into the equation:
-209 [the constant, b_0] $- 5.48x_1 + 0.29x_2 - 0.22x_3 + 7.83x_4 - 12.3x_5 + 16.4x_6 + 8.46x_7 - 9.17x_8 + 10.7x_9$

† Weight (kg) x 10/height (cm²); # No mass = 1, dubious = 2, diameter <6 cm = 3, diameter 6–12 cm = 4, diameter >12cm = 5; $ Well-formed = 1, soft = 2, watery = 3.

TABLE 7–6. IOIBD (Oxford) Index

Score 1 for each feature (where present)

1	Pain present
2	Bowels 6+/day or blood or mucus
3	Perianal complications
4	Fistula
5	Other complications
6	Mass present
7	Wasting/emaciation
8	Temperature above 38°C
9	Abdominal tenderness
10	Hb below 10 g/100 mL

TABLE 7–7. Perianal Disease Index 13

Perianal Disease Activity	Scale
Discharge	0–4 (none to gross fecal soilage)
Pain/restriction of activities	0–4 (none to severe pain, severe limitation)
Restriction of sexual activities	0–4 (no restriction to unable to do any)
Degree of induration	0–4 (none to gross fluctuance/abscess)
Type of perianal disease	0 = no perianal disease/skin tags
	1 = anal fissure or mucosal tear
	2 = <3 fistulae
	3 = >3 fistulae
	4 = sphincter ulceration or fistulae with significant undermining of skin

some to calculate. The IOIBD (International Organization for Inflammatory Bowel Disease), or Oxford Index (Table 7–6), was developed in reaction to the perceived complexity of the CDAI. It gives each of 10 items a weight of one as either present or absent. The score is thus simply the total number of items present at the time the patient is seen. The Oxford Index has not been subjected to tests of validity or reproducibility.

The French Groupe d'Etudes Therapeutiques des Affections Inflammatoires Digestives (GETAID) has devised and validated a Crohn's Disease Endoscopic Index of Severity (CDEIS) that is useful for recording and following the colonoscopic manifestations of Crohn's disease. However, GETAID found that endoscopic severity, as reflected in the CDEIS, correlated very poorly with either clinical activity (CDAI) or biological markers of inflammation.

Perianal Crohn's Disease

The general-purpose indexes often do not reflect the severity of illness due to perianal Crohn's disease. Therefore, a Perianal Disease Index was devised by the McMaster IBD Study Group (Table 7–7). As expected, scores on this index did not correlate with the CDAI, but there was a correlation with both patient and physician assessment of the patient's degree of illness.

Quality of Life in Inflammatory Bowel Disease

In contrast to the dismay expressed at the subjective elements of the CDAI, there recently has been recognition of the importance of instruments that measure the effect of IBD on patient quality of life. The most widely used of these is the IBDQ questionnaire devised by the McMaster group. It consists of questions covering four domains: bowel symptoms, systemic symptoms, emotional function, and social function. Response options are consistently presented as 7-point scales. This instrument has been extensively validated. Like the CDAI, the IBDQ is strongly affected by diarrhea-related symptoms. A self-administered form, suitable for mail-in responses, has been developed. Another successful approach has been use of visual analog scales in several dimensions of a patient's life, yielding an overall numeric score as well as scores for each dimension.

Inflammatory Bowel Disease Measurement in Practice

None of the instruments discussed above has been widely adopted by practicing gastroenterolgists in their everyday practice. All of them were devised for use in therapeutic trials. For clinical trials in Crohn's disease, the current instruments of choice are the CDAI and the IBDQ used together. For clinical trials in ulcerative colitis, the St. Mark's Index and a sigmoidoscopic scoring system would be a good choice. In a sense, every patient treated in clinical practice is part of a therapeutic trial. The quantitatively minded clinician might well consider keeping a record of patient responses to these therapeutic interventions using, for example, the Harvey-Bradshaw Index and the short-form IBDQ. These data could be collected with a minimum of expense and effort. The results, tabulated and graphed using one of several available software programs, would give a revealing longitudinal picture of a patient's battle with IBD.*

Suggested Readings

Best WR, Becktel JM, Singleton JW, Kern F Jr. Development of a Crohn's disease activity index: National Cooperative Crohn's Disease Study. Gastroenterology 1976;70:439–44.

Cellier C, Sahmoud T, Froguel E, et al. Correlations between clinical activity, endoscopic severity, and biological parameters in colonic or ileocolonic Crohn's disease. A prospective multicentre study of 212 cases. Gut 1994;35:231–5.

Groupe d'Etudes Therapeutiques des Affections Inflammatoires du Tube Digestif (GETAID), Mary JY, Modigliani R. Development and validation of an endoscopic index of the severity for Crohn's disease: a prospective multicenter study. Gut 1989;30:983–9

---

* Editor's Note: It is hoped that some effort will be made to quantify the responses to Remicade® (infliximab), as this type of therapy is being utilized by thousands of patients before thorough clinical trials have been conducted.

Guyatt G, Mitchell A, Irvine EJ, et al. A new measure of health status for clinical trials in inflammatory bowel disease. Gastroenterology 1989;96:804–10

Harvey RF, Bradshaw JM. A simple index of Crohn's disease activity. Lancet 1980;1:514–5.

Hyams JS, Ferry GD, Mandel FS, et al. Development and validation of a pediatric Crohn's disease activity index. J Pediatr Gastroenterol Nutr 1991;12:439–47.

Irvine EJ. Usual therapy improves perianal Crohn's disease as measured by a new disease activity index. J Clin Gastroenterol 1995;20:27–32.

Lichtiger S, Present DH, Kornbluth A, et al. Cyclosporine in severe ulcerative colitis refractory to steroid therapy. N Engl J Med 1994;330:1841–5.

Love JR, Irvine EJ, Fedorak RN. Quality of life in inflammatory bowel disease. J Clin Gastroenterol 1992;14:15–9.

O'Brien JJ, Bayless TM, Bayless JA. Use of azathioprine or 6-mercaptopurine in the treatment of Crohn's disease. Gastroenterology 1991;101:39–46.

Myren J, Bouchier IAD, Watkinson G, et al. The O.M.G.E. Multinational Inflammatory Bowel Disease Survey 1976–1982. A further report on 2,657 cases. Scand J Gastroenterol 1984;19(Suppl 95):1–27.

Powell-Tuck J, Brown RL, Lennard-Jones JE. A comparison of oral prednisolone given as a single or multiple daily doses for active proctocolitis. Scand J Gastroenterol 1978;13:833–7.

Present DH, Korelitz BI, Wisch N, et al. Treatment of Crohn's disease with 6-mercaptopurine: a long-term, randomized, double-blind study. N Engl J Med 1980;302:981–7

Sandler RS, Jordan MC, Kupper LL. Development of a Crohn's index for survey research. J Clin Epidemiol 1988;41:451–8.

Singleton JW, Hanauer S, Robinson M. Quality-of-life results of a double-blind, placebo-controlled trial of mesalamine in patients with Crohn's disease. Dig Dis Sci 1995;40:931–5.

Truelove SC, Witts LJ. Cortisone in ulcerative colitis: final report on a therapeutic trial. BMJ 1955;2:1041–8.

Van Hees PAM, Van Elteren PH, Van Lier HJJ, Van Tongeren JHM. An index of inflammatory activity in patients with Crohn's disease. Gut 1980;21:279–86.

CHAPTER 8

Computer Database for Patients with Inflammatory Bowel Disease

Jean-Frédéric Colombel, MD, PhD, Dominique Cochelard, PhD,
Antoine Cortot, MD, Jean-Marc Brunetaud, MD, PhD

At the dawn of this new century, inflammatory bowel disease (IBD) represents a considerable burden for the gastroenterologic community. The incidence of IBD has stabilized since the 1970s and prevalence is steadily increasing. It has recently been calculated that, extrapolating the results observed in Olmsted County to the projected Caucasian-American population in 2005, there may be as many as 580,000 cases of Crohn's disease (CD) among Caucasian Americans in the middle of the next decade. Revolution in the pharmacologic therapy of IBD is currently underway. New drugs, such as infliximab, are highly effective yet expensive. Most gastroenterologists will thus have to assume care for a large number of young IBD patients who will require life-long treatments of increasing complexity and cost.

On the other hand, IBD remains relatively rare and evidence has accumulated that they are heterogeneous and may represent a syndrome with multiple etiologies. Defining homogeneous clinical subgroups may help to identify the causes of IBD and to refine therapeutic approaches. For instance, it is possible that different susceptibility genes may underlie phenotypic differences in IBD. Identification of a particular phenotype will help the search for a corresponding gene. Aggressive therapeutic strategies should be restricted to patients at high risk for unremitting disease. Progress in this respect will require the creation of large national and international cross-sectional IBD data resources. The goal would be to characterize a large number of currently followed IBD patients according to validated clinical classification systems.

Use of a database system is now indispensable both at the individual (gastroenterologist) and collective (referral centers, national and international organizations) levels. The computer will allow the gastroenterologist to easily retrieve the history of each patient and to monitor other course in the context of other patients. Collection of large cohorts of patients using standardized diagnostic criteria and phenotypes would be critical to making further progress in various fields such as epidemiology, pathophysiology, and pharmacoeconomics.

Software Specifications

The computer system has to meet several requirements in order to be used both in daily practice and for clinical studies. In order to avoid possible errors and misinterpretations, all of the data should be entered during the consultation (in real time) by the clinician in charge of the patient. This means a fast software with a user-friendly interface. It may be necessary to compromise between completeness and swiftness. Collection of data according to standardized criteria and classifications will allow interplay between centers as well as summation of cases. Ethical guidelines and confidentiality rules should be followed.

Development of an Inflammatory Bowel Disease Software System

This software was created on the Microsoft Access® DataBase Manager, with the oriented object language V.B.A. (Visual Basic for Application) concept, allowing a great level of interactivity. The two main bodies of the software are data management and data processing.

Data Management

Data management comprises four main parts:
(1) Patient identification record, which deals with administrative data
(2) One or more patient evolution records, which describe the patient's history, clinical characteristics, and treatment. Data are entered using dialog boxes with a limited number of keyboard entries. These procedures minimize the risk of error during data entry
(3) Synthesis, which are summary files containing selected medical data
(4) Tools: this screen facilitates a patient's record search

Patient Identification Record

This part comprises one screen that only has to be completed once and may be printed (Figure 1).

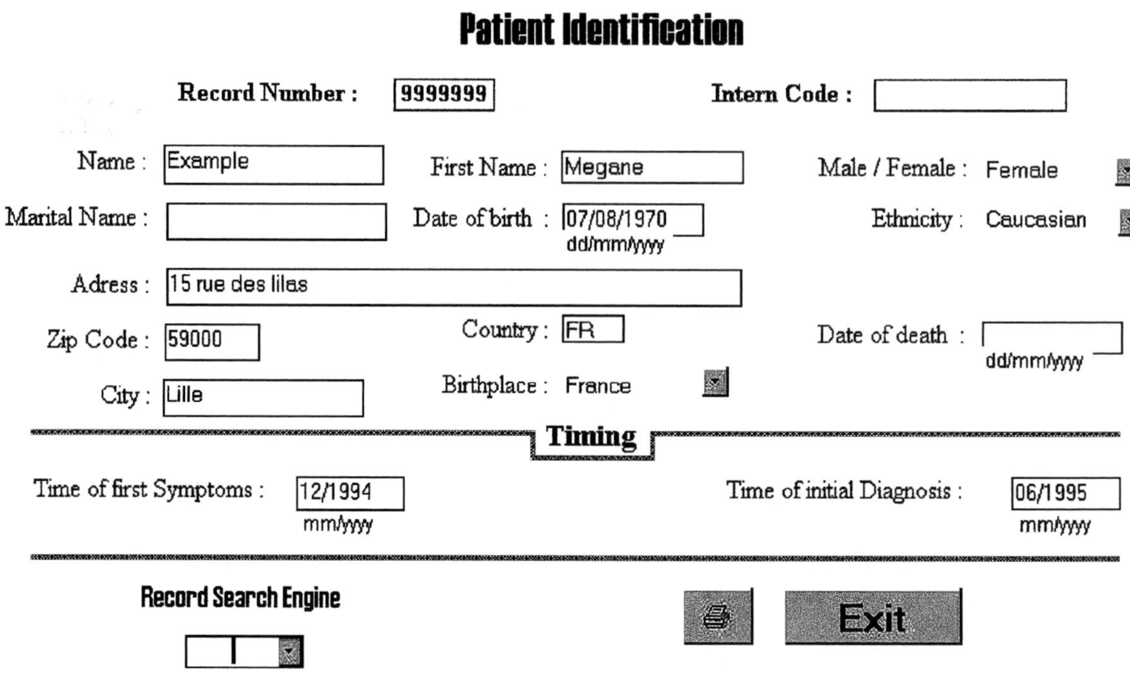

Patient Identification

Record Number : 9999999 **Intern Code :**

Name : Example   First Name : Megane   Male / Female : Female

Marital Name :   Date of birth : 07/08/1970   Ethnicity : Caucasian
                  dd/mm/yyyy

Adress : 15 rue des lilas

Zip Code : 59000   Country : FR   Date of death :
                                                    dd/mm/yyyy

City : Lille   Birthplace : France

Timing

Time of first Symptoms : 12/1994   Time of initial Diagnosis : 06/1995
                          mm/yyyy   mm/yyyy

Record Search Engine

Exit

FIGURE 8–1. Patient Identification Record. Age at diagnosis is the age at which the diagnosis of IBD was first definitively established using standard criteria (5).

PATIENT EVOLUTION RECORD
This portion permits one to monitor the patient on different occasions and is comprised of five different screens. Once the patient identification record has been created, as many follow-up sessions as wanted may be added. The data of each session will be kept in the computer's memory and can be recalled later (see synthesis). When a new session starts, data of the last session are

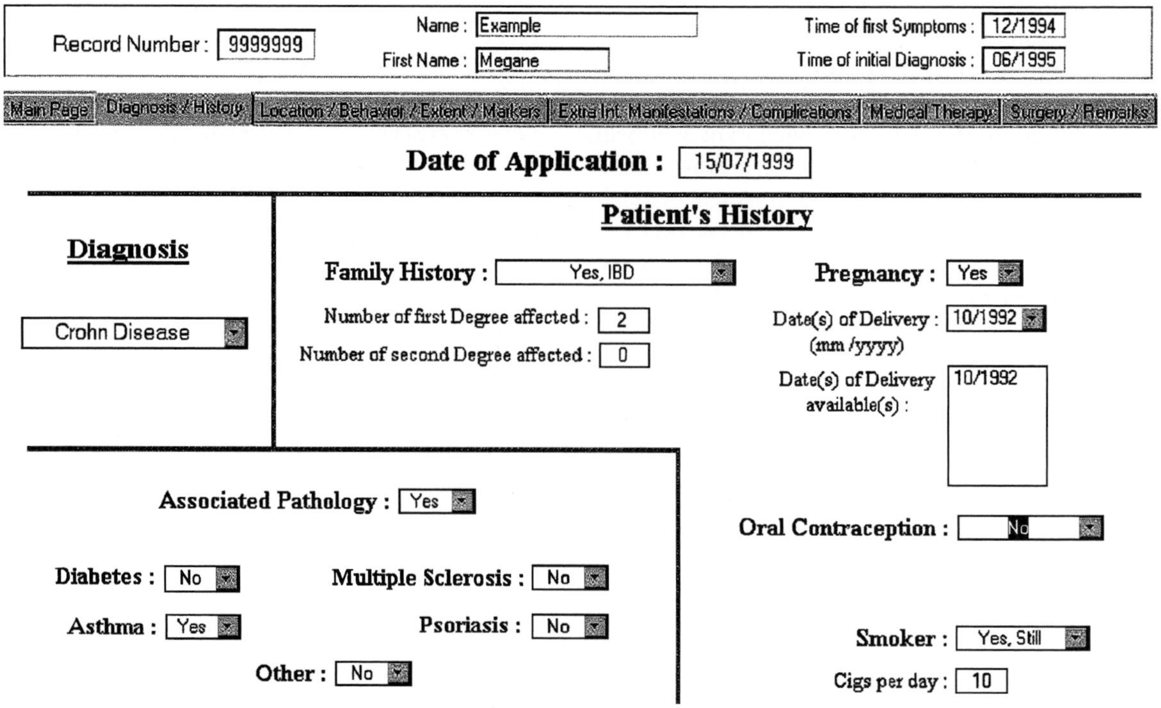

Record Number : 9999999   Name : Example   Time of first Symptoms : 12/1994
                           First Name : Megane   Time of initial Diagnosis : 06/1995

Main Page | Diagnosis / History | Location / Behavior / Extent / Markers | Extra Int. Manifestations / Complications | Medical Therapy | Surgery / Remarks

Date of Application : 15/07/1999

Diagnosis

Crohn Disease

Patient's History

Family History : Yes, IBD   Pregnancy : Yes

Number of first Degree affected : 2   Date(s) of Delivery : 10/1992
Number of second Degree affected : 0   (mm /yyyy)

                                        Date(s) of Delivery   10/1992
                                        available(s) :

Associated Pathology : Yes

Diabetes : No   Multiple Sclerosis : No   **Oral Contraception :** No

Asthma : Yes   Psoriasis : No

Other : No   **Smoker :** Yes, Still

                                        Cigs per day : 10

FIGURE 8–2. Patient Evolution Record. Screen 1: "Diagnosis/History." Inflammatory bowel disease diagnosis box has three entries: CD, ulcerative colitis, and indeterminate colitis, which represent 10% of patients in large epidemiologic studies (5).

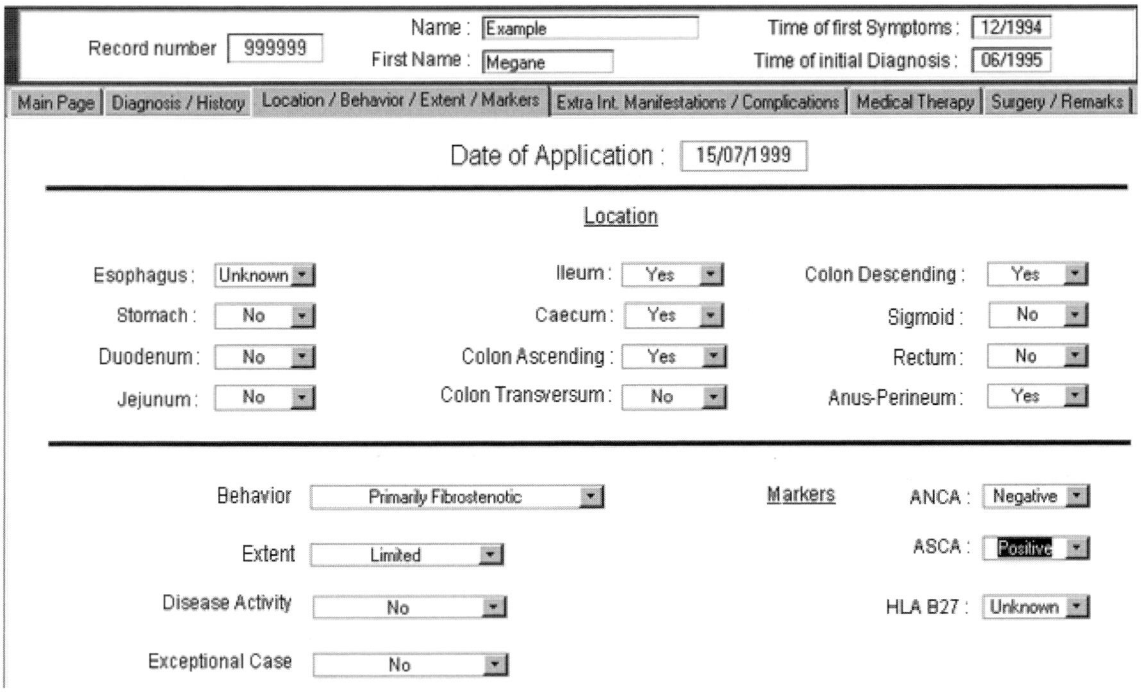

| Record number | 999999 | Name : | Example | Time of first Symptoms : | 12/1994 |
| | | First Name : | Megane | Time of initial Diagnosis : | 06/1995 |

| Main Page | Diagnosis / History | Location / Behavior / Extent / Markers | Extra Int. Manifestations / Complications | Medical Therapy | Surgery / Remarks |

Date of Application : 15/07/1999

Location

Esophagus :	Unknown	Ileum :	Yes	Colon Descending :	Yes
Stomach :	No	Caecum :	Yes	Sigmoid :	No
Duodenum :	No	Colon Ascending :	Yes	Rectum :	No
Jejunum :	No	Colon Transversum :	No	Anus-Perineum :	Yes

			Markers		
Behavior	Primarily Fibrostenotic		ANCA :	Negative
Extent	Limited		ASCA :	Positive
Disease Activity	No		HLA B27 :	Unknown
Exceptional Case	No			

FIGURE 8–3. Patient evolution record. Screen 2: "Location/Behaviour/Extent/Markers." Minimum involvement for a location is defined as any aphtous lesion or ulceration. Crohn's disease behavior and extent may be determined according to Vienna and Roma classification (6,7). Evaluation of disease activity should rely on the general evaluation by the clinician.

displayed on the screens and the gastroenterologist has simply to modify the items that have changed since the last consultation:

- Screen 1 is titled "Diagnosis/History" (Figure 2).
- Screen 2 is titled "Location/Behaviour/Extent/Markers" (Figure 3).
- Screen 3 is titled "Extra Intestinal Manifestations/ Complications" (Figure 4).

- Screen 4 is titled "Medical Therapy" (Figure 5).
- Screen 5 is titled "Surgery/Remarks" (Figure 6).

SYNTHESIS

The IBD software program permits the display of two screens that contain the most important data for the follow-up of the patient. The simple synthesis screen provides a summary of the six previous screens at first

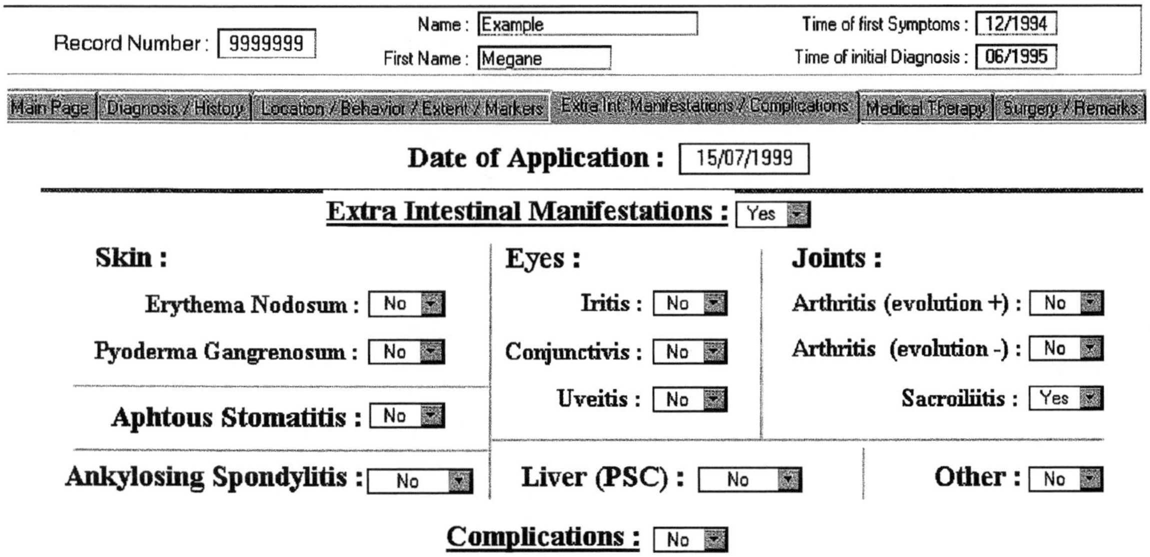

| Record Number : | 9999999 | Name : | Example | Time of first Symptoms : | 12/1994 |
| | | First Name : | Megane | Time of initial Diagnosis : | 06/1995 |

| Main Page | Diagnosis / History | Location / Behavior / Extent / Markers | Extra Int. Manifestations / Complications | Medical Therapy | Surgery / Remarks |

Date of Application : 15/07/1999

Extra Intestinal Manifestations : Yes

Skin :	Eyes :	Joints :
Erythema Nodosum : No	Iritis : No	Arthritis (evolution +) : No
Pyoderma Gangrenosum : No	Conjunctivis : No	Arthritis (evolution -) : No
Aphtous Stomatitis : No	Uveitis : No	Sacroiliitis : Yes
Ankylosing Spondylitis : No	Liver (PSC) : No	Other : No

Complications : No

FIGURE 8–4. Patient Evolution Record. Screen 3: "Extra Intestinal Manifestations/Complications." Complications comprise pouchitis, small bowel cancer, colon cancer, cholangiocarcinoma, and acute severe colitis.

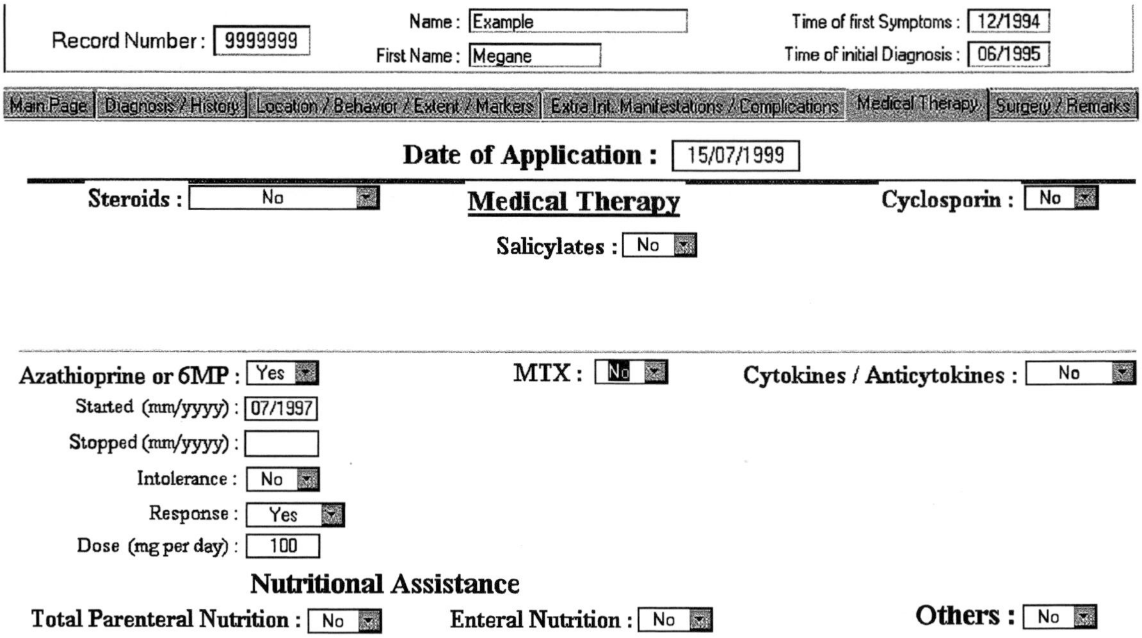

FIGURE 8–5. Patient Evolution Record. Screen 4: "Medical Therapy." For each treatment date of start and stop, dosage and response (yes, no, unknown) may be pointed.

diagnosis, at last visit, and at any consultation, allowing a brief review of the medical history of the patient. The event detection synthesis screen is focused on medical and surgical treatment. It lists the different therapeutic agents that the patient has received and the date and type of surgical interventions.

TOOLS

The search engine has a record number box search, a family name search (including marital name), and a first name box search. Keying in the first characters of the name or first name can start the patient's record search. Main data of the result search are displayed at the top of the tools screen.

Data Processing

This software portion is not in its final version, but we are developing standardized and detailed data processing. At present, the user builds step by step a Structured Query Language (SQL) request for the database interrogation. Some boxes, including all patients' record items, are proposed. The user must click into these boxes to ask for his/her request. The request result that can be shown or printed currently provides the record number, the name (with the marital name), the first name, and the dates of application found.

TECHNICAL SPECIFICATIONS

The software runs under the Windows® 9x environment. The source code is written with a Microsoft® Access 97 database and the software is compiled. The database is furnished with a run time of Microsoft® Access 97 (ie, it is not required to have Microsoft® Access 97 installed in the computer). The software's installation is easy to perform. The installation directory is C:\MITDSOFT and the software requires 3 megabytes on hard disk. It does not work with Apple platforms.

Prospects

This software has been successfully tested in different sites. It offers a useful method for the management of IBD data, with limited keyboard entries. Filling out a session takes between 3 and 5 minutes, which makes it usable by all practitioners. Its use, however, requires sufficient availability and motivation for clinicians to fill out the database in real time. To achieve this goal, clinicians must identify a clear interest for providing the effort.

The personal interest is immediate: files of patients with CD or UC are often thick and contain multiple events. The task of synthesizing the history of the patient will be accelerated, thus facilitating the goals of the current consultation.

The computer database will lead to agreement on a common language and standardization.

Another motivating factor is that the database may provide a precise report for the institution of the activity of a clinical unit devoted to IBD. The financial burden of IBD management, already heavy, will likely increase in the forthcoming years notably due to the occurrence of new biologic treatments. At least in Europe, the financial support of these new treatments must be discussed with

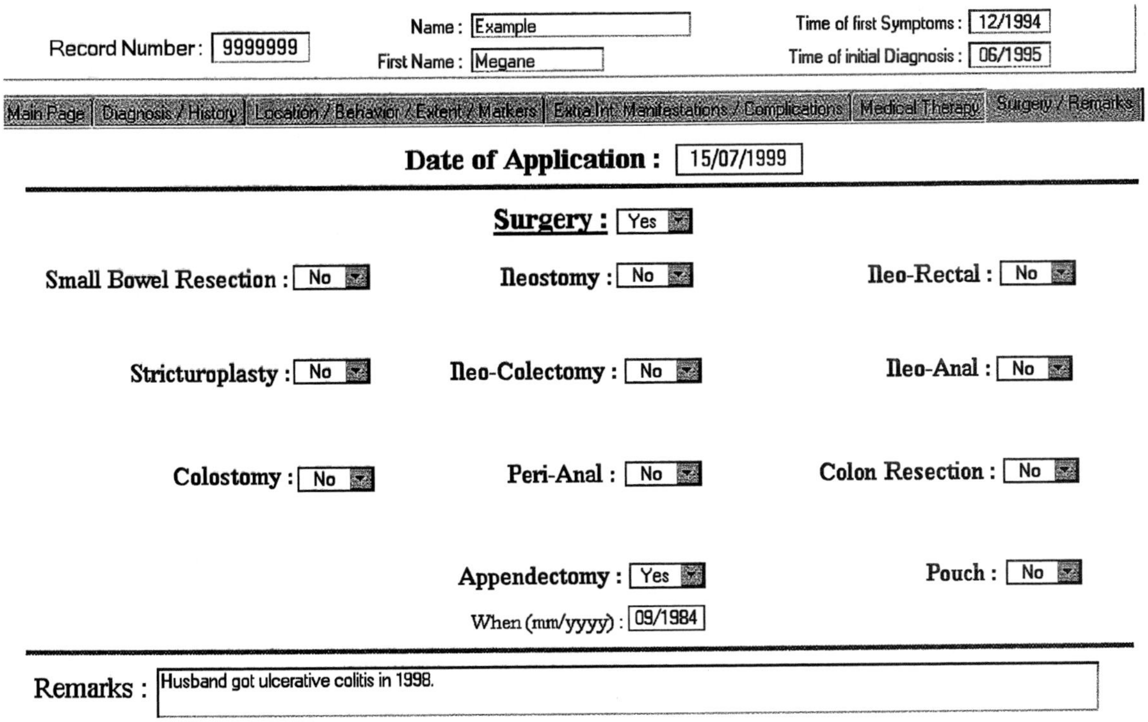

| Record Number : | 9999999 | | Name : | Example | | | Time of first Symptoms : | 12/1994 |
| | | | First Name : | Megane | | | Time of initial Diagnosis : | 06/1995 |

Main Page | Diagnosis / History | Location / Behavior / Extent / Markers | Extra Int. Manifestations / Complication | Medical Therapy | Surgery / Remarks

Date of Application : 15/07/1999

Surgery : Yes

Small Bowel Resection : No   Ileostomy : No   Ileo-Rectal : No

Stricturoplasty : No   Ileo-Colectomy : No   Ileo-Anal : No

Colostomy : No   Peri-Anal : No   Colon Resection : No

Appendectomy : Yes   Pouch : No
When (mm/yyyy) : 09/1984

Remarks : Husband got ulcerative colitis in 1998.

FIGURE 8–6. Patient Evolution Record. The date of each surgical session can be indicated. A free space at the bottom of this last screen allows mentioning of some special events occurring during the session.

institutional authorities. The availability of such a database will provide an objective basis for discussion.

An attractive but less immediate interest is the prospect of building up a network of data shared between different centers. These networks may be regional and thus can provide help by referral centers in the management of difficult cases followed in private or public practice. They could also be used nationally or internationally leading to the accumulation of a large amount of data that could provide new information on IBD.

In summary, an IBD Internet could offer new and exciting possibilities to everyone involved in the management of these difficult diseases, from the primary care personnel to the most experienced authorities in the field.

Supplemental Reading

Bayless TM, Tokayer, AZ, Polito JM II, et al. Crohn's disease: concordance for site and clinical type in affected family members—potential hereditary influences. Gastroenterology 1996;111:573–79.

Coche JC, Colombel JF. Heterogeneity of inflammatory bowel disease: clinical subgroups of patients. Research and Clinical Forums. IBD and Salicylates-3 1997;20:136–45.

Feagan BJ. Pharmacoeconomics and Crohn's disease. In: Mignon M, Colombel JF, eds. Recent advances in the pathophysiology and management of inflammatory bowel diseases and digestive endocrine tumors. Paris: John Libbey Eurotext, 1999:81–94.

Gasche C, Scholmerich J, Brynskov J, et al. A simple classification of Crohn's disease. Report of the Working Party for the World Congress of Gastroenterology, Vienna 1998. Inflamm Bowel Dis (In press).

Gower-Rousseau C, Salomez JL, Dupas JL, et al. Incidence of inflammatory bowel diseases in Northern France (1988–1990). Gut 1994;35:1433–8.

Loftus EV, Silverstein MD, Sandborn WJ, et al. Crohn's disease in Olmsted County, Minnesota, 1940–1993: incidence, prevalence, and survival. Gastroenterology 1998;114:1161–8.

Sachar DB, Andrews HA, Farmer RG, et al. Proposed classification of patient subgroups in Crohn's disease. Gastroenterol Int 1992;3:141–54.

Silverstein MD, Loftus EV, Sandborn WJ, et al. Clinical course and costs of care for Crohn's disease: Markov model analysis of a population-based cohort. Gastroenterology 1999;117:49–57.

CHAPTER 9

USEFUL BIOLOGIC MARKERS AS ACTIVITY INDICES

JEFFERY A. KATZ, MD

Interpretation of the cause of symptoms in a patient with inflammatory bowel disease (IBD) can be challenging. Although increased symptomatology commonly results from an increase in intestinal inflammation, other complications, such as strictures or bacterial overgrowth, may also be the cause. In addition, a variety of extrinsic factors including medication, infection, food, and emotional stress can lead to worsening diarrhea, abdominal pain, malaise, and fatigue. The differentiation between clinical relapse due to increased (inflammatory) disease activity or some other factor is critical in the management of IBD. Only active inflammation will be modified by therapy with anti-inflammatory or immunomodulatory drugs. In general, a combination of clinical, endoscopic, radiographic, and/or laboratory data are necessary to assess IBD activity.

There is currently no single laboratory test that defines either ulcerative colitis (UC) or Crohn's disease (CD) as active or determines disease severity. Instead, a series of composite instruments such as the CD Activity Index (CDAI), Harvey-Bradshaw index, or Van Hees activity index for CD and the Truelove-Witts classification or Powell-Tuck score for UC have been developed to classify "disease activity." Recently, quality of life assessments have also been adopted. These indices are reviewed in an earlier chapter. Although widely used and well validated over time, these indices rely to differing degrees on subjective patient assessment of symptom severity. However, an objectively obtained, cost-effective, and reproducible laboratory measure of disease severity and activity would be more useful. Likewise, a simple marker assessing risk of relapse also would be valuable. Ultimately, advances in our understanding of the pathophysiology of inflammation in IBD holds the potential that newer biologic markers will eventually provide a more objective assessment of disease activity. The value of both older and newer biologic markers of IBD disease activity will be discussed.

Biochemical Markers of Inflammation

Acute-phase reactants have been extensively evaluated as surrogates for disease activity in both UC and CD. Although affordable, easy to perform, and readily available, assays including erythrocyte sedimentation rate (ESR), C-reactive protein (CRP), and orosomucoid (an α1-acid glycoprotein) have shown variable levels of correlation with disease activity, generally better with CD than UC. The ESR is often elevated with active IBD but is not useful to discriminate patients with mild or moderate disease. The long half-life of proteins contributing to the ESR (and serum orosomucoid) limits the sensitivity to distinguish rapid clinical changes. C-reactive protein has a shorter half-life and corresponds better with clinical and pathologic assessment of relapse, remission, and response to therapy. However, like other acute-phase proteins, CRP is not specific for bowel inflammation. Multifactorial analysis has suggested that serum orosomucoid (not routine in the U.S.) more precisely correlates with clinical status of both UC and CD compared to ESR and CRP. Importantly, the combination of elevated orosomucoid, ESR, and α2-globulin has an 88 percent accuracy in predicting disease relapse of Crohn's disease within 18 months. Likewise, a persistently elevated ESR or CRP often predicts clinical relapse over 90 days. In clinical practice, an elevated ESR or CRP may be useful in the assessment of disease activity for individual patients if they were determined to be normal during a time of quiescent disease. Additionally, a return to baseline values of acute-phase reactants after a disease flare for individual patients may predict a longer lasting remission.

A variety of other biochemical markers of disease activity have been evaluated (Table 9–1), including serum markers of coagulation and fibrinolysis, cholinesterase, neutrophil elastase, urinary neopterin, fecal lysozyme, fecal calprotectin, and fecal lactoferrin. All of these have emerged more as nonspecific indicators of inflammation than markers of disease activity and have not correlated closely with clinical disease indices.

Markers of Intestinal Protein Loss and Permeability

The intestinal loss of serum proteins and blood cells is considerably increased in IBD and can be used as a quantitative measure of intestinal inflammation.* Fecal α_1-antitrypsin provides an assessment of enterocolonic

Editor's Note: Markers of intestinal protein loss and permeability can be useful for clinical research but are not clinically used in the majority of settings. (SBH)

TABLE 9–1. Potential Laboratory Markers of IBD Activity*

Biochemical Markers

In serum
 ESR
 CRP
 Orosomucoid
 Prothrombin fragment 1 + 2
 Fibrin degredation products
 Neutrophil elastase
 Cholinesterase

In Stool
 α1-antitrypsin
 Lysozyme
 Calprotectin
 Lactoferrin

In urine
 Neopterin

Permeability Markers

$_{51}$Cr-EDTA
Lactulose mannitol ratio

Radiographic Markers

^{111}*In-labelled leukocyte excretion*
^{99}*Tc-m-labelled leukocyte excretion*
Doppler ultrasound
PET scanning
Gadolinium MRI

Immunologic Markers

Cytokines and cytokine receptors
 IL-1β (stool)
 IL-1/IL-1RA (tissue and stool)
 sIL-2R (serum)
 IL-6 (serum)
 TNF-α (serum and stool)
 TNF receptors p55 and p75 (urine)
 IL-8 (rectal dialysate)

Adhesion molecules
 ICAM-1
 VCAM
 L-selectin

Eicosanoids (rectal dialysate)
 PGE_2
 $PGF_{2\alpha}$
 TxB_2
 LTB_4

Other
 Nitric oxide (tissue)

*Clinically useful markers are italicized.

protein loss and differentiates controls from IBD patients. The clearance of fecal α$_1$-antitrypsin (clearance = fecal α$_1$-antitrypsin concentration x 24-hour fecal volume/ serum concentration) is a more reliable marker of disease activity than fecal α$_1$-antitrypsin alone and may be an indicator of asymptomatic recurrence in CD but requires a 24-hour stool collection and does not correlate closely with clinical indices.

A variety of gut lavage fluid proteins have also been used to assess disease activity in IBD. Immunoglobulin

G concentrations in lavage fluid correlate closely with activity indices; α$_1$-antitrypsin and albumin concentrations apparently correlate less well. Although enteric protein loss should reflect intestinal inflammation, variations of segmental inflammation, protein exudation, lumenal loss of inflammatory cells, and lack of association with symptoms limit their discriminative capacity.

Another method of assessing intestinal inflammation involves assessing intestinal permeability using chromium-51-labeled EDTA or the lactulose-mannitol ratio. These examinations measure the transit of small nonmetabolized test molecules across the intestinal mucosa. As inflammation directly increases permeability, the latter may be expected to correlate with increased disease activity. Indeed, one study has shown a positive correlation between permeability, CRP, orosomucoid, and CDAI, but, in general, these evaluations have not proved useful as measures of disease activity. The tests do not reflect IBD-specific inflammation and may be altered by NSAIDs, other medications, or alcohol ingestion. In addition, these assays measure small bowel permeability and are not adequate measures of colonic inflammation. Increases in intestinal permeability may be useful as predictors of impending disease relapse in asymptomatic CD patients.

Radiographic and Ultrasonic Markers of Inflammation

Quantitative assessment of IBD location and activity has been attempted using a variety of radiographic techniques. Indium-111 or technetium-99m-labeled autologous leukocytes can be used to localize sites of inflammation and disease extent and correlate well with the results of standard radiologic or endoscopic imaging. An estimate of disease activity can be obtained by quantifying labeled leukocyte excretion in the stool or by comparing uptake in the inflamed intestine with uptake in the liver or spleen. Although such quantitative evaluations correlate (weakly) with clinical disease activity indices for both UC and CD, colonoscopy, and acute-phase reactants, studies have used small samples, lack standardized techniques, require specialized leukocyte labeling facilities and equipment, and increase radiation exposure. These have limited the widespread use of these radiologic techniques. Newer methodologies and isotopes may allow better evaluation and use of these tests that are highly specific for intestinal inflammation.

Ultrasound evaluation of bowel wall thickness and Doppler ultrasound of mesenteric flow have also been used as measures of disease activity. There is a chapter on ultrasound. Although duplex Doppler scanning appears to distinguish active CD from inactive CD, more subtle and specific assessments of disease activity are currently lacking. Positron emission tomography (PET) scanning also may be useful, in the future, to assess active disease as may gadolinium magnetic resonance imaging (MRI).

Immunologic Markers of Inflammation

Tissue injury in IBD is largely immune-mediated; therefore, cytokines, cytokine-receptors, and other mediators of inflammation should correlate with disease activity. Advances in molecular biologic techniques allow standardized, rapid evaluation of serum and tissue protein and mRNA levels to assess the production of inflammatory mediators and immune cell activation. Many cytokines and their receptors, including interleukin (IL) - 1, IL-1 receptor antagonist (IL-1RA), IL-2, soluble IL-2 receptor (sIL-2R), IL-4, IL-6, IL-8, IL-10, tumor necrosis factor (TNF-α), and interferon-γ, have been measured in IBD serum, stool, filter paper applied to mucosa, and tissue. When both pro- and anti-inflammatory cytokines have been simultaneously evaluated in vivo through analysis of stool samples or rectal dialysates from IBD patients, the level of IL-1β and the ratio of IL-1RA/IL-1β reflected active disease by multivariate factor analysis. Additionally, symptomatic response was correlated with an increase in anti-inflammatory cytokines IL-4 and IL-10. Such studies are valuable in illustrating the complex balance between specific mediators of inflammation and their antagonists, but suggest that identification of any single immune molecule as a reliable marker of disease activity may be difficult. The current best candidates as biologic measures of disease activity are discussed below.

Interleukin-2

When T cells are activated, IL-2 receptors (IL-2R) are expressed on the cell surface. In active CD, both serum and tissue concentrations of the soluble form of the dimeric IL-2R complex, sIL-2R, are significantly increased and reflect mucosal inflammatory activity. In CD, serum concentration of sIL-2R correlates with acute-phase reactants and the CDAI. In addition, with successful therapy, sIL-2R decreased in parallel with the CDAI and serum orosomucoid. High sIL-2R serum levels have also been predictive of risk of clinical CD relapse. In UC, data are more limited regarding correlations between sIL-2R and disease activity.

Interleukin-6

Circulating levels of IL-6, a broad-spectrum cytokine involved in the induction of acute-phase reactants, are elevated in active CD but not in patients with UC. However, tissue IL-6 is consistently elevated in most IBD patients and correlates with endoscopic and histologic inflammation. In CD, IL-6 shows greater elevation with colonic disease compared to isolated small intestinal disease. Circulating IL-6 levels inversely correlate with serum albumin and, compared to CRP, may be a better marker of disease activity in steroid naive patients. Other studies have reported no relationship between serum IL-6 and clinical symptoms. These inconsistent results could be due to methodologic differences of IL-6 measurement, influences of steroid therapy, or small sample sizes of the study populations. Recently, results of a longitudinal study of 136 CD patients found a significant elevation of IL-6 in CD patients with primarily inflammatory disease, compared to patients with fibrostenotic disease. A strong correlation to disease activity ($r = .72$; $p \leq .001$) was noted. Furthermore, longitudinally measured IL-6 directly reflected response during steroid therapy and predicted clinical relapse after steroid-induced remission. IL-6 levels also may be useful to stratify patients with a high risk of relapse.

Tumor Necrosis Factor

The clinical success of infliximab, a chimeric monoclonal antibody directed against TNF-α, in the treatment of CD points to TNF-α as a key regulator of inflammation. In contrast to most proinflammatory cytokines that are measurably elevated in IBD serum and mucosa, increases of TNF-α have been notoriously difficult to document. Elevated TNF-α in the sera of children with active UC and colonic CD and in the stools of children with both UC and CD have been reported and correlated with active disease. Isolated intestinal mononuclear cells from patients with active IBD secrete increased amounts of TNF-α compared to controls. The stimulated secretion of high levels of TNF-α and IL-1β by isolated human lamina propria mononuclear cells from CD patients in clinical remission after steroid therapy was predictive of disease relapse within 1 year. To date, however, these studies have yet to be replicated, and it is unlikely that measuring TNF-α directly in the serum or stool will be useful in assessing disease activity.

In contrast to the difficulty measuring TNF-α directly, soluble TNF receptors (sTNF-R) can be readily detected in the urine and serum of patients with CD. Levels of sTNF-R p55 and p75 were significantly elevated in 25 patients with active UC or CD, compared to patients with inactive disease or normal controls, and declined in parallel with the clinical response to therapy. The biologic implications of these changes are uncertain. In a recent study, patients treated with infliximab had a decrease in CDAI and significant clinical improvement; serum concentrations of soluble TNF receptors p55 or p75 did not change. More extensive studies of sTNF-Rs are necessary before these assays will be accepted as accurate markers of disease activity.

Adhesion Molecules

Circulating soluble intercellular adhesion molecule-1 is increased in IBD compared to controls but correlates only weakly with sIL-2R, CRP, and orosomucoid and does not increase the precision of activity assessment compared with clinical and endoscopic indices. Soluble vascular cell adhesion molecule-1 is also found at higher levels in the circulation of IBD compared to control subjects, but correlates poorly with disease activity. In UC, but not CD, L-selectin levels rise with worsening symptoms. Thus, significant overlap exists between IBD and controls for all of the cell adhesion molecules studied to date in both active and inactive disease, making it unlikely that this class of molecules will emerge as clinically useful markers of disease activity.

Additional immune and inflammatory mediators have been evaluated as potential markers of disease activity. Using rectal dialysis, prostaglandin E_2 and thromboxane B_2 have been found to be elevated, particularly in UC, and correlate with endoscopic estimates of disease severity. Interleukin-8 concentrations from rectal dialysates in active UC have been shown to be significantly higher than controls, as have colonic nitric oxide levels in active UC or colonic CD. These measurements of inflammation all have correlated poorly with clinical assessments of disease activity.

Conclusion

The accurate assessment of clinical disease activity in IBD is critical to appropriate and effective patient care. The availability of an accurate, rapid, easy to perform, and affordable biologic parameter of disease activity would be invaluable to physicians caring for IBD patients. Unfortunately, such a test does not currently exist. Despite our increasing knowledge of the pathophysiology of intestinal inflammation, we do not yet know all of the factors that control the worsening or improving of disease symptoms. Until we can fully identify the signals that initiate and accompany a flare of UC or CD, we must still rely on our clinical skills and nonspecific markers of inflammation to assess disease activity.

Despite their subjective components, clinical indices remain the mainstay for assessing disease activity in clinical trials. For the practicing physician, the addition of CRP and orosomucoid, if available, or ESR can be useful to support the diagnosis of a disease flare. A quantitative assessment of leukocyte excretion in the stool, if standardized, rapid, and easy to perform, would likely provide an adjunctive objective measure of intestinal inflammation. At present, labeled leukocyte scans remain restricted to specialty research centers. Measurement of a specific serum, tissue, or stool cytokine, eicosanoid, adhesion molecules, or other inflammatory molecule cannot presently be recommended as accurate, solitary tests of disease activity. However, as more is learned about the complex interactions between various proinflammatory and immunoregulatory molecules, it is conceivable that measurement of a panel of inflammatory mediators

could accurately reflect clinical disease severity. For now, careful and precise clinical evaluation must still complement the information provided by currently available biologic markers. A bibliography of 38 references is available upon request at *jak24@po.cwru.edu*.

Supplemental Reading

Boirivant M, Pallone F, Ciaco A, et al. Usefulness of fecal α_1-antitrypsin clearance and fecal concentration as early indicator of postoperative asymptomatic recurrence in Crohn's disease. Dig Dis Sci 1991;36:247–52.

Brignola C, Campieri M, Bazzocchi G, et al. A laboratory index for predicting relapse in asymptomatic patients with Crohn's disease. Gastroenterology 1986;91:1490–4.

Hadziselimovic F, Emmons LR, Gallati H. Soluble tumor necrosis factor receptors p55 and p75 in the urine monitor disease activity and the efficacy of treatment of inflammatory bowel disease. Gut 1995;37:260–3.

Jones SC, Banks RE, Haidar A, et al. Adhesion molecules in inflammatory bowel disease. Gut 1995;36:724–30.

Keshavarzian A, Fusunyan RD, Jacyno M, et al. Increased interleukin-8 (IL-8) in rectal dialysate from patients with ulcerative colitis: evidence for a biological role for IL-8 in inflammation of the colon. Am J Gastroenterol 1999;94:704–12.

Lauritsen K, Laursen LS, Bukhave K, Rask-Madsen J. In vivo profiles of eicosanoids in ulcerative colitis, Crohn's colitis, and *Clostridium difficile* colitis. Gastroenterology 1988;95:11–7.

Louis E, Belaiche J, Kemseke CV, et al. Soluble interleukin-2 receptor in Crohn's disease: assessment of disease activity and prediction of relapse. Dig Dis Sci 1995;40:1750–6.

Mishra L, Mishra BB, Bayless TM, et al. In vitro cell aggregation and cell adhesion molecules in Crohn's disease. Gastroenterology 1993;104:772–9.

Rachmilewitz D, Eliakim R, Ackerman Z, Karmeli F. Direct determination of colonic nitric oxide level—a sensitive marker of disease activity in ulcerative colitis. Am J Gastroenterol 1998;93:409–12.

Reinisch W, Gasche C, Tillinger W, et al. Clinical relevance of serum interleukin-6 in Crohn's disease: single point measurements, therapy monitoring, and prediction of clinical relapse. Am J Gastroenterol 1999;94:2156–64.

Saiki T, Mitsuyama K, Dyonaga A, et al. Detection of pro- and anti-inflammatory cytokines in stools of patients with inflammatory bowel disease. Scand J Gastroenterol 1998;33:616–22.

Schreiber S, Nikolaus S, Hampe J, et al. Tumor necrosis factor alpha and interleukin 1beta in relapse of Crohn's disease. Lancet 1999;353:459–61.

Welson MJ, Masoomi AM, Britten AJ, et al. Quantification of inflammatory bowel disease activity using technetium-99m HMPAO labeled leukocyte single photon emission computed tomography (SPECT). Gut 1995;36:243–50.

Wyatt J, Vogelsang H, Hubl W, et al. Intestinal permeability and the prediction of relapse in Crohn's disease. Lancet 1993;341:1437–9.

CHAPTER 10

IMAGING OF MUCOSAL INFLAMMATION

DINA F. CAROLINE, MD, SETH N. GLICK, MD, AND PATRICK L. O'KANE, MD

Although cross-sectional imaging modalities have become staples of abdominal imaging, barium studies remain preeminent for imaging abnormalities of the luminal gastrointestinal (GI) tract, particularly mucosal disease.* Whether the study is of the esophagus, stomach, and duodenum (upper GI), small bowel, or colon (barium enema), the depiction of mucosal abnormalities requires high-quality radiographic studies. Specifically, double-contrast technique is required for upper GI and barium enema examinations. The small bowel may be evaluated after catheter intubation with single- or double-contrast technique (enteroclysis or small bowel enema) or with a dedicated fluoroscopic examination using compression and distension techniques to evaluate the entire small bowel. Insufflation of air into the rectum when the cecum is opacified after oral administration of barium (peroral pneumocolon) often provides excellent visualization of the terminal ileum.

Ulcerative Colitis

Ulcerative colitis (UC) is an idiopathic inflammatory disease primarily confined to the mucosa of the rectum and colon. Although the barium enema is not a primary diagnostic procedure, it often is helpful for confirming a clinical diagnosis, evaluating extent and severity of disease, and detecting complications. Barium examination retains an important diagnostic role in the differentiation of UC from Crohn's disease.

The earliest visible abnormality on barium enema correlates with the endoscopic appearance of edematous hyperemic mucosa. On double-contrast barium enema, there is loss of the normally sharp, distinct edge of the barium–air interface. Instead, the interface appears as an indistinct, fuzzy mucosal line causing a fine granular pattern (Figure 10–1). This may be accompanied by blunting and broadening of the haustral clefts. Characteristically, these changes are contiguous, circumferential, and symmetric, beginning at the rectum and extending continuously for a variable distance proximally with no skip areas. The transition from abnormal to normal mucosa is gradual.

Crypt abscesses form when inflammatory cells in the crypts of Lieberkühn form ulcers and erode into the

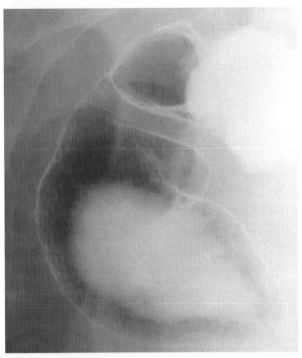

FIGURE 10–1. Early ulcerative proctitis with blurring of the normally sharp mucosal line.

lumen. Barium adheres to the surface of these small ulcerations, giving the mucosa a stippled appearance (Figure 10–2). As the disease progresses, the ulcerations erode through the muscularis mucosa into the loose submucosal tissues. As the less resistant submucosal tissue is undermined, the ulcers extend laterally, causing the development of flask-shaped or "collar-button" ulcers.

In severe cases of UC, there is severe ulceration of the mucosa and submucosa and much of the mucosa is denuded. Small residual islands of inflamed mucosa (inflammatory pseudopolyps) produce a polypoid appearance on barium enema examination (Figure 10–3).

---

* Editor's Note: Inflammation imaging with tagged leukocytes, gadolinium-enhanced magnetic resonance imaging (MRI), and positron emission tomography (PET) scanning are mentioned elsewhere, but it is recommended that other sources be sought for detailed information. (TMB)

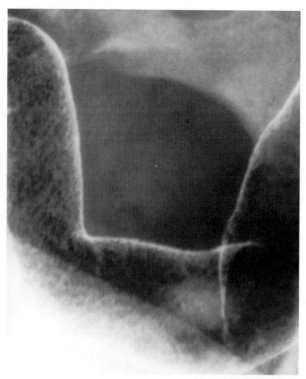

FIGURE 10–2. Barium flecks adhere to superficial ulcers producing mucosal stippling.

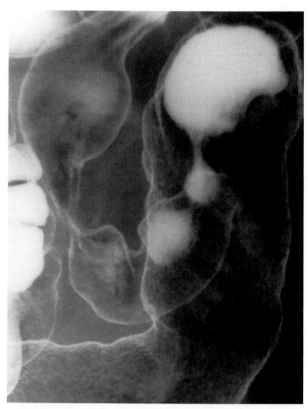

FIGURE 10–4. Coarse granular mucosal pattern with loss of the normal haustra in a patient with a 25-year history of CUC.

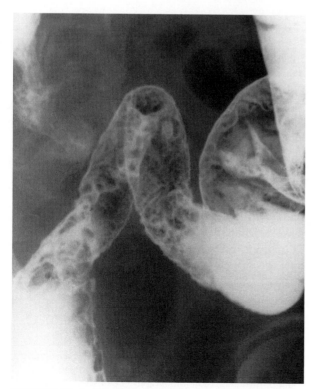

FIGURE 10–3. Severely inflamed mucosa with "collar-button" ulcers, and inflammatory pseudopolyps. Luminal narrowing, a feature of CUC, also is present.

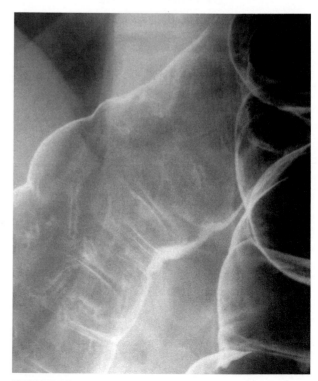

FIGURE 10–5. Filiform polyps in quiescent UC.

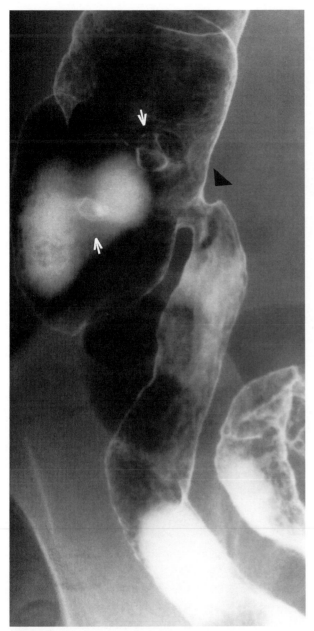

FIGURE 10–6. Backwash ileitis. The ileocecal valve is widely patent (*arrowhead*) and the ileum is dilatated with effaced folds. There is superficial ulceration of the cecum, and the haustra are abnormal. Nodular lesions (pseudopolyps) (*white arrows*) are radiographically indistinguishable from neoplastic polyps.

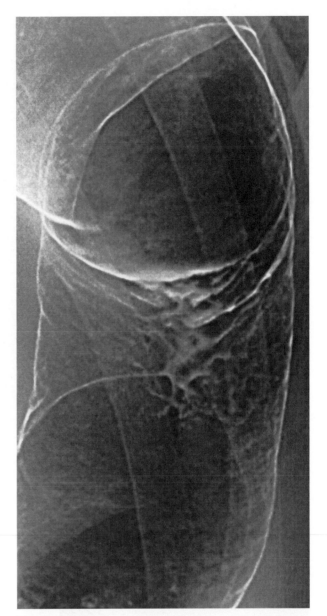

FIGURE 10–7. Colonic dysplasia. Focal plaque-like filling defect with small nodules in patient with CUC.

Chronic Ulcerative Colitis

In chronic ulcerative colitis (CUC), the bowel wall is thickened and the lumen is often narrowed. These changes frequently are seen by cross-sectional imaging. Healing of ulcerated mucosa with granulation tissue results in a granular mucosal pattern that resembles the granularity seen in early UC but usually has a somewhat coarser texture (Figure 10–4). Regenerated mucosa also may overgrow, forming a nodular or polypoid appearance (postinflammatory pseudopolyps). These may be filiform (long and thin), short, or mass-like (Figure 10–5). Nodular or mass-like pseudopolyps may be radiographically indistinguishable from neoplasms.

The terminal ileum is secondarily affected in about one-third of CUC patients with pancolitis. In these patients, a barium examination demonstrates a widely patent ileocecal valve and a dilated terminal ileum with a granular mucosa and loss of the normal fold pattern (Figure 10–6). Carcinoma arising in UC often is indistinguishable from benign strictures. Premalignant dysplastic mucosa occasionally is detected as focal areas of nodular or angular filling defects (Figure 10–7).

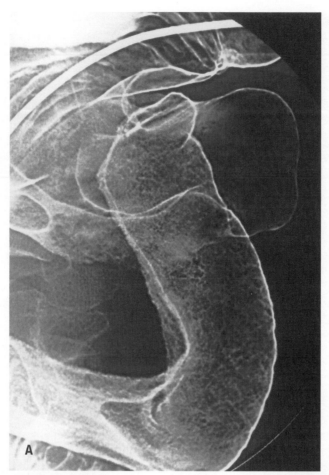

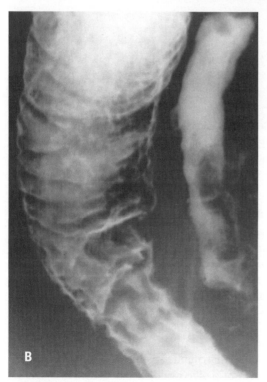

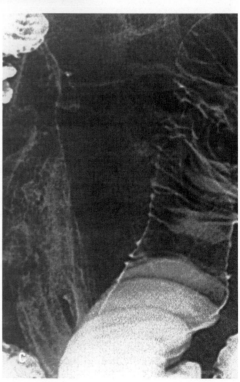

FIGURE 10–8. Early small bowel Crohn's disease. *A*, Coarse, thickened villous pattern with scattered aphthous ulcers; *B*, coarse villous pattern with thickened folds adjacent to a loop of bowel with more advanced disease; and *C*, stellate and linear erosions in terminal ileum.

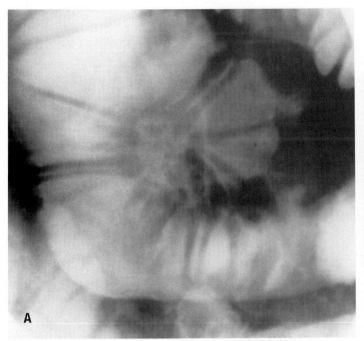
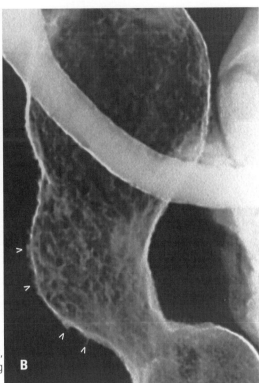

FIGURE 10–9. Progression of inflammation in Crohn's disease. *A*, Large, flat, stellate ulcer with radiating folds; and *B*, coarse, inflamed mucosa with fissuring ulcers (*arrowheads*).

Crohn's Disease

Crohn's disease is a granulomatous disease that can affect any portion of the GI tract. Unlike UC, which is predominantly a superficial disease confined to the colon, Crohn's disease is a process in which inflammation involves all layers of bowel wall and adjacent mesentery. The best imaging modality for evaluating the transmural features of the disease, including bowel-wall thickness, and mesenteric extension and complications of the disease, such as fistulae and abscesses, is computed tomography. Because Crohn's disease initially affects the mucosa and submucosa, high-quality barium studies are the imaging modality of choice for diagnosis of early disease.

The radiographic appearance of Crohn's disease of the small bowel is well described. Parallel findings are found in other portions of the GI tract. High-quality barium examinations depict early changes in the small bowel characterized by coarsening of the villous pattern, mucosal-fold thickening, and shallow mucosal erosions (aphthous ulcers) (Figure 10–8). These findings may be present alone or in combination, with the specificity of the diagnosis increasing with presence of more than one of these findings. Increasing submucosal edema causes further widening of folds, leading to their partial or complete effacement. Continued inflammatory infiltrate and submucosal fibrosis cause distortion and interruption of folds.

Aphthous ulcers enlarge and deepen, assuming a variety of configurations. Typical appearances include stellate,

linear, crescentic, and "rose-thorn" shapes (Figure 10–9). As the disease progresses, ulcers gradually extend through the bowel wall and into the adjacent mesentery. Once the disease process becomes transmural, cross-sectional imaging supersedes barium as the primary imaging modality.

Features of early Crohn's disease in the colon differ from those seen in the small bowel, because of underlying morphologic differences in early Crohn's disease. In the small bowel, edematous villi create a granular appearance. This pattern is not seen in the colon, where background mucosa typically is normal or near normal. Ulceration of inflamed lymphoid follicles forms the shallow aphthous erosions, which are the radiographic hallmark of early Crohn's colitis.

Mucosal features seen on double-contrast barium enema may provide important information to help distinguish UC from Crohn's colitis. Characteristically, in Crohn's colitis, the background colonic mucosa appears normal, whereas in UC, the entire surface of the involved colon is ulcerated. In Crohn's colitis, aphthous ulcers may be scattered, clustered, or involve the entire colon (Figure 10–10). Ulcerative colitis begins at the rectum and extends proximally as a contiguous symmetric, continuous process. Crohn's disease is discontinuous, sparing the rectum in 50 percent of cases with a patchy asymmetric distribution. In UC, the entire involved mucosal surface appears abnormal, with a granular or stippled appearance and diffuse deeper ulcers occurring in advanced disease. In early and intermediate Crohn's disease, ulcers are found

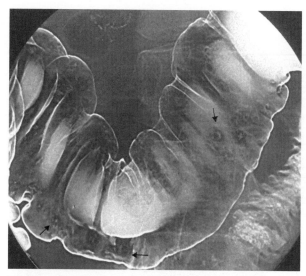

FIGURE 10–10. Early Crohn's colitis. Aphthous and small stellate erosions (*arrows*) with normal background mucosa.

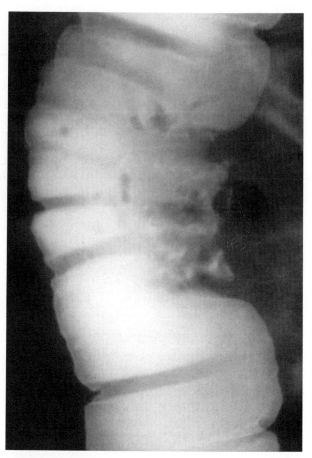

FIGURE 10–11. Asymmetric "skip" lesion with Crohn's disease. Deep ulcers are seen along one bowel wall. Several small polyps also are present. Both proximal and distal to this focal abnormality, the bowel is normal.

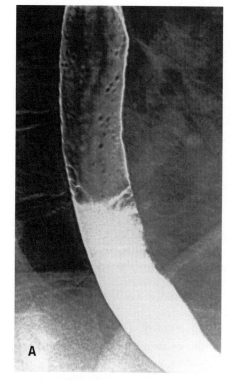

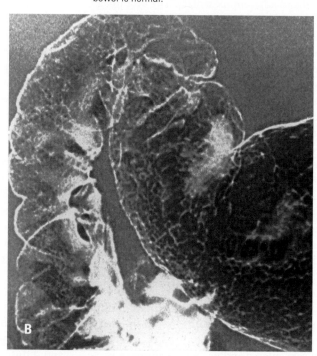

FIGURE 10–12. Crohn's disease may affect organs other than small bowel or colon. *A*, Aphthous ulcers scattered in mid-esophagus; *B*, antroduodenal Crohn's disease: coarse mucosa with aphthous ulcers and thickened folds.

adjacent to normal-appearing mucosa (Figure 10–11). Barium studies also may be helpful in distinguishing Crohn's disease from UC by demonstrating presence of disease elsewhere in the gut.

Inflammatory infiltrates and edema may cause focal mucosal protrusions, more commonly in the colon than in the small bowel. Polypoid protrusions in Crohn's disease, as in UC, result from a variety of pathologic processes. The familiar "cobblestone pattern" associated with relatively advanced Crohn's disease is caused by criss-crossing longitudinal and transverse linear ulcers, with edematous islands of mucosa forming the "cobblestones." Postinflammatory polyps are caused by overgrowth of granulation tissue.

Unlike UC, Crohn's disease also may affect the esophagus, stomach, and duodenum. These organs rarely are involved in the absence of small bowel or colon disease. Radiographic findings in early disease mimic the findings seen in the small bowel or colon (Figure 10–12).

In summary, high-quality barium studies can show mucosal abnormalities in exquisite detail with patterns that frequently can suggest specific diagnoses.

Editor's Note

Radionuclide-labeled white blood cells can be used for nuclear scintigraphy. For example, technetium 99m hexamethyl propylenamine oxime (HMPAO) can be helpful in assessing the presence of active inflammation. Information on extent and intensity of inflammation also can be derived (Arndt JW, Grootscholten MI, vanHogezand RA, et al. Inflammatory bowel disease activity assessment using technetium-99m-HMPAO leukocytes. Dig Dis Sci 1997; 42:387–93). Gadolinium MRI studies and PET scans also are being used in an attempt to assess inflammation and to distinguish active disease from fibrotic strictures. (TMB)

Supplemental Reading

Bartram CI, Laufer I. Inflammatory bowel disease. In: Laufer I, Levine MS, eds. Double contrast gastrointestinal radiology. 2nd Ed. Philadelphia: WB Saunders, 1992:580–645.

Cockey BM, Jones B, Bayless TM, Shauer AB. Filiform polyps of the esophagus with inflammatory bowel disease. AJR Am J Roentgenol 1985;144:1207–8.

Glick SN. Crohn's disease of the small intestine. Radiol Clin North Am 1987;25:25–45.

Gore RM, Laufer I. Ulcerative and granulomatous colitis: idiopathic inflammatory bowel disease. In: Gore RM, Levine MS, Laufer I, eds. Textbook of gastrointestinal radiology. Philadelphia: WB Saunders, 1994:1098–141.

Herlinger H, Caroline DF. Crohn's disease. In: Gore RM, Levine MS, Laufer I, eds. Textbook of gastrointestinal radiology. Philadelphia: WB Saunders, 1994:824–44.

Jones B, Abbruzzese AA. Obstructing giant pseudopolyps in granulomatous colitis. Gastrointest Radiol 1978;3:437–8.

Maglinte DDT, Chernish SM, Kelvin FM, et al. Crohn disease of the small intestine: accuracy and relevance of enteroclysis. Radiology 1992;184:1–6.

Orel SG, Rubesin SE, Jones B, et al. Computed tomography vs. barium studies in the acutely symptomatic patient with Crohn's disease. J Comput Assist Tomogr 1987;11:1009–16.

CHAPTER 11

CROHN'S DISEASE: COMPUTED TOMOGRAPHIC SCANNING IN CLINICAL DECISION-MAKING

KAREN M. HORTON, MD, AND ELLIOT K. FISHMAN, MD

Despite the availability and widespread use of endoscopy today, radiologic imaging studies continue to play a valuable role in the diagnosis and management of patients with Crohn's disease (CD). Contrast studies such as the upper gastrointestinal series, the small bowel series, and the barium enema are still important diagnostic tools to evaluate patients with inflammatory bowel disease (IBD) and allow excellent visualization of mucosal disease. These examinations, however, give only limited information about extraluminal extension of disease or extraintestinal manifestations.

Recent advancements and improvements in spiral computed tomography (CT) technology have made CT a valuable and necessary adjunct to traditional contrast examinations in patients with Crohn's disease. New spiral CT scanners allow faster data acquisition combined with more rapid contrast infusion and narrow collimation. The average CT examination of the abdomen and pelvis can be performed in less than 60 seconds. This speed and narrow collimation results in excellent evaluation of the entire gastrointestinal tract. Another distinct advantage of CT over contrast studies is its ability to accurately image the wall of the gastrointestinal tract as well as any extraluminal extension of disease and adjacent organs. This chapter will review the role of CT in the diagnosis and management of patients with CD.

Technique

Optimal CT imaging of the gastrointestinal tract requires attention to technique, adequate oral contrast, and intravenous contrast. Insufficient oral contrast can result in collapsed loops of normal bowel that can simulate disease or can result in misdiagnosis of diseased loops as normal undistended loops. We use the following protocol in patients with known or suspected IBD.

Approximately 750 to 1000 cc of a 3 percent oral iodinated contrast solution is administered 60 to 90 minutes before the scan and an additional 250 cc of oral contrast immediately before the start of the scan. This should provide adequate contrast opacification of the stomach and small bowel. If esophageal pathology is suspected, Esopho-Cat® paste (EZM Co, Westbury, New York) can also be administered immediately prior to the scan to coat the esophagus. If colonic involvement is suspected, the colon should be adequately opacified. In outpatients, oral contrast can be administered the night before the study as well as prior to the scan to ensure that the contrast opacifies the colon as well as the small bowel. Alternatively, in urgent cases, or in patients in whom limited colonic disease is suspected, 3 to 4 percent iodinated contrast solution can be administered gently through a rectal tube immediately prior to the scan.

The administration of intravenous contrast is necessary for complete evaluation of patients with IBD, especially if extra-intestinal disease or complications such as an abscess are suspected. We routinely administer 100 to 120 cc of iohexol (Omnipaque 350®, Nycomed, Princeton, New Jersey) at a rate of 2 to 3 cc/s injected through a peripheral vein using a mechanical injector pump. Imaging should begin 45 to 50 seconds after initiation of contrast injection.

The abdomen and pelvis should be routinely imaged from the level of the diaphragm through the perineum. It is important that CT scanning extend through the perineum. In a series of patients documented by Yousem et al, perirectal-perianal abnormalities are demonstrated in CT in up to 37 percent of Crohn's patients. Using spiral CT, 5 mm collimation can be performed with a table speed of 8 mm/s, with reconstruction every 5 mm. If necessary additional scans can be obtained through specific areas of concern utilizing thinner collimation (3 mm). Also, multiplanar reconstructions or three-dimensional (3-D) imaging can be helpful problem-solving tools in difficult cases. In a series of patients with CD reported by Raptopoulos et al (1997), multiplanar reconstruction improved observer confidence and was found to be complementary and often superior to conventional barium studies.

Primary Disease

The normal wall thickness of a loop of distended small bowel or colon is less than 3 mm. When it is distended and opacified with contrast agent, the normal bowel is not definable on CT. The esophageal wall should measure less than 3 mm when distended. The normal gastric wall can measure up to 5 to 7 mm.

The earliest perceptible change on CT in patients with CD is wall thickening, usually involving the distal small bowel and colon (Figure 11–1). Since contrast studies

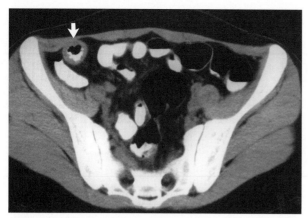

FIGURE 11–1. A 55-year-old male with Crohn's disease (CD). Spiral CT demonstrates circumferential thickening of a loop of ileum (*arrow*) in the right lower quadrant.

such as the small bowel series or enteroclysis are the most sensitive radiologic techniques for detecting the earliest mucosal changes of IBD, CT is usually reserved for the patients with a known diagnosis in whom the extent of disease or the presence of complications is suspected. However, CT may be the first modality to suggest the disease in patients presenting with nonspecific complaints.

The typical bowel thickness of a segment involved with CD is 5 to 15 mm. This bowel thickening is usually symmetric and diffuse and on thin-section CT scans, ulcerations in the mucosal surface can sometimes be detected (Figure 11–2). Eccentric thickening or "skip" areas can be present. Although bowel-wall thickening is a nonspecific finding that can occur in a variety of inflammatory and neoplastic diseases, the appearance and degree of wall thickening in CT can sometimes aid in diagnosis. For instance, in a study of colonic wall thickening in CT, Philpotts et al (1994) noted that the mean colon wall thickness in Crohn's colitis was 13 mm and the appearance was homogenous. This was significantly

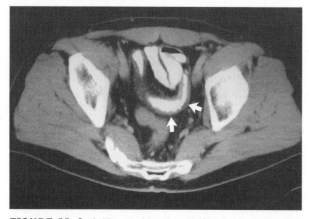

FIGURE 11–2. A 35-year-old male with CD. Contrast-enhanced spiral CT demonstrates circumferential thickening of a small bowel loop (*arrows*) in the pelvis. There is a slight scalloping of the bowel wall, compatible with ulceration.

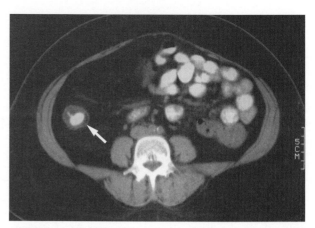

FIGURE 11–3. A 55-year-old female with longstanding CD. Spiral CT demonstrates minimal circumferential thickening of the wall of the right colon. There is a low attenuation halo (*arrow*) within the thickened wall compatible with fat deposition. There is also a proliferation of mesenteric fat in the right abdomen.

greater than in ulcerative colitis, where the mean wall thickness was 7.8 mm and the appearance heterogenous. In addition to wall thickening, CT may demonstrate a low-density zone or "halo" within a thickened bowel loop, either small bowel or colon. Usually, the low-density zone is of soft tissue density, representing submucosal edema, or it can be of fat density, due to submucosal fat deposition (Figure 11–3). This halo originally was thought to be specific for IBD but also can be seen in radiation enteritis, intestinal ischemia, and typhlitis.

The second area commonly involved in CD is the mesentery. The normal mesentery is homogeneous and has an attenuation similar to that of fat, measuring in the range of –90 and –130 Hounsfield units. The interface between the bowel and mesentery is usually sharply defined. The earliest inflammatory changes of CD are detected by inflammatory stranding in the mesentery adjacent to diseased bowel loops (Figure 11–4). With more advanced disease, mesenteric inflammation can increase with or without the formation of an abscess or phlegmon (Figure 11–5). Fistulae from the bowel may extend into the mesentery and appear as linear tracts.

In patients with longstanding CD, there may be increased fat around affected loops of large or small bowel. This increased fat can simulate a mass or abscess on small bowel series. The increased mesenteric or pericolonic fat seen on CT scan corresponds to the "creeping" mesenteric fat noted at surgery and pathologically (see Figure 11–3). Increased mesenteric fat is specific for CD. However, increased perirectal fat can be seen in patients with ulcerative colitis as well.

Mesenteric adenopathy can be present in patients with CD. Usually, the mesenteric nodes are small, ranging between 3 and 8 mm. Inflammatory nodes typically measure less than 1 cm in short axis. If mesenteric or retroperitoneal nodes measure greater than 1 cm in short

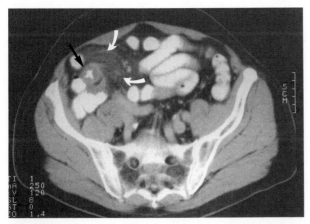

FIGURE 11–4. A 71-year-old male with CD and right lower quadrant pain. Contrast-enhanced spiral CT demonstrates moderate wall thickening of the distal ileum (*arrow*). There is also increased attenuation of the adjacent mesenteric fat (*curved arrows*) compatible with active inflammation.

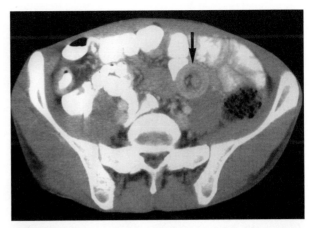

FIGURE 11–6. A 25-year-old male with CD and intermittent abdominal pain. Contrast-enhanced spiral CT demonstrates the classic CT appearance of an intussusception (*arrow*). There is thickening of a small bowel loop with a target appearance representing the intussuscepting mesenteric fat and vessels.

axis, the possibility of superimposed malignancy (adenocarcinoma or lymphoma) should be considered, as there is an increased incidence of malignancy in patients with CD.

Complications

Although CT may be the first modality to suggest the diagnosis of CD in patients presenting with nonspecific abdominal pain, the **major clinical application of CT is in the definition of the extent of disease and in the detection of complications such as abscesses and fistulae.** At our institution, patients with known CD are referred for CT when they experience a change in clinical course, such as increasing abdominal pain, diarrhea, or distention. Computed tomography is valuable in the evaluation of these patients and **can affect patient management in 28 percent of patients with symptomatic CD.** Computed tomography may reveal previously unexpected findings

that subsequently lead to a change in medical or surgical management.

Obstruction

Computed tomography is valuable in cases involving patients with suspected small bowel or colonic obstruction and can frequently determine the cause of obstruction and whether there is evidence of strangulation or ischemia. In patients with CD, small bowel obstruction can result from stricture, inflammatory masses, adhesions following surgical resections, or (rarely) intussusception (Figure 11–6). Computed tomography is also helpful in distinguishing obstruction from ileus. A definite advantage of CT over barium studies is its ability to detect additional diseased segments distal to the site of obstruction. The iodinated contrast material is also less problematic than barium in the possibly obstructed patient.

Fistulae

Although contrast studies can define the presence of enteric fistulae, the extent and involvement of adjacent organs or structures can be difficult to define on standard radiographs (Figure 11–7). Additionally, a fistulous tract may be edematous and therefore may not fill with contrast. In this case, the fistula may go undetected on conventional contrast studies but can still be visualized on CT. Finally, the fistulous tracts may be in an area such as the perianal, perirectal, or gluteal regions, which are technically difficult to evaluate on barium studies. Computed tomography, on the other hand, has none of these limitations. Regardless of the location of the fistulous tract, CT examination can define its presence as well as define, by direct visualization, its true extent. Extension into muscle, viscera, spine, or bladder all can be easily detected on CT using a properly designed examination with careful attention to scanning techniques. On CT, one potential limitation is that

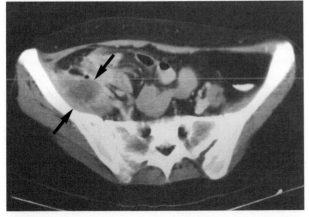

FIGURE 11–5. A 21-year-old female with CD, fever, and right hip pain. Contrast-enhanced spiral CT revealed a 4 cm low-density fluid collection in the iliac muscle compatible with abscess (*arrows*). The abscess is adjacent to a loop of inflamed small bowel.

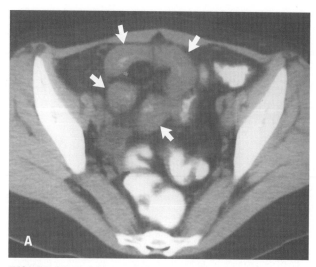 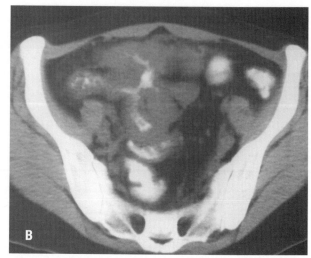

FIGURE 11–7. A 24-year-old female with CD and chronic pelvic pain. *A,* Spiral CT demonstrates moderate thickening of multiple small bowel loops in the lower abdomen (*arrows*). *B,* Several diseased loops form a "starburst" configuration compatible with enteroenteric fistulae.

although a fistulous tract may be detected, it is sometimes impossible to be certain whether the tracts are patent, unless contrast material actually opacifies the tract itself. In patients with enterocutaneous fistulae, contrast can be injected through the skin opening before the CT scan to opacify the tract and to evaluate its course.

The perirectal and perianal regions are reportedly involved in up to 60 percent of patients with colonic involvement of CD. The perirectal region is difficult to evaluate with other imaging modalities, except perhaps MRI. In a recent review we found that 81.5 percent of patients referred to us had perirectal and/or perianal disease. Computed tomography can provide very clear definition of the boundaries of the perirectal zone, allowing for the detection of small fistulous tracts and perirectal abscesses (Figure 11–8). Although most of these tracts extended only into the perirectal-perianal fat planes,

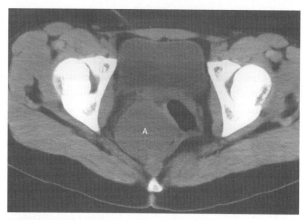

FIGURE 11–8. A 23-year-old female with CD, fever, and perirectal pain. Standard small bowel series was unremarkable (not shown). Spiral CT with oral contrast demonstrates a 4 cm abscess (A) collection between the rectum and uterus. Computed tomography or sonography can also be used for guidance during percutaneous drainage.

others extended into adjacent viscera (eg, prostate, vagina), muscle (obturator internus, gluteus maximus), or bone (hip joint). The full definition of the extent of fistulae is important in planning medical or surgical management.

Abscesses

The second major complication in the patient with CD is the development of an abscess. This can involve any of the major viscera, such as the liver and spleen, or can be deep in the retroperitoneal or pelvic cavities. Abscesses also can involve adjacent muscles or bone (see Figure 11–5). Computed tomography is ideally suited for evaluating all these regions in a single examination.

One of the more common areas for an abscess to develop is between loops of bowel, that is, an interloop abscess. Interloop abscesses are very difficult to diagnose on conventional contrast studies such as the small bowel series. Computed tomography with contrast opacification of bowel loops can help detect small abscesses and define their relationship to the bowel. A CT also can be used for planning the patient's therapy, such as choosing surgical versus percutaneous drainage under CT guidance. Van Sonnenberg and colleagues (1984) have shown that CT can be particularly helpful for patients who are not surgical candidates or in cases where surgery is delayed until the patient is in a better medical and nutritional state.

Cancer

Recent literatures supports the belief that there is an increased risk of small bowel adenocarcinoma, colorectal cancer, and possibly cholangiocarcinomas in patients with CD. Although colonoscopic examination and biopsies for dysplasia are the most useful surveillance methods, CT can play an important role in cancer detection and staging. Virtual colonoscopy, which is a 3-D CT scan

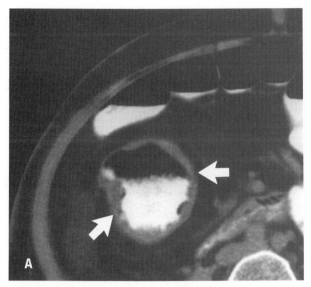 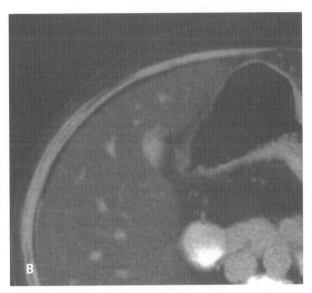

FIGURE 11–9. A 33-year-old female with CD. *A,* Spiral CT demonstrates minimal thickening of the cecum (*arrows*). *B,* Also, there is diffuse low attenuation throughout the liver compatible with fatty infiltration.

of the colon, is currently under investigation as a quick noninvasive tool for screening patients at increased risk for colon cancer. This technique has been evaluated in colonic polyps and colon cancer (Fenlon et al, 1999).

Extra-intestinal Complications of Crohn's Disease

Extra-intestinal complications in patients with CD also can be evaluated with CT. The most common areas of extra-intestinal involvement include the liver and biliary tree, the urinary tract, and the musculoskeletal system

Hepatobiliary Tract

The most common extra-intestinal manifestation of CD is fatty infiltration of the liver, which can be due to either the patient's poor nutritional state or use of steroids to treat the bowel disease. Fatty liver appears as diffuse low attenuation on CT (Figure 11–9). Pericholangitis and sclerosing cholangitis are rare but occur with increased frequency in the patient with CD. Primary bile duct carcinomas also occur with increased frequency but are very unusual. Magnetic resonance imaging is proving useful for biliary tract or liver. The presence of gallstones is common, particularly in patients following distal bowel resection or when there is extensive disease in the distal ileum. Although some gallstones can be visualized on CT, ultrasound is much more sensitive for evaluation of the gallbladder and for the detection of calculi.

Urinary Tract

The urinary tract can be involved in CD. Renal calculi are not uncommon and are often of the oxalate type due to involvement of the terminal ileum and resultant problems of malabsorption. Thin collimation (3 mm) noncontrast CT can be performed to detect renal calculi and obstructing ureteral stones in symptomatic patients. This quick, noncontrast scan often obviates the need for intravenous pyelography. At our institution, noncontrast CT currently is the first modality performed in patients with suspected ureteral obstruction.

Since CD often involves multiple loops of bowel with subsequent fibrosis and adhesions, the ureters can be involved, resulting in obstruction. The right ureter is typically involved more frequently than the left, since CD often occurs in the right lower quadrant. Finally, the bladder can be involved with thickening due to adjacent inflammation or in more severe cases to the development of enterovesical fistulae. A carefully performed CT examination should be able to detect the presence, extent, and etiology of the fistula. In addition to detecting the fistula, by defining its location and the affected zone of the bladder and bowel, surgical planning is facilitated. Of note: if an **enterovesical fistula is suspected, intravenous contrast should not be administered.** Then, if contrast is detected in the bladder, it must be oral contrast that entered the bladder through an enterovesical fistula.

In a series of 275 patients with CD, 22 patients had bladder abnormalities, 10 of which were enterovesical fistulae. In 8 of the 10 cases the fistulae were from small bowel to bladder, and in 2 cases they were from sigmoid colon to bladder. In all 10 patients, other imaging studies (cystoscopy, intravenous pyelography, barium enema) produced false-negative results. Crohn's disease is the second most common cause of enterovesical fistulae, the most common cause being diverticulitis. In our experience, fistulae between the small bowel and bladder in CD usually occur anteriorly on the right side of the bladder.

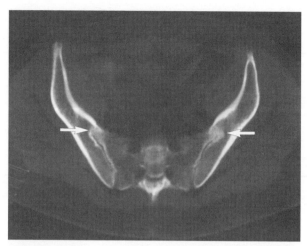

FIGURE 11–10. A 34-year-old male with CD and bilateral hip pain. Spiral CT demonstrates minimal sclerosis of both sacroiliac joints (*arrows*) compatible with mild sacroiliitis.

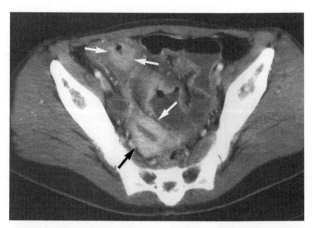

FIGURE 11–11. A 21-year-old female with CD and pain. Contrast-enhanced spiral CT with water as oral contrast demonstrates marked enhancement of a few small bowel loops in the right lower quadrant (*arrows*) compatible with active inflammation and hyperemia. The use of water as oral contrast allows better visualization of the enhancing bowel wall.

This is in contradistinction to the situation in patients with diverticulitis, in whom the involvement is usually posterior or posterior on the left side. This is one of the findings that helps us suggest the cause of an enterovesical fistula.

Musculoskeletal System

The musculoskeletal system is involved in up to 60 percent of patients with CD. The most common finding is sacroiliitis commonly resembling the human leukocyte antigen (HLA)-B27 antigen positive type (Figure 11–10). Sacroiliitis in CD tends to be bilateral with erosions and sclerosis on both sides of the joint space. Most are asymptomatic. In more severe cases, bony ankylosis may be seen. These patients may present clinically with back pain and findings suggestive of exacerbation of the primary disease process in the bowel. Computed tomographic scans using bone settings (window width 1776H, window center 176H) can detect the bone involvement. Computed tomography is more sensitive than plain films in detecting the presence of sacroiliitis.

One of the skeletal complications of CD not related to the primary process but to therapy is the development of avascular necrosis of the femoral heads. Although standard radiography can detect avascular necrosis, CT has been shown to be more sensitive than standard radiography in its early detection. We have seen several patients with **pelvic pain** suggesting either a pelvic abscess or perirectal disease who have had unsuspected avascular necrosis. The use of CT in these cases obviously has an impact on subsequent patient management.

Finally, we have seen several cases of sacral osteomyelitis secondary to enteric fistulae and subsequent abscesses. This should always be considered in patients with inflammatory bowel disease and back pain.

Future Directions

A definite limitation of the radiologic evaluation of CD has been determining the activity of disease. Although initial reports of contrast-enhanced CT scans suggested that enhancement could be used to determine disease activity, this has not proved reliable in any large series of patients to date. However, **multidetector-array CT**, the latest advancement in CT technology, may be useful in this regard. These new scanners combine multiple rows of detectors and faster gantry speeds, thus allowing examinations to be performed in a few seconds. This speed combined with faster intravenous injection rates (3 to 5 cc/s) should allow the acquisition of functional data. For instance, enhancement of a segment of small bowel can be evaluated over time. From these data, perfusion rates can be calculated that may help determine disease activity.

Another advancement in CT scanning of the gastrointestinal tract relates to oral contrast. Traditionally, high-density oral agents (dilute barium or iodinated agents) are used to opacify the gastrointestinal tract. However, these high-density agents limit visualization of the adjacent enhancing bowel. Investigations are underway assessing the use of alternative agents such as water as a potentially useful oral contrast agent as it allows better visualization of the enhancing wall (Figure 11–11). More research is necessary to determine the optimal oral contrast agent.

Three-dimensional volume rendering of CT data is becoming more available and may come to play a role in the evaluation of patients with CD. The ability to view the gastrointestinal tract in three dimensions with CT eliminates the problem of superimposed loops.

References

Fenlon HM, Nunes DP, Schroy PC III, et al. A comparison of virtual and conventional colonoscopy for the detection of colorectal polyps. N Engl J Med 1999;341:1496–503.

Philpotts LE, Heiken JP, et al. Colitis: use of CT findings in differential diagnosis. Radiology 1994;190:445–9.

Raptopoulos V, Schwartz RK, et al. Multiplanar helical enterography in patients with Crohn's disease. AJR Am J Roentgenol 1997;169:1545–50.

Van Sonneberg E, Mueller PR, et al. Percutaneous drainage of 250 abdominal abscess and fluid collections. I. Results, failures, and complications. Radiology 1984;151:337–41.

Yousem D, Fishman EK, et al. Computed tomographic findings in perirectal and perianal Crohn's disease. Radiology.

Supplemental Reading

Fishman EK, Wolf EJ, et al. CT evaluation of Crohn's disease: effect on patient management. AJR Am J Roentgenol 1987; 148:537–40.

Goldman SM, Fishman EK, et al. CT in the diagnosis of enterocutaneous fistulae. AJR Am J Roentgenol 1985;144:1229–33.

Gore RM, Balthazar EJ, et al. CT features of ulcerative colitis and Crohn's disease. AJR Am J Roentgenol 1996;169:1462–3.

Gossios KJ, Tsianos EV. Crohn's disease: CT findings after treatment. Abdom Imaging 1997;22:160–3.

Merine D, Fishman EK, et al. Bladder involvement in Crohn's disease: role of CT in detection and evaluation. J Comput Assist Tomogr 1989;13:90–3.

Meyers MA, McGuire PV. Spiral CT demonstration of hypervascularity in Crohn's disease: "vascular jejunization of the ileum" or the "comb sign." Abdom Imaging 1995;20:327–32.

CHAPTER 12

Transabdominal Bowel Sonography in Clinical Decision-making

Christoph Gasche, MD

Before offering therapeutic advice, the ultimate goal of inflammatory bowel disease (IBD) clinics is to understand the ongoing problem in a specific patient. Symptoms are important landmarks for the differentiation between active disease and remission. Symptoms such as diarrhea or abdominal pain, however, are nonspecific and do not suffice as a basis for relevant therapeutic decisions. Especially in Crohn's disease, it is necessary to update the information on the location pattern and the status of possible complications such as strictures, fistulas, or abscesses. All of this information can be easily obtained by a fast, inexpensive, noninvasive, safe, and radiation-free technique that does not require special preparation: transabdominal bowel sonography (TABS) is a key to a better perception of our patient's symptoms.

What Am I Talking About?

The term TABS specifies that this procedure is different from regular abdominal ultrasound, although the devices are the same and the investigation is also done through the abdominal wall. This distinction is important since the target is the bowel rather than other abdominal organs. During regular abdominal ultrasound procedures, bowel gas may hinder the examiner from viewing certain organs. Thus, examiners are trained to avoid "bowel views." In contrast, TABS targets primarily the bowel, and no attention is usually paid to other organs. By separating these two procedures, the average duration of a single TABS examination is about 15 minutes (including evaluation of the images and dictating the report).

How Does Transabdominal Bowel Sonography Work?

I perform TABS by using a 3.5-MHz, 78-mm curved array and a 10- to 5-MHz broadband, 38-mm linear array transducer (Ultramark 9, Advanced Technology Laboratories Inc., Bothel, Washington). The technical improvement of sonographic devices continuously increases image resolution. Together with growing investigators' experience, the quality of TABS has advanced over the past decade. TABS can be done at any time of the day without prior bowel preparation.

At the Vienna IBD Center, appointments are usually made for the morning, and patients are asked to have breakfast 2 hours beforehand. No special preparations such as overnight fasting, oral deflating drugs, or enemas are prescribed. I usually ask for the patient's diagnosis, their previous bowel resections, and their current clinical symptoms (particularly, location of pain). I start the procedure by identifying the ileocecal junction (Figure 12–1), which is located next to the right psoas muscle. From this point, I try to depict the downstream parts of the colonic frame until its visibility is lost in the deep pelvic portion of the distal sigmoid. The continuous identification of small bowel loops is more difficult. By following the terminal ileum from the ileocecal junction, visibility is often lost deep in the right side of the pelvis. Proximal small bowel loops are then screened without knowledge of continuity. The duodenum is examined last. Primarily I look for bowel wall thickening (≥ 3 mm). In such areas, I further evaluate for luminal narrowing, wrapping mesenteric masses, intra-abdominal fistulas, or abscesses and take pictures of all lesions. No evaluation of the stomach or the distal (deep pelvic) parts of sigmoid and rectum is intended.

In many European and Asian countries (eg, Japan, Korea), abdominal ultrasound is shared between radiologists and gastroenterologists. Gastroenterologists, however, have performed most TABS studies in IBD patients. The rational for this is twofold: first, a full understanding of TABS requires broad knowledge of the physiologic and pathologic bowel features. This is particularly true when dealing with IBD. Second, radiologists tend to focus more on computed tomography (CT), magnetic resonance imaging (MRI), or virtual endoscopy. I consider TABS to have the potential to become as important to gastroenterologists as echocardiography has become for cardiologists.

What Can We Expect to See by Transabdominal Bowel Sonography?

The thickness of the normal bowel wall depends on the degree of luminal distension and the current status of peristalsis. Collapsed or contracted loops show thicker

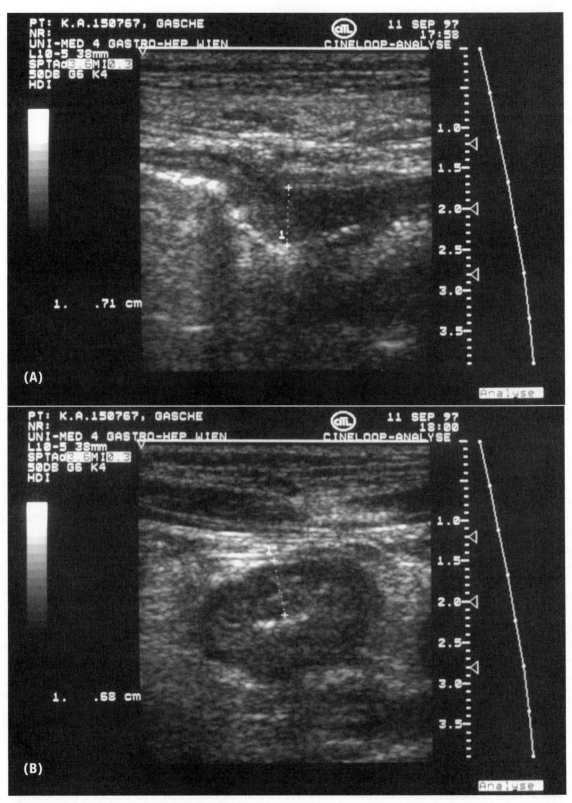

FIGURE 12–1. TABS findings at the ileocecal valve in Crohn's disease. The longitudinal section (*A*) shows bowel wall thickening of 7.1 mm at the position of the ileocecal valve. The homogenous hypoechoic wall of the terminal ileum is located on the right side of the measurement bar. There has already been a loss of the corresponding bowel layers. On the left side of the measurement bar, the adjacent portion of the cecum shows less wall thickening (which corresponds to less inflammation) and a preserved sonographic appearance of the five typical layers of the bowel wall. On a cross-section through the ileocecal valve (*B*), the bowel wall thickening is confirmed (6.8 mm). The collapsed bowel lumen is narrowed as shown by a short hyperechoic central band.

TABLE 12–1. What Clinical Questions Can Be Answered by Transabdominal Bowel Sonography?

Crohn's Disease	Ulcerative Colitis
What is the location pattern?	How proximal is the extent of disease?
Strictures (location, length, and functional severity)?	How thick (how sick) is the bowel wall?
Fistulas (size, configuration, relation to bowel strictures and to other organs)?	Is there evidence of severe disease (ie, pneumocolon or megacolon)?
Intra-abdominal abscesses (detection, guided drainage)?	
What is the cause of abdominal pain: stricture, abscess, lymphadenitis, pure inflammation, non–bowel-related (pancreatitis, urolithiasis, etc.)?	
Postoperative recurrence of disease	
Control of intestinal or fistula healing under immunosuppression	

muscular layers but do not exceed 3 mm in thickness. Transmural bowel inflammation in IBD is typically mirrored by an alteration of the echo-architecture of the bowel wall. The so-called target lesion correlates with distinct layers of the bowel wall (Figure 12–2A): hyperechoic (bright) central luminal gas, the hypoechoic (dark) mucosal layer, hyperechoic submucosa (which is the main contributor to bowel wall thickening in IBD), hypoechoic muscularis propria, and finally hyperechoic serosa, with possible fibrofatty proliferation of the mesentery (so-called "creeping fat"). During the progression of disease, these distinct layers become indistinct and can be completely lost (Figure 12–2B). Sonography not only visualizes intestinal lesions but even more importantly identifies peri-intestinal changes such as the creeping mesentery or local lymphadenopathy. In experienced hands, the value of TABS for detection of intra-abdominal fistulas and abscesses is even higher than with other imaging techniques such as CT or MRI.

Can Transabdominal Bowel Sonography Reliably Distinguish between Ulcerative Colitis and Crohn's Disease?

Every textbook gives distinct endoscopic and histologic features of ulcerative colitis and Crohn's disease, which helps to establish a precise diagnosis in up to 90 percent of IBD patients. These methods have withstood the test of time and are considered as the gold standard. TABS will not challenge endoscopy and histology in this regard, so I do not use TABS for diagnosing IBD. This does not mean that all TABS features are nonspecific. For example, TABS can easily recognize typical terminal ileitis. In cases of indeterminate colitis, the distribution of bowel wall thickening (right- versus left-sided) might nonspecifically suggest either Crohn's disease or ulcerative colitis. Keeping in mind that both colonic strictures and even fistulas may occur in ulcerative colitis, the presence of such complications cannot be regarded as 100 percent specific for Crohn's disease. Although it is not recommended for making an initial diagnosis, the value of TABS is greatest for the longitudinal management of IBD patients.

What Clinical Questions Can Be Answered by Transabdominal Bowel Sonography?

The primary yield of TABS procedures is the follow-up of IBD patients. Although ulcerative colitis-associated intestinal wall thickening is readily detected and can be used for estimation of the proximal extent of disease, most of the TABS applications focus on the management of patients with Crohn's disease (Table 12–1). For newly referred IBD patients, TABS is a convenient and reliable method to serially evaluate bowel morphology, in lieu of repeating endoscopy and small bowel series. At the primary examination, TABS might also provide insight into the symptoms of a particular patient (eg, abdominal pain and stricture). Another frequent TABS indication is steroid resistance or steroid dependence. In my experience, it is not unusual to detect previously unrecognized fistulas or cold abscesses in this population, since these lesions may not respond to steroids.

The applicability of TABS is not limited to the identification of intra-abdominal fistulas. TABS can be used further to watch the healing of fistulas using appropriate therapy (see also other chapters). When patients must undergo an intestinal resection, postoperative recurrences can be investigated with TABS. Thus far, there are only a few studies on this; future improvements of quality may increase the sensitivity. Previous research on superior and inferior mesenteric artery blood flow has also evaluated the ability of TABS to measure and predict clinical relapse.

How Can Transabdominal Bowel Sonography Detect Small Fistulas?

Fistulas in Crohn's disease have been regarded as tracks that connect two epithelial surfaces. The recognition of fistulization has been generally based on the radiologic appearance of the connecting track in barium studies or the observation of a fistulous orifice reaching the skin. Fistulas, however, may arise much earlier from deep intestinal fissures that penetrate the muscular coat and progress to small sinus tracks. They end as blind tracks in

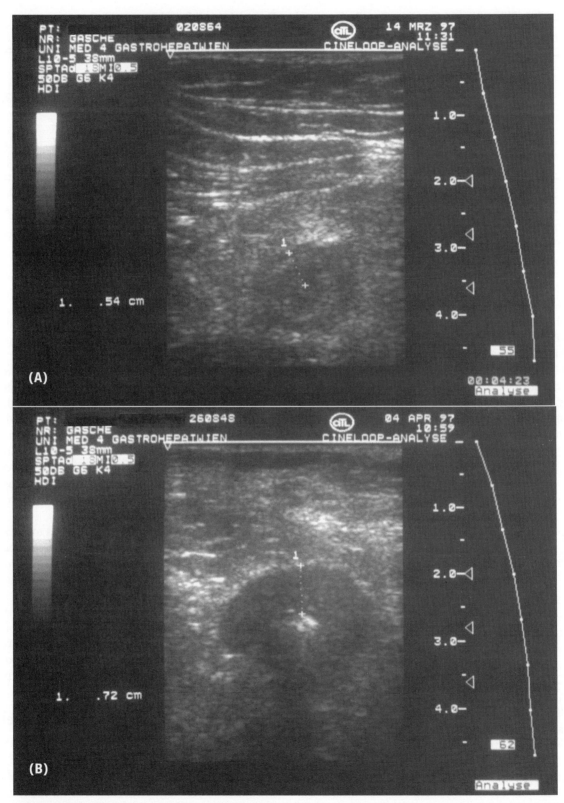

FIGURE 12–2. TABS confirms progression of Crohn's disease. (*A*), The so-called target lesion correlates to distinct layers of the bowel wall: hyperechoic (bright) central luminal gas content (not visible on *A*), hypoechoic (dark) mucosal layer, hyperechoic submucosa (which mainly contributes to bowel wall thickening in IBD), hypoechoic muscularis propria, and at the outside of the measurement bar, the hyperechoic serosa with fibrofatty proliferation of the mesentery. (*B*), During progression of disease, these layers are indistinct and can be completely lost. Massive bowel wall thickening (7.2 mm) relates also to significant luminal narrowing, which is reflected by a dot-shaped hyperechoic lumen.

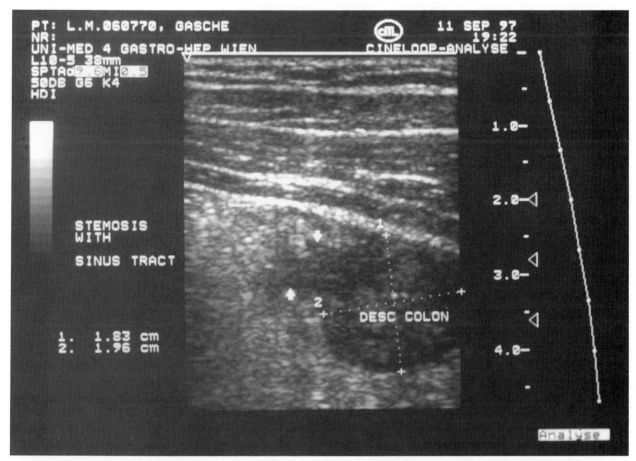

FIGURE 12–3. A sinus track arising from the descending colon in Crohn's disease. Note the intense bowel wall thickening (9 to 10 mm) and the lack of any identifiable central lumen, which is typical of a significant stricture. At the left side of the colon, a hypoechoic sinus tract (*arrows*) arises into the surrounding hyperechoic mesentery.

the mesentery, retain necrotic debris, and act as tiny abscesses (Figure 12–3). It may take months to years until such tracks reach the wall of an adjacent hollow-organ (mostly another bowel loop) or the skin. However, I consider the primary bowel penetration and blindly ending tracks to be more relevant for clinical practice than a complete connecting track between hollow organs: the blind tracks may give rise to huge abscesses with the potential of systemic bacterial complications, such as peritonitis or sepsis. Thus, it is important to detect fistulas before such complications arise.

We recently showed that TABS is very accurate even for detecting small fistulas (87 percent sensitivity, 90 percent specificity). During the TABS procedure, fistulas are sought in areas of bowel wall thickening where there are hypoechoic peri-intestinal lesions, usually surrounded by hyperechoic mesenteric fat (Figure 12–4). The cut off between fistulas and abscesses is arbitrary, since both lesions refer to the same pathologic event, that is, bowel penetration. We have chosen to make the diagnosis of abscess for lesions ≥ 2.0 cm in their cross-sectional diameter (Figure 12–5). The sensitivity for detection of intra-abdominal abscesses by TABS ranges somewhere between

95 and 100 percent. Thus, TABS is an appropriate method to confirm a clinically suspected abscess.

How Can Transabdominal Bowel Tomography Detect Bowel Strictures?

The transmural inflammation of the bowel wall in Crohn's disease is accompanied by tissue fibrosis, bowel wall thickening, and luminal narrowing. Bowel obstruction is one endpoint of chronic intestinal inflammation. TABS can identify bowel strictures by detecting severe luminal narrowing accompanied by destruction of wall layering and loss of peristaltic bowel movement, with or without prestenotic bowel dilatation (see Figures 12–2B and 12–3). It is important to know that a correlation exists between bowel wall thickening and the degree of intestinal stenosis: the thicker the bowel wall, the less the available luminal space. During real-time sonography, the clinical relevance of strictures can be estimated by observing intense peristaltic activity of more proximal bowel loops. Prestenotic dilatation of loops can be appreciated as well. This is why I ask my patients to eat breakfast before the examination. We should examine not only

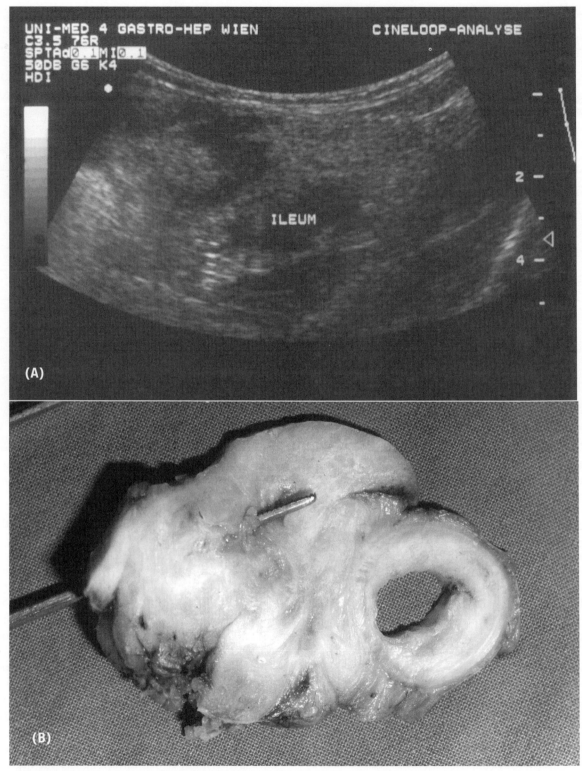

FIGURE 12–4. Correlation of TABS findings with the corresponding pathologic specimen. A blind-ended fistulous tract was detected in a patient with Crohn's disease who complained of right lower quadrant pain. Note the large hypoechoic lesion arising from the left side of the terminal ileum and creeping through the mesentery into the abdominal wall (*A*). After ileocecal resection, the pathology confirmed the sonographic finding (*B*). The tip of the forceps indicates the fistula surrounded by fibrosis and mesenteric fat.

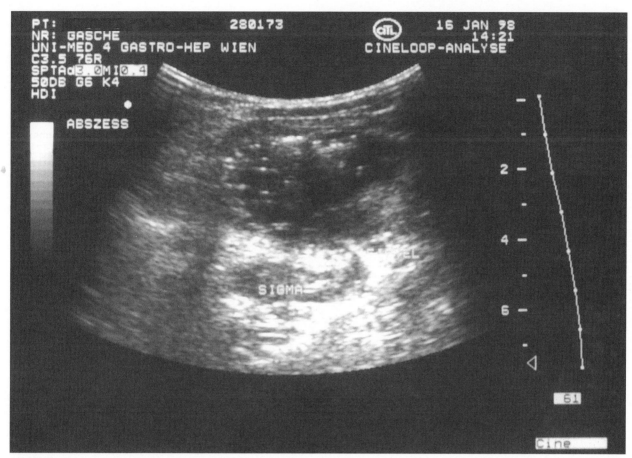

FIGURE 12–5. An intra-abdominal abscess arising from leakage in the sigmoid colon of a Crohn's patient. Besides the size of the lesion (approximately 5 cm), hyperechoic gas inclusions point to the diagnosis of abscesses. Acute pain and fever were relieved by ultrasound-guided drainage.

the luminal diameter but also the length of bowel obstruction to determine the severity of the mechanical barrier. Sequential lesions may add to the clinical symtomatology. Another dimension defining the significance of strictures is stool viscosity. This is particularly relevant in cases of left-sided colonic obstruction. Positron emission tomography scanning and gadolinium MRI may be helpful in distinguishing actual inflammatory strictures from fibrotic fixed strictures.

What Are the Shortcomings of Transabdominal Bowel Sonography?

The appropriate use of any imaging techniques in IBD depends on the specific goal in the individual patient. Each method has its limitations. For example, it is obvious that small bowel enteroclysis is not suitable to visualize sigmoid ulcers. Regarding TABS, it is important to recognize its anatomic limitations. The stomach, the deep pelvic portion of the sigmoid, and the rectum are difficult to study. Therefore, I do not attempt to detect lesions in these areas. TABS is not suitable for cancer surveillance in ulcerative colitis either. In general, abdominal ultrasound has been criticized because of high interobserver variability. This may also apply for TABS and is mainly due to the dynamic nature of sonography and to the lack of procedure standardization. When compared to CT or MRI scans, the dynamic nature of TABS also bears advantages: it allows the study of bowel motility and helps to determine the significance of strictures.

The Patient's Perspective

The understanding of both indications and limitations of TABS will give rise to a fruitful use of this method in future. TABS is a safe, inexpensive, noninvasive, and radiation-free technique that does not require special preparation. It is not associated with additional pain. This fact is appreciated by our patients, who are very tolerant of this methodology. Repeated measures and controls are possible without added risks. Providers of this technique will realize that it satisfies not only the physician, who will attain a better perception of the ongoing problem, but also the patient, who will profit from problem-specific care.

Supplemental Reading

Andreoli A, Cerro P, Falasco G, et al. Role of ultrasonography in the diagnosis of postsurgical recurrence of Crohn's disease. Am J Gastroenterol 1998;93:1117–21.

Gasche C, Moser G, Turetschek K, et al. Transabdominal bowel sonography for detection of intestinal complications in Crohn's disease. Gut 1999;44:112–7.

Kelly JK, Preshaw RM. Origin of fistulas in Crohn's disease. J Clin Gastroenterol 1989;11:193–6.

Ludwig D, Wiener S, Bruening A, et al. Mesenteric blood flow is related to disease activity and risk of relapse in ulcerative colitis: a prospective follow up study. Gut 1999;45:546–52.

Maconi G, Parente F, Bollani S, et al. Abdominal ultrasound in the assessment of extent and activity of Crohn's disease: clinical significance and implication of bowel wall thickening. Am J Gastroenterol 1996;91:1604–9.

Schwerk WB, Beckh K, Raith M. A prospective evaluation of high resolution sonography in the diagnosis of inflammatory bowel disease. Eur J Gastroenterol Hepatol 1992;4:173–82.

CHAPTER 13

MODE OF ACTION OF ANTI-INFLAMMATORY AGENTS

THEODORE KALOGERIS, PhD, AND MATTHEW B. GRISHAM, PhD

Despite several decades of extensive investigation, the etiology and specific pathogenetic mechanisms responsible for inflammatory bowel disease (IBD) (Crohn's disease [CD], ulcerative colitis) remain the subject of active investigation. Recent experimental and clinical studies suggest that the initiation and pathogenesis of these diseases are multifactorial involving interactions among genetic, environmental, and immune factors. Regardless of how exactly these interactions ultimately promote chronic gut inflammation, it is becoming increasingly apparent that the immune system plays a crucial role in disease pathogenesis.

Although several different etiologic theories have been proposed to account for this apparent immune activation, data obtained from a number of different experimental and clinical studies suggest that the chronic gut inflammation may result from a dysfunctional immune response to components of the normal gut flora. Inherent in this theory is the concept that intestinal and/or colonic inflammation is initiated and perpetuated by the absence or dysfunction of certain regulatory T lymphocytes that control the normal mucosal cell-mediated immune response to luminal antigens. The inability to downregulate cell-mediated immunity results in the sustained overproduction of T-helper cell 1 (Th1)-derived cytokines such as tumor necrosis factor-α (TNF-α), interferon-γ (IFN-γ), and α- or β-lymphotoxin. Th1-derived cytokines are known to activate resident macrophages inhabiting the mucosal interstitium. By virtue of their tissue distribution and ability either to produce or respond to local and circulating mediators, tissue macrophages occupy a central position in the inflammatory cascade. For example, activated macrophages will release a plethora of pro-inflammatory mediators including cytokines (TNF-α, interleukin (IL)-1β, IL-6, IL-8, IL-12), metalloproteinases (collagenase, gelatinase), arachidonate metabolites (prostaglandins, leukotrienes), lipid mediators (platelet activating factor), and reactive metabolites of oxygen and nitrogen (superoxide, hydrogen peroxide, nitric oxide).

Many of these macrophage-derived mediators will activate the venular endothelium to express endothelial cell adhesion molecules (ECAMs) and recruit additional inflammatory cells such as neutrophils and monocytes that amplify the inflammatory cascade by releasing copius amounts of TNF-α, IL-8, reactive oxygen, and nitrogen species and metalloproteinases. The net result of this dysregulation of cell-mediated immunity is a dramatic shift, or imbalance, in cytokine production within the intestinal interstitium such that a Th1 response predominates. Indeed, this is exactly what is observed in CD.

The objectives of this review are to summarize recent work investigating mechanisms by which certain pro-inflammatory cytokines (eg, TNF-α) promote chronic gut inflammation, discuss new therapeutic strategies evolving as a result of these findings, and to present new emerging concepts regarding mechanisms of action of established anti-inflammatory medications.

TNF-α, Anti-TNF-α Therapy, and Mechanisms of Inflammation

The importance of certain pro-inflammatory cytokines as critical mediators of chronic gut inflammation was established by a recent series of clinical studies demonstrating that immunoneutralization of TNF-α remarkably attenuated inflammation and tissue injury observed in CD. Tumor necrosis factor-α is synthesized and secreted by monocytes, macrophages, and T cells as an inactive precursor that is rapidly proteolyzed to a 17kD monomer. Monomeric TNF-α rapidly combines to form the biologically active 51kD trimeric cytokine that binds to either the 55kD or 75kD transmembrane TNF-α receptor located on the surface of a number of different cell types. Receptor-ligand interaction initiates signaling events that ultimately lead to the transcription of a number of genes involved in the inflammatory response. It is known, for example, that TNF-α promotes the upregulation of ECAMs, several different cytokines (including itself), and the inducible forms of nitric oxide synthase (iNOS or NOS 2) and cyclo-oxygenase 2 (COX 2). Because elevated levels of TNF-α have been found in the stool, serum, and tissue of patients with IBD, therapeutic strategies to inactivate or render this potent pro-inflammatory cytokine less effective were initiated several years ago. Recent breakthroughs in biotechnology and genetic engineering have allowed for the production of three new therapies for the treatment of CD. Infliximab

(Remicade®, Centocor, Malvern, Pennsylvania) is a chimeric monoclonal antibody (mAb) to human TNF-α assembled by linking the variable region of mouse anti-human TNF mAb to human immunoglobulin (Ig)G1. Infliximab binds both soluble trimeric TNF-α as well as transmembrane-bound TNF-α. This mAb acts as both a carrier and as a TNF antagonist. The mechanisms by which infliximab renders TNF-α biologically inactive are not known with certainty; however, there is growing evidence to suggest that it binds to and neutralizes free and transmembrane TNF as well as binding to transmembranal TNF and promoting cytolysis of TNF-producing cells via complement fixation antibody-dependent cellular cytotoxicity (ADCC), or apoptosis. The net result is a downregulation of Th1 cytokine production, ECAM expression, and serum metalloproteinases. Clinical trials administering infliximab for CD demonstrated that intravenous infusion of 5 mg/kg significantly reduced the Crohn's Disease Activity Index (CDAI) and attenuated histopathologic and endoscopic inflammation within 4 weeks of treatment. Infliximab also has been shown to reduce significantly drainage from abdominal or perianal fistulae in the majority of CD patients.

A second immune-based therapy targeting TNF-α is a humanized mAb to TNF-α, CDP571 (Therapeutics Ltd., Berkshire, UK). This mAb has been shown to bind soluble and membrane-bound TNF but does not fix complement or mediate ADCC. A relatively small, multicenter, double-blind, placebo-controlled and randomized Phase IIa study found that a single dose of CDP571 produced significant reductions in the CDAI in patients with CD with 30 percent of the patients experiencing clinical remission.[*]

Etanercept (Enbrel®, Immunex, Seattle, Washington) represents a third foray into anti-TNF-α therapy. Approved for rheumatoid arthritis and under study for CD, this fusion protein is a modified soluble TNF-α receptor constructed by linking the extracellular ligand-binding domain of the human p75 TNF receptor to the Fc portion of IgG1. Etanercept binds soluble trimeric TNF-α and competitively inhibits binding of TNF-α to membrane-bound TNF-α receptors, preventing TNF-α from exerting its biologic effects.

Although the mechanisms by which newer anti-TNF therapies attenuate chronic gut inflammation have not been completely defined, it appears that most, if not all, of the anti-inflammatory activity of these biologics result from the inhibition of TNF-induced transcriptional activation of a multitude of genes involved in acute and chronic inflammation. For example, TNF-α activates the nuclear transcription factor-kappa B (NF-κB), a ubiquitous transcription factor and pleiotropic regulator of numerous inflammatory and immune responses. Once activated, NF-κB translocates from the cytosol to the nucleus of the cell where it binds to its consensus sequence on the promoter-enhancer region of different genes, thereby activating the transcription (Figure 13–1). Nuclear transcription factor-κB regulates expression of several different pro-inflammatory cytokines (IL-1, IL-2, IL-6, IL-8, IL-12, TNF), ECAMs such as intercellular adhesion molecule 1 (ICAM-1), vascular cell adhesion molecule 1 (VCAM-1), E-selectin, and mucosal addressin cell adhesion molecule 1 (MAdCAM-1), as well as NOS 2 and COX 2.

Nuclear transcription factor-κB normally resides within the cytosol in its inactive state bound to its inhibitor protein κB (IκB). In addition to TNF-α, a large number of different bacterial and viral products, cytokines, and lipid mediators activate NF-κB. It is unlikely that each of these stimuli activates the cytoplasmic NF-κB-IκB complex via completely different pathways. Indeed, there is a growing body of experimental data to suggest that many, if not all, of these stimuli activate multiple signaling pathways that converge to enhance reactive oxygen metabolism within the cell (see Figure 13–1). This has been shown for the NF-κB activators TNF, IL-1, lipopolysaccharide, phorbol esters, ultraviolet light, radiation, anti-IgM, okadaic acid, and anti-CD28. Further supporting this concept is the recognition that certain lipophilic, membrane-permeable oxidants, such as H_2O_2 and oxidant-producing xenobiotics (eg, menendione), activate NF-κB. The identity of specific intracellular sources for this enhanced oxidative metabolism has not been identified; however, prostaglandin synthase, xanthine oxidase, mitochondria, NADPH oxidase, and cytochrome P-450 are likely candidates. Sources of exogenous oxidants in vivo that could activate NF-κB include activated phagocytic leukocytes (eg, polymorphonuclear neutrophil leukocytes [PMNs], monocytes, macrophages, and eosinophils.

Furthermore, NF-κB activation has been shown to be inhibited in vitro by a wide variety of structurally diverse enzymatic or nonenzymatic antioxidants, or free radical scavengers such as SOD, catalase, GSH peroxidase, N-acetylcysteine, vitamin E derivatives, α-lipoic acid, and certain dithiocarbamates. Furthermore, several recent studies have demonstrated that certain antioxidants inhibit NF-κB in vivo and attenuate inflammatory tissue injury. Indeed, it is intriguing to speculate that the observed protective effects of certain anti-inflammatory agents with known antioxidant activity in various models of IBD may be due to inhibition of NF-κB activation. As will be discussed later, the aminosalicylates represent one such class of anti-inflammatory drugs.

The exact mechanisms by which oxidants activate NF-κB are not yet known. However, it is thought that certain

---

[*] Editor's Note: Recently completed trials have further demonstrated clinical benefits and steroid–sparing, although additional supportive trials are necessary to clarify dose and administration schedules.

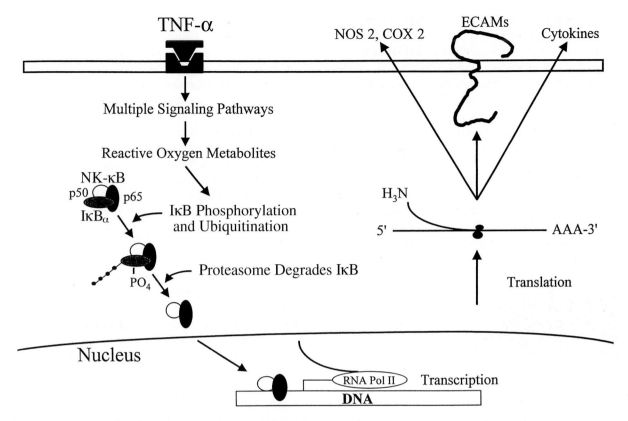

FIGURE 13–1. Tumor necrosis factor-α (TNF-α)-induced activation of nuclear transcription factor-kappa B (NF-κB). Cytokine-receptor interaction initiates multiple signaling pathways that converge to enhance intracellular reactive oxygen metabolism. These oxidants directly or indirectly activate one or more inhibitor-protein κB (IκB) kinases and ubiquitinating enzymes resulting in the phosphorylation and polyubiquitination of IκB. The 26S proteasome complex selectively degrades the post-translationally modified IκB, thereby liberating the transcriptionally active p50/p65 heterodimer. This transcription factor is transported into the nucleus, where it binds to its consensus sequence in the promoter/enhancer region, upstream of different genes, where it activates the transcription of a variety of genes known to be important in the inflammatory response, such as endothelial cell adhesion molecules (ECAMs), cytokines, and enzymes such as nitric oxide synthase (NOS 2) and cyclo-oxygenase 2 (COX 2). DNA = deoxyribonucleic acid; RNA Pol II = ribonucleic acid promoter region; MRNA poly A tail used for stability.

reactive oxygen species activate directly or indirectly one or more redox-sensitive kinases that specifically phosphorylate IκB. Once phosphorylated, IκB is selectively ubiquinated, then degraded via the non-lysosomal, ATP-dependent 26S proteolytic complex, thereby promoting nuclear translocation of the heterodimeric p50/p65 transcription factor (see Figure 13–1). Thus, pro-inflammatory cytokines such as TNF-α induce inflammation by activating NF-κB and inducing the expression of numerous pro-inflammatory genes. This relatively recent appreciation of the molecular events involved in regulation of the immune and inflammatory responses has prompted investigators to reevaluate the mechanisms by which established anti-inflammatory medications mediate their protective effects in patients with active IBD.

Glucocorticoids

Glucocorticoids are currently used to suppress inflammation in a wide variety of disorders, including IBD, allergic disorders, autoimmune diseases, and rheumatoid arthritis. In some cases, they are the most effective treatment available. Because of concern for potentially serious side effects, there has been considerable interest in the development of modified steroids and/or novel approaches to delivery of steroids (eg, "regional therapy") to take advantage of these compounds' anti-inflammatory activity, while minimizing deleterious side effects. These efforts will be facilitated by new data regarding molecular mechanisms of anti-inflammatory actions of steroids. There is a separate chapter on use of steroids and one on steroid nonresponsiveness.

Many steroid effects are mediated by a class of receptors normally resident in an unbound, inactive form in the cytoplasm of target cells. Steroids enter most cells by diffusion, whereupon they bind to, and thus "activate," their cytoplasmic receptors. The activated receptors then undergo structural changes, resulting in translocation to the nucleus, dimerization, and subsequent binding to specific control regions (termed glucocorticoid response elements, or GRE) of steroid-responsive genes, thus activating or repressing transcription of those genes. This classic mechanism of action of glucocorticoids may be involved in activation of certain anti-inflammatory proteins, such as lipocortin-1, secretory leukocyte protease inhibitor, IL-1 receptor antagonist, and IL-10. However, the precise role of glucocorticoid receptor/GRE interactions in stimulating production of these proteins is not clear and for some (lipocortin-1, IL-10), the effects appear to be indirect. Moreover, most anti-inflammatory and immunosuppressive effects of glucocorticoids appear to be due to inhibition rather than induction of gene expression.

Glucocorticoids inhibit transcription of several pro-inflammatory cytokines and chemokines, including (among others) IL-1β, IL-2, IL-6, TNF-α, IL-8, and MCP-1. However, none of these or other cytokines possess a negative GRE consensus sequence in their upstream promoters. Recent evidence indicates that glucocorticoids inhibit expression of inflammatory genes by effects on either synthesis or activity of inflammatory transcription factors, such as NF-κB and AP-1.

Two mechanisms have been proposed for the negative modulatory effect of glucocorticoid receptors on NF-κB: the first is dependent upon synthesis of IκBα, which binds to NF-κB in the cytoplasm preventing translocation to the nucleus and subsequent interaction with and stimulation of NF-κB-dependent genes. However, since IκBα does not have a GRE in its promoter, the precise mechanism of glucocorticoid's effects is obscure. The second mechanism of glucocorticoid-mediated inhibition of NF-κB involves direct binding of an activated glucocorticoid receptor to the DNA transactivation region of the RelA/p65 subunit of NF-κB, thus masking the site required for binding to and activation of NF-κB-dependent genes. A similar mechanism is thought to account for glucocorticoid's inhibitory influence upon AP-1 activation. In fact, excessive production of AP-1 (thus sequestering available activated glucocorticoid receptors) at inflammatory sites has been proposed as a possible mechanism for resistance to the anti-inflammatory effects of glucocorticoids in some patients. There is a chapter on steroid resistance in IBD.

Systemic side effects of steroid therapy, including hypothalamic-pituitary-adrenal axis insufficiency, osteoporosis, diabetes, steroid myopathy, and infectious and neuropsychiatric complications, limit the therapeutic use of classic glucocorticoid agonists for inflammatory diseases. However, most of the anti-inflammatory effects of glucocorticoids appear to be mediated by direct interaction between a single activated glucocorticoid receptor and inflammatory transcription factors. In contrast, the endocrine and metabolic effects are mediated by binding of receptor homodimers to GRE in glucocorticoid-responsive genes (transactivation). Thus, efforts are underway to develop novel compounds that selectively transrepress, thus reducing systemic complications during prolonged glucocorticoid therapy. Several compounds have greater transrepression than transactivation effects, including RU486, fluticasone propionate, and budesonide; of these, regionally administered budesonide (a 17-α substituted steroid) is considered ideal due to its high water solubility, extensive first-pass metabolism in the liver and intestine, and major metabolites possessing minimal systemic activity. Recently, another novel class of synthetic steroids (so-called "dissociated glucocorticoids") was described that exhibits potent transrepressive but little transactivation effects in vivo, suggesting that continued improvement in steroid development for treatment of inflammatory diseases with reduced risk of systemic side effects is possible. There are several chapters on budesonide and beclomethasone.

Aminosalicylates

Aminosalicylates (sulfasalazine, 5-aminosalicylate) have been a mainstay in the treatment of IBD for a number of years. Sulfasalazine (SZ) is composed of a sulfapyridine moiety covalently linked to 5-aminosalicylic acid (5-ASA) via an azo-bond. Pharmacokinetic studies have established that SZ passes unmodified through the upper gastrointestinal tract until it reaches the colon where it is metabolized by enteric bacteria to yield sulfapyridine and 5-ASA. Although several clinical studies have demonstrated that 5-ASA is the pharmacologically active moiety in SZ, there remains active debate as to whether the parent compound has some unique type of anti-inflammatory activity. A number of new-generation preparations of 5-ASA have been developed to avoid the side effects of sulfapyridine. Although the aminosalicylates, especially SZ, have been used for several decades in the treatment of IBD, the mechanisms by which these agents mediate their anti-inflammatory activity remain essentially unknown. Numerous pharmacologic activities have been attributed to the aminosalicylates, including antibiotic actions, inhibition of cyclo-oxygenase, thromboxane-A synthase, and platelet activating-factor synthase activies as well as inhibition of immunoglobulin production by plasma cells and downregulation of cellular functions of natural killer cells, mast cells, and neutrophils. One of the more popular mechanisms of action proposed to account for the potent anti-inflammatory activity of the aminosalicylates is inhibition of 5-lipoxygenase (5-LO)-mediated generation of the pro-inflammatory lipid mediator leukotriene B$_4$ (LTB$_4$). Recent clinical studies demonstrating the lack of clinical efficacy of two structurally distinct yet very specific 5-LO inhibitors (eg, zileuton, MK-519) in patients with active IBD suggest that the anti-inflammatory activity of the aminosalicylates is not due to their ability to inhibit 5-LO. Another possible mechanism by which these compounds may mediate their anti-inflammatory activity is by scavenging reactive oxygen and nitrogen species. It has been well documented that the aminosalicylates are potent antioxidants on par with ascorbic acid (vitamin C). The antioxidant properties of 5-ASA may make this compound especially well suited to inhibit NF-κB activation as described previously. Indeed, a recent series of investigations have shown that salicylates and their derivatives exhibit inhibitory effects on NF-κB activation. Sodium salicylate and acetylsalicylic acid both inhibit NF-κB-dependent transcription, possibly by directly inhibiting the activity of IκB kinase, which would normally phosphorylate IκBα, leading to its degradation and the subsequent translocation of NF-κB to the nucleus. In addition, both SZ and 5-ASA have been shown to inhibit activation of NF-κB activation as well, the former by inhibiting phosphorylation and degradation of IκBα, the latter by inhibiting phosphorylation of the p65 subunit of NF-κB, as well as having additional inhibitory effects on mitogen activated protein kinase (MAPK) pathways. There are separate chapters on metabolism of azathioprine and 6-mercaptopurine.

Acknowledgment

Some of the work reported in this chapter was supported by grants from the Crohn's and Colitis Foundation of America, the National Institutes of Health (DK47663 and DK43785), and the Feist Foundation of Louisiana State University Medical Center in Shreveport, Louisiana.

Supplemental Reading

Baeuerle PA, Henkel T. Function and activation of NF-kappa B in the immune system. Annu Rev Immunol 1994;12:141–79.

Barnes PJ. Anti-inflammatory actions of glucocorticoids: molecular mechanisms. Clin Sci 1998;94:557–72.

Flohe L, Brigelius-Flohe R, Saliou C, et al. Redox regulation of NF-kappa B activation. Free Radic Biol Med 1997;22:1115–26.

Grisham MB. Molecular and cellular aspects of intestinal inflammation: clinical implications in inflammatory bowel disease. Inflamm Bowel Dis 2000;1:1–14.

Hawkey CJ, Dube LM, Rountree LV, et al. A trial of zileuton versus mesalazine or placebo in the maintenance of remission of ulcerative colitis. The European Zileuton Study Group For Ulcerative Colitis. Gastroenterology 1997;112:718–24.

Miles AM, Grisham MB. Antioxidant properties of aminosalicylates. Methods Enzymol 1994;234:555–72.

Powrie F. T cells in inflammatory bowel disease: protective and pathogenic roles. Immunity 1995;3:171–4.

Roberts WG, Simon TJ, Berlin RG, et al. Leukotrienes in ulcerative colitis: results of a multicenter trial of a leukotriene biosynthesis inhibitor, MK-591. Gastroenterology 1997;112:725–32.

Sandborn WJ, Hanauer SB. Antitumor necrosis factor therapy for inflammatory bowel disease: a review of agents, pharmacology, clinical results, and safety. Inflamm Bowel Dis 1999;5:119–33.

Schmid RM, Adler G. NF-κB/Rel/IκB: Implications in gastrointestinal diseases. Gastroenterology 2000;11:1208–28.

CHAPTER 14

MANAGEMENT OF DISTAL COLITIS

MASSIMO CAMPIERI, MD

Distal colitis is defined as ulcerative colitis (UC) limited to the distal 30 to 50 cm of the large intestine (involving the rectum, sigmoid, and descending colon) and not extending beyond the splenic flexure. Distal colitis is the most common clinical scenario of UC accounting for 60 to 70 percent of outpatients. From the management perspective, and also due to other physiologic and prognostic features, it is best to separate "distal colitis" from "proctitis," in which the inflammatory process is confined to the rectum. Proctitis often demonstrates more extensive mucosal inflammation, both macroscopic and histologic, compared to more extensive disease and thus may require a more prolonged therapeutic approach.

Therapeutic Options

The clear-cut study by Azad Khan et al in 1977 demonstrated the therapeutic efficacy of 5-aminosalicylic acid (5-ASA) and opened the door for both rectal and oral formulations. Initially, high-dose (4 g) 5-ASA (mesalamine) enemas were adopted after demonstrating efficacy, the ability to spread up to the splenic flexure, and minimal systemic absorption or toxicity. Subsequently, dose-ranging trials have failed to demonstrate a dose-response between rectal administration of mesalamine 1 to 4 g daily.

Topical Mesalamine

The first line of approach to either first attacks or relapses of distal colitis has been the use of mesalamine enemas (2 g in 60 mL volumes) (Figure 14–1). We have observed a rapid improvement in symptoms within 1 to 2 weeks and clinical remission after 4 weeks in 65 to 90 percent of patients.[*] The duration of enema therapy may require 6 to 8 weeks or even longer to complete endoscopic healing. The demonstration of complete histologic disappearance of inflammation is a more precise marker of remission and bears a better prognosis by virtue of a lower risk of relapse. After induction of remission, treatment is usually continued for several additional weeks, then reduced to alternate-night enemas, particularly after prolonged or troublesome attacks.

IMPROVING COMPLIANCE WITH TOPICAL THERAPY

While topical mesalamine is the most effective means of controlling distal colitis, compliance may be difficult due to rectal administration of a product that must be used in bed and is associated with leakage and occasional abdominal discomfort. To overcome these problems, pharmaceutical formulations have been developed to improve patient adherence to rectal treatment.

Foams have been developed in Europe that have a propellant gas and that provide a uniform spread along the left colon similar to hydrocortisone foams available in the United States. Nevertheless, some patients still complain of gas, bloating, and abdominal discomfort. Gel formulations also are under development that appear to be easier to retain than foam with less intrusion on daily activities.[†]

In our practice we generally employ smaller volumes of suspension enemas (30 mL enema, suppositories, or foams) to reach the upper rectum and reserve the higher-volume (60 mL) suspensions for when more proximal spread to the sigmoid or descending colon is required. The use of small-volume enemas, anticholinergics, or warm baths before enema administration is discussed in the chapter on unresponsive distal disease.

Oral Aminosalicylates

While there is no agreed-upon regimen for oral aminosalicylates to treat distal colitis, most of our patients are on maintenance treatment with oral mesalamine at doses between 1.6 and 2 g daily after initiating rectal therapy with enemas or other topical formulations.

We usually start with topical treatment, alone, for a first attack and add oral mesalamine if there is no immediate response to (re-)introduction of enema therapy or in the case of relapsing disease. The combination of oral and topical mesalamine has been demonstrated to be superior to either treatment alone. However, in our clinical experience, we reserve this approach for patients with more severe disease or when topical therapy is not rapidly effective.

---

[*] Editor's Note: These proportions are higher than have been demonstrated in North American trials. (TMB)

[†] Editor's Note: Neither mesalamine foams nor gels are available in the United States. Mesalamine suppositories are available that reach the upper margin of the rectum and are easily retained on a bid or tid schedule. (TMB)

Topically Active Steroids

Rectal administration of glucocorticoids has been an established therapy for distal colitis for nearly 40 years. Unfortunately, systemic absorption and side effects can still accompany topical use of conventional steroids (eg, hydrocortisone, prednisone, methylprednisolone). Recently, a series of nonabsorbable corticosteroids (eg, beclomethasone dipropionate) or rapidly metabolized compounds (eg, budesonide) have become available outside of the United States' market. Administration of budesonide enemas (2 mg hs) thus far has not been associated with significant suppression of the hypothalamic-pituitary-adrenal axis. We have limited the use of topical corticosteroids in patients who cannot tolerate or fail to respond to topical mesalamine. There is a separate chapter on topically active steroid therapy in distal colitis.

The combination of rectal mesalamine and corticosteroid can be used and the combination may be more effective than either single compound. Alternatively, the administration of a topical steroid in the morning and topical mesalamine at night is another treatment strategy for patients who do not respond to the single drug approach.

Refractory Distal Colitis and Steroid Dependence

Patients who do not respond to topical mesalamine alone or in combination with topical corticosteroids are treated with oral steroids until they respond. If they fail to improve with oral steroids, they are admitted to the hospital for intensive management with high-dose, intravenous corticosteroids (methylprednisolone 60 mg). The intensive intravenous regimen usually is effective at inducing remission in the majority of patients with distal disease. However, if there are frequent relapses as steroids are tapered, despite combinations of oral and topical mesalamine, we have had success with azathioprine, 2 to 3 mg/kg daily. Most patients are able to taper off steroids, while maintaining oral and topical aminosalicylates, within 4 to 6 months. Patients for whom steroid tapering fails or those patients with persistent symptoms are candidates for colectomy.[‡] There is a chapter on immunomodulator use in distal colitis.

Maintenance Therapy

The vast majority of patients with distal colitis will require maintenance therapy on a long-term basis to prevent relapse. We prefer to continue with oral mesalamine maintenance therapy (1.6 to 2.4 g/d) supplement with tapering, then intermittent, topical therapy if patients continue to relapse.[§] In general, patient adherence to oral therapy has been better than with topical treatment alone.

Treatment of Proctitis

Mesalamine suppositories have been highly effective and well tolerated for patients with disease limited to the distal 20 cm of colon. We usually begin with 500 mg mesalamine suppositories administered twice daily for at least 1 month. Other centers prefer 1 g suppositories administered only at night. If the patient improves, we will taper to a single suppository for several months.

If the patient does not improve with mesalamine suppositories, we perform a sigmoidoscopy to assess whether the disease has progressed proximal to the rectum. If this is so and the disease remains distal, we substitute mesalamine enema therapy as used above. Again, as with distal disease, rectal therapy is more effective than oral mesalamine for proctitis and many patients with more proximal colitis fail to respond to oral therapy due to residual disease in the rectum. Again, in this group, the addition of mesalamine suppositories often is successful and combination oral/topical mesalamine may be necessary on a long-term basis.

If patients do not respond to topical therapy with mesalamine suppositories, combination therapy with mesalamine and corticosteroids, either as enemas, foams, or suppositories, can be very effective. Once patients improve, the corticosteroid is discontinued and the patient maintained using mesalamine suppositories, with or without oral mesalamine. It is not our practice to use oral corticosteroids for UC confined to the rectum.

Conclusions

Topical treatment is the initial therapy of choice for patients with distal colitis. Enemas are most effective for disease proximal to the rectum, whereas suppositories are both effective and well tolerated in the setting of proctitis. There remains significant controversy and differences of approach regarding dosing, available formulations, and duration of topical versus oral therapy in different parts of the globe.

Reference

Azad Khan AK, Piris J, Truelove SC. An experiment to determine the active therapeutic moiety of sulphasalazine. Lancet 1977;2:892–5.

[‡] Editor's Note: The indications for colectomy in distal colitis or proctitis are the same as for extensive disease. (SBH)

[§] Editor's Note: We commonly employ higher doses of oral mesalamine maintenance, up to 4.8 g/d, for patients who relapse on oral maintenance doses. (SBH)

Supplemental Reading

Bitton A, Peppercorn MA. Medical therapy of ulcerative procti- tis and proctosigmoiditis including refractory disease. Inflamm Bowel Dis 1995;1:207–19.

Campieri M, Gionchetti P, Belluzzi A, et al. Optimum dosage of 5-aminosalicylic acid as rectal enema in patients with active ulcerative colitis. Gut 1991;32:929–31.

Campieri M, Paoluzi P, D'Albasio G, et al. Better quality of therapy with 5-ASA colonic foam in active ulcerative colitis. A multicenter comparative trial with 5-ASA enema. Dig Dis Sci 1993;38:1843–50.

D'Albasio G, Paoluzi P, Campieri M, et al. Maintenance treat- ment of ulcerative proctitis with mesalazine suppositories: a double-blind placebo-controlled trial. The Italian IBD Study Group. Am J Gastroenterol 1998;93:799–803.

Dick AP, Holt LP, Dalton ER. Persistence of mucosal abnormal- ity in ulcerative colitis. Gut 1996;7:355–60.

Ekbom A, Helmick C, Zack M. The epidemiology of inflamma- tory bowel disease: a large population-based study in Sweden. Gastroenterology 1996;100:350–8.

Gionchetti P, Venturi A, Rizzello F, et al. Retrograde colonic spread of a new mesalazine rectal enema in patients with distal ulcerative colitis. Aliment Pharmacol Ther 1997;11:679–84.

Hanauer SB. Dose ranging study of mesalamine (Pentasa) ene- mas in the treatment of acute ulcerative proctosigmoiditis: results of a multicentered placebo controlled trial . The US Pentasa Enema Study group. Inflamm Bowel Dis 1998; 4:79–83.

Jenkins D, Goodall A, Scott BB. Ulcerative colitis: one disease or two? (Quantitative histological differences between distal and extensive disease.) Gut 1990;31:426–30.

Kornbluth A, Sachar DB. Ulcerative colitis practice guidelines in adults. Am J Gastroenterol 1997;92:204–11.

Safdi M, De Micco, Sininsky C, et al. A double-blind compari- son of oral versus combination therapy in the treatment of distal ulcerative colitis. Am J Gastroenterol 1997;8:515–40.

CHAPTER 15

Topically Active Corticosteroids for Colitis

GORDON R. GREENBERG, MD, FRCP(C)

Ulcerative colitis universally involves the rectum, but the proximal extent of the disease is variable. When inflammation is limited to the rectum (proctitis) or to the sigmoid colon (proctosigmoiditis), the symptoms of urgency, tenesmus, and bleeding cause substantial impact on daily activities, but systemic complications are lower when compared to panulcerative colitis. Topical administration of corticosteroids has been a mainstay of primary therapy for distal ulcerative colitis over several decades and also is a useful adjunct to oral therapy for more extensive disease. However, conventional corticosteroids may be associated with a spectrum of undesirable side effects and thus newer steroid formulations have emerged that provide advantages over conventional steroid preparations.

Mechanisms of Action

Corticosteroids are among the most potent anti-inflammatory and immunosuppressive agents used for the treatment of inflammatory bowel disease. All of their effects are mediated by binding to high-affinity intracellular glucocorticoid receptors anchored to a dimer of the 90 kD heat shock protein. Steroid binding leads to a dissociation of the receptor from this complex, translocation to the nucleus, and binding to glucocorticoid response elements located within the promoter regions of glucocorticoid target genes. Enhanced or reduced transcription of these genes causes alterations in messenger ribonucleic acid (mRNA) and thus modifies protein synthesis. The human glucocorticoid receptor is comprised of two highly homologous isoforms termed hGRα and hGRβ. Glucocorticoids bind to hGRα, which modulates the expression of steroid-responsive genes; hGRβ does not bind glucocorticoids and is transcriptionally inactive, but does have the ability to antagonize the effects of hGRα. The proposed mechanisms for the presence of steroid-refractory ulcerative colitis include (1) the presence of greater numbers of low-affinity steroid receptors and (2) an increased ratio of hGRβ to hGRα.

Both the early events of inflammation including increased vascular permeability, vasodilatation, and infiltration of neutrophils and the late manifestations such as vascular proliferation, granuloma formation, fibroblast activation, and collagen deposition are suppressed by corticosteroids. Glucocorticoids cause a decrease in leuko-

cyte traffic to inflamed tissue by inhibiting expression of adhesion molecules including endothelial leukocyte adhesion molecule-1 (ELAM-1) and intercellular adhesion molecule 1 (ICAM-1). Steroids reduce the synthesis and the actions of several pro-inflammatory cytokines (eg, interleukin [IL]-1β, tumor necrosis factor [TNF]-α) and block the synthesis of lipo-oxygenase and cyclo-oxygenase products by inducing the synthesis of lipomodulin. Lipomodulin reduces phospholipase A_2 production, thereby limiting the availability of arachidonate for the synthesis of leukotriene B_4, prostaglandins, and thromboxane A_2. Reduction of antigen presentation, lymphocyte proliferation, and thus cellular and humoral immunity are also important steroid effects. Other actions of corticosteroids include enhanced absorption of water and electrolytes from the gut and improved nutrient intake by stimulating appetite.

Topical Corticosteroid Preparations

Although a proportion of all topical steroid preparations used for distal ulcerative colitis are absorbed, their efficacy is determined primarily by the local anti-inflammatory potency and not by systemic activity. However, the adverse effects associated with steroid administration are related to absorption and the bioavailability in the circulation. As the liver is the major site of steroid metabolism, it is the magnitude of hepatic first-pass inactivation or clearance rate that determines systemic bioavailability.

Conventional Topical Steroids

The conventional group of corticosteroid preparations includes hydrocortisone liquid enemas (Cortenema®, Solvay Pharmaceuticals Inc., Marietta, Georgia), hydrocortisone foam (Cortifoam®, Schwarz Pharma, Mequon, Wisconsin) and the more potent betamethasone liquid enemas (Betnesol®, Glaxo Wellcome, Research Triangle Park, North Carolina)* and constitutes the group of topical steroid agents most often used in clinical practice. The systemic bioavailability of these compounds approaches 80 percent, as they all share the property of low hepatic first-pass inactivation. Hydrocortisone has the lowest affinity for the glucocorticoid receptor and is

---

* Editor's Note: Not available in the United States. (TMB)

the least potent of all topical steroid preparations. Steroid absorption is reduced by the foam formulation, contributing to a relatively greater topical anti-inflammatory activity in the rectum. In contrast, the enema preparations will reliably reach the splenic flexure for colitis involving the left colon. However, the rate of absorption is inversely related to the degree of inflammation. When the disease is limited to the sigmoid colon, absorption of liquid preparations may actually be facilitated by the presence of normal mucosa more proximally. Liquid squeeze bottle enemas also have the disadvantage of causing more rapid rectal distension, facilitating reflex contractions with involuntary expulsion, and thus resulting in a more limited contact time. Because the absorption of all rectally administered steroid preparations tends to increase as colonic inflammation is reduced, steroid-related side effects may be most prominent after 2 to 4 weeks of therapy.

Newer Topical Steroid Preparations

The newer formulations of corticosteroids provide a more optimal structure-activity profile through alterations of the basic hydrocortisone molecule. Enhanced topical anti-inflammatory potency is achieved by the introduction of lipophilic constituents into the 16α or 17α position of the corticosteroid D ring; esterification in the 17α position also substantially increases preferential glucocorticoid activity. Esterification at the 21 position of the D ring confers more rapid hepatic steroid breakdown to metabolites with little or no systemic bioactivity. This metabolic advantage of high first-pass hepatic metabolism markedly reduces systemic bioavailability and the potential for steroid-related side effects. Three new steroid preparations have been developed for rectal administration and include tixocortol pivalate, beclomethasone, and budesonide.† Each of these products shares the property of high first-pass metabolism, but varies in its topical anti-inflammatory potency, water and lipid solubility, and its absorption into the gut wall.

TIXOCORTOL PIVALATE

The first new steroid formulation to be clinically evaluated for distal ulcerative colitis was tixocortol pivalate (Rectovalone®), a synthetic steroid derivative of hydrocortisone. This agent has the property of high first-pass metabolism, but the potency is similar to hydrocortisone. In distal ulcerative colitis, clinical improvement after administration of tixocortol pivalate 250 mg/100 mL enemas is comparable to that with hydrocortisone enemas, but without a reduction in serum cortisol. However, because of the low topical anti-inflammatory potency,

there has been a limited role for this agent in clinical practice.

BECLOMETHASONE DIPROPRIONATE

Beclomethasone dipropionate, a 17α substituted glucocorticoid, has greater topical potency than hydrocortisone and is inactivated by hepatic first-pass metabolism but has low water solubility. The efficacy for distal ulcerative colitis after 3 mg beclomethasone dipropionate enemas is similar to that of 30 mg prednisolone 21-phosphate enemas and without suppression of cortisol levels. Because of its poor water solubility this formulation has not been developed for clinical use in ulcerative colitis.

BUDESONIDE

Of the newer steroid preparations, budesonide (Entocort®, Astra Draco, AB, Lund, Sweden) has the most optimal structure-activity steroid profile and is the most extensively evaluated preparation. Budesonide is a nonhalogenated glucocorticoid structurally similar to 16α-hydroxyprednisolone. When compared to other newer steroid formulations, budesonide has higher topical potency (about 200-fold > hydrocortisone), is water soluble, and undergoes about 85 percent hepatic first-pass metabolism (compared to about 20 percent metabolism observed with prednisolone). The relative instability of budesonide in a carbomer vehicle (used in 5-ASA enemas) requires that a 2.3 mg micronized budesonide tablet be added to a 115 mL isotonic saline vehicle, just prior to administration. The tablet also contains riboflavin as a yellow colorant to confirm dissolution. This enema preparation is designed to deliver 2 mg/100 mL budesonide.

Several controlled trials have shown that budesonide enemas are efficacious in the treatment of mild to moderate distal ulcerative colitis. After 6 to 8 weeks of treatment with budesonide 2.0 mg/100 mL enemas, 40 to 55 percent of patients show clinical improvement and about one-half of this group will achieve complete remission. In some studies a statistically insignificant benefit was observed by increasing the budesonide dose to 8 mg daily. When compared to conventional corticosteroid enemas (hydrocortisone 100 mg/d or methylprednisolone 20 mg/d), budesonide 2 mg/100 mL enemas achieve equivalent symptomatic, sigmoidoscopic, and histologic improvement, but without the plasma cortisol suppression observed after the conventional rectal steroid preparations. Evaluation of budesonide 2 mg/100 mL enemas against 5-ASA 4 g enemas for distal ulcerative colitis showed a similar endoscopic and histologic outcome, but the overall symptomatic improvement tended to favor 5-ASA. Budesonide (Entocort) enemas are available in Canada and some compounding pharmacists in the United States will prepare budesonide enemas.

‡ Editor's Note: Neither tixocortal, beclomethasone, nor budesonide have been submitted for FDA approval for use in IBD in the United States. (SBH)

Therapeutic Strategies with Topical Steroids

Initial Attack

For patients with an initial attack of mild to moderate distal ulcerative colitis, treatment alternatives include topical steroid or topical 5-ASA preparations. Although both types of agents are useful, the composite clinical experience indicates that 5-ASA rectal preparations are the more effective therapy for inducing symptomatic, endoscopic, and histologic improvement, as well as complete remission, and should be the initial agent of choice. For proctosigmoiditis, treatment to remission requires 1 to 4 g 5-ASA enemas daily for 3 to 6 weeks, which are well tolerated without side effects. The chapter on therapy of distal colitis provides information on this topic.

Although budesonide 2 mg/100 mL liquid enemas provide a comparable rate of remission, patient acceptance may be lower because the more viscous carbomer vehicle in 5-ASA enemas tends to facilitate a longer retention time. This difference may account for the slower response time to budesonide and the apparent requirement for a longer 6- to 8-week treatment period to achieve remission. For proctitis, a 5-ASA 500 mg suppository administered once or twice daily for 3 to 6 weeks usually is effective for symptomatic remission. Corticosteroid suppositories containing a therapeutic dose of 40 mg are less helpful and not easily available, but can be obtained from special-order pharmacies for 5-ASA refractory patients.

There are no controlled data to show an adjunctive effect between topical 5-ASA and corticosteroid enemas for distal ulcerative colitis. However, for patients with severe urgency and tenesmus, a twice-daily regimen comprising one application of hydrocortisone foam (Cortifoam) administered in the morning and a 5-ASA enema administered in the evening is often useful for providing more rapid improvement and symptomatic remission. A small proportion of patients with distal ulcerative colitis show a true exacerbation of the inflammatory process with increased bleeding and urgency to treatment with 5-ASA enemas, usually within 3 to 5 days of administration. This entity should be distinguished from the secretory diarrhea associated with oral 5-ASA preparations. When disease exacerbation occurs after rectal 5-ASA therapy, budesonide 2 mg/100 mL enemas administered daily for 6 to 8 weeks are usually effective in achieving remission.

Refractory Disease

Notwithstanding a combined treatment approach with topical 5-ASA and steroid enemas and an oral 5-ASA preparation, a proportion of patients with distal ulcerative colitis will remain refractory. After endoscopic confirmation that the disease has not extended, oral prednisone is usually considered the next treatment option. Because contact time is one of the prime determinants of efficacy to topical therapy, an alternate strategy is the employment of the Truelove method of a controlled rectal drip administered over 30 to 40 minutes in the left lateral position, usually prior to bedtime. Although a dose-response effect to budesonide disposable enemas has not been demonstrated in clinical trials, we have used budesonide 6.9 to 9.2 mg daily (3 to 4 tablets) in 150 mL of the liquid vehicle administered daily for 2 to 4 weeks as a rectal drip to induce a clinical response in refractory patients. While the cost of this approach may be a mitigating factor for some patients, budesonide at these higher doses is well tolerated and not associated with steroid-related side effects despite evidence of suppressed plasma cortisol levels in a proportion of patients.[‡] Betamethasone 5 mg/100 mL also may be administered by the rectal-drip technique with good clinical efficacy, but at the expense of clinically detectable steroid side effects.

Maintenance Therapy

After an initial response to treatment, 60 to 65 percent of patients with distal ulcerative colitis will relapse within 1 year. There is no role for topical conventional steroids as a maintenance therapy for distal ulcerative colitis; 5-ASA 4 g enemas administered 1 to 3 times weekly will maintain remission in the majority of patients. For distal ulcerative colitis patients who show exacerbation of their disease after topical 5-ASA preparations, budesonide 2 mg/100 mL enemas employed 1 to 3 times weekly are also beneficial for the maintenance of long-term remission, without steroid-related side effects. The use of oral mesalamine products and, if necessary, azathioprine is discussed in other chapters.

Newer Oral Steroid Preparations

Formulation of budesonide into enterocapsule preparations facilitates delivery of the drug to the terminal ileum and colon. One preparation (Entocort) is effective for the treatment of ileocecal Crohn's disease, but the distribution characteristics of this formulation do not allow for extension beyond the right colon. Therefore, Entocort enterocapsules are not helpful for the treatment of ulcerative colitis. Evaluation of a modified Entocort formulation with a coating designed to provide colonic delivery of 10 mg budesonide showed clinical improvement for extensive and left-sided ulcerative colitis, but this

---

[‡] Editor's Note: Prior to oral steroid therapy, our approach has been to combine topical steroids and 5-ASA. We add a 2 mg budesonide tablet into the 5-ASA suspension for nighttime administration or have a compounding pharmacist produce a combination 2 mg budesonide/500 mg 5-ASA suppository for hs or bid use in proctitis. (SBH)

preparation has not been developed for clinical use. A different formulation of 9 mg budesonide (Budenofalk®, Falk Pharma, Freiburg, Germany), available in Europe, has been shown to be effective for the maintenance of remission in previously steroid-dependent ulcerative colitis. Whether colonic-release preparations of oral budesonide alone or in combination with oral 5-ASA would be as effective as prednisone for more extensive ulcerative colitis, without the steroid-related side effects, remains a promising area for further study.

Conclusions

The symptoms associated with distal ulcerative colitis may significantly impact quality of life. Although topical conventional corticosteroid preparations are a useful treatment, the composite clinical experience indicates that topical 5-ASA preparations will usually provide greater efficacy for distal ulcerative colitis. However, in the patient who is refractory to 5-ASA therapy or shows true 5-ASA sensitivity, topical hydrocortisone foam or budesonide may prove to be useful. Further refinements of the colonic release systems for oral budesonide enterocapsules may be of benefit to patients with more extensive ulcerative colitis.

Supplemental Reading

Campieri M, Cottone M, Miglio F. Beclomethasone dipropionate enemas versus prednisolone sodium phosphate enemas in the treatment of distal ulcerative colitis. Aliment Pharmacol Ther 1998;12:361–6.

Danish Budesonide Study Group. Budesonide in distal colitis. Scand J Gastroenterol 1991;26:1225–9.

Greenberg GR. Budesonide for the treatment of inflammatory bowel disease. Can J Gastroenterol 1994;8:369–72.

Hamedani R, Feldman RD. Review article: drug development in inflammatory bowel disease: budesonide—a model of targeted therapy. Aliment Pharmacol Ther 1997;11 (Suppl 3):98–107.

Hanauer SB, Robinson M, Pruitt R, et al. Budesonide enema for the treatment of active, distal ulcerative colitis and proctitis: a dose-ranging study. U.S. Budesonide Enema Study Group. Gastroenterology 1998;115:525–32.

Keller R, Stoll R, Foerster EC, et al. Oral budesonide for steroid-dependent ulcerative colitis: a pilot trial. Aliment Pharmacol Ther 1997;11:1047–52.

Lofberg R, Danielsson A, Suhr O, et al. Oral budesonide versus prednisolone in patients with active extensive and left-sided ulcerative colitis. Gastroenterology 1996;110:1713–8.

Marshall JK, Irvine EJ. Rectal corticosteroids versus alternative treatments in ulcerative colitis: a meta-analysis. Gut 1997;40:775–81.

Mulder CJ, Fockens P, Meijer JW, et al. Beclomethasone dipropionate (3 mg) versus 5-aminosalicylic acid (2 g) versus the combination of both (3 mg/2 mg) as retention enemas in active ulcerative proctitis. Eur J Gastroenterol Hepatol 1996;8:549–53.

Richter F, Scheppach W. Innovations in topical therapy. Baillieres Clin Gastroenterol 1997;11:97–109.

Thiesen A, Thompson AB. Review article: older systemic and newer topical glucocorticosteroids and the gastrointestinal tract. Aliment Pharmacol Ther 1996;10:487–96.

CHAPTER 16

Pseudo-intractability of Inflammatory Bowel Disease

Arvey I. Rogers, MD, FACP

Introduction

Inability to produce or sustain a clinical remission or prevent frequent relapses should not lead us to make too early a presumption that the disease is truly intractable. Assigning the intractability label connotes a more serious form of inflammatory bowel disease (IBD), one that will require more time, more attention, more patient-family-physician distress, the likely inclusion of "big gun" pharmacotherapy, and even the consideration of surgical intervention.

The following definitions will be used in discussing **pseudo-intractability**:

- Remission usually implies overall resolution of clinical symptoms with endoscopic healing of the mucosa. There are no subjective or objective manifestations of inflammatory activity. **Activity indices**, that is, standard numerical scores (Crohn's Disease Activity Index [CDAI], UCAI), may be utilized by clinicians conducting research.
- Relapse: recurrence of subjective manifestations of clinical activity always accompanied by objective evidence (endoscopic, histologic, radiologic, laboratory) of active disease. Frequent relapses may be defined as intractability.
- Intractability: (1) hard to control or deal with; (2) difficult, stubborn (*Reader's Digest Oxford: Complete Wordfinder*). (1) Not easily governed, managed, or directed; (2) obstinate; (3) not easily relieved or cured (≈ pain) (*Webster's Ninth New Collegiate Dictionary*). Disease activity persists or relapses occur frequently despite what would ordinarily be considered effective therapy for a first-time occurrence or what previously had been effective in managing relapses and maintaining remission.
- Pseudo-intractability: persistence of symptoms in the absence of objective evidence of disease activity or persistence of inflammation not related to the usual pathophysiology of UC; may take the form of relapses (pseudo-relapses?), again not explained solely by the behavior of the disease.

Etiologies for Pseudo-intractability

When a patient with new-onset or a relapse of ulcerative colitis (UC) or Crohn's disease (CD) fails to respond to appropriate therapy, the clinician responsible for making critical management decisions is challenged to begin the process of "problem solving" the therapeutic failure, a process facilitated by seeking answers to several questions. Why have I been unable to induce or sustain a remission? What symptoms and/or signs are manifesting that might be caused by factors other than the IBD itself? Is the disease truly intractable? What other factors might be responsible for creating the mistaken impression of disease intractability, that is, pseudo-intractability? The answers to these questions will become clearer when the focus is on (a) the therapy, (b) aggravating factors, (c) imitating illnesses or factors, and (d) miscellaneous etiologies for diarrhea. Table 16–1 outlines the approach to use for distinguishing pseudo-intractability. Pseudo-intractability can pertain to either **therapy-resistant symptoms** of "active" disease or **frequent relapses during** maintenance regimen. It is prudent in both circumstances to consider these possibilities: (1) that the patient does not have IBD (highly unlikely, but worth considering); (2) that the symptoms are not caused by IBD or IBD alone; and (3) that persisting symptoms or relapse have been precipitated by factors extrinsic to the disease itself.

Therapy

The primary considerations for success at inducing and/or maintaining a remission are that (1) the patient be administered the proper (maximum, tolerated) dose of the medication(s); (2) the medication achieve the desired therapeutic blood or mucosal levels; (3) the medications be targeted to the site responsible for producing the most prominent/disturbing symptoms; (4) the medication(s) be administered for the appropriate length of time; and (5) the employment of combined approaches, that is, oral and rectal preparations, be considered when symptoms are stubborn and difficult to control. Often, the "super specialist" consulted to explain and treat "intractability" simply increases the dose of the drug(s) already on board (sometimes after obtaining a red blood cell count [RBC] level of a metabolite, ie, 6-thioguanine, in a patient

TABLE 16–1. Etiologic Considerations

1. Etiologies (explanations for) of pseudo-intractability

   A. Improper choice of therapy

   B. Inadequate dosage of medication(s) selected to induce remission

   C. Insufficient duration of therapy

   D. Imitating side effect of therapy
      (1) Diarrhea (and/or bleeding)
         (a) Mesalamine side effect
         (b) Antibiotic-related
         (c) Side effect of immunomodulator Rx

   E. Failure to administer concomitantly rectal preparations (when dictated by symptoms)

   F. Ineffectiveness of medications utilized
      (1) Noncompliance
      (2) Impaired absorption (diseased bowel, shortened bowel, drug interactions)
      (3) Failure to reach target organ ie, gastric outlet obstruction, bypass as by fistulae
      (4) Insufficient exposure time, ie, rapid transit
      (5) Failure to activate drug, ie, antibiotics + salicylazosulfapyridine

   G. Factors aggravating (or imitating) underlying IBD
      (1) NSAIDs
      (2) Smoking
      (3) Birth control pills
      (4) Associated irritable bowel syndrome
      (5) Narcotic addiction or dependency
         (a) Abdominal pain
         (b) Ileus
      (6) Food intolerance (lactose, sorbitol, fructose)
      (7) Superimposed infectious diarrhea
      (8) Steroid withdrawal
      (9) Incontinence
      (10) Rectal scarring with loss of compliance

   H. Multiple etiologies for diarrhea (other than active IBD)
      (1) Bacterial overgrowth (ileus, shortened bowel, fistulae, loss of ileocecal sphincter barrier)
      (2) Fistulae
      (3) Drug side effects, ie, antibiotics, masalamine, immunomodulators
      (4) Ileal scarring, resection, bypass
      (5) Bowel obstruction (paradoxical diarrhea)
      (6) Gastric acid hypersecretion consequent to massive small bowel resection
      (7) Malabsorption induced by "overdose" of cholestyramine

receiving azathioprine or 6-mercaptopurine), substitutes a pharmacologically related compound, (ie, mesalamine to reduce olsalazine-induced diarrhea; or sulfasalazine to simultaneously treat IBD-associated arthropathy), adds a preparation targeting a less-than-optimally accessed site (ie, the rectum, utilizing enemas or suppositories), or suggests a lengthier period of observation.

On occasion, persistent or even worsening symptoms (and sometimes even signs) attributable to the IBD being treated are related to the treatment itself. Diarrhea may be induced by aminosalicylates, olsalazine (Dipentum®) the most notable example. Frank allergic colitis has been attributed to mesalamine, and sulfasalazine may induce *Clostridium difficile*-associated diarrhea with or without accompanying colitis. It is worth recalling that erythema

nodosum may occur as an allergic reaction to sulfa preparations or azathioprine.

Monitoring compliance is difficult. Even pill-count components in clinical studies are no guarantee. Despite physicians' fantasies and sometimes lofty assumptions, patients are not always devoted adherents to their physician's recommendations. Gentle reminders and frequent reinforcement are integral elements to ensure a higher level of compliance, especially when therapeutic effectiveness has not been realized as quickly as the physician hoped and the patient assumed.

Failure to respond to an appropriate therapeutic regimen also may be the result of **impaired drug absorption** or **failure to reach or remain in the target organ**. Diffuse inflammation and/or prior resection of the small intestine, fistulization, gastric outlet obstruction, and rapid transit are factors compromising drug effectiveness. Tenesmus accompanying active rectal inflammation and/or reduced rectal compliance, the result of chronic inflammation, will shorten exposure time to rectal mucosa of orally or rectally administered therapies. Efforts to improve retention, that is, reduced enema volume, the use of suppositories, agents to reduce motor function, and mild sedation, may convert pseudo-intractability to tractability.

Inasmuch as the pro-drugs, sulfasalazine and olsalazine (containing azo-bonds), require cleavage by bacterially elaborated azo-reductases to release the active 5-ASA component, it is conceivable that co-administration of antibiotics that alter gut flora may interfere with this metabolic process, thereby reducing drug effectiveness.

Aggravating Factors

Smoking, especially in women with CD, concomitant use of nonsteroidal anti-inflammatory drugs (NSAIDs) (cyclo-oxygenase 2 [COX 2] inhibitors may be as risky), and oral contraceptives (more controversial) all should be considered as factors contributing to disease intractability and relapse. Spontaneously occurring infectious diarrheas precipitated by the use of antibiotics, (ie, *C. difficile*-related), or occurring as a complication of immunomodulatory therapy (ie, cytomegalovirus [CMV]), may, in addition to producing its own set of confusing or mimicking symptoms and signs, precipitate a relapse of previously quiescent colitis and resist conventional therapies. While CMV is infrequently diagnosed, and routine performance of fecal cultures, toxin assays, and colonic mucosal biopsies (looking for inclusion bodies of CMV) is not advocated, CMV should be considered as an explanation for refractory disease in the setting of immune suppression or presence of atypical features suggesting infectious mononucleosis.

Pseudo-arthritis is a frequent complication of steroid tapering and may mimic the arthritis associated with IBD. Re-institution of low-dose (5 mg/d) prednisone may be required to control symptoms. Some physicians even attribute headaches, worsening acne, abdominal cramps, and/or diarrhea to steroid tapering or withdrawal.

Imitating Illnesses (or Factors)

Estimates vary regarding the frequency with which irritable bowel syndrome (IBS) coexists with inflammatory bowel disorders. It is an accepted fact that it can mimic IBD long before the latter is finally diagnosed. Of more importance than the issue of frequency of concurrence is the fact that it is often difficult to differentiate one from the other exclusively on the basis of presenting or recurring symptoms. Compounding the problem of differential diagnosis is that objective evidence of CD, that is, aphthous ulcerations, is present frequently in the absence of subjective complaints or other objective evidence of clinically active disease. When uncertainty exists, it is reasonable to institute symptomatic therapy alone, assuming that IBS is imitating an IBD relapse and assuming there is no pressing urgency to initiate anti-inflammatory therapy.

Patients with active IBD may experience abdominal pain severe enough to require the use of narcotic-analgesic medications. Episodes of intestinal obstruction and prior surgeries set the stage for their use. The associated psychotropic properties of these medications create the potential for secondary gain and dependency, confounding both the interpretation and management of abdominal pain complaints. In addition to abdominal pain, drug-dependent patients will register other symptoms (sometimes simulated or as a consequence of drug withdrawal) attributed to IBD in order to obtain these medications. Furthermore, it is important to recall that the narcotic bowel may produce symptoms of diarrhea consequent to bacterial overgrowth, abdominal bloating mimicking intestinal obstruction, or weight loss—all symptoms that can mimic active IBD. On rare occasions, the overuse of motility suppressants and/or antispasmodics may cause similar symptom complexes.

Small bowel obstruction (secondary to chronic stenosis) not advanced enough to present itself in a classic form, may produce low-grade, recurrent symptoms suggestive of IBD relapse, that is, abdominal cramps, diarrhea, pseudo-anorexia (sitophobia), and consequent weight loss. A complete small bowel series may reveal ileal or jejunal luminal narrowing and associated proximal dilation without evidence of active inflammation.

Miscellaneous Etiologies for Diarrhea

Lactose intolerance, while no more prevalent in IBD patients than in the general population, can produce symptoms of diarrhea and abdominal bloating and present as a pseudo-relapse of IBD. Because some medications and elixirs contain sorbitol or fructose, they should be considered as contributing to diarrhea when it appears in the absence of other clinical features associated with active inflammation.

Especially challenging is the differential diagnosis of diarrhea in the patient who has CD and who has undergone prior surgery. Because choleraic diarrhea is generally easily managed by the use of bile acid–binding resins, it is always worth considering the possibility that ileal dysfunction is responsible for diarrhea after resections of less than 100 cm. Dysfunction may be the result of prior resection, spontaneously occurring (jejunocolonic) fistula, surgically induced bypass, or inflammation. Under usual circumstances, diarrhea is recognized early following surgery except when the initial resection is of an unusually short length of diseased ileum. Thereafter, if recurrent ileal inflammation ensues and ultimately heals, the "burned out" dysfunctioning length of ileal mucosa is effectively lengthened—resulting in diarrhea that often responds to binding resins like acid. Unless entertained as a possibility, unresponsive diarrhea will likely be attributed erroneously to intractable IBD.

Bacterial overgrowth complicating coloenteric fistulae, small intestinal strictures, or ileus complicating chronic narcotic use may produce imitating, intractable diarrhea, creating the impression of disease intractability. Unless this complication is considered, diagnosed, and managed specifically or treated empirically, unnecessary and inappropriate anti-inflammatory therapies will be introduced with no benefit to the patient.

On occasion, the ileum may fistulize to the sigmoid colon, resulting in intractable diarrhea because of the resulting colonic bypass. Such fistulae are not always easy to recognize, and the unsuspecting endoscopist will only diagnose "inflammation" in the sigmoid colon and prescribe, without benefit, local and/or systemic therapy to manage intractable IBD-related symptoms.

Conclusions and Recommendations

Before embarking on a course of management, whether medical or surgical, for assumed intractability, it is reasonable to consider the alternative: that factors other than the IBD itself may account for recurrent, poorly or incompletely responsive, or even intractable symptomatology. It is easy to diagnose active inflammation but not always as easy to attribute the convincing and supportive objective features to a wide range of associated subjective complaints and objective findings. Because of this, pseudo-intractability or pseudo-relapse must always be considered a possible explanation for sometimes discordant subjectivity and objectivity. Factors possibly responsible for aggravating or mimicking disease activity should be sought, modified, or eliminated whenever possible. Initiating, prolonging, or modifying therapies with potential for the occurrence of both short-term and long-term adversities is serious business and any decision to do so should be considered carefully when managing what is thought to represent intractability or the inability to maintain disease remission.

Supplemental Reading

Bartlett JG, Laughon BE, Bayless TM. Role of microbial agents in relapses of inflammatory bowel disease. In: Bayless TM, ed. Current management of inflammatory bowel disease. Philadelphia: B.C. Decker, Inc., 1989:86–92.

Blackwell B. Drug therapy: patient compliance. N Engl J Med 1973;289:249–52.

Cottone M, Rosselli M, Orlando A, et al. Smoking habits and recurrence in Crohn's disease. Gastroenterology 1994;106: 643–8.

Cuffari C, Theoret Y, Latour S, Seidman G. 6-Mercaptopurine metabolism in Crohn's disease: correlation with efficacy and toxicity. Gut 1996;39:401–6.

D'Albasio G, Pacini F, Camarri E, et al. Combined therapy with 5-aminosalicylic acid tablets and enemas for maintaining remission in ulcerative colitis. Am J Gastroenterol 1997; 92:1143–7.

Hanauer SB, Meyers S. Management of Crohn's disease in adults. Am J Gastroenterol 1997;92:559–66.

Kornbluth A, Sachar DB. Ulcerative colitis practice guidelines in adults. Am J Gastroenterol 1997;92:204–11.

National Pharmaceutical Council. Emerging issues in pharmaceutical cost containment. Reston, VA: National Pharmaceutical Council. US Department of Health and Human Services, 1994.

Safdi M, DeMicco M, Sninsky C, et al. A double-blind comparison of oral versus rectal mesalamine versus combination therapy in the treatment of distal ulcerative colitis. Am J Gastroenterol 1997;92:1867–73.

Shabsin HS. Behavioral pain management. In: Bayless TM, ed. Current management of inflammatory bowel disease. Philadelphia: B.C. Decker, Inc., 1989:349–53.

Stotland BR, Cirigliano MD, Lichtenstein G. Medical therapies for inflammatory bowel disease. Hospital Practice. May 15, 1998.

CHAPTER 17

REFRACTORY DISTAL COLITIS

PHILIP B. MINER, JR., MD

Patients with refractory distal colitis suffer unrelenting or episodic symptoms of colonic inflammation despite maintenance therapy. Evaluation is approached in terms of the symptoms that disrupt their lives and the extent and severity of mucosal inflammation. Although these two issues are integrally related with a positive therapeutic response improving both, optimal management addresses each individually. Refractory colitis is a term with numerous possible interpretations: failure to respond to conventional therapy, partial therapeutic response, extension of the disease, persistent symptoms despite apparent mucosal healing, or control of disease only with doses of medication that induce toxicity. The principal persistent symptoms are rectal bleeding, pain, tenesmus, constipation, increased number of stools, nocturnal diarrhea, fecal incontinence, perineal pain, and systemic symptoms such as fatigue and fever.

Directing the Evaluation of the Patient Toward Treatment Options

History and Physical Examination

A patient referred for a second opinion to manage distal colitis requires a complete evaluation to confirm the diagnosis and assess the extent of disease. The most common identifiable causes of relapse are infection (enteric and systemic), seasonal variation, allergies, and nonsteroidal anti-inflammatory drugs (NSAIDs). Each of these risk factors can be modified to improve disease outcome. Other issues occasionally arise, such as a change in medication or a change in smoking status, that can influence the course of the disease.

Nocturnal diarrhea is a particularly useful clinical clue since intense physiologic stimulation is necessary to arouse a patient from sleep. This implies either marked mucosal inflammation or eosinophil predominant mucosal inflammation. Eosinophils are an important component of the mucosal inflammatory response, and their function has a diurnal variation with eosinophils being most active between 11 pm and 2 am. Tenesmus is a rectal symptom dependent on rectal inflammation with important therapeutic implications. The inflammatory component can be modified by topical rectal medications

(mesalamine or glucocorticoids) that focus on this anatomic site. Adjunctive therapy with antihistamines is often useful as histamine plays an important physiologic role in rectal contractility and in the relaxation of the internal anal sphincter (IAS). Constipation in left-sided ulcerative colitis is a perplexing observation for the patient who is complaining of 10 to 15 stools a day. Patients need to be questioned carefully to distinguish between bloody, mucoid discharge and the passage of stool elements. In distal colitis, the spasm of the rectum and sigmoid colon induces stasis of colonic contents in the colon proximal to active inflammation. This problem is often exacerbated by the use of antidiarrheal agents. Constipation can be a factor in mesalamine failure.

Physical examination highlights three important areas. Tenderness in the distribution of suspected disease suggests the length of the left colon that is involved with inflammation with the intensity of discomfort related to the active inflammation. Perineal dermatitis reflects the extent and severity of diarrhea and seepage. Right lower quadrant pain one-third of the way from the umbilicus to the anterior iliac crest correlates directly with the number of ileal mast cells. This is a reflection of the extent of intestinal inflammation as well, carrying the important therapeutic implication of symptomatic improvement with antihistamine therapy. Systemic manifestations of disease are less common in distal colitis than in pancolitis or Crohn's disease, and their presence suggests intense focal inflammatory disease (or possibly disease extension).

Laboratory Findings

In distal colitis, the laboratory findings parallel the abnormalities of pancolitis but usually are less intense related to the extent of mucosal involvement. The general indices of inflammation (erythrocyte sedimentation rate, albumin, C-reactive protein, platelet count, white blood cell count) are related to the nature and intensity of the inflammatory response. The diagnostic and prognostic value of tests of intensity of inflammation is limited in distal ulcerative colitis. More useful are laboratory tests that focus on treatable aspects of colitis: bacterial infection (enteric and systemic), *Clostridium difficile* toxin, fecal leukocytes, fecal eosinophils, and Charcot-Leyden crystals in the stool. Considerable debate flourishes regarding the importance of bacterial infection in inducing disease relapse since most studies lack the scientific rigor necessary to be confident about the relationship of infection to relapses in disease activity. Epidemiologically, the association of nonenteric infection with colitis relapse in children supports the role of systemic infection and disease activity. The best explanation for this association is a general upregulation in the immune system. This induces the activity of the gastrointestinal immune system to a level of activity above the threshold of mucosa tolerance. This results in disease activation. This logical construct does not require that specific infections be identified, only that an immune response be increased. If this is accepted for systemic infection, then enteric infection as a cause of disease relapse is easily explained by both generalized as well as gastrointestinal mucosal immune induction. Recent interest in luminal influences on initiation of inflammatory bowel disease and on disease relapses supports this mechanism.

A second luminal mechanism related to changes in mucosal permeability may be more important. An increase in intestinal permeability will enhance the presentation of antigenic constituents of the intestinal lumen to the immune system with subsequent immune upregulation. Increased permeability occurs with allergies, eosinophil activation, NSAID use, and infection. One of the most remarkable examples of an increase in intestinal permeability is caused by *C. difficile*. This observation provides a mechanism of *C. difficile* disease activation in the absence of a concentration of toxin sufficient to damage the mucosa. I usually prescribe an empiric course of metronidazole (750 to 1000 mg a day for 7 days) in patients with a clinical presentation implicating *C. difficile* by history (antibiotic exposure, flares in disease following preparation for colonoscopy) or consistent laboratory findings (rapid development of hypoalbuminemia with normal potassium or a positive *C. difficile* toxin). If the patient responds to this antibiotic trial, I follow treatment with a week of bile acid binding resin to diminish the risk of a recurrence of *C. difficile*. Since metronidazole has no recognized therapeutic role in the treatment of ulcerative colitis, a response to empiric therapy suggests (1) *C. difficile* infection, (2) a metronidazole susceptible infection as a contributing cause of the colitis, or (3) the presence of indeterminant colitis with a high probability of Crohn's colitis.

Cytomegalovirus (CMV) has also emerged as an important infectious cause of disease exacerbation. The postulated pathophysiology is susceptibility to CMV due to immunosuppression. Although this is often the situation, there are cases of CMV-induced disease relapses in patients not being treated with immunosuppressive drugs, which should alert the clinician to seek CMV as a cause for disease activation in clinically appropriate situations.

Flexible Sigmoidoscopy

Flexible sigmoidoscopy provides important information about the severity and the extent of the inflammation. Although it was once felt that the extent of colitis did not progress, epidemiologic evidence supports the progression of proctitis in 46 percent of patients and in progression to pancolitis in 70 percent of patients initially diagnosed with left-sided colitis. In patients with refractory colitis, sigmoidoscopy determines whether progression of disease has occurred. In addition, visible changes suggesting different forms of colitis can be determined. Focal edema and ulceration suggests Crohn's disease, pseudomembranous colitis, or solitary rectal ulcer syndrome (SRUS). Biopsies of areas of mucosal inflammation should be obtained. Occasionally, the mucosa appears normal in the presence of clinical symptoms of colitis. Biopsy evaluation for collagenous colitis, lymphocytic colitis, microscopic colitis, or eosinophilic gastroenteritis is particularly important in these patients. Sigmoid biopsies are most reliable for collagenous colitis.

Histology

The histology may suggest that Crohn's colitis, collagenous colitis, or microscopic colitis is the reason the patient has not responded to treatment. Particular interest should be directed toward the intensity and location of eosinophil infiltration. The relative number of eosinophils is important since eosinophilic crypt abscesses carry greater clinical significance. Also, documentation of eosinophils migrating through the mucosal surface suggests that eosinophils are playing a pivotal role in the inflammatory process. When eosinophils are prominent by histologic assessment or confirmed indirectly by the presence of Charcot-Leyden crystals in the stool, short-term high-dose steroids often induce remission.

Another important histologic finding is the pathognomonic volcanic eruption appearance of the surface mucosal inflammation in *C. difficile* colitis. Since metronidazole has no primary role in the treatment of ulcerative colitis, its best use is in the treatment of *C. difficile*. Another misleading diagnosis is SRUS. This ischemic lesion is usually misdiagnosed as Crohn's proctitis rather than ulcerative colitis because of the deep ulcerations and mucosal edema, which usually accompanies symptoms of distal colonic inflammation. The disrupted muscle fibers that form a chaotic pattern below the mucosal surface create a pathognomonic pathologic lesion.

Treating Symptoms of Distal Colitis

Symptoms of proctitis are the driving force that brings patients to the physician. Although the intent of treatment is to decrease mucosal inflammation, patient symptoms must also be addressed. In fact, in some of the patients who are considered refractory, the problem is continued symptoms of disease rather than persistent colonic inflammation.

Rectal Bleeding

Rectal bleeding is one of the few symptoms of ulcerative colitis for which the only management strategy is to decrease the mucosal inflammation. Howevere, assessment of anemia and the degree of iron deficiency should lead to iron replacement when necessary, and if the anemia does not respond to iron replacement, an iron absorption test should be done. Ferrous sulfate (300 mg) is given with blood drawn for iron at time zero, 1 hour, 2 hours, and 4 hours. If the iron level does not increase two fold in one of the samples, the patient will probably require parenteral iron. An increase in the iron without a corresponding increase in the hemoglobin or hematocrit after 30 days of iron replacement suggests low erythropoetin. If low erythropoetin is documented, replacement should be instituted. This is discussed in the chapter on hematologic complications.

Pain

A variety of pain problems occur in ulcerative colitis including abdominal, perineal, and somatic pain. Visceral pain can be treated with antihistamines that block one of the primary visceral pain pathways. Clonidine, which also has a primary effect on visceral pain (generally a dose of 0.1 mg bid is well tolerated), can form the basis for initial therapy. Tricyclic antidepressants act by a peripheral mechanism (H1-receptor antagonism) as well as centrally to block pain perception (amitriptyline 25 to 50 mg hs). Anticholinergics can decrease the discomfort associated with intestinal cramps, although I am hesitant to use antimotility agents in left-sided ulcerative colitis due to the possibility of increasing the problem of constipation. NSAIDs should be avoided for the symptomatic treatment of pain as they are one of the principal cases for disease relapse. Instead, I use acetaminophen, tramadol, propoxyphene, and occasionally codeine derivatives with the same caution I employ with other antimotility agents.

Tenesmus

Tenesmus is a complex pelvic floor symptom related to rectal contractility associated with IAS relaxation. Topical rectal therapy is useful in decreasing the symptoms, but antihistamines modulate the relaxation of the IAS and decrease rectal contractility without inducing impaired colonic motility.

Constipation

Constipation arises from the spasm of the pelvic floor, impaired transit through the inflamed left colon, and decreased motility of the proximal normal-appearing colon. The best strategy is to prevent the dessication of stool in the proximal colon. This can be accomplished by using water retention agents such as magnesium hydroxide or polyethelene glycol (Miralax, Colyte, etc.), olsalazine as a small bowel secretory agent, or bulk laxatives such as Metamucil. The latter normalize stool consistency whether the patient has too little water or an excess of water in the colon. Care should be taken to interpret this symptom carefully as patients occasionally mistakenly attribute constipation to the symptom of tenesmus with nonproductive straining at stool.

Increased Number of Stools

Usually, the increase in the number of stools correlates with the symptom of tenesmus and should be treated by modifying pelvic floor reactivity rather than attempting to use antimotility agents to decrease stooling as this may complicate the clinical course by inducing proximal constipation.

Nocturnal Diarrhea

Nocturnal diarrhea may be due to intense rectal inflammation but more often is related to the diurnal variation in eosinophil function (greatest activity between 11 pm and 2 am) and the relationship of eosinophils to the inflammatory process. An attempt should be made to document an eosinophil component by biopsy or fecal eosinophils and Charcot-Leyden crystals. Antihistamines often suppress the nocturnal diarrhea, but if Charcot-Leyden crystals are present in the stool, then the eosinophil concentration in the intestinal mucosa is sufficient to cause tissue damage and short-term high-dose steroids should be part of the treatment protocol (prednisone for 6 days, beginning with 60 mg taken at 8 am with a decrease by 10 mg a day for 6 days).

Fecal Incontinence

Fecal incontinence is also related to the problem of pelvic floor instability and can be managed as detailed in the paragraphs above. An additional approach is to use bile acid binding drugs that solidify the stool while decreasing the effect of bile acids on the stimulation of rectal contractility and IAS relaxation. I begin with 1 g colestipol tablets, three once or twice a day, and adjust the dose to maximize control.

Perineal Pain

Perineal pain has two components: the first is due to pelvic floor instability and the second is related to chemical dermatitis from leakage of liquid stool. In addition to the treatment of the pelvic floor, the use of a lotion to protect the skin provides most patients with symptomatic relief. I ask patients to practice gentle and compulsive perineal hygiene with minimal trauma drying techniques (patting dry, not rubbing, or preferably a hair dryer on a low heat setting) then using a perineal lotion such as Balneol, which neutralizes the colonic fluid pH (to decrease the injury to the skin) while helping to replace the oils in the skin.

Systemic Symptoms (eg, Fatigue and Fever)

Problems with systemic symptoms are less frequent with left-sided ulcerative colitis than with pancolitis or Crohn's disease because the cytokine drive is less due to the smaller amount of inflammation. Unfortunately, these problems are difficult to manage with our current approaches and require suppression of the active inflammatory process.

Management of Distal Colitis by Improving Mucosal Inflammation

Mesalamine

The recommended dosing of mesalamine was established in an arbitrary way related to the known pharmacophysiology of sulfasalazine. The decision was based on the 4 g sulfasalazine dose (equivalent to 1536 mg mesalamine). In managing refractory colitis, the dose of oral mesalamine should be pushed to at least 4 grams with supplementation by topical rectal therapy of at least 4 grams as well. Duration of therapy should be for several weeks before considering the patient mesalamine resistant. Olsalazine is particularly useful in left-sided colitis, especially when constipation is a clinical feature. Since olsalazine increases small bowel fluid secretion, it can be used to increase the fluid content in the colon and offset the problem of hard stools.

Specific, careful inquiry should seek assurance that medication compliance is not an issue, although this is usually not relevant in refractory disease since patients with active disease will increase the mesalamine dose, often without medical advice, in an attempt to gain control over their symptoms. There is a separate chapter on compliance.

Distribution of Mesalamine

Mesalamine is a topically active drug that must be distributed over the inflamed mucosa before it can be effective. Principles of anorectal physiology influence the distribution of topically active drugs. With left-sided colitis, there is relative stasis of colonic contents in the right colon; thus, oral drugs may not reach the active inflammation in the left colon, and topical rectal therapy more effectively applies medication to the inflamed mucosa. In refractory disease, topical rectal therapy should always be tried. Often pelvic floor instability makes retention of mesalamine enemas difficult. Several tricks, including suppositories or partial enemas, can be tried to reduce these symptoms. Rectal contractility and IAS pressure are

directly proportional to the volume infused into the rectum. Mesalamine suppositories are easier to retain because of their volume and more viscous state. The distribution of the suppository is limited to approximately 20 cm. A 500 mg mesalamine suppository twice a day allows rapid improvement of the distal mucosa and improved ability to accommodate the enema. A partial enema can also be used with completion of the dose 20 to 30 minutes later since the lower volume will stimulate less rectal contractility and minimize the relaxation of the IAS. Antihistamines help enema retention by inhibiting relaxation of the IAS and decreasing rectal spasm, decreasing the risk of fecal incontinence. Finally, a pre-enema helps to clear the rectum and permit retention of the volume of the enema. The physiologic changes of the pre-enema are complex and include decreasing the volume in the rectum and sigmoid colon and exchanging stool for the less stimulating enema fluid.

Sensitivity to Mesalamine

The final concern related to mesalamine is chemical sensitivity. The characteristic pattern of mesalamine sensitivity is the development of abdominal pain and diarrhea, which has less blood than a usual disease flare. Flexible sigmoidoscopy reveals an edematous and erythematous mucosa, occasionally with broad ulceration. Often the clinical impression is that the patient has indeterminate colitis with a progression from typical ulcerative colitis to Crohn's disease. The patient often goes into remission with glucocorticoids. We have been unable to identify any characteristic histologic features to assist in the diagnosis. Discontinuing the mesalamine provides symptomatic relief within 72 hours, and the symptoms will increase with a rechallenge. It is imperative to understand that the colitis that was present before beginning the mesalamine will continue to be a medical problem and needs to be managed by alternative medications. The improvement after discontinuing the mesalamine documents the chemical colitis but often is a short-lived remission. In documented mesalamine sensitivity, all of the related drugs should be avoided.

Glucocorticoids

The role of glucocorticoids in chronic refractory left-sided ulcerative colitis is uncertain. I am cautious about glucocorticoid use in all patients with inflammatory bowel disease. When eosinophils play a role in the inflammatory process (see histology section above), high-dose, short-term steroids are useful for inducing remission. Rarely, glucocorticoids need to be given for a prolonged period of time (eg, waiting for 6-mercaptopurine [6-MP] to be effective). In these instances, I try to use steroids every other day to decrease the systemic toxicity of steroids. Rectal steroids have the advantage of aggressively modulating the gastrointestinal immune system with less systemic effect than oral steroids. In the absence of mesalamine sensitivity, nearly all studies show that rectal mesalamine is superior to rectally administered steroids. Steroids with high first-pass clearance such as budesonide may be particularly useful in refractory left-sided ulcerative colitis but only when in contact with the diseased mucosa. The principles for management with topical rectal steroids are the same as with topical mesalamine with the additional caveat that the normal colonic mucosa efficiently absorbs glucocorticoids while mesalamine is minimally colonic absorbed. There are anecdotal reports that combining topical steroids and topical mesalamine is effective in some patients. Some advise adding budesonide powder to a mesalamine enema.

6-Mercaptopurine and Azathioprine

6-Mercaptopurine and azathioprine have moved from the experimental arena to accepted medications for management of inflammatory bowel disease. In patients with refractory disease unresponsive to mesalamine and not explained by one of the reversible causes of disease relapse, I use 6-MP or azathioprine. Details of management with these drugs are discussed elsewhere.

Methotrexate

Methotrexate is a folate inhibitor that has immunosuppressive properties that likely are mediated through antagonism to interleukin-1. Initial response to 15 to 25 mg by intramuscular injection weekly is reasonable, but the relapse rate after 3 to 6 months is high. Despite the reports of failure to maintain remission in all patients, many of my patients have been maintained in remission for prolonged periods of time. The oral dosing regimen does not seem to be as effective as parenteral administration. Liver toxicity with methotrexate is a concern since cirrhosis may not be reflected by tests other than liver biopsy and firm data are not available.

Nicotine

Epidemiologic studies support a protective role for smoking in ulcerative colitis. This is a complicated pharmacologic issue that provides some insight into the neuroimmune control of gastrointestinal immunity, motility, and secretion. Nicotine patches may be helpful in some patients, but they do not seem to be as effective as smoking. A few patients have made the decision to return to smoking with marked improvement in refractory ulcerative colitis that did not respond to any other therapeutic approach.

Metronidazole

With the exception of ulcerative colitis patients with concurrent *C. difficile* infection, metronidazole plays no role in the management of ulcerative colitis. Recent recognition that the mucosa of patients with ulcerative colitis is sensitive to levels of *C. difficile* toxin not detected by the conventional laboratory tests has led to my use of an empiric trial of metronidazole in some patients with refractory disease. These patients have one or more of the following clinical characteristics: (1) an event sufficient to change their colonic bacterial flora (eg, antibiotics, preparation for colonoscopy), (2) right lower quadrant abdominal pain, (3) watery diarrhea atypical for a flare of the patient's usual disease, and (4) hypoalbuminemia in the face of normal serum potassium. If a clinical response to metronidazole treatment occurs, then I continue treatment with metronidazole (750 to 1000 mg/d) for 14 days and follow with 7 to 10 days of a bile acid binding resin (eg, colestid 3 g bid).

Heparin

Heparin is a fascinating drug with immunologic and anticoagulant properties. The preliminary reports of its effectiveness led to a multicentered trial that is modestly encouraging. In my unblinded experience, 10,000 units heparin SQ twice a day was effective as a mechanism to induce remission in patients with refractory disease. My enthusiasm for this innovative approach will be modulated until the final data analysis is available.

Cyclosporine

Intravenous cyclosporine induces rapid and complete remission in ulcerative colitis and Crohn's disease. In my experience with cyclosporine, it is a bridge for surgery as all of the patients I have treated ultimately required surgery. Rather than risk the complications of cyclosporine in left-sided colitis, I favor alternative medical management or proceeding directly to surgery.

Other Drugs

Several other drugs have been used in the treatment of ulcerative colitis, but few data support their use at this time. These include omega-3 fatty acids, 5-lipoxygenase inhibitors (zileuton), cromolyn, bismuth, clonidine, antibiotics, and acemannan. The specific cytokine agonists and antagonists have also not proven to be useful in ulcerative colitis. More data will be needed to support the use of these drugs. There is a separate chapter on bismuth and other mucosal protective strategies.

Surgery

Surgical intervention is an important aspect of disease management. A few patients with left-sided ulcerative colitis are disabled by their symptoms and do not respond to medical therapy. The improved surgical outcome following ileoanal anastamosis following a total colectomy makes this approach reasonable in a majority of patients with truly refractory colitis with less health risk than long-term glucocorticoid therapy.

CHAPTER 18

COEXISTENCE OF INFLAMMATORY BOWEL DISEASE AND IRRITABLE BOWEL SYNDROME

STEPHEN M. COLLINS, MBBG, FRCP (UK), FRCPC

Irritable bowel syndrome (IBS) is a chronic abdominal symptom complex for which no structural underlying abnormality can be demonstrated. It is a common disorder that affects all age groups with an increased frequency in females. Few if any of the clinical features of IBS can confidently distinguish it from inflammatory bowel disease (IBD). The multiplicity and chronicity of symptoms and their relationship to altered bowel habit can be helpful hints. A psychoneurotic disposition, evidence of anxiety or depression, and a tendency to somatize symptoms referable not only to the gut but other organ systems are pointers in favor of IBS. However, when IBS occurs in a patient with established IBD, this can be a difficult diagnosis. Since IBS is a very common disorder, it is not unexpected to find patients with both IBS and IBD. However, the question is whether there is a special relationship between these two disorders.*

On the Relationship of Irritable Bowel Syndrome and Inflammatory Bowel Disease

Very large-scale clinical epidemiologic studies would be required to determine confidently whether IBS occurs more commonly in IBD patients and to determine whether IBD leads to IBS. The author is not aware of such data at the time of writing. In the absence of this information, one must look to basic scientific studies in order to test the concept that inflammation predisposes to gut irritability and hypersensitivity. A relationship between experimental colitis and motor activity in cats was first described by MacPherson and Pfeiffer, who found that the in vivo recorded motility changes persisted after resolution of the inflammation in the colon. Studies in small animals with intestinal inflammation induced by nematode infection show quite clearly that motility is altered during the acute infection, which lasts 2 to 3 weeks, but, more importantly, the motor changes persist for at least 6 weeks following resolution of the infection and the

accompanying inflammation. A recent extension of this work shows that while infection and the inflammatory response were restricted to the proximal small intestine, motor changes were also found in the colon after recovery from infection. Thus, if these data can be extrapolated to humans, small intestinal involvement by Crohn's disease (CD) could conceivably induce persistent motility changes in the colon in the absence of overt inflammation.

Other Inflammatory Conditions Associated with IBS

Recently, much attention has been paid to an entity called "post-infectious IBS" (PI-IBS). This term was first coined by Chaudhary and Truelove in the 1960s when they undertook a review of their large IBS patient group in Oxford, England. They found that about one-third of their patients experienced the onset of IBS following what appeared to have been an acute episode suggestive of gastroenteritis. In the past decade, several outbreaks of food poisoning have been followed, and it has been found that at least 20 percent of these patients go on to develop an IBS-like syndrome. In some of these patients, anorectal motility was performed showing abnormalities reminiscent of IBS. Thus, these findings may be interpreted in light of animal studies cited above as the following: transient infection/mucosal inflammation in the small bowel leads to persistent sensory-motor dysfunction in the distal colon as a basis for symptom generation in PI-IBS (Figure 18–1).

Is the Gut Physiologically Normal in IBD Patients in Remission?

It is well known that active colitis is accompanied by altered motility, but the relevant question is whether abnormal motility reverts to normal once the IBD is in remission. A study by Loening-Baucke et al (1989) studied rectosigmoid motility in patients in histologically proven remission from ulcerative colitis (UC). They measured spontaneous and meal-induced changes and while they found spontaneous motility to be normal, meal-stimulated activity (the gastrocolic reflex) was reduced in some of the UC patients in remission. In addition they found the sensory perception threshold for rectal distension to be lower than in controls.

---

* Editor's Note: I had written on this topic in the 1989 edition. Dr. Collins has added some new interesting twists in 2000 but some of the ideas in my original chapter are still very useful clinically. We have therefore reproduced my original manuscript as the next chapter. (TMB)

IBS IN IBD

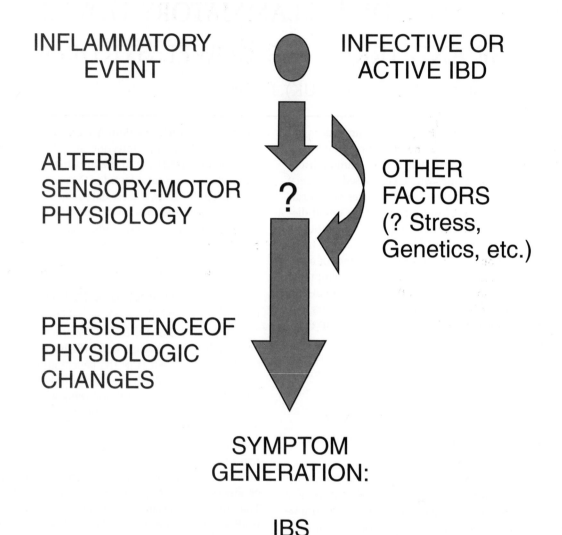

FIGURE 18–1. The putative mechanism underlying the expression of IBS in IBD patients. This diagram describes how an acute inflammatory event, such as an exacerbation of IBD or an episode of gastroenteritis, may lead to IBS. The acute event is accompanied by motor-sensory changes that, in some patients, do not resolve with the inflammation and provide a theoretic basis for symptom generation.

Using a radio-labeled meal, Rao et al (1987) studied gastrointestinal transit and stool output in UC patients with different degrees of disease activity and extent. Although not the focus of their studies, they noted that gastric emptying and small bowel transit were abnormal in patients with quiescent UC.

Thus, the presence of abnormal sensory-motor function in the rectosigmoid, as well as more proximal changes in transit, could be a basis for IBS-like symptom generation in patients in remission from UC.

Do Patients in Remission from Inflammatory Bowel Disease Express Irritable Bowel Syndrome-Like Symptoms?

There has been only one study evaluating this subject. Isgar et al (1983) showed that UC patients shown at sigmoidoscopy to be in remission exhibited IBS-like symptoms with a higher-than-expected frequency. They found that on studying 98 patients in each group, only 7 percent of non-IBD patients exhibited three or more IBS symptoms. This occurred in 30 percent of UC patients in remission. This finding, when taken in conjunction with physiologic studies performed on such patients, provides evidence of an association between IBD and IBS. If one can extrapolate on data from animal studies, it is evident that previous inflammation leaves the gut physiologically disturbed, providing a cause-and-effect relationship. If one may extend this to humans, then IBD leads to IBS in susceptible individuals.

Clinical Dilemma

The management problem is that of the **symptomatic** patient who appears to be in remission from IBD. Is this due to unidentified inflammation or to altered physiology, and hence IBS? Should the patient be investigated? Should the patient receive more anti-inflammatory or immunomodulatory therapy? Should the patient be told he or she has another, separate problem and should receive treatment directed at that?

Diagnosis of Irritable Bowel Syndrome in Ulcerative Colitis

Diagnosis of IBS is clearly an easier problem to address in UC than in CD. If one knows the patient's pattern of disease and the corresponding symptoms, it is a small matter to evaluate the rectosigmoid mucosa for evidence of active disease, with or without a biopsy—depending on the appearance of the mucosa. If constipation, a sense of incomplete evacuation of stool, and bloating are present, and if there is no evidence of proctosigmoiditis, then IBS is likely. Cramping, abdominal pain, and diarrhea are less easily distinguished from IBD: here one would really need to know that there is no histologic evidence of inflammation. Care should be taken to biopsy appropriate areas, particularly if the patient has been taking anti-inflammatory enemas. In most instances, except in indeterminate colitis, a sigmoidoscopy rather than a full colonoscopy should suffice.

Diagnosis of Irritable Bowel Syndrome in Crohn's Disease

Diagnosing IBS in CD is obviously a more difficult task, depending upon the distribution of the disease in the patient. It is wise to step back and review the patient's history to determine whether there is any suggestion of an IBS-like history present for several years before IBD was diagnosed, accepting that such symptoms could have been reflecting undetected IBD (compare symptoms with those associated with active disease in the same patient). If the CD is restricted to the colon, a colonoscopy may help. If the disease is more extensive, a small bowel radiograph may be required if some time has elapsed since the previous examination. A leukocyte count, C-reactive protein, and erythrocyte sedimentation rate [ESR] would be helpful particularly if these indices have been

increased in the past during *bona fide* relapses. Calculation of a Crohn's Disease Activity Index (CDAI) is not often helpful in this instance as the scoring incorporates subjective measures (that might reflect IBS). The physical examination might be helpful if the patient's previously active CD was restricted to the terminal ileum with tenderness in the right lower quadrant of the abdomen. The finding of mild tenderness over the sigmoid colon might be more suggestive of IBS. If the patient has strictures or extensive small bowel disease, one must consider the development of lactose intolerance, bile acid malabsorbtion, or bacterial overgrowth as a factor contributing to current symptoms, particularly cramping and diarrhea.

Cautionary Notes

Stress is traditionally implicated in IBS relapses and the clinical evidence regarding its role in causing relapses of IBD is controversial. Again, one must look to basic science for guidance. Just as human IBD can be aggravated by nonsteroidal anti-inflammatory drugs, so can experimental forms of IBD. Thus, it is worth noting a recent study in which stress was able to induce colitis in animals. Thus, the presence of stressful circumstances should not necessarily lead one to suspect IBS over IBD; in this situation, each case should be evaluated on its own merit.

Treatment of Irritable Bowel Syndrome in Inflammatory Bowel Syndrome Patients

In all instances, patients should be made aware of the fact that IBS and IBD coexist, and that the former is a benign disorder that has no implications for the prognosis of their IBD. Patients should be well informed in this respect so that, over the course of time, they will come to recognize whether their symptoms most likely reflect IBS or IBD. This should help patients cope with their condition.

With a few reservations, IBS symptoms should be treated in a manner similar to that used with IBD patients. A high-fiber diet or bulking agents should not be recommended in a patient with CD and a history of obstruction due to strictures. Anti-spasmodics should not cause concern in most IBD patients except those who have had upper gastrointestinal symptoms with gastric outlet obstruction, or those with strictures and a history of small bowel obstruction, as anticholinergic medication will undoubtedly slow transit further. There are similar concerns regarding prokinetics and opiates in such patients.

While anxiety and depression should systematically be treated if present, there is no reason for not using low-dose tricyclic antidepressants to treat functional abdominal pain or diarrhea. Patients who have had serious complications such as toxic megacolon should be treated cautiously, although they are unlikely to present with disease in remission, and thus warrant consideration of a diagnosis of IBD. Such patients are highly sensitive to opiate-based medication. With the advent of newer ligands to treat IBS, such as 5-HT (serotonin) agonists or antagonists and sensory modulators such as kappa opiate agonists, it remains to be determined if such drugs have the ability to influence inflammatory processes in any deleterious way. The pharmacologic effects of such drugs need to be tested first in animal models of IBD.

Summary

There is good scientific evidence that inflammation of the gut alters its physiologic performance, and this may persist after resolution of the inflammation. This has obvious implications for the relationship of IBD and IBS. It is this author's belief that IBS occurs with greater frequency in certain patients in remission from IBD, and this is more easily appreciated in UC than in CD. Symptoms of IBS in the context of IBD are no different from those typical for that condition. An awareness of this relationship is of key importance in making a confident diagnosis, as is a good knowledge of the patients' history and the characteristic behavior of their IBD. In some complicated IBD patients, extensive investigation by colonoscopy with or without small bowel radiography may be required. For most patients, treatment of IBS should follow the usual guidelines with notable exceptions in the case of patients with histories of obstruction.[†]

References

Chaudhary NA, Truelove SC. The irritable bowel syndrome. Q J Med 1962;31:307–22.

Isgar B, Harman M, Kaye MD, Whorwell PJ. Symptoms of irritable bowel syndrome in ulcerative colitis in remission. Gut 1983;24:190–2.

Loening-Baucke V, Metcalfe AM, Shirazi S. Rectosigmoid motility in patients with quiescent and active ulcerative colitis. Am J Gastroenterol 1989;84:34–9.

MacPherson BR, Shearin NL, Pfeiffer CJ. Experimental diffuse colitis in cats: observation on motor activity. J Surg Res 1978;25:42–9.

Rao SSC, Read NW, Brown C, et al. Studies on the mechanism of bowel disturbance in ulcerative colitis. Gastroenterology 1987;93:934–40.

Supplemental Reading

Barbara G, Vallance BA, Collins SM. Persistent intestinal neuromuscular dysfunction after acute nematode infection in mice. Gastroenterology 1997;113:1224–32.

Bergin AJ, Donnelly TC, McKendrick MW, Read NW. Changes in anorectal function in persistent bowel disturbance following salmonella gastroenteritis. Eur J Gastroenterol Hepatol 1993;5:617–20.

Duffy LC, Zielezny MA, Marshall JR, et al. Lag time between stress events and risk of recurrent episodes of inflammatory bowel disease. Epidemiology 1991;2:141–5.

Duffy LC, Zielezny MA, Marshall JR, et al. Relevance of major stress event as an indicator of disease activity prevalence in inflammatory bowel disease. Behav Med 1991;17:101–10.

Garrett JM, Sauer WG, Moertel GC. Colonic motility in ulcerative colitis after opiate administration. Gastroenterology 1967;53:93–100.

Garrett VD, Brantley PJ, Jones GN, McKnight GT. The relation between daily stress and Crohn's disease. J Behav Med 1991;14:87–96.

Gwee KA, Leong YL, Graham C, et al. The role of psychological and biological factors in postinfective gut dysfunction. Gut 1999;44:400–6.

Neal KR, HJ, SR. Prevalence of gastrointestinal symptoms six months after bacterial gastroenteritis and risk factors for development of the irritable bowel syndrome: postal survey of patients. BMJ 1997.

McKendrick MW, Read NW. Irritable bowel syndrome—post salmonella infection. J Infect 1994;29:1–3.

North CS, Alpers DH, Helzer JE, et al. Do life events or depression exacerbate inflammatory bowel disease? Ann Intern Med 1991;114:381–6.

North CS, Clouse RE, Spitznagel EL, Alpers DH. The relationship of ulcerative colitis to psychiatric factors: a review of findings and methods. Am J Psychiatry 1990;147:974–81.

Qui B, Vallance B, Blennerhassett P, Collins SM. The role of CD^4+ve lymphocytes in the susceptibility of the mice to stress-induced relapse of colitis. Nat Med 1999;5:1178–82.

[†] Editor's Note: The following chapter covers some of the clinical applications of the overlap of IBS and IBD. (TMB)

CHAPTER 19

Coexistent Irritable Bowel Syndrome and Inflammatory Bowel Disease[*]

Theodore M. Bayless, MD

The irritable bowel syndrome is a quite common combination of symptoms. It accounts for one-third to one-half of all patients seen in many digestive disease clinics and practices. Other individuals who do not seek medical attention have a similar tendency to certain symptoms or pathophysiologic motor responses and probably also have undiagnosed irritable bowel syndrome. This tendency to irregular bowel habits and/or diarrhea or abdominal pain with stress is thought, according to Drossman and co-workers, to occur in 10 to 15 percent of college-age students. The tendency to irritable bowel disease symptoms may be inherited in some patients or, at the least, be a response to common familial and environmental stresses.

Irritable bowel syndrome is much more common than idiopathic inflammatory bowel disease. Thus, it should not be surprising that many people with inflammatory bowel disease are initially told that they have irritable bowel syndrome before the inflammatory bowel disease diagnosis is firmly established. Conversely, in the patient with irritable bowel syndrome, once the additional diagnosis of inflammatory bowel disease is firmly established, the physician and the patient either may forget a preexisting irritable bowel syndrome or one or both parties may assume that the preexisting irritable bowel syndrome symptoms were actually the unappreciated (and undiagnosed) onset of inflammatory bowel disease. The negative influence of this type of assumption on the physician-patient relationship is not measurable but is certainly possible to imagine.

It is proposed here that a number of people have both irritable bowel syndrome and inflammatory bowel disease. This coexistence is examined from several aspects: (1) How does one make the diagnosis of irritable bowel syndrome in a patient with definite inflammatory bowel disease? (2) Can some of the stress and psychologically related symptoms in inflammatory bowel disease patients be due to underlying irritable bowel syndrome? (3) Can irritable bowel syndrome be the cause of some symptoms in a patient with inflammatory bowel disease? (4) Can inflammatory bowel disease or its treatment aggravate irritable bowel syndrome? (5) Can some of the interactions between these two conditions be prevented, (eg, avoiding formation of the ileoanal pouch in a patient with both irritable bowel syndrome and ulcerative colitis)? Some of the discussion focuses on the treatment of the manifestations of irritable bowel syndrome, including patient education as to the existence of both problems.

Definitions

Irritable bowel syndrome, the most common gastrointestinal condition encountered by physicians, is usually diagnosed on the basis of abdominal pain, altered bowel habits, and the absence of detectable pathology. Painless (or "nervous") diarrhea affects about 10 percent of irritable bowel syndrome patients and may be a separate variant because the patients seem to have different personality types and the course of the illness seems to be more directly affected by emotional stress. The symptoms of irritable bowel syndrome usually begin in the teenage years or in the early twenties, although abdominal pain in childhood may also be related to the later appearance of irritable bowel syndrome. At least half of adult patients have the onset of symptoms before the age of 35. In fact, approximately one-third of patients can remember symptoms as far back as adolescence.

It is not unusual when obtaining a family history to hear of disordered bowel habits in a close relative. Hearing that a relative has irritable bowel syndrome, spastic colon, mucous colitis, or constipation alerts one to consider the presence of irritable bowel syndrome. It is easiest to obtain an accurate history when the propositus is a child. Along these lines, recurrent abdominal pain of childhood is most common in children whose parents give a history of bowel disorders. Whether this is genetic or environmental is not clear.

Is there a pathognomonic motor abnormality in patients with irritable bowel syndrome? There are a number of pathophysiologic alterations from normal that can be demonstrated in many irritable bowel syndrome patients. These changes include increased basal colon motility that may correspond with the spasticity seen on x-ray and endoscopic examinations. These changes are accentuated by the distention produced by these diagnostic

---

[*] Editor's Note: This chapter was written in 1989 for the first edition. Please see accompanying chapter by Collins for more recent views.

examinations. Eating produces a delayed but prolonged change in myoelectric activity in patients with irritable bowel syndrome. Exaggerated sigmoid contractions after food ingestion, especially after large fatty meals, may account for some of the left lower quadrant pain so commonly noted by irritable bowel syndrome patients. Narcotic medications can also produce a hyperactive response in the sigmoid, perhaps creating a vicious cycle of increased colonic pain in a patient with irritable bowel syndrome. Emotional interviews can also produce bowel contractions in susceptible individuals, some of whom have the irritable bowel syndrome. Are these motor and myoelectric alterations essential for the diagnosis of irritable bowel syndrome? It is estimated that 85 percent of irritable bowel syndrome patients have some of these changes. Another important question is whether one can recognize these irritable bowel syndrome related alterations in motility and motor function in someone with ulcerative colitis, which also produces colonic motor changes. Does the increased rate of transit through the left colon in patients with active ulcerative colitis create more motility problems for the (coexisting) irritable bowel syndrome?

What constitutes a sufficient patient history to determine that a patient has irritable bowel syndrome? Is nervous diarrhea with major stress enough? Is a history of teenage constipation enough? What percentage of individuals with colonic motor alterations categorically deny any bowel habit changes?

Prevalence of Irritable Bowel Syndrome

In the United States, two-thirds of the patients seeking medical attention for irritable bowel syndrome are women. Interestingly, in other cultures such as India, where men make more frequent use of the medical care system than women, irritable bowel syndrome is seen more often in men than in women. Sandler, Drossman and his colleagues in North Carolina reported that 15 percent of apparently healthy college students stated that they had had altered bowel habits or nervous diarrhea that seemed to be compatible with irritable bowel syndrome. Only 6 percent had sought medical attention for those symptoms. This group of "patients" (as opposed to the healthy questionnaire respondents) had a history of seeing a physician in response to symptoms in other systems. Thompson and Heaton reported a 13 percent incidence of symptoms of irritable bowel syndrome in an apparently healthy population in England. In the United Kingdom study, 7 percent of controls fulfilled the criteria for irritable bowel syndrome. As mentioned earlier, in terms of prevalence of irritable bowel syndrome, gastroenterologists usually state that one-third to one-half of the patients attending a digestive disease practice or clinic have irritable bowel syndrome. It should, therefore, not be surprising if one encounters some patients who have both inflammatory bowel disease and irritable bowel syndrome. Some families have both conditions. In a study seeking the frequency of the symptoms of irritable bowel syndrome in ulcerative colitis patients in remission, Isgar and co-workers felt that 33 percent of their patients met the criteria used for irritable bowel syndrome compared with 7 percent of their healthy controls. Interestingly, these symptoms of irritable bowel syndrome were not restricted to the ulcerative colitis patients with distal disease. Constipation was also very common, occurring in 31 percent of the ulcerative colitis group.

Examples of Clinically Relevant Pathophysiology

There are several pathophysiologic alterations found in the small bowel and colon of patients with irritable bowel syndrome that could be aggravated or brought to the level of clinical awareness by inflammatory bowel disease or its treatment.

Pain or Diarrhea after Ileo-Right Colon Resection

PATHOPHYSIOLOGY

Balloon distention of the rectum and rectosigmoid (which mimics the arrival of stool in the rectum after a meal) induces spastic, often painful contractions in irritable bowel syndrome patients that are significantly greater than those encountered in normal subjects. This hyperresponsiveness to distention can also be documented in the small bowel.

CLINICAL CORRELATE

This experimental situation of rectosigmoid distention can be mimicked by the increased volume of fluid and stool that may enter the left colon after a meal in a patient with Crohn's disease who has had an ileo-right colon resection. Bile salt wasting and the resulting increased fluid volume can cause spasm and pain in the left colon of a patient with irritable bowel syndrome and inflammatory bowel disease. If narcotics are prescribed for this left sigmoid colon pain, the vicious cycle of chronic pain described earlier may ensue. This is discussed in the chapter on post-resection diarrhea.

MANAGEMENT

Knowing that the patient with Crohn's disease had irritable bowel syndrome prior to bowel resection aids in the evaluation of postoperative diarrhea and left-sided pain. This then becomes a more attractive alternative than the assumption that Crohn's disease has now (immediately postoperatively) spread into the previously normal-appearing left colon. Although this concept seems straightforward, it was often not considered by some physicians who have referred patients for consultation. Management would include trying to lessen steatorrhea and stool volume as well as prescribing dicyclomine

10 mg or loperamide 2 mg or 4 mg before meals, plus perhaps polycarbophil tablet (500 mg) or a teaspoon of psyllium or a half-packet of cholestyramine.

Active Proctosigmoiditis

PATHOPHYSIOLOGY

We are all familiar with the splenic flexure syndrome in which there is a postprandial contraction of the sigmoid colon, followed by often painful distention of the proximal colon, especially in the area of the more cephalad bowel. Since the colons of some patients with irritable bowel syndrome are more sensitive to this distention, the pain produced in the left upper quadrant can be quite severe. Creating constipation even in healthy subjects can cause one or more symptoms of irritable bowel syndrome.

CLINICAL CORRELATE

Active proctitis or *proctosigmoiditis* can cause severe spasm in the sigmoid area, thereby producing either constipation, or perhaps in the patient with coexistent irritable bowel syndrome, left upper quadrant pain.

MANAGEMENT

Again, alerting patients to the coexistence of two syndromes—inflammatory bowel disease and irritable bowel syndrome—helps them to understand the need to lessen their intake of carbonation, to utilize dietary bulk such as polycarbophil or psyllium in small quantities, and possibly to use antispasmodics such as dicyclomine, 10 mg, 15 or 30 minutes before meals. Treating the proctosigmoiditis also lessens the colon spasm.

STRESS-RELATED SYMPTOMS

Since altered rectosigmoid motility can be elicited in irritable bowel syndrome patients (and also in some non-irritable bowel syndrome patients) by stressful interviews, one wonders if some of the inflammatory bowel disease patients, especially those with proctitis, who seem to become much more symptomatic with psychological stress, might also have coexistent irritable bowel syndrome. Is this one of the reasons why earlier psychologists and psychiatrists studying a few individuals became convinced that ulcerative colitis was psychologically induced? Other "modern" views of *IBS*, *Stress Management, Relaxation Therapy*, and *Psychiatric Complications* are discussed in separate chapters.

Ileal Pouch Procedures

A loop of grossly normal small intestine is used to produce a Kock pouch (continent ileostomy) or an ileal pouch for an ileoanal anastomosis. These pouches are expected to store about 300 mL of ileal effluent prior to catheterization or evacuation. Although the normal ileum gradually adapts to this new role, patients' pouches

have differing capacities and therefore they have differing numbers of bowel movements. The smaller the ileal pouch capacity, the more bowel movements one would expect in a 24-hour period.

It is now clear that the small intestine in patients with irritable bowel syndrome is hyperreactive to meals and distention. The spasm created can be painful. Therefore, it would seem, theoretically, that if a patient with irritable bowel syndrome and ulcerative colitis underwent an ileoanal anastomosis, the ileal pouch might be quite hyperactive. Such patients might have relatively more bowel movements or even painful spasm when the pouch is distended. They can only expel half the contents of the already small pouch. We have seen three young women with preexisting irritable bowel syndrome and relatively limited but painful "unresponsive" ulcerative colitis who underwent total colectomy and ileoanal anastomoses. All three subsequently had to undergo conversion to an ileostomy because of severe and continuous pain (without pouchitis) when their ileoanal pouches were in continuity. The symptoms immediately stopped when their pouches were defunctionalized and then recurred when ileoanal reanastomosis was performed. Permanent ileostomies were later created in at least two of these patients. Based on this experience, I usually advise patients with definite histories of painful irritable bowel syndrome who are about to undergo a total colectomy and ileostomy alternative to avoid an ileoanal pouch anastomosis. Please see the chapter on high output ileoanal pouches.

Exaggeration of Response to Secretagogues

CAFFEINE

Oral caffeine (75 to 300 mg) presumably causes transient net secretion in the jejunum and ileum of "all" healthy individuals. Most do not have diarrhea because the colon can reabsorb this increased fluid load. However, if one combines excessive caffeine intake (such as 1,000 mg per day) with irritable bowel syndrome, then severe diarrhea results. Treating a person by giving nothing by mouth (intravenous fluids only) often lessens or eliminates this type of diarrhea. If an inflammatory bowel disease patient who is very sensitive to caffeine undergoes a bowel resection procedure, modest amounts of caffeine, such as are found in tea or cola drinks or proprietary analgesic compounds, may cause (potentially correctable) diarrhea.

POSTCHOLECYSTECTOMY DIARRHEA

Similarly, we have encountered postcholecystectomy diarrhea due to excessive bile salt wasting in a few patients with coexisting irritable bowel syndrome. They responded to cholestyramine plus loperamide or deodorized tincture of opium. Since patients with Crohn's disease may undergo cholecystectomy for gallstones, it is not surprising that we have also encountered a few patients with multiple small bowel resections and severe postcholecystectomy diarrhea. A few had their gallbladders removed earlier but did not become symptomatic in terms of watery diarrhea until a modest ileal resection was performed. They have also responded to a combination of cholestyramine and loperamide or deodorized tincture of opium.

LACTOSE INTOLERANCE

Some irritable bowel disease patients seems to be quite symptomatic after the ingestion of only modest amounts of lactose. With extensive ileal resections for Crohn's disease, lactose intolerance may be further exacerbated. Lactose-hydrolyzed milk, lactase enzyme, and yogurt- and lactose-restricted diets are sometimes helpful.

Patient-Physician Relationship

I have found it very helpful to explain to the patient with irritable bowel syndrome and inflammatory bowel disease that he or she has two disorders and that each may cause its own symptoms. Explaining the pathophysiology of the symptoms seems to help the patient adjust medications and understand and accept symptoms caused by meals or by stress. Some patients are relieved to learn that their original physician was not wrong when he or she made the diagnosis of irritable bowel syndrome years before the apparent onset of inflammatory bowel disease.

The anxiety created by symptoms of irritable bowel syndrome in a young person whose sibling or parent has inflammatory bowel disease can be quite troublesome. Thus, an important service has been to help evaluate family members when one sibling had inflammatory bowel disease but the parents or other siblings had irritable bowel syndrome. Since inflammatory bowel disease may appear at different ages in different siblings, one may have to reevaluate some individuals several times.

Although the thesis of coexistence of irritable bowel syndrome and inflammatory bowel disease is a simple one, I have rarely seen it mentioned in articles or textbooks. I have found this concept very helpful in evaluating and advising "complicated" patients with inflammatory bowel disease.

Editor's Note

This chapter was written for the first edition in 1989. Please see the accompanying chapters on IBS and IBD plus chapters on post-resection diarrhea and on excess bowel movements after ileoanal pouches (Chapter 44).

Supplemental Reading

Isgar B, Harman M, Kaye MD, et al. Symptoms of irritable bowel syndrome in ulcerative colitis in remission. Gut 1983;24:190–2.

Kellow JE, Phillips SF. Altered small bowel motility in irritable bowel syndrome is correlated with symptoms. Gastroenterology 1987;92:1885–93.

Marcus SN, Heaton KW. Irritable bowel-type symptoms in spontaneous and induced constipation. Gut 1987;28:156–9.

Sandler RS, Drossman DA, Nathan HP, McKee DC. Symptom complaints and health care seeking behavior in subjects with bowel dysfunction. Gastroenterology 1984;87:314–8.

Thompson WG, Heaton KW. Functional bowel disorders in apparently healthy people. Gastroenterology 1980;79:283–8.

Wald A, Back C, Bayless TM. Effect of caffeine on the human small intestine. Gastroenterology 1976;71:738–42.

CHAPTER 20

Infectious Agents as Aggravating Factors in Inflammatory Bowel Disease

Scott D. Lee, MD, and Christina M. Surawicz, MD

When patients present with diarrhea, one of the first questions is whether it is an infection or an attack of inflammatory bowel disease (IBD). Initial symptoms may be very similar, including diarrhea (with or without blood), abdominal pain or cramps, fever, and even arthralgias. Clinical features that favor infection are acute onset of diarrhea (often greater than 10 bowel movements per day) and fever early in the course. Conversely, IBD usually has a more insidious onset, fewer than 6 bowel movements daily, and early fever is uncommon.

Colonoscopic features can suggest infection or ulcerative colitis (UC), but are rarely diagnostic. Mucosal biopsy, however, can be useful in distinguishing acute self-limited colitis or infectious-type colitis from IBD. Preservation of normal crypt architecture is typical with infection. In contrast, chronic architectural changes and basal inflammation are present early in the course and are more indicative of IBD. However, to further complicate matters, infections sometimes can precipitate IBD, and intercurrent infections can mimic or induce flares of IBD.

Infections That Mimic Inflammatory Bowel Disease

Bloody diarrhea, the hallmark presenting symptom of UC, is mimicked by infectious dysentery. In Washington state, *Campylobacter jejuni* is the most common pathogen isolated from stools of patients with bloody diarrhea—followed, in order, by *Salmonella*, *Shigella*, and *Escherichia coli* 0157:H7. These pathogens are all characterized as "ileocolonic" invasive organisms.

Campylobacter, *Salmonella*, and *E. coli* 0157:H7 can affect the right colon and mimic appendicitis or Crohn's disease (CD). Initial watery diarrhea is more common for all pathogens except *Shigella*—the latter often presents with bloody diarrhea and tenesmus due to rectal and left colon involvement—symptoms that mimic UC. *Escherichia coli* 0157:H7 has a predilection for the right colon, and thus may be mistaken for IBD or ischemic colitis at initial presentation.

All of these pathogens are food- or water-borne. *Campylobacter* infection often is associated with poultry. Home cooks may place grilled chicken back on the platter where uncooked chicken has rested—into potentially infectious poultry juices. *Salmonella* also is associated with poultry and undercooked or raw eggs. Our state (Washington) is famous for its *E. coli* 0157:H7 outbreaks associated with undercooked hamburger meat. Other epidemics have been associated with venison, contaminated swimming pool or lake water, basil pesto, unpasteurized apple juice, and even sprouts. If other family members or close contacts are ill, an epidemic should be suspected, appropriate cultures taken, and the health department notified.

Aeromonas hydrophila (a water-borne pathogen) and *Plesiomonas shigelloides* (from shellfish, most frequently raw oysters) can cause acute colitis: cases of chronic colitis following infection with either of these pathogens have been described. Since the chronic colitis mimics UC, it is unclear whether the organisms cause chronic colitis or precipitate the onset of UC.

Amebic Colitis

We do not see many cases of **amebic colitis**—most occur in returned travelers, truck drivers, or migrant workers from endemic areas. Homosexual practices are sometimes involved in transmission. Typical symptoms of amebic colitis are diarrhea and rectal bleeding. However, not all patients are from endemic areas. Cases of amebic colitis mimicking UC have been "unmasked" by steroid therapy precipitating fulminant colitis and bowel perforation. Serology is the most accurate test as stool studies or colonoscopy with biopsy sometimes may miss organisms. Serology will be negative in asymptomatic cyst carriers. Detecting a liver abscess in a sexual partner has been the diagnostic clue in a few patients.

Chronic Infectious Colitides

Most infectious colitides are acute, but some can have a more chronic picture including *Entamoeba histolytica*, tuberculosis, and *Yersinia*. *Yersinia enterocolitica* and *Y. pseudotuberculosis* are uncommon in the United States but their predilection for the terminal ileum may mimic appendicitis and CD in endemic areas. Diarrhea may last for several months, and can be accompanied by a large joint arthropathy simulating the "colitic" arthritis of IBD. Diagnosis requires either stool culture on a special cold enrichment medium or serology. Other infections that cause granulomas can mimic CD, including *Chlamydia trachomatis* proctitis, an uncommon sexually transmitted pathogen in homosexual men.

Cytomegalovirus (CMV) is a more common opportunistic pathogen causing colitis in immunosuppressed individuals. We and others have reported cases of CMV colitis—some with self-limited rectal involvement after rectal intercourse. Patients have been described who presented with simultaneous onset of CMV colitis and IBD—some with UC, some with CD—suggesting that the IBD was precipitated by the acute infection.[*]

Clostridium difficile colitis occurs either as a hospital-acquired infection or as a complication of antibiotics that alter the fecal flora and allow overgrowth of *C. difficile* and production of its toxins. The diarrhea is usually watery, but blood can occur in severe cases. Typical pseudomembranes on the colon are not always present and the diagnosis usually is confirmed by detection of toxin in the stools.

Infections That Aggravate Inflammatory Bowel Disease

There is no evidence that a single infectious agent is responsible for the onset of CD or UC, although both have been diagnosed after an episode of infectious diarrhea. However, multiple infectious agents can mimic IBD and have been implicated in relapse of disease. A list of infectious pathogens and treatments is presented in Table 20–1.

Campylobacter jejuni

Although *C. jejuni* is not a frequently encountered pathogen in recurrent IBD, there are case reports of patients with IBD in whom exacerbation of their baseline disease was associated with this organism. Some required treatment with antibiotics for resolution of their symptoms. Patients with IBD are not at increased risk or susceptibility for infections with *C. jejuni*.

Salmonella

Although previous retrospective studies had postulated that *Salmonella* infections occurred more frequently in patients with IBD, patients with IBD are probably not at an increased risk for acquiring *Salmonella*. Although rare, when *Salmonella* infection does occur in IBD patients it can exacerbate symptoms and result in a severe relapse.

---

[*] Editor's Note: Cytomegalovirus colitis is an important cause of unresponsive colitis, especially in patients on steroids or immunomodulators. CMV mononucleosis is a presentation to keep in mind. In such patients, cytomegalovirus presenting as pouchitis in an ileal pouch-anal anastomosis also has been described in another chapter. (TMB)

TABLE 20–1. Infectious Pathogens in IBD and Treatments

Infectious Pathogen	Treatment
Campylobacter jejuni	Ciprofloxacin 500 mg PO bid for 5 to 7 days
Shigella	Ciprofloxacin 500 mg PO bid for 5 to 7 days
Salmonella	Ciprofloxacin 500 mg PO bid for 5 to 7 days
Escherichia coli	Ciprofloxacin 500 mg PO bid for 5 to 7 days
Clostridium difficile	Metronidazole 250 mg PO qid for 10 days
Mycobacterium	Need to check type and sensitivities
Entamoeba histolytica	Metronidazole 750 mg PO tid for 10 days
Herpes simplex virus	Acyclovir 200 mg/q4h 5 times a day for 10 days
Cytomegalovirus	Ganciclovir 5.0 mg/kg Q12° for 14 to 21 days

Shigella

Currently there is no evidence that *Shigella* plays a major role in exacerbations of IBD. However, as with any other group of patients, if an infectious etiology is suspected, routine stool cultures for *Shigella* should be taken.

Escherichia coli

None of the many different pathogenic types of *E. coli* has been consistently implicated in relapses of UC. Enteroadherent forms have been found in tissue of patients with CD but their exact role is unclear because similar enteroadherent strains can be found in patients without IBD. (There is some preliminary evidence that some forms of *E. coli* may be responsible for relapses in IBD.)

PROBIOTICS

Nonpathogenic strains of *E. coli* have been used as probiotics to reduce the number and severity of relapses in IBD patients. Rembacken et al (1999) found that giving patients nonpathogenic strains of *E. coli* was as effective as mesalamine in preventing relapse. This supports the theory that intestinal microorganisms play a role in relapse of symptoms and that modifying the bowel flora can prevent relapse of symptoms. There are discussions of probiotics in several other chapters, including preventing pouchitis.

Clostridium difficile

Although reports in the early 1980s implicated *C. difficile* toxin in relapses of IBD, subsequent studies do not support this. Burke et al (1987) found that only 2 of 62 patients admitted for UC relapse were *C. difficile*–toxin positive and this was related strongly to previous antibiotic use. Rolny et al (1983) also found that only 5 percent of hospitalized IBD patients were toxin positive and none required any treatment for *C. difficile*. Presumably these patients in the hospital became colonized with *C. difficile* but did not have *C. difficile*–associated diarrhea.

Hyams and McLaughlin (1985) found *C. difficile* toxin in only 3 of 128 stool studies in a pediatric IBD population. None required specific treatment for *C. difficile* and all resolved spontaneously within 3 weeks. The three patients with *C. difficile* were clinically indistinguishable from other IBD patients.

Patients with IBD are not more likely to be *C. difficile*–toxin positive nor is *C. difficile* a major factor in relapse of IBD, except in patients who recently have received antibiotics. Sulfasalazine therapy is not a risk factor for the development of *C. difficile* disease. Diagnosis is made by detecting toxin in the stools: toxin B by cytopathic assay or enzyme immunoassay (EIA) tests to detect toxins A, B, or both. Mucosal biopsy can be helpful but usually is not needed.

Cytomegalovirus

The association of IBD and CMV infrequently has been reported in patients with IBD and often was associated with toxic megacolon. In a recent case series, nine patients with refractory symptoms had CMV, diagnosed in surgical specimens in two, and by endoscopic biopsies in seven. Five of seven responded to ganciclovir. The two who did not respond to ganciclovir therapy required intravenous cyclosporin therapy as the colitis progressed. Some patients have improved spontaneously as steroids were withdrawn, whereas others have gone on to colectomy.

Herpes Simplex Virus

There has been only one reported case of herpes simplex virus (HSV) exacerbating IBD. The patient had CD and developed toxic megacolon and the HSV was found in the surgical specimen. Numerous Cowdry A and multinucleated ground-glass cells were found in the epithelial cells. The patient tested negative for human immunodeficiency virus and previous colonic biopsies did not show any evidence of HSV.

Herpes simplex virus colitis is itself a rare entity. IFN alpha-2a has been tried in 16 patients with IBD in whom there was PCR evidence of HSV I in intestinal biopsies. There was slow improvement of clinical symptoms in 12 of 16, requiring an average of 8 weeks to become symptom free and an average of 6 months to become virus free in the affected tissue. There was also a remission of the extra-intestinal manifestations. Further investigation is needed and it should be noted that this was a select group of patients.

Parasites

There have been sporadic reports of *Entamoeba histolytica* and *Giardia lamblia* exacerbating IBD, especially in individuals who live in or have traveled to an area endemic for *E. histolytica*. Their symptoms often will respond to appropriate antiparasitic therapy.

Mycobacterium: A Special Situation

There is a large body of literature evaluating mycobacteria as a cause of Crohn's disease. *Mycobacterium paratuberculosis* is known to cause Johne's disease, a chronic granulomatous enteritis in animals. This has led to the hypothesis that CD may be secondary to *M. paratuberculosis* infection. Sanderson et al (1992) used polymerase chain reaction to evaluate the presence of *M. paratuberculosis* DNA in patients with CD and found that they had a higher prevalence than controls. However, the balance of evidence does not support the association and there is no current evidence that mycobacteria play a role in the recurrence of symptoms in IBD patients.[†‡]

References

Burke D, Axon A. *Clostridium difficile*, sulphasalazine, and ulcerative colitis. Postgrad Med 1987;63:955–7.

Hyams JS, McLaughlin JC. Lack of relationship between *Clostridium difficile* toxin and inflammatory bowel disease in children. J. Clin Gastroenterol 1985;7:387–90.

Rembacken B, Snelling A, Hawkey P, et al. Non-pathogenic *Escherichia coli* versus mesalazine for the treatment of ulcerative colitis: a randomised trial. Lancet 1999;354:639.

Rolny P, Jarnerot G, Mollby R. Occurrence of *Clostridium difficile* toxin in inflammatory bowel disease. Scand J. Gastroenterol 1983;18:61–4.

Sanderson J, Moss M, Tizard M, Hermon-Taylor J. *Myobacterium paratuberculosis* DNA in Crohn's disease. Gut 1992;33:890–6.

Editor's Note

A copy of the 56-item reference list can be obtained from the author at *surawicz@u-washington*.

Supplemental Reading

Begos D, Rappaport R, Jain D. Cytomegalovirus infection masquerading as an ulcerative colitis flare-up: case report and review of the literature. Yale J Biol Med 1996;69:323–8.

Campieri M, Gionchetti P. Probiotics in inflammatory bowel disease: new insight to pathogenesis or a possible therapeutic alternative? Gastroenterology 1999;116:1246–60.

Dumonceau J, Van Gossum A, Adler M, et al. No *Mycobacterium paratuberculosis* found in Crohn's disease using polymerase chain reaction. Dig Dis Sci 1996;41:421–6.

El-Serag H, Zwas F, Cririllo N, Eisen R. Fulminant herpes colitis in a patient with Crohn's disease. J Clin Gastroenterol 1996;22:220–3.

Klauber E, Briski LE, Khatib R. Cytomegalovirus colitis in the immunocompetent host: an overview. Scand J Infect Dis 1998;30:559–64.

---

† Editor's Note: Further, there is no good evidence that therapy for *M. paratuberculosis* is effective for treating CD. (SBH)

‡ Editor's Note: Cattlemen in several countries, spurred into action by a recent NIH/NIAID consensus conference <http://www.niaid.nih.gov/dmid/crohn's.htm>, which stated that the relationship is not yet disproven, decided to remove *Mycobacterium paratuberculosis*-carrying cattle from their herds; the remaining cattle herds are advertised as "Johnesfree." This is because of the public's perception of a potential problem. We may not think the relationship is proven but the cattlemen do not want to risk another blow to the beef industry. (TMB)

Kruis W, Schutz E, Fric P, et al. Double-blind comparison of an oral *Escherichia coli* preparation and mesalazine in maintaining remission of ulcerative colitis. Aliment Pharmacol Ther 1997;11:853–8.

Malchow H. Crohn's disease and *Escherichia coli*. A new approach in therapy to maintain remission of colonic Crohn's disease? J Clin Gastroenterol 1999;25:653–8.

Ng FH, Chau TN, Cheung TC, et al. Cytomegalovirus colitis in individuals associated with onset of inflammatory bowel disease. Dig Dis Sci 1993;38:2307–10.

Rachima C, Maoz E, Apter S, et al. Cytomegalovirus infection associated with ulcerative colitis in immunocompetent individuals. Postgrad Med 1999;74:486–9.

Rowbotham D, Mapstone N, Trejdosiewicz L, et al. *Mycobacterium paratuberculosis* DNA not detected in Crohn's disease tissue by fluorescent polymerase chain reaction. Gut 1995;37:660–7.

Ruther U, Nunnensiek C, Muller H, et al. Interferon alpha (IFN alpha 2a) therapy for herpes virus–associated inflammatory bowel disease (ulcerative colitis and Crohn's disease). Hepatogastroenterology 1998;45:691–8.

Schultsz C, Moussa M, van Ketel R, et al. Frequency of pathogenic and enteroadherent *Escherichia coli* in patients with inflammatory bowel disease and controls. J Clin Pathol 1997;50:573–9.

Shumacher G, Sandstedt B, Kollberg B. A prospective study of first attacks of inflammatory bowel disease and infectious colitis. Clinical findings and early diagnosis. Scand J Gastroenterol 1994;29:265–74.

Stolk-Engelaar VM, Hoogkamp-Korstanje JA. Clinical presentation and diagnosis of gastrointestinal infections by *Yersina enterocolitica* in 261 Dutch patients. Scand J Infect Dis 1996;28:571–55.

Surawicz CM, Haggitt RC, Husseman M, McFarland LV. Mucosal biopsy diagnosis of colitis: acute self-limited colitis and idiopathic inflammatory bowel disease. Gastroenterology 1994;107:755–63.

Willoughby JM, Rahman AF, Gregory MM. Chronic colitis after *Aeromonas* infection. Gut 1989;30:686–690.

CHAPTER 21

USE OF NICOTINE AND TOBACCO IN COLITIS

ELENA RICART, MD, AND WILLIAM J. SANDBORN, MD

Sulfasalazine, mesalamine, and oral corticosteroids are the standard first-line therapies for ulcerative colitis (UC). However, a considerable number of patients are candidates for immune modifier therapy because of refractory symptoms or toxic effects of these drugs. Thus, there is a need for alternative treatments. Nicotine may fulfill such a role. Previous epidemiologic observations suggested a beneficial effect of smoking in patients with UC and led to the investigational use of nicotine as a therapeutic agent.

Ulcerative colitis is largely a disease of nonsmokers. This epidemiologic observation, reported first by Harries et al in the early 1980s, has been consistently confirmed in other case-control studies of hospital and community-based populations worldwide. The risk for disease is reduced in current smokers and increased in non-smokers, with the greatest risk in ex-smokers. Approximately two-thirds of former smokers with UC develop the disease after giving up smoking, with a particularly high incidence in the first few years. Several studies have related smoking with UC disease activity, showing a more favorable clinical course in patients who smoke, and highest rates of hospitalization and colectomy for active UC in ex-smokers. Smoking also seems to be protective against pouchitis after colectomy and ileal pouch-anal anastomosis for UC, and against primary sclerosing cholangitis.

Mechanisms of Action

Since the etiology of inflammatory bowel disease (IBD) remains unknown, the possible mechanisms of action for a beneficial effect of smoking in UC are speculative.

Nicotine appears to be at least one of the agents in cigarette smoke that is beneficial for UC. Nicotine has many physiologic and pharmacologic actions. Its receptors are distributed ubiquitously and stimulation may affect the central, peripheral, and autonomic nervous systems, as well as the immune, inflammatory, and neuroendocrine pathways.

The potential mechanisms of action of nicotine in UC include suppression of humoral and cellular immunity (decreases in IgA concentration in colonic lavage fluid in smokers and changes in IL-1β, IL-2, IL-8, IL-10, and TNF-α concentrations in controls and patients with UC

have been observed); modulation of eicosanoid-mediated inflammation (through inhibition of thromboxane synthetase, cyclo-oxygenase, and lipoxygenase); stimulation of endogenous cortisol release (which may have beneficial effects in UC); decrease of rectal blood flow to a normal range (which is increased in UC); and probably inhibition of oxygen free radical production by neutrophils. Colonic mucus is decreased in patients with UC, and smokers with UC have increased mucus production. However, nicotine has minimal to no effect on mucus production in controls or patients with UC.

Treatment with Nicotine

TRANSDERMAL NICOTINE

Initial studies with nicotine administered as chewing gum were inconclusive and poorly controlled, but with the introduction of transdermal nicotine it has been possible to perform controlled trials to determine the safety and efficacy of nicotine therapy for UC.

The first randomized, double-blind placebo-controlled study of transdermal nicotine in 72 nonsmokers with active colitis showed positive results, with a significantly higher remission rate in patients treated with nicotine (15 to 25 mg/d) compared to the placebo group (48.6% vs. 24.3%, respectively, $p = .03$). Another double-blind placebo-controlled study in 64 nonsmokers with active UC showed clinical improvement in 39 percent of patients treated with nicotine (11 to 22 mg/d) versus 9 percent of patients receiving placebo ($p = .007$). Both studies began with the lower nicotine doses to improve patient tolerance, with subsequent dose escalation after 1 or 2 weeks. Adverse events were more common among the patients receiving nicotine in the two studies. In contrast, a randomized double-blind study comparing 15 mg/d of prednisolone with 15 to 25 mg/d of transdermal nicotine showed that nicotine produced side effects more commonly than prednisolone with a trend toward lower efficacy. Results in maintenance of remission have been less promising. A placebo-controlled study demonstrated that a lower dose of transdermal nicotine (15 mg/16 h) was not efficacious for maintenance of remission in UC when given alone for 6 months.

It appears that there may be a dose-response relationship between the transdermal nicotine dose and both plasma concentrations of nicotine and clinical response. In the two placebo-controlled trials where nicotine demonstrated efficacy for the treatment of active UC, the mean trough serum nicotine concentration was 11.3 ± 8.4 ng/mL for the 22 mg/24 h dose, and 8.2 ± 7.1 ng/mL for the 25 mg/24 h dose. In contrast, in the placebo-controlled trial where transdermal nicotine did not demonstrate efficacy for maintaining remission in UC, the 15 mg/16 h dose resulted in a mean trough plasma nicotine concentration of 5.3 ng/mL.

In summary, clinical studies show that transdermal nicotine is beneficial in the treatment of active UC, but long-term low-dose treatment is not efficacious and is limited by frequent side effects.

In our clinical practice, we use transdermal nicotine to control a flare-up of symptoms in patients who have limited medical options, having had no success with sulfasalazine, mesalamine, low-to-moderate dose of corticosteroids, and in many cases azathioprine or 6-mercaptopurine, and who are being considered for semi-elective surgery. Such patients are treated with nicotine patches at an initial dose of 7 to 11 mg/d for 7 days and then changed to patches of 21 to 25 mg/d for 21 days. If intolerable side effects develop while using the large patch, the patients resume using the smaller patch. Patients who wear the smaller patch and develop intolerable side effects are discontinued from nicotine therapy. Concurrent therapies with oral/topical 5-aminosalicylate compounds (sulfasalazine, mesalamine), and/or oral/topical corticosteroids are maintained. After remission, the nicotine often is tapered and the patient is continued on maintenance therapy with another agent such as mesalamine. However, some of our patients have continued with 21 to 25 mg/d of transdermal nicotine for up to 22 months with apparent good results. If there is no response and the patient has exhausted all of the medical alternatives, then surgery is recommended.

TOPICAL ADMINISTRATION OF NICOTINE TO THE COLON

In an attempt to avoid side effects of transdermal nicotine and to determine the effectiveness of nicotine in left-sided UC, two pilot clinical studies of nicotine tartrate and nicotine carbomer liquid enemas were performed. Both studies demonstrated a significant reduction in clinical activity and endoscopic inflammation, and one study demonstrated a significant reduction in histologic inflammation. Peak and trough concentrations of nicotine as determined at 4 weeks were low or undetectable, suggesting that nicotine administered directly to the colon can result in a local treatment effect in the absence of therapeutic serum nicotine concentrations. However, the nicotine tartrate liquid enemas were difficult to

TABLE 21–1. Side Effects of Transdermal Nicotine

Skin irritation, erythema, contact dermatitis
Lightheadedness, dizziness
Nausea, vomiting
Headaches
Sleep disturbance, violent/sexual dreams
Central nervous system stimulation
Diaphoresis, sweating
Shakiness, tremor
Tachycardia
Hypertension

retain, and both enema formulations are only useful for patients with distal UC. A dose-ranging pharmacokinetic study in healthy volunteers demonstrated that delayed-release oral nicotine tartrate capsules containing 3 mg or 6 mg of nicotine base have low systemic absorption due to first-pass hepatic metabolism and are well tolerated. Placebo-controlled trials with this formulation of nicotine for the treatment of UC are warranted.

At present, we do not use nicotine enemas or other topical delivery systems in clinical practice, reserving them instead for clinical trials.

Adverse Events

Adverse events with transdermal nicotine are frequent (77 percent of nicotine-treated patients) and in some cases severe enough to necessitate discontinuation of the treatment (13 percent of nicotine-treated patients). This is an important limiting factor for transdermal nicotine therapy. The most frequent adverse events reported with transdermal nicotine are shown in Table 21–1. Side effects occur more often in life-long nonsmokers than in ex-smokers, although nonsmokers have fewer nicotine-associated side effects if they are initially administered a low-dose rather than a high-dose patch. In contrast, there are few side effects associated with nicotine enemas.

In addition to short-term dermatologic and neurological side effects of nicotine, the long-term complications associated with smoking must be taken into consideration. These include addiction, cardiovascular disease, osteoporosis, and, theoretically, cancer.

Nicotine administered via a transdermal patch results in a gradual rise in plasma nicotine concentrations and peak concentrations are lower than those that occur during smoking. Thus, transdermal nicotine is not addictive and no nicotine addiction was observed after a 6-month trial of 15 mg/d of transdermal nicotine administered for UC remission.

Treatment with nicotine results in hemodynamic effects through the activation of the sympathetic nervous system, but does not seem to enhance thrombosis; in one study, nicotine actually lowered plasma fibrinogen concentrations and did not affect markers of platelet activation, endothelial damage, or serum lipids.

Nicotine itself is not a carcinogen but is a precursor of *N*-nitrosamines (such as 4-[methylnitrosamino]-1-[3-pyridyl]-1-butanone [NNK]) that are recognized carcinogens. Whether there is an endogenous formation of these *N*-nitrosamines with exposure to non-tobacco sources of nicotine is unknown.

Finally, whether nicotine accelerates the hepatic metabolism of estrogens and thus contributes to osteoporosis has not been determined but it is plausible given that nicotine is metabolized in the liver via the cytochrome P-450 enzyme pathway. This point is especially important in women with IBD, in whom smoking is an independent risk factor for osteoporosis.

Conclusion

Ulcerative colitis is a disease of nonsmokers. Treatment with transdermal nicotine appears to be efficacious for active UC at the highest tolerated dose of nicotine (22 to 25 mg/24 h) but it is not effective at low doses as maintenance therapy. Uncontrolled pilot studies showed that nicotine enemas may be of clinical benefit for left-sided colitis. Controlled studies with topical nicotine treatment (enemas or delayed-release oral capsules) are awaited. Adverse reactions are a limiting factor for long-term transdermal nicotine therapy, particularly in life-long nonsmokers, whereas nicotine enemas have low systemic absorption and are well tolerated. At present, transdermal nicotine is not a first-line therapy for UC and should be reserved for patients who have failed other medical therapies. Although smoking is reported to be beneficial for the course of UC, prescription of smoking must be tempered by the significant and potentially fatal consequences of its effects on other body systems and in our clinical practice we strongly discourage patients from smoking.

Supplemental Reading

Cohen RD, Hanauer SB. Nicotine in ulcerative colitis. How does it work and how can we use it? Clin Immunother 1996;3:169–74.

Green JT, Thomas GAO, Rhodes J, et al. Nicotine enemas for active ulcerative colitis—a pilot study. Aliment Pharmacol Ther 1997;11:859–63.

Harries AD, Baird A, Rhodes J. Non-smoking: a feature of ulcerative colitis. BMJ 1982;284:706.

Pullan RD, Rhodes J, Ganesh S, et al. Transdermal nicotine for active ulcerative colitis. N Engl J Med 1994;330:811–5.

Sandborn WJ. Nicotine therapy for ulcerative colitis: a review of rationale, mechanisms, pharmacology, and clinical results. Am J Gastroenterol 1999;94:1161–71.

Sandborn WJ, Tremaine WJ, Offord KP, et al. Transdermal nicotine for mildly to moderately active ulcerative colitis: a randomized, double-blind, placebo-controlled trial. Ann Intern Med 1997;126:364–71.

Sandborn WJ, Tremaine WJ, Leighton JA, et al. Nicotine tartrate liquid enemas for mildly to moderately active left-sided ulcerative colitis unresponsive to first-line therapy: a pilot study. Aliment Pharmacol Ther 1997;11:663–71.

Thomas GA, Rhodes J, Mani V, et al. Transdermal nicotine as maintenance therapy for ulcerative colitis. N Engl J Med 1995;332:988–92.

Thomas GA, Rhodes J, Ragunath K, et al. Transdermal nicotine compared with oral prednisolone therapy for active ulcerative colitis. Eur J Gastroenterol Hepatol 1996;8:769–76.

Editor's Note: Since smoking is theoretically harmful for patients with small bowel Crohn's disease, what does one conclude when a patient with "indeterminant colitis" responds to nicotine patches?

Also, we should have "smoking cessation" in one's list of causes of relapses in ulcerative colitis. (TMB)

CHAPTER 22

Immunomodulator Use in Patients with Distal Colitis

Stephen P. James, MD

This chapter outlines an approach to the use of immunomodulators for distal colitis, including both ulcerative colitis (UC) and Crohn's disease (CD). The discussion reviews the decision-making whether to use an immunomodulator, what modulators are available, how to implement and monitor therapy, and duration of therapy. The accumulated evidence and experience demonstrating the effectiveness of immumodulators over the last 25 years has led to their widespread use to the benefit of many patients with inflammatory bowel disease (IBD). Therefore, it is important for every gastroenterologist treating patients with IBD to become well educated regarding this class of medications and to develop an efficient approach for their use. There are separate chapters on immunomodulator use in UC and in CD.[*]

Immunomodulators

The list of effective immunomodulator agents currently available for use in IBD is very limited (Table 22–1). Use of azathioprine for IBD was first reported in the 1960s, but for many years concern about safety and efficacy resulted in very slow acceptance of azathioprine or 6-mercaptopurine (6-MP) by gastroenterologists. In major reviews in the early 1970s, use of azathioprine in IBD was still considered experimental. Currently, these medications should be considered mainstream therapy. The long-term safety profile is excellent and probably better than that for corticosteroids. The toxicities limiting therapy are now well defined, and with proper patient selection, patient education, and monitoring there should be no reluctance to initiate therapy. For reasons that are entirely unclear from the scientific standpoint, methotrexate seems to have more limited efficacy in IBD,[†] compared to rheumatoid arthritis, where it is a mainstay of therapy. Recent data in rheumatoid arthritis suggest that methotrexate may have important synergy with monoclonal anti-tumor necrosis factor (TNF) therapy. Hence, the use of methotrexate in IBD may need to be re-examined as a component of combination therapy. Cyclophosphamide, an important agent

for treatment of vasculitis, has had minimal efficacy in IBD, although most available information is anecdotal. Cyclosporin is effective in severe extensive UC, but the need for this potentially toxic and risky immunosuppressive drug for distal UC should be very limited. Cyclosporin enemas have been used by some practitioners, although a randomized controlled trial showed no efficacy, and therefore I do not advocate its use. Infliximab (Remicade®, Centocar, Malbern, Pennsylvania), chimeric monoclonal anti-TNF antibody, is effective for treatment of CD, but it is presently unknown whether this agent is effective in UC, and more trials are needed. Although the list of immunomodulators for use in proctitis is currently very limited, this situation may change considerably in the future. A wide range of immune modifying drugs, including cytokines, antibodies against cell surface molecules, antisense oligonucleotides, and neurotransmitter antagonists and agonists, are in various stages of testing in IBD, and it is likely that in the not too distant future, many more selective immune modulating agents will be available to the IBD practitioner.

Indications for Use of Immunomodulators

Table 22–2 lists the most common indications for the use of immunomodulators in IBD including frequent relapse requiring corticosteroids, corticosteroid dependence, presence of corticosteroid complications, significant contraindications to corticosteroid use, and active disease despite optimal medical management with nonimmunomodulator drugs. Outside the United States, where budesonide is available, corticosteroid complications may be diminished. However, similar considerations should be used to decide whether a patient should be treated with an immunomodulator. For CD, there is evidence that use of azathioprine or 6-MP may change the natural history of the disease and in the long run may have fewer complications than corticosteroid therapy. Some authorities recommend azathioprine or 6-MP as initial therapy, and studies are underway to evaluate the efficacy of this approach. At present, I do not institute azathioprine or 6-MP as initial therapy, but reserve their use for the scenario listed in Table 22–2.

---

[*] Editor's Note: This chapter contains practical information on the actual use of azathioprine and 6-MP that is not in other chapters. (TMB)

[†] Editor's Note: Methotrexate is less effective in UC than CD.

TABLE 22–1. Commonly Used Immunomodulator Agents for Treatment of Distal Colitis

Agent	Typical Dose	Side Effects/Limitations
Azathioprine	2.0–2.5 mg/kg/d	Fever, rash, lymphopenia, pancreatitis
6-Mercaptopurine	1.0–1.5 mg/kg/d	Same
Methotrexate	15–25 mg/weekly	Leukopenia, hepatic fibrosis, nausea, vomiting, diarrhea, hypersensitivity pneumonitis
Infliximab (Crohn's only)	5 mg/kg/variable interval	Infusion reaction, high cost

Patient Evaluation

Historical Aspects

Prior to initiating immunomodulator therapy, the factors listed in Table 22–3 need to be assessed. By far, the most important step is to obtain an accurate and thorough history. For decision-making, the diagnosis of CD or idiopathic UC or proctitis must be established. The duration of disease is an important consideration. For patients with recent onset of disease, it is not possible to accurately prognosticate regarding response to therapy or frequency of relapse, and I often delay implementing immunomodulator therapy until I have followed the patient for some period of time. In addition, the patient with recent onset of disease may suffer from progressive extension of disease and may no longer fit into the category of distal colitis. There are three other chapters on distal colitis and unresponsive distal disease.

I often find that patients with recent onset of IBD have received insufficient education about the disease and have high anxiety levels about their symptoms. This, in turn, leads the patient to report frequent, severe, or medically refractory symptoms that may not correspond to the severity of endoscopic findings. It is critical to reassure patients with clear explanations about the cause of their symptoms and their significance. This may even obviate the need to use immunomodulators in patients with minimal disease. As indicated in two separate chapters, the presence of coexistent irritable bowel syndrome (IBS) must be kept in mind in evaluating the patient who has persistent symptoms or steroid-dependent disease.

For the patient with longer duration disease, a careful history regarding prior therapies provides helpful information about which therapies have worked in the past and which ones have failed. In particular, if a patient reports a failure of prior immunomodulator therapy, I

TABLE 22–2. Common Indications for Use of Immunomodulators in Distal Colitis

Frequent relapse requiring corticosteroids

Corticosteroid dependence

Corticosteroid complications

Contraindication to corticosteroid use (severe diabetes, psychosis)

Active disease refractory to optimal therapy with oral, topical 5-ASA, corticosteroids

Crohn's disease: consider early use to modify natural history or as primary therapy

attempt to determine whether past dosing or duration of therapy was adequate to conclusively consider the patient a treatment failure. Comorbid conditions significantly interact with IBD and modify the interpretation of symptoms or the approach to therapy. In contrast, severe obesity, hypertension, diabetes, or cardiovascular disease may be reasons to consider early institution of immunomodulator therapy as an alternative to corticosteroids. An accurate medication history is essential, particularly since patients may receive medications from multiple different physicians and forget to list all of their current therapies. The family history may reveal IBD in other family members, and often the relatives' pattern of disease helps to predict the patient's prognosis. Determining a family history of colorectal cancer is important for planning colorectal cancer screening. The social history is invaluable for long-term management of patients in whom subjective issues are often very important. The level of education, family support, and maturity are important issues when embarking on therapy where compliance is essential. In considering immunomodulator therapy, it is important to determine whether the

TABLE 22–3. Information Useful in Decision-making for Immunomodulator Therapy

History
  IBD: Diagnosis, duration, extent, severity of symptoms, frequency of relapse, prior therapy, and response to therapy
  Comorbid conditions
  Medications
  Family history: clues for possible prognosis in familial IBD; cancer history
  Occupation, support system, patient needs and expectations
  Medications
  Family planning considerations (female and male)

Physical examination
  Evidence of active IBD
  Evidence of comorbid conditions

Routine laboratory studies
  CBC, electrolytes, creatinine, BUN, glucose, LFTs
  Stool *C. difficile* toxin

Flexible sigmoidoscopy
  Diagnosis: UC, Crohn's, indeterminate
  Extent, severity
  Complications: stricture, fistulae

Possibly useful adjuncts
  ANCA/ASCA antibody testing
  Thiopurine S-methyltransferase polymorphism

patient is planning to have children in the immediate future because of the potential impact of medications on conception or pregnancy.

Clinical Assessment

The physical examination and routine laboratory studies should assess clues of active disease or complications that could modify choice of therapy. The chapters on resistant proctitis, pseudorefractory colitis, and coexistent IBS are also useful. Prior to instituting immunomodulator therapy I perform flexible sigmoidoscopy to determine the correlation between endoscopic severity and symptoms. It is also important to exclude the presence of strictures, for example, that could cause persistent symptoms not amenable to immunomodulator therapy. If there is doubt about the diagnosis, presence of more proximal CD, or if colorectal cancer screening is indicated, a colonoscopy should be performed. At the present time, I do not routinely obtain ANCA/ASCA antibody determinations to evaluate patients with refractory distal colitis pending additional studies that indicate utility in management.‡ Likewise, I do not routinely test for thiopurine S-methyltransferase (TPMT) gene polymorphisms as a predictor of patients at risk for adverse events following treatment with azathioprine or 6-MP. However, it is possible that further clinical studies of this type of testing will provide prospective utility and allow more cost-effective management.

Optimization of Conventional Therapy

Before proceeding to immunomodulator therapies, it is important to determine that full therapeutic benefit of primary therapies have been exhausted and that other explanations for persistent symptoms have been excluded (Table 22–4). In particular, topical therapies for distal colitis often are highly effective; however, many patients are reluctant to administer rectal preparations. This is discussed in the chapters on distal colitis and UC in children. If it is not clear that the patient is really a treatment failure on topical therapy, I make an attempt with strong support and encouragement to have the patient use rectal preparations while reviewing the risks and benefits of immunomodulator therapies with them. Likewise, escalation of oral aminosalicylate preparations should be considered. In patients with Crohn's colitis, antibiotic therapy can be used in conjunction with other therapies. There is a chapter on this topic. In patients who have pain as a major symptom, with or without IBS components to their clinical picture, it may be helpful to use analgesics or antidepressants in addition to therapies directed at mucosal disease.

‡ Editor's Note: In select cases, the presence of ASCA may be important to confirm CD that would allow consideration of methotrexate or anti-TNF approaches. (SBH)

TABLE 22–4. Common Situations Where Immunomodulators Can Potentially Be Avoided

Treatment failure due to suboptimal dosing of topical, oral salicylates

Treatment failure due to reluctance of patient to use prescribed rectal preparations

Symptoms due to IBS dominate the syndrome with minimal or mild IBD

Symptoms predominantly due to anxiety related to symptoms caused by minimal disease

Symptoms predominantly due to depression

Unrealistic expectations of patient to be free of all disease

Initiating Immunomodulator Therapy

Having determined the indications for an immunomodulator, I initiate therapy with 6-MP unless the patient has previously used azathioprine and is familiar with this drug. The clinical outcome with the two agents does not appear to differ except that a generic azathioprine is available. Therapy with 6-MP is initiated at 1 to 1.5 mg/kg/d. There is no rationale for initiating therapy with a suboptimal dose unless it is known that the patient has TPMT deficiency. I always confirm that the patient has a normal total lymphocyte count prior to initiating therapy. When initiating therapy, it is important to review the issues outlined in Table 22–5. The patient must understand the slow onset of action, possibility of failure, and potential toxic side effects. I warn patients not to attempt to adjust the dose of immunomodulator themselves, particularly since many patients are accustomed to adjusting their corticosteroid dose without informing their physicians. The controversial risk of birth defects associated with use of azathioprine or 6-MP needs to be discussed with the patient. There are two chapters on IBD and pregnancy.

The patient needs to adhere to the monitoring program. I obtain CBCs after 2 weeks for the first month, then monthly for 3 months, and then at least every 3 months for as long as the patient continues the medication. I obtain LFTs every 3 months. For the patient who is

TABLE 22–5. Implementation of Azathioprine/ 6-Mercaptopurine Therapy

Discuss and implement the following with the patient:

Expected benefit: slow onset, probability of response 65%, reduction or discontinuation of corticosteroids

Prohibit patient self-medication or dose adjustment

Risks: immediate allergic drug reaction, pancreatitis, leukopenia, hepatitis

Discuss pregnancy considerations

Outline and implement monitoring program: CBC, LFTs

Discuss long-term plan for concurrent medications (ASA, corticosteroids), duration of therapy

Refer patient to CCFA Website: ccfa.org for resource information (books) and Website information on immunomodulators: http://www.ccfa.org/medcentral/library/meds/

corticosteroid dependent, I usually delay tapering corticosteroid for about 3 months after initiating 6-MP therapy. I do not routinely evaluate the response to therapy by repeated flexible sigmoidoscopy in patients in whom a reliable history can be obtained. There is no indication to modify immunomodulator therapy based on the presence of histologic remission. I inform the patient that if they have a good response, therapy will generally be continued for a protracted period of time, usually 2 years, before I will consider discontinuing therapy.

Failure of 6-Mercaptopurine/Azathioprine Therapy

If patients fail initial therapy with standard doses of 6-MP, and the total lymphocyte count is adequate, I institute a dose escalation of 50 percent for 6-MP. In the future, it is possible that measurement of drug metabolite levels will be useful in decision-making. If after 6 months of therapy there is no discernible improvement in the patient's clinical situation, I will consider alternative therapies, such as methotrexate. Initial therapy with subcutaneous injection (probably as effective as intramuscular) is generally more effective, but I will accept the patient's preference for oral therapy if he or she has significant concerns about injections.[§] I initiate therapy at 25 mg/wk. Patients should receive supplemental folic acid

to diminish side effects. If therapy is effective, tapering of corticosteroids can be initiated within 4 to 8 weeks. The long-term safety of methotrexate in IBD is unknown.[//] Precautions regarding hepatic toxicity should be exercised as for all patients receiving methotrexate. Patients with abnormal LFTs, concurrent viral hepatitis or alcoholism, and possibly diabetes or significant lung disease should be excluded. There is a separate chapter on methotrexate.

As indicated above, for the patient with distal colitis due to CD, infliximab is an option as described in a chapter on anti-cytokine therapy. Cyclosporine is usually not required for management of distal UC, and efficacy in CD is uncertain. Likewise, surgery is usually not required for distal colitis but may be required for Crohn's colitis, as discussed in a separate chapter .

Supplemental Reading

George J, Present DH, Pou R, et al. The long-term outcome of ulcerative colitis treated with 6-mercaptopurine. Am J Gastroenterol 1996;91:1711–4.

Hawthorne AB, Logan RF, Hawkey CJ, et al. Randomised controlled trial of azathioprine withdrawal in ulcerative colitis. BMJ 1992;305:20–2.

Kozarek RA. Methotrexate and ulcerative colitis: wrong drug? Wrong dose? Or wrong disease? Gastroenterology 1996;110:1652–6.

Stein RB, Hanauer SB. Medical therapy for inflammatory bowel disease. Gastroenterol Clin North Am 1999;28:297–321.

[§] Editor's Note: I consider the data on parenteral methotrexate to be much stronger than for oral dosing. (SBH)

[//] Editor's Note: Recent maintenance trials have demonstrated benefits of 15 mg weekly for CD over 1 year. (SBH)

CHAPTER 23

MUCOSAL PROTECTIVE AND REPAIR AGENTS IN THE TREATMENT OF COLITIS

PROFESSOR JOHN RHODES, AND GARETH A.O. THOMAS, MD, BSc, MRCP

The terms "mucosal protection and repair" in relation to colitis are based on the concept that mechanisms involved in mucosal defence may at times be overwhelmed and the mucosa damaged. An appreciation of some of the features that protect colonic mucosa may help identify how certain therapeutic agents produce their effect. Among the agents that will be discussed are carbomers, bismuth, nicotine, lignocaine, probiotics, and short-chain fatty acids.

Colonic Mucosal Barrier

The colonic mucosal barrier is somewhat analogous to the barrier that protects the stomach. Both are lined by a continuous layer of mucus gel adherent to the mucosa that serves as an interface between luminal contents and surface epithelium. It also provides a lubricating and protective physical barrier between the mucosal surface and luminal contents. The layer is not seen on conventional histologic preparations of tissue but can be seen by phase contrast illumination on thickly cut sections of mucosa, without fixation. It is an easily distinguished layer about 150 μm in depth, which stains readily with the periodic acid–Schiff (PAS) reaction. An equilibrium is maintained by freshly secreted mucus replacing that which is lost from the luminal surface by enzymatic digestion and mechanical shear (Figure 23–1). The surface gel is composed of mucus glycoproteins consisting of a central protein backbone with large numbers of attached oligosaccharides, which account for glycosylation of the molecule. The carbohydrate chains are attached to the protein core to produce a structure resembling a bottle brush, with the surface or peripheral regions of the carbohydrate chains showing a variable degree of substitution with sialic acid and sulfate groups.

The thickness and integrity of this adherent layer probably are central to its role in mucosal protection, while the viscous gel-forming property of the mucus, in turn, depends on the degree of glycosylation. Fecal bacteria produce enzymes that digest the mucin protein core (proteases) and the released carbohydrate fragments.

Mucus Barrier in Colitis

Disruption of the surface gel would leave the epithelium open to luminal assault from bacterial enzymes, allergens, and toxins. We have measured the depth of the mucus

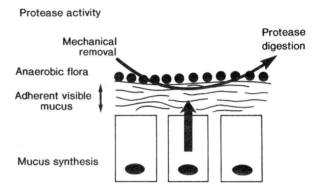

FIGURE 23–1. A continuous layer of mucus gel adheres to the colonic epithelium and forms an interface between mucosa and the lumen. Surface mucus is removed by protease activity and mechanical shear.

layer in freshly resected surgical specimens and compared 'normal' mucosa from patients with carcinoma of the bowel with that of patients with ulcerative colitis (UC) and Crohn's disease (CD). In UC, there was no visible mucus layer in areas that were inflamed while, elsewhere, values were normal. In contrast, the mucus thickness was increased in CD, even in areas of inflamed mucosa.

FECAL ENZYMES

We have also measured the fecal protease activity in stool and found significantly raised levels in active colitis with mean activity three times greater than normal. There is also increased mucin sulfatase activity in UC, particularly in active disease. Although these changes in enzymatic activity may be secondary to mucus breakdown, they also may play a primary role in disrupting the mucus layer.

TREFOIL PEPTIDES

Trefoil peptides, a group of cysteine-rich peptides, also may play an important role in the mucus layer. Three human trefoil peptides have been identified and are referred to as trefoil factor family (TFF) peptides, of which TFF3 is found throughout the small and large intestine. They appear to have important roles in epithelial protection and mucosal healing. They also may play a part in mucus stabilization by interacting or cross-linking with mucins, to aid formation of the gel layer. With mucosal injury, there is rapid upregulation of trefoils that facilitate repair by a process of epithelial restitution. In a number of animal models and cell lines, trefoils have been shown to promote mucosal healing and cell migration across damaged areas.

Metabolic Requirements of the Colonic Mucosa

The colonic epithelium has high metabolic demands. The short-chain fatty acids (SCFA) propionate, acetate, and n-butyrate are products of bacterial fermentation of complex carbohydrates such as fiber and starch in the colon. n-Butyrate is the dominant and preferred energy source for colonic epithelium. It is essential for maintenance of the epithelium since a marked reduction in its supply leads to mucosal atrophy, impaired barrier function, and inflammation. This is seen in diversion colitis where luminal nutrients are absent due to discontinuity of the fecal stream—the inflammation is indistinguishable from UC. It even has been suggested that UC may be an energy-deficient disease of the large bowel epithelium.

Therapeutic Implications

Based on the concept that the mucosal barrier plays a pivotal role in UC, it should be possible to target different factors in this relationship that may have a beneficial therapeutic effect. To focus attention on the mucosa and epithelial barrier leads conceptually to a different management approach from that conventionally taken. Such an approach almost certainly will improve our understanding of the disease and permit the development of alternative and perhaps more effective therapeutic strategies to induce remission and prevent relapse. We will discuss how modification of the barrier with mucosal protective and repair agents has been attempted, and place the results in a clinical context. In many instances, the specific mode of action of the drug or compound remains unclear and proposals are largely speculative.

Enhancing the Protective Mucus Gel Barrier

Based on the finding that the mucus layer is either thinner or absent in active UC compared with healthy controls, various attempts have been made to protect the underlying epithelium by improving the quantity and quality of the adherent mucus layer. The maintenance of a healthy mucus layer depends on the equilibrium between synthesis and secretion of normal mucus and its degradation by protease enzymes principally produced by luminal bacteria.

CARBOMER

Polyacrylic carbomers are synthetic long-chain polymers characterized by multiple carboxyl side-chains. Although relatively insoluble, with sodium hydoxide they form viscous gels that adhere both to mucosa and surface mucus; they bind to the mucus gel, strengthen its physical structure, and inhibit fecal protease activity. Although the concept of using carbomers for inflammatory bowel

disease is attractive, we have no clinical evidence for their efficacy when used alone.

More interest has been focused on the effect of carbomer coupled with other potentially active agents such as bismuth, nicotine, or lignocaine. In this situation, the carbomer probably serves a dual function by enhancing the mucus layer and acting as a vehicle or carrier for other compounds. In theory at least, the adherent properties of carbomers should prolong the active compound's contact with the mucosa.

Carbomer Coupled to Other Compounds

BISMUTH CARBOMER

Bismuth has been coupled with carbomer with an intent to inhibit bacterial degradation of mucus. Two compounds of bismuth—tripotassium dicitratobismuthate and subsalicylate—have been shown, in small uncontrolled trials, to be efficacious in active UC. When coupled with carbomer in a randomized trial of 63 patients with active left-sided colitis, 450 mg bismuth citrate carbomer enemas were similar in efficacy to 2 g of mesalazine enema. They are well tolerated and may be worth considering for patients who are refractory to, or intolerant of, mesalazine.

NICOTINE CARBOMER

Transdermal nicotine has been shown to be effective in active UC but its benefits are limited by side effects in a significant number of patients. There is a chapter on nicotine usage in UC. Some animal data suggest that nicotine may enhance the adherent layer of mucus in the large bowel, while in vitro work with explants of colonic mucosa has shown increased mucus synthesis in the presence of nicotine. Carbomer has been successfully combined with nicotine and used with effect as a topical treatment in a small pilot study of active UC. The enemas were well tolerated and associated with low systemic levels of nicotine. A randomized trial has not yet been performed. At present, we would reserve use for patients failing conventional treatment who improve on transdermal nicotine but suffer systemic side effects from the nicotine. Topical use of nicotine is also discussed in the other chapter cited.

LIGNOCAINE CARBOMER

Topical lignocaine has been reported to benefit patients with UC. Encouraged by this, we coupled lignocaine with carbomer and tested it in a small pilot study of 18 patients with active UC. Disappointingly, we did not find convincing evidence of improvement. Controlled trials are needed to establish a role for local anesthetics as topical therapy in UC.*

---

* Editor's Note: The therapeutic benefit of topical anesthetic agents in some patients with UC may be due either to sensory nerve involvement or a direct anti-inflammatory effect of the anesthetic. (TMB)

Other Ways of Enhancing or Reducing Disruption of the Protective Mucus Gel Barrier

SUCRALFATE

In addition to carbomers, the mucus layer may be strengthened by sucralfate, a sulfated disaccharide complexed with aluminium hydroxide. Sucralfate forms a viscous protective layer that adheres to gastric and, presumably, rectal mucosa. In an early open study, there appeared to be benefit in active disease. However, in two controlled trials, sucralfate enemas were inferior to steroids and 5-aminosalicylates.

PROBIOTICS

An alternative approach to enhance or strengthen the mucus layer is to decrease the rate of degradation of the mucus by protease-producing bacteria. This can be done with carbomer and/or bismuth preparations, but another approach involves probiotics or antibiotics to change the mucosal associated flora. Although an attractive concept, in practice it is difficult to achieve. There have been anecdotal reports of success with fecal broths of bacteria, but there have been no controlled trials to confirm the efficacy of this approach. In addition, there have been no studies showing convincing benefit from antibiotics in UC. Probiotics and antibiotics are discussed in separate chapters.

Enhancing the Colonic Mucosal Metabolic Requirements

SHORT-CHAIN FATTY ACIDS (SCFAS)

Under normal circumstances, both mucosal inflammation and a leaky barrier should heal. Failure to heal in UC probably lies with defective downregulation of immunoinflammatory events—a problem that usually is addressed by using anti-inflammatory drugs or immunosuppressive agents. Alternatively, it may be due to an inadequate epithelial repair process, which may be due in part to an energy-deficient epithelium that is slow to heal and regenerate. The epithelium has high metabolic requirements supplied by short-chain fatty acids (SCFAs), propionate, acetate, and *n*-butyrate produced from bacterial fermentation of complex carbohydrates in the colon. *n*-Butyrate is the dominant and preferred energy source for colonic epithelium. Initial observations with a mixture of SCFAs and butyrate monotherapy, given as enemas, produced clinical benefit. However, more recently, three randomized, placebo-controlled studies have been less convincing in showing real differences between placebo and SCFAs. In the largest study, SCFA enema was compared with placebo in more than 100 patients. There was no difference in clinical or histologic measurements between groups. However, in a subgroup of patients with a short current episode of colitis, those receiving SCFAs showed dramatic clinical improvement far superior to placebo.

In summary, enemas of butyrate or a combination of SCFAs are an attractive option since they offer a physiologic approach to treatment, and adverse events are uncommon. The unpleasant odor associated with combined SCFAs enema has been less of a problem when fatty acids are given individually. Although some patients seem to benefit, the results of recent placebo-controlled trials are less encouraging and more work is required to identify whether certain subgroups of patients should be targeted. In practice, we do not use them.

The Place of Mucosal Protective and Repair Agents in Clinical Practice

Although an approach to treatment based on the colonic mucosal barrier is superficially attractive, the therapeutic agents that have been examined have not achieved either proven value or commercial availability. With standard therapy of topical or oral 5-aminosalicylates and/or steroid preparations, remission can be achieved in approximately 80 to 90 percent of patients with distal UC. It is difficult for new alternative treatments to compete with the impressive rate of first-line therapy. A new treatment would have to be at least as effective, better tolerated, and perhaps more economical in order to replace conventional therapy. One possible application for newer agents would be use in those patients who are resistant to conventional therapy or have difficulty because of side effects. At present, it is our clinical practice to reserve agents such as bismuth and nicotine carbomer for such patients, or for clinical trials. In the long term, however, alternative approaches to therapy offer hope of new effective therapy for patients with UC.

Editor's Note

The use of growth hormone and a high-protein diet has been reported to be helpful in patients with Crohn's disease in the small bowel and colon (Slonim AE, Bulone L, Damore MB, et al. A preliminary study of growth hormone therapy for Crohn's disease. N Engl J Med 2000; 342:1633–7).

Selected Reading

Bjorck S, Dahlstrom A, Johansson L, et al. Treatment of the mucosa with local anaesthetics in ulcerative colitis. Agents Actions 1992;10:C61.

Bruer RJ, Soergel KH, Lashner BA, et al. Short-chain fatty acid rectal irrigation for left-sided ulcerative colitis: a randomized, placebo-controlled trial. Gut 1997;40:485–91.

Green JT, Evans BK, Rhodes J, et al. Lignocaine carbomer enemas for ulcerative colitis—a pilot study. Gut 1997;41:224A.

Green JT, Thomas GAO, Rhodes J, et al. Nicotine enemas for active ulcerative colitis—a pilot study. Aliment Pharmacol Ther 1997;11:859–63.

Hutton DA, Allen A, Pearson JP, Foster SNE. Mucolysis of the colonic mucus barrier by faecal proteinases: inhibition by interacting polyacrylate. Clin Sci 1990;78:265–71.

McCaffert DM, Sharkey KA, Wallace JL. Beneficial effects of local or systemic lidocaine in experimental colitis. Am J Physiol (Gastrointestinal Liver Physiol) 1994;266:G560.

Pullan RD, Ganesh S, Mani V, et al. Comparison of bismuth-citrate and 5-aminosalicylic acid enemas in distal ulcerative colitis: a controlled trial. Gut 1993;34:676–9.

Pullan RD, Thomas GAO, Newcombe RG, et al. Thickness of adherent mucus gel on colonic mucosa in humans and its relevance to colitis. Gut 1994;35:353–9.

CHAPTER 24

Therapeutic Expectations: Medical Management of Ulcerative Colitis

Stephen B. Hanauer, MD

Therapeutic expectations for ulcerative colitis (UC) must take into consideration the chronic, medically incurable nature of inflammatory bowel disease (IBD), the varied mucosal extent, potential severity, and disease- or therapy-related complications. It is most useful to consider the therapeutic expectations with regard to inducing remission, maintaining remission, treating symptoms, and treating or preventing complications. In addition, with the advent of pelvic pouch procedures, an additional goal of medical therapy is to treat, and eventually prevent, pouchitis.

Induction of Remission

The primary goal of therapy for UC is to induce a clinical remission. An important characteristic of UC is the capacity of the mucosa to "regenerate" an intact epithelial lining. Independent of the severity of acute mucosal inflammation, neutrophils that invade the epithelial crypts can be replaced by normal, chronic inflammatory cells associated with distortion of the crypt architecture. In some situations of long-term remission, the mucosa can heal to the point that pathologists cannot discern any abnormalities. The presence of postinflammatory "pseudopolyps" bears no relation to symptoms or risk of chronic (eg, neoplastic) complications.

From an endoscopic viewpoint, remission is defined by the presence of an intact epithelium with a visible submucosal vascular pattern without ulceration, significant friability, or granularity. Pseudopolyps, mucosal bridging, and areas of "atrophic mucosa" with distorted vasculature represent prior episodes of severe inflammation. Radiographic correlates include resolution of the mucosal ulceration, and granularity and restoration of haustrations.[*]

Clinical remission implies resolution of inflammatory symptoms of bleeding, urgency, passage of mucopus, and diarrhea. Inflammatory symptoms must be distinguished from common variations in bowel habits related to diet or irritable bowel syndrome (IBS) manifestations (eg, looser stools, cramps, bloating) in the setting of a healed mucosa. The absence of urgency and tenesmus implies improved rectal compliance and renewed ability to distinguish gas from feces. A chapter on IBS and IBD discusses post-IBD symptoms.

It is common for symptomatic remission to precede endoscopic healing and for the latter to occur prior to histologic remission. Furthermore, topical therapy for UC can heal the rectum, allowing normal or near-normal bowel function despite residual, proximal inflammatory changes. Although, intuitively, it would make sense that complete colonic healing should improve the long-term prognosis, no data exist that support differences between distal healing in an asymptomatic patient and complete colonic healing.

Typically, after induction of remission there is a transitional phase into maintenance therapy. It must be emphasized that, to successfully begin maintenance therapy, it is necessary to complete inductive treatment. Failure to complete induction virtually guarantees failure of maintenance. Patients who are discharged from the hospital while still symptomatic often require rehospitalization for reinstitution of intensive therapy or more aggressive inductive treatment owing to premature cessation of inductive therapy. The same admonition applies to outpatients who begin withdrawing from steroids prior to complete clinical recovery or patients with distal colitis who stop topical (rectal) therapy prematurely.

Maintenance of Remission

The second priority of therapy for UC is to sustain a clinical remission. Usually, this entails maintenance of an intact mucosa with absence of ulceration, friability, or significant granularity at endoscopy and absence of neutrophils in the epithelial crypts. From a prognostic standpoint, it has been demonstrated that the presence of residual polymorphonuclear leukocytes in the epithelium bears a worse prognosis, although it is not customary to perform endoscopic biopsies to confirm histologic remission.[†]

It has become clear that maintenance therapy for UC depends upon the therapy necessary to induce remission. There is no "cookbook" approach to transitioning from

---

[*] Editor's Note: I would argue that loss of haustrations could represent an irreversible change secondary to injury and loss of mucosa and submucosa. Restoration of haustra might be an impossible goal in terms of remission. (TMB)

[†] Editor's Note: Finding polymorphonuclear leukocytes in a biopsy has been thought by some to be a predictor of a relapse. (TMB)

inductive to maintenance therapy; however, the intensity of acute therapy necessary to induce remission and the duration of therapy required to complete resolution of clinical symptoms can be clues to the prognosis. Experience (in the absence of controlled trial data) dictates that steroids should be tapered according to the duration of time required to induce remission, that patients who require cyclosporine benefit from the addition of long-term immunomodulation with azathioprine (AZA) or 6-mercaptopurine (6-MP), and that many patients with distal colitis who require topical mesalamine continue to need topical therapy (albeit at reduced frequency) to maintain remissions.

Expectations for maintenance therapy require more participation from the patient to comply with (adhere to) the treatment regimen. A significant contributor to relapse is nonadherence to maintenance treatment. Patients require education regarding the long-term goals of maintenance therapy (eg, preventing relapse, reducing long-term complications of disease activity, or risks of acute therapy with steroids). In addition, patients should be warned against the use of nonsteroidal anti-inflammatory drugs (NSAIDs) and discuss means of smoking cessation, when applicable, because of the potential risks of relapse or chronic activity. Routine follow-up appointments should be scheduled to enhance and review compliance and to monitor for long-term complications of UC or therapy. There is a separate chapter on compliance with therapy.

Treatment of Symptoms

In addition to anti-inflammatory therapy to heal colonic inflammation, many patients benefit from recommendations to minimize residual symptoms related to diet or colonic irritability. Although there are no dietary factors that have been recognized to induce colitis, to ignore diet obviates a component of therapy that contributes to symptoms. Therefore, discussions regarding a patient's nutritional intake are important to avoid intensifying potential complications of anti-inflammatory therapy. Factors that contribute to symptoms, such as lactose intolerance, excessive intake of sorbitol or fructose, or stimulants (eg, caffeine), should be sought. Patients with distal colitis often are constipated, and addition of fiber may help to improve bowel function. In addition, review of a patient's diet exposes risks to the patient of complications associated with IBD that are attributable to inadequate intake of protein, hematopoietic requisites (iron or folate), and calcium. It is essential to ensure that patients with lactose intolerance who take corticosteroids have adequate calcium intake.

Symptomatic therapy is available for treating common symptoms not directly related to active inflammation. It should be obvious that active disease should be excluded by thorough evaluation of the patient (including endoscopy to assess mucosal disease activity) before ascribing symptoms to concurrent IBS. Even in the presence of active disease, symptomatic therapy can reduce frequency and urgency of bowel function and may even improve tolerance for anti-inflammatory therapy. For instance, patients with mild to moderate colitis may benefit from loperamide prior to application of topical therapy to minimize rectal urgency and improve anal sphincter tone. Antispasmodics also can be used to treat abdominal cramping in the setting of mild disease, because antidiarrheal agents can alleviate some stool frequency. However, antimotility agents should be prescribed for patients with severe disease to avoid risks of inducing megacolon. Tricyclic antidepressants can be helpful to reduce bowel frequency associated with spasm and to assist in improving sleep by reducing nocturnal symptoms. Likewise, alternative psychotherapeutic agents may be beneficial to treat concurrent symptoms of anxiety or depression that are primary or secondary to corticosteroids.

Prevention of Complications

An important expectation of therapy for UC is the prevention (or treatment) of complications related to the disease or therapy. Ulcerative colitis can be complicated by intestinal or extra-intestinal complications. Intestinal complications, such as bleeding and associated anemia, hypoproteinemia, or electrolyte abnormalities require prompt control with inductive therapies. Thereafter, supplementation with iron and folic acid (with sulfasalazine) should treat and prevent further development of anemia during maintenance therapy. Other intestinal complications, such as toxic megacolon or perforation, can be prevented with aggressive inductive therapies, according to the severity of presentation. Patients should be warned against the use of NSAIDs and to alert their physician when primary care physicians or other specialists prescribe antibiotics or other medications, to be certain they do not induce diarrhea (Clostridium difficile) and are compatible with UC therapy.

Controlling colonic inflammation usually prevents extra-intestinal complications, such as peripheral arthritis and cutaneous manifestations. Again, patients should be warned against use of nonprescription NSAIDs. In the presence of arthritic symptoms, skin lesions, or sclero-conjunctivitis, patients should be reassessed, to exclude subtle colon inflammation that would benefit from more intensive maintenance dosing. Central arthritis (sacroiliitis, ankylosing spondylitis) or uveitis requires the input of a specialist to control inflammatory features that are "out of synch" with colitis. Communication with the rheumatologist or ophthalmologist should coordinate therapeutic approaches, to minimize the risk of interference with therapy for colitis. There are chapters on ocular skin and joint complications of IBD.

The primary long-term complications of UC are dysplasia and colon cancer. It remains to be determined whether and how these can be prevented with medical therapy, although there are preliminary indications that aminosalicylate therapy and folic acid supplementation may reduce the risk. In any event, surveillance for dysplasia should be considered a component of therapy for UC to prevent the risk of invasive cancer. There are three chapters on this topic.

Both inductive and maintenance therapy for UC can be associated with preventable or treatable complications. Corticosteroids are associated with a spectrum of complications, including metabolic derangements (hypokalemia, hyperglycemia), hypertension, osteoporosis, cataracts, acne, and psychological disorders. Minimizing exposure can prevent the long-term complications of steroids. This can be accomplished by beginning inductive therapy at optimal doses (eg, 40 to 60 mg of prednisone) with a more rapid taper once clinical remission has been achieved. Attempting to start therapy at low or moderate doses "to prevent side effects" often is counterproductive in that there is an incomplete response necessitating higher doses of steroids over prolonged intervals. During initiation of steroid therapy, patients are monitored for electrolyte disorders and blood pressure determinations. Many young patients are troubled by steroid-induced acne that can be treated with topical therapy or antibiotics. Psychological sequelae are not uncommon and range from modest sleep disorders to steroid-induced psychoses. Counteractive therapies, range from short-term use of hypnotics to psychiatric consultation and prescription of antidepressants or antipsychotics.

Metabolic bone disease has been recognized more commonly as a complication of IBD as well as of steroid therapy. With the advent of dual photon absorptiometry, scanning baseline bone density assessments are advocated for patients at risk for osteoporosis. These include postmenopausal females and patients requiring or having received chronic steroid therapy. Although steroids are not advocated for long-term use, there are patients with chronic exposure attributable to steroid dependence. Supplementation with calcium and vitamin D has become a standard recommendation for most patients on steroids, and treatment to improve bone mineralization with biphosphonates, including alendronate (Fosamax®, Merck Research Laboratories, West Point, New Jersey), risedronate (Actonel®, Procter & Gamble, Cincinnati, Ohio), or calcitonin (Miacalcin®, Novartis Pharmaceutical Corp., Basel, Switzerland), should be considered for patients with documented osteopenia.

The application of immunomodulator therapy is accompanied by additional therapeutic expectations for acute and maintenance therapy. Potent immunosuppressants, such as cyclosporine or tacrolimus, require experienced application and monitoring for hyperkalemia, nephrotoxicity, hypertension, and opportunistic infection. Most patients receiving immunotherapy with steroids and cyclosporine or tacrolimus should be considered for prophylaxis against *Pneumocystis* with trimethoprim-sulfamethoxazole. Use of AZA or 6-MP requires short- and long-term monitoring of blood counts to prevent leukopenia or bone marrow suppression. Whether therapeutic monitoring of genetic polymorphisms of thiopurine methyltransferase activity or 6-thioguanine and 6-methylmercaptopurine levels will add therapeutic benefits for patients receiving AZA or 6-MP remains to be established.

Aminosalicylates are the most commonly employed agents for short- and long-term use in UC. Although these agents normally are considered safe, there are potential complications that require monitoring, including sulfa-related hemolysis, bone marrow suppression, hepatitis, and folate deficiency related to sulfasalazine; idiosyncratic nephrotoxicity related to mesalamine; and rare examples of pancreatitis, pulmonitis, or hepatitis attributable to any of the aminosalicylates.

Even supportive, symptomatic therapies require monitoring for abuse (narcotics or anxiolytics) or risks of developing megacolon (antimotility agents).

Supplemental Reading

Ardizzone S, Petrillo M, Imbesi V, et al. Is maintenance therapy always necessary for patients with ulcerative colitis in remission? Aliment Pharmacol Ther 1999;13:373–9.

Hanauer SB. Review articles: drug therapy: inflammatory bowel disease. N Engl J Med 1996;334:841–8.

Hanauer SB. Medical therapy of ulcerative colitis. In: Kirsner JB, ed. Inflammatory bowel disease. 5th Ed. Philadelphia: WB Saunders, 2000:529–77.

Hanauer SB, Stathopoulos G. Risk-benefit assessment of drugs used in the treatment of inflammatory bowel disease. Drug Saf 1991;6:192–219.

Irvine EJ. Quality of life issues in patients with inflammatory bowel disease. Am J Gastroenterol 1997;92(Suppl):18S–24S.

Kornbluth A, Sachar DB. Ulcerative colitis practice guidelines in adults. American College of Gastroenterology. Practice Parameters Committee. Am J Gastroenterol 1997;92:204–11.

CHAPTER 25

SEQUENTIAL AND COMBINATION THERAPY OF ULCERATIVE COLITIS

WILLIAM J. TREMAINE, MD

Therapy Strategies

Ulcerative colitis is a chronic inflammatory disease of unknown cause and incurable with current medications. For palliation, the clinician must choose from an array of oral, per-rectal, and intravenous treatments with many dosing options. The medications, doses, and routes of delivery for treatment of active disease may be different from those used for maintenance of remission. The clinician cannot rely entirely on evidence-based data to define the course of treatment because most therapeutic trials assess a single drug given at a fixed dose. No controlled trial can address the changing needs of patients over time through the spectrum of changes in disease activity and extent. Many unresolved issues remain regarding optimal therapy for UC: for example, whether sequential or combination therapy is best.

Pros and Cons of Sequential Therapy

Initial treatment of every patient with one drug at a single dose and delivery route is the traditional and least complicated way for clinicians and patients to judge the efficacy and tolerability of a treatment. Most controlled trials are designed in this manner, providing evidence-based data about the outcome of treatment. The compliance with using a single drug is likely to be better than with multiple drugs or delivery routes and the cost probably will be less. If the initial treatment is not effective or tolerable, then the dose can be adjusted, with or without starting other drugs. The main drawback to sequential therapy is that the trial and error method of adding medications may prolong the time to response, compared to starting multiple drugs together, so this approach is most attractive for mildly active disease when controlling symptoms quickly is less critical.*

---

* Editor's Note: I do not concur with the "trial and error" concept of sequential therapy. After any evidence-based therapy fails, the subsequent course is likely to have less of an evidence base. Nevertheless, all therapy of human disease is "trial and error." (SBH)

† Editor's Note: The "paucity of data" often infers negative data—that combination therapy was not statistically superior to either single agent. (SBH)

Pros and Cons of Combination Therapy

Starting multiple treatments at once, either with the same drug or by different delivery routes, or using two or more drugs may give a combined effect with more prompt onset of action and better efficacy than starting with a single drug and adding others later. This intuitive logic is well accepted by clinicians who have seen the apparent benefit of using two or more treatments at once, such as mesalamine and prednisone. The approach is most commonly used for moderate or severe disease when there is urgency to get the symptoms controlled promptly. "Downsides" to combination therapy are the paucity of data from controlled trials to confirm the benefits, difficulty identifying the offending drug if an adverse effect occurs with multiple drug therapy, lower patient compliance, and probably higher cost.†

Sequential Therapy

DISTAL DISEASE

Mesalamine enemas are my first choice for treatment of ulcerative proctitis and distal ulcerative colitis to the splenic flexure (Table 25–1). The 4 g dose given nightly for 3 weeks is effective in 80 percent of patients with active disease, and most patients can retain the enemas

TABLE 25–1. Sequential Therapy for Ulcerative Colitis

Rectosigmoid Disease
Mesalamine enemas
Mesalamine enemas + oral
Mesalamine (enemas + oral) + prednisone
Mesalamine enemas + oral + prednisone + nicotine
Stop mesalamine and observe
Azathioprine if steroid-dependent
Surgery if quality of life is poor

Extensive Disease
Mesalamine oral
Mesalamine oral + enemas
Mesalamine (oral + enemas) + prednisone
Mesalamine (oral + enemas) + prednisone + nicotine
Stop mesalamine and observe
Azathioprine if steroid-dependent
Intravenous steroids
Surgery if refractory to medications
Cyclosporine if severe disease and surgery declined

through the night. For the patient who responds, I switch to oral mesalamine 2.4 g daily for maintenance therapy at 3 weeks. If episodes of worsened symptoms recur no more than once or twice a year, I repeat the mesalamine enemas for 3-week courses, in addition to continuing oral mesalamine 2.4 g daily. If flares recur more frequently, I increase the dose of oral mesalamine to 4.8 g daily for maintenance therapy.

When symptoms are not controlled with high-dose oral mesalamine plus mesalamine enemas, prednisone 40 mg daily is added for 10 days. If there is a good response with prednisone plus mesalamine, the same dose of prednisone is continued for the balance of 3 weeks then the dose is reduced by 10 mg weekly down to 20 mg daily, then the dose is reduced by 5 mg weekly, until the prednisone is stopped. The mesalamine enemas and tablets are continued for an additional 3 weeks, and the enemas stopped, and oral mesalamine 4.8 g daily is continued for another 6 months. For the patient who continues to do well, the oral mesalamine is reduced by one tablet per day, monthly until the patient is again at a dose of 2.4 g daily. For the patient who responds to oral prednisone but promptly worsens as the dose is reduced, I add azathioprine 2.5 mg/kg daily and after 2 months begin to taper the prednisone for another 6 weeks.[‡]

If the response to prednisone is unsatisfactory, I start nicotine patches at an initial dose of a 7 mg patch daily for a week, then a 14 mg patch daily for a week, and then use the 21 mg patch for 4 weeks.[§] If there is a good response with the combination of mesalamine and nicotine patches, I taper the patches to the next lowest dose for 2 weeks until the patches are discontinued. There is a separate chapter on the use of nicotine in UC. For patients who have not responded adequately to any of these measures, I recommend colectomy with ileal J-pouch to anal anastomosis if the patient is under age 65 and in general good health, or end ileostomy if the patient is older. There are several chapters on surgery for ulcerative colitis.

EXTENSIVE DISEASE

For disease that extends proximal to the splenic flexure, oral mesalamine is the first choice of therapy. For mild symptoms, an initial dose of sulfasalazine, a pro-drug of mesalamine with sulfapyridine as the relatively inactive carrier, 1 g three or four times daily can be effective. I start sulfasalazine at 1 g daily and increase the dose by a gram each day up to 4 g daily and check the CBC after 1 week

on the full dose to look for toxicity. If the patient has had previous adverse effects with sulfasalazine or other sulfa drugs, or if the patient has coverage on an insurance prescription payment plan for other mesalamine compounds, I start the pH-sensitive mesalamine tablets (Asacol®, Procter & Gamble Pharmaceuticals, Cincinnati, Ohio) in a dose of 2.4 g (3 tablets twice daily). If the patient reports recurrent passing of pH-sensitive tablets unbroken in the stool, I use the slow-release mesalamine capsules (Pentasa®, Ferring-Shire Pharmaceuticals Inc., Florence, Kentucky) in an initial dose of 2.5 g daily. Occasionally, a patient tolerates olsalazine (Dipentum®, Pharmacia & Upjohn Inc., Peapack, New Jersey) but not the oral mesalamine drugs, and it can be given as 250 mg four times daily.[//] If the symptoms are not controlled in 10 days, I increase the mesalamine dose to 4.8 g/d. For the patient who started on sulfasalazine initially, and who has not responded to 4 g daily, I switch to Asacol 4.8 g daily or Pentasa 4.5 g daily. Some patients have good relief with oral mesalamine except for persistent urgency and occasional blood streaks with mucus or stools: the addition of mesalamine suppositories (Rowasa®, Solvay Pharmaceuticals Inc., Marietta, Georgia, or Fivasa) or mesalamine enemas (Rowasa)—one nightly—may control the lingering symptoms.

For moderate symptoms, I start high-dose oral mesalamine with Asacol 4.8 g daily or Pentasa 4 g daily. If symptoms do not improve in a week, I add prednisone 40 mg as a single morning dose. If the symptoms come under control, then prednisone can be tapered after 2 weeks, with reductions of 10 mg per day each week down to a dose of 20 mg daily, then reductions of 5 mg daily each week thereafter until prednisone is discontinued. If there is initial improvement but then worsening of symptoms either while tapering prednisone or within a few weeks of stopping, I increase the dose and taper again. For patients whose symptoms flare as the prednisone dose is tapered, I increase prednisone to the dose that controlled the symptoms and add azathioprine 2.5 mg/kg daily, then begin to taper the prednisone after another 2 months. For patients who do not improve with prednisone, nicotine patches are a consideration, gradually increasing to a dose of 21 mg daily. If major symptoms persist despite these measures, I recommend surgery with proctocolectomy and ileal J-pouch to anal anastomosis for the patient who is under age 65, or end-ileostomy for older patients and those with anal sphincter incompetence.

Severe worsening of colitis may be due to medications such as antibiotics, NSAIDs, or sometimes to sulfasalazine or mesalamine, even in the patient who has tolerated sulfasalazine or mesalamine for months or

---

[‡] Editor's Note: Several additional options can be considered. We prefer to maintain the dose of oral mesalamine at 4 to 4.8 g daily. We also continue mesalamine enemas until patients have completely tapered off steroids. (SBH)

[§] Editor's Note: There is no published data that nicotine patches will improve steroid-unresponsive disease. (SBH)

[//] Editor's Note: Safety and efficacy data for oral mesalamine support dosing up to 4.8 g daily and for olsalazine up to 2 to 3 g daily. (SBH)

TABLE 25–2. Treatment of Severely Active Ulcerative Colitis With Intravenous Cyclosporine A: Response

Author of Study	Number of Patients	CyA Alone	Steroids + CyA	Steroids Alone	p Value
Lichtiger	20	—	82%	0%	<.001
D'Haens	20	70%	—	60%	NS
Svanoni	30	67%	93%	—	NS

years.[#] Patients with severe flares usually require hospitalization and intravenous corticosteroids. It is worthwhile suspending the sulfasalazine or mesalamine to make certain the flare is not an adverse reaction to the drug. At the same time, cultures should be obtained in order to check for intercurrent infection. If symptoms do not improve with 3 to 5 days of intravenous steroids such as Solu-Medrol 40 mg every 8 hours,[**] then proctocolectomy or intravenous cyclosporine should be considered. I recommend surgery as the best choice in this situation, but some patients are unwilling to proceed with surgery and cyclosporine is a reasonable alternative after thorough discussion of the risks and benefits. Improvement with cyclosporine mandates starting azathioprine or 6-mercaptopurine for maintenance therapy, overlapping cyclosporine and azathioprine for 3 to 6 months. I use antibiotic prophylaxis for *Pneumocystis carinii* with trimethoprim 160 mg /sulfamethoxazole 800 mg (one double-strength tablet) daily while the patient is on cyclosporine. For the patient who maintains remission, I will continue azathioprine and mesalamine for years.

Combination Therapy

Most controlled trials use single drug therapy, so there is not much evidence-based data to support the initial use of combination therapy for ulcerative colitis. However, the end result of sequential therapy is often combination therapy, so starting with two or more agents is a reasonable, if unproved, strategy. Combination oral and rectal mesalamine appeared more effective than either oral mesalamine 2.4 g/d or mesalamine enemas 4 g nightly. However, this may have been simply a dose-response effect, with the cumulative 6.4 g of mesalamine given with combination therapy being more effective than the lower oral doses. It is reasonable to start with combination oral and enema therapy, but the choice must be individualized; compliance may be low for some patients if both oral and rectal drugs are given initially, before it has been demonstrated to the patient that single therapy alone is not effective.

I am not enthusiastic about initial combination treatment with mesalamine and prednisone; for mild to moderate disease, the majority of patients respond to mesalamine without steroids and for most patients steroids are unnecessary. When the patient fails to respond to mesalamine and steroids are indicated, the question arises whether combination therapy with azathioprine or 6-mercaptopurine should be started along with prednisone or intravenous steroids.[††] This combination approach has been used in Crohn's disease because most patients become steroid-dependent and eventually require an immune modulator. However, patients with UC most often can be maintained on mesalamine once a flare is controlled with prednisone. The exception is the patient intolerant of mesalamine in whom azathioprine could be started along with prednisone to maintain remission after prednisone is discontinued.

For severe disease, high-dose steroids are indicated. The addition of mesalamine is not likely to increase the outcome and carries the risk of adverse effects with worsening symptoms that can mask the response to the steroids. Combination treatment with steroids and cyclosporine and cyclosporine alone have been tested (Table 25–2). Single therapy using intravenous cyclosporine, perhaps in the patient with a history of steroid-induced psychosis, avascular necrosis, or other severe side effects from corticosteroids, is reasonable in severe disease. There is a chapter on immunomodulator use in UC.

Conclusion

Sequential therapy for ulcerative colitis is supported by evidence from prospective trials and clinical experience. Combination therapy should be tested in additional clinical trials and ideally clinical use of combination therapy should be evidence based. The key concepts are still to achieve a remission and then to institute maintenance therapy.[‡‡]

[#] Editor's Note: I do not share the experience that patients develop mesalamine intolerance after months or years. However, concurrent steroid therapy can "mask" mesalamine intolerance that becomes apparent as steroids are tapered. (SBH)

[**] Editor's Note: There is more variation in practice than evidence for steroid-dosing in severe UC. We prefer 40-60 mg of Solu-Medrol as a continuous infusion. In clinical trials, 1 g was no more effective than 60 mg. (SBH)

[††] Editor's Note: A similar question requiring clinical data is whether patients starting azathioprine or 6-MP also require maintenance mesalamine. (SBH)

[‡‡] Editor's Note: Institutions with a lot of experience with ileoanal J-pouch surgery may go directly to that option, while others may offer cyclosporine in an effort to delay or avoid surgery in exchange for prolonged immunosuppressant use and long-term colonoscopic surveillance. The chapter on immunomodulator use in UC describes those options. (TMB)

Supplemental Reading

D'Haens G, Lemmens L, Hiele M, et al. Intravenous cyclosporine (Cya) monotherapy versus intravenous methylprednisolone (MP) monotherapy in severe ulcerative colitis: a randomized, double-blind controlled trial. Gastroenterology 1998;114:963A.

Hyde GM, Thillainayagam AV, Jewell DP. Intravenous cyclosporin as rescue therapy in severe ulcerative colitis: time for a reappraisal? Eur J Gastroenterol Hepatol 1998;10:411–3.

Lichtiger S, Present DH, Kornbluth A, et al. Cyclosporine in severe ulcerative colitis refractory to steroid therapy. N Engl J Med 1994;330:1841–5.

Marshall JK, Irvine EJ. Rectal aminosalicylate therapy for distal ulcerative colitis: a meta-analysis. Aliment Pharmacol Ther 1995;9:293–300.

Safdi M, DeMicco M, Sninsky C, et al. A double-blind comparison of oral versus rectal mesalamine versus combination therapy in the treatment of distal ulcerative colitis. Am J Gastroenterol 1997;92:1867–71.

Sutherland LR, Roth DE, Beck PL. Alternatives to sulfasalazine: a meta-analysis of 5-ASA in the treatment of ulcerative colitis. Inflamm Bowel Dis 1997;3:65–78.

Svanoni F, Bonassi U, Bagnolo F, et al. Effectiveness of cyclosporine A (CsA) in the treatment of active refractory ulcerative colitis (UC). Gastroenterology 1998;114:1096A.

CHAPTER 26

ULCERATIVE COLITIS: A DIVERSE DISEASE WITH DIVERSE QUESTIONS AND DIVERSE SOLUTIONS

KEVIN T. GERACI, MD

Ulcerative colitis (UC) presents a spectrum. What is studied as one disease is, in fact, a blend of several conditions whose final common denominator is diffuse inflammation of the colon associated with distortion of crypts on microscopic examination. There are multiple variables at work. Under certain circumstances, UC involves the entire colon; under other circumstances, it involves only the left colon. What variables lead to pancolitis as opposed to distal colitis and proctitis? Is it the agent or the host that determines extent of disease? Regardless of why it happens, why should each be considered the same? There are clinical trials for pancolitis and left-sided colitis as distinct from proctosigmoiditis. The assumption of diversity of disease is seldom considered beyond this anatomic distinction.

A particular colitis may respond more favorably to therapy at a given stage of disease than at another stage. Altering the gut flora by antibiotic therapy has not been effective in established UC. Probiotic therapy early in the disease shows promise. A type of colitis might respond to therapy more readily when certain host conditions exist compared to when these conditions are absent. The cytokines that begin intestinal inflammation may be "primed" by certain events intrinsic to the person or occurring in the gut lumen of an individual about to have an acute attack. The question of what makes one person respond to a given therapy whereas another person fails it remains unanswered. Seventy percent of patients with proctosigmoiditis respond to 5-aminosalicylic acid (5-ASA). What is it about the nonresponding 30 percent that makes them different?* Clinical trials are challenged by the diversity of UC. Each type might respond differently to various events that occur in the host or to different therapies at different stages, as if each is a different disease.

Spectrum of Therapy

Clinicians move from one therapy for colitis to another as if UC is a spectum. First, 5-ASA is tried for one type of UC; if this therapy fails, corticosteroids, either local or systemic, follow for what unspokenly is another type of UC. 6-Mercaptopurine or azathioprine enters therapy for a third type of UC and, finally, surgery cures all.

Indeterminate Colitis

Diseases that inflame the colon are mimickers. Indeterminate colitis, for one, eludes the best diagnosticians. After a patient who has had UC for years undergoes colectomy, the pathologist may find that the inflammation in the colon is transmural. How could so many years of endoscopy with endoscopic biopsies that confirmed a diagnosis of UC be preempted by assessment of the complete surgical specimen? If Crohn's disease and UC are indeed distinct diseases, what is indeterminate colitis? Therapeutic options available for indeterminate colitis are considered in two chapters.

Bacterial Immunologic Interactions

Where do collagenous colitis, lymphocytic colitis, and microscopic colitis mesh into the disease model of UC? Ulcerative colitis in the setting of recurring *Clostridium difficile* may be another distinct form of colitis. Patients with known UC who become infected with *C. difficile* respond to metronidazole or vancomycin. This subgroup of patients may be treated with *Lactobacillus* with expectation of prolonging remission of both *C. difficile* culture-positive and culture-negative UC. Studies support altering intestinal flora as valid therapy both for active UC and for maintenance of remission. There may be a distinct subgroup of patients with UC who respond to probiotics. Clinical trials whose design strongly considers diversity of cause, duration, and stage of disease will bring clarity to a complex problem. Practitioners await tools of microbiology and immunology to help distinguish various causes and mechanisms of disease for this spectrum of colonic inflammation called ulcerative colitis.

RELATION TO IRRITABLE BOWEL SYNDROME

The premise that UC is, in fact, a group of ulcerative colitides leads to questions:

---

* Editor's Note: Answers to this question may relate to mucosal genetic differences in acetylating enzymes in responsive and nonresponsive patients. (TMB)

Is a subset of distal UC related to irritable bowel syndrome? Animal and human studies have shown that the enteric nervous system modulates gastrointestinal inflammation (Collins et al, 1999). There may be a subset of patients with irritable bowel syndrome whose stressful environment may influence colon mucosal endothelia or epithelia and lead to inflammation. At times, proctitis and proctosigmoiditis do not respond to systemic corticosteroid therapy. These same cases frequently improve when therapy for irritable bowel syndrome is added to conventional therapy for proctitis. Effective treatment of proctitis and proctosigmoiditis without systemic steroids includes use of local mesalamine and systemic 5-ASA. When 5-ASA fails to bring complete remission, addition of antispasmotics and bulking agents and stool softeners may help. 5-Hydroxytriptamine (5HT) antagonists, such as Alosetron (Glaxo Wellcome, Research Triangle Park, North Carolina), are possibly useful agents whose efficacy needs to be tested in clinical trials of proctosigmoiditis. There is a chapter by Collins in this text that further explores IBS and IBD interrelations.

Cyclosporine Therapy

Refractory Colitis

Treatment of refractory colitis requires careful study of subgroups. Truelove stated that severity of disease is related to the length of one's colon that is involved by inflammation. This comment does not convey the problems that refractory distal disease can give (Edwards, 1964). Fifteen percent of patients requiring colectomy for UC have solely left-sided disease. What therapy is appropriate for this subgroup? Clinical trials vary in conclusions about cyclosporine. Intravenous use of cyclosporine has delayed colectomy in refractory pancolitis in 50 to 80 percent of cases. Cyclosporine, despite its risks of renal, hematologic, and neurologic untoward effects, stops disease activity effectively in at least 50 percent of cases. Cohen and colleagues (1999) reviewed the 5-year experience at the University of Chicago, showing a greater success rate of avoiding colectomy when cyclosporine therapy was followed by 6-mercaptopurine or azathioprine therapy. The least cyclosporine therapy provides is time for the patient and his or her physician to prepare for colectomy when the next relapse occurs. The most cyclosporine therapy provides is a better quality of colectomy-free life. In the author's experience, 9 of the first 10 patients for whom cyclosporine was prescribed in 1993 have undergone colectomy, even though azathioprine therapy followed its use.

The efficacy of cyclosporine seems to be similar for refractory distal colitis and for pancolitis. Trials of various doses of oral cyclosporine added to prednisone and 5-ASA to treat patients with proctosigmoiditis would be of interest. Lowering the therapeutic range but lengthening duration of treatment might lessen the untoward effects of infection, renal failure, seizures, and anemia. The preferred therapy in stubborn distal colitis begins with high doses of systemic 5-ASA, local 5-ASA, and finally systemic steroids and cyclosporine. Chlordiazepoxide, clidinium bromide, omega-3 fatty acids (fish oil), or a leukotriene inhibitor can be added if the proctosigmoiditis remains refractory. Once remission is achieved, 6-mercaptopurine or azathioprine might be considered for long-term maintenance.

Heparin

Trials of low molecular weight heparin, both short and long term, are needed in UC regardless of extent of disease. Gaffney and co-workers (1991) showed that intravenous heparin had promise in treatment of refractory UC. Torkvist and colleagues (1999) used low molecular weight heparin in a small case-controlled study of refractory mild-to-moderate UC with improvement noted in 11 of 12 subjects and complete remission in 50 percent. Controlled studies of low molecular weight heparin would clarify the question of efficacy of its use. Heparin trials are reviewed in the chapter on hematology and the chapter on the new approaches.

Corticosteroids

When should systemic corticosteroids be stopped? The quick answer to this question is "after the disease has been in remission for 6 months." Frequently, corticosteroids are tapered early arbitrarily with no recurrence of disease. At other times, corticosteroid therapy with doses as low as 5 or 10 mg/d is continued indefinitely, because the colitis flares as prednisone is tapered from 10 mg/d to zero. A clinical trial studying various schedules of tapering corticosteroids would be interesting. Improvement in disease activity would be measured against side effects of corticosteroid therapy, such as osteoporosis, diabetes, weight gain, infection, and sleeplessness. A Cortisyn stimulation test can be used during the tapering period to ensure normal function of the adrenal glands prior to stopping therapy or maintaining prednisone at 5 mg/d indefinitely. The decision of which method is chosen depends upon the clinical response of the patient.[†]

Osteoporosis remains a concern in long-term steroid use in inflammatory bowel disease (IBD). Patients with IBD, especially CD, develop osteoporosis even without corticosteroid therapy. Those with UC about to embark on a course of corticosteroids should have a screening bone density test. Fosamax® (Merck, West Point, New

---

[†] Editor's Note: A single report describing use of alternate-day steroids in patients in whom 4 mg of sulfasalazine was inadequate to maintain remission presumably is obsolete with higher doses of mesalamine and/or azathioprine. Perhaps controlled ileal release budesonide will find some role in this setting. (TMB)

Jersey), Actonel (Procter & Gamble, Cincinnati, Ohio) and other similar agents prevent accelerated osteoporosis in IBD. These are discussed in a separate chapter on osteoporosis. Clinical improvement has been shown in preliminary studies with pentoxifylline, a phosphodiesterase, in Crohn's disease.

Cancer Risk

Until molecular characteristics of cancer-prone colonic inflammation are defined, surveillance of inflamed colons by means of periodic colonoscopy is the standard of care. Alternatives are needed to the present schedule of surveillance colonoscopy and biopsy to screen for cancer in UC. A popular recommendation is for patients with pancolitis of 8 to 10 years duration to have colonoscopy every 2 years to look for dysplasia. At 20 years duration of disease, the interval changes to annually.[‡] A clinical trial of the presently recommended intervals for surveillance colonoscopy compared to longer screening intervals is needed. The longer intervals between colonscopies seem to be appropriate after an initial surveillance colonoscopy shows no dysplasia but trials are weak.

A family history of colon cancer raises the risk of developing colon cancer in UC. Cancer risk is increased in pouches after colectomy with ileoanal anastamoses. This is also true in patients whose UC is complicated by sclerosing cholangitis. Options for dealing with varying degrees of dysplasia are outlined in two separate chapters.

Dysplastic associated lesions are sessile masses that harbor atypia. Adenomatous polyps proximal to inflamed bowel and not surrounded by dysplasia are not to be considered dysplastic lesions and may not require colectomy. Rubin and colleagues (1999) have shown that patients with chronic colitis who have adenomatous polyps in inflamed mucosa may be treated in a similar fashion as long as the flat mucosa adjacent to it is not dysplastic. This is outlined in a chapter in this book and discussed in two other chapters. Rubin and others suggest that adenomatous polyps in colitic colons should not be treated by total colectomy. Even polyps located in inflamed segments should not, in his opinion, be treated as dysplastic associated lesions and should not require colectomy. If dysplasia exists in flat mucosa near the polyp or elsewhere, colectomy is advised.

Conclusion

Ulcerative colitis presents, responds to therapy, and has a natural history that suggests that it is a spectrum. The host, the luminal environment, the mucosal border, and the immune system of the lamina propria and vascular walls participate in molding this spectrum. Clinical trials that approach UC with these distinct participants in mind may yield more success than outcomes obtained in the past two decades.

References

Cohen RD, Stein D, Hanauer SB. Intravenous cyclosporine in ulcerative colitis: a five-year experience. Am J Gastroenterol 1999;94:1587–92.

Collins SM, Barbara G, Vallance B. Stress, inflammation and the irritable bowel syndrome. Can J Gastroenterol 1999;13 (Suppl A): 47A–49A.

Gaffney PR, O'Leary JJ, Doyle CT, et al. Response to heparin in patients with ulcerative colitis. Lancet 1991;337:238–9.

Edwards FC, Truelove SC. The course and prognosis of ulcerative colitis. II. Long-term prognosis. Gut 1964; 309.

Rubin PH, Friedman S, Harpaz N, et al. Colonoscopic polypectomy in chronic colitis: conservative management after endoscopic resection of dysplastic polyps. Gastroenterology 1999;117:1295–300.

Torkvist I, Thorlacius H, Sjoqvist U, et al. Low molecular weight heparin as adjuvant therapy in active ulcerative colitis. Aliment Pharmacol Ther 1999;10:1323–8.

Supplemental Reading

Katz J, Willis J, Cooper G, et al. Treatment of Crohn's disease with pentoxifylline: lack of correlation between clinical improvement and mucosal cytokine levels. Am J Gastroenterol 1999;94:270. (Abstr)

Merger M, Croitoru K. Infections in the immunopathogenesis of chronic inflammatory bowel disease. Semin Immunol 1998;10:69–78.

Messmann H, Knuchel R, Baumler W, et al. Endoscopic fluorescence detection of dysplasia in patients with Barrett's esophagus, ulcerative colitis, or adenomatous polyps after 5-aminolevulinic acid-induced protoporphyrin IX sensitization. Gastrointest Endosc 1999;49:97–101.

Rembacken BS, Snelling AM, Hawley PM, et al. Non-pathogenic *Escherichia coli* versus mesalazine in the treatment of ulcerative colitis: a randomized trial. Lancet 1999:354;635–9.

[‡] Editor's Note: A chapter in this book advocates shortening the interval to 1 year at age 50. Please see the three chapters on this topic for details. (TMB)

CHAPTER 27

Aminosalicylates Therapy for Ulcerative Colitis

Stephen B. Hanauer, MD

Aminosalicylates have been a mainstay of therapy for ulcerative colitis (UC) for over 40 years. The various delivery systems for 5-aminosalicylic acid (5-ASA) are first-line inductive agents for mild to moderate active disease, the primary maintenance therapy for remitted UC, and used in conjunction with corticosteroids during transition from inductive to maintenance therapy.

Sulfasalazine is the prototype aminosalicylate, and an original "designer drug." Sulfasalazine was developed by Nana Svartz and colleagues at the Karolinska Institute with the concept of combining an antibacterial agent (sulfapyridine) with an anti-inflammatory (5-ASA: mesalamine in North America, mesalazine in Europe). The efficacy of sulfasalazine for UC was serendipitous despite the original concepts that the inflammation in the colon in UC was similar to the inflammation in the joints of rheumatoid arthritis and that both diseases were caused by a similar bacteria found in the stool of afflicted patients. Subsequent elucidation of the metabolism of sulfasalazine by colonic bacterial azo-reductases into sulfapyridine (primarily absorbed, metabolized by genetically determined hepatic acetylation, and excreted in the urine) and 5-ASA (metabolized in a nongenetically[*] determined manner by colonic epithelium and re-excreted into the colonic lumen) led to studies that defined 5-ASA as the active moiety. Sulfapyridine now is recognized as primarily a "carrier" for 5-ASA to prevent proximal absorption and to allow luminal delivery to distal sites of colonic inflammation. These pharmacologic and early clinical trials opened the door to a variety of delivery systems for both oral and topical (rectal) 5-ASA available in different countries around the world.

5-Aminosalicylic Acid Formulations

Recognition of the pharmacology of sulfasalazine and the requisite need to protect 5-ASA against proximal absorption has led to the development of a series of mesalamine analogues. These include topical formulations of mesalamine as suppositories, enemas, or foam; oral mesalamine coated with various pH-dependent polymers (eg, Asacol®, Procter & Gamble Pharmaceuticals, Phoenix, Arizona; Salofalk®, Axcan Pharma Inc., Minneapolis, Minnesota); oral mesalamine encapsulated into ethylcellulose microgranules (Pentasa®, Ferring-Shire Pharmaceuticals, Florence, Kentucky); or alternative azo-bond derivatives that combine two 5-ASA moieties into a dimer (olsalazine, Dipentum®, Pharmacia & Upjohn Inc., Peapack, New Jersey) or attach 5-ASA to an alternative, inert carrier (balsalazide, Colazide®, AstraZeneca, Wayne, Pennsylvania). Most of the oral aminosalicylates have been compared in controlled clinical trials in Europe to equimolar concentrations of sulfasalazine and have been found to be equally efficacious, but better tolerated.

Rectal formulations of mesalamine include suppositories, enemas, and (outside the United States) foams. Suppositories are effective for treatment of disease up to 15 to 20 cm; enemas and foams reach disease margins up to the splenic flexure. The dose-response of topical mesalamine for active UC appears to plateau at about 1 g/d, although conventional therapies include 4-g enemas.

Aminosalicylic Dosing Issues in Ulcerative Colitis

Clinical trials have demonstrated a dose-response for sulfasalazine up to 4 g/d whereas experienced clinicians became accustomed to using doses up to 6 to 8 g/d in selected individuals. In retrospect, those who tolerated higher doses were fast acetylators of sulfapyridine, since slow acetylators have greater side effects, owing to higher plasma concentrations of free sulfapyridine. In clinical trials, up to 30 to 40 percent of patients were unable to tolerate sulfasalazine at doses of 4 g/d. Additional patients developed allergic reactions to the sulfa.

With the advent of non–sulfa-containing aminosalicylates, most of these agents have been compared, head-to-head, with sulfasalazine. Since sulfasalazine is composed of approximately 40 percent 5-ASA, most trials examined 1.5- to 3.0-g doses of sulfasalazine compared to 800 mg to 1.5 g of mesalamine. Of interest, in most studies, sulfasalazine was numerically, but not statistically, superior to the agent to which it was compared, suggesting some

---

[*] Editor's Note: There may be genetically determined differences in intracellular acetylation (n-acetyltransferase) in the colonic mucosa. (TMB)

possible therapeutic activity from the sulfa moiety.[†] In contrast, placebo-controlled trials in the United States have explored higher doses of oral mesalamine, up to 4.8 g/d, comparable to 12 g of sulfasalazine. These trials have demonstrated that, in contrast to sulfasalazine, the dose-response to oral mesalamine is divorced from dose-related side effects, at least up to 4 to 5 g/d.

Careful attention is necessary in interpreting clinical trials of the aminosalicylates in UC, because of variations in indications (active disease vs maintenance), therapeutic end-points and indices, and duration of treatment. In addition, response rates in trials using active agents for comparison have been significantly higher than therapeutic response in placebo-controlled trials. To date, despite a few studies comparing specific aminosalicylates, insufficient data exist to conclude that any oral aminosalicylate is superior to another in any specific scenario for UC.

Adverse Effects of Aminosalicylates

As discussed, the clinical usefulness of sulfasalazine is compromised by a significant rate of side effects attributable to the sulfapyridine molecule. As many as 30 or 40 percent of patients are not able to tolerate the doses required to provide optimal inductive or maintenance benefits. There are three overlapping categories of adverse effects related to sulfasalazine and each can be managed differently. The most common category, intolerance, includes nausea or dyspepsia, myalgias or arthralgias, and headaches, which primarily are attributed to the sulfapyridine moiety and are more common in slow acetylators of sulfapyridine. These effects can be minimized by gradually titrating the starting dose upward and administering sulfasalazine with food or via an enteric-coated formulation.

Hypersensitivity to sulfasalazine can be either to the sulfapyridine (common) or mesalamine (rare). In the past, allergic manifestations of fever or rash were managed by gradually desensitizing patients with gradually increasing doses. Currently, most patients with sulfa allergies can be managed by an alternative, non-sulfa, formulation. Other sulfapyridine or sulfasalazine hypersensitivities include rare cases of hepatitis, pancreatitis, pneumonitis, hemolytic anemia, or bone marrow suppression. Reversible sperm abnormalities (hypomotility and abnormal morphology) are common in males. Sulfasalazine impairs the absorption of folic acid; thus, supplementation with folic acid (1 mg/d) is recommended.

Although hypersensitivity reactions can occur with any mesalamine compound, they are far less common than the sulfa-related toxicities. Rare cases of pneumonitis,

pericarditis, pancreatitis, and idiosyncratic nephritis have been described. Despite the theoretic potential for salicylate-like interstitial nephritis, at doses up to 5 g/d, there is no predictable nephrotoxicity in adults receiving mesalamine formulations.

Finally, mesalamine rarely can cause worsening of colitis. This may be masked when patients are receiving concurrent steroids and can appear as "refractory colitis." Generally, it is recommended that patients who are unable to taper steroids despite high doses of mesalamine be given a trial off mesalamine to rule out unanticipated hypersensitivity colitis. One clue may be seen if patients do not tolerate topical mesalamine enemas. In this situation, one should have a raised suspicion that mesalamine may exacerbate symptoms. The worsening of colitis is distinguishable from loosening of stools or diarrhea related to increased ileal secretion induced by olsalazine. The latter is a dose-related phenomenon that usually improves as the colitis heals.

Indications for Aminosalicylates in Ulcerative Colitis

Distal Colitis

Topical mesalamine is the most effective agent for the *induction of remission* in mild to moderate UC and has been an important adjunct for patients who have not responded to oral aminosalicylates or oral or topical steroids. Mesalamine enemas (1 to 4 g/hs) have been more effective than topical steroids for inducing remission in distal colitis. Mesalamine suppositories 1.0 to 1.5 g/d (Rowasa®, Solvay Pharmaceuticals Inc., Marietta, Georgia; FIV-ASA®, Axcan Pharma Inc., Minneapolis, Minnesota), either nightly or in divided doses, are highly effective for patients with proctitis up to 20 cm and may be adjunctive to oral therapy for patients who cannot retain enemas.[‡] Foam mesalamine products (not available in the United States) also may afford improved tolerability compared to mesalamine enemas. There are separate chapters on distal colitis and on topical 5-ASA use.

Oral aminosalicylates also are effective *inductive agents* for patients with distal disease. In clinical trials, response rates with oral aminosalicylates for patients with distal UC are the same as response rates for extensive colitis. However, when compared to topical mesalamine, oral agents, although often preferred for convenience and compliance, are not as effective as topical mesalamine. This may be owing to right-sided "constipation" in contrast to rapid transit through the left colon as occurs in distal colitis. These features culminate in mesalamine

---

[†] Editor's Note: The intact sulfasalazine molecule itself presumably has some activity when given as an oral solution for esophagogastric disease or as an enema. The portion that influences arthritis is discussed below. (TMB)

[‡] Editor's Note: I assume other people also prescribe 500-mg suppositories nightly. Perhaps we are underdosing. I commonly suggest Cortofoam® (Solvay Pharmaceuticals Inc.) in the morning plus mesalamine suppositories at night. (TMB)

being present in the feces proximal to the margin of inflammation and reduced concentrations in the inflamed distal colon. The dose-response for oral aminosalicylates improves at levels between 1 and 5 g/d. In active disease, there is no evidence of superiority of one agent compared with another. However, if a patient is constipated, olsalazine, which produces dose-related loosening of stools, may be preferable. Unfortunately, at doses above 3 g/d with olsalazine, most patients report diarrhea.

Topical mesalamine also is the most effective *maintenance therapy* to prevent relapse of distal colitis. In this situation, it is not the dose but the *frequency* of administration that is of primary importance. Patients who prefer not to continue on long-term rectal therapy can attempt transitioning to an oral maintenance regimen. However, many patients who require topical therapy to improve will require some frequency of topical therapy to maintain remissions. Usually, an attempt is made to gradually reduce the frequency of topical therapy: initially nightly, then every other night, every third night, and so on, according to the difficulty in achieving the initial response. Most patients then continue on the lowest frequency that maintains their well-being (quality of life, absent urgency and bleeding, ability to pass gas without getting to the toilet).§ If patients flare, oral aminosalicylates can be added at doses up to 5 g/d of mesalamine (or equivalent of 5-ASA). Predictable nephrotoxicity has not been observed with combined doses up to 8.8 g/d of mesalamine (4 g enemas + 4.8 g oral).

Topical mesalamine also can be used to wean patients with distal colitis off steroids. In the situation of steroid dependence, topical therapy should be continued nightly, until steroids are completely weaned. Only then should the frequency of topical therapy be reduced. Topical mesalamine also can be combined with topical corticosteroids to enhance the efficacy of both agents for patients with refractory distal disease. Topical therapy should be used for rectal symptoms regardless of the extent of disease in the remainder of the colon.

Extensive Colitis

Oral aminosalicylates are the most commonly prescribed agents to *induce remission* in mild to moderate UC. Sulfasalazine in divided doses totaling 2 to 6 g/d, mesalamine at 1.6 to 4.8 g/d, or olsalazine at 1 to 3 g/d is effective in approximately 70 percent of patients. Those who do not respond to the lower end of the dose range within a few weeks should receive doses at the upper end prior to moving on to steroid therapy, as long as they are not worsening and continue with mild symptoms. The addition of topical mesalamine or a topical steroid can

help to alleviate troublesome distal symptoms (urgency, tenesmus) until the oral therapy "kicks in." Although patients should begin to respond within weeks, several months may be necessary before the patient is in total remission.

Maintenance Therapy

Oral aminosalicylates also are the primary *maintenance therapy* to prevent relapse of colitis after remission has been achieved. Again, there are practical considerations that differentiate sulfasalazine from the non–sulfa-containing aminosalicylates. There is dose-related efficacy for the maintenance effects of all oral aminosalicylates. With sulfasalazine, the maintenance dose of 2 g/d is often selected as the best "balance" between efficacy and side effects. This has led to previous recommendations to reduce the active dose down to 2 g/d as a maintenance dose. Unfortunately, this precludes use of a more efficacious maintenance dose. In contrast, in the absence of dose-related side effects with mesalamine, the optimal maintenance dose (with respect to efficacy) is the same as the inductive dose. The only constraints are cost and compliance. Typically, administration of oral aminosalicylates on a twice-daily schedule is recommended, to enhance compliance. Because of variations in gastric emptying and colonic motility among patients, there is no rationale to require administration of oral mesalamine compounds in more than two doses per day.

As with distal colitis, there often is a period of transition between inductive therapy with corticosteroids and maintenance treatment with aminosalicylates. Within the tertiary practice setting, the majority of patients who require steroids to induce remission require doses of mesalamine at the higher end of the dose range (2.4 to 4.8 g/d). The maintenance dose usually is not reduced from the inductive dose. However, after at least 1 year of stable remission, with the patient off steroids, the dose may be tapered gradually down to the equivalent of 1.5 g/d of mesalamine. Studies from the United Kingdom have demonstrated benefit from 800 mg/d of mesalamine (equivalent to 2 g sulfasalazine); however, the majority of patients require higher doses (possibly related to the tertiary practice setting).

One setting in which sulfasalazine may be preferable to mesalamine is with associated arthritic manifestations. In contrast to the gastroenterologic trials demonstrating that 5-ASA is the active moiety of sulfasalazine to treat colitis, rheumatologic trials comparing oral sulfapyridine, oral mesalamine, and oral sulfasalazine have suggested that the sulfapyridine moiety contributes more to the improvement of arthritis. Therefore, sulfasalazine is preferred in the treatment of patients with arthritic symptoms, including peripheral arthritis as well as ankylosing spondylitis and sacroiliitis.

---

§ Editor's Note: The author and co-editor (SBH) makes the point that the inability to distinguish gas from stool is a symptom of active proctitis. (TMB)

Supplemental Reading

d'Albasio G, Paoluzi P, Campieri M, et al. Maintenance treatment of ulcerative proctitis with mesalazine suppositories: a double-blind placebo-controlled trial. The Italian IBD Study Group. Am J Gastroenterol 1998;93:799–803.

Diav-Citrin O, Park YH, Veerasuntharam G, et al. The safety of mesalamine in human pregnancy: a prospective controlled cohort study. Gastroenterology 1998;114:23–8.

Gionchetti P, Campieri M, Venturi A, et al. Systemic availability of 5-aminosalicylic acid: comparison of delayed release and an azo-bond preparation. Aliment Pharmacol Ther 1996;10:601–5.

Gionchetti P, Rizzello F, Venturi A, et al. Comparison of oral with rectal mesalazine in the treatment of ulcerative proctitis. Dis Colon Rectum 1998;41:93–7.

Green JR, Gibson JA, Kerr GD, et al. Maintenance of remission of ulcerative colitis: a comparison between balsalazide 3 g daily and mesalazine 1.2 g daily over 12 months. ABACUS Investigator group. Aliment Pharmacol Ther 1998;12:1207–16.

Hanauer S. Medical therapy for ulcerative colitis. In: Kirsner J, ed. Inflammatory bowel disease. Philadelphia: WB Saunders, 2000:529–77.

Kruis W, Brandes JW, Schreiber S, et al. Olsalazine versus mesalazine in the treatment of mild to moderate ulcerative colitis. Aliment Pharmacol Ther 1998;12:707–15.

Miner P, et al. The effect of varying dose intervals of mesalamine enemas for the prevention of relapse in distal ulcerative colitis. Presented at the 10th World Congress of Gastroenterology, 1994.

Sutherland L, et al. The use of oral 5-aminosalicylic acid for maintenance of remission in ulcerative colitis (Cochrane Review). The Cochrane Library. Oxford: Update Software, 1998;3.

Sutherland L, et al. Systematic review of the use of oral 5-aminosalicylic acid in the induction of remission in ulcerative colitis (Cochrane Review). The Cochrane Library. Oxford: Update Software, 1998;3.

CHAPTER 28

Systemic Corticosteroids in Inflammatory Bowel Disease

Humphrey J.F. Hodgson, MD, FRCP

After antibiotics, most physicians would accept corticosteroid therapy as the second major advance in drug therapy during the last century, and with reference to ulcerative colitis (UC) they are the first. Following the demonstration of their dramatic effects in rheumatoid arthritis in the late 1940s, corticosteroids were rapidly tested in UC. By good fortune, early investigation of their value was performed in the setting of controlled therapeutic trials, and the central importance of these drugs in the treatment of UC relies on the firmest of scientific grounds. While advances in general medical care and surgical expertise undoubtedly played a role, the dramatic reduction in mortality of an acute attack of UC, observed between studies before the 1950s, and those since the 1960s, falling from 31 percent to 1 percent, is predominantly a manifestation of the corticosteroid effect.

Any therapy in UC must be considered with respect to its use in acute relapse, maintenance, and with chronic continuous (chronic active colitis) or frequently relapsing colitis. Corticosteroid therapy in UC may be initiated topically or systemically, and systemic treatment may be given orally or parenterally. Systemic administration may be combined with local therapy; systemic corticosteroids may be combined with 5-ASA preparations, again either topically, orally, or both, and occasionally with immunosuppression. Different systemic corticosteroid preparations are available, with similar anti-inflammatory effects, but with some differences in potency and tendency to cause side effects. Despite the relative homogeneity of patients in UC as a clinical group (at least in comparison with Crohn's disease), there are different scenarios of disease onset, activity, severity, and distribution. With this substantial number of variables, despite a number of clinical trials performed since those that initially established the value of corticosteroids, there remain extensive areas in which there is no firm evidence to guide management. Deciding exactly what should be done and when to do it remain domains where the physician's judgment (and prejudice) is of prime importance.

This chapter will survey briefly those corticosteroids available for systemic use before considering practicalities of use in patients with various categories of UC. While the mode of action of corticosteroids lies outside the scope of this chapter, it is worth re-emphasizing that the drugs as a class have a very wide variety of actions. There are two other chapters that discuss the modes of action of corticosteroids as well as steroid-resistant patients. There is a broad spectrum of activity on pro-inflammatory processes (decrease in T and B cell function; decrease in production of monokines, lymphokines, and chemokines such as TNF-α, IL-1, IL-6, and IL-8; decreased release of proteolytic enzymes from neutrophils; decrease in leukotrienes and prostanoid formation). Additionally, corticosteroid effects that are largely irrelevant to the treatment of inflammation and lead to undesirable side effects include sodium and water retention and potassium loss (mineralocorticoid effects), impaired glucose handling, decreased calcium absorption, decreased protein synthesis, increased protein catabolism, and diminished tissue repair, as well as sustained inhibition of the pituitary-adrenal axis and loss of endogenous adrenocortical activity. While in the future corticosteroid structures may be modified to diminish some of the undesirable actions, with current preparations, the systemic anti-inflammatory (glucocorticoid) action only can be achieved in practice with some propensity to develop undesirable side effects.

Corticosteroid Preparations

Initial controlled studies were performed with the natural compound cortisone, which is rapidly metabolized by hepatic hydroxylation to hydrocortisone. Prednisone and prednisolone are synthetic glucocorticoids with a similar relation—prednisone, the prodrug, is hydrolyzed to prednisolone by the liver. The modification of the hydrocortisone molecule to prednisolone diminishes (but does not abolish) mineralocorticoid activity, but increases its glucocorticoid potential four- to fivefold. Methylprednisolone has 20 percent more glucocorticoid activity than prednisolone. An advantage of prednisolone is increased bioavailability after oral administration compared with hydrocortisone (80% vs. 60% bioavailability). The intravenous preparation of prednisolone, extensively used in the 1970s and 1980s, is no longer readily available. Thus, for intravenous use, most physicians use hydrocortisone or methylprednisolone. For oral use, prednisolone and prednisone generally are employed.

The practice of using ACTH to stimulate endogenous corticosteroid production has fallen into disuse, although there was controlled evidence of its effectiveness in colitis especially in patients who had not received prednisone (a rare event these days). Despite the advantage of avoiding adrenal suppression, the combination of the necessity for parenteral use, mineralocorticoid side effects, reports of occasional anaphylactic reactions, and adrenal hemorrhage contributed to the obsolescence of ACTH.

Approaches to the Use of Systemic Steroids

Severe Acute Colitis

The well-recognized clinical criteria for a severe attack of UC (diarrhea more than six times a day, prominent bleeding, elevated pulse [higher than 100/min], elevated temperature [>100°F], elevated ESR [> 30 mm/h], hemoglobin less than 11 g/dl) are generally accepted as defining a group of patients who need admission, acute rapid assessment, and immediate initiation of high doses of corticosteroid therapy. Debate continues as to whether all criteria need to be present to define a severe attack and there are those who maintain that only one is all that is required. Any three of the four clinical signs are enough to place patients in this category. These criteria also dictate a group of patients who almost certainly have extensive colitis.

These are the patients in whom systemic steroids are potentially life-saving. Popular intensive protocols such as the "Oxford regime" add antibiotics, local corticosteroids, and a nothing-by-mouth regime to systemic steroids. It seems clear from various trials that the overwhelming critical factor is the use of systemic corticosteroids, and each of those additional factors has been omitted without making matters worse. I prefer to use hydrocortisone 100 mg q6h IV reflecting its ready availability. Intravenous methylprednisolone (60 mg) once a day in a single morning dose is an alternative regime*, which has advantages: less mineralocorticosticoid activity and less likely to induce edema and hypertension during the first few days. In fact, in such ill patients, hypertension is only rarely a problem, although hypokalemia and fluid retention (particularly likely because of the probable presence of a low serum albumin) can be troublesome. A "bolus" regime using a single 1 g dose of methylprednisolone intravenously, as used in "hematologic" practice, was not shown to be effective.

Some authorities suggest oral usage—60 to 80 mg prednisolone—in acute colitis if there is no problem with gastric emptying. There are no direct clinical comparisons of oral versus systemic administration. It is my bias that if a patient is sick enough to be admitted to hospital, he or she is sick enough for the physician to make certain that the prime therapeutic drug definitely is being administered by using it, at least initially, via the intravenous route.

Acute Severe Ulcerative Colitis Treated with Steroids

It is to be expected that within a few days—sometimes indeed overnight—there will be a rapid decrease in temperature and diarrhea. Reported figures indicate that 60 to 70 percent of patients should be in remission by 5 days, with a further 10 to 15 percent improving. Clearly, whether and how much improvement occurs is the central issue in defining further intervention, and a variety of courses may emerge.

Progressive Rapid Improvement in All Clinical Parameters

In these patients, intravenous treatment may be changed to oral therapy with an equivalent dose after 3 days or so. It is essential to ensure, if shifting from hydrocortisone to oral prednisolone, that there is no dip in blood levels as may occur, for example, when the intravenous preparation is stopped in the evening and the oral preparation is not administered until the next morning.† I advocate a period of overlap of about 12 hours to avoid this. With persistent improvement, patients should have their systemic steroids tapered off over about 10 weeks. I follow a pattern such as intravenous steroids (100 mg hydrocortisone q6h) for 3 days, then 60 mg prednisolone orally for 3 days, 45 mg for 3 days, 40 mg for 3 days, and 30 mg for 3 days, and then decrease by 5 mg weekly to 10 mg and then by 2.5 mg weekly to zero.

Failure to Improve

Twenty to thirty percent of patients with severe colitis will experience neither rapid remission nor improvement. Defining the appropriate action is one of the most difficult problems in UC management, and new therapeutic opportunities such as adjunctive therapy with cyclosporine A both have helped and complicated these decisions. The identification of the "failing-to-improve" patient, although generally obvious on clinical grounds, can be helped by laboratory assessment. Failure to decrease circulating CRP levels significantly by the third day, or the clinical sign of failing to reduce stool frequency to below three times a day each, has been associated with the subsequent necessity for colectomy. The efficacy of cyclosporine A (4 mg/kg/IV) in "failed-to-improve" acute colitis was demonstrated in a clinical trial with small numbers. Though borne out in clinical practice, this regime does not commonly achieve the 85 percent or so remission rate of the initial trial. In practice

---

* Editor's Note: We prefer 40 to 60 mg as a continuous infusion over 24 hours. (SBH)

† Editor's Note: We prefer to make certain the patient is having forming bowel movements without blood or urgency prior to substituting oral for parenteral steroids. (SBH)

about three out of five patients seem to improve. It seems reasonable practice to add cyclosporine A if there is no clear trend to improvement on the third or fourth day after initiating treatment, providing that there is an appropriate back-up service, including blood cyclosporin level monitoring, and experience with the drug in the hospital. For the 40 percent of those so treated who do not improve rapidly after the addition of cyclosporine A, as indeed for the 30 percent of all patients with severe colitis in general who are not improving, the most important issue is how long to persist in the hope that medical treatment will "turn the corner." There is a separate chapter on management of severe colitis.

It is worth recalling that the pioneering first-rate series—from pre-cyclosporine A days—in which mortality was all but eliminated, were those in which the decision to proceed to colectomy was taken if significant improvement was not observed within 5 days. There often are pressures to extend this time period: the patient's unwillingness to accept surgery, the physician's hope that things may still improve, and surgical issues in scheduling operating room time. There is now further opportunity for delay waiting for cyclcosporine A treatment, if it has been initiated, to work. Thus, the timing of surgery has become perhaps a more difficult judgment. All would agree that failure to show any improvement at all, if corticosteroid treatment alone is being used, after 4 to 5 days should lead to surgery (earlier if there are additional features of megacolon or peritoneal findings, or if worsening occurs). Most would agree that in patients with severe colitis, failure to show an improvement by 8 to 9 days, even if cyclosporine A has been used, should lead to surgery. It is worth considering that prolonged steroid therapy may trouble the patient and the surgeon in the postoperative period with poor wound healing and a propensity to infection.

Relapse After Initial Control

Perhaps 15 percent of patients will relapse while corticosteriod therapy is being reduced, and provide, though less commonly, a parallel to those patients with Crohn's disease whose disease activity is steroid-dependent. They present a difficult management problem in the absence of clear guidelines from prospective trials. It is necessary always to remember that UC can be cured by surgery, and of course restorative proctocolectomy has made this option significantly more acceptable over the last three decades. Thus, the patient's informed appreciation, expectation, and choice are essential components of the decision. Sensible guidelines for such patients include:

First, defining steroid-response versus steroid dependence. Continual improvement in local treatment, advances in 5-ASA medications for delivery to the colon, and the tendency to use progressively higher doses of 5-ASA as better delivery vehicles become available all

mean that "steroid-dependency" needs to be reprobed by dose reduction after optimization of all other treatments.

Second, considering whether adjunctive immunosuppression is necessary. If more than 7.5 to 10 mg prednisolone is required to maintain control, the addition of azathioprine or 6-mercaptopurine—drugs with which the greatest experience is available—is helpful. From series of patients requiring more than 10 mg prednisolone, there is good anecdotal evidence of the steroid-sparing effects of azathioprine. A trial in which patients in remission on azathioprine and corticosteroids had the azathioprine withdrawn proved that such combined therapy makes a given dose of corticosteroid more effective in maintaining remission.

Third, alternate-day prednisolone. Alternate-day prednisolone also can be used to maintain steroid-induced remission. The controlled evidence for this involved the use of 40 mg prednisolone on alternate days, but it did not avoid induction of steroid-induced side effects, and extended only to 3 months treatment. Thus, while this approach has proven to be effective, the prospect of long-term treatment with this regime is somewhat daunting.[‡] The use of a lower dose of alternate-day prednisolone, together with daily azathioprine, as pioneered in the treatment of pediatric Crohn's disease, is a slightly different approach that probably is quite commonly and effectively used in this recalcitrant group of chronic steroid-dependent colitis.[§]

Other Considerations in Acute Disease

In a patient with a previous diagnosis of UC, there is little anxiety in starting systemic corticosteroid therapy on the above indications when relapse occurs. There is of course a possibility that an infectious agent also may be present (eg, *Clostridium difficile*) in about 10 percent of patients at relapse, and such important information needs to be sought by immediate fecal culture, and by assay for *C. difficile* fecal toxin on admission. However, there is little evidence that corticosteroids in this setting lead to systemization or worsening of coexisting infection. Cytomegalovirus infection may be an issue in patients on corticosteroids and/or immunomodulators.

The position is more problematic in the initial attack. While in clinical practice it generally transpires that most patients who *seem* after initial history, examination, and sigmoidoscopic examination to have UC *do* have UC, other conditions, notably *Campylobacter* colitis and

---

[‡] Editor's Note: In the absence of data, I do not consider steroids to have a maintenance role for the vast majority of UC patients. (SBH)

[§] Editor's Note: In the past, I have used low-dose alternate-day steroids along with maximum doses of 5-ASA or sulfasalazine in patients who could not tolerate azathioprine. In the future, sustained-release budesonide or methotrexate may be helpful in such patients. (TMB)

amebic colitis, remain problematic. Should one withhold steroids until those possibilities have been excluded? Should one cover the infective possibility with antibiotics and if so, with what? I am not aware of evidence that 24 to 48 hours of high-dose corticosteroid will lead to a more complicated course of these infections (provided they are subsequently treated) but urgent assessment of both rectal histology seeking to differentiate UC from acute infectious colitis, and stool culture and examination to identify pathogens, must urgently be performed. If the undiagnosed patient has signs and symptoms of UC sufficient to place them in the severe category, systemic steroid therapy should be started forthwith, and addition of antibiotics to cover possible infections seems pragmatic and sensible. The use of a quinoline such as ciprofloxacin is a sensible option due to its proven effect on *Campylobacter*, and if epidemiologic considerations (eg, recent return from Central or South America, the Indian subcontinent, Southeast Asia) favor amebiasis, metronidazole also can be added. If the criteria for severe disease are not fulfilled, and suspicion of infection is high, the results of bacteriologic studies can be awaited before corticosteroid therapy is started. Under those circumstances, it would be sensible to initiate some treatment for IBD by using 5-aminosalicylate.

Other Adjunctive Therapy

Although the association between corticosteroids and peptic ulceration has been rethought over the years and is currently best established as predisposing to the development of complications from preexisting ulceration, the incidence of steroid-related dyspepsia makes the simultaneous administration of an H2 antagonist, such as rantidine, sensible.

MAINTENANCE OF REMISSION

Systemic steroids were not found—unless doses of the equivalent of 20 mg prednisolone were used—to be effective in preventing relapse if commenced in UC in remission. The approach in those patients whose recent steroid-induced remission relapses has already been discussed.

OBVIATING THE SIDE EFFECTS OF CORTICOSTEROIDS

During continued therapy, hypokalemia, hyperglycemia, and hypertension should be looked for and treated if necessary. Short-term oral potassium supplementation, oral hypoglycemics or insulin, and antihypertensives may be required temporarily. After a short course of corticosteroids, long-term sequelae are not recognized with the exception of those patients whose steroid-induced diabetes persists, who currently are regarded as having had a previous diabetic tendency unmasked by the glucocorticoid. Of more concern are long-term consequences of steroid therapy: bone disease (both osteoporosis and osteonecrosis), skin atrophy, and cataract formation. In the majority of cases with UC, such issues are not a cause for concern, as long-term therapy is not required. However, it is helpful to remember that local corticosteroids, particularly as enemas, if used longterm occasionally can induce systemic effects. Up to 50 to 80 percent of steroid enemas are absorbed, equivalent to 10 to 20 mg of prednisone. Hence, even in patients on longer-term rectal therapy with systemic steroids, awareness of bone disease, the ability to screen for decrease in bone density, and the ability to reverse bone density changes (if not necessarily fracture frequency in osteoporosis) are required.[//]

Most gastroenterologists now urge the use of hormone replacement therapy and/or regular calcium supplementation in female patients with Crohn's disease (CD). In CD, the necessity for this advice is compounded by the added propensity for malabsorption of calcium, the higher life-time steroid dosages in CD compared with UC, as well as evidence that systemic cytokines activation in CD, independent of corticosteroid treatment, can induce osteoporosis. In UC, the risks are less, but preventable bone disease is an area that merits more attention than it generally receives. It would seem advisable that if a patient has needed two or more 10-week courses of high-dose steroids within a couple of years, and definitely if a patient has a long-term steroid-dependent remission, a DEXA scan should be performed. Normal bone density would indicate only future vigilance, with a repeat scan after 2 to 3 years time if further corticosteroid therapy is needed and perhaps advice on modest calcium supplementation (1 g per day, with vitamin D (800 IU daily)). If, however, a decreased bone mineral density is found, the use of bisphosphonates now offers the possibility of not only halting but reversing the damage.

MILD TO MODERATE DISEASE

Patients with active disease not fulfilling the "severe" criteria fall into the easily understood but poorly defined mild or moderate group. Most mild disease, often distal in distribution, does not require systemic steroids, although it may well be that the local administration of steroid enemas twice daily is in part effective by a systemic effect—particularly when more proximal colitis is responding to local treatment administered rectally.

In moderate disease, oral corticosteroids as used by an outpatient are clearly effective, have been proven to be superior to salicylazosulfapyridine, and are also more

---

[//] Editor's Note: Biphosphonate therapy (etidronate, alendronate, and risendronate) have been shown to have a significant effect on bone mineral density by preventing bone loss and increasing bone mass in patients receiving corticosteroids, such as 20 mg in rheumatoid arthritis. Risedronate (Actonel) causes significantly less esophageal injury than alendronate (Fosamax). This can be advantageous in terms of drug safety. Fracture risk is known to be decreased. (TMB)

rapid in effect than the newer 5-ASAs. An early study by Baron et al (1962) showed that the effects of corticosteroids were dose-related, with 20 mg of prednisolone being less effective than 40 or 60 mg, and 40 mg slightly slower though producing fewer side effects than 60 mg of prednisolone.

Some authors advocate the use of 20 mg of prednisolone for mild disease and 40 mg for moderate disease. It is my impression that although this approach is often effective, there may sometimes be a loss of the effectiveness of steroids if a slow escalation of dose is used (eg, 20 mg for 2 weeks—not better—try 30 mg—not better— try 40 mg). Occasionally, this approach seems to lead to failure to improve when higher doses are eventually given to a patient who fails to respond at lower doses. I am aware as I write that there is both anecdotal and ascertainment bias to that statement![#]

It is interesting, however to note that there is an evolving concept of glucocorticoid unresponsiveness that may be definable by in vitro studies of glucocorticoid receptors on lymphocytes taken before treatment is initiated. There is a separate chapter on steroid unresponsiveness. While this approach is not likely to find its way into clinical practice, the concept emphasizes the importance of defining early on whether patients with UC respond to corticosteroids, a concept only achieved by giving a sufficient dose. Because the vast majority of patients who need corticosteroid therapy are expected to have a short course and not require maintenance, I follow the maxim that if systemic corticosteroids are required, the dose should be adequate, and thus I advocate the use of 45 to 60 mg daily if oral treatment is initiated for moderately active disease. It is important to note that even though a patient may be well enough to be treated as an outpatient, if systemic corticosteroid treatment is required, he or she

should certainly be reviewed within 7 days to see if improvement is indeed occurring; failure to improve after 2 weeks as a outpatient, or worsening at any time, is an indication for admission, further assessment, and the initiation of intravenous corticosteroids.

Supplemental Reading

Baron JH, Connell AM, Kanaghinis TG, et al. Outpatient treatment of ulcerative colitis. Comparison between three doses of oral prednisolone. BMJ 1962;2:441–3.

Campston JE. Management of bone disease in patients on long-term glucocorticoid therapy. Gut 1999;44:770–2.

Chakravarty BJ. Predictors and the rate of medical treatment failure in ulcerative colitis. Am J Gastroenterol 1993;88:852–5.

Hawthorne AB, Logan RF, Hawkey CJ, et al. Randomised controlled trial of azathioprine withdrawal in ulcerative colitis. BMJ 1992;305:20–2.

Hearing SD, Norman M, Probert CSJ, et al. Predicting therapeutic outcome in severe ulcerative colitis by measuring in vitro steroid sensitivity of proliferating peripheral blood lymphocytes. Gut 1999;45:382–8.

Langholz E, Munkholm P, Davidsen M, Binder V. Course of ulcerative colitis: analysis of changes in disease activity over years. Gastroenterology 1994;107:3–11.

Powell-Tuck J, Bown RL, Chambers TJ, Lennard Jones JE. A controlled trial of alternate-day prednisolone as a maintenance treatment for ulcerative colitis in remission. Digestion 1981;22:263–70.

Travis SPL, Farrant JM, Nolan DJ, et al. Predicting outcome in severe ulcerative colitis. Gut 1996;38:905–10.

Truelove SC, Willoughby CP, Lee EG, et al. Further experience in the treatment of severe attacks of ulcerative colitis. Lancet 1978;ii:1086–8.

Truelove SC, Witts LJ. Cortisone in ulcerative colitis. Final report on a therapeutic trial. BMJ 1955;2:1041–8.

[#] Editor's Note: I concur that doses should begin high, 40 mg prednisone, with rapid taper for responders, rather than starting with low to intermediate doses that may require dose-escalation and prolonged symptoms and steroid exposure. (SBH)

CHAPTER 29

Steroid Unresponsiveness in Inflammatory Bowel Disease

Miquel A. Gassull, MD, PhD, and Maria Esteve, MD

Although systemic glucocorticoid treatment is associated with a large number and sometimes severe side effects, this is still the first and most useful therapeutic tool in treating patients with both acute (moderate-severe) ulcerative colitis (UC) and Crohn's disease (CD). In these clinical situations, glucocorticoids are both rapidly acting, within 48 hours, and effective, with a response rate of about 80 percent. Unresponsiveness to steroid treatment leads to the need for therapeutic decisions including surgical resection or the use of immunosupressive drugs.

Steroid Refractoriness

Steroid refractoriness is defined as the lack of clinical and biologic response to steroid treatment within an established period. Setting this time period (5 to 7 days) in advance is crucial, since as the time passes, especially in those patients who are not getting worse, but are not getting better, severe complications may develop, masked by the administered steroids. Rectal sparing can occur even with severe pancolitis so that the sigmoidoscopic appearance of the diseased bowel is not generally taken into account. In addition, patients with severe disease seldom undergo total colonoscopic examination.

Frequency of Steroid Resistance and Dependence

The frequency of "true" steroid refractoriness in severe UC ranges from 25 to 57 percent. In CD, steroid resistance occurs in about 20 percent of patients. However, another 35 percent of patients with CD will develop steroid dependence, which may be considered an important form of refractoriness. This subgroup of patients is discussed in other chapters.

Pseudorefractoriness

Before establishing the diagnosis of primary steroid resistance, it is important to rule out the existence of "pseudo" refractoriness to steroids, as described in another chapter. This includes patients with previous ileocolonic resections, bacterial overgrowth, abdominal pain due to fibrous strictures, and an abdominal abscess in febrile patients with known CD.

Another steroid refractoriness challenge is patients with mild to moderately active left-sided UC and right colon constipation. These patients present with abdominal pain and increased number of bowel movements, sometimes even loose movements containing small amounts of blood. These symptoms usually are relieved with bulking laxatives.

Opportunistic gastrointestinal (GI) infection, such as cytomegalovirus, can also lead to refractoriness. This is discussed in a separate chapter

Molecular Basis of Steroid Resistance

The molecular basis of steroid resistance has been widely assessed in other inflammatory conditions, including asthma and rheumatoid arthritis. The anti-inflammatory effect of glucocorticoids is produced by inhibiting the promoter regions of the genes expressing inflammatory molecules (eg, cytokines, enzymes, adhesion molecules). This is not done by a direct action of the complex steroid-receptor upon these genes but by interfering with the activity of the intracellular transcription factors promoting such genes (nuclear factor [NF]-κB, activator protein-1 [AP-1]). Investigations have been focused on reduced glucocorticoid receptors (GCR), decreased binding affinity for GCR, or poor DNA binding affinity of GCR to the DNA glucocorticoid response element (GRE). The interfering mechanism may involve direct interaction on one of the protein components of the transcription factors or may occur by promoting the expression of I-κB, which maintains these transcription factors in an inactive form. The latter mechanism seems to be important in chronic inflammation (Figure 29–1).

Steroid resistance most frequently is observed in those patients with severe disease. It has been suggested that in this situation, the anti-inflammatory capacity of corticosteroids is probably overwhelmed by an excessive synthesis of proinflammatory cytokines, owing to an excessive activity of various intracellular transcription factors, which in turn may reduce the affinity of the steroid-receptor complex to its intracellular ligand. Both mechanisms favor an excess expression of inflammatory molecules and a positive feedback system with perpetuation of the inflammatory response.

In inflammatory bowel disease (IBD), the pathophysiology of the steroid resistance has not yet been clarified. Knowledge of these mechanisms could lead to early

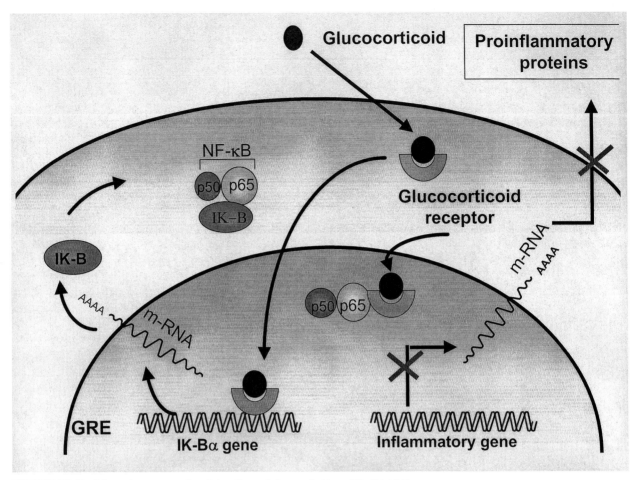

FIGURE 29–1. Schematic representation of the effects of glucocorticoids on NF-κB inhibition.

identification of those patients who will not respond to steroids, avoiding an unnecessary and dangerous prolonged exposure to these drugs. It has been suggested that glucocorticoid refractory acute UC arises in patients in whom T-cell proliferation is relatively resistant to glucocorticoid inhibition. Proliferation of peripheral blood T cells from patients with UC who failed to respond to steroid therapy was inhibited by less than 60 percent by therapeutic glucocorticoid concentrations, whereas in complete responders inhibition of T-cell proliferation was 60 percent or higher. Since proliferation assays are relatively inexpensive and the results may be available in 48 hours, they might be helpful in the diagnosis of steroid unresponsiveness. Further research is needed to clarify the value of measuring in vitro steroid sensitivity of proliferating peripheral blood lymphocytes or other factors contributing to refractoriness, such as the number and affinity for glucocorticoid receptors. It is not yet known if any of these procedures will be useful in routine clinical practice for the early detection of steroid refractory patients.*

Therapeutic Alternatives to Steroids

Therapeutic alternatives to steroids are discussed in the chapters on refractory disease. They include azathioprine, 6-mercaptopurine, cyclosporine, and, perhaps, mycophenolate mofetil, methotrexate, and infliximab (Figure 29–2).

Azathioprine and 6-Mercaptopurine

The most widely used drugs to control inflammation in refractory patients, both in UC and CD, are azathioprine (AZA) or 6-mercaptopurine (6-MP). In Crohn's disease, both have demonstrated their usefulness in the control of inflammation in active disease, steroid sparing in steroid dependence, maintenance of remission, and closure of fistulae. The usual recommended doses are 2 to 2.5 mg/kg/d of AZA or 1.5 mg/kg/d of 6-MP. Some patients who are nonresponsive to AZA may respond to higher than usually administered doses. The assessment of erythrocyte thiopurine methyltransferase (TPMT) activity or following 6-thioguanine (6-TG) levels may be helpful to avoid severe myelotoxicity. Further research is needed to

---

* Editor's Note: An additional genetic factor in determining glucocorticoid responsiveness may lie in elevated levels of multidrug-resistant (MDR) genes. These MDR genes code for a drug efflux pump, p-glycoprotein 170, and may transport glucocorticoids and other drugs as well as proinflammatory cytokine out of lymphocytes and epithelial cells. (TMB)

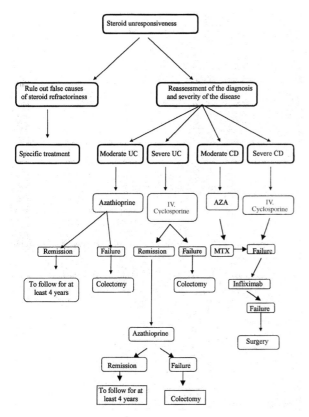

FIGURE 29–2. Steroid unresponsiveness: schematic of therapeutic approach.

establish whether the levels of TPMT enzyme activity may predict the therapeutic response to AZA

Adverse Reactions

Adverse reactions may appear in 15 percent of the patients on AZA, and 3 percent may be severe. Most of the hematologic or hepatic side effects of AZA may be easily detected and prevented. Hypersensitivity reactions such as pancreatitis cannot be prevented. Macrocytosis, as indicated by a high MCV (106 μ^3 or more), also can be observed; there is no indication to discontinue this treatment because of it. When markers of potential AZA or 6-MP toxicity, such as leukopenia between 3,000 and 3,500 cells/mm^3, total absolute neutophil count lower than 1,500, or a lymphocyte count below 700, as well as mild derangement in the liver function tests (LFTs), are found, treatment should not be discontinued, but a second test should be performed. If confirmed, decreasing the doses administered by one-third should effect stabilization. Usually, there is no need to return to the previous dose, but if necessary, the dose can be slowly increased with monitoring of 6-TG levels.

Cyclosporine A

CROHN'S DISEASE

High-dose cyclosporin A (CsA) may be a good alternative in severe steroid refractory patients; it has a rapid thera-

peutic effect, with improvement usually occurring within 1 to 2 weeks. There are chapters on cyclosporine use in UC and in CD. Uncontrolled trials in refractory patients with CD indicate a variable response to intravenous administration of CsA, ranging from 44 to 100 percent of partial or complete response, with a high rate of relapse after drug discontinuation if AZA is not added. Uncontrolled experience with the use of high-dose intravenous CsA in patients with CD supports the use of this drug in the management of steroid refractory or dependent patients with IBD. Results with fistula and perianal disease are discussed in other chapters.

ULCERATIVE COLITIS

In steroid refractory UC, controlled experience with CsA 4 mg/kg/d by continuous intravenous infusion demonstrated an 82 percent response in the CsA-treated group versus 0 percent in the placebo group. Uncontrolled trials have confirmed that intravenous CsA avoids colectomy in a high percentage of refractory patients with UC who experience severe attacks. Limited information using the new oral CsA formulation, called Sandimmune Neoral (Sandoz Pharmaceuticals Corp., Basel, Switzerland), suggests that orally administered CsA may be as effective as intravenous administration. However, there are no controlled trials in severely refractory patients. The details of cyclosporine toxicity are discussed in other chapters.

COLECTOMY AVOIDANCE

Intravenous CsA may only postpone but not avoid colectomy in severely refractory patients with UC. Since the relapse at 1-year follow-up is common, a maintenance regimen should be administered to try to avoid disease relapse and, hence, colectomy. Azathioprine, administered after stopping intravenous CsA while slowly tapering corticosteroids, is useful in maintaining long-term remission induced by intravenous CsA in steroid refractory patients with severe UC. Some authors have recommended oral CsA for 3 to 6 months after intravenous CsA in combination with AZA therapy and tapering dose of steroids, to allow the therapeutic action of AZA to start. However, overlapping three immunosuppressive drugs for several months increases the probability of opportunistic infections. To prevent such complications, trimethoprim-sulfamethoxazole prophylaxis (2 tablets, 160 to 800 mg 3 times/wk) has been proposed. There is some concern that this antibiotic may worsen the myelotoxicity related to AZA. Overlapping three immunosuppressors is unnecessary since remission achieved using intravenous CsA, as seen in the controlled and uncontrolled series, may remain for months. On the other hand, the refractoriness to steroids probably is not a permanent or established situation. After achieving CsA-induced remission, the milieu of T-cell and other inflammatory cell changes and a certain degree of steroid sensitivity may be restored.

Duration of Azathioprine Maintenance

It is not yet known how long AZA therapy must be maintained to prolong remission after intravenous CsA treatment. There is limited information about how long to wait before discontinuing AZA or 6-MP given for steroid refractoriness.[†] These drugs should not be discontinued before 6 months of treatment have been completed.

Mycophenolate Mofetil

Mycophenolate mofetil is another immunomodulator, similar to AZA, with promising therapeutic efficacy in the management of refractory patients. Information about the efficacy of mycophenolate mofetil is limited but a recent randomized trial in patients with CD with a high-risk relapse rate, suggests that, administered at doses of 15 mg/kg/d, it may be as effective as AZA in the control of inflammation. It also becomes therapeutically effective more quickly (1 mo after starting the drug) in patients with severe disease. There is much less experience with this agent than with AZA.

Methotrexate

Methotrexate is another alternative to be administered to steroid refractory patients with CD who are intolerant of or resistant to AZA. No specific data exist regarding patients refractory to steroids but steroid-sparing has been documented in CD. This is outlined in a separate chapter. Based on the available information on steroid-dependent patients, 25 mg/wk intramuscularly for 16 weeks followed by maintenance with weekly oral doses of 7.5 to 15.0 mg/wk may be a reasonable schedule in patients requiring more than 20 mg of prednisone to maintain remission, expecting a 40 percent remission rate. Importantly, long-term efficacy seems to be limited, since the 1-year relapse rate is higher than 50 percent. A CD trial, using 15 mg once a week IM for 10 months also maintained a remission rate of about 70 percent. There are no controlled data on UC maintenance.

Adverse Events

The severity of some methotrexate-related adverse events may overshadow its possible therapeutic benefit. Hepatotoxicity, related to cumulative doses, may be severe in 3 percent of the treated patients. Severe hepatotoxicity has been seen mainly in patients with other possible causes of liver damage including alcohol abuse, viral hepatitis, diabetes, and obesity. Bimonthly assessment of liver enzymatic profile should be performed. High-risk patients should probably be excluded from methotrexate

therapy. Although folate supplements have been advocated for reducing adverse reactions, there is no established schedule that is proven to be effective in either preventing or lessening side effects without influencing therapeutic efficacy. Folinic acid at 1 mg every 8 weeks is one suggested but unproven dose. The reader is referred to the chapter on methotrexate use.

Infliximab

Infliximab is a murine monoclonal antibody directed against tumor necrosis factor-alpha (TNF-α), a key cytokine initiating a cascade of events leading to an inflamed bowel and its clinical manifestations. Results with CD are described in several chapters in this book.

Results in severely steroid refractory CD patients have led to enthusiasm in both patients and doctors because of the rapid therapeutic action, potential improvement in patient's quality of life with less hospital admissions, and avoidance of steroid side effects.

Unanswered Questions

There are several questions to be answered due to the lack of adequate long-term trials. What is the significance of the development of antibodies to anti-murine monoclonal antibody anti-TNF-α (human anti-chimeric antibodies [HACA]) after repeated treatments? These antibodies develop in 4 percent of the patients, and they tend to appear more often when long periods have elapsed between treatments than when treatments are scheduled every 6 to 8 weeks. The HACA may not be present in the patient's plasma before administering one of the repetitive treatments, but it may be found after the infusion. An HACA assay may not be available in many hospitals. Alternatively, to prevent anaphylactic reactions, it has been suggested by some that before any repeated intravenous infusion of infliximab, a bolus of 40 mg of prednisone should be administered, or that these patients should be treated on a maintenance basis with AZA or methotrexate. These suggestions are based only on personal observations but without enough data to make firm recommendations. In addition, anti–double-stranded DNA antibodies, which may be a prelude to drug-induced lupus erythematosus in a small percentage of patients, appear in 12 percent of cases.

How often can this treatment be administered? Little is known about the long-term effects of TNF-α blockade. There is concern about the possibility of non-Hodgkin's lymphoma developing in some patients with Crohn's disease or rheumatoid arthritis. There is also the question whether long-term treatment with infliximab is cost-efficient and improves the quality of life of patients. There is a chapter on anti-cytokine therapy.

Little is known about the possible maintenance effect of AZA or methotrexate once the patient has achieved remission with infliximab. Also, the potential role of other

---

[†] Editor's Note: One report suggests that a 4-year remission lessens the likelihood of relapse after discontinuing AZA. Patients with small bowel CD seem to be more likely to relapse than those with active colonic or perianal disease. Discontinuing AZA or any immunosuppressive drug may lead to a severe relapse, at times with perforation. (TMB)

immunosuppressive drugs, such as mycophenolate mofetil, as maintenance treatments has not been explored.

Summary

When a patient presents with steroid resistance, it is important to rule out false causes of refractoriness, such as bile-salt malabsorption, bacterial overgrowth, and coexistent irritable bowel syndrome. It also is important to detect the existence of viral or bacterial gastrointestinal infections that may enhance the synthesis of inflammatory mediators perpetuating the disease process. The molecular basis of genuine steroid resistance is unclear but an understanding will allow earlier diagnosis and treatment. Therapeutic alternatives to steroids should be individualized but a personal schematic approach is illustrated in Figure 29–2.

Supplemental Reading

Farrell RJ, Murphy A, Long A, et al. High multidrug resistance (p-glycoprotein 170) expression in inflammatory bowel disease patients who fail medical therapy. Gastroenterology 2000;118:279–88.

Feagan BG, Fedorak RN, Irvine EJ, et al. A comparison of methotrexate with placebo for the maintenance of remission in Crohn's disease. N Engl J Med 2000;342:1627–32.

Feagan BG, Rochon J, Fedorak RN, et al. Methotrexate for the treatment of Crohn's disease. N Engl J Med 1995; 332:292–7.

Fernández-Bañares F, Bertrán X, Esteve-Comas M, et al. Azathioprine is useful in maintaining long-term remission induced by intravenous cyclosporine in steroid refractory severe ulcerative colitis. Am J Gastroenterol 1996;91:2498–9.

Hearing DA, Norman M, Probert CSJ, et al. Predicting therapeutic outcome in severe ulcerative colitis by measuring in vitro steroid sensitivity of proliferating peripheral blood lymphocytes. Gut 1999;45:382–8.

Kornbluth A, Present DH, Lichtiger S, Hanauer S. Cyclosporine for severe ulcerative colitis: a user's guide. Am J Gastroenterol 1997;92:1424–8.

Munholm P, Langholz E, Davidsen M, Binder V. Frequency of glucocorticoid resistance and dependency in Crohn's disease. Gut 1994;35:360–2.

Neurath MF, Wanitschke R, Peters M, et al. Randomised trial of mycophenolate mofetil versus azathioprine in chronic active Crohn's disease. Gut 1999;44:625–8.

Schottelius AJG, Balwin AS. A role for transcription factor NF-κB in intestinal inflammation. Int J Colorectal Dis 1999;14:18–28.

Thiele K, Bierhaus A, Autschbach F, et al. Cell-specific effects of glucocorticoid treatment on the NF-κBp65/IκBα system in patients with Crohn's disease. Gut 1999;45:693–704.

Vega R, Bertran X, Menacho M, et al. Cytomegalovirus infection in patients with inflammatory bowel disease. Am J Gastroenterol 1999;94:1053–6.

West SC. Methotrexate hepatotoxicity. Rheum Dis Clin North Am 1997;23:883–914.

CHAPTER 30

IMMUNOMODULATORS IN ULCERATIVE COLITIS

ASHER KORNBLUTH, MD

The immunomodulators, 6-mercaptopurine (6-MP), azathioprine (AZA), and cyclosporin A (CSA), are of value in the management of the ulcerative colitis (UC) patients who are dependent on, or refractory to, oral steroids. CSA is effective as a short-term intravenous (IV) and oral agent for achieving remission in patients with severe colitis refractory to IV steroids. 6-Mercaptopurine and AZA, but not CSA, also are effective as maintenance agents for patients who have required steroids, 6-MP/AZA, or CSA to achieve remission.

Indications for 6-Mercaptopurine/Azathioprine Use

Steroid-Refractory Patients

6-Mercaptopurine/AZA should be considered in the UC patient with active inflammatory disease despite maximal medical therapy (with oral aminosalicylates, topical aminosalicylates and steroids, and high doses of prednisone of 40 to 60 mg/d), who is not so acutely ill as to warrant hospitalization for a course of intravenous steroids and/or cyclosporine therapy. A key determinant is whether the patient can tolerate an additional 3 months of UC symptoms and potential steroid toxicity while awaiting a therapeutic response to 6-MP/AZA.

Steroid-Dependent Patients

A subset of UC patients who respond to high doses of oral steroids will promptly and predictably experience a flare-up of symptoms when steroids are tapered below a threshold prednisone dose—typically 15 to 20 mg daily. This is an unacceptable long-term steroid dose for patients with a curable disease, and 6-MP/AZA should be considered to facilitate a successful steroid taper. While any chronic prednisone use in UC generally is unacceptable, lessons learned from our rheumatology colleagues suggest that doses of ≥ 7.5 mg daily are particularly inimical and should prompt either use of 6-MP/AZA or discussions regarding the merits of a curative colectomy. Dose ranges from reported series have been 1 to 1.5 mg/kg for 6-MP and 1.5 to 2.5 mg/kg for AZA. No comparisons of dose-ranging trials have been performed. The response rates with AZA/6-MP for either steroid-

refractory or steroid-dependent UC in controlled and uncontrolled series approximate 65 to 70 percent.

Initiating Therapy and Monitoring for Efficacy and Toxicity

When initiating 6-MP/AZA, the relative risks and benefits should be discussed and documented in the patient chart, but it has not been my custom in practice to list each of the individual risks or benefits in detail, or to have the patient sign an informed consent document.

Potential 6-MP/AZA toxicities to be discussed include the risk of bone marrow suppression, particularly leukopenia, and the need for vigilant compliance to CBC monitoring. A patient who has a history of poor adherence to medical therapy or physician follow-up should not be treated with 6-MP/AZA.

Serious infections fortunately occur infrequently and often, but not always, are related to leukopenia. Patients are advised to call immediately with the development of fevers or any focal signs or symptoms of infection. For minor infections (eg, herpes zoster, sinusitis, bronchitis, etc.), and in the absence of leukopenia, appropriate antibiotics are prescribed and 6-MP/AZA is continued. For more serious infections, appropriate antibiotics are begun and 6-MP is discontinued regardless of the white blood cell count. Most, but not all, patients who develop serious infections on 6-MP do so while also still on substantial steroid doses.

Liver enzyme elevations representing either drug-induced or viral-induced hepatitis occur in less than 2 percent of patients and may require 6-MP/AZA dose reduction or discontinuation. Liver test abnormalities may take the form of either hepatocellular or cholestatic changes. With minor elevations of liver enzymes (less than 2 normal), 6-MP/AZA generally can be continued without dose reduction with frequent monitoring. If more significant liver enzyme abnormalities develop, 6-MP/AZA should be discontinued, allowing the enzymes to return to normal, prior to reinitiating 6-MP/AZA at a lower dose. Elevated RBC levels of 6-MMP are associated with a 15 percent risk of abnormal liver function tests. Allergic reactions occur in approximately 2 to 3 percent of patients, who typically present with fever, rash, or arthralgias and usually in the first 3 weeks of starting or of increasing the dose. In approximately 2 percent of patients, acute pancreatitis may develop as a hypersensitivity reaction and resolves when the drug is discontinued.[*] Rechallenge with either 6-MP or AZA should be avoided due to inevitable recurrence of pancreatitis. Some patients develop fatigue, arthralgias, or myalgias without other evidence of an allergic or hypersensitivity reaction and are able to tolerate continued drug use, although a dose reduction may be required.

Risk of colonic malignancy or other solid tumors is not increased in UC patients treated with 6-MP/AZA. Similarly, the risk of lymphoma is not increased in IBD patients on 6-MP/AZA, although isolated case reports probably represent an underlying higher incidence of lymphoproliferative disease in IBD.

I begin with 6-MP 50 mg daily, although a higher initial dose is advocated by others. A CBC and chemistry profile are measured at baseline and the CBC is checked weekly for the next 4 weeks, then monthly. I generally do not increase the 6-MP/AZA dose within the first 3 to 4 weeks; dose increases after this time are made by 25 mg increments. Any dose increase is followed by a weekly CBC for the next 2 weeks.[†] Liver function tests are followed monthly for the first several months and then approximately 3 times annually.

If the white blood cell count falls below 4,000, 6-MP is held until the white blood cells recover; then it is restarted at a lower dose, again following the CBC closely. In order to ensure patient compliance with monthly labs, I prescribe only a 1-month supply of 6-MP, and refills are not dispensed unless the patient's monthly labs have been checked.

The mean time to therapeutic response to 6-MP/AZA is 3 to 4 months. Some patients may not demonstrate full benefits for 6 to 9 months. On the other hand, some patients with UC will note improvement as early as 1 to 2 months. By 3 or 4 months, the steroid dose should have been substantially tapered or discontinued, allowing the 6-MP/AZA benefit to be evident.

When tapering prednisone, I generally taper in 10 mg decrements down to approximately 20 to 30 mg and then by 5 mg or smaller amounts based upon the patient's response. Although it is, in most institutions, a mandatory goal to wean all UC patients from steroids, a too-rapid taper may trigger a disease relapse. In general,

steroids in UC should be tapered over weeks to months, not months to years.[‡]

Controversy exists whether raising 6-MP/AZA doses to levels sufficient to provoke mild leukopenia increases efficacy. Certainly, for a patient who has not improved after a 3-month course of 6-MP/AZA at a submaximal dose, the dose should be raised so long as the white blood cell count remains acceptable.

Measurements of 6-MP/AZA metabolites may be a helpful guide in patients who have not achieved their response to a maximum dose of 6-MP or AZA, that is, 1.5 mg/kg/d or 2.5 mg/kg/d, respectively.[§] Therapeutic response appears to be greater in patients with 6-thioguanine (6-TG) levels >230 pmol/8×10^8 red blood cells. Elevated levels of 6-methyl-mercaptopurine (6-MMP) increase the risk of hepatotoxicity. No correlation has been found between 6-TG and 6-MMP levels. Low or absent 6-TG levels do support a suspicion of poor drug compliance. There is a chapter on the use of 6-TG levels to monitor AZA/6-MP dosages without producing leukopenia.

Maintenance of Remission

Patients with severe UC who achieve remission with either steroids or CSA still face a daunting short-term prognosis—the likelihood of colectomy over the ensuing 6 to 12 months is as high as 50 percent. These patients, as well as patients who have achieved remission with the use of 6-MP/AZA, benefit from long-term 6-MP/AZA to maintain remission. A controlled withdrawal study of AZA patients found that patients who continued on AZA had a 50 percent greater likelihood of maintaining remission than patients in whom AZA was withdrawn.

The optimal duration of treatment with 6-MP/AZA to maintain remission is unknown. Generally, the drug is continued for at least 1 to 2 years. Even beyond this point, we and others have observed that patients who discontinue 6-MP have higher relapse rates than patients continuing on longer-term therapy.

I usually revisit the issue of continued 6-MP/AZA use on an annual basis after 2 years of 6-MP therapy. For the patient who has endured a long, stormy course prior to achieving remission, a longer duration of 6-MP/AZA may be preferred. On the other hand, patients with a milder course who promptly were tapered from steroids and brought into remission with 6-MP/AZA may be

---

[*] Editor's Note: Our experience is 5 to 10 percent risk of pancreatitis. (SBH). Our experience is 2 percent, perhaps because we also start with 1 to 1.5 mg/kg plus high-dose mesalamine, which affects TPMT enzyme levels. (TMB)

[†] Editor's Note: We check the CBC at 2-week intervals after a dosing change, then monthly as the patient is tapering from steroids, then quarterly for the duration of the therapy. We obtain liver enzymes at 1 month, 3 months, then on a 6 to 12 month basis. (SBH)

[‡] Editor's Note: We taper to an alternate-day dose before discontinuing steroids. (TMB)

[§] Editor's Note: No prospective trials have defined optimal metabolite levels or demonstrated superiority versus monitoring of white blood cells. (SBH)

[||] Editor's Note: In most clinical series, an aminosalicylate has been maintained in conjunction with AZA/6-MP—we also have used AZA/6-MP alone, for patients intolerant of, or allergic to, aminosalicylates. (SBH) It is possible that continuing an aminosalicylate enhances the effect of AZA/6-MP by influencing TPMT levels. (TMB)

given the option of discontinuing the drug after a 2-year period of use and reinstituting it promptly should a significant relapse occur.[//]

Cyclosporine

Commercially available formulations of CSA include an IV concentrate, a liquid oral solution, or gelatin capsule (Sandimmune, Novartis Pharmaceutical Corp., Basel, Switzerland) or a newer oral liquid or capsule micro-emulsion formulation with enhanced bioavailability (Neoral, Novartis Pharmaceutical Corp.). It is important to note that dosing and pharmacokinetic differences exist between Sandimmune and Neoral.

Indications for Cyclosporine A Use

The most common indication for cyclosporine use is severe UC refractory to a 7- to 10-day course of intra-venous steroids. Less frequently, cyclosporine may be used for selected patients refractory to, or dependent on, oral steroids. In such a setting, CSA is usually reserved for those patients who either do not respond to 6-MP/AZA or cannot tolerate these agents. The protocol for CSA use is identical, however, for each of these indications.

Initiating Cyclosporine A Therapy

Earlier series that initiated therapy with the Sandimmune formulations as either oral therapy or as bolus IV therapy failed to produce satisfactory results. Subsequently, Lichtiger and Present pioneered the use of *continuous* IV CSA infusion for severe steroid-refractory colitis. Cyclosporine A now is considered an alternative option to colectomy for patients with severe disease refractory to conventional medical therapy. As with 6-MP/AZA, the risks and benefits of CSA therapy should be reviewed in detail. In our practice, we document that this dialogue has occurred, but do not have the patient sign "informed consent."

Baseline history, and physical and laboratory results are reviewed before initiating CSA. As with 6-MP/AZA, non-compliant patients should not be treated with CSA. Patients with a past history of seizures must be on adequate anti-seizure medications. A past history of malignancy other than a treated basal or squamous cell carcinoma is a relative contraindication to CSA use.

When initiating CSA, there must be no evidence of active infection. Hypertension must be adequately controlled. Calcium channel blockers may offer protection against CSA-induced nephrotoxicity but increase CSA blood levels. Other drugs that increase blood CSA levels include metoclopramide, ketoconazole, fluconazole, erythromycin, and corticosteroids, while drugs such as rifampin, phenobarbital, phenytoin, and carbamazepine lower blood CSA levels.

Baseline laboratory data include measurement of serum creatinine since the primary short- and long-term toxicity of CSA is nephrotoxicity. Serum potassium should be monitored for CSA-induced hyperkalemia. Both

hypocholesterolemia (serum cholesterol < 120 mg/dL) and hypomagnesemia (serum magnesium of < 1.5 mg/dL) significantly increase the risk for seizures in patients treated with CSA. While hypomagnesemia may be promptly corrected with parenteral magnesium, hypo-cholesterolemia, which may frequently occur in these malnourished, hypoalbuminemic patients, can be far more difficult to correct. Accordingly, serum cholesterol levels should be checked early in potential candidates for intravenous CSA.

Before initiating IV CSA therapy, curative surgical options are reviewed and we generally consult our surgical colleagues for an introductory meeting with the patient. We initiate 4 mg/kg/d of intravenous CSA[#] as a continuous infusion over 24 hours, except for elderly patients or patients with mildly impaired creatinine clearance for whom a lower dose is selected, that is, approximately 2 mg/kg/d. In patients with borderline or low serum cholesterol levels, we may choose to start the CSA in very low dose, that is, 1 mg/kg/d, anticipating that CSA will elevate serum cholesterol levels to a safer range (ie, > 120mg/kg/d), before increasing the CSA to full dose. During the first hour of infusion, the patient should be closely monitored for signs of very infrequent allergy or anaphylaxis. Patients are continued on IV steroids for their severe colitis. If the patient has been on 6-MP/AZA, these are temporarily held during the initial IV CSA phase to reduce the risk of potent "triple immuno-suppression." However, the addition of 6-MP/AZA after hospital discharge is essential to maintain a long-term response to CSA (see below).

Daily Monitoring

Patients with severe colitis should be closely monitored as described in the chapter on that topic. Whole blood CSA levels should be measured every 2 days with the aim of achieving a level of 300 to 500 mg/mL during the acute IV continuous infusion phase using either the monoclonal radioimmunoassay or the high-performance liquid chromatography (HPLC) assay.[**]

The CSA dose is reduced by 25 percent if drug levels are elevated for 2 consecutive days or if serum creatinine increases by 30 percent over baseline, if serum liver enzymes double, or if diastolic blood pressure exceeds 90 mm Hg or systolic blood pressure exceeds 150 mm Hg despite antihypertensive treatment. The CSA dose is decreased by even larger amounts, or is held temporarily,

---

[#] Editor's Note: No dose-ranging data are available. Other experienced clinicians begin at 2 mg/kg with similar monitoring and blood level goals. (SBH)

[**] Editor's Note: No therapeutic range has been established for UC. The 300 to 500 mg/mL level is via monoclonal antibody radioimmunoassay. Most centers use the HPLC assay with an intended therapeutic range of 200 to 400 mg/mL. (SBH). Because the author describes a 24-hour infusion, these are not "trough" levels. (TMB)

if a more significant rise in serum creatinine occurs. Daily inquiries should be made regarding symptoms of CSA toxicity such as headache, nausea, or paresthesia. During the short-term IV phase, these have not been found to be dose-limiting side effects. Careful attention is paid to evidence of infection, especially at the site of central intravenous catheters.

Assessment of Outcome and Switching to Oral Cyclosporine

Decisive clinical improvement is generally noted within 4 to 5 days and intravenous CSA is continued for 7 to 10 days. Patients who have not demonstrated improvement with a significant decline in diarrhea and rectal bleeding within 7 days of IV CSA, or any patient whose condition worsens during CSA therapy, are referred for surgery. Sigmoidoscopy is rarely necessary to guide decision-making; rather, a clinical decision should be based on the patient's clinical response.

For the patient who is on a course of IV CSA, the oral dose prescribed prior to hospital discharge is twice the daily IV dose, for example, a patient who maintained therapeutic blood levels on 200 mg/d of IV CSA is treated with 200 mg of oral CSA[††] every 12 hours in addition to prednisone (I use 60 mg daily with the goal of a rapid taper) and aminosalicylate maintenance.

Upon hospital discharge, patients are followed weekly for the first 2 to 4 weeks and then at 2- to 4-week intervals. Outpatient CSA levels should only be measured as a 12-hour trough level and we aim for levels of 100 to 300 mg/mL during the outpatient phase. The oral dose is never increased above 8 mg/kg/d and in our experience all UC patients achieve therapeutic levels with this dose and generally require somewhat lower doses. Nephrotoxicity can occur even with therapeutic levels and serum chemistries must be vigilantly monitored during the entire outpatient phase.

Cyclosporine A dose reductions are based upon the CSA level reduction desired. For example, in a patient with a level of 400 mg/mL, the dose is reduced by at least 25 percent. The pharmacokinetics of CSA absorption and metabolism are variable and so any dose change should be followed by a repeat CSA level after 1 week.

We have learned the importance of adding 6-MP/AZA during the outpatient phase. Approximately 60 to 80 percent of patients requiring CSA continue in remission up to 3 to 5 years if 6-MP/AZA is added. In the absence of 6-MP/AZA use, long-term remission rates fall to as low as 10 percent. The ideal timing for the addition of 6-MP/AZA is not yet known, but it is our practice to add 6-MP/AZA shortly after hospital discharge to allow a prompt steroid

withdrawal within the ensuing 3 months. This "triple-drug" immunosuppression with CSA, prednisone, and 6-MP/AZA increases the risk of opportunistic infections and we now routinely add trimethoprim-sulfamethoxazole, 1 double-strength tablet three times a week as *Pneumocystis carinii* prophylaxis. Cyclosporine is generally tapered by reducing the dose by 50 percent for 2 weeks followed by complete CSA withdrawal after 6-MP/AZA has been used for at least 3 months.

Monitoring for Toxicity

As with 6-MP/AZA, patients on CSA are informed to promptly report any fevers or focal signs of infection. If they are minor, and the CSA levels are therapeutic, the infection is treated without changing the CSA dose. However, with more serious infections, the CSA dose is reduced or held while the infection is treated. More frequent though less worrisome adverse effects are headaches, hirsutism, paresthesias, and gingival hyperplasia. These latter adverse effects have not required dose reduction in outpatient CSA use. In the limited 6- to 9-month duration of CSA use in UC, no lymphomas are known to have occurred either during active treatment or in follow-up of up to 12 years. There are chapters on immunomodulator use in distal colitis and Crohn's disease that provide additional information and other references on these agents.

Supplemental Reading

Cuffari C, Theoret Y, Latour S, Seidman G. 6-Mercaptopurine metabolism in Crohn's disease: correlation with efficacy and toxicity. Gut 1996;39:401–6.
Feagan BG, Fedorak RN, Irvine EJ, et al. A comparison of methotrexate with placebo for the maintenance of remission in Crohn's disease. N Engl J Med 2000; 342:1627–32.
George J, Present DH, Pou R, et al. The long-term outcome of ulcerative colitis treated with 6-mercaptopurine. Am J Gastroenterol 1996;91:1711–4.
Hawthorne AB, Logan RFA, Hawkey CJ, et al. Randomized controlled trial of azathioprine withdrawal in ulcerative colitis. BMJ 1992;305:20–2.
Kornbluth A, Present DH, Lichtiger S, Hanauer S. Cyclosporine for severe ulcerative colitis: user's guide. Am J Gastroenterol 1997;92:1424–8.
Present DH, Meltzer SJ, Krumholz MP, et al. 6-Mercaptopurine in the management of inflammatory bowel disease: short- and long-term toxicity. Ann Intern Med 1989;111:641–9.
Sandborn WJ. A critical review of cyclosporine therapy in inflammatory bowel disease. Inflamm Bowel Dis 1995;1:48–63.
Sandborn WJ. A review of immune modifier therapy for inflammatory bowel disease: azathioprine, 6-mercaptopurine, cyclosporine and methotrexate. Am J Gastroenterol 1996;91:423–33.
Yoon C, Kornbluth A, George J, et al. Is cyclosporine as effective in chronic ulcerative colitis as in severe ulcerative colitis? Gastroenterology 1998;114:G4586.

[††] Editor's Note: The microemulsion formulation Neoral provides a more consistent blood level. Careful attention is needed if oral formulations are substituted. (SBH)

CHAPTER 31

MANAGEMENT OF SEVERE ULCERATIVE COLITIS

GUNNAR JÄRNEROT, MD, PhD, FRCP

Severe or fulminant ulcerative colitis (UC) is a potentially fatal disease that was associated with a 30 percent mortality rate prior to the introduction of corticosteroids and, in steroid-refractory cases, early surgery. The mortality rate should be less than 2 percent in specialist centers. During recent years, the trend has changed from saving lives to improving the quality of life of patients by saving colons or using modern surgical methods.

Etiology

The reason that an episode of UC becomes severe is uncertain. The first episode can follow this course. Usually, such patients have had bowel symptoms for some time before they seek medical advice, ascribing it to a temporary abdominal upset. In some cases, an incorrect medical diagnosis has been made initially, which has delayed adequate treatment.

In patients who already have a diagnosis of UC and later develop a severe episode, superimposed problems include infectious gastroenteritis, antibiotics, smokers who have discontinued smoking, or discontinuing maintenance therapy. A moderate relapse can be made more severe by antidiarrheic medications, agents affecting gastrointestinal motility, or by preparation for colonoscopy or large bowel enema. That emotional events could be of paramount importance is often cited but has seldom been proven.

Differential Diagnosis

Before a definite diagnosis is made, infectious causes must be ruled out by fecal culture, examination for ova and parasites, *Clostridium difficile*, and rectal biopsy for cytomegalovirus.

Antibiotics, including penicillin V, ampicillin, and amoxicillin, sometimes can cause another form of severe enterocolitis, possibly attributable to a hypersensitivity reaction. This inflammation usually is most pronounced in the right colon. Nonsteroidal anti-inflammatory drugs (NSAIDs) can cause an exacerbation of existing UC. They can also cause idiopathic colitis, at times indistinguishable from UC, that responds to withdrawal of the drug. Neutropenic enterocolitis is a necrotizing life-threatening disease, mainly affecting the terminal ileum, cecum, and ascending colon, usually seen in patients with hemato-

TABLE 31–1. Criteria for Classification of Severity of Ulcerative Colitis[*]

Parameter	Severe Attack	Mild Attack
Diarrhea	≥ 6 times 24 h	≤ 4 times 24 h
Blood in stool	Obvious	None or slight
Fever	> 37.5°C (morning)	Normal
Pulse	≥ 90/min	Normal
Anemia	Hb ≤ 100 g/L	No
ESR, CRP	≥ Doubled	Normal

[*] A moderately severe attack has criteria between a severe and mild attack. ESR = erythrocyte sedimentation rate; CRP = C-reactive protein.

logic or other malignancies treated with cytostatics. Radiation can induce proctocolitis, which, however, rarely becomes severe.

The most difficult differential diagnosis is between UC and Crohn's colitis. However, the initial treatment usually is similar for both diseases.[*]

Definition

The criteria established by Truelove and Witts (1955) still are useful (Table 31–1). It was later determined that bloody diarrhea ≥ 6 times 24 h in combination with one or more of the other signs is sufficient to classify the attack as severe. Carbonnel and colleagues (1994) substantiated this approach by a colonoscopic study, showing that, of 46 patients with endoscopically severe colitis, only 8 fulfilled all of the criteria of Truelove and Witts, but 30 fit the modified criteria. The endoscopic appearance can be an adjunct to the clinical history. Only 2 of 39 patients with moderately severe colitis had all of the original severe criteria of Truelove and Witts and only 16 had the modified criteria. This means that some patients with moderate or mild disease as judged from the clinical history in fact have severe colitis as evaluated endoscopically, which is important, because the degree and depth of the colonic ulcerations have profound impact on the outcome of treatment. Therefore, patients with severe inflammation at rigid sigmoidoscopy should be hospitalized even if they only have a moderately severe attack according to the

---

[*] Editor's Note: Pathologists have difficulty distinguishing UC from Crohn's disease in colons removed for fulminant colitis because of the deep transmural ulcers. Many of the "new" diagnoses of Crohn's disease in patients with ileal pouch-anal anastomosis are based on this difficulty. (TMB)

clinical history. If the sigmoidoscopy tube is continuously filled from above with loose, watery, blood-stained feces, it is almost certain that the patient has extensive and probably significant inflammation. Solid feces indicates distal disease.[†]

Patients with definite or strongly suspected severe colitis must be admitted to hospital for intensive treatment.

General Management Measures

The immediate steps after admission are fecal cultures, blood tests for hematology, electrolytes, serum proteins, and liver function tests. A plain abdominal radiograph is essential for evaluation of free gas, toxic colonic dilatation, fecal contents, mucosal islands, and air-filled small bowel loops.

Free gas in the abdomen indicates colonic perforation, which requires surgical treatment. Toxic dilatation of the colon is a dreaded complication in fulminant colitis. It is potentially reversible, and during strict monitoring by a staff trained to care for these patients, conservative treatment for 24 hours can be allowed. If no improvement has been achieved after 24 hours, surgical intervention is advisable. Some gastroenterologists use a thin, soft rubber catheter introduced into the rectum and a nasogastric or intestinal suction tube in combination with changing positions of the patient in an attempt to deflate the colon.

A colonic diameter of more than 5.5 cm often is called colonic dilatation. That may be so, but to be a toxic colonic dilatation, signs of atonia are required. Radiographs taken with 20- to 30-minute intervals show abscence of peristalsis by a constant air-filling of the same colonic segment. This indicates transmural inflammation with neuromuscular degeneration, causing loss of peristalsis. If the left colon contains solid feces, the probability of substantial colitis is low; a distal colitis is more plausible. Retention of stool in the right colon is a more serious sign.

Mucosal islands can sometimes be seen on a plain abdominal radiograph. They are caused by ulcerations into the muscle layers, indicating severe inflammation and a high risk of a poor response to medical treatment. The mucosal islands can be even better visualized by very cautious insufflation of 500 to 800 mL air into the rectum. In expert hands, this air enema is a safe procedure of great value.[‡]

The severity of the inflammation also can be assessed by sigmoidoscopy or colonoscopy, even on an unprepared bowel. A left-sided sigmoidoscopy or colonoscopy is usually sufficient. This procedure is safe in skillful hands and often helps to differentiate at an early stage between UC and Crohn's colitis.[§] However, the author has found that colonoscopy is more useful somewhat later in the evaluation of patients who have not responded and those with only partial response to treatment, to improve decision-making for continuing therapy. Three or more air-filled small bowel loops suggest that there will be an impaired response to medical therapy.

These preliminary measures are sufficient at this stage of disease. It is important to evaluate the extent of the disease early, as the response to medical therapy is poorer in more extensive diseases. The sooner this can be evaluated, the sooner the psychological preparation of the patient for the possibility of surgery can be initiated.

In this context, it is important to emphasize that the surgeon is an essential part of the medical team from the beginning of the hospitalization.

Special Treatment

The mainstay of the medical treatment is corticosteroids, taken orally with nothing except small sips of water, and total parenteral nutrition.[||] In the original Oxford model, antibiotics were given. Currently, antibiotics are prescribed only if the sigmoidoscopy shows prominent mucopurulent exudate, in which case, either metronidazole, 400 mg twice a day, or ciprofloxacin, 500 to 750 mg twice a day, is recommended.[#] For a week or two, it usually is possible to avoid a central venous catheter and all its potential complications by daily relocating the intravenous needle. These principles of treatment are disputable, owing to the lack of controlled trials.

Corticosteroids

The optimal dose of corticosteroids never has been settled in controlled trials. The only dose-ranging study compared 20, 40, and 60 mg of orally administered prednisolone in patients with mild to moderately severe UC: 40 mg was better than 20 mg and almost as good as

---

[†] Editor's Note: Although there are several reports cited in this chapter as to the safety of colonoscopy during an acute episode of colitis, many physicians initially rely on abdominal radiographs and unprepared flexible sigmoidoscopy, and perhaps computed tomography to evaluate the extent of severe colitis. (TMB)

[‡] Editor's Note: Do we need this information enough to risk distending the bowel in an acutely ill patient? It is cheaper than computed tomography. (TMB)

[§] Editor's Note: Finding unsuspected cytomegalovirus colitis sometimes explains unresponsiveness. This and other issues are discussed in the chapter on unresponsive colitis. (TMB)

[||] Editor's Note: Although I also restrict oral feedings in the severely ill patient, my co-editor (SBH) does feed such patients. Some authors believe that unabsorbed carbohydrates are a source of short-chain fatty acids (SCFAs), which, theoretically, are helpful for the colonic mucosa. (TMB)

[#] Editor's Note: If there is an impending perforation (fever, tenderness, leukocytosis), I usually employ adequate coverage for peritonitis. (TMB)

60 mg, but with fewer side effects. Usually, corticosteroids are administered intravenously in severe colitis, but even in acute colitis, corticosteroids given orally are absorbed completely but somewhat more slowly than those administered intravenously.

However, most centers use high-dose intravenous steroids (eg, hydrocortisone 100 mg/d or methylprednisolone 16 mg qds). Once-daily administration of betamethasone (60 mg) induces fewer corticosteroid side effects; there is no proof that multiple doses or continuous drip is more effective and megadoses of corticosteroids have not been found better in a controlled trial.[††] One small unconfirmed study showed that patients who had been on corticosteroids earlier responded better to hydrocortisone, whereas those who had not had corticosteroid therapy responded better to adrenocorticotropic hormone (ACTH).[‡‡] Rectal corticosteroids can be administered as adjunct therapy, but this has never been tested in a controlled setting.

Corticosteroid treatment in patients with suspected fulminant UC should not be delayed by waiting for fecal culture results. Although case reports can be found in the early literature about disasters following steroid treatment of patients with infectious colitis, the author has never seen this happen during 40 years of clinical practice. The only exception may be a suspicion of amebic colitis. Hemorrhagic colitis, caused by *Escherichia coli* 0157:H7 verotoxins, also should be diagnosed quickly and treated early. It is so important to gain control of a severe attack of UC that the benefits of early treatment outweigh possible drawbacks.

The duration of corticosteroid therapy has been discussed for years. Truelove and Jewell (1974) favored surgery for patients who had not responded after 5 days of intravenous treatment. The patients who had done well or were improved were switched to oral feeding and steroids by mouth. If the bowel symptoms recurred, surgery was recommended. A similar policy has been in effect at the Örebro Medical Center Hospital for many years, with the same results as in Oxford; however, the intravenous corticosteroid was used slightly longer (7 to 10 d).

Colonoscopy, rather than food challenge, is relied on to improve decision making in patients with incomplete or poor response to treatment; however, this protocol has not been proven in a controlled trial.

Bowel Rest

Although bowel rest is of value in Crohn's colitis, its benefit in UC has not been proven. Two controlled trials could not show any difference in colectomy rate between patients on a normal hospital diet and those on bowel rest. Nevertheless, bowel rest and total parenteral nutrition are believed to be of value in these patients, who often have a poor appetite. Furthermore, it makes it easier to prepare the patient if a colonoscopy is indicated after 5 to 7 days in patients with poor or incomplete response.

Antibiotics

In the original Oxford model, tetracycline was included. However, controlled trials with intravenous metronidazole or intravenous tobramycin in acute severe colitis showed no benefit. On the other hand, in mild to moderately severe attacks, oral vancomycin failed to have a statistically significant effect, and oral tobramycin (120 mg 3 times/d) showed symtomatic remission in 74 percent after 3 to 4 weeks, in comparison to 43 percent in the placebo group. The majority of patients had moderately severe disease. Metronidazole (400 mg orally twice a day) is recommended only in patients with a marked purulent exudation at sigmoidoscopy. There is a chapter on antibiotic use in UC.

5-Aminosalicylic Acid

5-Aminosalicylic acid (5-ASA)-based drugs should be withdrawn during the intensive steroid therapy, because combined use has not been tested in clinical trials.[§§]

Immunosuppressives

Although azathioprine (AZA) and 6-mercaptopurine (6-MP) have not been widely studied in UC, they are being used for unresponsive disease and for maintaining remission. One controlled withdrawal study has supported their use as maintenance therapy, although most of the patients were also on a 5-ASA-based drug.[// //] As AZA and 6-MP take 7 to 16 weeks to achieve a remission, they are not usually considered as treatment for acute colitis but are the treatment of choice after cyclosporine use. Whether intravenous AZA could shorten the response time in UC to 4 weeks has not been proven. One trial in patients with Crohn's disease suggested a 4-week response, whereas another minimized the 4-week response.

[†] Editor's Note: Co-editor SBH describes continuous steroid infusions in his writings. (TMB)

[‡‡] Editor's Note: Concerns about adrenal hemorrhage plus the rarity of patients being admitted before the use of prednisone seemingly have diminished the use of adrenocorticotropic hormone. (TMB)

[§§] Editor's Note: If the patient is able to take oral medications, I tend to continue high-dose mesalamine as well as topical mesalamine or topical corticosteroid. (TMB)

[// //] Editor's Note: The "conventional wisdom" is that it is difficult to withdraw patients with UC from AZA or 6-MP if they really needed it to achieve a remission. (TMB)

Intravenous cyclosporine in a dose of 4 mg/kg body weight has been used in patients who have not improved after 7 to 10 days of corticosteroid therapy. This was supported by a small controlled trial in which 9 of 11 patients responded (82%), compared to 0 of 9 patients who received a placebo. Later uncontrolled studies indicate that 2 mg/kg might be as effective. Other reports suggest that steroids may not be necessary for there to be a response to cyclosporine.

Although cyclosporine is dramatically effective over the short perspective, the risk of side effects must be considered, as well as the long-term benefit. Little is published about the long-term results. The largest series, from Oxford, England, describes 132 patients with severe colitis: 84 did not respond to conventional treatment with corticosteroids and 34 proceeded to colectomy directly. Fifty patients were treated with cyclosporine 4 mg/kg; remission was achieved in 28 (56%), and they were switched to oral cyclosporine (5 mg/kg). The remaining 22 were operated. During a mean follow-up of 19 months, 8 of the 28 responding patients relapsed and had surgery. Thus, during this fairly short observation period, only 40 percent of the cyclosporine-treated patients escaped colectomy. It is likely that 6-MP or AZA would be better for maintenance treatment, as reports indicate that 60 percent of patients who respond to cyclosporine remain in remission.

In Sweden, cyclosporine as rescue therapy in corticosteroid-resistant patients has not been adopted. This is because of the fear that the morbidity and possibly the mortality caused by the drug might be greater than that caused by the disease. Furthermore, modern surgical alternatives work fairly well and also "eliminate" the disease. However, it is fair to state that the quality of life is better in patients with an intact colon than in those who have undergone colectomy.

General Care and Assessment of Response

Beyond the pharmacologic therapy, the patient must be monitored carefully. Temperature and pulse frequency are recorded twice daily. The patient records time of bowel movement, fecal consistency, and blood in feces. Hemoglobin, leukocytes, platelets, C-reactive protein, or erythrocyte sedimentation rate, are measured daily. Corticosteroids can cause leukocytosis and possibly thrombocytosis, which can be confusing.

Palpation and auscultation of the abdomen are done several times each day to note tenderness and to evaluate peristalsis to detect impending dilatation. The physician who is inexperienced with these cases is advised to take daily plain abdominal radiographs. Three or 4 days after initiating therapy, a sigmoidoscopy is of further help in monitoring the response and a biopsy helps to rule out cytomegalovirus.

Assessment of response is made mainly on clinical and laboratory grounds, although repeat plain abdominal radiography during ongoing treatment can show signs of impending perforation or definite toxic dilatation that requires surgery. Several analyses have been made on prognostic factors. An early multivariate analysis of 189 admissions for active colitis showed that a maximum body temperature > 38.0°C during the first 24 hours after admission indicated medical failure in 56 percent, and more than 12 bowel movements in 55 percent (Lennard-Jones et al, 1975). A temperature > 38.0°C on day 4 indicated an 88 percent failure rate. Mucosal islands or dilatation on an abdominal radiograph both indicated a 75 percent failure rate.

A prospective study at Oxford of 51 episodes in 49 patients showed that pancolitis was less common in complete responders (19%) than in incomplete responders (54%) or patients who underwent colectomy (60%). It also confirmed the importance of mucosal islands seen on plain abdominal radiographs

Patients with more than eight bowel movements on day 3 or with three to eight bowel movements and a C-reactive protein level > 45 mg/L had an 85 percent chance of needing a colectomy on the same admission.##

The importance of the extent of disease was shown in a retrospective study with complete clinical and endoscopic remission in 47 percent of patients with total colitis compared to 88 percent in those with less extensive disease (Järnerot et al, 1985). It is possible to predict the likely outcome of corticosteroid treatment on day 3, and then either add cyclosporine or mentally prepare the patient for surgery.

References

Carbonnel F, Lavergne A, Lemann A, et al. Colonoscopy of acute colitis: a safe and reliable tool for assessment of severity. Dig Dis Sci 1994;39:1550–7.

Järnerot G, Rolny P, Sandberg-Gertzén H. Intensive intravenous treatment of ulcerative colitis. Gastroenterology 1985;89:1005–13.

Lennard-Jones JE, Ritchie JK, Hilder W, Spicer CC. Assessment of severity in colitis: a preliminary study. Gut 1975;16:579–84.

Truelove SC, Jewell DP. Intensive intravenous regimen for severe attacks of ulcerative colitis. Lancet 1974;1:1067–70.

Truelove SC, Witts LJ. Cortisone in ulcerative colitis. Final report on a therapeutical trial. BMJ 1955;2:1041–8.

Editor's Note: Persistence in tachycardia, rising sedimentation rate, hypokalemia despite supplementation, hypothermia, and pain requiring narcotics are considered signs of deteriorating condition and of impending perforation. (TMB)

Supplemental Reading

Alemayehu G, Järnerot G. Colonoscopy during an attack of severe ulcerative colitis is a safe procedure and of great value in clinical decision making. Am J Gastroenterol 1991;86:187–90.

Almer S, Bodemar G, Franzén L, et al. Use of air enema radiography to assess depth of ulceration during acute attacks of ulcerative colitis. Lancet 1996;347:1731–5.

Hyde GM, Thillainayagam AV, Jewell DP. Intravenous cyclosporine as rescue therapy in severe ulcerative colitis: time for a reappraisal? Eur J Gastroenterol Hepatol 1998;10:411–3.

Lichtiger S, Present DH, Kornbluth A, Gelernt I. Cyclosporine in severe ulcerative colitis refractory to steroid therapy. N Engl J Med 1994;330:1841–5.

Travis SPL, Farrant JM, Ricketts C, et al. Predicting outcome in severe ulcerative colitis. Gut 1996;38:905–10.

CHAPTER 32

USE OF ANTIBIOTICS AND OTHER ANTI-INFECTIOUS AGENTS IN ULCERATIVE COLITIS

PIERRE MICHETTI, MD, AND MARK A. PEPPERCORN, MD

Abundant evidence suggests that an imbalance between luminal bacteria and the host inflammatory and immune response plays a central role in the pathogenesis of inflammatory bowel disease (IBD). Development of ulcerative colitis (UC) has been observed after enteric infection with *Salmonella, Shigella*, and *Yersinia* species. While these specific pathogens are not considered etiologic agents of UC, a transient infection may initiate a cascade of inflammatory events that, in predisposed individuals, can lead to UC. Similarly, although many enteric pathogens have been associated with relapse of UC, there is no evidence that persistence of these infections is a cause of the disease.

The hypothesis that UC was due to bacteria was an integral part of the rationale of Dr. Nanna Svartz when she developed sulfasalazine. She had observed increased concentrations of diplostreptococci in the feces of patients with UC and rheumatoid arthritis, and reproduced arthritic lesions in rats by injection of streptococci isolated from these patients. When sulfapyridine became available in 1938, Dr. Svartz conceived of combining the sulfa drug, known for its action against streptococci, with a compound that would concentrate in the connective tissues of joints or in the submucosa of the colon.

5-Aminosalicylic acid (5-ASA) was chosen for its tissue tropism action. Sulfasalazine was indeed effective in inducing and maintaining remission of UC; however, the active component of the molecule later was shown to be the 5-ASA, and not the sulfa moiety, and led to the development of new aminosalicylates.

Recent data from genetically engineered rodent models of IBD also suggest a prominent role of the intestinal microflora in both Crohn's disease (CD) and UC. Mice with targeted mutations in various genes encoding cytokines or T lymphocyte markers develop colitis when raised in conventional conditions and colonized with normal intestinal flora. However, these animals do not develop intestinal inflammation when maintained in germ-free conditions. Recent studies in these models have shown that antibiotics that selectively inhibit defined subsets of luminal bacteria prevent colitis. A similar preventive effect was obtained by rectal administration of probiotics or by oral administration of lactulose to favor the growth of lactobacilli.

In recent UC clinical trials, administration of live non-pathogenic *Escherichia coli* or a mixture of bifidobacteria, lactobacilli, and streptococci was equivalent to mesalamine in maintenance of remission. Taken together, these data suggest that the beneficial effect of antibiotics may not result from a long-term reduction in total bacterial load but rather from a qualitative alteration of the resident bacterial population. The recent human data further suggest a role for probiotics in the maintenance therapy for UC patients. This topic is also discussed in the chapter on the role of bacteria in CD and the chapter on pouchitis.

Several randomized controlled trials evaluating antibiotic regimens in patients with active UC gave inconsistent results. The first trial compared vancomycin given for 7 days with placebo in 33 patients with active UC also receiving intravenous prednisolone. The absence of infection, including *Clostridium difficile*, was verified. No overall difference in outcome could be shown, but a trend toward a reduction in the need for colectomy was observed in patients receiving vancomycin. Intravenous metronidazole, as an adjunct to steroids or to sulfasalazine, also failed to improve the outcome in active UC patients.

In contrast to these negative studies, a 1-week course of oral tobramycin was more effective than placebo in a study that included 84 patients. The benefit observed, however, was short-lived. Indeed, in a follow-up study, the patients who entered remission on tobramycin and were maintained on this medication showed a relapse rate comparable to controls. The combination of tobramycin and metronidazole was also disappointing when tested in acute, severe UC patients. Rifaximin, a nonabsorbable form of rifampicin, was shown to improve stool frequency and rectal bleeding in patients with moderate to severe UC, but the global analysis of the patients remained negative. Finally, a short course of ciprofloxacin also failed to improve outcome of patients with acute UC.

Clinical Settings for Possible Antibiotic Use

The lack of antibiotic benefits in randomized trials should not completely preclude their use in the management of selected UC patients. In clinical practice, these drugs may benefit patients with an acute flare of the disease, toxic patients with or without megacolon, and subsets of patients with refractory disease.

Acute Relapse

In selected patients with an acute relapse of disease activity, antibiotics may have a role, as many of these relapses are caused by treatable infectious organisms.* *Clostridium difficile* is the most common pathogen associated with UC relapses. This agent has been reported as a cause of UC relapse even in the absence of recent exposure to antibiotics. In these situations, pseudomembranes may be absent on flexible sigmoidoscopy, and some experts suggest obtaining *C. difficile* culture and toxin assay to rule out infection. Other investigators, however, have been unable to establish a *C. difficile* infection as a cause of UC exacerbations in the absence of recent antibiotic usage.

A careful history is thus still useful to orient the investigations and should cover recent travel history as well as contact with patients with diarrhea. Indeed, other enteric pathogens, including cytomegalovirus (CMV) bacteria and parasites, also can mimic or trigger relapses of UC. We recommend stool samples for bacterial culture, ova and parasites, *C. difficile* toxin and studies for CMV be obtained from all patients with a major flare of UC. These tests should be obtained before a course with systemic steroids is initiated. When very ill patients require steroids before the results of the stool evaluations are available, the authors may initiate coverage with ciprofloxacin and metronidazole. The antibiotics can be withdrawn once the absence of infection is confirmed. In patients who fail to respond to conventional therapy directed at the colitis after 1 week, repeat stool studies for *C. difficile* should be obtained.†

Severe Disease with Toxicity

Severely ill UC patients usually are treated with parenteral corticosteroids in a hospital setting. If these patients have signs of transmural colitis, systemic toxicity, or fulminant colitis with or without megacolon,‡ most "experts" add antibiotics to the treatment regimen, although no controlled trials have confirmed the benefit of antibiotics in this setting. The authors use a combination of intravenous ampicillin, gentamicin, and metronidazole or a third-generation cephalosporin and metronidazole in these patients.

Severe Nontoxic Colitis

In addition, there is a subset of patients with severe disease but no toxic signs who occasionally benefit from antibiotic therapy. As a group, these are patients who have failed to improve after 1 week of high-dose parenteral corticosteroids. Although not toxic, they run a low-grade fever despite steroid therapy, and show excessive bands on peripheral blood smear. We described a series of seven patients in whom broad-spectrum antibiotic therapy with ampicillin, gentamicin, and metronidazole was followed by a striking resolution of diarrhea and rectal bleeding. A simultaneous defervescence and disappearance of the bandemia was observed.

The mechanisms by which antibiotics contribute to the improvement of this subgroup of patients remain unclear. Several situations may contribute to the maintenance of colonic inflammation in severe UC. It is possible that the persisting symptoms were due to unrecognized enteric infection, including *C. difficile* with a false-negative toxin assay. Alternatively, broad-spectrum antibiotic coverage may induce a transient reduction in luminal bacteria antigen production, decrease transmural bacteria translocation, or even treat an unrecognized microperforation. Although the benefit of this strategy has not yet been tested in a prospective study, the authors continue to add antibiotics to the treatment regimen of this type of severe nontoxic UC patient refractory to steroid therapy.§

Chronic Active Ulcerative Colitis

Finally, antibiotics were recently reported, in a less-than-ideal study, to be useful in some outpatients with chronic active UC refractory to conventional therapy. In this study, 83 patients responding poorly to conventional therapy were randomly assigned to therapy with ciprofloxacin or placebo for 6 months. The investigators observed a failure rate of 21 percent in the ciprofloxacin group versus 44 percent with the placebo ($p < .02$), with corresponding endoscopic and histologic improvements. This study suffered from several methodologic flaws and its results should be regarded with caution. The definition of refractory disease was not based on response to therapy but on evaluation by the referring physician, resulting in inclusion of patients with suboptimal pre-entry therapy. As a result, a large proportion of the patients were not on oral mesalamine or steroids at inclusion. Mesalamine therapy was introduced in 70 percent of patients at the time of inclusion and may have confounded the outcome of the study. In addition, the group randomized to ciprofloxacin contained an excess proportion of smokers, which may have contributed to their clinical remissions.

*† Editor's Note: We do not advocate antibiotics for all flare-ups of colitis. The number of exacerbations related to identifiable pathogens remains small. We advocate cultures for pathogens and *C. difficile* for acute flare-ups, after travel to endemic areas, or for patients with exposure to antibiotics. (SBH)

‡ Editor's Note: Transmural and fulminant colitis are inferred from abdominal tenderness, fever leukocytosis, or "thumbprinting" on abdominal radiography. (SBH)

§ Editor's Note: This is not a generally accepted policy. We do not routinely add antibiotics in the absence of transmural or fulminant colitis. (SBH)

Taken together, the results of all of these studies fall short of convincingly demonstrating a benefit of antibiotics in patients with UC. A ciprofloxacin trial, however, may be justified for patients who have failed all other therapies or are steroid-dependent and may be facing colectomy.[//]

Supplemental Reading

Burke DA, Axon ATR, Clayden SA, et al. The efficacy of tobramycin in the treatment of ulcerative colitis. Aliment Pharmacol Ther 1990;4:123–9.

Dickinson RJ, O'Connor HJ, Pinder I, et al. Double-blind controlled trial of oral vancomycin as adjunctive treatment in acute exacerbations of idiopathic colitis. Gut 1985;26:1380–4.

Gionchetti P, Rizzello F, Ferrieri A, et al. Rifaximin in patients with moderate or severe ulcerative colitis refractory to steroid treatment: a double-blind, placebo-controlled trial. Dig Dis Sci 1999;44:1220–1.

Kruis W, Schutz E, Fric P, et al. M Double-blind comparison of an oral *Escherichia coli* preparation and mesalazine in maintaining remission of ulcerative colitis. Aliment Pharmacol Ther 1997;11:853–8.

Mantzaris GJ, Archavlis E, Christoforidis P, et al. Prospective randomized controlled trial of oral ciprofloxacin in acute ulcerative colitis. Am J Gastroenterol 1997;92:454–6.

Mantzaris GJ, Hatzis A, Kontogiannis P, Triantafyllou GA. Intravenous tobramycin and metronidazole as an adjunct to corticosteroids in acute, severe ulcerative colitis. Am J Gastroenterol 1994;89:43–6.

Peppercorn MA. Are antibiotics useful in the management of nontoxic severe ulcerative colitis? J Clin Gastroenterol 1993;17:14–7.

Rembacken BJ, Snelling AM, Hawkey PM, et al. Nonpathogenic *Escherichia coli* versus mesalazine for the treatment of ulcerative colitis: a randomised trial. Lancet 1999;354:635–9.

Svartz N. Sulfasalazine: II. Some notes on the discovery and development of salazopyrin. Am J Gastroenterol 1988;83:497–503.

Turunen UM, Färkkilä MA, Hakala K, et al. Long-term treatment of ulcerative colitis with ciprofloxacin: a prospective, double-blind, placebo-controlled study. Gastroenterology 1998;115:1072–8.

Venturi A, Gionchetti P, Rizzello F, et al. Impact on the composition of the faecal flora by a new probiotic preparation: preliminary data on maintenance treatment of patients with ulcerative colitis. Aliment Pharmacol Ther 1999;13:1103–8.

[//] Editor's Note: Both ciprofloxacin and metronidazole are thought to have some immunosuppressant properties in addition to their anti-bacterient actions. However, a recent trial of a compound similar to ciprofloxacin but without antibiotic activity was reportedly not significantly effective in a trial in IBD patients. Probiotic maintenance therapy of colitis and of pouchitis is receiving increasing attention. (TMB)

CHAPTER 33

Management of Ulcerative Colitis in Children

Harland S. Winter, MD

Inflammatory bowel diseases (IBDs) in children are chronic illnesses with symptoms that wax and wane. Although some children may experience a prolonged remission, many have recurrent exacerbations that require ongoing medical evaluation and therapy. In a recent study, children with ulcerative colitis (UC) were diagnosed more rapidly than children with Crohn's disease (CD); however, in both diseases, a significant time elapsed prior to the start of effective therapy. This delay of over 6 months from the time of onset of symptoms to initiation of treatment indicates that more awareness of these diseases is needed among primary care providers.

Quality of Life

Quality of life is reduced in children with IBD; however, children and adolescents with CD may have different responses to their illness than children with UC. Pediatric patients with UC are more concerned about bowel symptoms, whereas children with CD seem more bothered by changes in body image and the impact of the disease on school function and activities. Although all children with IBD experience frustration, children with UC express more anger and embarrassment. In caring for children with IBD, pediatric gastroenterologists are aware of these psychological patterns and integrate psychosocial support into the treatment plan. Many adolescent who are in remission are unwilling to participate in group activities that focus on discussion of illness, and adolescents whose disease is flaring often feel too ill to attend support groups. Finding the proper way to support the adolescent often is a challenge for the pediatric subspecialist.

The Internet provides such an opportunity. Adolescents often are willing to communicate with others using chat rooms that have been established by organizations such as the Crohn's and Colitis Foundation of America (CCFA). This medium provides the independence and anonymity demanded by most teenagers. Physicians also can use the Internet to communicate with patients in college. Students are well versed in how to use e-mail and feel comfortable contacting their physicians in this way. E-mail provides the clinician with an opportunity not only to adjust medication but also to learn how the student is adjusting to the rigors of school. There are two chapters on dealing with pediatric and teenage patients with IBD and their families.

Pharmacologic Therapy

Deciding which medication to use to induce remission in a child with new-onset UC depends on the severity of the disease. Children who have mild disease characterized by bloody diarrhea or abdominal cramps, without fever, anemia, or hypoalbuminemia, usually respond to sulfasalazine, mesalamine, or olsalazine. The efficacy of sulfasalazine is equivalent to moderate doses of mesalamine, but the toxicity is greater. Untoward events associated with sulfasalazine include headache, anemia, pruritis, fever, bloody diarrhea, neutropenia, thrombocytopenia, and oligospermia. In children, headache often is the most troublesome side effect, but the symptom usually responds to dose reduction. For children who are allergic to sulfa, olsalazine and mesalamine are reasonable alternatives. However, in a blinded trial, children who were treated with olsalazine had a higher rate of diarrhea and eventually required steroid therapy more often than children who received sulfasalazine. Over 90 percent of children with mild disease activity experience resolution of symptoms within 6 months of starting therapy, and over half maintain that remission for 1 year.

Some children with mild disease have inflammation limited to the distal colon and respond to topical therapies. One should suspect distal disease in the child who has blood per rectum, tenesmus, and urgency but a normal sedimentation rate and normal hematocrit. Many adolescents prefer foam products to liquid enemas for delivery of topical corticosteroids. Rectal steroid suppositories also are available. Mesalamine can be delivered in either suppository or enema formulations and is often beneficial in controlling proctitis. Although many adolescents rebel at the thought of rectal administration of medication, discussing the benefits of fewer side effects may enable some to overcome their hesitancy.[*]

---

[*] Editor's Note: Proctitis commonly extends to left-sided or pancolitis in young people. The rapidity of extension and increase in severity can be alarming to all concerned. (TMB)

Moderate to Severe Disease

In contrast to children with mild disease at presentation, about 70 percent of children with moderate to severe disease require corticosteroids in the first year of treatment. Characteristics of moderate to severe disease include more than six bloody stools daily, abdominal cramps, awakening at night to defecate, fever, anemia, or hypoalbuminemia. Most children with these symptoms are started on corticosteroids. The decision whether to use oral or intravenous steroids is made according to the clinical severity of the disease and guided by the patient's ability to tolerate oral medication. Although the value of restricting food and fluid in children has not been evaluated in controlled studies, temporarily eliminating oral nutrition may decrease abdominal cramps and mucosal bleeding by keeping mesenteric blood flow at baseline levels. When intravenous corticosteroids are used, it is at a dose of 1 to 2 mg/kg/d of prednisone divided into two doses (maximum dose 40 mg/d). Keeping the hematocrit over 30 and the serum albumin in the low normal range theoretically may enhance mucosal healing, possibly by decreasing edema and improving delivery of oxygen to the inflamed mucosa.

For the child who does not respond to therapy after 14 days, additional therapeutic interventions should be sought. If the child or family members are reluctant to consider surgery, adding cyclosporine or tacrolimus induces remission in some children who have disease unresponsive to steroids and bowel rest. Most children respond to these potent inhibitors of interleukin (IL)-2 and interferon-gamma (IFN-γ) within 10 days of initiation of treatment; however, with prolonged follow-up, over 50 percent eventually require total colectomy. The addition of 6-mercaptopurine (6-MP) or azathioprine (AZA) may help maintain a long-term remission when immunoregulatory agents are discontinued and corticosteroids are decreased. Newer agents, such as mycophenolate mofetil, have had little usage in the pediatric population.

Maintenance

Mesalamine, sulfasalazine, or olsalazine most often is prescribed for maintenance of remission in children with UC. Although the optimal dosage has not been determined in published pharmacologic trials involving pediatric patients, standard therapy is 50 to 60 mg/kg/d in three or four divided doses of sulfasalazine and 30 to 40 mg/kg/d in three divided doses of mesalamine. Olsalazine produces increased diarrhea in patients; therefore, this medication is used less commonly.

Immunomodulator Therapy

Many children require the addition of an immunoregulatory agent such as AZA or 6-MP to reduce disease activity, sustain remission, and permit corticosteroid reduction. The safety of 6-MP and AZA in children with either UC or CD recently was reviewed by Kirschner (1998). Either medication was well tolerated in over 80 percent of children, and almost 90 percent were able to achieve some degree of prednisone reduction. Nevertheless, the medication was stopped in about one in five children because of hypersensitivity or infectious complications. In another pediatric study, which was restricted to children with UC, 75 percent of patients were able to discontinue corticosteroids with a median time of 8.4 months (Kader et al, 1999). Although the amount of time these patients were followed up after stopping corticosteroids was relatively short, the speculation is that 6-MP or AZA is beneficial in maintaining remission with relatively few side effects. Pancreatitis, leukopenia, and self-limited hepatitis are the most commonly observed side effects. Clinical experience suggests that flares of disease in children treated with 6-MP or AZA may be less severe and may not require prolonged corticosteroids to control. Clearly, for the adolescent population, any medication that avoids or minimizes the use of corticosteroids is to be considered preferable.

Surgical Intervention

The decision to perform a colectomy in a child with UC should be made by the patient, family, and health care providers all working together to reach consensus. Guidelines for treatment of UC in children and adolescents are listed in Table 33–1. In contrast to a condition such as polyposis, UC allows the patient only limited control over how long to wait before consenting to surgical therapy.

Although the function of ileoanal pouches is good, over 11 percent of children experience some complications. In a pediatric series of over 600 children with UC, polyposis, or Hirschsprung's disease, the average number of daily bowel movements 6 months after surgery was 4.8 (Fonkalsrud and Bustorff-Silva, 1999). About 3 percent of children eventually required pouch removal and permanent ileostomy. However, in other series with shorter duration of follow-up, reversal of the pouch is not as frequent and quality-of-life assessment following ileoanal pullthrough is excellent (Shamberger et al, 1999). The main negative factor was the presence of a surgical scar.

Recent advances in surgical techniques in children have permitted restorative proctocolectomy with rectal mucosectomy and hand-sewn ileoanal anastomosis without the placement of a temporary diverting ileostomy. Although experience with this type of procedure is positive, children seem to take longer to recover and adapt to the pouch. However, once the adaptation has occurred, the children are pleased that they can avoid another surgery. The concern about long-term function of pouches made in childhood seems to be unfounded. The

TABLE 33–1. Guidelines for Treatment of Ulcerative Colitis in Children and Adolescents

Proctitis	Topical therapy 5-ASA: enema or suppository Corticosteroids: foam, suppository, or enema
Mild to moderate colitis	Oral aminosalicylates Sulfasalazine 50–60 mg/kg/d divided qid with 1 mg/d folic acid Olsalazine 30–40 mg/kg/d divided tid Mesalamine 30–40 mg/kg/d divided tid Oral corticosteroids 1–2 mg/kg/d, maximum dose 40 mg/d
Severe colitis	Methylprednisolone or prednisone: 1–2 mg/kg/d divided bid po or iv Cyclosporine or tacrolimus Colectomy
Fulminant colitis	Total nutritional support Maintenance of electrolyte balance Avoid anemia or hypoalbuminemia Psychiatric support If no response to treatment of severe colitis, colectomy required
Maintenance	Oral aminosalicylates Sulfasalazine 50–60 mg/kg/d divided qid with 1 mg/d folic acid Olsalazine 30–40 mg/kg/d divided tid Mesalamine 30–40 mg/kg/d divided tid For refractory or steroid-dependent disease: Azathioprine 1.5–2.0 mg/kg/d 6-MP 1.0–1.5 mg/kg/d
Conditions requiring surgery	Intractable symptoms: diarrhea, blood loss Steroid dependency and growth delay Intolerable side effects of corticosteroids Uncontrollable hemorrhage Colonic perforation Carcinoma

5-ASA = 5-aminosalicylic acid; 6-MP = 6-mercaptopurine

question of potential dysplasia is always of concern, but a recent retrospective review of 58 pediatric patients with a mean follow-up of 5 years did not reveal any evidence of dysplasia (Sarigol et al, 1999). There is a chapter on ileal pouch-anal anastomosis (IPAA) in children, one on long-term results with IPAA, and another on dysplasia in pouches.

As surgical techniques improve and more is learned about the adaptation of pouches in growing children, patients and providers will be better prepared with information upon which to base a decision. Some pediatric gastroenterologists believe that offering potent immunosuppression to a child with a disease that is cured by colectomy is wrong. They argue that the potential for

serious complications from prolonged immunosuppression is greater than the risks of surgery. They point to the excellent quality of life most children with ileoanal anastomosis enjoy as evidence to avoid medical therapy that has significant morbidity. As children are followed up and evaluated, these issues will be resolved.

Conclusion

The balance between medical and surgical therapy for UC depends upon the tempo of the disease. In most children, 5-aminosalicylic acid (5-ASA) products are beneficial in maintaining remission. Issues of compliance in the adolescent population require special attention by health care providers. For those pediatric patients in whom surgery becomes an option, the child or adolescent must be an active participant in the decision. The risks of using potent immunosuppressive agents must be balanced against the potential complications of surgery and the possibility for cure.

References
Fonkalsrud EW, Bustorff-Silva J. Reconstruction for chronic dysfunction of ileoanal pouches. Ann Surg 1999; 229:197–204.

Kader HA, Mascarenhas MR, Piccoli DA, et al. Experiences with 6-mercaptopurine and azathioprine therapy in pediatric patients with severe ulcerative colitis. J Pediatr Gastroenterol Nutr 1999;28:54–8.

Kirschner BS. Safety of azathioprine and 6-mercaptopurine in pediatric patients with inflammatory bowel disease. Gastroenterology 1998;115:813–21.

Sarigol S, Wyllie R, Gramlich T, et al. Incidence of dysplasia in pelvic pouches in pediatric patients after ileal pouch-anal anastomosis for ulcerative colitis. J Pediatr Gastroenterol Nutr 1999;28:429–34.

Shamberger RC, Masek BJ, Leichtner AM, et al. Quality-of-life assessment after ileoanal pull-through for ulcerative colitis and familial adenomatous polyposis. J Pediatr Surg 1999;34:163–6.

Supplemental Reading
Dolgin SE, Shlasko E, Gorfine S, et al. Restorative proctocolectomy in children with ulcerative colitis utilizing rectal mucosectomy with or without diverting ileostomy. J Pediatr Surg 1999;34:837–9.

Griffiths AM, Nichols D, Smith C, et al. Development of a quality-of-life index for pediatric inflammatory bowel disease: dealing with differences related to age and IBD type. J Pediatr Gastroenterol Nutr 1999;28:S46–52.

Heikenen JB, Werlin SL, Brown CW, Balint JP. Presenting symptoms and diagnostic lag in children with inflammatory bowel disease. Inflamm Bowel Dis 1999;5:159–60.

CHAPTER 34

INDETERMINATE COLITIS

RICHARD P. MACDERMOTT, MD

The vast majority of patients with inflammatory bowel disease (IBD) can be classified as having either ulcerative colitis (UC) or Crohn's disease (CD). However, approximately 10 to 15 percent of patients are not readily characterized and are diagnosed as having indeterminate colitis, until the natural course of the disease makes it more clear whether either UC or CD is the actual disease entity. Indeterminate colitis is most commonly associated with patients with acute colitis, due to either severe UC or severe Crohn's colitis, because of the extensive nonspecific mucosal damage that occurs with intense colonic inflammation.

A definitive diagnosis of UC or CD also can be elusive in patients who have features suggestive of CD, such as inflammation of the terminal ileum and/or features inconsistent with classic UC, such as rectal sparing. Patients with UC may have mild involvement of a small portion of the terminal ileum (backwash ileitis). Relative rectal sparing can be seen in patients with UC who have received rectal 5-aminosalicylic acid (5-ASA) or steroid enemas and patients with UC also can have perirectal disease. Either UC or CD can present with intestinal bleeding. Pseudopolyps can be seen in patients with either longstanding UC or Crohn's colitis. In some patients who come to urgent colectomy, pathologic examination of the resected colon may not be diagnostic of either UC or CD. Granulomas are the hallmark of CD, but in a small number of patients with UC, granulomas can be found. Pathologic interpretation also can be confounded by the fact that transmural inflammation occasionally can be seen in very severe UC. Thus, the clinical criteria by which the diagnosis of UC or Crohn's colitis is made are not absolute. Because of this, patients whose diagnosis is unclear are classified as having indeterminate colitis.

Clinical Characteristics

The incidence of indeterminate colitis in southeastern Norway has been evaluated by Moum and colleagues, who determined that in a 3-year period, there were 525 new cases of ulcerative colitis and 93 new cases of indeterminate colitis. This resulted in an annual incidence rate of 13.6/100,000 for UC and 2.4/100,000 for indeterminate colitis. Stewenius et al determined that the average annual incidence of definite or probable UC in Malmo, Sweden,

was 7.3/100,000 while that of indeterminate colitis was 1.6/100,000. They observed a relapse rate within 10 years of diagnosis of 70 percent for definite UC and 77 percent for indeterminate colitis. These studies indicate that indeterminate colitis occurs in small but nevertheless significant numbers and has a relapse rate similar to UC.

The natural history of indeterminate colitis has been evaluated by Wells et al, who followed a group of 46 patients with a pathologic diagnosis of indeterminate colitis made by examination of resected colon. Seventy-five percent of the indeterminate colitis patients had undergone an urgent colectomy (either partial or complete). By taking all preoperative clinical and diagnostic features into account, 19 patients could be classified as having CD and 11 as having UC. This left 16 of 46 patients with a pathologic diagnosis of indeterminate colitis who also were classified clinically as having indeterminate colitis. These 16 patients were followed for a minimum of 2.5 years and a median of 10 years, during which time three patients were reclassified as having UC, and one patient as having CD, and 12 remained classified as having indeterminate colitis. Kangas et al followed six patients who had both a preoperative clinical as well as a postoperative pathologic diagnosis of indeterminate colitis. After a median follow-up of 5.5 years, three of the six patients were reclassified as having CD, while the other three patients remained classified as having indeterminate colitis. Even after careful clinical and diagnostic evaluation, complete pathologic examination, and long-term follow-up, a small subgroup of patients remain who have IBD of the colon, which cannot be categorized as either UC or Crohn's colitis.

Overall Approach to the Patient with Indeterminate Colitis

Indeterminate colitis most likely represents either UC or Crohn's colitis.[*] Therefore, any therapy that is effective in either UC or CD may prove useful in the treatment of indeterminate colitis. The choice of therapy will depend upon the extent and severity of the indeterminate colitis.

---

[*] Editor's Note: Having seen families with indeterminate colitis, I think this may be a separate disorder. (TMB)

If medically induced remission cannot be achieved and maintained, then a colectomy should be considered.

Medical Treatment of Indeterminate Colitis

Mild Distal Indeterminate Colitis

Although distal colitis usually is ulcerative proctitis or ulcerative proctosigmoiditis, distal colitis also can be an early manifestation of CD. Therefore, distal colitis, in some patients, may initially be indeterminate in nature. Topical 5-ASA enemas and/or suppositories are the therapy of choice for proctitis and proctosigmoiditis, because of their ability to both induce and maintain remission as well as their low side-effect profile. Topical steroid preparations in the form of suppositories, foams, and enemas also are very effective in treating indeterminate proctitis and proctosigmoiditis. Topical steroids, in contrast to topical 5-ASA products, are only moderately effective in maintaining distal indeterminate colitis remission. Details of therapy of distal colitis, including oral mesalamine, are given in separate chapters.

Moderately Active Indeterminate Colitis

Although oral steroids can be very effective in moderately active indeterminate colitis, there is no proven benefit of oral steroids in maintaining remission in colitis. Steroid-dependent and/or steroid-refractory patients are at a high risk for long-term steroid side effects and every effort must be made to find a way to treat their indeterminate colitis without steroids.

The use of 5-ASA products is very important in patients with moderately active indeterminate colitis, because many patients can achieve both induction and maintenance of remission through the optimal use of oral and topical 5-ASA products. Because many patients with indeterminate colitis eventually prove to have UC, sulfasalazine is appropriate for use in moderately active indeterminate colitis. Sulfasalazine often takes 4 to 6 weeks to effectively control colonic inflammation. After 5 to 6 months of therapy, when the indeterminate colitis is in remission, a maintenance dose of 3 to 4 g per day can be used. Details of sulfasalazine therapy are presented in a separate chapter.

Oral mesalamine (5-ASA) preparations (Asacol®, Procter & Gamble Pharmaceuticals, Cincinnati, Ohio; Pentasa®, Ferring-Shire Pharmaceuticals Inc., Florence, Kentucky) have proven to be of benefit in inducing and maintaining remission in UC. For patients with moderately active indeterminate colitis, the oral mesalamine agents need to be used in high doses to achieve maximal effect. The effective daily dose ranges usually are 3.6 to 4.8 g for Asacol and 3 to 4 g for Pentasa, given in 3 to 4 divided doses per day. Once a successful therapeutic effect

has been achieved, usually in 6 to 8 weeks, the dosage of oral mesalamine used to achieve remission should be continued in the same range in order to maintain remission. In patients with chronic refractory indeterminate proctitis, indeterminate proctosigmoiditis, or left-sided indeterminate colitis, optimal doses of both oral mesalamine combined with 5-ASA enemas and/or suppositories may be needed in order to successfully provide maximal topical 5-ASA delivery throughout the colon.

5-Aminosalicylic acid agents are effective at maintaining medical remission and preventing relapses, but only if the patient continues to take the 5-ASA medications in optimal dosages. Details of mesalamine therapy are presented in chapters on UC management.

The value of antibiotics has been demonstrated in treating CD. Because many patients with indeterminate colitis eventually turn out to have CD, it is appropriate to treat active indeterminate colitis patients with antibiotics. Metronidazole (Flagyl) can be effective in inducing remission in active Crohn's colitis. Ciprofloxacin has been used successfully in the treatment of both CD and UC with improvement in symptoms. Prantera and his colleagues have shown that ciprofloxacin 500 mg twice daily plus metronidazole 250 mg 4 times daily led to clinical remission in up to 46 percent of patients with active refractory CD. Therefore, this combination may be useful in patients with moderately active indeterminate colitis.

Steroid-Refractory, Steroid-Dependent Chronic Indeterminate Colitis

6-Mercaptopurine (6-MP), Purinethol, and azathioprine (Imuran) have been used successfully for over 30 years in patients with either UC or Crohn's colitis who are refractory to standard therapy and who have not been able to taper off their corticosteroids. Both have also proven to be effective in maintaining remission in UC and Crohn's colitis. It is very appropriate to use immunomodulators in treating steroid-refractory, steroid-dependent indeterminate colitis. These agents often take 3 to 4 months to demonstrate their full effect, although some patients respond more quickly. Once a desired therapeutic effect is achieved, Imuran or Purinethol usually are continued for 3 to 4 years, before gradual reduction of the dose for long-term maintenance. There are chapters on immunomodulator therapy in distal colitis, UC and Crohn's colitis.

Infliximab (Remicade®, Centocor Inc., Malvern, Pennsylvania) is a monoclonal antibody directed against tumor necrosis factor-alpha (TNF-α) and recently approved for the therapy of CD. The infusion of infliximab leads to a marked reduction of CD activity within 4 weeks. The effect of a single infusion of infliximab lasts at least 8 weeks and in some cases longer. A multicenter international trial of infliximab demonstrated that 5 mg/kg dose resulted in 81 percent of the CD patients having a good clinical response, and 48 percent of the patients achieving clinical remission within 4 weeks. Because indeterminate colitis often ultimately turns out to be CD, it seems appropriate to use Remicade in chronic steroid-refractory, steroid-dependent, indeterminate colitis patients who have not responded to conventional therapy. It should be emphasized that one of the initial goals is to taper the patient off steroids. Therefore, if there is an adequate response to infliximab, steroids should gradually be reduced and eventually stopped. It is possible that repeated infusions of Remicade will be needed to maintain responses. The role of other medications to aid in long-term remission maintenance may include 6-MP, Imuran, or methotrexate as well as the 5-ASA products. Information on anti-TNF therapy is detailed in a separate chapter. Whether patients with indeterminant colitis will respond similarly to some patients with Crohn's colitis remains to be determined.

Severe Acute Indeterminate Colitis

Patients with severe acute colitis require hospitalization whether or not the exact nature of the colitis has been determined. At the time of admission, evaluation by surgery is mandatory because 20 to 30 percent of severely ill patients with acute colitis will ultimately require a colectomy. Details of management of severe fulminant colitis are presented in separate chapters, including a discussion of cyclosporine therapy.

Subtotal Colectomy Specimen Diagnoses

Because of deep transmural ulceration that occurs with fulminant colitis, pathologists will not uncommonly be unable to place the patient in a specific category, that is, UC or Crohn's colitis. These patients are classified as indeterminate colitis. Many of the difficult decisions as to use of an ileoanal pouch anastomosis or the possibility of ileal recurrence and the need for prophylactic therapy arise in this group of patients.

Implications of a Diagnosis of Indeterminate Colitis

Many patients with indeterminate colitis require a colectomy either due to severe acute colitis refractory to therapy or steroid-dependent, steroid-refractory colitis. Koltun and colleagues evaluated 288 patients who had undergone ileal pouch-anal anastomosis. Of 235 patients with chronic UC, only 8 (3%) experienced complications requiring operative therapy. In contrast, of 18 patients with indeterminate colitis, 9 (50%) experienced complications requiring an operative procedure. McIntyre et al observed a higher failure rate following ileal pouch-anal anastomosis in patients with indeterminate colitis (19%) than in patients with chronic UC (8%). Similar findings were made by Atkinson et al who observed a success rate for restorative proctocolectomy of 95 percent in patients with UC, but only 81 percent in patients with indeterminate colitis. These studies have led to the conclusion that patients with indeterminate colitis are more likely to have perianal complications and a higher likelihood of pouch failure following ileal pouch-anal anastomosis. Some surgeons prefer to perform an ileorectal anastamosis in such patients. This is discussed in the surgery section of this text.

The role of colonoscopic surveillance for dysplasia in order to detect colons at a high risk of developing colorectal cancer is well documented for UC. The risk with Crohn's colitis is high enough that surveillance is being utilized in those patients as well. Stewenius and colleagues observed an incidence of colorectal cancer in UC of 1.4/1000 person years and an incidence of colorectal cancer in indeterminate colitis of 2.4/1000 person years. Therefore, patients with indeterminate colitis involving either the entire colon or the left colon are at the same increased risk for developing colonic cancer as are UC patients and so should be included in a surveillance program.

Conclusion

Indeterminate colitis is a type of IBD involving the colon that cannot be definitively categorized as either UC or CD. Indeterminate colitis may be merely part of a spectrum, somewhere in between UC and CD. However, it is also possible that indeterminate colitis in the setting of a continued diagnosis of indeterminate colitis after long-term follow-up is a separate disease process, which should be categorized as a specific type of IBD. Therapeutic approaches useful for indeterminate colitis are similar to those for UC or Crohn's colitis. Once medically induced remission has been achieved, long-term medical maintenance of remission for indeterminate colitis includes oral and rectal mesalamine and/or immunomodulators (6-mercaptopurine or Imuran). Although a diagnosis of indeterminate colitis is not an absolute contraindication to an ileal pouch-anal anastomosis, both patient and physician should be aware of the increased risk of complications and the lower success rate that can occur. Patients with indeterminate colitis should undergo yearly or bi-yearly colonoscopic surveillance beginning 8 years after the initial onset of disease symptoms.

Supplemental Reading

Atkinson KG, Owen DA, Wankling G. Restorative proctocolectomy and indeterminate colitis. Am J Surg 1994;167: 516–8.

Kangas E, Matikainen M, Matilla J. Is indeterminate colitis Crohn's disease in the long-term follow-up? Int Surg 1994;79:120–3.

Koltun WA, Schoetz DJ, Roberts PL, et al. Indeterminate colitis predisposes to perineal complications after ileal pouch-anal anastomosis. Dis Colon Rectum 1991;34:857–60.

McIntyre PB, Pemberton JH, Wolff BG, et al. Indeterminate colitis: long-term outcome in patients after ileal pouch-anal anastomosis. Dis Colon Rectum 1995;38:51–4.

Moum B, Vatn MH, Ekbom A, et al. Incidence of ulcerative colitis and indeterminate colitis in four counties of southeastern Norway, 1990–93. Scand J Gastroenterol 1996;31:362–6.

Peppercorn MA. Antibiotics are effective therapy for Crohn's disease. Inflamm Bowel Dis 1997;3:318–9.

Prantera C, Zannoni F, Scribano ML, et al. An antibiotic regimen for the treatment of active Crohn's disease: a randomized, controlled clinical trial of metronidazole plus ciprofloxacin. Am J Gastroenterol 1996;91:328–32.

Stewenius J, Adnerhill I, Anderson H, et al. Incidence of colorectal cancer and all cause mortality in non-selected patients with ulcerative colitis and indeterminate colitis in Malmo, Sweden. Int J Colorectal Dis 1995;10:117–22.

Stewenius J, Adnerhill I, Ekelund G, et al. Ulcerative colitis and indeterminate colitis in the city of Malmo, Sweden. A 25-year incidence study. Scand J Gastroenterol 1995;30:38–43.

Stewenius J, Adnerhill I, Ekelund G, et al. Risk of relapse in new cases of ulcerative colitis and indeterminate colitis. Dis Colon Rectum 1996;39:1019–25.

Wells AD, McMillan I, Price AB, et al. Natural history of indeterminate colitis. Br J Surg 1991;78:179–81.

CHAPTER 35

Dietary Recommendations for Active and Inactive Ulcerative Colitis

Geoffrey Gibson, MD

This chapter discusses the role of diet and nutritional support in ulcerative colitis (UC) in which the catabolic effect (breakdown or loss of body tissue) of inflammation, impaired nutrient absorption, and gastrointestinal (GI) dysfunction can rapidly lead to malnutrition.

Inactive Ulcerative Colitis

Inactive UC is a chronic disorder and may be associated with malnutrition, specific elemental deficiencies, and specific food intolerances.

Inadequate Intake

Patients may not eat enough to meet their nutritional requirements because of anorexia, drug side effects (eg, nausea, headache, and anorexia), food-induced diarrhea, or pain. Specific elemental deficiencies necessitating oral replacement include iron deficiency, secondary to blood loss; folate deficiency associated with sulfasalazine therapy; calcium deficiency, associated with steroid usage; and dietary restriction (eg, avoidance of dairy products).

Lactose Intolerance

Failure of absorption of lactose allows colonic bacteria to produce short-chain fatty acids, particularly acetate, butyrate, and propionate, and release of hydrogen. In lactose-intolerant people, production of hydrogen produces bloating, nausea, and flatulence and unabsorbed short-chain fatty acids produce diarrhea. Lactose intolerance may be primary (racial or congenital) or secondary (eg, due to bacterial overgrowth or intestinal mucosal disease or injury). The incidence of lactose intolerance varies widely among races and ethnicities (Table 35–1).

The incidence of UC is not increased in lactose intolerant people, and the incidence of lactose intolerance is not increased in patients with UC. In quiescent disease, lactose restriction is important to control symptoms only in those patients documented to have lactose intolerance, presumably on a genetic basis.

Short-Chain Fatty Acids

It has been demonstrated that short-chain fatty acids, particularly butyrate, are the main source of energy for colonocytes. The suggestion is that in UC there is an impairment within the mitochondria of colonocyte oxidation of short-chain fatty acids, particularly butyrate.

TABLE 35–1. Incidence of Lactose Intolerance in Healthy Individuals of Various Races and Ethnicities

Race or Ethnicity	Incidence (%)
Scandinavian	5
Western European	7–20
Hispanic	50
Ashkenazi Jew	70
Mediterranean	70
African or African American	70–90
Native American	80–90
Asian	90–95

Whereas it has been demonstrated that patients with localized proctitis, with mild activity, respond in placebo-controlled studies to butyrate enemas, there have been no scientific studies demonstrating any advantage of altered oral intake of fat in the treatment of inactive UC. However, clinical experience would suggest that reduction of oral intake of fat may be associated with some lessening of diarrhea. This may be of particular importance for patients who have undergone cholecystectomy, for those consuming large quantities of poorly absorbed fats (eg, olestra) for the purpose of dieting, and for those with a coexistent irritable bowel syndrome.

Low-Sulfide Diet

Sulfide is required for anaerobic bacteria to produce short-chain fatty acids such as butyrate. Reduced sulfides inhibit oxidation of butyrate in the mitochondria of the colonocytes, with accumulation of butyrate for cellular energy production. Sulfides appear to act at both a luminal and an intracellular level. In UC, levels of anionic sulfide may be elevated, and these patients have more hydrogen sulfide in fecal samples than control cases.

Institution of a low-sulfide diet in patients with inactive UC may be beneficial in reducing recurrence of disease (Table 35–2). Although controlled, double-blind trials are needed, the author's clinical impression is of an improvement in disease and possibly a reduction of recurrence in patients who adhere to this diet.[*]

---

[*] Editor's Note: The author is providing an "impression" and emphasizes the need for clinical trial data to support this concept. (SBH)

TABLE 35–2. Stipulations of a Low-Sulfide Diet*

Avoid Completely	Diminish	Use
Eggs	Red meat	Chicken
Cheese		Fish
Whole milk		Skimmed milk
Ice cream		All other vegetables and complex fiber
Mayonnaise		
Cruciferous vegetables		
Cabbage		
Broccoli		
Cauliflower		
Brussel sprouts		
Sulfite		
Wines		
Cordials		
Dried fruit		

*A low-sulfide diet is designed to diminish the intake of sulfur-containing amino acids, which when ingested in excess are transferred back into the intestine where toxic sulfides may form.

It has been suggested that withdrawal of foods that are high in sulfides (eg, milk, eggs, and cheese) confers a therapeutic benefit on UC patients. Institution of a sulfide-reduced diet is associated with clinical improvement about 6 weeks after initiation of the diet. This is a restrictive diet to most people in Western society. It is important that medication be continued coincidentally with institution of the diet.

Dietary Fiber

Fiber is a nutrient produced by breads, cereals, and fruit and vegetables. Dietary fiber is the component of plant and vegetable food that is not digested in the human intestine. There are two types of fiber: (1) lignins and cellulose from cereals (especially wheat) and (2) pectins and gums from fruits, vegetables, and oats.

In the human colon, lignins and cellulose produce a bulky soft stool by reducing reabsorption of water in the colon. When the bowel is acutely inflamed, fiber intake should be limited. However, patients with proctitis and minimal distal disease need to have fiber as part of the regimen to prevent constipation.

There is no therapeutic role for dietary fiber in inactive disease, but an adequate diet containing fiber and fluid are recommended to maintain regular bowel function either in patients with inactive disease or in those entering a period of recovery from more active disease.

Plantago ovata seeds are degraded in fecal homogenates to yield butyrate and acetate and, theoretically, could be of benefit for the treatment of UC. The Spanish group for the study of Crohn's disease and UC suggested that 10 g of *Plantago ovatum* twice a day was equally as effective as mesalamine (500 mg 3 times a day) for maintaining remission of UC (Fernandez-Banares et al, 1999). It should be noted that psyllium husk (ispaghula) consists only of the epidermis of dried *P. ovata* seeds, and theoretically, whole seeds should be preferable to psyllium as a form of dietary fiber. This interesting study needs to be repeated, and further studies on the role of fiber need to be performed so that more definitive recommendations can be made.

Fish Oils

Although possibly of some value in acute disease, the role, if any, of fish oils in preventive therapy in inactive disease has not been established.

Enteral or Parenteral Feeding

The aim of nutritional therapy is to prevent or treat malnutrition, and these therapies play no role in inactive disease.

Active Ulcerative Colitis

Active UC involves pathologic and physiologic changes both within the colonic mucosa and systemically. The colonic mucosa is inflamed and associated with loss of fluid, electrolytes, proteins and immunoglobulins, albumin, and hemoglobin.

Systemic manifestations of fever and anorexia are associated with reduced oral intake of nutrients. However, the body is in a catabolic state, with increased nutritional requirements and increased energy needs as a result of fever, associated infections, and steroid therapy. In these situations, nutritional support is essential. In such cases, parental or enteral nutrition not only may be of value but may be essential in patient management.

Specific Elemental Deficiency

Adequate caloric intake may be achieved by a high intake of carbohydrate and fat, but, as mentioned, an increase of dietary fat may exacerbate diarrhea and abdominal pain. It is difficult to increase dietary fat in patients who have severe anorexia due to resulting decreases in the rate of gastric emptying. Iron and nutritional supplements are necessary to compensate for blood loss and increased erythropoeitic activity, but the side effects of iron given orally, such as abdominal pain or diarrhea, may limit its use.

Deficiency of zinc, calcium, folic acid, electrolytes, and protein may be acute and severe. Replacement is essential, either orally or by intravenous infusion. Transfusion of blood and blood products may be necessary.

Lactose

If there is a history of, or question regarding, lactose intolerance, restriction of milk products is advisable and should continue for at least 6 weeks.

Short-Chain Fatty Acids

There is no proven indication for the use of short-chain fatty acids in acute or active colitis, and their limited role in the form of rectal enemas in inactive or localized proctitis previously has been discussed.

Low-Sulfide Diet

In active colitis, there is almost certainly accelerated mitochondrial oxidation of butyrate and reduced energy production in the colonocytes. Increasing the intraluminal substrate, using short-chain fatty acid enemas, gives a variable response, but it has been noted that an increase in dietary and, hence, luminal sulfide significantly reduces mitochondrial oxidation of butyrate. The institution of a low-sulfide diet and avoidance of lactose, as previously suggested, are an adjunct to drug therapy and nutritional support, but should *not* be envisaged as an *alternative* to drug therapy.[†]

Fiber

Fiber increases stool bulk and softens the stool by reducing water absorption by the colon. In fulminant or severe active colitis, total colonic rest is thought to be important and fiber is contraindicated.

As the colon recovers and stool frequency decreases, the introduction of small amounts of fiber, such as ispagula, may reduce stool frequency and fluid loss. However, no advantages of the use of soluble or insoluble fiber have been demonstrated with clinical trials.

Parenteral Nutrition

More than 25 years ago, it was observed that Crohn's disease refractory to medical therapy improved with bowel rest and total parenteral nutrition (TPN), as assessed by both nutritional status and disease symptoms. However, in 1980, 20 patients with acute severe UC were given either oral feeding or TPN while continuing intravenous corticosteroids; TPN did not appear to offer any therapeutic advantages (Dickinson et al, 1980). A subsequent study from St. Mark's Hospital in London and Rouen, France, compared oral feeding with total bowel rest and TPN in 27 patients on 60 mg daily of intravenous prednisolone (McIntyre et al, 1986). Again, as judged by the necessity for colectomy and clinical recovery, bowel rest offered no advantage.

Many subsequent studies have failed to demonstrate any therapeutic effect of parenteral nutrition in UC, but the above-mentioned studies and others confirmed a significant nutritional benefit in these patients. It must be noted that there is a significant increased risk of major sepsis in these sick patients with UC on steroids and parenteral nutrition.

Enteral Nutrition

Enteral nutrition refers to a liquid formula diet taken orally or by nasoenteric feeding. These diets may be

---

[†] Editor's Note: The concepts should be considered personal recommendations and have not been tested in controlled trials. (SBH)

elemental (nitrogen as free amino acids), oligomeric (nitrogen as specific short peptides), or polymeric (nitrogen as whole proteins). The amount of fat and medium-chain triglyceride (MCT) may also be varied.

Enteral feeding is expensive but does not have the serious septic side effects associated with parenteral nutrition. The dosage is limited by diarrhea and nausea, the latter associated with delayed gastric emptying. Enteral nutrition is effective as a nutritional supplement where oral nutrition fails, but there is no evidence that enteral nutrition has any therapeutic value in the treatment of active UC. In fulminant UC, in which the patient often requires surgery, enteral nutrition is an important adjunct to drug and surgical therapy, particularly during the perioperative period.

Fish Oils

Several investigations have studied the therapeutic effect of dietary fish oils in experimental colitis in rats and hamsters. In many of these studies, oils containing eicosapentaenoic acid attenuated colitis, suggesting that fish oils may be involved in the maintenance of the integrity of the mucosal cell membrane or in suppression of the inflammatory response. In humans, a diet of high n-3 fatty acids (alpha-linolenic acid) produced a reduction in blood mononuclear cell TNF and interleukin production. In a controlled clinical study in patients with UC, Aslan and Triadasilopoulos (1992) observed a 53 percent reduction in disease activity in refractory UC, compared with 4 percent in controls, when these patients were fed fish oil fatty acids. No known studies have confirmed the above findings; further studies are needed before this therapy can be recommended. This therapy also is subject to poor compliance due to side effects and a fishy odor.

Exclusion Diets

Some adults have a degree of intolerance to naturally occurring chemicals and additives in foods. In such cases, excessive intake of these substances may cause pain, nausea, bloating, diarrhea, and other gastrointestinal symptoms. Symptoms usually are of sudden onset and transient. Although chemicals, such as salicylates, monosodium glutamate (MSG), flavor enhancers, preservatives, food coloring, and others certainly cause asthma, migraine, and gastrointestinal symptoms, they do not cause inflammatory bowel disease. Exclusion diets play no role in the therapy of UC.

Alternative Medicine

This discussion would not be complete without reference to alternative medical therapy instituted particularly by patients, physicians, chiropractors, pharmacists, natural therapists, iridologists, and others. There is a separate chapter on alternative medicine. Many of these therapies are herbal, such as slippery elm, Swedish Bitters, marshmallow root, horseradish root, ginger, ginseng, St. John's wort, and others. Many of these may contain naturally occurring salicylates, and, certainly, some patients do seem to derive significant clinical benefit from these therapies. In Chinese and Asian culture, herbs have been used for centuries, and physicians should respect this culture. In the author's clinical practice, such therapy is not discouraged; however, it is essential that patients both inform their physician of the therapy and agree to continue the medication that has been prescribed.

Yogurt, acidophilus, lactobacillus, and other related products are widely used by patients with chronic UC. Unless allergy to milk protein is suspected, patients may continue these therapies. Soy-based products are discouraged because of the high sulfide content. Antioxidants and evening primrose oil also are widely used.

Further studies need to be done on a scientific basis before physicians are able to confidently assure and advise patients of the role of these therapies in UC, their benefits, and their disadvantages. The chapter on alternative approaches does provide additional information.

References

Aslan A, Triadasilopoulos G. Fish oil fatty acid supplementation in active ulcerative colitis. Am J Gastroenterol 1992; 87:432–7.

Dickinson RJ, Ashton MG, Axon ATR, et al. Controlled trial of intravenous hyperelementation and total bowel rest as an adjunct to routine therapy in acute colitis. Gastroenterology 1980;79:1999–204.

Fernandez-Banares F, Hinojoso J, Sanchez-Lombrana JL, et al. Randomized clinical trial of *Plantago ovata* seeds (dietary fiber) as compared with mesalamine in maintaining remission in ulcerative colitis. Am J Gastroenterol 1999; 94:2:427–33.

McIntyre PB, Powell-Tuck J, Wood SR, et al. Controlled trial of bowel rest in the treatment of severe acute colitis. Gut 1986;27:481–4.

Supplemental Reading

Bayless TM, Rosenswerg NS. A racial difference in incidence of lactase deficiency. A survey of milk intolerance and lactase deficiency in healthy adult males. JAMA 1966;197:968–72.

Grisham MB, DeMichele SJ, Garleb KA, et al. Sulphasalazine or enteral diets containing fish oil or oligo-saccharides attenuate chronic colitis in rats. Inflamm Bowel Dis 1996;2:178–98.

Hallert C, Kaldma M, Petersson BG. Ispaghula husk may relieve gastrointestinal symptoms in ulcerative colitis in remission. Scand J Gastroenterol 1991;26:747–50.

Paige DM, Bayless TM, Huang SS, Weber R. Lactose hydrolyzed milk. Am J Clin Nutr 1975;28:818–22.

Wright R, Truelove SC. A controlled therapeutic trial of various diets in ulcerative colitis. BMJ 1965;2:138–41.

Yernia P, Cittadini M, Caprilli R, Torsoli A. Topical treatment of refractory distal colitis with 5-ASA and sodium butyrate. Dig Dis Sci 1995;40:305–7.

CHAPTER 36

Novel Manipulations of Inflammatory Mediator Pathways

Bruce R. Yacyshyn, MD, FRCPC, FACG

Advancing knowledge of inflammatory mediator pathways is providing new options for management of Crohn's disease (CD) and ulcerative colitis (UC).* Compounds currently completing late-stage clinical trials in UC and CD can be divided into three groups: *cytokines*, including interleukin (IL)-10 and, potentially, IL-12 and IL-11; *anti-adhesion molecules*, including antisense to intracellular adhesion molecule-1 (ICAM-1) and monoclonal antibodies to integrins β_7 and $\alpha_4\beta_7$; and *anti-cytokine therapies*, such as infliximab or etanercept that target tumor necrosis factor-α (TNF-α).

Four new biologic agents recently have been approved: two antibodies to the IL-2 receptor, for prophylaxis of acute renal transplant rejection (daclizumab, Zenapax®, Roche Laboratories Inc., Nutley, New Jersey; basiliximab, Simulect®, Novartis Pharmaceutical Corp., East Hanover, New Jersey); a TNF-α chimeric antibody (infliximab, Remicade®, Centocor Inc., Malvern, Pennsylvania), for CD; and a TNF-α p75 receptor-IgG1Fc fusion protein (etanercept, Enbrel®, Immunex Corp., Seattle, Washington), for rheumatoid arthritis. These new agents offer the potential for more effective and specific therapy and less toxicity. Their individual and collective definitive assessment of safety and efficacy awaits more extensive and long-term clinical experience.

Another theoretic approach to therapy has focused on the role of leukapheresis in the treatment of inflammatory bowel disease (IBD). This aspect of IBD therapy proposes removal of T cells from the circulation. In contrast, another potential approach to treatment of IBD invokes parasites or vaccines to skew the T-helper (Th) cell response (Figure 36–1). This mechanism also may have therapeutic applications by using probiotic bacteria, such as *Lactobacillus* or nonpathogenic *Escherichia coli* to modify the immune response. Finally, the role of the coagulation cascade as an arm of the inflammatory pathway has been well described. There are ongoing studies in UC with heparin as a novel method of interrupting the immune-coagulation pathway.

---

* Editor's Note: The reader is referred to a millennial review of the therapy of IBD by Sands. Gastroenterology 2000;118: S68–82. (TMB)

Agents Influencing Inflammatory Response

Probiotic Effects

It is hypothesized that bacteria are important regulators of the immune response in IBD, functioning both as initiators of inflammation and as regulators and potential therapeutic delivery systems. Recent work has shown that nonpathogenic *E. coli* may have benefits similar to those of mesalamine in the treatment of UC. Administration of *E. coli* strain Nissle 1917 induced clinical remission in 39 (68%) of 57 patients taking a 2.5×10 bacteria per capsule dose of two tablets a day compared to 44 (75%) of 59 patients who received 800 mg of mesalamine twice a day. The mean time to remission was comparable, 42 days and 44 days, respectively. The downregulation of inflammation may be secondary to the "probiotic effect," that is, ingestion of a living organism to favorably affect the health of a host.

As the effector cell of the immune response in IBD is the T lymphocyte, one rational approach to modify the inflammatory response is to remove the T-cell population from the periphery. The removal of T-effector cells results in clinical improvement in other conditions. T-cell apheresis was championed by Bicks as a method to decrease active inflammation in CD. His chapter in the first edition of this text documents his pioneering work. More recently, investigators, primarily in Japan, have described clinical benefits from leukacytapheresis therapy for UC.

T-Lymphocyte Manipulation

To assess the ingestion of the worm *Trichuris suis* to reduce inflammation in patients with UC or CD, researchers administered 2,500 worm eggs to patients orally. Improvement was noted in clinical indexes of both UC and CD, with no adverse effects. Although the exact mechanism of this response is uncertain, it is hypothesized to normalize the Th response in the inflammation of both diseases. However, because CD and UC have discordant Th responses (CD is Th1, and UC is most consistent with a Th2 response), it is unknown how these differing immune responses could both be resolved. In

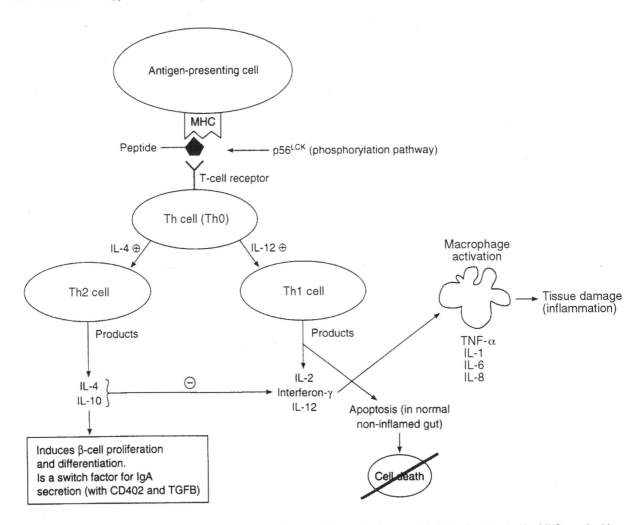

FIGURE 36–1. The Th1/Th2 paradigm and intestinal cytokine regulation. IgA = immunoglobulin A; IL = interleukin; MHC = major histocompatibility complex; Th = T helper; TNF = tumor necrosis factor; + and – indicate an effect on response. (Reproduced with permission from Yacyshyn BR. New biotechnological therapies for Crohn's disease: where are we now? Biodrugs, Adis International Ltd. 1998;10:301–16.)

experimental models of Th1-induced inflammation, a parasite-induced Th2 response blocked development of inflammation. Although this form of treatment may benefit patients, its mechanism requires further clarification.

Heparin

Inflammation results in hypercoagulability, and the clinical benefit of heparin, first observed by clinicians working in Russia, has been further studied in an uncontrolled trial in Ireland. Other groups have reported benefits in extraintestinal manifestations of IBD, including arthritis and pyoderma gangrenosum. Recently, a double-blind randomized trial of heparin in UC demonstrated a trend to improvement of symptoms. Using a starting dose of heparin of 10,000 units twice a day subcutaneously and increasing the frequency to three times per day in patients with a normal partial thromboplastin time after initiation of therapy, by 6 weeks, 1 of 35 patients who received

placebo and 6 of 33 who received heparin went into remission. Overall, 7 of 35 placebo and 14 of 33 heparin-treated patients were in remission or improved (p = .046). Owing to the intrinsic risk of bleeding, initiation of heparin therapy is not advocated at this time except in hospitalized patients. More interest in heparin therapy can be anticipated if current clinical trials of oral heparin demonstrate efficacy for other conditions. This topic is discussed in the chapter on hematologic complications in IBD.

Tumor Necrosis Factor-α

An understanding of the effects of immunomodulators and biodrugs on the intestinal immune system in homeostasis as well as in IBD requires knowledge of the two mechanisms that the gut uses to maintain its integrity: the epithelial surface, which provides a physical barrier to bacteria in the intestinal lumen, and the intestinal immune system, in which the intestinal lamina propria mucosal cells play a key role in antigen processing and eradication of pathogens.

A measure of epithelial integrity is intestinal epithelial permeability. Cytokines implicated in the pathogenesis of CD and capable of inducing increased intestinal permeability include interferon (IFN)-γ, IL-4, and TNF-α. Tumor necrosis factor is a 157-amino acid protein produced by monocytes, T cells, and macrophages, and TNF-α plays an important role in the development of increased intestinal permeability. Animal studies have shown benefit after anti-TNF antibody administration, and measurement of stool TNF-α correlates with intestinal inflammation. These and other findings linking TNF-α to intestinal inflammation led to the first uncontrolled study of anti-TNF antibodies in the therapy of CD, reported in 1995, in which 9 of 10 corticosteroid-dependent patients achieved a clinical response (Crohn's Disease Activity Index [CDAI] decline of >70) within the first 4 weeks of therapy with infliximab, and clinical remission occurred in 40 percent after 4 weeks. Details of this and subsequent trials are presented in the chapter on anticytokine therapy in CD.

In a 12-week, multicenter, double-blind, placebo-controlled trial of infliximab in 108 patients with moderate to severe CD (CDAI 220–400) resistant to standard medical therapy, including steroids, patients received a single dose of placebo or infliximab at 5 mg/kg, 10 mg/kg, or 20 mg/kg. Clinical response or remission at week 2 occurred in 61 percent of treated patients compared with 17 percent of patients receiving placebo. Significant differences in response were found between all treatment groups and placebo at weeks 2, 4, and 12. Thirty-four percent of nonresponders improved after a subsequent open-label infusion 10 mg/kg. Adverse effects were similar in study and placebo groups.

Additional studies of infliximab have shown that histologic improvement in ileocolonic biopsies of patients with CD parallels the improvement of a number of markers of immune activation. Although relatively large numbers of patients have been treated with infliximab, the long-term effects of treatment and re-treatment on the immune responsiveness of these patients or their risk of developing adverse reactions, including lymphoma, are not known. There is a great deal of observational experience with Remicade® (Centocor Inc., Malvern, Pennsylvania) now that over 30,000 patients have been treated. Brief preliminary work presented in 1996 evaluating a limited number of patients with UC did not support improvement in anti-TNF-α antibody treatment, but abstracts at DDW in 2000 suggest efficacy in some UC patients.

Interleukin-10 in Inflammatory Bowel Disease

The role of increased intestinal permeability contributing to the pathogenesis of IBD is supported by animal models, such as IL-10-deficient mice that demonstrate intestinal permeability defect before the development of enterocolitis. Recombinant human IL-10 administered over 7 consecutive days in a placebo-controlled, dose escalation trial in corticosteroid-resistant CD induced similar improvement in the CDAI in patients treated with IL-10 and those receiving placebo. Improvement in treated patients was sustained beyond the second week of therapy, whereas patients receiving placebo showed a trend toward relapse. No dose–effect relation could be observed. Clinical adverse effects were seen in 18 percent of patients and consisted primarily of headache, anemia, nausea, leukocytosis, and fatigue. Although this study was not powered to demonstrate efficacy of IL-10 therapy, 81 percent of IL-10-treated patients experienced clinical remission or response in contrast with 46 percent of placebo-treated patients. There were no differences in the Endoscopic Index of Severity (EIS) score on colonoscopy with ileoscopy on days 1 and 28. A follow-up study of IL-10 in CD yielded only equivocal data at best. This drug, like many biologics, does not have a standard dose-response curve. Moreover, some patients treated with IL-10 developed severe, pronounced, and protracted periods of thrombocythemia that normalized with the withdrawal of the drug. Results to date in limited unpublished clinical experience have not supported its use for UC, with only transient effect being shown. Because of this mixed clinical experience, the potential role of IL-10 in the future management of IBD is ambiguous.

Phase I–II Trial Experience of ISIS 2302 (Antisense to ICAM-1)

The molecule ISIS 2302 hybridizes to sequence at the 3′ untranslated region of human ICAM-1 messenger ribonucleic acid (mRNA) (Figure 36–2). Although preliminary studies looked promising, recent larger trials failed to demonstrate efficacy compared with placebo in chronic active CD. A large, 300-patient, double-blind, crossover, placebo-controlled multicenter study that ended its recruitment phase in August 1999 is being conducted to validate clinical experience using antisense to ICAM-1. A trial of topical enema preparation of ISIS 2302 for distal UC is planned. Although no human experience is yet available for this formulation, animal models suggest that this approach is feasible and potentially efficacious.

Future Directions

Most clinical studies of biologic drugs targeting inflammatory mediators have enrolled populations of patients refractory to treatment with conventional therapies. It is not known if these patients represent the same population for each drug or whether they are not responsive to single therapy using a specific compound. This has led to interest in both identifying markers to predict response in different patients and in developing combinations of drugs that will induce rapid, predictable clinical

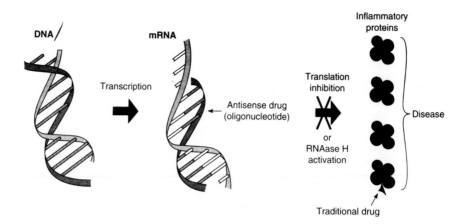

FIGURE 36–2. Antisense technology: the antisense drug binds to mRNA and activates RNAase H, which destroys the complex or, alternatively, binds to mRNA and inhibits its translation. (Reproduced with permission from Yacyshyn BR. New biotechnological therapies for Crohn's disease: where are we now? Biodrugs, Adis International Ltd. 1998;10:301–16.)

responses in patients while not compromising safety. This type of research has led to interest in P-glycoprotein-170 (P-gp-170) as a mediator of cyclosporine A transport from effector lymphocytes in IBD. The purpose was to determine whether transport by molecules, such as P-gp-170, could account for the lack of efficacy of cyclosporine A in CD as well as the varied clinical response seen in UC. The highest expression of P-gp-170 was found in CD lymphocytes in contrast to UC (low) and normals. This finding is consistent with the UC-like lesions identified in the colons of P-gp knockout mice. The mechanism of action of other drugs could be similarly studied.

Conclusion

Understanding the pathophysiology of IBD has led to a number of new candidate drugs and therapeutic modalities. Of these, the anti-TNF antibody is currently the only one to enter clinical practice, and only for CD. Other, less conventional, candidates include heparin therapy for UC, probiotics, leukacytopheresis, antisense to ICAM-1, and *Trichuris suis*. Other contenders that hold promise include IL-11, IL-12, and antibody to integrin $\alpha_4\beta_7$, as well as others. The rapid expansion of knowledge of inflammatory mediators doubtless will produce more experimental therapeutic approaches.

Editor's Note

A complete 64-item bibliography prepared by the author can be requested at *bruce.yacyshyn@ualberta.ca*. Some of the references appear in the Supplemental Reading sections of other chapters.

Supplemental Reading

Ayabe T, Ashida T, Kohgo Y. Centrifugal leukocyte apheresis for ulcerative colitis. Ther Apher 1998;2:125–8.

Day R, Forbes A. Heparin, cell adhesion, and pathogenesis of inflammatory bowel disease. Lancet 1999;354:62–5.

Dugas B, Mercenier A, Lenoir-Wijnkoop I, et al. Immunity and probiotics. Immunol Today 1999;20:387–90.

Folwaczny CN, Wiebecke B, Loeschke K. Unfractioned heparin in the therapy of patients with highly active inflammatory bowel disease. Am J Gastroenterol 1999;94:1551–5.

Korzenik JR, Robert ME, Bitton A, et al. A multi-center, randomized, controlled trial of heparin for the treatment of ulcerative colitis. Gastroenterology 1999;116:G3264.

Musso A, Condon TP, West GA, et al. Regulation of ICAM-1 mediated fibroblast T-cell reciprocal interaction: implications for modulation of gut inflammation. Gastroenterology 1999;117:546–56.

Rembacken BJ, Snelling AM, Hawkey PM, et al. Non-pathogenic *Escherichia coli* versus mesalazine for the treatment of ulcerative colitis: a randomised trial. Lancet 1999;354:635–9.

Sasaki M, Tsujikawa T, Fujiyama Y, Bamba T. Leukocytapheresis therapy for severe ulcerative colitis. Ther Apher 1998; 2:101–4.

Sawada K, Ohnishi K, Kosaka T, et al. Leukocytapheresis with leukocyte removal filter as new therapy for ulcerative colitis. Ther Apher 1997;1:207–11.

Schreiber S, Fedorak RN, Wild G, et al. Safety and tolerance of rHu IL-10 treated in patients with mild/moderate active ulcerative colitis. Gastroenterology 1998;114:G4424.

Summers RW, Urban J, Elliott D, et al. Th2 conditioning by *Trichuris suis* appears safe and effective in modifying the mucosal immune response in inflammatory bowel disease. Gastroenterology 1999;116:G3592.

Targan SR, Hanauer SB, van Deventer SJH, et al. A short-term study of chimeric monoclonal antibody cA2 to tumor necrosis factor alpha for Crohn's disease. N Engl J Med 1997;337:1029–35.

Tracey KJ, Cerami A. Tumor necrosis factor: a pleiotropic cytokine and therapeutic target. Annu Rev Med 1994; 45:491–503.

Van Deventer SJ, Elson CO, Fedorak RN. Multiple doses of intravenous interleukin-10 in steroid refractory Crohn's disease. Gastroenterology 1997;113:383–9.

Vincenti F, Kirkman R, Light S, et al. Interleukin-2-receptor blockade with daclizumab to prevent acute rejection in renal transplantation. Daclizumab Triple Therapy Study Group. N Engl J Med 1998;338:161–5.

Yacyshyn BR. New biotechnological therapies for Crohn's disease: where are we now? Biodrugs, Adis International Ltd. 1998;10:301–16.

Yacyshyn B, Maksymowych W, Bowen-Yacyshyn MB. Differences in P-glycoprotein-170 expression and activity between Crohn's disease and ulcerative colitis. Hum Immunol 1999;60:677–87.

Yacyshyn BR, Bowen-Yacyshyn MB, Jewell L, et al. A placebo-controlled trial of an ICAM-1 antisense oligohucleotide in the treatment of Crohn's disease. Gastroenterology 1998;114:1133–42.

CHAPTER 37

THERAPEUTIC EXPECTATIONS: SURGICAL MANAGEMENT OF ULCERATIVE COLITIS

KEITH A. KELLY, MD

This chapter focuses on what patients can expect after surgery for medically refractory ulcerative colitis. Almost all patients will be better off after operation than before operation. The operation is safe. Their colitis will be "cured," their colitis medications will be discontinued, and their intestinal symptoms will subside. Their physiologic and social functions will generally be preserved or improved, and a feeling of good health and a satisfactory quality of life will return. However, the outcome may not be perfect, and long-term complications can occur. Physicians do their best to achieve an excellent outcome and avoid complications, while providing compassionate, cost-effective, surgical care.

Currently, most patients who undergo elective surgery for ulcerative colitis have a proctocolectomy and an ileal pouch-anal canal anastomosis. However, proctocolectomy and Brooke ileostomy, proctocolectomy and continent ileostomy (Kock pouch), and colectomy and ileorectostomy still are used, and are also explained to the patient. Indeed, these operations still are the operations of choice for selected patients.

Proctocolectomy and Ileal Pouch-Anal Canal Anastomosis

Operative Management

In proctocolectomy and ileal pouch-anal canal anastomosis (IPAA), the entire diseased colon and rectum are removed, but the anal sphincters are preserved. A new rectum is formed from the terminal ileum—an ileal pouch. The pouch provides a new reservoir for stool. Anastomosing the pouch to the anal canal restores transanal defecation. Furthermore, the combination of the new reservoir and the preserved anal sphincters results in satisfactory fecal continence.

A proximal loop ileostomy is put into place during their operation to divert stool temporarily away from the pouch and pouch-anal anastomosis. This enhances healing of the pouch and anastomosis and helps to avoid leak and sepsis in the early postoperative period. The stoma is closed at a second operation 2 months later. Young patients with minimal rectal inflammation, not on steroids, and with a tension-free anastomosis and

a good blood supply to the pouch may not need the ileostomy.

This operation most often is done at open celiotomy, but it has sometimes been accomplished using laparoscopic techniques. These techniques are purported to lessen postoperative discomfort and speed recovery; however, it has not been proven that these advantages ensue with laparoscopic techniques, which take longer and are more expensive. The well-tested, open approach is recommended.

Patients are advised that they will have abdominal pain and discomfort in the early postoperative period after surgery, but that pain can be almost completely controlled with epidural analgesia supplemented with intravenous and oral analgesic agents. Epidural analgesia has the added advantage of shortening the duration of postoperative ileus.

Most patients are discharged from the hospital at about 7 days following the first operation and about 5 days after the second operation, for a total length of hospital stay of about 12 days. They can expect to return to office work by 1 month after the first operation and 2 to 3 weeks after the second operation.

Safety of Surgery

Open proctocolectomy with IPAA is a safe operation. Only three postoperative deaths occurred in the first 1,000 patients who underwent this procedure at the Mayo Clinic. Immediate postoperative complications, including bleeding, intestinal obstruction, wound infection, wound hernia, venous thrombosis, urinary retention, intra-abdominal and pelvic abscess, and intestinal fistulae, occur in about 25 percent of patients, but almost all of them respond readily to therapy with medications and other nonoperative means. Intestinal obstruction is the exception; one of three patients with this complication requires reoperation.

Cure of Colitis

Patients are assured that they will never have colitis again after the operation. The entire diseased large intestine is removed, and so colitis can never recur in it. However, some surgeons leave in place a small, 1- to 3-cm area of ulcerative colitis just proximal to the dentate line. They believe this prevents damage to the anal sphincters during the operation and so enhances postoperative continence. The inflammation in this retained mucosa may remain quiescent in most patients, but there is a possibility of a flare-up of inflammation and even the development of cancer in this area. For these reasons, complete excision of this mucosa along with the rest of the diseased large intestine is advisable. Satisfactory continence is achieved in most cases.

Extra-intestinal manifestations of the colitis may or may not subside after operation or may even appear after the large intestine has been removed. Peripheral arthritis, thromboembolic phenomena, and uveitis usually subside, while cutaneous lesions, such as erythema nodosum and pyoderma gangrenosum, may or may not resolve. In contrast, sclerosing cholangitis, central arthritis, and rheumatoid spondylitis will not subside. In fact, these latter conditions may appear for the first time in the postoperative period. In a global sense, the patients are instructed that an operation on the large intestine may not "cure" all aspects of their disease.

Discontinuation of Medication

The patient is assured that after operation, all medications that have been taken in an effort to treat the colitis can be discontinued. Prednisone or other corticoids must be decreased gradually over a several-month period, but all other anticolitic drugs can be stopped immediately. Some side effects and complications of the drugs that have already occurred prior to the operation, such as cataracts and aseptic necrosis of the hip, may need additional therapy after operation, whereas steroid-induced hypertension and diabetes mellitus usually spontaneously improve. Loperamide, which thickens bowel movements, decreases fecal output, and strengthens the anal sphincter, may still be required in some patients after surgery.

Subsidence of Symptoms

Abdominal cramps, hematochezia, anemia, weight loss, and a feeling of poor health rapidly subside after the operation. By 2 months after ileostomy closure, patients who have undergone IPAA can expect to have 5 to 6 bowel movements per day. This stool frequency is much better than the 12 stools per day experienced by the average patient with colitis before surgery. Women, especially, find a stool frequency of 5 stools per day not a problem. They simply empty their pouch at the time of urination. Moreover, the fecal urgency, tenesmus, and incontinence before surgery are less troublesome after the operation. After IPAA, patients are able to defer defecation for 30 minutes or more, whereas this often is impossible in the patient with active colitis. After surgery, the frequency of defecation also can be controlled by oral intake: deferring intake decreases the frequency of bowel movements.

Preservation of Function

Proctocolectomy and IPAA preserves transanal defecation, avoids a long-term stoma, and provides reasonable fecal continence, especially during the day. Some fecal spotting occurs at night that may require a pad for protection, but this is not needed by the majority of patients. Most patients pass one bowel movement per night or one every other night.

Sexual function, including erection and ejaculation in males and orgasm in both males and females, is satisfactory in all but a small percentage of subjects. The older the patient, the more likely the dysfunction. However, women may have more difficulty with conception, because of the development postoperatively of adhesions around the ovaries and fallopian tubes. Nevertheless, many women have conceived successfully after surgery and delivered healthy babies either vaginally or by cesarean section. If labor is prolonged or causing excess stress on the anal sphincters, cesarean section is advisable.

The abdominal and ileostomy wounds usually heal well and allow patients to resume full social and physical function after the sixth postoperative week. Younger patients can resume strenuous activity, such as bike racing, wrestling, and mountain climbing at that time; older patients can begin golf and swimming. The patients can expect an excellent quality of life after surgery.

Long-Term Complications

Long-term complications can occur; about 10 percent of patients develop intestinal obstruction, and of these, one-half require operative relief. Use of a sodium hyaluronate and carboxymethylcellulose bioresorbable membrane (Seprafilm®, Genzyme Inc., Boston, Massachusetts) at operation may decrease the long-term risk of intestinal obstruction, but this is as yet unproven. Inflammation in the pouch (pouchitis) occurs more commonly. One or more episodes have occurred in about half of the patients by 8 years after surgery. When pouchitis occurs, medical therapy with antibiotics or other medications is effective in controlling it in nearly all patients; only 1 percent need pouch excision or diverting ileostomy to control it. The long-term consequences of pouchitis, including the risk of dysplasia and even cancer, are as yet unknown. Because of these risks, patients, especially the older ones, should consider surveillance proctoscopy with biopsy of the pouch beginning 3 to 5 years after surgery.*

Pouchitis, anal stricture, anal fistulae, perianal abscesses, and anal incontinence may develop as the months and years go by after operation. They usually respond to surgical and nonsurgical therapy, but they do

---

* Editor's Note: The patient who, preoperatively, had dysplasia or cancer in the rectum or who develops atrophic mucosa in the pouch seemingly is at greater risk of dysplasia. Further studies are needed. (TMB)

account for loss of the pelvic pouch and conversion to a Brooke ileostomy or a continent ileostomy in some patients. Such conversions have occurred in about 5 percent of patients by 5 years after surgery, but reach 8 percent by 8 years after operation. Whether this trend will continue is unknown.

Patients are at increased risk for urinary stones postoperatively. Urine output is scant because of the loss of water and salt in the stool. The large intestine in health absorbs water and salt efficiently, but after proctocolectomy these functions are lost. The ileum adapts and takes over these functions to some extent, but it does not completely compensate. Hence, patients must drink plenty of water and use table salt. Patients also may be at risk for gallstones. However, because almost all of the ileum, the site of bile salt absorption, is preserved, this may not be the case. Bile salts, secreted by the liver into bile, help to solubilize cholesterol in bile and so prevent gallstones. After the operation, the ileal pouch does absorb vitamin B_{12}, so that parenteral administration of this vitamin usually is not needed.

Other Operations

Proctocolectomy and Brooke Ileostomy

Patients older than 65 years of age should consider proctocolectomy and Brooke ileostomy instead of IPAA. The anal sphincter begins to lose its strength in the seventh decade of life. A strong anal sphincter is required to prevent fecal incontinence after an ileoanal operation. Some older subjects with a strong anal sphincter demonstrated by anal manometry might still be candidates for an ileoanal procedure, but this is rare. Patients who have lost their rectum at a previous operation and patients who have a damaged anal sphincter because of previous surgery, childbirth, or disease also usually require a Brooke ileostomy or a continent ileostomy.

Patients undergoing proctocolectomy and Brooke ileostomy must wear an appliance over the incontinent stoma day and night to collect fecal discharge. There may be skin irritation, noises and odors from the stoma, the possibility of leakage, and an unsightly appearance of the stoma. Nevertheless, with good stomal care, almost all patients make a satisfactory adjustment to the stoma and experience an excellent quality of life after surgery.

Proctocolectomy and Continent Ileostomy (Kock Pouch)

Patients with proctocolectomy and continent ileostomy have an ileal pouch that acts as a reservoir for stool, just as with IPAA. However, in these patients, a section of ileum leads from the pouch to a stoma placed in the right lower quadrant of the abdomen. A valve, also made of ileum, is placed between the stoma and the lumen of the pouch to keep the pouch continent. The patient must intubate the pouch through the stoma and valve about four times per day to empty the pouch. Intubation usually is not required at night. In the majority of patients, adjustment to the intubations is rapid and satisfaction is high. The advantages of this procedure over Brooke ileostomy include fecal continence without the need to wear an ileostomy bag and that no gas or stool escapes from the pouch between intubations. However, revision of the pouch is necessary in about one of every seven patients to keep the pouch continent and to maintain easy intubation over the months and years following surgery. Pouchitis develops with the same frequency in these pouches as it does in ileal pouches joined to the anal canal.

Colectomy and Ileorectostomy

Colectomy and ileorectostomy is a procedure that is seldom recommended, because it leaves the rectal disease in place where it can cause continued symptoms, require treatment, and mandate the need for surveillance to guard against the development of rectal cancer in future years. However, this operation does have the advantage of no stoma, continued transanal fecal discharge, reasonable fecal continence, and minimal risk of urologic and sexual dysfunction postoperatively. These advantages persuade a few younger patients, especially those who do not wish to accept even a minimal risk of impotence, to choose this operation rather than the IPAA procedure. However, most patients are better served by one of the other surgical options.

Supplemental Reading

Gullberg K, Stahling D, Liljequist L, et al. Neoplastic transformation of the pelvic pouch mucosa in patients with ulcerative colitis. Gastroenterology 1997;112:1487–92.

Kelly KA, Pemberton JH, Wolff BG, Dozois RR. Ileal pouch-anal anastomois. Curr Probl Surg 1992;29:57–131.

Kohler LW, Pemberton JH, Zinsmeister AR, Kelly KA. Quality of life after proctocolectomy: a comparison of Brooke ileostomy, Kock pouch, and ileal pouch-anal anastomosis. Gastroenterology 1991;101:679–84.

McLeod RS. Quality of life after surgery for ulcerative colitis. Probl Gen Surg 1999;16:158–66.

Morimoto H, Cullen JJ, Messick JM Jr, Kelly KA. Epidural analgesia shortens postoperative ileus after ileal pouch-anal canal anastomosis. Am J Surg 1995;169:79–83.

Wexner SD, Salum MR. Laparoscopic surgery for inflammatory bowel disease. Probl Gen Surg 1999;16:88–99.

CHAPTER 38

INDICATIONS FOR COLECTOMY AND CHOICE OF PROCEDURES

JAMES M. BECKER, MD

Indications for Surgery

Nearly half of patients with chronic ulcerative colitis (CUC) undergo surgery within the first 10 years of their illness, mainly because of the chronic nature of the disease and the tendency for relapse.[*] In addition, occasional fulminant complications occur, and a significant risk of malignant degeneration exists. The indications for surgery vary widely, and these differing indications have varied implications for the timing of surgery and the choice of operative procedure. Indications for surgical intervention include (1) massive unrelenting hemorrhage, (2) toxic megacolon with impending or frank perforation, (3) fulminating acute ulcerative colitis (UC) unresponsive to steroid therapy, (4) obstruction owing to stricture,[†] (5) evidence of dysplasia or colonic cancer, (6) systemic complications, (7) intractability, and (8) in children, an additional indication for surgery is failure to grow or develop secondary sexual characteristics at an acceptable rate.

Perforation

Acute perforation occurs infrequently, with the incidence directly related to both the severity of the initial attack and the extent of bowel disease. Although the overall incidence of perforation during a first attack is less than 4 percent, if the attack is severe, the incidence rises to about 10 percent. Although free colon perforation occurs more frequently in the presence of toxic megacolon, it is important to remember that toxic megacolon is not a prerequisite for the development of perforation. In the presence of colonic perforation, the operation should be definitive without being overly aggressive. Abdominal colectomy with ileostomy and Hartmann closure of the rectum is the procedure of choice.

Hemorrhage

Massive hemorrhage secondary to UC is rare, occurring in fewer than 1 percent of patients and accounting for about 10 percent of urgent colectomies performed for UC. Prompt surgical intervention is indicated after hemodynamic stabilization. Uncontrollable hemorrhage from the entire colorectal mucosa may be the one clear indication for emergency proctocolectomy. If possible, the rectum should be spared for later mucosal proctectomy with ileoanal anastomosis, realizing that about 12 percent of patients will have continued hemorrhage from the retained rectal segment.

Toxic Megacolon

Acute toxic megacolon occurs in 6 to 13 percent of patients with UC. Initial treatment for toxic megacolon includes intravenous fluid and electrolyte resuscitation, nasogastric suction, broad-spectrum antibiotics to include anaerobic and aerobic gram-negative coverage, and total parenteral nutrition to improve nutritional status. Although the therapeutic role of steroids in toxic megacolon is controversial, most patients presenting with a severe attack of UC are already on steroid therapy and, thus, need stress doses of corticosteroids to prevent adrenal crisis.[‡] When toxic megacolon is promptly treated, subsequent surgery is not inevitable. Even among patients in whom prompt resolution has occurred, about half require surgery within a year, and most eventually require colectomy.

In the presence of acute toxic megacolon caused by UC, surgery can be associated with high operative morbidity and mortality. Postoperative complications, including sepsis, wound infection, abscess, fistula, or delayed wound healing, have been reported in up to half of patients. In older series, postoperative mortality rates ranged between 11 and 16 percent and, for the subset of patients with perforation, 27 to 44 percent. The overall

---

[*] Editor's Note: The author's indication of 50 percent of patients is considerably higher than the expectation of the editors and of most other centers of approximately 20 to 25 percent. (SBH)

[†] Editor's Note: Chronic strictures in CUC are usually neoplastic, especially if duration of CUC is over 8 years, if the strictures are proximal to the splenic flexure, or if the patient presents with colonic obstruction. (SBH and TMB)

[‡] Editor's Note: Intestinal intubation and rotating the patient, as popularized by Present et al, are discussed in the chapter on fulminant colitis. Cyclosporine use is discussed in several chapters. (TMB)

[§] Editor's Note: These statistics are from older series; currently, the overall mortality rates for emergent surgery should be less than 5 percent. (SBH)

mortality rate after emergency surgery is 8.7 percent; the mortality rate is 6.1 percent for total abdominal colectomy and 14.7 percent for proctocolectomy.§ This observation suggests that more conservative surgery is appropriate in the acute setting. With the popularity of anal sphincter-sparing procedures, the surgeon should usually consider leaving the rectum intact, allowing subsequent mucosal proctectomy and ileoanal anastomosis.

For most patients with UC, a colectomy is performed when the disease enters an intractable, chronic phase and becomes a physical and social burden to the patient. With sphincter-sparing operations available for UC, it has become critically important to avoid proctectomy when possible and to distinguish diagnostically patients with UC from those with Crohn's disease.

Surgical Approaches

Proctocolectomy and Ileostomy

Chronic ulcerative colitis is cured once the colon and rectum are removed; therefore, single-stage total proctocolectomy with Brooke ileostomy has historically been the operation of choice for elective surgical treatment. A decision tree for surgical options in UC is included in the chapter on Brooke ileostomy. Despite the fact that this operation eliminates all diseased tissue and the risk of malignant transformation, it has been poorly accepted by some patients. This reluctance is primarily because a permanent abdominal ileostomy is required. Immediate maturation of the stoma eliminates many of the mechanical problems associated with ileostomy.

Although 90 percent of patients with a Brooke ileostomy are able to adequately adjust to the stoma, between 25 percent and 50 percent of patients with ileostomies complain of appliance-related problems. These include skin irritation or excoriation, discomfort, leakage, and odor, as well as the financial burden and the time and effort involved in caring for an ileostomy with modern disposable stomal devices. There is a separate chapter on Brooke ileostomy and another by an ostomy nurse. Perhaps more important than these problems are the significant psychologic and social implications of a permanent ileostomy, particularly for young and physically active patients.

Until about 20 years ago, single-stage total proctocolectomy with ileostomy was the elective operation of choice for complications of UC. Currently, proctocolectomy is the procedure of choice in relatively few patients. The operation carries the advantages that it is curative, there is no anastomosis to heal, and it requires only a single operation. It provides the patient with a predictable functional result and eliminates the fear of anal incontinence.

The disadvantage of total proctocolectomy is that it results in permanent fecal incontinence. Patients require an external ileostomy device, which may need emptying four to eight times per day, and significant complications are associated with the operation. Among patients with UC, 10 to 25 percent require stoma revision, 10 to 20 percent have perineal wound problems, and 7 to 13 percent develop postoperative bowel obstruction at some point. Of major concern are bladder and sexual dysfunction associated with parasympathetic nerve injury. Impotence is reported to occur in to up to 5 percent of male patients after proctectomy for benign disease.

Subtotal Colectomy

Subtotal colectomy, Brooke ileostomy, and Hartmann closure of the rectum or ileorectal anastomosis have been employed in the surgical treatment of UC for decades. The operation eliminates an abdominal stoma if ileorectal anastomosis is performed and, because the pelvic autonomic nerves are not disturbed, impotence and bladder dysfunction are not a risk. (There is a chapter on ileorectal anastomosis.) Subtotal colectomy with ileostomy is the procedure of choice in the emergency setting or if the diagnosis of UC as opposed to Crohn's disease cannot be clearly established. (See the chapters on indeterminate colitis.) Abdominal colectomy with ileorectal anastomosis usually leaves the patient with full continence but has not gained wide popularity because it is not a curative operation. The inflammatory process persists in the retained rectum, and there is an ongoing risk of malignancy that may be as high as 17 percent after 20 years.

Continent Ileostomy

In 1969, Kock described the continent ileostomy, made entirely of terminal ileum and consisting of an intestinal pouch serving as a reservoir for stool, with an ileal conduit connecting the pouch to a cutaneous stoma. The operation was modified several years later to include an intestinal nipple valve between the pouch and the stoma. Patients empty the pouch by passing a soft plastic tube through the valve via the stoma. The advantage of this operation is that it is a curative procedure that offers a potentially new life style by making the ileostomy continent and avoiding an external appliance. There is a separate chapter on this operation and its complications.

The continent ileostomy has been associated with a high complication rate. Most of the complications are related to displacement of the nipple valve, producing fecal incontinence or difficulty intubating and emptying the pouch. Valve failure has been reported to occur in between 4 to 40 percent of patients. Although the Kock ileostomy has advantages over the Brooke ileostomy, its high rate of mechanical, functional, and metabolic complications has limited its clinical usefulness. In centers that offer all surgical alternatives to patients with UC requiring colectomy, few Kock pouches are being constructed. The continent ileostomy may be useful in patients who have already undergone total proctocolectomy and ileostomy and, after careful counseling, demand an attempt at a continence-restoring procedure.

Ileoanal Anastomosis

Rather than ablating the entire rectum, anus, and anal sphincter, in CUC, the physician can selectively dissect out and remove the rectal mucosa down to the dentate line of the anus. This preserves an intact rectal muscular cuff and anal sphincter apparatus. Continuity of the intestinal tract can be reestablished by extending the ileum into the pelvis endorectally and circumferentially suturing it to the anus in an end-to-end fashion. The potential advantages of this approach are (1) it eliminates all diseased tissue; (2) it is as definitive an operation as total proctocolectomy; (3) it preserves parasympathetic innervation to the bladder and genitalia and eliminates the problem of urinary dysfunction or impotence, because the pelvic dissection is confined to the endorectal plane; (4) it avoids a long-term draining perineal wound, because the abdominal perineal proctectomy is eliminated; (5) a permanent abdominal stoma is unnecessary, because of the ileoanal anastomosis; and (6) it preserves the anorectal sphincter and maintains continence.

In the past two decades, there has been increasing development of the ileoanal pullthrough procedure; in part because other alternatives, such as the Kock pouch, were not as successful as originally hoped. In addition, important technical advances have been made. It was found that there was an inverse correlation between ileal compliance and capacity and stool frequencies in patients after the end-to-end ileoanal anastomosis. This process of ileal adaptation and dilatation could be hastened by the surgical construction of an ileal pouch or reservoir proximal to the ileoanal anastomosis. Several types of ileal reservoirs have been proposed, including the J pouch, S pouch, W pouch, and lateral side-to-side isoperistaltic pouch. Several studies have compared the functional result after ileoanal anastomosis with and without an ileal reservoir and have demonstrated a reduction in stool frequency in adult patients in whom an ileal pouch was constructed, particularly in the early postoperative period. There are two other chapters on the ileoanal J pouch.

Another important technical addition to the operation is a temporary diverting loop ileostomy. This allows fecal diversion during the early weeks of ileal pouch and ileoanal anastomotic healing, thereby reducing the incidence of pelvic sepsis and ileal pouch and ileoanal anastomotic dehiscence. Some surgeons have eliminated the loop ileostomy in good-risk patients.

Although it was thought initially that only patients who were young and had relatively quiescent disease were candidates for ileoanal anastomosis, the indications have been considerably liberalized during the past 10 years. Patients are not candidates if other medical problems or the severity of the colitis preclude a 4- to 6-hour operation. Although some series have reported that younger patients have a superior result compared with older patients, others have not found this to be the case. Many surgeons are comfortable in offering ileoanal anastomosis to patients in their sixth or seventh decade if they are in relatively good health and have adequate anal sphincter function. Disease severity has neither been found to be associated with enhanced operative morbidity nor to correlate with subsequent functional results. However, Crohn's disease is a contraindication to the operation. The most important criterion for electing to perform ileoanal anastomosis is that the patient fully understands the nature of the operation and has realistic expectations about the outcome.

The postoperative morbidity and functional results from most large series after ileoanal pullthrough have been encouraging. In my experience, 82 percent of 500 patients underwent surgery for UC and 18 percent for familial polyposis. The mean age was 36 years (range, 11 to 76 yr). Sixty-two percent of the patients were male. Experience with ileal pouch-anal anastomosis (IPAA) supports the absence of mortality and low morbidity that can be achieved with this operation if it is performed frequently, carefully, and with a standard operative technique. No operative deaths occurred in the series, and the overall operative morbidity after the IPAA portion of the operation was about 10 percent. The major operative morbidity was bowel obstruction, both after the initial operation and after loop ileostomy closure. The bowel obstruction rate requiring reoperation compared favorably with the incidence of reoperation reported after proctocolectomy and ileostomy. Pelvic and wound infections have been reported to occur in 10 to 20 percent of patients undergoing ileoanal anastomosis, although the overall infection rate was reduced to about 5 percent in several more recent large series. A 5 to 10 percent failure rate, necessitating conversion to permanent ileostomy, has been reported in several series, although in my own experience it is closer to 10 percent.

Although results with mucosal proctectomy and IPAA have been excellent, divergent points of view have arisen regarding the operative technique and its effect on anal physiology and functional result. In recent years, a number of surgeons have advocated an alternative approach to conventional endoanal rectal mucosal dissection that eliminates distal mucosal proctectomy altogether. The distal rectum is divided near the pelvic floor, leaving the anal canal largely intact. The ileal pouch is then stapled to the top of the anal canal. The rationale for this approach is that, by preserving the mucosa of the anal transition zone, the anatomic integrity of the anal canal would be preserved and the rate of fecal incontinence improved. Although several studies have suggested that patients have improved sensation and better functional results following preservation of the anal transition zone, this has not been documented by prospective controlled study. There is a chapter describing the stapled approach and a chapter on the problem of pouchitis. Furthermore there is concern that leaving disease-bearing mucosa in the anal canal exposes patients to a life-long risk of persistent inflammatory disease and the potential for malignant transformation necessitating lifetime surveillance of the residual rectal mucosa. Mucosectomy must be recommended in patients with rectal dysplasia, proximal rectal cancer, diffuse colonic dysplasia, and familial polyposis. The view favoring the stapled approach is presented in the chapter on the ileoanal pouch.

The functional result after ileoanal anastomosis has been consistent in the larger series with adequate late follow-up data. These studies have demonstrated that the number of bowel movements was in the range of four to nine daily, with an average of six per day. Nocturnal bowel movements occurred one to two times nightly with a mean of slightly over one. Nocturnal seepage of stool or staining was observed in 20 percent of patients in the early postoperative period, but by 1 year it was infrequently observed.

Conclusion

A significant proportion of patients with UC require operation, with the realization that colectomy does not reflect a therapeutic failure but rather a permanent cure. Colectomy with mucosal proctectomy and endorectal IPAA is the operation of choice for young patients and for most adults requiring elective proctocolectomy for CUC. Total proctocolectomy with Brooke ileostomy should be reserved for patients who are not candidates for ileoanal anastomosis or who, after careful counseling about all of the surgical alternatives, elect that alternative. Subtotal colectomy with ileostomy and Hartmann closure of the rectum should be performed when emergency colectomy is indicated or if the diagnosis of UC, as opposed to Crohn's colitis, is uncertain. Because of the added morbidity of this staged approach and the possibility of a less optimal functional result, attempts should be made to prepare the patient for a single-stage colectomy, mucosal proctectomy, and IPAA. The continent ileostomy should be considered in patients desirous of an attempt to restore continence who are not candidates for IPAA or in whom total proctocolectomy with ileostomy has already been performed.

Editor's Note

A complete 21-item reference list can be obtained on request. Fax: 617 638-8607.

Supplemental Reading

Ambroze WL, Pemberton JH, Dozois R, et al. The historical pattern and pathological involvement of the anal transition zone in patients with ulcerative colitis. Gastroenterology 1993;104:514–8.

Becker JM. Ileal pouch-anal anastomosis: current status and controversies. Surgery 1993;113:599–602.

Becker JM, Raymond JL. Ileal pouch-anal anastomosis: a single surgeon's experience with 100 consecutive cases. Ann Surg 1986;204:375–83.

Block GE, Moossa AR, Simonowitz D, Hassan SZ. Emergency colectomy for inflammatory bowel disease. Surgery 1977;82:531–6.

Dozois RR, Kelly KA, Beart RW, Beahrs OH. Improved results with continent ileostomy. Ann Surg 1980;192:319–24.

Meagher AP, Farouk R, Dozois RR, et al. Ileal pouch-anal anastomosis for chronic ulcerative colitis: complications and long-term outcome in 1310 patients. Br J Surg 1998;85:800–3.

Pemberton JH. The problem with pouchitis. Gastroenterology 1993;104:1209–11.

Pemberton JH, Kelly KA, Beart RW, et al. Ileal pouch-anal anastomosis for chronic ulcerative colitis. Ann Surg 1987;206:504–13.

Sugerman HJ, Newsome HH, DeCosta G, Zfass AM. Stapled ileoanal anastomosis for ulcerative colitis and familial polyposis without a temporary diverting ileostomy. Ann Surg 1991;213:606–17.

Trickson W, Tavery I, Fazio V, et al. Manometric and functional comparison of ileal pouch anastomosis with and without anal manipulation. Am J Surg 1991;161:90–6.

CHAPTER 39

ROLE OF THE ENTEROSTOMAL THERAPY NURSE

JANICE C. COLWELL, RN, MS, CWOCN

The enterostomal therapy (ET) nurse is an advanced practice clinician with postgraduate certification in the fields of wound, ostomy, and continence nursing. The ET nurse provides education, clinical management, and support to ostomy patients and their families as well as to the staff that work with ostomy patients who are learning to live with inflammatory bowel disease (IBD). Stoma and skin care management as well as methods for integrating the stoma into daily living are some of the skills that the ET nurse brings to the health care team.

Preoperative Management

Once a patient is informed that the creation of a stoma is an option, the ET nurse becomes part of the health care team. At this point, the patient and family, if appropriate, are provided with information that demonstrates how a stoma is incorporated into daily life. Most people have no understanding of how a stoma works, how it looks, or how it is managed. Depending upon the patient and the disease, creation of a stoma may be viewed as a relief of symptoms or as a failure of medical treatment and something to be avoided. Determining the patient's expectations from surgery is important. This provides a stepping stone to planning education and support. The ET nurse will spend time discussing the patient's concerns and describing the appearance of the stoma, how it works, and how it is managed. Printed and audiovisual information is available and useful to many patients and families. Some patients benefit from talking with other people who have made the adjustment to living with a stoma, and referrals can be made for this. The United Ostomy Association, a national support group of persons with ostomies, can be contacted to help with ostomy visitation.

Stoma Criteria

Stoma Placement

The placement of a stoma is one of the critical factors in patient adjustment. The stoma must be located in an area that maintains the pouching system seal despite activity and clothing. After interviewing and examining the patient, the ET nurse selects the stoma site based upon the available ostomy pouching systems and familiarity

with individual surgical techniques. The following factors are considered when siting an abdominal stoma:

1. Away from dominant creases, folds, and bony prominences
2. Within the rectus abdominis muscle
3. Visible to the patient
4. At the crest of the infraumbilical abdominal bulge

The sitting position is optimal for stoma siting. A stoma marking disc or skin barrier is held up to the patient's abdomen noting the above considerations. The patient bends forward so that all creases and folds are noted. An additional factor to consider is the belt line of the patient's clothes. If possible, the stoma site should be selected below the belt line to facilitate concealment of the pouching system. Once the site is selected, it is marked with a surgical pen and covered with a transparent dressing. The marked site will be maintained for up to 2 weeks with this method. Including the patient in the decision regarding stoma placement is an important component of the adaptation process. The next chapter on the Brooke ileostomy provides additional details.

Stoma Creation

Stoma construction is the second critical factor for maintaing a pouching system seal. Ileostomies should be created to protrude 2 to 2.5 cm above the skin so that the effluent will be discharged directly into the pouch and not undermine the adhesive seal. A flush stoma level with the skin allows the output to undermine the seal, denude the peristomal skin, and cause pouching adhesive failure. Temporary loop ileostomies, performed to protect the ileoanal anastomosis, are frequently less than optimal stomas due to tension that produces a flush or retracted stoma. A support rod rests under the loop that stays in place for 1 to 14 days such that the skin barrier must be fitted around the stoma and the support rod. Loop stomas require advance pouching techniques as well as pharmacologic management of the high effluent volumes.

Postoperative Management

At the conclusion of surgery, a drainable, transparent ostomy pouch is placed over the stoma allowing staff to visualize the stoma and the presence of output. Stoma

TABLE 39–1. Resources

Ostomy Product Manufacturers	Professional Nursing Organization	Ostomy Patient Support Group
Coloplast 1955 West Oak Circle Marietta, GA 30062 1-800-533-0464 www.coloplast.com	Wound, Ostomy and Continence Nurses Society 1550 S. Coast Hwy., Suite 201 Laguna Beach, CA 92651 1-888-224-WOCN www.wocn.org	United Ostomy Association 36 Executive Park Suite 120 Irvine, CA 92714 1-800-826-0826 www.uoa.org
Convatec P.O. Box 5254 Princeton, NJ 08543 1-800-631-5244 www.convatec.com		
Hollister Incorporated 2000 Hollister Drive Libertyville, IL 60048 1-800-323-4060 www.hollister.com		
NuHope Laboratories, Inc. P.O. Box 331150 Pacoima, CA 91333 1-800-899-5017 www.nu-hope.com		

function generally begins 48 to 72 hours after surgery. One of the first indications of returning peristalsis is the presence of flatus that, since the pouch is air tight, inflates the pouch. Since the stoma is edematous, the gas may cause some noise when released. The patient should be assured that this noise is temporary and will disappear as the stoma edema recedes.

The stoma is assessed for signs of mucosal necrosis every 8 hours for the first 48 hours. If necrosis is suspected, the stoma is intubated with a small lubricated test tube, a pen light is directed into the center of the test tube, and the level of intestinal viability is noted. The stoma mucosa also can be pricked with a needle to determine blood flow. A normal postoperative stoma should be edematous, red, shiny, and moist. The mucocutaneous junction and the peristomal skin should be intact. Patients with IBD receiving corticosteroids may develop a mucocutaneous junction separation. If found, the area should be evaluated for depth of separation, and the treatment consists of filling the site with a skin barrier powder and fitting the solid skin barrier seal up to the stoma. The separation should heal in a 2- to 3-week period.

Patient Education

Due to decreasing postoperative hospitalization time, teaching of stoma management must begin as soon as possible. Because of limitations of time and patients' attention span, educating family members is important. The patient first is taught how to empty the pouch, and by postoperative day 3 should be independent with this activity. Pouch changing usually begins on postoperative days 2 to 4 with the patient assisting as much as possible. Home care is reviewed on day 5: topics include obtaining supplies, problem solving (checking on the seal, decreasing the diameter of the pouch to accommodate the shrinking stoma, treating denuded skin), and adjustment issues (how to wear clothes, how to talk about the "new" stoma). Again, family members can be helpful for the assimilation of this new information. A referral to a home care nursing service also may be indicated. The most important referral is to schedule the ET nurse outpatient clinic/office visit approximately 2 weeks after discharge to evaluate patient management, reassess stoma size and function, and to support the patient in the adjustment period. Subsequent outpatient visits are scheduled as necessary.

Pouching Options

The goals for choosing a pouching system are maintenance of a seal around the stoma for at least 3 days and protection of the peristomal skin. Important considerations are the patient's preference and acceptance. See Table 39–1 for manufacturer information.

Skin Barriers

All pouching systems consist of a solid skin barrier and odorproof pouch. The solid skin barrier, a thin flexible material manufactured of gelatin, pectin, and carboxymethylcellulose sodium, provides protection from stomal output and adheres the pouching system to the patient's skin. It is resistant to fecal output and maintains shape and adhesive properties for 3 to 7 days. Standard barriers last up to 4 days, while extended-wear barriers can be worn up to 7 days. Solid skin barriers are available as solid wafers, cut to fit the stoma; attached to the pouch, cut to fit or precut round openings; or precut washers, placed directly around the stoma.

Skin barriers also are available in three other formulations: liquid, paste, and powder. Liquid skin barriers are plasticized agents that place a barrier on the peristomal skin and are utilized to seal skin against stripping from aggressive adhesives or to seal denuded peristomal skin. Two types of liquid skin barriers are available, one with alcohol as a vehicle (which will cause burning if used on denuded skin) and "no sting," alcohol-free wipes. Paste skin barrier is used as a "caulking" agent around stomas to prevent migration of effluent under solid skin barriers and to fill uneven peristomal planes. Powder skin barriers are used to absorb moisture on the peristomal skin. A light dusting of the powder is placed upon the irritated area, rubbed into the area, and then sealed with the "no sting" barrier wipe. The pouching system then will adhere.

Pouches

While all currently manufactured pouches are odor proof, several pouch types are available. The type and style depend upon stoma location and construction, stoma output (volume and consistency), patient preference, and cost.

LENGTH OF 8″, 10″, OR 12″

The shorter the pouch used, the more often a patient must empty the pouch. A pouch never should be more than one-third full; otherwise, the weight of the pouch will loosen the adhesive seal. The 12″ ileostomy pouch is the standard size and, on average, allows emptying four to five times per day.

POUCH FILM

There are clear and opaque films. As previously noted, a clear pouch is used postoperatively, allowing the staff to visualize the stoma and pouch contents. Subsequently, the majority of patients switch to an opaque pouch.

ONE- OR TWO-PIECE SYSTEM

A one-piece system has the pouch and solid skin barrier attached as one unit. The two-piece system consists of the solid skin barrier wafer with body-side adhesive and a top-side flange that accepts the pouch. The pouch can be changed as required without disturbing the skin barrier seal. This allows wearing a shorter pouch for certain activities (eg, swimming) and substitution of a standard size pouch for "normal" wear time. The shorter pouch is snapped on the adhesive wafer for the activity and then popped off and replaced.

DRAINABLE OR CLOSED END

When stomal output reaches 200 cc, the pouching system must be emptied. It is advisable for patients to wear a drainable system that will allow them to empty the pouch

into the toilet, tissue off the end, and replace the clamp. Occasionally, patients will utilize a closed-end pouch on a two-piece system, pop the pouch off, throw it away, and replace it. Technically, this can be a problem as the patient must remove the pouch before it becomes more than one-half full (to avoid spilling the contents), and they must be in a location where they can discard the pouch.[*] Cost can be an issue when pouches are thrown away more than every 3 days.

PRECUT VERSUS CUT-TO-FIT

The peristomal skin must be protected from the damaging effects of the stomal output. This is achieved by snugly fitting the solid skin barrier against the stoma base. If a stoma is round, a precut pouching system can be utilized. Oval or uneven stomas are accommodated with a "cut-to-fit" pouching system.

Adjustment Issues

Adjustment to living with a stoma is a process that occurs over time as patients gain confidence in the ability to live life without fear of stoma-related issues. Information that will make adjustment as easy as possible includes dietary management, clothing considerations, daily activities, and intimacy issues.

Postoperatively, the patient should follow a low-residue diet until stoma edema has resolved. New foods should be introduced slowly and the patient advised to chew all foods thoroughly. Certain foods will thicken or loosen the output, making emptying the pouch easier. Postoperative gas may be an issue for approximately 1 week. Subsequently, most ileostomy gas is due to swallowing air (eg, during smoking or drinking carbonated beverages through a straw) or if the patient is lactose or fructose intolerant.

Clothing should not need to be significantly altered to accommodate an ostomy pouch. Snug undergarments help to flatten pouches against the abdomen by allowing the effluent to be equally distributed along the length of the pouch.

The outer adhesive on all ostomy pouches is water-resistant, allowing the patient to shower and bathe while wearing the pouch. Alternatively, the stoma and peristomal area can be exposed to a shower without harm. When the patient is engaging in prolonged water activity, a waterproof tape can be applied along the perimeter of the tape on the pouching system.

Sexual Activity

Return to sexual activity can pose problems for some patients with an ostomy. People should be encouraged to be honest with their partners and be certain they under-

---

[*] Editor's Note: Not in the toilet! Plastic bags are not biodegradeable. (SBH)

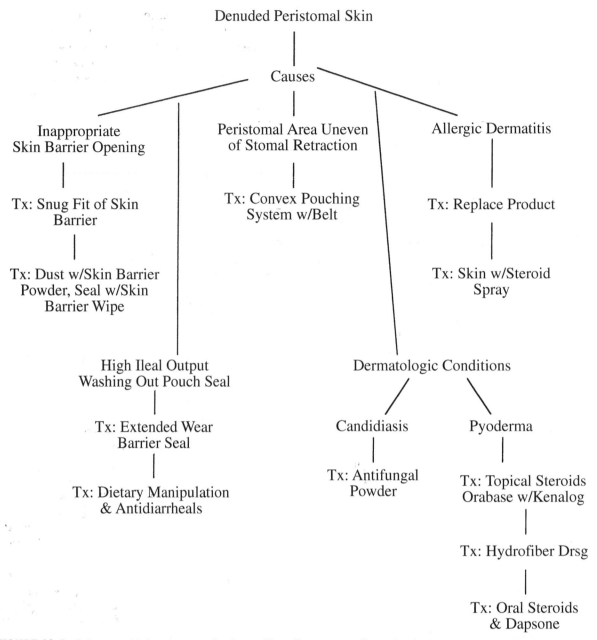

FIGURE 39–1. Reference guide for treatments of various problems. Tx = treatment; Drsg = dressing.

stand that the stoma has no feeling and that pressure exerted against the stoma or the pouch will not cause harm. Practical suggestions include emptying the pouch prior to sexual activity and using a mini pouch (on the two-piece system), which is a short pouch that hangs no longer than 2 inches and will not be in the way. Pouch covers are available from manufacturers in materials similar to lingerie. There is a chapter by an enterostomal therapy (ET) nurse on body image, sexuality, and IBD.

Emergency Kit

A person with an ostomy should carry an "emergency" kit with them at all times that includes adhesive tape (for emergency pouch saves), a precut ready-to-go pouch,

premoistened towelettes, several paper towels, and a medium-sized plastic bag. The emergency kit will allow the person to save a loosened pouch or to do an emergency change if necessary.

Problem Solving

Skin Problems

Peristomal skin problems are related to failure to maintain an adequate seal around the stoma. The stoma should be assessed for size, protrusion, type and quantity of output, and patency of the lumen. The peristomal skin should be examined with the patient in both the standing and sitting positions; contours should be checked for skin retraction. The size of the stoma must be duplicated on the solid skin barrier; if more than ⅛″ of skin is exposed to the stomal output, the skin will become denuded. Treatment consists of a proper-fitting skin barrier opening to cover the exposed, denuded skin and treatment of the denuded skin with barrier powder, sealed with barrier liquid wipes. Severely denuded, inflamed skin can be treated topically with sparingly applied steroid spray. Creams or ointments are too moist to maintain the pouch seal.

If the skin is uneven or has folds or deep scars, a flat pouching system may not make contact with the skin, necessitating a convex pouching system that protrudes into the uneven peristomal skin area to enhance the pouching seal. A stoma that does not protrude above the skin level also can be managed with the use of a convex pouching system. The convexity will apply gentle pressure around the stoma, causing the effluent to be discharged into the ostomy pouch.

Peristomal contact dermatitis resulting from pouching systems can induce reddened, weepy skin and inability to maintain a seal. Once the offending product is identified, it is replaced and a steroid spray is utilized until healing.

Candidiasis

Presentation of a diffuse, red, moist rash with satellite lesions on the peristomal skin is likely to be candidiasis. Topical treatment consists of securing a snug skin barrier seal to prevent moisture/leakage onto the peristomal skin and use of an antifungal powder at pouch change (every 3 days to provide treatment). If the area does not demonstrate evidence of healing in three pouch changes, oral antifungal medication is recommended.

Pyoderma

The incidence of pyoderma gangrenosum in patients with ulcerative colitis is as high as 12 percent and can occur in the peristomal area. Ulcers usually present as small painful lesions. The perilesional area displays a purplish hue surrounded by a halo of erythema. Moisture from ulcers can disrupt the ostomy seal. Systemic treatment includes corticosteroids and dapsone.† Topical treatment includes a topical steroid in a paste base (Orabase with Kenalog) and absorbent dressings/preparations (skin barrier powder and/or hydrofiber dressings). If the ulcers have significant depth, a thin layer of steroid paste is applied to the ulcer base and a piece of hydrofiber dressing is placed to fill the ulcer and absorb wound drainage so the solid skin barrier of the pouching system can be placed over the dressed ulcer. Pouch change depends upon the integrity of the seal; a 2- to 3-day seal

is desirable. The management of peristomal pyoderma is multidisciplinary with the gastroenterologist and ET nurse working together with the patient.

High Stomal Output

High stomal output can erode the solid skin barrier causing the pouching seal to leak. An important assessment of stomal function includes the amount of output. Patients can relate this by describing the amount of times the pouch is emptied in 24 hours and by describing the consistency of output. Normal ileostomy output should be approximately 1,000 cc/24 h with pasty consistency comparable to loose oatmeal. Temporary diverting loop stomas typically have an increased output because of shortened absorptive intestinal surface. If a patient is encountering high liquid output, an extended-wear barrier should be used with the pouching systems. Dietary counseling such as decreasing caffeine, lactose, and fat intake may assist in decreasing output; antidiarrheal medications such as loperamide may be needed.

Stomal Patency

Stomal patency should be assessed yearly by digital examination. The stoma should easily accommodate a lubricated finger; the ring of scar tissue at the mucocutaneous junction should not be very snug, and the fascial ring should not be tight. A snug, retracted stoma can cause intermittent obstructive symptoms. See Figure 39–1 for a quick reference guide.

Supplemental Reading
Bass EM, Del Pino A, Tan A, et al. Does preoperative stoma marking and education by the enterostomal therapist affect outcome? Dis Colon Rectum 1997;49:440–2.

Colwell JC. Enterostomal care in inflammatory bowel disease. In: Kirsner JB, Shorter RG, eds. Inflammatory bowel disease. 4th Ed. Baltimore: Williams & Wilkins, 1995:888–97.

Erwin-Toth P, Barret P. Stoma site marking: a primer. Ostomy Wound Mgmt 1997;43:18–25.

Erwin-Toth P, Doughty DB. Principles and procedures of stomal management. In: Bryant R, ed. Ostomies and continent diversions: nursing management. St. Louis: Mosby-Year Book, 1992:29–103.

Fleshman JAW, Lewis MG. Complications and quality of life after stoma surgery: a review of 16,470 patients in the UOA data registry. Semin Colon Rectal Surg 1991;2:66–72.

Golis AM. Sexual issues for the person with an ostomy. J Wound Ostomy Continence Nurs 1996;23:453–6.

Hull T. Ileoanal procedures: acute and long term management issues. J Wound Ostomy Continence Nurs 1999;26:201–6.

Pieper B, Mikols C. Predischarge and postdischarge concerns of person with an ostomy. J Wound Ostomy Continence Nurs 1996;23:105–9.

† Editor's Note: Cyclosporine is mentioned in the next chapter and is discussed, along with pulse steroids, in the chapters on skin problems in IBD. (TMB)

CHAPTER 40

BROOKE ILEOSTOMY

JASON H. BODZIN, MD

The Brooke ileostomy is the procedure of choice for the termination of the remaining bowel after the removal of the colon and rectum. It provides a safe and effective conduit for the bowel contents, which then empty unimpeded into an appropriate collection device. The main feature separating Brooke ileostomies from any precursors is eversion of the terminal bowel to coapt the serosal surface outside of the abdominal cavity such that serositis and ileal stenosis do not occur. Prior to this technique, ileostomy dysfunction was a physiologic consequence of ileostomy stenosis that occurred regularly in stomas. The Brooke ileostomy has stood the test of time such that surgeons today continue to utilize this operation as the procedure of choice for small bowel end stomas.

Surgical Options

The Brooke ileostomy is the procedure against which all other operations for ulcerative colitis (UC) and Crohn's colitis must be compared. The algorithms in Figures 40–1 and 40–2 depict the options for surgery in UC (Figure 40–1) and Crohn's disease (CD) (Figure 40–2). The continent ileostomy is an option before or after the creation of

a Brooke ileostomy for patients with UC but is generally contraindicated for patients with CD. In addition, the Brooke ileostomy may be a temporary procedure preceding a staged operation to restore bowel continuity. Conversely, the Brooke ileostomy may be a salvage procedure when one of the other alternative operations has been performed as the primary procedure. In CD, an ileoproctostomy can be converted to a Brooke ileostomy if the result is not satisfactory. Total proctocolectomy with Brooke ileostomy also is the operation for Crohn's colitis with the lowest rate of ileal recurrence.

As depicted in the UC surgical decision tree (see Figure 40–1), patients with advanced age, poor anal sphincter function, perianal disease, or other contraindications to sphincter-saving operations should be offered total proctocolectomy with Brooke ileostomy as the primary procedure. If any of the other alternatives fail, they can be salvaged with the Brooke ileostomy. In addition, other patients choose the Brooke ileostomy over alternative procedures because it is a single operation that provides predictable control of their lives plus an excellent state of health in the overwhelming majority of the patients.

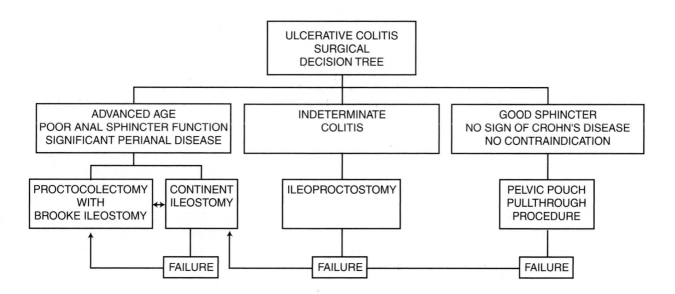

FIGURE 40–1. Surgical options for ulcerative colitis.

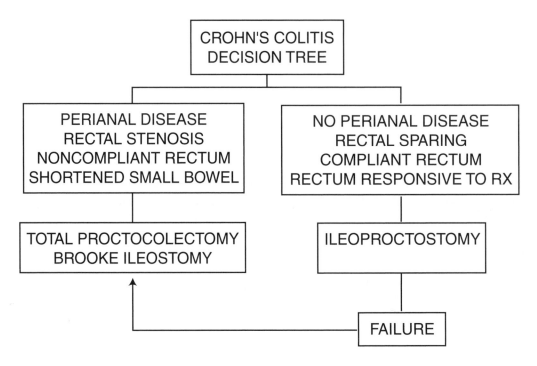

FIGURE 40–2. Surgical options for Crohn's disease. RX = prescriptions.

Preoperative Preparation

Preparation of the patient for the Brooke ileostomy is an important part of the procedure. Patients should talk to other patients who have had this procedure for the same disease and who have had a satisfactory result. Bowel preparation is carried out at home. Preparation of the gastrointestinal tract for proctocolectomy always consists of mechanical emptying of the bowel using a sodium phosphate solution or citrate of magnesia. Others have found success with polyethylene glycol preparations. Oral antibiotic preparation is controversial. I use a modified Nichols-Condon regimen that utilizes 1 g of neomycin and 1 g of erythromycin base every 4 hours, for four doses beginning at noon on the day before surgery. Patients who are already having significant diarrhea are usually given a single bottle of citrate of magnesia as the entire mechanical preparation. The preparation should be modified to the patient's clinical bowel pattern to avoid dehydration. Because nausea is a frequent accompaniment when antibiotics are used, I prescribe an antiemetic routinely.

Enterostomal Therapist Consultation

Patients are seen by an enterostomal therapist prior to surgery either by separate appointment a few days before the surgical procedure or in the preoperative holding area on the day of surgery. It is important to mark the patient when he or she is fully awake and cooperative. The appropriate site should be selected after noting the abdominal anatomy with the patient sitting, standing, and preferably wearing street clothes. In the operating room, the site should be scratched or otherwise indelibly marked on the patient, since ink markers may be rubbed off during the operation itself and be invisible at the end of the procedure when the stoma is actually constructed.

Operative Procedure

The procedure begins with the creation of the stomal site. The terminal ileum has been clamped or stapled off during the operation. The creation of the stoma usually follows the completion of the operation and is completed in two parts. While the abdomen is open, the stomal site is created. A circle of skin is excised using the stomal marking as the center of the circle. The diameter is approximately 15 to 20 mm for the average stoma. Even though this circle is quite small when it is created, it readily enlarges and easily accommodates the bowel. For obvious reasons, it is better to make an opening too small than too large. Using sharp dissection or electrocautery, a cylinder of subcutaneous fat is removed until the fascia is approached. Retractors are placed to provide exposure and an X-shaped incision is made in the rectus fascia without injury to the muscle below. The size of the X roughly fits the size of the original circle made in the skin. The edges of the incision in the fascia should clearly be demarcated and the muscle visualized below. With a finger in the peritoneal cavity, on the peritoneum opposite the opening, a clamp is inserted by the other hand spreading the rectus muscle in line with its fibers and down to the peritoneum. The clamp then pushes the peritoneum against the operators' finger of the opposite hand, and if the peritoneum cannot be readily penetrated, cautery or a small incision can be performed on the tip of the clamp to assist penetration. The peritoneum then is spread by the clamp and a finger is inserted between the jaws of the clamp and through the peritoneum up into the opening that has been created. A second finger inserted from the skin side of the stomal opening then can be inserted next to the finger coming up from the peritoneal cavity, and eventually the opening is widened to two finger widths. Further incision of the peritoneum is not necessary and may be detrimental.

Attention then is turned to the bowel itself. The end of the ileum to be matured should be denuded of its mesentery for a distance of about 3 cm. If there is any question about the viability of the end, it should be trimmed back to healthy, pink bowel. The bowel is then brought through the newly created stomal opening and should protrude 2 to 3 cm above the skin without any tension or pulling of the bowel inward. The skin with the bowel protruding should remain flat once the bowel has been pulled through. If there is any tension on the bowel itself, the mesentery should be freed, such that the tension is relieved. No sutures are placed between the peritoneum and the bowel or the fascia and the bowel. Some surgeons close the right gutter between the lateral abdominal wall and the stomal mesentery while others feel this is unnecessary. The stoma remains in its position, unopened and unmatured until the abdominal wound is closed.

The maturation of the stoma is performed by the use of an absorbable suture such as Vicryl® or similar suture in an interrupted fashion. Generally, eight individual stitches are placed starting with the four quadrants and then one stitch between each of those stitches, making a total of eight. Each stitch is a maturing stitch that consists of a full-thickness bite of the end of the bowel, a seromuscular bite of the corresponding portion of the bowel at the skin level, followed by a subcuticular bite in the corresponding portion of the skin. These stitches are placed individually and hemostats are placed to hold each individual suture to keep the entire wound open and visible until all of the stitches are placed. They then are tied individually and the knots are cut closely. A bag is cut to fit the stomal size and the patient leaves the operating room with a suitable collection pouch in place.

End-Loop Modification

In obese patients or those with very frail mesenteric vessels, the end of the stoma may not survive the trip through the subcutaneous tissues. Patients with circulatory disorders may have a poor pulse pressure and the end of the ileum that has been denuded of vessels may not be able to survive. In such instances or others in which the vitality of the stoma is in question, an end-loop modification is appropriate. In this variety of stoma, the end of the ileum is brought as a loop and the mesentery is left in place. The loop is matured with the unopened end of the stoma in the subcutaneous tissue. The maturation of this end-loop ileostomy is technically more challenging than the standard Brooke variety. However, when properly constructed, this type of stoma will look and function exactly like the typical Brooke ileostomy. For a complete discussion of the technique for the construction of an end-loop ileostomy, please see the description by Oakley and Fazio (1993).

Stoma Maintenance

Maintenance of the stoma takes some practice and a lot of common sense. Patients should be instructed by a qualified enterostomal therapist who remains available for later questions. Most minor problems produced by the geography of the pouch and its proximity to the abdominal wound, wrinkles and curves in the skin, and the bony prominences can be managed by the choice of a suitable ostomy pouch. Convex pouching systems are useful when the height of the stoma is a problem.

Complications

Complications of the Brooke ileostomy may be a mere nuisance or may be so severe as to require revision or translocation of the stoma. Superficial slough of the mucosa or full-thickness necrosis of the stoma usually occurs shortly after stomal construction. Necrosis that does not go below the fascia may frequently improve over time, and if pouching is not a significant problem, observation may be appropriate. Necrosis below the fascia requires immediate operation to revise and essentially redo the stomal construction. Superficial slough will nearly always heal on its own and generally does not require reconstruction of the stoma.

Stomal Obstruction

Stomal obstruction can occur at several levels and is most common at the level of the fascia. The diagnosis is by radiography, which usually shows an air ileogram up to the level of the obstruction or by careful manual examination of the stoma. This problem usually can be remedied by percutaneous laceration of the fascia with a finger in the stoma to guide the action of the scalpel and preserve the integrity of the bowel.

Volvulus

Volvulus of the small bowel around the stoma can occur. This requires operation, sometimes on an urgent basis. In such cases, the right gutter space between the mesentery of the stoma and the lateral and posterior peritoneal walls should be closed to prevent recurrence.

Crohn's Disease in Ostomy

Recurrent CD in an ileostomy is a not uncommon phenomenon. A number of patients who were operated on for "ulcerative colitis" many years ago are now presenting with pre-ileostomy strictures, indicative of CD. These strictures occasionally are asymptomatic but should be treated as any Crohn's recurrence. Occasionally, surgery is necessary to resect a strictured segment and create a new stoma from healthy bowel. In my practice, such patients are placed on life-long prophylactic therapy after surgery.[*]

Metabolic Complications

Metabolic problems after ileostomy may be troublesome. Many patients do not encounter any metabolic difficulties after colonic resection and ileostomy output may be formed and resemble normal feces. On the other hand, many patients, particularly those with CD, have a very watery or liquid output that may be troublesome. For the first 6 months after an ileostomy creation, patients should be encouraged to increase their salt and fluid intake. This is particularly true when patients complain of lightheadedness or postural hypotension symptoms. Electrolyte-containing solutions should be suggested such as soups, Gatorade, Pedialyte, and similar drinks. Occasionally, antidiarrheal agents such as loperamide or diphenoxylate with atropine are necessary. If portions of the terminal ileum have been resected prior to construction of the stoma, dietary supplementation may be necessary as for any patient who has undergone ileal resection.

Peristomal Fistula

Peristomal fistula may occur shortly after ileostomy construction (as a technical complication) or it may occur much later, in which case it is indicative of CD. When the fistula is due to obstruction distally, the stoma should be revised and often will require transfer to the opposite side. When there is no associated obstruction, and the fistula can be pouched within the ordinary stomal opening, medical treatment such as immunosuppressive therapy or infliximab (Remicade®, Centocor, Malvern, Pennsylvania) may be utilized. Branching fistulae will nearly always require stomal reconstruction.[†]

Pyoderma Gangrenosum

---

[*] Editor's Note: Pentasa® (Ferring-Shire Pharmaceuticals, Florence, Kentucky) would be a minimum. Since azathioprine or 6-MP are excellent maintenance medications, some patients are placed on these medications but trials of efficacy and dosage are needed. (TMB)

[†] Editor's Note: My preliminary experience is to have peristomal fistulae recur after Remicade is discontinued. (TMB)

Pyoderma in the peristomal distribution is not unusual and can be troublesome. There are many different treatments for pyoderma, such as local application of steroid preparations or cyclosporine paste, steroid injections into the base of the pyoderma, or oral or intravenous cyclosporine in resistant cases. Translocation of the stoma is to be discouraged since pyoderma is likely to occur at the site of the new stoma. When pyoderma creates excess granulation tissue and pouching becomes a problem, the hypertrophic tissue can be leveled with the use of the CO_2 laser.

Prolapse

Prolapse of an ileostomy usually can be repaired by an outpatient procedure in which the ileostomy is carefully freed from the skin, the prolapsed bowel resected, and a new ileostomy created from the remaining bowel 2 to 3 cm above skin level. This can be done under local anesthesia, and the procedure has minimal morbidity in experienced hands.

Bleeding

Bleeding from the ileostomy itself may be caused by a misplaced or traumatic pouch or may be related to portal hypertension. In the latter case, a "caput medusae" may occur around a stoma. This should be treated by local injection of sclerosing agents, which are utilized in a manner similar to esophageal or gastric variceal injection. Hypertrophic granulation tissue may grow on a stoma and may bleed in response to minor trauma. These granulations can be cauterized safely with silver nitrate sticks in the office or removed by the CO_2 laser in the operating room. The ileal mucosa readily regenerates after laser ablation of stomal granulation tissue even when significant tissue is removed.

Quality of Life

The role of the enterostomal therapist in the management of ileostomy difficulties cannot be overemphasized. Each ileostomy patient should have available to him or her the means of contacting a knowledgeable enterostomal therapist to help with day-to-day problems. In addition, complications can be presented to the stomal therapist for appropriate triage.

The quality of life of patients following ileostomy surgery is nearly always better than that prior to surgery. Comparisons of quality-of-life issues usually are made between the Brooke ileostomy and other rectal-sparing procedures such as the ileoproctostomy or ileoanal pull-through. Studies that have looked at these issues have always shown high levels of satisfaction with whatever operation was chosen by an individual patient.

It should be kept in mind that a well-constructed and well-located stoma is a requirement for patient satisfaction.

The construction of the stoma should not be relegated to the least experienced surgeon and should remain the focus of the operation until the last stitch is placed and the stomal pouch is carefully applied.

Reference

Oakley J, Fazio V. Ileostomy. In: Fielding LP, Goldberg SM, eds. Rob and Smith's operative surgery. Alimentary track and abdominal wall-colon, rectum and anus. 5th Ed. London: Butterworth Heinemann, 1993:257–60.

Supplemental Reading

Brooke BN. The management of ileostomy including its complications. Lancet 1952;2:102–4.

McLeod RS, Lavery IC, Leatherman JR, et al. Factors affecting the quality of life with conventional ileostomy. World J Surg 1986;10:474–80.

Roy PH, Sauer WG, Behars ON, et al. Experiences with ileostomies: evaluation of long-term rehabilitation in 497 patients. Am J Surg 1970;119:77.

Todd IP. Intestinal stomas. London: Heinemann, 1978.

CHAPTER 41

Continent Ileostomy (Kock Pouch)

Sandy L. Fogel, MD

It is generally recognized that the Brooke ileostomy was the major advance in the treatment of any disease that required removal or diversion of the entire colon. The Brooke ileostomy should still be considered the gold standard in terms of health, functional abilities, and stability. It gives more freedom from further medication and less need for further surgical procedures. However, the Brooke ileostomy is still viewed by many as less than ideal, and the majority of people facing proctocolectomy would rather do without the bag and without storage of stool on the outside of the body.

The first reasonably successful procedure that was developed to overcome this objection was the continent ileostomy, or Kock pouch. The second alternative is the ileoanal pouch procedure, which is discussed elsewhere.

Continent Ileostomy

The continent ileostomy was popular in the late 1970s through the 1980s but has justifiably fallen into disfavor despite its successes. As well as discussing these successes, there will be a lengthy discussion of the failures, especially the late ones. Late complications are a continuing cause of surgical referral.*

The continent ileostomy or Kock pouch is based in part on the concept of a reservoir of bowel with a reverse intussusception to create a valve. This procedure has gone through multiple slight alterations and improvements, especially in the construction of the valve, but basically remains unchanged.

Technique

The continent ileostomy requires the use of approximately 45 cm of distal small bowel. Two 15-cm segments are folded upon themselves and a long side-to-side anastomosis is formed along the adjacent walls of the ileum. The terminal 15 cm is then used to form a valve, which prevents leakage. This is done by creating a reverse intussusception of 5 cm in length, thereby using 10 cm of bowel. The remaining 5 cm is used to reach the abdominal wall as a stoma. This can be placed flush with the skin and be lower in the right lower quadrant than a Brooke

ileostomy because it does not leak stool and does not require a bag. The pouch is completed by folding the remaining looped bowel and closing the pouch. The valve projects into the lumen of the pouch and creates continence. As stool fills the pouch and pressure increases, it presses on the outer portion of the valve, squeezing it shut. Defecation is accomplished by passing a tube through the stoma into the pouch, overcoming the resistance of the valve. This allows stool to flow out through the tube, emptying the pouch.

Valve Stability

The major technical problem that needed to be solved was stability of the valve. It is held in place by a series of sutures and/or staples along the length of the valve. Since there is a double layer of bowel, there are also two layers of mesentery. The sutures placed along the valve need to be away from the mesentery or bleeding and/or ischemia may result. The peritoneum and excess fat is stripped from the mesentery to decrease the volume in the intussusception and to add to the fixation. The serosal surface of the bowel is scored with electrocautery, also to improve fixation as the two opposed serosal surfaces hopefully fuse. A fascial collar is wrapped around the outflow tract to prevent dilation. At one time, mesh was used as a collar but the problem of erosion was too great.

Despite these maneuvers, the valves are not always stable. Several other manipulations have been attempted, the most prominent of which is the *Barnett adaptation*. This pouch is made with a reversed, isoperistaltic valve, which is discussed later. It also replaces the piece of fascia with an additional length of bowel used as a collar around the outflow tract.

Immediate Postoperative Period

In the immediate postoperative period, the drainage tube is placed into the pouch and secured in place. In the early years, this was done for up to 6 weeks, but more recently for 10 days to 2 weeks. This is still important because the valve creates a small bowel obstruction, which would lead to an unacceptable risk of leak from the long suture lines proximal to the point of obstruction. Upon removing the tube, patient education must take place immediately. The person with a new continent ileostomy must be able to

---

* Editor's Note: This chapter is longer than many others, which were edited to avoid duplication. This information seemed unique and largely survived the editorial blade. (TMB)

intubate the pouch from day 1; otherwise, this will again be a functional small bowel obstruction. Initially, the pouch is emptied very frequently, but over the next 4 to 6 months it will dilate and become the reservoir that is intended. Eventually, the pouch is emptied anywhere from two to six times a day. The patient perceives a sense of fullness, but no sense of urgency. Between emptying, the stoma is covered with a small absorbent dressing to keep the moisture from the mucosa off the skin and clothes. Some need to irrigate because the stool is too thick to flow through the tube, but this is the exception. Overall, people with a working continent ileostomy find it very satisfactory and usually preferable to the alternative of a Brooke ileostomy.

Patient Selection

A continent ileostomy may be made in people with a diagnosis of ulcerative colitis (UC) or familial adenomatous polyposis. It can be done at the time of colectomy or subsequently. It also can be done in some who have had a failed ileoanal pouch procedure or in the rare case of removal of the colon and rectum for other reasons.

Contraindications

A continent ileostomy should not be done for Crohn's disease (CD). The risk of recurrence of CD in the pouch is too high. It should not be done for the diagnosis of *indeterminate colitis*. Some feel that exceptions can be made in people who have had indeterminate colitis and have had a stable ileostomy with no evidence of recurrent CD in the small bowel for 5 years. It should not be made in people undergoing colectomy on an urgent or emergent basis, or in those on a prolonged course of high-dose steroids. Patients who have a failed ileoanal pouch procedure secondary to severe pouchitis should not be given this operation since pouchitis will recur in the continent ileostomy. Exceptions include the obese, the very young, or the elderly. It should not be done in patients who lack the psychological or physical ability to care for themselves. Lastly, it should not be done by those surgeons who rarely perform the procedure.

Early Problems

Besides the usual complications of any major surgical procedure, there are a number that are specific to continent ileostomy procedures.

Ischemia of the Pouch or Outflow Tract

This rare complication usually is noted early and has the same clinical syndrome as ischemic bowel from any other source. If it involves the outflow tract, it can be seen by direct inspection of the stoma. It usually results in the loss of the pouch, requiring creation of a Brooke ileostomy. It is an understandable risk because of the twists and turns made in the mesentery during creation of the continent ileostomy.

Anastomotic Leak

This usually is noticed due to drainage of stool from the closed suction drain that should be placed in the right lower quadrant at the time of creation of the pouch. It can occur anywhere from the 4th to the 10th postoperative day. It usually can be managed without loss of the pouch. The drainage catheter is left in place within the pouch and converted to a sump drain. The patient is to take nothing by mouth and is started on total parenteral nutrition. With time, this fistula will close. Proximal diversion rarely is needed, but is another option.

Transvalvular Fistula

This is noticed due to incontinence anywhere from 1 to 3 weeks postoperatively and usually after removal of the catheter. It can also occur early with leakage of stool around the catheter. The fistula allows stool from the pouch to bypass the valve and exit directly to the outflow tract. It is the result of very focal ischemia and may be caused by injury to the small mesenteric vessels during defatting of the mesentery or by sutures in the valve. It also may arise from over-vigorous use of cautery in an attempt to stabilize the intussusception. It also may occur later by erosion of the mesh in those who have had a mesh collar. In any event, this invariably requires reoperation with creation of a new valve.

Stomal Stenosis

Stenosis can occur anywhere from several months after surgery onwards, and usually is at the skin level. This type of stenosis is relatively easy to fix with dilatations, local excision of scar, or more frequently with a small advancement V-Y plasty. However, in those prone to vigorous scar formation, it may recur. If the stenosis includes any significant length of the outflow tract, the flap can be lengthened and advanced as far down the outflow tract as is needed, even through the level of the anterior fascia.

Valve Disruption

This also may occur at any time and also is a complication that requires reoperation. It is manifest by near total incontinence, which cannot be left untreated. The flush stoma and low position does not allow adequate placement of an external appliance. This subject is discussed later.

Pouchitis

Pouchitis is related to stasis of stool within a small bowel reservoir. It can occur early or late, and depending upon the specific definition one accepts, may occur in most or all pouches. Not all pouches with histologic changes of either acute or chronic inflammation have clinically relevant pouchitis, and not all pouches with the typical clinical syndrome have severe acute inflammation. Pouchitis can be defined as being present only when it creates symptoms sufficient to require treatment. Clinically relevant pouchitis is rare, but does occur in those who have pouches for polyposis. Most who develop clinically significant pouchitis have the onset within 2 years, with the median time to onset of only 5 months. Early pouchitis usually is more severe and includes low-grade fever, malaise, pain and tenderness over the pouch, and increased stool output, which occasionally contains blood. Those who experienced extra-intestinal manifestations of their UC, especially the bone and joint complaints, may have these symptoms recur.

Pouchitis can be intermittent or continuous and responsive to treatment or unresponsive. The treatment usually consists of metronidazole, ciprofloxacin, or tetracycline. Some need continuous treatment, perhaps with patients rotating antibiotics on an alternate-week basis. Pouchitis usually is not the cause of either reoperation or loss of the pouch.

Summary

During the initial discussion with a person contemplating a continent ileostomy, a figure of approximately 20 percent early complication rate requiring some form of surgical intervention should be quoted along with another 20 percent incidence of pouchitis. However, over the years it has become clear that late complications occur and we do not as yet know what the final percentage of reoperation or pouch loss will be. There have been people with perfect pouch function for 20 years or more who then present with their first problems.

Late Problems

Most of the literature reports complications within 1 or 2 years of the procedure, but it is clear that several continue to occur, with unknown frequency, 5, 10, 15, or 20 years later. Most disturbing are reports of dysplasia and development of cancer within the pouch. This is rare, and other problems are far more frequent. Although stenosis of the outflow tract and transvalvular fistula, in theory, may occur at any time, I have not seen stenosis past the relatively early stages, and I have seen only one late fistula in the absence of a mesh collar. Pouchitis, valve prolapse, and valve disruption are the problems that continue to occur. Patients with these problems complain of slowly increasing difficulty intubating the pouch, progressive incontinences, or both. They occur with varying degrees. Many put up with these problems for quite some time before calling. They are seldom of sudden onset and do not represent complete cessation of function of the pouch. Few have other complaints to help in distinguishing one from the other, but it is crucial to do so because the treatments are very different.

Late Pouchitis

Late pouchitis in a continent ileostomy is clinically different from early pouchitis or pouchitis found in ileoanal pouches. It presents mostly with incontinence, with the relative absence of any other symptom. There is very little pain or tenderness, no fever, and no diarrhea or blood. There is little or no difficulty intubating the pouch, although a few individuals report this. Pouch endoscopy does not reveal the typical changes of acute inflammation with erythema, friability, or ulceration. There is chronic inflammation, but this occurs with almost all pouches. It seems to be a variety of pouchitis because usually it responds well to antibiotics. A few patients who have had several months or years of slowly increasing incontinence have the incontinence disappear in several days to a week. Some responses last several months after a 2-week course of antibiotics but virtually all recur and require intermittent repeated courses at times for many years.

Valve Prolapse

Valve prolapse occurs with the intussusception intact. The entire double thickness of the bowel remains together and prolapses to a varying degree through the outflow tract. In order for this to occur, the outflow tract must be relatively dilated, from the fascial collar outward. The prolapse may be partial or complete.

Complete prolapse, with the entire valve being visible on the abdominal wall outside the mucocutaneous junction, occurs mainly in those in the third trimester of pregnancy. This is possible because of the progesterone-induced softening of fibrous tissue that allows abdominal and pelvic expansion, coupled with increased intra-abdominal pressure. It is relatively easy to manually reduce, and is managed with an indwelling catheter for the duration of the pregnancy. Within weeks of delivery, things return toward normal and the prolapse ceases. These women seldom have subsequent prolapse. Complete prolapse also may occur without pregnancy, but this is very unusual.

Most often, prolapse is partial, with the tip of the valve being present somewhere within the outflow tract, not visible outside the stoma. If one would look down the tract, the prolapsed valve would resemble the uterine cervix, with a small central path leading to the interior of the pouch, and a circular cul-de-sac surrounding it. This appearance explains the difficulty experienced in intubation of the pouch. The tube must hit the central tract exactly to enter the pouch. Anything slightly off-center will result in the catheter hitting a blind-folded end of bowel. Those with this situation will report difficulty intubating the pouch—requiring multiple attempts—but eventually will accomplish the task when the tube suddenly and effortlessly enters the pouch. Pushing does not help. It only creates local trauma, in which case small amounts of blood may be seen. Occasionally, the inability to intubate the pouch causes a small bowel obstruction. However, when prolapse occurs, the functional part of the valve shortens. The pressure increases and incontinence usually occurs. This is akin to overflow incontinence of the urinary bladder.

DIAGNOSIS

Upon examination of such a pouch, digital examination of the outflow tract occasionally reveals an obvious palpable prolapse. This can be reduced manually as a temporary measure. More often it cannot be felt with the fingertip, and other diagnostic methods are needed. I have found that careful palpation with the tip of a Kelly clamp inserted through the stoma usually identifies the typical anatomy, suggesting prolapse. The last maneuver is pouch endoscopy. This may visualize the prolapse, and often reduces it. It also rules out valve disruption. There is a chapter on pouch endoscopy.

REPAIR

The repair of valve prolapse has been fairly problematic. The techniques range from laparotomy with opening the pouch and staple fixation within, to cautery-induced scarification of the subcutaneous tissue around the outflow tract. A newer technique involves ultrasonic fragmentation of the adjacent mucosal surfaces within the pouch to induce additional fixation. We now perform a simple outpatient procedure under local anesthesia consisting of separation of the mucocutaneous junction at the antimesenteric portion of the outflow tract for about 180° of the circumference. This is dissected along the bowel wall to the fascia. A single heavy polypropylene suture is placed in the fascia to narrow the outflow tract at this location. A series of silk Lembert sutures then are placed from this location outward along the bowel wall to narrow the remaining outflow tract. This is all done with the drainage catheter in place to ensure a snug fit, but to avoid creating stenosis. At the conclusion of the repair, the catheter is removed and normal intubation of the pouch resumes immediately. In a small group of patients, only one has had a recurrence of prolapse with this procedure.

Valve Disruption

Valve disruption is the worst of the complications to haunt a continent ileostomy. Despite the numerous maneuvers designed to create a stable valve, some valves still come apart. The frequency is unknown, because there is no literature reporting 20- or 30-year follow-up. It is not inevitable, and likely does not occur in most. I estimate that late disruption occurs in anywhere from 5 to 20 percent of pouches. Its most typical presentation is incontinence that usually comes on gradually because of slow, progressive loss of valve length and symmetry. As the valve shortens, the length of bowel lost from the valve projects out of the pouch toward the abdominal wall. Since this is a fixed location, the bowel will kink to the side, creating an acute angulation. This then accounts for the second complaint, that of difficulty intubating the pouch. The degree of incontinence usually is significant, creating a need for surgical repair. The stoma is low on the abdominal wall and flush with the skin and is very difficult to treat with a bag, although this is a reasonable short-term maneuver. Repair involves laparotomy and complete mobilization of the pouch and outflow tract. The old valve and outflow tract are resected and discarded. The small bowel is divided 15 cm proximal to the pouch and this is used to create a new valve and outflow tract. The pouch is turned 180° and the proximal small bowel is anastomosed to the defect in the pouch created by removal of the old valve. This is called an isoperistaltic reversal procedure. It can be done once. Any further major problems should be treated with removal of the pouch and conversion to a Brooke ileostomy. Another pouch should not be made. The length of small bowel lost or potentially lost during this procedure is too likely to create problems with ileal function and diarrhea.

Summary

When I receive a phone call concerning late dysfunction of a continent ileostomy, it invariably involves incontinence, difficulty with intubation, or both. Those who have only slowly increasing incontinence usually have late pouchitis treatable with antibiotics. Those with only difficulty intubating usually have valve prolapse. And in those with significant components of both, one would fear valve disruption.

In the case of predominantly difficult intubation, the diagnosis of prolapse can be made in the office without endoscopy or contrast study. The repair is relatively easy.

In the case of patients with both incontinence and difficulty with intubation, I give antibiotics prior to the visit. A few of these people also appear to have a significant component of pouchitis and improve sufficiently to remain satisfied without further surgical intervention. If there is no significant improvement with antibiotics, local examination of the outflow tract will reveal prolapse if present, but this usually represents valve disruption. This is confirmed by pouch endoscopy with retroflexion of the scope.

Once valve disruption is confirmed, one may proceed directly to a discussion with the patient concerning either repair by isoperistaltic reversal or by conversion to a Brooke ileostomy. Since there are even less data on long-term stability of a reversed valve, a few people are reluctant to do this if faced with yet another major operation in 10 or 20 more years. However, most with working continent ileostomies are so satisfied with them that they will go through any number of major operations to keep them and to keep them properly functioning.

Supplemental Reading

Barnett WO. Current experiences with continent intestinal reservoir. SG&O 1989;168:1–5.

Cohen Z. Pouch inflammation following reservoir procedures. In: Bayless TM, Hanauer SB, eds. Advanced therapy of inflammatory bowel disease. Hamilton: BC Decker, 1990: 137–4.

Curtis RD, Sweeney WB, Denobile JW, Hurwitz E. Kock pouch dysfunction during pregnancy. Management of a case. Surg Endosc 1996;10:775–7.

Ecker KW, Hildebrandt U, Haberer M, Feifel G. Biomechanical stabilization of the nipple valve in continent ileostomy. Br J Surg 1996;83:1582–5.

Fazio VW, Tjandra JJ. Technique for nipple valve fixation to prevent valve slippage in continent ileostomy. Dis Colon Rectum 1992;35:1177–9.

Gottlieb LM, Handelsman JC. Treatment of outflow tract problems associated with continent ileostomy (Kock pouch). Dis Colon Rectum 1991;34:936–40.

Hulten L. Proctocolectomy and ileostomy to pouch surgery for ulcerative colitis. World J Surg 1998;22:335–41.

Kohler LW, Pemberton JH, Zinsmeister AR, Kelly KA. Quality of life after proctocolectomy. A comparison of Brooke ileostomy, Kock pouch, and ileal pouch-anal anastomosis. Gastroenterology 1991;101:679–84.

Svaninger G, Nordgren S, Oresland T, Hulten L. Incidence and characteristics of pouchitis in the Kock continent ileostomy and the pelvic pouch. Scand J Gastroenterol 1993;28: 695–700.

CHAPTER 42

ILEOANAL POUCH ANASTOMOSIS

FEZA H. REMZI, MD, AND VICTOR W. FAZIO, MB, MS, FRACS, FACS

Restorative proctocolectomy (RP) with ileoanal anastomosis (IPAA) has become the gold standard of surgical treatment for ulcerative colitis (UC). In many series, 90 percent plus of procedures for UC involve RP/IPAA. This may be performed as a primary two-stage procedure, of total proctocolectomy (TPC) and IPAA, with temporary loop ileostomy, or multistaged with subtotal colectomy oversew of rectal stump and end ileostomy, followed by completion proctectomy IPAA and loop ileostomy, with the final (third) procedure being closure of loop ileostomy. Figure 42–1 outlines indications for surgery.

Single-Stage Procedure

In a few cases (up to 10% of RP cases), the procedure is done in one stage, TPC and IPAA without loop ileostomy. This is an alternative we will use in well-motivated and informed patients who are:

- aware of the 10 percent leak rate from the pouch anal anastomosis and the possibility that an urgent ileostomy may be required in the early postoperative period; and*
- aware that recovery—both hospital stay and recovery time (return of stamina) to return to work and social activities may be double that of the usual 6- to 7-day hospital stay and the 2 months normal recovery time. This is due to the combination of recovering from a major abdominal procedure as well as from the obligatory early excessive stool frequency accompanying a one-stage operation.

Thus, we will consider the one-stage operation:
- where there is no toxicity or feature adverse to tissue healing (prednisone dose < 20 mg/d, diabetes, immunosuppressive therapy);
- where the operation has proceeded effortlessly with minimal blood loss (no transfusion requirement) and hemostasis is considered excellent;
- where there has been no difficulty in getting the pouch to reach the anus without excessive tension;

---

* Editor's Note: One also should be aware that a pouch that has leaked or been infected may heal with a smaller capacity, thus increasing the number of bowel movements per day for that individual patient. (TMB)

- where intact tissue rings (doughnuts) have been obtained using the double-stapled technique; and
- where during the operation pouch/anastomotic testing with air has shown no anastomotic or pouch leak.

Paradoxically, this may be the procedure of choice in obese patients who cannot lose weight preoperatively. In those individuals, addition of a temporary ileostomy may produce such tension on the superior mesenteric artery (the determining factor for the ease of reach of the pouch to the anus) that we believe the completed IPAA may be excessively vulnerable to leak or disruption.

Other Procedures for Ulcerative Colitis Patients

Subtotal or Total Colectomy and Ileostomy

This is preferred in cases of:

- a diagnostic dilemma ("indeterminate colitis")—this includes features that are ambiguous for Crohn's disease (CD) versus UC (eg, patchy colonic disease, backwash ileitis);
- patients on very large doses (eg, 50 to 60 mg/d) of prednisone;
- patients with toxic colitis or megacolon;
- gross obesity, where ability to lose weight is precluded by high-dose steroids; or
- malnutrition, especially hypoalbuminemia.

Following subtotal colectomy (STC) and ileostomy, and favorable histologic review, patients may undergo completion proctectomy and IPAA some 5 to 6 months later.

Total Colectomy and Ileorectal Anastomosis

This may be the procedure of choice in two situations, both requiring absence of florid or significant rectal disease: (1) patients with distant metastases (liver, lung) where colon cancer complicates UC and (2) the younger woman who is anxious to maximize her chances of child bearing. There is evidence that RP/IPPA, with its necessary pelvic adhesions postoperatively, will diminish fertility due to peritubal and periovarian adhesions. Additionally, we will apply hyaluronidase/methylcellulose film (Seprafilm-Genzyme®) to the gonadal structures to limit such

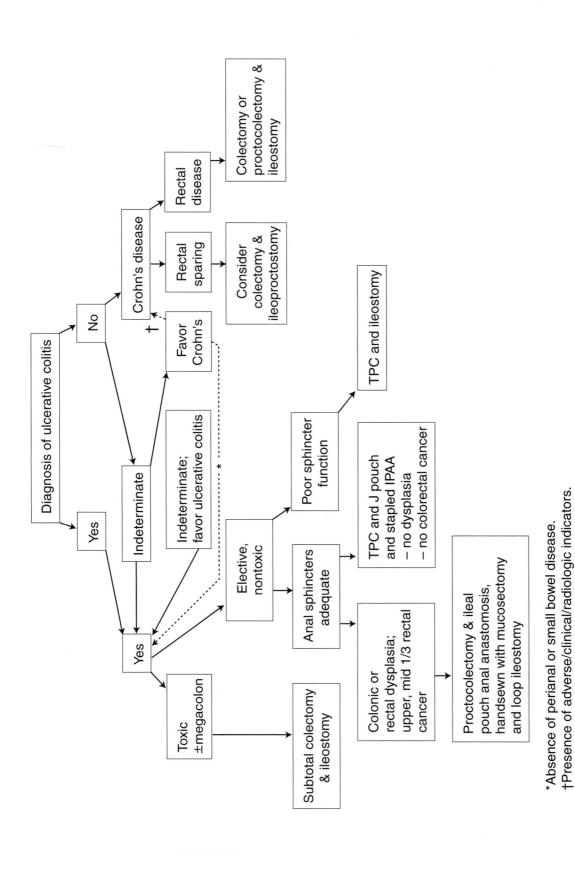

FIGURE 42–1. Indications for surgery. TPC = total proctocolectomy; IPAA = ileal pouch-anal anastomosis; * = absence of perianal or small bowel disease; † = presence of adverse/clinical/radiologic indicators.

*Absence of perianal or small bowel disease.
†Presence of adverse/clinical/radiologic indicators.

adhesions. Patients may undergo rectal resection and conversion to a pelvic pouch in 30 to 50 percent of cases—should disabling proctitis occur or rectal cancer risk become significant with future pregnancies. Following RP and IPAA, we recommend cesarean section due to the risk of sphincter injury from episiotomy or prolonged or difficult labor. Although data from several sources attest to the early good pouch function with vaginal delivery, the studies are flawed by the lack of adequate follow-up of pouch function in the middle-aged woman, many years after IPAA. There is a chapter on ileorectal anastomosis and two chapters on pregnancy and IBD.[†]

Total Proctocolectomy and Ileostomy

This has been the standard surgical treatment of UC and is appropriate when:

- the patient is not unduly concerned about having a permanent ileostomy;
- anal sphincter function is poor (we note, however, that preoperative anal incontinence may be due to very active rectal disease reflecting urgency, rather than true sphincter deficiency. Such patients merit anal physiology testing, with particular emphasis on resting pressure. Values above 35 to 40 mm of mercury do not contraindicate RP when the concern is preoperative sphincter function);
- cancer of the lower third of the rectum is present;
- there is a history of radiation to the abdomen; or
- the patient is elderly. When patients over the age of 70 years undergo RP/IPAA, although they perceive quality of life to be good/satisfactory, pad usage and incontinence are considerably greater than in their younger counterparts. Careful discussion must be had with these older patients before offering them RP.

Restorative Proctocolectomy and Ileal Pouch-Anal Anastomosis

Indications

It follows that RP/IPAA is a suitable and preferred operation for patients where subtotal colectomy or TPC and Brooke ileostomy are not indicated. In general, these are patients who are in good condition mentally and physically; have had no previous small bowel resections; have good anal sphincter function; are without evidence of CD such as perianal fistula—past or present; may be diagnosed of indeterminate colitis; have no history of radiation to the abdomen; may undergo restorative proctocolectomy with curative intent if colorectal cancer is present; and, are particularly eligible if portal hypertension is present in association with UC.

Pouch Construction

A variety of pouch techniques and configurations have been described, including the J, S, W, and lateral isoperistaltic (H) types. We prefer the J pouch as it is simple to make using a linear stapler cutting technique, can be done rapidly (in 5 minutes or less), and has no obstructive defecation sequelae. The S pouch is occasionally used when excessive anastomotic tension is predictable in a given patient. Care is exercised to limit the exit conduit to 2 cm or less, as obstructive defecation—necessitating pouch emptying by periodic catheter intubation—may ensue.

Anastomotic Issues

The two main ways in which the pouch can be joined to the anal canal are by stapling and by hand-sutured techniques. We believe that the major complication of pouch surgery is sepsis secondary to anastomotic dehiscence; this in turn is due to excessive anastomotic tension. In our experience, the least septic complication rates occur when the ileal pouch is stapled to the top of the anal columns, 1 to 2 cm above the dentate line.

RETAINED MUCOSA

The above procedure leaves a zone, usually referred to as the anal transitional zone (ATZ), which commonly or usually harbors some colonic-type epithelium.[‡] This potentially is vulnerable to neoplastic and/or acute symptomatic inflammatory change. In the absence of synchronous colonic carcinoma at the time of index TPC and IPAA for UC, we found that so far the risk of dysplasia is low (two patients) and cancer in the ATZ has yet to be reported. From an oncogenic standpoint, our current view is that stapled IPAA is a reasonable approach if accompanied by a surveillance program. We recommend ATZ surveillance and biopsy every 2 to 3 years. Further data are needed before this examination frequency can be relaxed, in our view. There is a chapter on this same issue from the same institution by a pathologist interested in dysplasia.

ANAL MUCOSECTOMY

For patients with synchronous colorectal cancer, rectal dysplasia, or primary sclerosing cholangitis, postoperative ATZ dysplasia is a substantial risk and complete anal mucosectomy is recommended at the time of RP. If a patient has undergone stapled IPAA for cancer complicating UC (usually first diagnosed in the colectomy specimen) then

---

[†] Editor's Note: The views on cesarian section and avoidance of IPAA in patients with potential fertility problems should be considered carefully since this is a very experienced and thoughtful group. Other chapters are less specific on this topic. (TMB)

[‡] Editor's Note: Others refer to the columnar epithelium in naming this junctional zone. There are fingers of columnar epithelium that reach down into this junctional area. I do not think the risk of residual colitis and dysplasia should be minimized.(TMB)

close follow-up (eg, annual or biannual biopsies) is recommended. We were successful in preserving the pelvic pouch in two patients who underwent late transanal mucosectomy and pouch advancement for late development of ATZ dysplasia.

So why not do mucosectomy in every case? We believe that anal sphincter stretch is considerable and protracted (20 to 30 minutes) when hand-sewn techniques with mucosectomy are used, and that this produces significant and prolonged reduction in resting sphincter tone that is associated with higher rates (compared to stapled IPAA) of nocturnal *incontinence* and pad usage by patients. In the patients without risk factors for ATZ dysplasia (synchronous cancer or dysplasia in the rectum), the continence factor is a compelling reason to advocate stapled IPAA. In our opinion, when the risk factors for ATZ dysplasia **are** present, the balance of risk/benefit comes down in favor of complete mucosectomy.

A final point on this issue: if we see a patient whose body habitus suggests that anastomotic tension will be excessive with a hand-sewn anastomosis, we will lay out the pros and cons of a stapled alternative even if adverse oncologic indicators are present. We believe the patient should be given full data on this issue to allow a measured decision to be made along with the caveats (ATZ surveillance) attendant with a decision to pursue restorative proctocolectomy.[§]

"Cuffitis" or Inflammation of the Anal Transitional Zone

"Cuffitis" rarely reaches significant proportions and can be managed by topical agents such as corticosteriods or 5-aminosalicylic acid preparations. In the senior author's experience of 1005 pelvic pouch operations, only once has mucosectomy been required for this complication.

Bowel Obstruction

Small bowel obstruction is the most common reason for unplanned major reoperation on RP patients, occurring in 10 to 20 percent of cases, half of whom require surgery to release the adhesion(s) causing the obstruction. So far, the only factor associated with lessening this risk is ileostomy avoidance at the time of pouch construction—but at the price of possible sepsis and symptomatic anastomotic leak with ileostomy avoidance.

Evacuation Disorders

- Short strictures at the anastomosis: these generally respond to careful dilatation. Transanal stricture lysis is occasionally necessary for recurrent short strictures.

Long strictures (> 1 to 2 cm) require stricture excision and neopouch anal anastomosis either transanally or by abdomino-anal approach. Ischemia and sepsis are the two commonest causes.

- Long exit conduit of S or H pouches: these obstructions are managed by intermittent catheter intubation—about four times a day. If this is deemed disabling by the patient or if perforative complication occurs, repeat IPAA or ileostomy usually is needed.
- Paradoxical puborectalis contraction: this is an infrequent cause of evacuation disorder—often associated with pouchitis. Diagnosis is readily made with EMG or pouchography. Biofeedback usually is successful but requires four to six sessions.

Sepsis

Early in the postoperative period, pelvic abscess may be drained by computed tomographic guidance. Sepsis may be due to an infected pelvic hematoma or may be secondary to anastomotic leak. After drainage, prolonged fecal diversion often will allow repair of the leak. When healing is confirmed on pouch contrast enema, usually at 6 to 12 months post-IPAA, the ileostomy can be closed successfully.

Anastomosis fistulae or sinuses emanating from the pouch may require repeat IPAA or permanent ileostomy. Sepsis or fistulae, such as pouch anastomotic vaginal fistulae that appear late (over 6 months) from IPAA, often are indicative of CD, although not always.[//] The management ranges from intermittent antibiotic therapy—ciprofloxacin and metronidazole with or without local seton drainage—through to repeat IPAA with fistula exclusion. The latter is used if the former is unsuccessful.

Pouchitis

"Pouchitis" covers a spectrum of symptomatic inflammatory conditions of the ileal pouch mucosa. We understand this to be a syndrome combining histopathologic evidence of ileal pouch mucosal inflammation with clinical features characterized by one or more of the following: significant increase in stool frequency above the patient's usual base level, low-grade fever and malaise, bleeding, and dull pelvic pressure/pain. Most cases respond to metronidazole, with or without ciprofloxacin, given over a 5- to 10-day period. A chronic variety of pouchitis is much less common. We usually will treat such patients with initial long-term (6 months plus) metronidazole therapy. If there is little or no response, we will use either alone or in combination 5-ASA orally and by enema. There is a detailed chapter on pouchitis,

---

[§] Editor's Note: I believe this is a balanced view of a controversial topic. There are other surgical groups who still use mucosectomy, but stapling with a follow-up surveillance program is gaining popularity. (TMB)

[//] Editor's Note: Review of the pathology slides from the original colectomy specimen may reveal CD but if the colectomy was done for fulminant colitis, the differential diagnosis may be difficult. This is discussed in the chapter on pouch histology. (TMB)

including a discussion of CD in IPAA. Occasionally, ileostomy with pouch excision is necessary.

Postoperative Management

After RP and IPAA with loop ileostomy, patients invariably have high ileostomy outputs—from 1,000 to 2,000 + cc/24 h. Effectively the "high" ileostomy bypasses 20 percent or more of the distal small bowel and this sets the stage for dehydration. Patients are advised to:

- be aware of added risk factors for dehydration (hot weather, exercise, air conditioning);
- be aware of symptoms of dehydration (lassitude, fatigue, headache, nausea);
- maintain intake of adequate oral liquids, especially salty soups, electrolyte supplements;
- avoid high solid fiber/indigestible foods for 6 weeks (as with all new ileostomates);
- use bulking agents in liquid form (eg, Konsyl®, Citrucel®, Metamucil®);
- use liquid diphenoxylate plus atropine (Lomotil®) dosed on a weight basis to thicken enteric output;
- be aware of the fact that external ileostomy pouches may stay on for only 2 days or so (compared with 5 to 7 days for end ileostomies). Loop ileostomies tend to be flush with the skin;
- follow the steroid tapering schedule prescribed on discharge; and
- recognize symptoms of post-discharge bowel obstruction.

After the ileostomy is closed, a similar program is instituted. However, antidiarrheal medications can and should be given more forcefully, often combining all three preparations of a bulking agent, Lomotil (diphenoxylate and atropine) and Imodium® (loperamide).

Long-Term Follow-Up

Theoretically, if the patient has undergone mucosectomy as part of the RP and remains well, no follow-up is necessary after bowel function has stabilized—usually within 6 to 12 months.

In patients with ATZ preservation, recommendations for follow-up surveillance are outlined earlier. It should be noted that *not all* patients reported to have total mucosectomy have, in fact, had this done. Thus, these patients may be vulnerable to ATZ neoplasia development as monitoring is rarely done, least of all with biopsy surveillance. Additionally, patients with a chronic type of pouch inflammation, characterized by severe villous atrophy and crypt hyperplasia ("type C"), may be vulnerable to the complications of pouch "colon-ization"—namely, dysplasia. This is discussed in the chapter on pouch histology. Thus, we recommend to *all* of our patients that they have pouch surveillance *and* biopsy at regular intervals. There is no real evidence that indicates how frequently this

should be done, but every 3 to 5 years seems reasonable unless risk factors for dysplasia in the preserved ATZ are significant, in which case prudence dictates a closer surveillance schedule.

Conclusion

Our long-term follow-up of pouch function and quality of life indicates a very high degree of acceptance and happiness level of the patients undergoing restorative proctocolectomy. This is on a par with age- and sex-matched United States citizens using the SF36 assessment tool. Bowel movement frequency ranges from four to nine/24 h, averaging six times/d. This, however, is not a good indication of success as many patients will evacuate their pouches when it is convenient to do so, rather than defer defecation. Urgency, defined as inability to defer defecation for 15 minutes, is a major concern for many patients preoperatively. Invariably, this is negated by the pouch procedure; the exception is when patients develop pouchitis.

Pad use, either due to need or for a sense of security, increases with age, episodes of pouchitis, and the patients with mucosal stripping of the anal canal as well as decreasing sphincter function. Operative mortality remains under 0.5 percent and we have reported impotence rates of less than 1 percent. Although dyspareunia may occur post-pouch construction, overall, there is an improvement in female sexual function post-pouch compared to pre-pouch. Perhaps the most singled out problem of the pelvic pouch procedure is that of pouchitis—by eliminating one disease, the patient is set up for another. Yet this has to be viewed with the perspective that 90 percent of pouchitis cases are transient and easily treated, and that fewer than three-quarters of patients are subject to repeated episodes. Patients, in their quest for preservation of their anal function, understand and generally believe they "get a good deal" with the trade-off of RP.

Supplemental Reading

Bambrick M, Fazio VW, Hull TL, et al. Sexual function following restorative proctocolectomy in women. Dis Colon Rectum 1996;39:610–4.

Fazio VW. What is the better surgical technique in ileal pouch-anal anastomosis? Stapled anastomosis. Inflamm Bowel Dis 1996;2:148–50.

Fazio VW, O'Riordain MG, Lavery IC, et al. Long-term functional outcome and quality of life after stapled restorative proctocolectomy. Ann Surg 1999;230:578–86.

Fazio VW, Tjandra JJ. Transanal mucosectomy; ileal pouch advancement for anorectal dysplasia or inflammation after restorative proctocolectomy. Dis Colon Rectum 1994; 37:1008–11.

Fazio VW, Wu JS, Lavery IC. Repeat ileal pouch-anal anastomosis to salvage septic complications of pelvic pouches: clinical outcome and quality of life assessment. Ann Surg 1997;228:588–97.

Fazio VW, Ziv Y, Church JM, et al. Ileal pouch-anal anastomosis: complications and function in 1005 patients. Ann Surg 1995;222:120–7.

Gullberg K, Stahlberg D, Liljeqvist L, et al. Neoplastic transformation of the pelvic pouch mucosa in patients with ulcerative colitis. Gastroenterology 1997;112:1487–92.

Hull TL, Fazio VW, Schroeder T. Paradoxical puborectalis contraction in patients after pelvic pouch construction. Dis Colon Rectum 1995;38:1144–6.

Juhasz ES, Fozard B, Dozois RR, et al. Ileal pouch-anal anastomosis function following childbirth: an extended evaluation. Dis Colon Rectum 1995;38:159–65.

Kartheuser AH, Dozois RR, LaRusso NF, et al. Comparison of surgical treatment of ulcerative colitis associated with primary sclerosing cholangitis: ileal pouch-anal anastomosis versus Brooke ileostomy. Mayo Clin Proc 1996;71:748–56.

Marchesa P, Lashner BA, Lavery IC, et al. The risk of cancer and dysplasia among ulcerative colitis patients with primary sclerosing cholangitis. Am J Gastroenterol 1997;92:1285–8.

O'Riordain MG, Fazio VW, Lavery IC, et al. Dysplasia of the anal transitional zone (ATZ) after ileo-pouch anal anastomosis (IPAA): 5–10 year follow up. Dis Colon Rectum 1998;41:26A.

Tjandra JJ, Fazio VW, Milsom JW, et al. Omission of temporary diversion in restorative proctocolectomy—is it safe? Dis Colon Rectum 1993;36:1007–14.

Tuckson WB, Lavery IC, Oakley J, et al. Manometric and functional comparison of ileal pouch-anal anastomosis with and without anal manipulation. Am J Surg 1991;161:90–6.

Wexner SP, Rothenberger DA, Jensen L, et al. Ileal pouch vaginal fistulas; incidence, etiology and management. Dis Colon Rectum 1989;32:460–5.

CHAPTER 43

LONG-TERM RESULTS WITH ILEOANAL POUCH

JOHN H. PEMBERTON, MD

Ileal pouch-anal anastomosis (IPAA) is a complex, sophisticated operation, and complications occur frequently. The overall rate of morbidity for all patients still hovers between 25 and 30 percent. Failure, however, is rare, even in those who suffer a postoperative complication. At the Mayo Clinic, 94 percent of patients have a successful outcome. It is just as important to understand the complications of restorative proctocolectomy, how to avoid them, and what to do if they occur as it is to know how to select appropriate patients and how to perform the procedure rapidly and accurately. Although it is not discussed any further here, the key to a successful outcome is a surgeon who performs the operation effortlessly; the operation struggled through is the one fraught with complications and sometimes failure.

Mayo Clinic Experience with Ileal Pouch-Anal Anastomosis

From January 1, 1981, to September 14, 1999, 1,990 IPAA operations had been performed at Mayo; 1,218 patients were operated upon between January 1, 1981, and September 15, 1998. The standard operation consisted of abdominal colectomy, proximal proctectomy, and distal endorectal mucosal resection to the dentate line, construction of a J-pouch, and a pouch-anal anastomosis. In addition, since 1994, double-stapled IPAA also has been performed. Most patients had a diverting ileostomy constructed, which was closed 2 to 3 months later. The ratio of men to women was 1:1, and the mean age of the group was 32 years.

Early Clinical Results

Ninety-six percent of patients had a protecting ileostomy established at the first operation; of these, 97 percent were loop ileostomies. On discharge from hospital after ileostomy closure, 79 percent of patients were "completely continent," 19 percent were "mostly continent" (occasional daytime and nighttime soilage), and 2 percent were incontinent. Ninety-four percent of the patients had 10 or fewer stools per day and 96 percent had 2 or fewer stools at night within 10 days of ileostomy closure. Stool bulkers were given to 47 percent of the patients on discharge from hospital, and agents to slow transit were prescribed for 49 percent. Two patients died postoperatively.

Morbidity

Overall, 30 percent of patients had a postoperative complication. Most complications occurred in the early postoperative period and did not result in loss of the pouch or long-term disability.

PELVIC INFECTION

Pelvic infection was a serious complication, occurring in the early postoperative period in about 5 percent of patients with ulcerative colitis (UC). Computed tomography (CT) was useful for demonstrating pelvic fluid collection or phlegmon. Patients with pelvic phlegmon usually responded to conservative treatment with broad-spectrum antibiotics and bowel rest. Patients with a pelvic abscess underwent CT-guided drainage, if technically feasible, or laparotomy and drainage. The incidence of pelvic sepsis is declining owing to increased experience with the procedure and to the construction of a shorter rectal muscular cuff.

ABDOMINAL SEPSIS

The incidence of *abdominal sepsis* was 6 percent and it was an ominous development. Ultimately, 41 percent of patients who underwent laparotomy for control of this sepsis required pouch excision. Moreover, normal function was achieved in only 29 percent of patients requiring operation. However, among septic patients who did not require reoperation, but rather had aggressive nonsurgical management, 92 percent had satisfactory pouch function over the long term.

SMALL BOWEL OBSTRUCTION

Small bowel obstruction occurred in 17 percent of the patients, 8 percent of whom required surgical intervention.

CLOSURE OF ILEOSTOMY

Closure of temporary ileostomies was also associated with complications. Peritonitis occurred in 4 percent and postoperative obstruction in 12 percent of patients. Proximal and distal serosal tears during stoma mobilization, in addition to anastomotic leaks, are important causes of peritonitis. If all extraperitoneal bowel (afferent and efferent limbs and the stoma itself) is resected, however, the chance of leaving an unrecognized perforation is nearly eliminated.

ANAL STRICTURE

Nearly all patients had a web-like stricture of the ileoanal anastomosis on returning for ileostomy closure. This stricture was dilated digitally without difficulty. If the pouch retracts under anastomotic tension, heavy scarring and a long, fibrotic stricture result. This type of stricture is manifested by increased difficulty with straining a stool, a sensation of incomplete pouch evacuation, or a high stool frequency (> 10 to 12 stools/d). Repeated anal dilatation may prevent progression of the stricture.

Late Clinical Results

STOOL FREQUENCY

The average stool frequency during the day was six stools, with one stool at night. Importantly, daytime and nocturnal stool frequency and the ability to discriminate flatus from stool has remained stable over time, whereas the need for stool bulkers and hypomotility agents has declined. This has been confirmed by others. Several large series have reported similar stool frequencies. The lower stool frequencies 6 months after surgery compared to frequency in the early postoperative period are likely attributable to increased pouch capacity developing over time.

INCONTINENCE

Major fecal incontinence (more than twice/wk) occurred in 5 percent of patients during the day and 12 percent during sleep. In contrast, minor episodes of nocturnal incontinence occurred in up to 30 percent of patients at least 1 year after the operation. A pad was worn by 28 percent of patients for protection against seepage. Interestingly, up to 60 percent of fully continent women wore a pad for fear of accidental fecal soilage. Minor perianal skin irritation was reported by 63 percent of patients.

INFLUENCE OF AGE

Not surprisingly, patients over 50 years of age had a higher daytime stool frequency than patients younger than 50 years (< 50 yr: 6 ± stools/d vs > 50 yr: 8 ± 4 stools/d). Men and women had similar stool frequencies postoperatively, but women had more episodes of fecal soilage during the day and night.

TEN-YEAR FOLLOW-UP

Regarding long-term function after IPAA, functional results at 1 year in a group of 75 patients after IPAA were compared with functional results in the **same** patients after 10 years. Stool frequency remained unchanged. In addition, 78 percent of those patients with excellent continence at 1 year after surgery remained unchanged at 10 years, 20 percent developed minor incontinence, and

one patient developed poor control. Forty percent of these patients with initial minor incontinence remained unchanged, 40 percent improved, and 20 percent worsened. Nocturnal fecal spotting increased during the 10-year period, but not significantly (38% increased to 52%).

Late Complications

POUCHITIS

The principal late complication after IPAA is nonspecific reservoir inflammation or pouchitis. A complete discussion of pouchitis appears elsewhere in this volume. The incidence of pouchitis has increased as follow-up has lengthened. At the Mayo Clinic, the incidence of pouchitis among patients with chronic UC is 60 percent. The mean interval from operation to first occurrence is 17 months. A second episode has been identified in about two-thirds of patients. The incidence is not affected by the type of pouch constructed, presence or absence or perioperative pelvic sepsis or backwash ileitis, or the age or sex of the patient. Higher recurrence rates occur in patients with extra-intestinal manifestations of UC (39%) than in those without manifestations (26%). Furthermore, exacerbations of extra-intestinal manifestations often have been related temporarily to flares of pouchitis.

The traditional treatment of pouchitis has consisted of oral antibiotics directed against anaerobic bacteria, with prompt response usually seen with 24 to 48 hours of starting therapy. Those patients refractory to antibiotics may respond to sulfasalazine or steroid enemas. In addition, there is recent evidence that bismuth subsalicylate (Pepto-Bismol®, Procter & Gamble Pharmaceuticals, Cincinnati, Ohio) is efficacious in the treatment of antibiotic-resistant pouchitis. In approximately 10 percent of patients with pouchitis, chronic pouchitis develops, requiring low-dose prophylactic oral antibiotics or enema administration. Ultimately, a small number of patients with pouchitis require either pouch revision or excision owing to pouchitis (< 2% of all patients after IPAA). Details of treatment are presented in a separate chapter.

SEXUAL DYSFUNCTION

Impotency and retrograde ejaculation developed in 1.5 percent and 4 percent of men, respectively. Dyspareunia developed in 7 percent of women postoperatively. Interestingly, 49 percent of women noted sexual dysfunction preoperatively yet sexual activity increased dramatically after IPAA because of an improvement in general health.

FAILURE

Six percent of patients ultimately require pouch excision or construction of a permanent ileostomy. Other large series have reported failure rates between 2 and 12 percent. The most frequent causes of failure, either alone or in combination, include pelvic sepsis, high stool volumes, Crohn's disease, and uncontrollable fecal incontinence. Pouchitis was the sole cause in 2 percent of all patients. Importantly, of the patients who failed, 75 percent failed within 1 year, 12 percent by 2 years, and 12 percent by 3 years. Thus, failure after IPAA is manifested within several years after the operation and is the result of a combination of early or late complications of the procedure.

Quality of Life

Issues of quality of life often are the deciding factors for patients choosing a particular operation for UC. Several studies that analyzed the outcome of surgery for UC have demonstrated that most patients are satisfied with the operation and lead a normal life style regardless of the procedure.

The quality of life following Brooke ileostomy and IPAA for UC and familial adenomatous polyposis have been studied. Patients were highly satisfied following either operation (Brooke ileostomy, 93%; IPAA, 95%). However, daily activities (sexual life, participation in sports, social interaction, work, recreation, family relationships, travel) were more likely to be adversely affected with a Brooke ileostomy than by IPAA.

Controversies

Which Pouch Design is Best?

Of all of the pouch designs championed in the literature ("S," "H," "W," "K," and "J"), the J-shaped pouch is easiest to construct and has functional outcomes identical to those of the more complex designs. It is the pouch design of choice at the Mayo Clinic.

Two Stages or One? Role of Defunctioning Ileostomy

The most feared complication of IPAA is pelvic sepsis, and therefore, a defunctioning ileostomy after pouch construction usually is performed to minimize its occurrence. Whereas pelvic sepsis complicates 6 percent of IPAA procedures at the Mayo Clinic, the rates reported in the literature vary between 0 and 25 percent. Moreover, disturbingly high rates of pelvic sepsis have been reported in patients undergoing a one-stage procedure (no ileostomy). Although the incidence of pelvic sepsis is low at the Mayo Clinic, when it occurs, it is responsible for a significant proportion of the failed pouches.

Protagonists of defunctioning ileostomies argue that diverting stomas allow the anal sphincter and ileal mucosa to recover before restoration of intestinal continuity, and that patients have a short-lived experience of a stoma to fully appreciate the ultimate benefit of IPAA. Use of loop ileostomy does not appear to protect the patient fully from pelvic sepsis; however, it is easier to manage a patient with sepsis if an ileostomy is in place.

Among the patients at the Mayo Clinic who required laparotomy to control sepsis, 41 percent lost the pouch ultimately and only 29 percent ever recovered ileoanal function. However, if no reoperation was required, 92 percent of patients with sepsis eventually had a functioning pouch. This is an important observation.

A reasonable approach to this dilemma is to use a defunctioning ileostomy in those patients receiving steroid treatment at the time of surgery and in patients who are nutritionally compromised or undergoing an urgent operation. Additionally, if there are concerns about pouch blood supply or anastomotic tension, a diverting stoma is almost mandatory. Using these criteria, 56 of 1,800 patients who underwent IPAA at the Mayo Clinic between 1980 and 1996 had a one-stage procedure performed.

Double-Stapled versus Hand-sewn Anastomosis

Much of the debate as to whether to staple the anastomosis or not has evolved because functional outcomes should be improved if the anal transition zone (or more recently "columnar cuff" [CC]) is preserved. Does preserving the CC enhance continence after IPAA? Stapled anastomosis in nonrandomized trials has been equated with better outcome, which in turn has been attributed to less injury to the anal sphincters, with preservation of the CC and hence anal sensory discrimination, and with preservation of the rectoanal inhibitory reflex. In order to determine if stapled IPAA conferred any advantage over hand-sewn IPAA, we conducted a randomized study (Reilly et al, 1997); 41 patients at the Mayo Clinic were randomized to double-stapled (n = 17 patients) or hand-sewn (n = 15 patients) techniques. In the stapled group, 1.5 to 2.0 cm of CC was preserved, whereas complete mucosectomy was performed in the hand-sewn group. Overall, complications were the same in the two groups. Stool frequency and rates of fecal incontinence during the day and night were similar between the groups. However, fewer patients treated with the double-stapled technique had incontinence at night. Moreover, resting and squeezing pressures were better preserved after double stapling. Both hand-sewn and double-stapled IPAA improved the quality of life dramatically. Double-stapled IPAA has further benefits because it may preserve the anal canal better than does the hand-sewn anastomosis and thus, for the first time, enable older and perhaps overweight patients to be candidates for IPAA.

Lingering Issues

Risk of Cancer

Patients with chronic UC are at risk of developing adenocarcinoma of the colon. This risk increases as the duration of disease and the extent of colonic involvement increases.

Any surgery that leaves behind diseased colonic mucosa puts the patient at risk of developing dysplasia or neoplasia in the residual colonic mucosa. The risk of developing a carcinoma in the residual colonic mucosa may be related directly to the amount of residual mucosa remaining in situ.

Complete excision of the rectum during IPAA decreases the risk of dysplasia significantly. With the widespread acceptance of stapled IPAA, the residual cuff epithelium (CE) is reduced to less than 1 cm or eliminated nearly completely. Studies, such as that by Tsunoda et al (1990), which demonstrated the presence of dysplasia in mucosectomy specimens, have been used as evidence to support the use of routine complete mucosal resection.

To make this topic even more complex, several studies report that viable mucosa is present in the rectal muscular cuff *after* mucosal resection. In one study, islands (rests) of mucosa were present despite "complete" mucosal resection (Haray et al, 1996). The incidence of dysplasia in the retained rectal mucosa, or distal rectal doughnut, after double-stapled ileoanal anastomosis is approximately 1 percent. Histologic analysis of mucosectomy specimens includes one report of a carcinoma, which had been undetected clinically, in a patient who had dysplasia in the rectal mucosa. Despite this, no patient has developed a rectal cancer in the retained rectal cuff after IPAA and endorectal mucosal resection. One patient did develop an adenocarcinoma in the retained CE. This area has the potential for dysplasia, neoplasia, and continuing inflammation after IPAA. However, interestingly, the four patients with carcinoma reported in a pouch all have been patients who underwent total mucosectomy as part of their original surgery.

The question of follow-up of the CE has been addressed by several investigators. The Cleveland Clinic reported its experience with 254 patients who underwent double-stapled IPAA and who had follow-up by undergoing annual postsurgical CE biopsy (Ziv et al, 1994). During a mean follow-up of 2 years, low-grade dysplasia was found in eight patients (3%). Repeat biopsies confirmed dysplasia in only two of these eight patients.[*] Significant correlation was seen between CE dysplasia and concurrent dysplasia or cancer of the large bowel *before* surgery. There was no association with age, sex, duration of disease, anastomotic technique, or length of rectal cuff. The risk of dysplasia in the residual columnar epithelium was 25 percent in patients who had cancer, but only 10 percent in patients who had dysplasia in the original proctocolectomy specimen.

Detection of neoplastic change in the pouch itself is a further reason to perform follow-up in patients with IPAA. Reports of dysplasia and carcinoma in the pouch mucosa have prompted some investigators to perform close follow-up in all patients by means of endoscopic surveillance and routine pouch biopsy. A subgroup of patients has been identified, in whom the mucosa of the pelvic pouch develops severe villous atrophy. These patients seem to have a significantly higher incidence of dysplasia compared with patients without villous atrophy (71 vs 0%). The former group may be at greater risk of developing carcinoma and may require more intensive follow-up with regular pouch endoscopy and biopsy.

Dysplasia

The presence of dysplasia in the pouch, rectal cuff, or CE should not be ignored. Routine endoscopic surveillance with biopsy after IPAA shows dysplastic changes in as many as 3 percent of patients. Low-grade dysplasia should prompt the surgeon to follow the patient closely and perform repeated multiple endoscopic biopsies of the cuff. Repeat biopsies are likely to be normal in the majority of patients, and continued surveillance of these patients is likely to be sufficient. Persistence of dysplastic mucosa or the presence of high-grade dysplasia is an indication for more aggressive intervention. Completion mucosectomy or laser ablation may be sufficient if the dysplastic mucosa involves the CC. In more refractory cases, pouch excision may be considered, but this is uncommon.[†]

Pregnancy

We and several other centers have observed that women who become pregnant and deliver a child after IPAA have few long-term problems with pouch function. However, the fertility rate of women after IPAA is unknown.

Psychological Factors

Some progress has been made toward identifying subgroups of patients who are more at risk than others of developing pouch dysfunction or complications. Several studies, during long-term follow-up, confirm that functional results are poor in patients who had adverse personality factors before surgery. Personality traits were measured before surgery in 53 patients undergoing surgery for chronic UC, and the traits correlated with psychological adjustment at a mean of 17 months after surgery. Findings suggested that the assessment of the patient's long-term sexual functioning and satisfaction before surgery, the importance attached to his or her appearance, level of alexithymia, and general capacity to tolerate frustration and setbacks in life should alert the surgeon to potential risk factors for poor adjustment after surgery.[‡]

References

[†] Editor's Note: We do not have enough experience with dysplasia in the setting of chronic status in an IPAA to be dogmatic. I usually urge against an IPAA in the presence of rectal dysplasia. If low-grade dysplasia developed in a Kock pouch or in an IPAA, this should be a matter of great concern. (TMB)

---

[*] Editor's Note: Dysplasia once is still dysplasia and is the greatest risk for development of cancer. (TMB)

Reilly WT, Pemberton JH, Wolff BG, et al. Randomized prospective trial comparing ileal pouch-anal anastomosis (IPAA) performed by excising the anal mucosa to IPAA performed by preserving the anal mucosa. Ann Surg 1997;225:666–77.

Tsunoda A, Talbot IC, Nicholls RJ. Incidence of dysplasia in the anorectal mucosa in patients having restorative procto-colectomy. Br J Surg 1990;77:506–8.

Ziv Y, Fazio VW, Sirimarco MT, et al. Incidence, risk factors, and treatment of dysplasia in the anal transition zone after ileal pouch-anal anastomosis. Dis Colon Rectum 1994;37:1281–5.

Supplemental Reading

Ambroze JWL, Pemberton JH, Dozois RR, et al. The histological pattern and pathologic involvement of anal transition zone in patients with ulcerative colitis. Gastroenterology 1993;104:514–8.

Haray PN, Amarnath B, Weiss EG, et al. Low malignant potential of the double-stapled ileal pouch-anal anastomosis. Br J Surg 1996;83:1406–8.

Lohmuller JL, Pemberton JH, Dozois RR, et al. Pouchitis and extraintestinal manifestations of inflammatory bowel disease after ileal pouch-anal anastomosis. Ann Surg 1990;211: 622–9.

McIntyre PB, Pemberton JH, Wolff BG, et al. Comparing functional results one year and ten years after ileal pouch-anal anastomosis for chronic ulcerative colitis. Dis Colon Rectum 1994;37:303–7.

Pemberton JH, Kelly KA, Baert RW Jr, et al. Ileal pouch-anal anastomosis for chronic ulcerative colitis. Ann Surg 1987;206:504–13.

Pemberton JH, Phillips SF, Ready RR, et al. Quality of life after Brooke ileostomy and ileal pouch-anal anastomosis. Ann Surg 1989;209:620–8.

Sugarman HJ, Newsome HH. Stapled ileoanal anastomosis without a temporary ileostomy. Am J Surg 1994;167:58–65.

Thompson-Fawcett MW, Warren BG, Mortensen NJ. A new look at the anal transition zone with reference to restorative proctocolectomy and the columnar cuff. Br J Surg 1998;85:1517–21.

Veress B, Reinholt FP, Lindquist K, et al. Long-term histomorphological surveillance of the pelvic ileal pouch: dysplasia develops in a subgroup of patients. Gastroenterology 1995;109:1090–7.

‡ Editor's Note: It is my view that the existence of irritable bowel syndrome before the development of UC is a potential harbinger of excessive evacuation and pain, because the pouch capacity often is reduced owing to spasm and the patient is able to evacuate only about half of the pouch contents. (TMB)

CHAPTER 44

Ileoanal Pouch: Evaluation of Excessive Bowel Movements

Laurence J. Egan, MD, and Sidney F. Phillips, MD

Proctocolectomy with ileal pouch-anal anastomosis (IPAA) is the preferred surgical option when colonic resection is necessary for the treatment of intractable ulcerative colitis (UC) and familial adenomatous polyposis. However, after IPAA, patients always defecate more frequently than do healthy people. Thus, after proctocolectomy, whether surgical continuity is restored with a terminal ileostomy or with a pouch, daily fecal volumes will be 500 to 700 mL. In health, fecal volumes do not often exceed 200 mL. Moreover, the reservoir of an ileoanal pouch is smaller than that of a normal rectum. Patients who complain of frequent bowel movements after IPAA must recognize their symptoms in this context; they will never have only one or two solid stools daily. Although patients who complain of frequent defecation after IPAA may have no identifiable pathology, they can, nevertheless, be helped to accept a new lifestyle by being taught to understand the postoperative physiology. Moreover, simple antidiarrheal therapy may significantly improve their lifestyle.

Evacuation Expectations

The majority of patients with normally functioning IPAAs should evacuate between four and eight times per day and once or twice at night. From most large series, the average rates are five and one bowel movements per 24 hours. Most patients need to defecate 30 to 60 minutes after eating. After the initial postoperative phase, patients should not have extreme fecal urgency and should be able to distinguish between the urges of flatus and feces. Approximately 10 to 20 percent of patients who undergo IPAA experience minor leakage of stool, especially at night, when they may need to wear a pad. However, they should be continent during the day. Passage of stools should be painless, should not be accompanied by the need to strain, and should feel complete. In taking the history, the features of "diarrhea" need to be defined precisely; increased fecal frequency needs to be distinguished from urgency, fecal leakage, or gross incontinence.

Importance of an Adequate History

Key to helping patients after IPAA who complain of excessive bowel movements is to make an accurate diagnosis. Disorders of the pouch outlet (the anal sphincter seg-

ment), the pouch itself, or the ileum proximal to the pouch may be the cause of increased stool frequency. In many patients, a careful history provides the astute clinician with a short list of diagnostic possibilities. The most important element of the history is to determine precisely what it is about pouch function that is unsatisfactory to the patient. A typical complaint might be of having to "go all the time." The physician must then determine exactly what the patient means. Is the patient having true watery diarrhea, or is the main complaint urgency or leakage? Is an inability to completely empty the pouch with consequent leakage of retained stool the real problem? Careful evaluation of the patient's complaints, in conjunction with a knowledge of the likely causes of symptoms, should point to the correct diagnosis.

Not all examples of excessive fecal frequency, urgency, or incontinence are attributable to the pouch or its dysfunctions. After proctocolectomy, diarrhea may be attributable to extraneous causes. In practice, it is advantageous to distinguish between patients who are seen after surgery and those who present later.

Excessive or Uncontrolled Bowel Movements in Patients with Newly Formed Pouches

Table 44–1 summarizes the diagnostic approach to and treatment of excessive bowel movements in the first 6 months after IPAA.

General Approach

Problems occurring soon after the operation (0 to 6 months) present more often to surgeons, but gastroenterologists also need to be aware of these issues. It is helpful to consider the time of onset of increased bowel frequency in relation to the age of the pouch. The first few weeks after closure of the temporary ileostomy and restoration of the fecal stream to the pouch often are marked by frequent loose stools, to which the pouch and the patient must be helped to adapt. The sensation of a full ileal pouch may be qualitatively different from that of a full rectum, and patients must learn to recognize those sensations that indicate that they need to empty the pouch.

TABLE 44–1. Approach to Patients Who Experience Excessive Bowel Movements in the First 6 Months After Pouch Reanastomosis

Cause	Diagnostic Approaches	Treatment
Unrealistic expectations	Exclude pathology by physical examination; consider endoscopy or pouchogram	Education and reassurance Fiber supplements, antidiarrheals
Anastomotic leak	Endoscopy; pouchogram	Intestinal diversion, abscess drainage, pouch revision (late decision)
Defective sphincter function and anal incontinence	Physical examination; anal manometry	Antidiarrheals, fiber supplements, biofeedback
Anastomotic stricture	Physical examination; endoscopy	Dilatation
Cuffitis	Pouchoscopy and biopsy	Mesalamine, steroids

Thus, some patients, if they have not received adequate preoperative counseling, have unrealistic expectations about the functional outcomes after "curative" IPAA surgery. They need to be educated; they will always have a high fecal volume, and their stools will never be fully formed. Moreover, it is important to reassure patients that a healthy pouch and anal sphincter gradually will adapt postoperatively, and consequently, bowel function should be expected to improve. In addition to reassurance and education, simple measures can significantly help patients with a new IPAA to learn to compensate. For example, fiber supplements, such as methylcellulose or psyllium, 1 g in a large glass of water once or twice a day, increases the consistency of stools. Loperamide (2 to 4 mg, taken 30 min before meals) reduces postprandial urgency. Although many patients who have undergone IPAA find that certain foodstuffs increase stool output, and they should learn to be circumspect or to pay the consequences, it is not particularly helpful to counsel individual patients on the consumption of specific foods. One patient's experience is likely to differ so much from another's. Rather, patients should experiment, be moderate, and be guided by their own experience in choosing a lifestyle that minimizes any negative impacts of the pouch. It is important not to promote compulsivity in dietary or other habits.

Although many patients who complain of excessive bowel frequency, diarrhea, or leakage soon after IPAA ultimately will be found not to have a structural or organic basis, one must not overlook the possibility of a postoperative complication. Small bowel obstruction occurs in the first weeks after pouch formation in 6 to 20 percent of patients. Though pain is the expected symptom of obstruction, increased fecal volumes can be the major complaint. However, half or less of the patients experiencing small bowel obstruction require reoperation.

Anastomotic Leakage

Fortunately, leakage at the pouch-anus anastomosis is rare, less than 10 percent in most surgical series, especially when the anastomosis is protected by a diverting ileostomy. Anastomotic leakage typically causes pelvic pain and abscess. Pouch dysfunction is exemplified by painful, incomplete evacuation and excessive frequency. Demonstration of a leak with a retrograde barium contrast study (pouchogram) usually is diagnostic. Occasionally, a pouch-vaginal or pouch-perineal fistula may develop in association with anastomotic leakage; this should always raise the question of unrecognized Crohn's disease. However, further investigation should be delayed until after the initial postoperative period. Treatment is surgical and may require intestinal diversion, drainage of an abscess, if present, and possibly revision of the pouch.

Defective Sphincteric Continence

Innervation of the internal anal sphincter may be disrupted during the perineal dissection and construction of the pouch-anus anastomosis. Consequently, resting pressures of the internal anal sphincter usually are reduced, at least for 6 to 12 months postoperatively. After this, there is a gradual return of basal anal tone; fortunately, function of the external sphincter, which is usually preserved, helps compensate for any lowering of internal sphincter pressures. Exceptions may be seen in elderly patients and multiparous women whose anal pressures were low before pouch construction. In this situation, defective anal continence can lead to leakage, which may be described by the patient as excessive bowel movements (diarrhea) after IPAA. Indeed, even patients who subsequently develop excellent pouch function may experience soiling, incontinence, and some degree of urgency soon after ileostomy closure.

Physical examination of the sphincter in these patients reveals low resting tone and sometimes low squeeze pressures, findings that can be confirmed by anal manometry if necessary. Effective management involves the judicial use of antidiarrheals such as loperamide (2 to 4 mg 30 minutes before meals) and fiber supplements, to increase stool consistency. Biofeedback may be helpful later, for those patients whose sphincter function returns only slowly or incompletely; retraining of patients to use the external anal sphincter to greater advantage can be helpful. In a minority of patients who have undergone IPAA, incontinence attributable to poor sphincter tone persists and is occasionally sufficient to require permanent ileostomy. This is one of the reasons for pouch failure.

TABLE 44–2. Approach to Patients Who Complain of Excessive Bowel Movements 6 or More Months After Reanastomosis

Cause	Diagnostic Approaches	Treatment
Normal pouch	Exclude pathology; consider unrelated causes of diarrhea; preexisting irritable bowel syndrome; stool culture; microscopy; endoscopy with or without pouchogram	Treat intercurrent diseases; reassurance; fiber supplements, antidiarrheals
Defective anal continence	Physical examination; anal manometry	Fiber supplements, antidiarrheals; biofeedback
Pouch outlet obstruction	Physical examination	Dilation
Cuffitis	Pouchoscopy and biopsy	Mesalamine, steroids
Pouchitis	Pouchoscopy and biopsy	Antibiotics, mesalamine
Crohn's disease	Pouchoscopy and biopsy; pouchogram	Antibiotics, azathioprine, infliximab

After the IPAA procedure, pouch excision, for all causes, ranges from 3 to 13 percent.

Pouch Outlet Obstruction

In the early postoperative period, before takedown of the diverting ileostomy, a thin web-like stricture often forms at the ileal pouch-anal anastomotic line. After the fecal stream into the pouch is restored, persistence of this stricture obstructs the pouch outlet, leading to incomplete evacuation, somewhat analogous to bladder outlet obstruction in prostatism. The patient complains of diarrhea because of incomplete emptying of the pouch that results in overflow leakage and fecal frequency. Digital examination of the anus demonstrates a narrowing of the upper anal canal. These strictures usually can be dilated easily with the finger or a rubber dilator. In some patients, anastomotic strictures can progress to become chronic, recurrent, and fibrotic and to require regular dilation.

Residual Inflammatory Bowel Disease

Pouch surgery with a double-stapled anastomosis leaves behind only a small cuff of rectal mucosa, 1 or 2 cm at most. No rectal mucosa should remain when the anastomosis is hand-sewn in conjunction with a distal rectal mucosectomy. However, in some cases, for example in obese patients when it is difficult to bring the small bowel deep into the pelvis, the surgeon may need to leave behind a more substantial cuff of rectal mucosa to which the pouch is anastomosed. The term "cuffitis" has been used to describe persistent inflammatory bowel disease (IBD) in the remnant of rectal mucosa. Most often it occurs in patients who had active disease before surgery. Symptoms are proportional to the amount of rectal mucosa that remains and to the severity of the inflammation. Patients complain of fecal frequency and urgency; the movements commonly are watery, with mucous and blood. Urgency and leakage occur, especially at night. Rarely, if several centimeters of rectum remain, systemic symptoms of malaise, low-grade fever, or weight loss may be experienced. Initial treatment with standard topical anti-inflammatory agents, such as mesalamine suppositories or hydrocortisone enemas, may be sufficient. Patients who do not respond to locally applied agents, and who require systemic steroids to control cuffitis, occasionally require a further operation to remove the inflamed rectal mucosa and to anastomose the pouch to the upper anal canal, if technically feasible.

Excessive Bowel Frequency in Patients with Established Pouches

Table 44–2 summarizes the diagnostic approach to and treatment of excessive bowel movements 6 months or longer after IPAA.

General Approach

Several large series have reported excellent long-term functional outcomes of IPAA for ulcerative colitis. Thus, 10 years after IPAA, incontinence never occurred during the day in 73 percent of patients, nor at night in 48 percent. However, many patients, at some time after construction of a pouch, experience increased bowel frequency, urgency, or incontinence, all symptoms that may be described as diarrhea. Inflammatory bowel disease of the pouch, known as pouchitis, is the most common but not the only cause of these symptoms. Pouchitis and its therapy are reviewed in another chapter in this book. Disorders of the pouch other than pouchitis include disorders of pouch emptying, diseases in the pre-pouch ileum, and any of the causes of diarrhea that may occur in patients with an intact bowel. In the majority of cases, a correct diagnosis should provide a management strategy that brings about improvement. Ten years after IPAA surgery, pouch failure requiring pouch excision or permanent ileostomy occurs in less than 10 percent of patients.

Problems with the Outlet

Pouch outlet obstruction, usually attributable to anastomotic scarring and stricture, leads to incomplete evacuation. This not only increases stool frequency but also prompts complaints of the need to strain; defecation may be painful, and there may be a recognition that the pouch has not been completely emptied. Incomplete evacuation often results in leakage of liquid stool around retained material in the pouch and the constant desire to defecate.

212 / Advanced Therapy of Inflammatory Bowel Disease

The patient makes repeated and frustrating trips to the toilet. Typically, pouch outlet obstruction may cause a feeling of pelvic fullness or bloating, but systemic symptoms, such as weight loss and malaise, are absent. Many patients have mild degrees of anal stenosis. It should be possible to insert the index finger easily into the pouch through a rather snug anastomosis. Inability to pass the examining finger easily into the pouch, and marked tenderness on attempting to do so are indicative of an anastomotic stricture.

It is usually possible to pass an endoscope through the stricture; this should be done to exclude a coexistent inflammation of the pouch. Indeed, incomplete emptying is thought to predispose to pouchitis. If pouchitis is present, it should be treated as described in a separate chapter on pouchitis. Dilation of the stricture relieves pouch outlet obstruction, thereby improving the ease and completeness of defecation. If the stricture is tight or tender, dilation is best done under general anesthesia. Thereafter, anal dilation can be repeated as needed, possibly with conscious sedation. A small number of patients with tighter and recurrent strictures need frequent dilation, even once or twice per week. These individuals may be trained to perform self-anal dilation using a rubber dilator. The need for more definitive surgical treatment of stubborn strictures needs to be a constant consideration of gastroenterologists and surgeons.

Problems with the Pouch

Defective function of the pouch is probably the commonest reason for excessive bowel frequency in patients who have undergone IPAA. Pouch inflammation, from pouchitis, unrecognized Crohn's disease, or infectious causes, often is the cause of true diarrhea (ie, passage of an abnormally high volume of feces). Patients complain of fecal frequency; the movements commonly are loose and watery and may contain mucus and blood. Urgency and leakage, especially at night, are common. In addition, depending on the severity of pouch inflammation, the presence of associated fistulae, Crohn's disease, or concurrent pouch outlet obstruction, pelvic pain may be present. Systemic symptoms of malaise, low-grade fever, or weight loss often are present in the more severe cases of pouch inflammation. Physical examination in patients with pouch inflammation often is normal. However, individuals with marked inflammation of the pouch from any cause may have the general features of patients with IBD, with low-grade fever, weight loss, and pallor. Crohn's disease is suggested by signs of small bowel obstruction, abdominal mass or tenderness, or perineal sepsis.

In most cases, endoscopy with biopsy of the pouch is diagnostic. Flexible upper gut endoscopes are recommended to examine ileal pouches, because of their narrower caliber and superior flexibility compared to sigmoidoscopes. It must be recognized that even in a healthy pouch, the ileal mucosa undergoes metaplasia to a more colonic type; accordingly, normal ileum is not seen endoscopically or histologically. The presence of edema, erythema, mucous exudates, and ulceration suggests pouch inflammation. If endoscopic changes are confined to the pouch and do not extend into the pre-pouch ileum, pouchitis is the likely diagnosis. However, if aphthous or deep ulcerations and other mucosal abnormalities extend proximally from the pouch, or are seen solely in the pre-pouch ileum, Crohn's disease is more likely. Occasionally, a linear series of shallow ulcerations is observed extending along the divided pouch septum. This appearance is suggestive of pouch ischemia, a complication that may occur if the mesenteric vessels have been stretched too deeply into the pelvis. Inflammation of the cuff of rectal mucosa that remains in some patients after IPAA (cuffitis) also can be visualized endoscopically. There is a separate chapter on pouch endoscopy.

Severe microscopic inflammation can be found in a pouch with a relatively normal endoscopic appearance. Thus, biopsy and histologic evaluation of the mucosa are essential. An experienced pathologist should be able to distinguish between pouchitis, Crohn's disease, and mucosal ischemia. There is a separate chapter on pouch pathology. Pouchography detects pouch leaks, fistulae, and strictures and, thus, can be helpful if these complications are suspected or if pouchitis needs to be differentiated from Crohn's disease.

Most cases of acute pouchitis promptly respond to a course of antibiotics, such as metronidazole (250 to 500 mg 3 times a day) or ciprofloxacin (500 mg twice a day) for 10 to 14 days. Occasionally, pouchitis becomes chronic and refractory to standard therapy. Further discussion of pouchitis can be found in the chapter on chronic pouchitis.

Approximately 5 percent of IPAA procedures are performed in patients whose primary diagnosis is revised at some point after surgery from ulcerative colitis to Crohn's disease. Crohn's disease may be the cause of chronic pouch and pre-pouch inflammation and fistulae. Once the diagnosis is confirmed, therapy is no different from that of pelvic and perianal Crohn's disease in patients still with a rectum. Infected cavities must be drained, obstruction must be excluded, and medical therapy with antibiotics, such as metronidazole (250 to 500 mg 3 times a day) or ciprofloxacin (500 mg twice a day), should be begun. Immunosuppressive therapy with azathioprine (2 to 2.5 mg/kg/d) or 6-mercaptopurine (1.5 mg/kg/d) is recommended in patients with Crohn's disease whose condition does not warrant immediate pouch excision. Open-label experience with tumor necrosis factor-alpha (TNF-α) antibody (infliximab, Remicade®, Centocor Inc., Malvern, Pennsylvania) for Crohn's disease of pouches has been published (Ricart et al, 1999). A single infusion of infliximab (5 mg/kg) resulted in a rapid and favorable response in most patients.

Despite the use of powerful immunosuppressive medications in patients with pouchitis, Crohn's disease of the pouch, or cuffitis, a minority do not respond. The resulting chronic inflammation leads to a scarred, noncompliant pouch. In such patients, it may become futile to continue attempts at medical therapy, because the quality of life will clearly be much better after pouch excision and permanent ileostomy.

Diarrhea Unrelated to the Pouch

After IPAA, patients are not immune to any of the more than 100 causes of diarrhea to which those with an intact bowel are equally susceptible. However, local symptoms, bleeding, incontinence, and urgency tend to focus attention toward a local cause in the pouch. It must be recognized, though, that increased fecal volumes, from any generalized osmotic or secretory form of diarrhea, will, of necessity, stress pouch function and focus attention on pouch dysfunction, perhaps inappropriately. Thus, any of the infectious diarrheas including cytomegalovirus must always be considered and excluded in patients with IPAA diarrhea. Moreover, patients lacking a colon are more sensitive to the fluid losses that accompany any common infectious diarrhea that increase fecal volumes. Thus, consideration must always be given to small bowel diseases, such as celiac sprue, lactase deficiency, Crohn's disease of the proximal bowel, and bacterial overgrowth. If a positive diagnosis of a pouch-related cause cannot be made, etiologies outside the pouch must be sought.*

Finally, approximately 10 percent of the general population suffer from one of the functional bowel disorders (eg, irritable bowel syndrome [IBS]), of which diarrhea is a prominent symptom. The coexistence of IBS and IBD must be anticipated in a minority of patients with preexisting IBS; some of these are thought to have dysfunction of an ileal pouch. When structural or infective causes can be excluded, these patients must be recognized because they need education, support, and symptomatic treatment.†

Supplemental Reading

Dean PA, Dozois RR. Surgical options: ileoanal pouch. In: Allan RN, Rhodes JM, Hanauer SB, et al, eds. Inflammatory bowel diseases. 3rd Ed. London: Churchill Livingston, 1997:761–72.

de Silva HJ, Kettlewell MGW, Mortensen NJ, Jewell DP. Acute inflammation in ileal pouches. Eur J Gastroenterol Hepatol 1991;3:343–9.

Levitt MD, Kuan M. The physiology of ileo-anal pouch function. Am J Surg 1998;176:384–9.

Meagher AP, Farouk R, Dozois RR, et al. Ileal pouch-anal anastomosis for chronic ulcerative colitis: complications and long-term outcome in 1310 patients. Br J Surg 1998;85:800–3.

Metcalf AM, Phillips SF. Ileostomy diarrhea. In: Krejs GJ, ed. Clinics in Gastroenterology. London: WB Saunders, 1986:705–22.

Phillips SF. IBD and irritable bowel syndrome: similar symptoms, different treatments? In: Monteiro E, Tavarela Velosa F, eds. Inflammatory bowel diseases: new insights into mechanisms of inflammation and challenges in diagnosis and treatment. Lancaster, UK: Kluwer Academic Publishers, 1995:139–45.

Ricart E, Panaccione R, Loftus EV, et al. Successful management of Crohn's disease of the ileoanal pouch with infliximab. Gastroenterology 1999;117:429–32.

Stryker SJ, Kelly KA, Phillips SF, et al. Anal and neorectal function after ileal pouch-anal anastomosis. Ann Surg 1986;203:55–61.

Thompson-Fawcett MW, Mortensen NJ, Warren BF. "Cuffitis" and inflammatory changes in the columnar cuff, anal transitional zone, and ileal reservoir after stapled pouch-anal anastomosis. Dis Colon Rectum 1999;42:348–55.

---

* Editor's Note: Caffeine intake, as little as 60 mg in a glass of cola or a cup of instant coffee, produces net small bowel secretion. Patients with any type of ileostomy may have their ostomy output increased by excessive caffeine ingestion. (TMB)

† Editor's Note: Among a group of patients with more than six evacuations per day, a third had a history of IBS for years before UC appeared. Radiographic pouch studies showed that their capacity was less than 100 mL and they could only expel less than half that volume, owing to a spasm of the pouch. We have urged some patients with a history of painful IBS before the diagnosis of UC to consider a Brooke ileostomy rather than an ileoanal pouch. (TMB)

CHAPTER 45

Ileoanal Pouch Surgery in Childhood

Eric W. Fonkalsrud, MD

Introduction

Total colectomy with the ileoanal pouch procedure (IAPP) is currently the most favorable option for the surgical management of ulcerative colitis (UC) in patients of all ages. Although the majority of published reports regarding the IAPP for UC have focused on the clinical experience with adult patients, this chapter will be directed to the operation and details of management for children.

Medical Management

Medical therapy for severe UC is nonspecific and based on measures to provide symptomatic relief. Although most patients will experience a transient remission with medical therapy, it is uncommon for the ultimate course of severe colitis to be altered in the majority of children or for a cure to be achieved without surgical treatment. In our experience, complications following surgical management of UC in children increase with the duration of the disease and the length and dosage of corticosteroids and immunosuppressive medications. Furthermore, aggressive or protracted medical therapy for UC in childhood has increased the frequency of emergency staged colectomy, with a resulting increase in morbidity, hospital stay, and less optimal functional results.

Surgical Management

Operation should be seriously considered for any child with UC before severe disability and major complications develop. Elective surgery is performed for children with persistent symptoms of UC despite medical therapy, children with growth failure, severe limitation of activities, and an unacceptable quality of life. Children with symptomatic UC often miss many days of school and must limit participation in physical and social activities. Urgent or emergency surgery (approximately 17 percent) is indicated for children with acute fulminant disease, extensive rectal bleeding, or toxic megacolon. Children with UC are more likely to have pancolitis, with an acute onset and more severe symptoms from UC than are adults. For children, the severely diseased colon should be removed while the epiphyses are still open to allow for optimal growth.

Surgical recommendations should be discussed in detail with the patient and parents. It is often helpful for the patient to speak to another child who has undergone operation previously in order to alleviate fears and concerns about hospitalization and a major operation with a temporary ileostomy. Preoperative discussion with an enterostomal therapist will help prepare the child and parents for an ileostomy. Although a permanent ileostomy for a child with UC is rarely necessary, care of an ileostomy is usually easily mastered by children. Impotence and bladder dysfunction after proctocolectomy in children are uncommon; however, these concerns have caused many children, parents, and physicians to defer surgery until the colitis becomes debilitating and the steroid therapy causes systemic complications.

Preoperative Preparation

Corticosteroid therapy is maintained until operation in order to avoid an acute flare-up. Oral intake is restricted to clear liquids for 48 hours before surgery; however, cathartics and hyperosmolar solutions such as Golytely are not used. Cleansing enemas are avoided since they may stimulate an acute flare-up of colitis. Oral antibiotics (erythromycin and neomycin) are given the night before surgery, and intravenous antibiotics (gentamicin and clindamycin) are started shortly before operation.

Surgical Options

Total proctectomy with permanent ileostomy, the standard operation for UC for more than 40 years, cures the disease, has a relatively low rate of complications, and produces good long-term results. Nevertheless, children often find the idea of needing to wear an ileostomy appliance for life very disturbing. Furthermore, approximately 30 percent of patients with an ileostomy experience appliance-related problems, including skin irritation, leakage, and odor. Currently, it is rare for a child to select proctocolectomy with permanent ileostomy when given a choice of other surgical alternatives. The continent ileostomy (Kock pouch) has been used rarely in UC in childhood because of the high incidence of complications requiring reoperation, and the need for frequent stomal catheterization. Subtotal colectomy with ileorectal anastomosis is currently used only in the very rare patient with UC who has rectal sparing. Active colitis persists in the rectum of most children and almost invariably requires total surgical removal.

Ileoanal Pouch Procedure

Because UC is primarily a disease of the mucosa, colectomy with rectal mucosectomy and the IAPP has become the most frequent operation for treatment of children with UC that is refractory to medical therapy. Removal of the entire rectal mucosa down to the dentate line does not appreciably interfere with function of the anal sphincter or the ability to discriminate between gaseous, liquid, and solid contents. The IAPP for UC in children has undergone many modifications since the report by Martin and associates in 1977. The early operations used a straight endorectal ileal pullthrough technique; however, many patients experienced stool frequency, urgency, and varying degrees of incontinence. Although a few surgeons still use the straight pullthrough technique, most surgeons construct an ileal pouch above the ileoanal anastomosis to reduce peristalsis in the distal ileum and to allow for fecal storage. Regardless of the type of reservoir used, as long as the lower 4 cm of the rectal muscle is not damaged, the resting and squeeze pressure of the anal sphincter often approaches normal values within 3 months.

Early experience with the IAPP demonstrated that a protecting ileostomy that completely diverts the fecal stream for approximately 3 months minimizes the risk of pelvic infection and pouch leak by 50 percent. The one-stage IAPP, however, has been performed successfully for many years on patients with polyposis coli and Hirschsprung's disease. Children with chronic UC who receive long-term steroids or other medications are often malnourished and frequently have a suppressed immune response. The one-stage IAPP should be considered only in children with UC who are in good health, adequately nourished, taking no steroids, on minimal immunosuppressive drugs, not obese, and who have minimal rectal inflammation. Recovery often is protracted when the ileostomy is omitted. A completely diverting end ileostomy is preferred in children to avoid the many complications in management of loop ileostomies reported by enterostomal therapists.

Although several different pouch configurations have been used clinically, the J-shaped pouch has been used most widely, is the simplest to construct, and produces the fewest long-term complications in children as well as adults. In the past, the lateral ileal reservoir has been used extensively for children and has achieved good long-term results, provided that the ileal spout between the lower end of the pouch and the anus was short. The lateral pouch currently is reserved for children in whom it is difficult to obtain sufficient length on the ileal mesentery for a J-shaped pouch, to reach the anus without tension. Reservoir configuration is relatively unimportant as long

as the pouch is made short (under 12 cm), which allows for most efficient function. A spout should be avoided if possible since a conduit between the pouch and the anal anastomosis may cause functional obstruction.

Ileoanal Pouch Construction

For most children, IAPP is performed in two stages. During the first operation, the patient is given general anesthesia and placed on the operating table in the lithotomy position. A nasogastric tube and bladder catheter are placed. Through a lower midline incision extending to slightly above the umbilicus, the entire colon and omentum are removed. If there is any inflammation present in the distal ileum, one should suspect Crohn's disease (CD), which would preclude the IAPP, in which case the colon would be removed and a Hartmann's rectal pouch and cutaneous ileostomy would be performed until the final pathology report was available. The rectum is thoroughly irrigated with antibiotic solution from below. The peritoneal reflection is incised circumferentially, and the rectum is mobilized with needle tip cautery dissection down to within 4 cm from the dentate line, where it is divided. The specimen is examined to rule out the presence of CD. A Parks retractor is placed into the rectum and the mucosa is mobilized from the rectal muscles using scissor and needle tip cautery dissection. Dilute epinephrine solution is injected between the mucosa and muscularis to facilitate the plane of dissection. All mucosa is removed down to the dentate line, and meticulous hemostasis is achieved. A few surgeons perform the mucosectomy from the pelvis rather than the perineum.

The ileal mesentery is mobilized adjacent to the superior mesenteric vessels extending into the upper abdomen to provide sufficient length for the distal ileum to reach the anus without tension. The distal 10 to 12 cm of ileum is doubled back on itself, which places the antimesenteric surfaces adjacent to each other. A small incision is made through the apex of the loop, and a GIA stapling device is inserted through the incision to construct the pouch. The upper end of the pouch is closed with inverting absorbable sutures. A second layer of absorbable suture is placed around the pouch staple and suture lines. The pouch is brought through the pelvis and rectal muscle canal with gentle traction taking care to avoid twisting the mesentery (Figure 45–1). The open apex of the pouch is sutured to the anoderm and rectal muscularis at the level of the dentate line with interrupted absorbable sutures. The ileum is transsected approximately 15 to 20 cm proximal to the upper end of the ileal pouch and the proximal end of the divided ileum is constructed into an end ileostomy stoma. The distal ileum is stapled closed and the pelvis is drained transabdominally for 3 to 4 days.

Intravenous steroids are tapered rapidly after operation; oral prednisone usually can be discontinued within

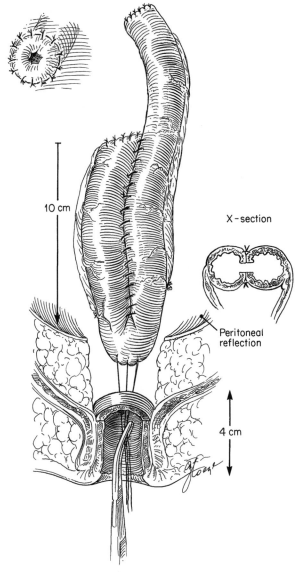

FIGURE 45–1. The completed J-pouch is drawn through the pelvis and rectal muscle canal with traction sutures. The open apex of the ileal pouch is sutured to the anoderm and rectal muscularis at the level of the dentate line with interrupted absorbable sutures. A completely diverting end ileostomy is used for approximately 3 months.

3 weeks. Intravenous antibiotics are given for 4 days and oral metronidazole is given for an additional 5 days. Most children are discharged from the hospital by the sixth day after operation. A Gastrografin (meglumine diatrizoate) contrast enema is performed within 2 months to ensure that the ileal pouch has no leaks or sinus tracts. Most children resume full activities within 3 weeks.

Approximately 3 months after the first operation, the child is rehospitalized for laparotomy with ileostomy closure and sigmoidoscopy. The ileoanal anastomosis is dilated under anesthesia. The patient is hospitalized for 5 to 6 days. When oral feedings are resumed, spicy foods, chocolate, and vinegar salad dressings are reduced in the

diet to minimize diarrhea. Low-dose metronidazole is given for approximately 6 weeks to reduce inflammation of the ileal mucosa caused by fecal storage in the ileal pouch. Medications to reduce peristalsis counteract the normal stimulus to pouch contraction, thereby promoting stasis, and thus rarely are necessary except for occasional frequency of nocturnal defecation during the first few weeks after surgery. Bulking agents rarely are helpful. Daily dilatation of the ileoanal anastomosis with a large Hegar's dilator (size 18) is initiated by the fourth postoperative day in those patients who have ileoanal stenosis or stricture and is continued at least twice weekly during the ensuing few weeks.

Clinical Experience

During the past 20 years, 151 children younger than 19 years of age (118 with UC, 23 with polyposis, 8 with Hirschsprung's disease, and 2 with colonic inertia) have undergone colectomy and IAPP at the UCLA Medical Center. Eighteen patients were younger than 10 years of age. During the same period, an additional 574 patients who were 19 years of age or older with UC, polyposis, or colonic interia underwent IAPP.

Long-term follow-up with J-shaped and lateral pouches has shown that the average number of bowel movements per day at 3 months is 5.9, whereas at 6 months it decreases to 4.2. Nocturnal staining or soiling more than twice weekly was present in 15 percent at 3 months, particularly in the very young patients. By 6 months, the incidence had decreased to only 5 percent of patients. None of the patients have experienced bladder dysfunction, and none of the 69 males has had impotence. Many of the patients participate in vigorous athletic activities including football, competitive sports, and marathon racing.

Fecal bile salts and serum B_{12} levels have been within the normal range in the 19 children in whom these studies were evaluated. Within several months, the ileal pouch mucosa began to function similar to that of the normal colon. A detailed review of the last 85 consecutive children shows that all but 2 are currently functioning well, indicating a decreased number of complications as our clinical experience has increased. Functional results and quality of life have been considered to be very good to excellent in 95 percent of the patients.

Complications following the IAPP have been reported to occur in 35 to 65 percent of patients (41% in our series of children, Table 45–1). Pouchitis is most common within the first 2 years after the IAPP and causes watery diarrhea, fever, malaise, and occasional arthralgias. Episodes are more frequent and severe in children than in adults. Liberal rectal dilatation after an IAPP and aggressive surgical correction of outflow obstruction have resulted in a less than 10 percent incidence of pouchitis in our overall series of 631 UC patients. Treatment for

TABLE 45–1. Complications Following Ileoanal Pouch Procedure in 151 Children

Complication	Percent
Anorectal strictures	17
Pouchitis	15
Adhesions, internal hernias	9
Wound infections	5
Pelvic sinus tracts	3
Ileostomy obstruction	2
Rectovaginal fistula	1.3
Retraction of ileoanal anastomosis	0.7
Bleeding	0.7
Pelvic abscess	0

16 patients had more than one complication.

pouchitis includes metronidazole, and daily pouch washouts with tap water or Rowasa enemas. For persistent cases, oral mesalamine and hydrocortisone retention enemas are used. A diverting ileostomy rarely may become necessary for children in whom chronic pouchitis may cause delayed growth and development. There is a chapter on chronic pouchitis management.

For symptomatic patients (from our early clinical experience) who developed dysfunction with the IAPP from mechanical causes, we have performed reconstructive operations on most with good success. Seven children who had a straight ileal pullthrough procedure had conversion to a J-shaped pouch with excellent results.

Controversy surrounds the benefits of hand-sewn ileal pouch-anal anastomosis versus the double-stapled pouch-low rectal anastomosis. The stapled anastomosis is technically easier and minimizes trauma to the rectal muscle complex. Patients with UC, however, often have severe rectal disease, which can interfere with healing of the rectal anastomosis and cause fistulae or obstruction to pouch outflow. The stapled pouch-rectal anastomosis is best suited for patients in whom tension is necessary to bring the ileal pouch down to the anus. Severe rectal UC, synchronous colon cancer, or mucosal dysplasia contraindicate anal mucosal preservation in patients of any age. Children with the onset of UC under the age of 16 years are at much higher risk for developing carcinoma of the colon or rectum than are older patients, and those with the stapled anastomosis will require a lifetime of annual surveillance sigmoidoscopy.

Conclusion

Ulcerative colitis is more severe in children than in adults and often has more acute symptoms. A child's growth may be markedly delayed by the UC as well as by long-term steroids and immunosuppressive medications. If colectomy is not performed until late adolescence, the child may never experience "catch-up" growth. Total colectomy with IAPP is a safe operation with approximately 95 percent of children functioning well more than 5 years after operation. The majority of postsurgical complications are correctable.

Supplemental Reading

Coran AG. A personal experience with 100 consecutive total colectomies in straight ileoanal endorectal pull-throughs for benign disease of the colon and rectum in children and adults. Ann Surg 1990;212:242–8.

Fonkalsrud EW, Loar N. Long-term results after colectomy and endorectal ileal pull-through procedure in children. Ann Surg 1992;215:57–62.

Fonkalsrud EW. Long-term results after colectomy and ileoanal pull-through procedure in children. Arch Surg 1996;131:881–6.

Fonkalsrud EW, Bustorff-Silva J. Reconstruction for chronic dysfunction of ileoanal pouches. Ann Surg 1999; 229:197–204.

Martin L, LeCoultre C, Schubert WK. Total colectomy and mucosal proctectomy with preservation of continence in ulcerative colitis. Ann Surg 1977;186:477–80.

CHAPTER 46

CHRONIC POUCHITIS

DAVID A. SCHWARTZ, MD, AND WILLIAM J. SANDBORN, MD

Introduction

Abdominal colectomy with ileal pouch-anal anastomosis (IPAA) has become the surgical treatment of choice for most patients with uncontrolled ulcerative colitis (UC). The most frequent long-term complication of this procedure is nonspecific inflammation of the ileal pouch, commonly referred to as pouchitis. At the Mayo Clinic, the cumulative number of patients with UC with IPAA who developed at least one episode of pouchitis is 32 percent, though other centers have shown incidences of up to 50 percent. Of these patients, approximately two-thirds have at least one recurrence of pouchitis. For many of these patients, pouchitis recurs frequently enough to cause a chronic problem. In fact, 15 percent of patients with pouchitis (5% of all patients with IPAA) require maintenance suppressive therapy and have been labeled as having chronic pouchitis. Of the patients with chronic pouchitis, almost 50% will require surgical excision or exclusion of the pouch for medically refractory disease. The following will be a review of the treatment options and the algorithm we use to treat chronic pouchitis.

Diagnosis and Definition of Pouchitis

A clinical diagnosis of pouchitis is made based on the symptoms of increased stool frequency, rectal bleeding, abdominal cramping, rectal urgency and tenesmus, incontinence, and fever in patients with an IPAA for UC. This should be confirmed by pouch endoscopy and biopsy. Endoscopy is essential in the initial assessment of pouchitis. It helps to evaluate contributing factors for pouchitis including outlet obstruction and allows for histologic information. Endoscopically, pouchitis manifests as edema, granularity, contact bleeding, loss of vascular pattern, mucosal hemorrhage, and ulceration within the pouch. Histologically, the acute changes of neutrophil infiltration and mucosal ulceration are superimposed on a background of chronic changes including villous atrophy, crypt hyperplasia, and chronic inflammatory cell infiltration. Biopsies from the posterior wall are more likely to show changes of pouchitis. However, these changes are patchy. Therefore, we recommend four quadrant biopsies, two pieces per site, placed in one bottle. In addition, any site of obvious inflammation also should be biopsied. The mucosa of the neoterminal ileum above the pouch should appear normal. This approach to diagnosis avoids the misdiagnosis of pouchitis in patients with other causes of pouch dysfunction. The Mayo pouchitis index was described by Sandborn et al. There is a chapter on pathology findings in pouches including a discussion of dysplasia.

Perinuclear Antineutrophil Cytoplasmic Antibody and Pouchitis

Before embarking on a discussion of the treatment of chronic pouchitis, a brief comment should be made regarding the predictive value of perinuclear antineutrophil cytoplasmic antibody (pANCA). Initial studies suggested an association between the presence of pANCA and pouchitis following IPAA for UC. This includes the initial report from our institution. However, the three follow-up studies failed to confirm this association. A recent follow-up study by Panaccione and colleagues from the Mayo Clinic re-examined the patients presented in the initial 1995 study. All 19 patients with chronic pouchitis were found to be pANCA-positive. In addition, five of the nine patients who were initially pANCA-positive but were found not to have pouchitis now have developed at least one episode of pouchitis during 5 years of follow-up. Of the 51 patients in this study, only 14 percent of pANCA-positive patients with UC and an IPAA have not developed pouchitis. In the studies from our institution, the pANCAs were drawn postcolectomy. This study appears to show a strong association between pANCA and the risk of developing pouchitis following IPAA for UC. To date, there have been no studies that have looked at pANCA positivity as a predictor of chronic pouchitis in a prospective manner.

While confirmatory studies are needed, pANCA may be useful for identifying patients at risk for chronic pouchitis after IPAA. The threshold for beginning suppressive medical therapy (as opposed to operation) might be lower in these patients given their risk of recurrent symptoms of inflammatory bowel disease (chronic pouchitis).

Medical Treatment of Chronic Pouchitis

The medical therapy used for chronic pouchitis is vast and varied. A list of agents reported to be of benefit is shown in Table 46–1 and discussed below. (See treatment algorithm—Figure 46–1.)

TABLE 46–1. Treatments Reported to be Efficacious for Pouchitis

Class	Example
1. Antibiotics	A. Metronidazole B. Ciprofloxacin C. Amoxicillin/clavulanic acid D. Erythromycin E. Tetracycline
2. 5-Aminosalicylates	A. Mesalamine enemas B. Sulfasalazine C. Oral mesalamine
3. Corticosteroids	A. Conventional corticosteroid enemas B. Budesonide enemas C. Oral corticosteroids
4. Immune modifier agents	A. Azathioprine
5. Oral probiotic bacteria	A. VSL-3
6. Nutritional agents	A. SCFA enemas or suppositories B. Glutamine suppositories
7. Other agents	A. Bismuth subsalicylate B. Bismuth carbomer enemas
8. Surgical options	A. Ileal pouch exclusion B. Ileal pouch excision

SCFA = short-chain fatty acids.

Modified with permission from Sandborn WJ. Pouchitis following ileal pouch-anal anastomosis: definition, pathogenesis, and treatment. Gastroenterology 1994;107:1856–60.

ANTIBIOTICS

The mainstay of therapy for pouchitis (acute or chronic) is an antibiotic with anaerobic activity. The most commonly used antibiotic for this purpose is metronidazole. Alternative antibiotics to metronidazole include ciprofloxacin, amoxicillin/clavulanic acid, erythromycin, and tetracycline. The majority of patients with pouchitis initially respond to metronidazole at doses of 10 to 20mg/kg/d and will continue to respond to metronidazole with subsequent flares. Clinical response typically is seen within 1 to 2 days.

Two placebo-controlled trials using metronidazole to treat pouchitis have been performed. McLeod et al conducted a single-patient randomized trial using either oral metronidazole or placebo to treat a patient with chronic pouchitis in a Kock continent ileostomy. Ten 14-day treatment episodes occurred. The patient's clinical course was significantly worse when receiving the placebo than when receiving metronidazole therapy. Madden and colleagues conducted a randomized double-blind, placebo-controlled crossover trial of oral metronidazole or placebo. They studied 13 patients with chronic pouchitis of whom 11 completed the trial. The mean stool frequency decreased significantly in these patients during metronidazole therapy. Side effects occurred in up to one-half of patients taking metronidazole therapy. The possible side effects of metronidazole include nausea, abdominal discomfort, headache, skin rash, and peripheral neuropathy.

TOPICAL METRONIDAZOLE

In an effort to reduce the side effects of oral metronidazole therapy, two studies have used topical metronidazole preparations for pouchitis. Nygaard et al used liquid metronidazole suspension (40 mg) instilled into the reservoir in an open-label study of 11 patients, 8 of whom had chronic pouchitis and 3 who were intolerant to oral metronidazole. All 11 improved on this therapy and 9 of 11 have continued to improve on either continuous (n = 3) or intermittent (n = 8) topical treatment. None of the patients experienced side effects from the medication. Of the 8 patients tested, serum levels of metronidazole were low in 4 and undetectable in 4. Isaacs and colleagues used vaginal preparations of metronidazole instilled through the anus to treat pouchitis in six patients with pouchitis, three of whom had recurrent disease and four of whom were intolerant to oral metronidazole. Like the Nygaard study, all patients improved on this treatment. One patient developed gastrointestinal intolerance similar to that occurring with oral metronidazole.

Patients with relapsing or chronic pouchitis are treated initially with oral metronidazole 250 mg tid for 10 days. If patients have a recurrence after discontinuing therapy, they are treated similarly. Those who fail treatment with metronidazole are given a course of ciprofloxacin or amoxicillin/clavulanic acid. As shown in previous studies, our experience has been that the majority of patients will respond to the second antibiotic. If the pouchitis occurs a third time within a short period of time, then maintenance therapy with the effective antibiotic (usually metronidazole) at the lowest clinically effective dose is indicated. For the patients who are on maintenance therapy and develop apparent bacterial resistance, cycling of multiple (three or four) antibiotics at 1-week intervals can be helpful. We occasionally use topical metronidazole therapy with the vaginal suppository formulation.

Because the majority of patients respond to antibiotics, if treatment with several antibiotics is unsuccessful, one should reconsider the diagnosis of chronic pouchitis. We have seen at least two patients with cytomegalovirus (CMV) infection of the pouch that was misdiagnosed as chronic pouchitis. The diagnosis is difficult unless the clinical suspicion is high or the pathologist recognizes the viral inclusion bodies. In order to make the diagnosis, pouch biopsies must be examined using monoclonal immunofluorescent staining for CMV. This is a crucial step before beginning immune-modifying therapy.

5-AMINOSALICYLATES

Several uncontrolled studies and anecdotal experiences have suggested the benefit of topical mesalamine, oral mesalamine, and sulfasalazine for pouchitis. A recent study has shown that the bacterial concentrations in the ileal pouch are sufficient to cleave the azo bond of

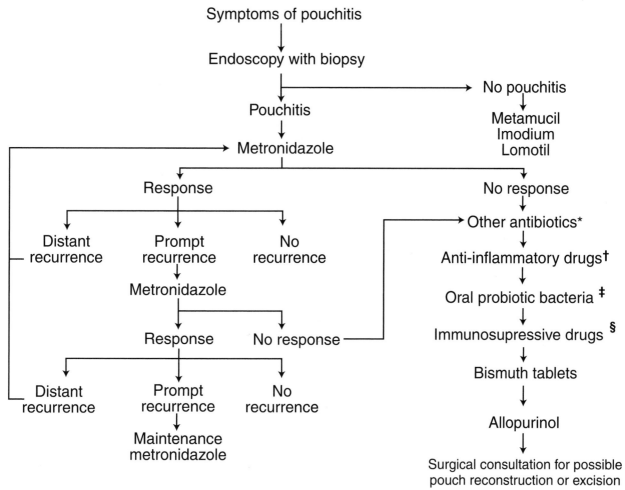

FIGURE 46–1. Treatment algorithm.

sulfasalazine. It is reasonable to assume that the Pentasa® (Ferring-Shire Pharmaceuticals Inc., Florence, Kentucky) formulation of mesalamine will result in some release of mesalamine into the ileal pouch. In our practice, we use the 5-aminosalicylates as a second-line agent for the treatment of chronic pouchitis. Typically, we start with the topical preparations first and reserve oral sulfasalazine or oral mesalamine in the form of Pentasa for the more refractory cases.

IMMUNOSUPPRESSIVE DRUGS

Corticosteroids have been reported anecdotally to be beneficial for pouchitis. The side effects associated with long-term oral steroid use makes repeated or chronic usage impractical. Topical preparations have the theoretical benefit of decreased systemic side effects. One study that utilized budesonide suppositories reported improvement in all of the 10 patients studied. Budesonide suppositories are not commercially available in the United States. We occasionally use corticosteroid enema or suppositories to treat acute pouchitis but rarely have used it

for chronic pouchitis because a significant amount of corticosteroid is absorbed systemically.

Another immune-modulating agent, azathioprine, has been reported to be of benefit. However, two studies involving a total of 11 patients with both IPAA for UC and liver transplantation for primary sclerosing cholangitis have reported chronic pouchitis in 5 (45%) of these patients despite heavy immunosuppression. These experiences suggest that immune modifiers may not be of great benefit for pouchitis. Therefore, we rarely use these agents unless the patient's diagnosis is changed to Crohn's disease.

ORAL PROBIOTIC BACTERIA

Recently, a single randomized, double-blind, placebo-controlled study of 40 patients with chronic pouchitis found an oral probiotic bacterial formula (VSL-3) to be beneficial in maintaining remission. All of the patients were in remission at the start of the study. The VSL-3 preparation contains multiple strains of lyophilized lactobacilli and other probiotic bacteria. Patients were given either preparation or placebo for 9 months. Only 15 percent of the treatment group suffered a flare of pouchitis compared to 100 percent of the placebo cohort. Another probiotic preparation has been found to be as effective as oral mesalamine for maintenance therapy in UC. Based on the available data, we would consider probiotic bacterial preparations as a potential adjuvant agent to maintain remission in patients with chronic pouchitis. We are awaiting confirmatory studies before adopting probiotic therapy in our clinical practice.

NUTRITIONAL AGENTS

A nutritional replacement approach to treatment using short-chain fatty acid (SCFA) enemas has been purposed for pouchitis because these patients may have decreased fecal SCFA concentrations. However, SCFAs seem to be more important in colonic mucosal homeostasis than in small bowel. The three studies utilizing this approach have shown little if any improvement with these agents. We do not advocate their use as therapy.

OTHER AGENTS

Bismuth carbomer enemas have been used with varying results. One open-label study reported benefit in 83 percent of patients with chronic pouchitis treated. However, a randomized double-blind placebo-controlled study from our institution found no difference compared with placebo. A recent report showed benefit using chewable bismuth subsalicylate tablets to treat pouchitis. Eleven of the 13 patients improved on this program during a 4-week treatment trial. We utilize bismuth to treat patients who have failed antibiotic and 5-ASA therapy. In general, the chewable bismuth tablets are the preferred method of delivery with an initial dose of two 262-mg tablets 4 times per day.

Allopurinol may prevent the production of oxygen free radicals by inhibiting xanthine oxidase. One study utilized this mechanism of action to treat chronic pouchitis and reported improvement in 7 of 14 patients treated.

Treatment Algorithm

It is important to separate patients with chronic pouchitis into groups of those with treatment-responsive pouchitis and those with treatment-resistant pouchitis. In general, the vast majority of patients fall into the treatment-responsive category and do very well on intermittent antibiotic therapy. Those who have frequent relapses (ie, > 2 in a short period of time) are classified as having chronic pouchitis and are put on maintenance antibiotics. If resistance to one antibiotic develops, rotating multiple antibiotics seems to lessen this problem.

The great difficulty lies in the small minority of patients who fall into the treatment-resistant category. We typically try topical treatment with mesalamine and/or steroids as the initial second-line agent in these patients. In refractory cases, sulfasalazine, oral mesalamine in the form of Pentasa, or oral steroids are utilized. However, only a few patients will ultimately respond to these agents. In countries where these are available, oral probiotic bacteria may be a useful adjuvant therapy for these patients, especially in order to maintain remission. Some patients may require combination therapy with multiple agents to maintain remission.

If a patient with chronic pouchitis does not respond to either antibiotics or 5-ASA/steroids and/or oral probiotic bacteria, it is reasonable to try some of the alternative agents as a last resort. These include chewable bismuth tablets and allopurinol. Despite exhaustive therapeutic attempts, some patients will be refractory to all forms of medical therapy and will need to be referred to a surgeon for either permanent ileostomy or pouch revision. (See Figure 46–1.)

Surveillance

Lastly, we want to stress the importance of annual surveillance for patients with an IAPP. The issue of risk of dysplasia within the pouch has been raised from studies by Gullberg et al. Their group has shown that dysplasia can occur anywhere within the pouch in the setting of chronic pouchitis. Therefore, we recommend annual surveillance for our patients with an IPAA who have chronic pouchitis. At the time of endoscopy, systematic four quadrant biopsies from the pouch with two pieces per site should be taken and placed in one bottle. This initially is done every 2 to 3 years. If dysplasia is noted, the surveillance program is intensified. If high-grade dysplasia is found, we would recommend that the pouch be excised.

Supplemental Reading

Gionchetti P, Rizzello F, Venturi A, et al. Maintenance treatment of chronic pouchitis: a randomized placebo-controlled, double-blind trial with a new probiotic preparation [abstract]. Gastroenterology 1998;114:985A.

Gullberg K, Stahlberg D, Liljeqvist L, et al. Neoplastic transformation of the pelvic pouch mucosa in patients with ulcerative colitis. Gastroenterology 1997;112:1487–92.

Hurst RD, Molinari M, Chung P, et al. Prospective study of the incidence, timing, and treatment of pouchitis in 104 consecutive patients after restorative proctocolectomy. Arch Surg 1996;131:497–500.

Isaacs K, Klenzak J, Koruda M: Topical metronidazole for the treatment of pouchitis. Gastrointest Endosc 1997;45AB108.

Madden MV, McIntyre AS, Nicholls RJ. Double-blind crossover trial of metronidazole versus placebo in chronic unremitting pouchitis. Dig Dis Sci 1994;39:1193–6.

Editor's Note: A very useful chapter. (TMB)

McLeod RS, Taylor DW, Cohen Z, Cullen J. The single patient randomized clinical trial: its use in determining optimal treatment for a patient with inflammation in a Kock continent reservoir ileostomy. Lancet 1986;1:726–9.

Nygaard K, Bergan T, Bjorkneklett A, et al. Topical metronidazole treatment in pouchitis. Scand J Gastroenterol 1994;29:462–7.

Panaccione R, Sandborn WJ, Tremaine WJ, et al. P-ANCA is associated with chronic pouchitis and predicts the future occurrence of acute pouchitis following ileal pouch-anal anastomosis [abstract]. Gastroenterology 1998;116:791A.

Sandborn WJ, McLeod R, Jewell DP. Medical therapy for the induction and maintenance of remission in pouchitis: a systematic review. Inflamm Bowel Dis 1999;5:33–9.

Sandborn WJ, Tremaine WJ, Batts KP, et al. Pouchitis after ileal pouch-anal anastomosis: a pouchitis disease activity index. Mayo Clin Proc 1994;69:409–15.

CHAPTER 47

ENDOSCOPY IN EVALUATING ILEAL POUCHES

ROBYNNE K. CHUTKAN, MD, AND JEROME D. WAYE, MD, FACP

The Continent Ileostomy

The continent ileostomy or Kock pouch is an alternative to the standard Brooke type of end-ileostomy. In fashioning the continent ileostomy, an internal pouch is constructed by bending a section of terminal ileum into a "U" loop. The antimesenteric borders of the two limbs are approximated and incised, then the outer and inner edges are sewn together to create the pouch. The inflow tract of ileum (afferent limb) enters the pouch in an unimpeded manner, whereas continence of the outflow tract (efferent limb) is achieved by invaginating a portion of the terminal-most ileum into the pouch, forming a two-layer "nipple" that protrudes into the pouch. The nipple valve, about 5 cm long, is kept in place by sutures and by mechanical abrasion of the apposing serosal layers, to promote adhesions. The outflow tract is the portion of ileum traversing the nipple and extending up to the skin surface.

The pouch can be fashioned at the time of the initial surgery or as a subsequent conversion from a Brooke ileostomy. Although ileoanal pouch surgery largely has supplanted the continent ileostomy operation, over the past 30 years, in thousands of cases worldwide, continent ileostomies have been fashioned, and for various reasons, the endoscopist may be requested to examine this type of pouch.

Most patients with a continent ileostomy have had a colectomy performed for ulcerative colitis or familial polyposis. This procedure also is indicated for patients who require proctocolectomy but are poor candidates for an ileal pouch-anal anastomosis (IPAA) and those with a failed IPAA. Like the IPAA, this procedure is generally avoided in Crohn's patients because of the risk of recurrent disease in the pouch. Although the continent ileostomy allows the patient to forgo an external appliance, the complexity of the surgical construction and the need to intubate the pouch actively several times a day for drainage increases the likelihood of complications compared to an end-ileostomy. When difficulties do arise with the continent ileostomy, endoscopy is the most expedient method of evaluation.

Endoscopic Anatomy of the Kock Pouch

A slim caliber instrument with an acutely angulating bending section is required, usually a gastroscope.

Intubation into the stoma is easily accomplished, after the patient has been on a clear liquid diet for 24 hours and has recently emptied the pouch. The outflow tract may contain a few erosions related to catheter intubation trauma. The pouch usually is football-shaped, with the nipple near one end. A U-turn is necessary to fully visualize the nipple, which appears as a smooth, slightly tapered, cylindrical mound that surrounds the scope. The junction with the pouch is smooth and devoid of any sharp angles. The inflow tract is near the nipple and can be intubated by making a large loop in the pouch or by pulling the scope to the edge of the nipple and twisting the shaft with the tip acutely angulated. The inner lining of the pouch is smooth, and because of the surgical construction, peristalsis is absent or may progress in different directions in various portions of the pouch.

Common Problems with the Kock Pouch

Four relatively common problems occur in patients with a mature continent ileostomy and may be encountered at any time after the operation, from the postoperative period to several years later. *Inability to intubate* the pouch for drainage constitutes a medical emergency. Other problems include *leakage* of gas or stool, *bloody discharge*, and *pain* in the area of the pouch. There is a separate chapter on the continent ileostomy and its complications.

INABILITY TO INTUBATE

The most dramatic complication occurs when the drainage catheter cannot be placed into the pouch. Most patients are aware of intermittent but increasing difficulty with intubation over weeks to months. In almost every case, this problem is caused by slippage or intussusception of a well-formed normal nipple into the outflow tract. The normal nipple protrudes into the pouch approximately 5 cm and acts as a flap-valve, impeding the outflow of pouch contents. As pressure within the pouch increases, so does coapting pressure on the lips of the nipple-valve, to ensure absolute continence of both gas and liquid. Intussusception of the nipple occurs as a result of two factors: (1) the pressure within the pouch and (2) the distensibility and caliber of the outflow tract.

The surgical success of the continent ileostomy is dependent upon the maintenance of blood supply to the portion of ileum that traverses the abdominal wall. Therefore, care is taken to avoid placing sutures or staples through the vascular supply of the efferent limb; this requirement leads to a relatively distensible outflow tract as it traverses the abdominal wall. However, the nipple is a fixed-diameter, firm, cylindrical protruberance into the pouch, and it can, with increased pressure, slide into the wider-caliber outflow tract. As the nipple intussuscepts into the portion of the outflow tract that traverses the abdominal wall, it rotates on its mesenteric attachment, causing the long axis of the nipple to become misaligned with the long axis of the outflow tract, resulting in difficulty with catheter intubation of the pouch.

When nipple slippage occurs, the angulation between the two parts of the outflow tract, the intranipple portion and the segment traversing the abdominal wall, may be up to 90 degrees. Fortunately, nipple intussusception usually occurs gradually, with the patient complaining of intermittent difficulty with intubation over days or weeks. Symptoms may develop acutely if the pressure in the pouch suddenly increases and "pops" the nipple into the outflow tract. The generally slow development of this complication results in the patient developing different adaptive techniques to successfully intubate and drain the pouch, such as changing body position or catheter angle. When intussusception of the nipple occurs, intubation may not be possible with the regular drainage catheter since entry into the nipple portion may be at quite an angle to the outflow tract. Occasionally, a Foley catheter may be pushed into the outflow tract and through trial and error gain access to the pouch for decompression. The distance between the abdominal wall and the intussuscepted nipple is too long to permit its de-intussusception using a finger passed through the stoma.

Endoscopy in the partially slipped nipple may permit identification of the angulated orifice, but when the nipple lies at 90 degrees or greater to the portion that traverses the abdominal wall, no orifice may be visible. When that occurs, the scope is advanced as far as possible, and with maximal tip deflection, rotation of the shaft will corkscrew the tip into the transversely lying nipple to enter the pouch. Once in, air and fluid are evacuated, and the instrument is exchanged over a guidewire with a drainage catheter that is taped in place until definitive surgery can be scheduled. An intussuscepted nipple usually can be identified because it sits in a circumferential depression around its base, or only a small portion of the nipple may be seen if the intussusception is of high grade. An endoscopist who is inexperienced in examining a continent ileostomy may mistake the angulated orifice for a fistula.

A fistula can occur in the nipple and is another cause of incontinence, as is intussusception. Fistulae may occur where tight sutures result in localized ischemia and a through and through slough occurs, usually at the nipple

base or occasionally in the body of the nipple. The entire basal portion of the nipple may be difficult to fully inspect, but acute tip angulation and shaft rotation will permit full visualization. Pouchitis is readily identified as erythema or ulceration within the pouch, although unrecognized Crohn's disease may have a similar appearance.

Ileal Pouch-Anal Anastomosis

The IPAA has become the procedure of choice for patients with ulcerative colitis and is now performed routinely by many surgeons. The ileal pouch uses the distal 30 to 35 cm of ileum and several different configurations are possible, including the J-shaped (most common), S-shaped, and W-shaped.

Endoscopic Anatomy of the Ileal Pouch-Anal Anastomosis

As with endoscopic examination of stomas, the ileoanal pouch is more easily examined with a gastroscope, owing to the greater tip deflection and the shorter bending radius. Although the inflow portion of the ileum may be acutely angulated, the pouch is intubated easily under most circumstances and the ileoanal anastomosis may be identified just beyond the anal verge at the level of the dentate line. The presence of neovascularity, a white edge, or adjacent scarring at the anastomosis may aid in its identification. Nodularity at the suture line may be evident in hand-sewn anastomoses. Bilateral small blind pouches just distal to the anastomosis correspond to the surgically created "dog ears" in stapled anastomoses and need to be carefully examined for residual rectal mucosa. In the absence of pouchitis or peripouch inflammation, the pouch is easily distensible with air insufflation. The normal ileal mucosa has a granular appearance and characteristic contractile pattern with a generally less pronounced vascular pattern relative to normal colonic mucosa. However, "colonization" of the pouch may occur over time with the ileal mucosa developing a more pronounced vascular pattern and glistening surface. A U-turn can and should be performed in the most distal aspect of the pouch, unless there is evidence of pouchitis or peripouch inflammation, where the risk of perforation with this maneuver is increased.

Common Problems with the Ileal Pouch-Anal Anastomosis

Dysplasia Surveillance

The endoscopist may be called on to examine the pouch for routine dysplasia surveillance purposes, because there is a risk of neoplastic degenerative residual rectal mucosa, particularly when a double-stapled IPAA is employed. The stapled technique leads to the formation of small bilateral blind pouches or "dog ears" of rectal mucosa as a result of the combined technique of linear transection of the anorectum and a circular stapled anastomosis, but preserves the anal transition zone, leading to better discrimination of gas and feces and fewer anastomotic complications. Although cancer in this setting is rare, cases have been reported in the literature of dysplasia and cancer in ileal pouches after IPAA. This is most likely in unrecognized residual rectal mucosa but can occur in atrophic ileal mucosa; therefore, annual examination with biopsies is warranted. The chapter on pouch pathology reviews this issue, as does the chapter on neoplasia in ulcerative colitis.

COMPLICATIONS

Complications after IPAA include pelvic sepsis due to leakage at the anastomosis, small bowel obstruction, pouchitis, stricture formation, incontinence, and fistulae.

Pelvic Sepsis

Fever, leukocytosis, and perineal pain and tenderness may suggest a pelvic phlegmon or abscess. Although these are generally extraluminal lesions diagnosed with the aid of imaging techniques such as computed tomography (CT), endoscopy may be useful in excluding other conditions, such as pouchitis. Peripouch inflammation secondary to anastomotic leakage has been detected with endoscopic ultrasound (EUS); this may be a useful modality in the patient with a dysfunctional pouch and no evidence of pouchitis on endoscopic evaluation, particularly if CT and contrast studies (pouchography) are unrevealing. EUS in this setting often demonstrates a thickened anal canal wall and external sphincter.

Small Bowel Obstruction

Small bowel obstruction occurs more commonly in the early postoperative period before ileostomy closure, but also can be seen as a late complication. Endoscopic decompression and passage of a rectal decompression tube, as with a sigmoid volvulus, may be useful, although persistent high-grade partial mechanical obstruction usually requires operative intervention.

Pouchitis

As many as 30 percent of patients experience one or more episodes of pouchitis after IPAA. The clinical diagnosis is based on a constellation of symptoms, including abdominal cramping; frequent loose stools, which often contain blood; urgency; tenesmus; incontinence; and fever. Although the etiology remains unclear, the endoscopic findings are characteristic and include diffuse reddening of the lining of the pouch, friability, nodularity, and ulceration. Ulcers range from small aphthous-type ulcerations scattered throughout the extent of the pouch to larger, more extensive linear ulcers that may resemble Crohn's disease. The endoscopic differential is generally between pouchitis and Crohn's disease, and histologic examination may be helpful in this regard.

Stricture Formation

Strictures at the anal anastomosis are encountered in approximately 5 percent of patients after IPAA and may be caused by infection, excessive tension at the anastomosis, or ischemia. Historically, the patient may complain of difficulty or pain with defecation and narrow caliber stool; digital rectal examination will confirm the diagnosis. Overflow diarrhea can occur as described in the chapter on output from IPAA. Gentle finger dilation of the stricture (with or without sedation depending on the patient's level of discomfort) may be possible, but often endoscopic dilation is required. Balloon dilation, using a "through-the-scope" dilator or Savary dilators over a guidewire, usually is required for symptomatic relief. Repeated dilations may be needed, although long, dense strictures often require surgical management.

Incontinence and Fistulae

Factors that determine continence after IPAA primarily are related to technical aspects of the surgery, although patient age, prior function, and severity of disease also play a role. Preservation of the anal transition zone is thought to be important in discriminating between solids, liquids, and gas. The decrease in anal sphincter pressure after IPAA may be attributable to a combination of neurogenic and morphologic damage as a result of intraoperative anal dilation, endoanal mucosectomy, and anastomosis. Some degree of nocturnal incontinence or spotting is common. In cases of significant daytime incontinence, endoscopy may be useful in diagnosing pouchitis or fistulae, both common causes of pouch leakage.

Pouch-perineal and pouch-vaginal fistulae often are associated with pelvic sepsis. A sinus tract may be visible on endoscopy, although the diagnosis usually is made clinically, based on history and CT or pouchogram.

Supplemental Reading

Church JM, Fazio VW, Lavery IC. The role of fiberoptic endoscopy in the management of the continent ileostomy. Gastrointest Endosc 1987;33:203–9.

Waye JD, Gelernt IM, Kreel I. Endoscopy of the continent ileostomy [abstract]. Gastroenterology 1974;66:829.

Waye JD, Kreel, I, Bauer J, Gelernt IM. The continent ileostomy: diagnosis and treatment of problems by means of operative fiberoptic endoscopy. Gastrointest Endosc 1997; 23:196–8.

CHAPTER 48

ROLE OF THE PATHOLOGIST IN EVALUATING CHRONIC POUCHES

ROBERT E. PETRAS, MD

Pouch Dysfunction and Review of the Original Colectomy Specimen

Evolving surgical techniques have changed the pathologist's role in the analysis of inflammatory bowel disease (IBD). Patients with ulcerative colitis (UC) have several surgical options that either create continence in an ileostomy (Kock pouch) or preserve anal sphincter function and restore continuity to the bowel (ileal pouch-anal anastomosis [IPAA]). These operations have in common the creation of a reservoir or pouch, formed by interconnecting loops of terminal ileum. In general, these pouch procedures are contraindicated in patients with Crohn's disease (CD) because of increased morbidity including fistula and abscess.

Pouch complications include inflammation, fistula, obstruction, incontinence, and anastomotic leaks. Although many complications result from surgical and mechanical difficulties, and others relate to the development of "primary" inflammation in the pouch (pouchitis), some of these complicated cases likely represent pouch recurrence of initially undiagnosed CD. In our experience, there is nothing quite like a pouch to bring out the Crohn's in someone!* These cases illustrate the inability to reliably differentiate UC from CD especially in severe colitis, even after examination of the colectomy specimen. Virtually all reports of surgical experience with IPAA for presumed UC contain approximately 2 to 7 percent of patients in whom the actual diagnosis proved to be CD. These cases usually present as late pouch abscesses or fistulae. Patients with these complications should be investigated with pouch biopsy to look for evidence of CD and also should prompt "re-review" of the original colectomy specimen, considering it from the viewpoint of the following classification system.

Pathologic Classification

We have adopted a four-tiered pathologic classification system for primary IBD in colectomy specimens: (1) ulcerative colitis; (2) Crohn's disease; (3) indeterminate colitis,

probably ulcerative colitis; and (4) indeterminate colitis, probably Crohn's disease.

Ulcerative Colitis

The definitive diagnosis of UC requires all of the following features: diffuse disease limited to the large intestine, involvement of the rectum, more proximal colonic disease occurring in continuity with an involved rectum (ie, no gross or histologic skip lesions), no deep fissural ulcers, no mural sinus tracts, no transmural lymphoid aggregates, and no granulomas.

Crohn's Disease

The definitive diagnosis of CD requires histologic verification with the demonstration of transmural lymphoid aggregates in an area not deeply ulcerated or the presence of non-necrotizing granulomas. In cases in which the gross and clinical features suggest CD (eg, skip lesions, linear ulcers, cobblestoning, fat-wrapping, terminal ileal inflammation), we advocate extensive histologic sampling to find the definitive histologic features of CD.

Indeterminate Colitis

The term "indeterminate colitis" is used for cases of idiopathic colonic IBD having ambiguous pathologic features that are inconclusive for a diagnosis of UC or CD. These cases usually are accompanied by fulminant clinical colitis, a setting in which the transmural inflammation and fissural ulcers (features usually associated with CD) are found in patients with a clinical course that indicates UC. Following our institutional policy, patients without clinical, endoscopic, or radiologic evidence suggestive of CD in whom the final pathology is indeterminate, will, in general, be considered suitable for IPAA.†

Several studies have apparently concluded that indeterminate colitis clinically acts like UC. Several limitations surround these analyses of indeterminate colitis, making such a firm conclusion premature. The limitations include the retrospective nature of the studies, the

---

* Editor's Note: Besides being a poor song title, this statement harkens back to Sartor's chapter on the role of bacteria in CD. (TMB)

† Editor's Note: Other institutions follow a similar policy with the understanding that if the intraoperative findings suggest the possibility of CD, a Hartmann's pouch of rectum will be left for a later IPAA if the pathology review supports a UC diagnosis. (TMB)

undefined criteria for indeterminate colitis, and the unknown influence of patient selection. A report by Pezim et al (1989) included 25 patients with a pathologic diagnosis of indeterminate colitis who had been operated on for UC. Two patients were lost to follow-up. Two of the remaining 23 patients (9 percent) developed abdominal wall and perianal fistula and eventually lost their pouches (vs 4 percent in the proven UC group) within a relatively short follow-up period (38 months ± 18 months). In an update of this cohort, two additional patients had pouch failure requiring pouch removal, and three other patients, including one originally lost to follow-up, are now thought to have CD, although their pouches still function satisfactorily. This report from the Mayo Clinic (McIntyre et al, 1995) also details a significantly higher rate of pouch failure (19 percent) in their group of indeterminate colitis when compared to their UC cases (8 percent). Wells et al (1991) reported 46 patients with a pathologic diagnosis of indeterminate colitis who they reclassified as probable CD (19 patients, 41 percent), probable UC (11 patients), and indeterminate colitis (16 patients).[‡]

Histologic Ileitis

Some authors report an increased incidence of histologic pouchitis in patients with extensive colitis or with terminal ileal active and chronic inflammation as identified pathologically in the colonic resection specimen. Since these authors correlated their colectomy findings with histologic, not clinical, pouchitis, the importance of their observations in clinical practice remains unknown. We do not recommend that the surgeon alter his/her decision for creation of an ileal pouch based on histologic findings in the terminal ileum or on the inflammatory pattern of the resection specimen, except for a definitive diagnosis of CD.

Pouches and Pouchitis Syndromes

A late complication of a Kock pouch and IPAA is the development of "primary" inflammation in the pouch with its associated clinical syndrome termed "pouchitis." The reported incidence ranges widely from 8 to 46 percent as a result of the lack of an accepted definition. Clinical, endoscopic, and histologic criteria for diagnosis have varied.

Pouch Biopsy

Pouch biopsy may be performed to confirm the presence of inflammation or to evaluate the possibility of CD.

[‡] Editor's Note: The issue of indeterminate colitis, which some pathologists invoke more readily than in the past, is **still a real problem**. Someone commented that "the national flower of the pathologist is the hedge." As outlined in two surgical chapters, some surgeons prefer an ileorectal anastomosis if the preoperative pathologic consensus is indeterminate colitis. (TMB)

TABLE 48–1. Pouchitis Disease Activity Index

Criterion	Score
I. Clinical	
A. Stool frequency	
1. Usual	0
2. 1 to 2 stools/d more	1
3. >3 stools/d more	2
B. Bleeding from pouch	
1. None or rare	0
2. Present	1
C. Urgency/cramping	
1. Never	0
2. Occasional	1
3. Frequent	2
D. Fever >100°F	
1. Absent	0
2. Present	1
II. Endoscopy	
A. Edema	1
B. Granularity	1
C. Friability	1
D. Loss of vascular pattern	1
E. Exudate	1
F. Ulcer	1
III. Histology	
A. Polymorph infiltration	
1. Mild	1
2. Moderate (crypt abscess)	2
3. Severe (crypt abscess)	3
B. Ulcer per low magnification field	
1. <25%	1
2. 25 to 50%	2
3. >50%	3

Classic pouchitis is defined as a total score >7.
Adapted from Sandborn WJ. Pouchitis following ileal pouch-anal anastomosis: definition, pathogenesis, and treatments. Gastroenterology 1994;107:1856–60.

Pouch biopsy specimens obtained from nondysfunctional pouches can show mild villus shortening and increased chronic inflammation with increased crypt proliferation, but in our experience most specimens appear similar to normal terminal ileum. A few neutrophils within surface epithelium and in the lamina propria are commonly seen in pouches that are functioning well. In contrast, pouches with classic pouchitis often have decreased epithelial mucin and decreased or absent lymphoid follicles. The most consistent finding in this classic form of pouchitis has been ulcers with granulation tissue and patchy accumulations of neutrophils within crypt epithelium and within the lamina propria with deep crypt abscess formation. Sandborn (1994) has proposed a "Pouchitis Disease Activity Index," which includes histologic findings (Table 48–1).

Biopsy Sites

There are no set guidelines as to where in a pouch to obtain a biopsy specimen. One assumes that the morphologic information in the literature is based either on directed biopsy (directed toward an endoscopic

TABLE 48-2. Pouchitis Syndromes: Proposed Classification

Antibiotic-responsive "pouchitis" syndromes
    Classic pouchitis (chapter 46)
    Proximal jejunal bacterial overgrowth

Chronic and refractory pouchitis syndromes
    Short-strip (segment) pouchitis
    Crohn's disease (refractory pouchitis with Crohn's-like histology)
    Chronic primary refractory pouchitis (chapter 46)

abnormality) or totally random biopsy. In the few studies that have addressed locational variation of histology in pouches, it appears that inflammation tends to be either diffusely distributed or more severe distally and posteriorly. In the absence of a focal lesion, it is suggested that a biopsy taken 5 cm from the ileoanal anastomosis may be the most sensitive for detecting pouchitis.

An inconsistent relationship between endoscopic and histologic changes in the pouch and a patient's symptoms has been noted. Therefore, many clinicians diagnose pouchitis exclusively on clinical criteria and reserve endoscopic examination with biopsy for those patients with refractory pouchitis or possible CD. This leads to inconsistency in both diagnosis and therapeutic responses. There are no reliable endoscopic or histologic criteria to differentiate most examples of pouchitis from CD in the pouch.

In my view, the clinical syndrome of pouchitis probably represents at least five different conditions (Table 48–2). There are two variants of antibiotic-responsive "pouchitis" syndromes: classic pouchitis and jejunal bacterial overgrowth. Classic pouchitis demonstrates endoscopic and histologic findings that support the pouch as the source of clinical symptoms. Patients with classic pouchitis usually respond to antibiotics such as metronidazole. Occasional patients with clinical symptoms of pouchitis have had endoscopically and histologically negative pouches, but have responded to antibiotics. Although rare, some of these patients have had proximal jejunal bacterial overgrowth, probably as a result of pouch distention causing an "ileal brake" phenomenon that decreases motility in the proximal intestine. This decreased motility may predispose some individuals to proximal small bowel bacterial overgrowth.

Pouchitis syndromes refractory to antibiotic therapy include short-strip pouchitis, CD, and chronic primary refractory pouchitis. To obtain a better functioning pouch, many surgeons, as described in this text, have abandoned the rectal mucosectomy IPAA. In short-strip pouchitis, clinical symptoms may be caused by exacerbation of UC in the small retained rectal segment and some respond to topical corticosteroids.

Although debated, missed CD is much more likely to present as a late pouch fistula or abscess than as refractory pouchitis. We have, on rare occasions, seen refractory pouchitis in which pouch biopsy specimens contain granulomas or in which the excised pouch shows histologic criteria for CD. Invariably, the original colectomy showed either missed CD or indeterminate colitis. Patients with chronic pouchitis should be investigated with endoscopy and biopsy to rule out CD or cytomegalovirus infection, which has been linked to some cases of refractory pouchitis.

Some patients with refractory pouchitis have required surgical removal of the pouch. After careful pathologic evaluation, no specific infection and no criteria for CD can be found in either the excised pouch or in the original colectomy specimen. We believe these cases represent primary refractory pouchitis. The causes of classic pouchitis and primary refractory pouchitis are unknown, but probably are related to a combination of stasis, bacterial overgrowth, the abnormal immune response of patients with IBD, or perhaps colonic-type metaplasia that occurs in some pouches.

Mucosal Adaptation

Histologic patterns of mucosal adaptation in pouches have been identified. Approximately 60 percent of patients exhibit type A mucosa with normal small bowel biopsy histology or only mild mucosal atrophy with minimal or no inflammation. The type B mucosa, characterized by transient atrophy with temporary moderate-to-severe inflammation followed by normalization of the intestinal mucosa, is seen in 30 percent of patients. The type C mucosa with permanent persistent atrophy and severe inflammation occurs in approximately 10 percent of pouches. Colonic-type features have been reported at least focally in pouches of all types by routine morphology, mucin histochemistry, immunohistochemistry, lectin binding, or electron microscopy. This colonic-type metaplasia is most well developed in the type C mucosa but is never complete. All pouches seem to retain mostly small bowel properties regardless of mucosal type or the duration of the pouch.

Pouchitis and Dysplasia

With long-term follow-up, it appears that epithelial dysplasia can develop in the pouch. This rare complication seems to be limited to the subgroup of patients (< 10 percent) in whom refractory pouchitis and colonic-type metaplasia develop (type C mucosa). Most investigators suggest yearly pouch surveillance once type C mucosa is established. However, until further information on cancer risk is available, it would seem prudent to survey types A and B mucosa as well, perhaps every other year.

Dysplasia also can develop in the small retained rectal segment (often incorrectly referred to as the "anal transitional zone") in patients who have had restorative proctocolectomy and stapled IPAA. We recommend annual endoscopic surveillance with biopsy for these rectal segments. The incidence of dysplasia is rare (< 3 percent of patients) and can be safely treated by completion mucosectomy.[§]

Editor's Note

The supplemental reading lists at the end of each chapter have been edited to avoid duplication. A complete 50-item bibliography for this chapter can be requested at <petrasr@ccf.org>.

References

McIntyre PB, Pemberton JH, Wolff BG, et al. Indeterminate colitis: long-term outcome in patients after ileal pouch-anal anastomosis. Dis Colon Rectum 1995;38:51–4.

Pezim ME, Pemberton JH, Beart RW Jr, et al. Outcome of "indeterminate" colitis following ileal pouch-anal anastomosis. Dis Colon Rectum 1989;32:653–8.

Sandborn WJ, McLeod R, Jewell DP. Medical therapy for induction and maintenance of remission in pouchitis: a systematic review. Inflamm Bowel Dis 1999;5:33–8.

Wells AD, McMillan I, Price AB, et al. Natural history of indeterminate colitis. Br J Surg 1991;78:179–81.

Supplemental Reading

Deutsch AA, McLeod RS, Cullen J, et al. Results of the pelvic-pouch procedure in patients with Crohn's disease. Dis Colon Rectum 1991;34:475–7.

Goldstein NS, Sanford WW, Bodzin JH. Crohn's-like complications in patients with ulcerative colitis after total proctocolectomy and ileal pouch-anal anastomosis. Am J Surg Pathol 1997;21:1343–53.

Gullberg K, Stahlberg D, Liljeqvist L, et al. Neoplastic transformation of the pelvic pouch mucosa in patients with ulcerative colitis. Gastroenterology 1997;112:1487–92.

Koltun WA, Schoetz DJ Jr, Roberts PL, et al. Indeterminate colitis predisposes to perineal complications after ileal pouch-anal anastomosis. Dis Colon Rectum 1991;34:857–60.

Munoz-Juarez M, Pemberton JH, Sandborn WJ, et al. Misdiagnosis of specific cytomegalovirus infection of the ileoanal pouch as refractory idiopathic chronic pouchitis. Dis Colon Rectum 1999;42:117–20.

Petras RE, Oakley JR. Intestinal complications of inflammatory bowel disease: pathologic aspects. Semin Colon Rectal Surg 1992;3:160–72.

Sandborn WJ. Pouchitis following ileal pouch-anal anastomosis: definition, pathogenesis, and treatment. Gastroenterology 1994;107:1856–60.

Sarigol S, Wyllie R, Gramlich T, et al. Incidence of dysplasia in pelvic pouches in pediatric patients after ileal pouch-anal anastomosis for ulcerative colitis. J Pediatr Gastroenterol Nutr 1999;28:429–34.

Schmidt CM, Lazenby AJ, Hendrickson RJ, Sitzman JV. Preoperative terminal ileal and colonic resection histopathology predicts risk of pouchitis in patients after ileoanal pull-through procedure. Ann Surg 1998;227:654–65.

Setti Carraro PG, Talbot IC, Nicholls JR. Patterns of distribution of endoscopic and histological changes in the ileal reservoir after restorative protocolectomy for ulcerative colitis. Int J Colorectal Dis 1998;13:103–7.

Shepherd NA, Healey CJ, Warren BF, et al. Distribution of mucosal pathology and an assessment of colonic phenotypic change in the pelvic ileal reservoir. Gut 1993;34:101–5.

Swan NC, Geoghegan JG, O'Donoghue DP, et al. Fulminant colitis in inflammatory bowel disease: detailed pathologic and clinical analysis. Dis Colon Rectum 1998;41:1511–5.

Veress B, Reinholt FP, Lindquist K, et al. Long-term histomorphological surveillance of the pelvic ileal pouch: dysplasia develops in a subgroup of patients. Gastroenterology 1995;109:1090–7.

Ziv Y, Fazio VW, Sirimarco MT, et al. Incidence, risk factors, and treatment of dysplasia in the anal transitional zone after ileal pouch-anal anastomosis. Dis Colon Rectum 1994;37:1281–5.

[§] Editor's Note: Surveillance for dysplasia in Kock pouches and IPAA is beginning to get increasing attention. Unfortunately, most patients are not in a registry, as some people maintain for UC and Crohn's colitis. A national registry, perhaps maintained by the CCFA, could provide a reminder to individuals and their current caregivers of the need for regular surveillance. This is potentially a life-saving mission. (TMB)

CHAPTER 49

SUPPORT FOR PATIENTS WHO UNDERGO OSTOMY AND POUCH SURGERY

KATHLEEN L. POTTER, RN, BSN, COCN

Is being cured or relieved of symptoms of chronic ulcerative colitis (UC) or Crohn's disease (CD) enough to ensure complete recovery? Are people so grateful to be rid of crampy abdominal pain, bloody frequent stools, fatigue, or urgency that they calmly, easily exchange these symptoms for an ileostomy, colostomy, or internal pouch? Certainly persons with inflammatory bowel disease (IBD) often experience a sense of relief after surgery, and many focus on return of physical health, regaining strength, getting good nutrition, and learning to care for an ostomy. But, the emotional aspects cannot be ignored. There are varying degrees of feeling physically disfigured, losing control, and feeling alone and helpless.

The person does need to gain confidence in his ability to care for his own ostomy through education and practice. Education in how to change and empty the appliance, to prevent leakage, to manage odor and gas, to care for the skin, where to purchase supplies, signs and symptoms of postoperative complications, and dietary issues is a critical first step in the adjustment after surgery. An enterostomal therapy (ET) nurse usually is the one best involved in this teaching. Once the patient has perfected these techniques, he or she is on the road to feeling safer and "more in control."

Walsh and colleagues (1995) found that ongoing support, attention, and reassurance should come from various sources. It is supportive for the physician to explain in clear terms the need for surgery, an overview of the surgery, and resulting body changes. Postoperatively, professionals are available to assist with problems, monitor symptoms, and provide interventions as appropriate. Long term, the patient needs a physician who can be counted on to knowledgeably diagnose and treat problems that may develop. When physical needs are properly met, psychosocial adjustments usually are smoother. For example, the person who has a large peristomal hernia will probably not be eager to pursue a love for swimming. Untreated Crohn's disease of the skin, which interferes with pouch adherence, would halt social adjustments.

The ET nurse who is available on an ongoing basis to answer questions, suggest products that will solve particular problems, examine the stoma area for potential problems, and evaluate the care being given plays an important role in supporting the person with an ostomy.

The specifics of this role are discussed in an earlier chapter in this section.

Friends, family, clergy, social workers, or mental health professionals also are available to listen and help. The level of support received from others helps patients accept themselves. The person with an ostomy should be encouraged to seek out those people with whom they can talk and have nurturing relationships. There are 11 chapters on patient support services in this volume.

Support Groups

For many, a group or specific individual in the group is the answer. Support groups, which usually are led by health care professionals, are found in some communities, meeting at various locations, such as hospitals or churches. A survivor of a disease generally facilitates self-help groups, and leadership is shared by the members.

United Ostomy Association

In the United States, the United Ostomy Association (UOA) is the organized self-help group for ostomates. It officially formed in 1962, but the groundwork was laid as early as 1949 when ostomy patients met for support. Its mission states that the UOA is "a volunteer-based health organization dedicated to providing education, information, support, and advocacy for people who have had or will have intestinal or urinary diversions." Self-help goes beyond just helping yourself, on to joining with others who have a mutual interest to be helped in a support situation, and then to remaining to help others. It makes people feel better to help someone else, and then usually their own coping is easier. Ostomies, CD, and UC are the types of conditions in which people could feel isolated, as though no one really understands what they are going through. The feelings of being out of control, disfigured, or dirty and fear of pouch leakage and odor are not easily discussed with just anyone. Joining one of the over 400 chapters throughout the United States and participating in local meetings may benefit an individual by meeting some of the goals of self-help groups: (1) to promote fellowship and dispel a sense of isolation; (2) to give support and encouragement to others; (3) to share coping strategies; (4) to release negative feelings, such as guilt; (5) to strengthen self-esteem; (6) to concentrate on abilities, not disabilities; (7) to exchange ideas and resources; and (8) to meet new friends.

Local chapter meetings are held monthly or as the group determines and usually consist of a business meeting, a program, and a time for socializing. The program could be a speaker of interest, small-group discussions, or an appliance fair.

PATIENT VISITING SERVICES

Another activity of the local chapter is the patient visiting service. Trained and certified visitors, upon request, provide either preoperative or postoperative visits. Efforts are made to match visitor by diagnosis, type of ostomy, age, and sex. The benefit of this contact is often not immediately realized, but, later (maybe weeks or months) that favorable impression often resurfaces. Visits can be arranged by calling the national office at 1 800 826-0826 or by calling the local chapter.

OTHER SUPPORT ACTIVITIES

A local newsletter and the *Ostomy Quarterly* (*OQ*), an excellent 60- to 80-page magazine, are part of the UOA membership benefits. Ostomates, physicians, nurses, and others write feature articles. Other sections in the *OQ* include Ask the ET, Ask the Doctor, Hints, Diet and Nutrition, and Pen Pals. Many ostomy product advertisements are displayed.

An annual 4-day national conference is an opportunity to meet with several hundred ostomates and their families for business meetings, educational sessions, support, socializing, and fun. The exhibit hall features numerous booths. Stoma clinics, where an ET nurse will examine the person's stoma and evaluate stoma and appliance needs, are a popular part of the conference. Appearances by celebrities with ostomies (Rolf Beniersche and Barbara Barrie) have been recent highlights. A separate youth rally for 11 to 14 year olds also is held each summer. It is a beneficial 5-day program, attended by approximately 100 youth, with past attendees as counselors and ET nurses to coordinate the rally.

Within the UOA, the Parents of Ostomy Children (POC) group has formed in recent years. The annual conference has sessions just for this group. There is a POC article in each *Ostomy Quarterly* geared toward education and support for children with ostomies. A POC newsletter, a directory of families, and a library of articles and books are available to assist families. This group can be contacted through the national office.

The Gay-Lesbian Ostomates Committee (GLO) is a group within the UOA and can be contacted through the national office or e-mail at *GLOContact@aol.com*.

With the increase in continent diversion surgeries has come the UOA's Continent Diversion Network. It began in Kansas and, in 1993, became an official UOA chapter. There is an outreach to the entire country with a news-letter, the *Continent Connection*, a library of information, a telephone registry, and a Website: *www.ostomyalternative. org*.

International Association

There also is an International Ostomy Association (IOA), founded in 1945 in the Netherlands. Their biannual magazine, called *Ostomy International*, includes educational articles, information from around the world about issues concerning people with ostomies, human-interest stories, and ostomy product advertisements. In the year 2000, a 10th World Congress will be held in the Netherlands. This 4-day conference has the theme "A Normal Life."

Ileoanal Reservoir Surgery

Many persons with UC are choosing an ileoanal reservoir procedure over the previously standard total proctocolectomy and permanent ileostomy. With this surgery comes its own set of acute and long-term issues. Other chapters in this book address issues specific to this surgery.

In addition to the UOA Continent Connection Network, centers where large numbers of these procedures have been performed have often formed their own support groups for the ileoanal reservoir patient. As with the ostomate, talking with a person who has had the same surgery can be invaluable.

Internet Information and Support

In addition to the changes in the types of surgeries done for IBD, there have been changes in the ways people receive support. For some, computers are an appealing avenue for medical and technical information and psychological support. There is growing use of the World Wide Web among ostomates. The UOA Website address is *www.uoa.org*, and this official organization can be reached by e-mail at *UOA@deltanet.com*. Plans are underway to further expand the Website. Currently, there is basic information: ostomy definitions, UOA membership information, the UOA history, and a list of local chapters and services available. One also finds a list of printed materials available for purchase, along with advertisements of ostomy equipment. For those contemplating ostomy surgery or who are new ostomates, the section "Twenty of the Most Frequently Asked Questions Following Ostomy Surgery" is helpful. Reassuring answers are given to questions, such as Who should I tell? What should I say about my surgery? Will there be odor coming from the pouch? What about sex and intimacy? Are there restrictions? Does the pouch get in the way?

Links to other sites provide more information of interest to the person with a colostomy, ileostomy, or ileoanal reservoir. Of the over 400 chapters, about 35 have their own Websites. Canadian and international chapter sites also can be reached through the UOA Website. The "Related Helpful Sites" links one to support groups where one can view questions, comments, and answers on ostomy-related topics or post one's own comments. These groups are the International Ostomy Association Web Forum, Ostomy Bulletin Board, Ostomy News Group, and Crohn's-Colitis Support News Group. Another helpful link is "Pouch Clip Board," which can be found via "Newsletters and Journals." Also, there are several chapters in this book dedicated to the support services offered by the Crohn's Colitis Foundation of America (CCFA).

Piwonka and Merino (1999), in studying factors that contribute to the postoperative adjustment to a colostomy, found that education for ostomy self-care was the most important factor, followed by psychological support and social support. The person who feels supported perceives a more positive adaptation to an ostomy. Those in a position to facilitate support should be aware of the great importance social support has in the recovery of persons undergoing these extensive bowel surgeries. Encouraging positive interactions with significant others, including those having the same surgery, is a part of the role of the health care professionals.

References

Piwonka MA, Merino JM. A multidimensional modeling of predictors influencing the adjustment to a colostomy. JWOCN 1999;26:298–305.

Walsh BA, Grunert BK, Telford GL, et al. Multidisciplinary management of altered body image in the patient with an ostomy. JWOCN 1995;22:227–35.

Supplemental Reading

Favreau A. Working together to preserve UOA. Ostomy Q 1999;1:54–6.

Illy KE. 10th International Ostomy Association. World Congress. Ostomy International 1999;21:47–8.

Mowdy S. The role of the WOC nurse in an ostomy support group. JWOCN 1998;25:51–4.

Steiner P, Banks PA, Present DH, eds. People not patients. New York: Crohn's and Colitis Foundation of America, 1985.

Other Sources

Crohn's and Colitis Foundation of America. *www.ccfa.org.*

International Ostomy Association. *www.ostomyinternational.org.*

J-Pouch Group. *www.j-pouch.org.*

National Institute of Diabetes and Digestive Kidney Diseases. *www.niddk.nih.gov.*

American Society of Colon and Rectal Surgeons. *www.fascrs.org.*

Shaz's ileostomy page (a page for persons with anostomy or J-pouch. *www.ostomy.50megs.com.*

United Ostomy Association. *www.uoa.org.*

Wound Ostomy and Continence Nurses Society. *www.wocn.org.*

CHAPTER 50

ILEORECTAL ANASTOMOSIS

IAN C. LAVERY, MD

Currently, the most popular choice of surgical treatment for ulcerative colitis (UC) is a *proctocolectomy* and a *pelvic pouch ileoanal anastomosis*. Other alternatives are a *proctocolectomy* and *ileostomy*, or a *colectomy* and *ileorectal anastomosis*. The construction of a *continent ileostomy* has fallen into disfavor because of a high complication rate, and it has been superceded by the pelvic pouch anal anastomosis. None of these operations is ideal, with each having some disadvantages. For a proctocolectomy and ileostomy, the obvious disadvantage is an ileostomy, but the procedure does remove all of the disease. It restores the patient to good health and eliminates the possibility of the development of a cancer in longstanding disease. The disadvantages of an ileal pouch-anal anastomosis (IPAA) are the less than perfect bowel function, both with respect to frequency of defecation and continence, and the possibility of pouchitis. It also requires more than one operation to perform the definitive procedure. However, it has become the most widely accepted procedure, because the functional results are acceptable and the patient's quality of life is good, without an ileostomy. There are several chapters on ileoanal pouches.

Ileorectal Anastomosis

Indications

Ileorectal anastomosis is an operation that should be considered under certain conditions. The most common indication is for the patient who has had a subtotal colectomy for toxic colitis, in whom the pathologist is not able to distinguish the features of mucosal UC or Crohn's disease (CD) (*indeterminate colitis*). A high percentage of patients who are operated on urgently for toxic colitis have had the disease for less than 3 months. There is no long history with previous biopsies or any pattern on which to come to any firm conclusion on the clinical course of the disease.

Performing an IPAA on large or obese patients can be technically demanding or impossible, from the standpoint of either doing the anastomosis or constructing the proximal ileostomy. Weight reduction is the first choice under these circumstances, but in more than a few instances, this is not achieved, for a host of reasons, and

surgery is necessary. Ileorectal anastomosis should be considered under these circumstances.

Another indication is for patients who have a cancer arising in the colitis with metastases. An ileorectal anastomosis is a good palliative procedure, in that it removes the colon with the colitis and the colonic cancer. It allows normal bowel function without an ostomy.

Suitability for Ileorectal Anastomosis

Not all patients are suitable candidates for an ileorectal anastomosis. The foremost consideration for suitability is the distensibility of the rectum. If the rectum is distensible, it will probably be usable for an ileorectal anastomosis and provide acceptable bowel function. If the rectum is fibrotic, narrow, and rigid and has no compliance, it is unable to store contents, so that it acts as a conduit giving unacceptable function.

The appearance of the mucosa of an out-of-circuit rectum bears no relation to how it will function. This is particularly so if examination is performed at the time of or soon after a subtotal colectomy for acute colitis, when the mucosa is still inflamed, not having had time to heal. On the other hand, when the bowel has been excluded for some time, diversion colitis may be evident. The mucosa is hyperemic and bleeds on contact just as in mucosal UC. Biopsies taken from out-of-circuit bowel are completely unreliable and cannot be used as a basis for making a diagnosis. Thus, the most important factor is the ability of the rectum to distend and act as a reservoir.

Manometric studies can be performed to measure compliance, but a simple digital examination to feel the rectum and assess its walls is more effective. After a subtotal colectomy for an exacerbation, the patient's health is restored and then the rectum heals. This phenomenon is most obvious in patients who have short-term disease. This is another reason to condemn performing a proctocolectomy in acute colitis. Even if the disease is shown to be CD and the rectum is usable, ileorectal anastomosis is an option if IPAA is not. After a subtotal colectomy, if the pathology is UC and the rectum is not usable, the choice of operation in most patients is a proctectomy and IPAA. If the rectum is usable in young patients, an IPAA reduces or eliminates the long-term risk of developing cancer in the rectum, even though this risk is small. In older patients whose sphincter may not be as functional, an ileorectal anastomosis may be more acceptable. Anal manometry should be performed whenever there is a question about sphincter function.

After an ileorectal anastomosis there is no ileostomy, and because there has been no pelvic dissection, there is no risk of autonomic nerve damage that would compromise bladder or sex function. There is a normal route of evacuation. This is particularly important in children and adolescents during their physical and emotional developmental years. Bowel function is adequate. There is no incontinence day or night, and the operative procedure is technically uncomplicated.

Anastomosis

The anastomosis is performed between the distal ileum, just proximal to the ileocecal valve, and the upper rectum (not distal sigmoid colon), 12 cm from the anal margin. The anastomosis may be hand-sewn or stapled. If the rectum is too inflamed to use staples or to function immediately, the anastomosis may be hand-sewn or a proximal loop ileostomy may be constructed. In many cases, the ileorectal anastomosis is a second-stage procedure following a subtotal colectomy, with the ileorectal anastomosis being performed after the rectum has healed. Most patients have a satisfactory result. In the event that the rectum does not function satisfactorily, a proctectomy can be performed with all of the options still available, depending on the evolution of the disease and the pathologic interpretation of the biopsies at the time. The only contraindication to an ileorectal anastomosis is a strictured, rigid rectum that acts as a conduit with no storage capacity, or if there is destruction of the anus, which could leave the patient incontinent.

Outcome

The disadvantages of an ileorectal anastomosis are somewhat theoretic rather than practical. The mucosa remains, which may develop proctitis in the same way the exacerbations and remissions occur when the entire colon is present. Medications may be necessary to induce or maintain remission. Most patients have four to five bowel movements a day. The number of bowel movements tolerated varies with individuals. This situation is similar to that following a pelvic pouch operation. The patient's tolerance relates to the number of bowel movements before the surgery and how strong the desire is to avoid an ileostomy, for example, for a patient who has been ill for a long time and having possibly 15 bowel movements per day with urgency, having the number reduced to four or five bowel movements per day may be acceptable. On the other hand, if the procedure is being done for cancer prophylaxis when bowel function may be normal, the increase to four or five bowel movements per day may not be accepted as readily. The number of bowel movements with an ileorectal anastomosis compares favorably with the numbers associated with an IPAA.

Operative Results

Questions regarding ileorectal anastomosis relate to the safety of the operation, the failure rate, how good the functional results are, and the cancer risks. Between 1965 and 1985, 145 patients (85 male, 60 female), with a mean age of 30.4 years (range, 9 to 72 yr) had an ileorectal anastomosis performed at The Cleveland Clinic. This was 26 percent of 555 patients who had surgery for UC in that time period. The mean duration of colitis before the ileorectal anastomosis was 11 years (7 to 14 years). At follow-up, which was 6 to 22 years, (mean, 8.2 yr), 114 (79%) had a functioning ileorectal anastomosis. Eighteen had had a proctectomy, four remained defunctionalized, and two had died postoperatively of pulmonary embolus. There was no in-hospital mortality. There were nine deaths, three from cancer of the colon present at the time of ileorectal anastomosis, and six of unrelated causes. Complications of surgery included two patients who had a postoperative pulmonary embolus, five who developed an abscess, three who developed a small bowel obstruction, and three who developed anastomotic leaks. All of the patients who developed anastomotic leaks were on steroids. Two required a diverting loop ileostomy for 3 months, and one of the leaks closed as a result of nonoperative treatment.

Cancer Risk

The development of carcinoma is a risk in UC. This is a small risk, but it cannot be ignored. In the Cleveland series, five patients (3%) developed cancer of the rectum. One patient was treated with local fulguration, because of the patient's age and general medical condition. She lived another 5 years before dying of another condition without evidence of cancer of the rectum. Three patients had a proctectomy. Two patients had a Dukes' A cancer (one found incidentally after proctectomy for proctitis). Another had disseminated disease and died after 14 months. The fifth patient was found to have dysplasia, refused surgery, developed cancer and refused surgery, and died of the carcinoma. This patient's ileorectal anastomosis had been present for 14 years. Importantly, most of the follow-up on these patients was before the benefit of the knowledge of dysplasia was available. Surveillance and annual biopsies should further reduce the risks. In the group, the mean duration of colitis before the diagnosis of carcinoma was 20 years, with a wide range of 13 to 30 years. After removal of the colon, the incidence of carcinoma is less than the incidence of carcinoma in the entire colon and rectum. The presumption is that this is because of the smaller area of mucosa at risk.

Quality of Life

In the patients' own assessment of their quality of life, 92 patients with a functioning ileorectal anastomosis were assessed. Eighty-four percent assessed themselves as being greatly improved, 15.2 percent as improved but not 100 percent, one patient felt unchanged, and two considered that they were worse off than before the ileorectal anastomosis. At follow-up, patients had an average of 4.3 bowel movements per day (range, 1 to 10). Five percent had nocturnal bowel movements. Fifty-five percent of patients were having between one to three bowel movements in 24 hours, and 85 percent had one to six bowel movements in 24 hours. There was no incontinence reported, and no dietary restrictions were prescribed. Twenty-three percent were taking antidiarrheal medication either intermittently or regularly. Thirty-three percent were taking sulfasalazine, and 8 percent were taking steroids.

Summary

With the proper selection of patients, the results of ileorectal anastomosis can be satisfactory. The procedure is not as technically complicated as some other operations for UC. It is a safe operation with minimal mortality and morbidity and, importantly, does not prevent other operations from being performed should the operation not work out as well as anticipated. The functional results are as good as or better than those with an IPAA or an ileostomy, and the risk of cancer in the retained rectum is small. Ileorectal anastomosis should be considered for patients who are not suitable for an IPAA or if there is a possibility of Crohn's disease.

Supplemental Reading

Grundfest SF, Fazio VW, Weiss RA, et al. The risk of cancer following colectomy and ileorectal anastomosis for extensive mucosal ulcerative colitis. Ann Surg 1981;193:9–14.

Jagelman DG, Lewis CB, Rowe-Jones DC. Ileorectal anastomosis. Appreciation by patients. BMJ 1969;1:756–67.

Lavery IC, Michener WM, Jagelman DG. Ileorectal anastomosis for inflammatory bowel disease in children and adolescents. Surg Gynecol Obstet 1983;157:553–6.

Longo WE, Oakley JR, Lavery IC, et al. Outcome of ileorectal anastomosis for Crohn's colitis. Dis Colon Rectum 1992;35:1066–71.

Oakley JR, Jagelman DG, Fazio VW, et al. Complications and quality of life after ileorectal anastomosis for ulcerative colitis. Am J Surg 1985;148:23–8.

Pastore RL, Wolff BG, Hodge D. Total abdominal colectomy and ileorectal anastomosis for inflammatory bowel disease. Dis Colon Rectum 1997;40:1455–64.

Soravia C, O'Connor BI, Berk T, et al. Functional outcome of conversion of ileorectal anastomosis to ileal pouch-anal anastomosis in patients with familial adenomatous polyposis and ulcerative colitis. Dis Colon Rectum 1999;42:903–8.

Thomas DM, Filipe MI, Smedley FH. Dysplasia and carcinoma in the rectal stump of total colitics who have undergone colectomy and ileorectal anastomosis. Histopathology 1989;14:289–98.

CHAPTER 51

Indeterminate Colitis: Surgical Approaches

Ian Lindsey, MBBS, FRACS, Bryan F. Warren, MB, ChB, MRCPath, and Neil J. McC. Mortensen, MD, FRCS

Although the medical treatment for ulcerative colitis (UC) and Crohn's disease (CD) is quite similar, restorative proctocolectomy (or ileal pouch-anal anastomosis), now considered the gold standard surgical treatment for UC, usually is contraindicated in known cases of CD due to the high probability of a poor outcome. Some have recently suggested that restorative proctocolectomy may be justified in carefully selected patients with CD, those without anoperineal or small bowel disease, as the results of surgery do not seem to be any worse than those for other restorative operations in CD. However, patients in this series may well have had indeterminate colitis, and it is generally agreed that ideally the surgeon should have a clear diagnosis of UC before undertaking restorative proctocolectomy. Originally, the term "indeterminate colitis" was coined by Price based on examination of colectomy specimens. It has fallen into common use now when a decision cannot be made on the basis of colonscopy and biopsy appearances.

Preoperative Strategies

Q. *What do you do if your pathologist cannot commit to a preoperative diagnosis?*

A. **Obtain optimum clinical, radiologic, and pathologic information.**

It is important to remember that a histology report of "indeterminate colitis" from colonoscopic biopsies reflects the presence of features of both UC and CD histologically, and the pathologist is unable to commit to either diagnosis. At this point, one must place such a report in its proper context, taking into account all features of inflammatory bowel disease including clinical and radiologic evidence. A lack of rectal biopsies is one reason pathologists will invoke an indeterminate diagnosis. A careful review of further discriminating features after initial pathologic uncertainty will allow many cases of indeterminate colitis to be reclassified as either UC or CD with reasonable confidence. It is important to be aware of any clinical features that are suspicious for CD that, in the setting of indeterminate colitis, will predict a poor outcome for restorative proctocolectomy compared to those without such features. The patient with a short history presents a particular difficulty.

When considering clinical features of CD, the most important factors include the absence of rectal disease and the presence of small bowel or anal disease. A past history of perianal fistula or fissure was found in a substantial proportion of patients who eventually turned out to have CD. However, anal disease does not necessarily mean CD. In our experience, around 10 percent of patients with UC coming to restorative proctocolectomy have an anal lesion—often a low fistula or a fissure. Nevertheless, a high fistula, rectovaginal fistula, or anal ulcer is more suspicious for CD.* There must be a thorough examination of the patient, including a search for any extra-intestinal manifestations.

The small and large bowel needs to be examined carefully to exclude any features of CD. If the pathologist is not happy with the adequacy of the specimens received, then colonoscopic and rectal biopsies should be repeated. Information from all other possible sources should be strenuously and thoroughly pursued, including biopsy and surgical specimens for pathologic review as well as clinical, endoscopic, and radiologic information from other doctors or hospitals. If the surgeon is uncertain about the colonoscopy, he should repeat the procedure for himself. Intubation of the terminal ileum at colonoscopy and biopsy is mandatory. Usually, the small bowel will have been imaged at some stage, but if not or if not for some time, then an up-to-date small bowel enema provides important information.

Q. *What if you still do not have a firm preoperative diagnosis of ulcerative colitis?*

A. **Stage the surgery, delay reconstruction, and biopsy the rectal stump.**

Where there is no particular doubt about the diagnosis, the surgeon and the pathologist should conduct a combined intraoperative macroscopic "confirmation" of the preoperative diagnosis of UC in the opened colectomy specimen prior to proctectomy. However, if there is any preoperative suspicion of CD, regardless of what the biopsies have shown, then it is unwise to proceed directly

---

* Editor's Note: Other authors are more dogmatic about all perianal fistulae being a harbinger of CD. (TMB)

to restorative proctocolectomy and the patient should undergo three-stage surgery. A colectomy with ileostomy is performed, giving the pathologist a better opportunity to make an accurate diagnosis. Restorative proctocolectomy still may be performed later, or if CD seems more likely or is confirmed, then completion proctectomy with ileostomy or ileorectal anastomosis, if the rectum is spared, may be contemplated. There is little evidence as to whether three-stage surgery reduces the incidence of a false-positive diagnosis of UC or whether surgical morbidity or pouch function is adversely affected. Some surgeons recommend routine staging of surgery in order to be as sure as possible of the diagnosis.

However, the situation may not become any clearer after colectomy. This is the case particularly when emergency colectomy has been performed for fulminant colitis. The severity of the pathologic changes frequently obscures any discriminating histologic features of either of the two diseases. A sizeable proportion of CD patients undergoing inadvertent restorative proctocolectomy previously have undergone emergency colectomy for fulminant colitis.

Once the colectomy has been performed, the rectal stump may yield further useful information. In general terms, the defunctioned rectum in UC causes worsening of the proctitis, as opposed to CD where the disease activity is more quiescent when the fecal stream is diverted. Multiple biopsies of the rectum should be undertaken. It is important to be aware that the diverted UC rectum can develop histologic features of CD, and that a previously spared rectum in CD may become inflamed, underlining the importance of the preexisting mucosal state.

Occasionally, the surgery cannot be staged preferentially. For example, the patient may wish to avoid a stoma at all costs. If there is diagnostic doubt, careful intraoperative macroscopic inspection of the opened colon prior to proctectomy with or without frozen section may be valuable. Pathologists usually decry the use of frozen section in the assessment of inflammatory bowel disease. We would maintain, however, that there is a limited but important role for frozen section in selected circumstances.

In circumstances when the macroscopic appearances of the opened colon lead to diagnostic doubt, we would recommend frozen section from:

- *The largest lymph node.* The presence of well-formed granulomas would support a diagnosis of CD. Poorly formed granulomas are not enough.
- *A transmural section of the most severely affected area.* This will assess the presence and pattern of transmural inflammation. Characteristically in CD, there are multiple discrete lymphoid aggregates throughout the full thickness of the bowel wall, particularly on the external border of the muscularis propria. In fulminant UC, inflammation may be seen deep to the mucosa, but this is a diffuse inflammatory cell infiltrate at the sites of severe ulceration and discrete lymphoid aggregates are not seen here.
- *Macroscopically normal bowel between focal lesions.* this is to look for continuity of mucosal disease. This is often the most useful sample. The only recognized and acceptable "skip" lesions in UC are in the appendix and the cecal patch lesion.

Minor changes should be ignored and the pathologist should be prepared to give one of three firm answers: "definite ulcerative colitis," "definite Crohn's disease," or "I do not know." Given that the appearances of the defunctionalized rectum in UC may be confused with CD, there is no role for frozen section of a diverted proctectomy specimen to determine whether a pouch should or should not be constructed. In tertiary colorectal referral centers, there is a high proportion of one- and two-stage pouch procedures. In this setting, the careful intraoperative macroscopic evaluation with or without frozen section becomes more important.

Q. What do you do if you are still left with a diagnosis of "indeterminate colitis?"

A. Talk to the patient and offer them restorative proctocolectomy.

Sometimes after seeking and reviewing all available information, the diagnosis still is not clear-cut, leaving a small proportion of patients overall (reported as 2 to 8% in series from major centers) with the label "indeterminate colitis." It is essential to grasp what the natural history of this group is. The majority of such cases behave like UC, and the risk of manifesting as CD is small (6 to 11%).

It must be remembered that a diagnosis of CD generally is considered a contraindication to restorative proctocolectomy. The risk of recurrent CD in the pouch, with loss of distensibility and function, the risk of abscess formation and fistulization, and the risk of subsequent pouch excision and short bowel syndrome, has been documented from experience with both the Kock pouch and ileal pouch.

What happens when restorative proctocolectomy is performed for indeterminate colitis? It appears that operative morbidity and pouchitis are similar to those in UC. Failure of the pouch (diversion or excision) is about twice as likely, according to the Mayo series, relating to the manifestation of CD in the anus or small bowel in a minority of these patients. The patients who retain their pouches have similar function to those with UC. This is generally supported in the literature, although one series from the Lahey Clinic has suggested an increased risk of perineal complications in indeterminate colitis pouches. This may reflect differences in defining indeterminate colitis histologically.

What happens when a pouch is made inadvertently for CD? The Cleveland Clinic experience has shown that

Management Algorithm

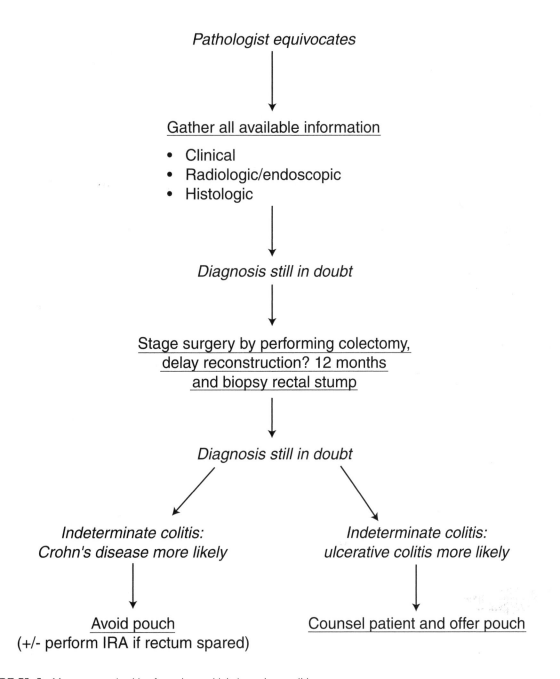

Pathologist equivocates

Gather all available information

- Clinical
- Radiologic/endoscopic
- Histologic

Diagnosis still in doubt

Stage surgery by performing colectomy,
delay reconstruction? 12 months
and biopsy rectal stump

Diagnosis still in doubt

*Indeterminate colitis:
Crohn's disease more likely*

*Indeterminate colitis:
ulcerative colitis more likely*

Avoid pouch
(+/- perform IRA if rectum spared)

Counsel patient and offer pouch

FIGURE 51–1. Management algorithm for patients with indeterminate colitis.

patients fall into two distinct groups. Those who demonstrated clinical features suspicious for CD preoperatively did poorly, with poor function and a very high rate of pouch excision (up to 45%). However, those who did not have features suspicious for CD managed to keep their pouches and had function similar to that of UC patients. In other words, they behave much like patients with indeterminate colitis.

Thus, patients with indeterminate colitis can be offered restorative proctocolectomy fairly confidently, knowing that as long as all of the aforementioned steps are taken, their outcome will be similar to UC patients. Even if the patient ends up having CD, the outcome usually is good if the surgeon diligently avoids restorative proctocolectomy on those indeterminate colitis patients with any clinical suspicions of CD. It is still possible that they do have CD and should be counseled accordingly. Mention should be made of the possibility of underlying CD, with an increased risk of sepsis, pouch failure, and pouch excision with permanent ileostomy.

Q. What is the role of ileorectal anastomosis for indeterminate colitis?

A. This is an option if the diagnosis is more likely to be Crohn's disease.

A diagnosis of indeterminate colitis may sway the surgeon toward performing an ileorectal anastomosis. This is made on the basis that if the patient has UC, then restorative proctocolectomy is still feasible, and if CD develops, then this is a reasonable therapeutic option. A precondition is a supple and spared (or relatively spared) rectum. The advantages are the avoidance of a stoma, subsequent biopsy of the rectum without the confounding superimposed effects of diversion on the rectal disease, and the chance to keep one's options open. The disadvantages are the risk of anastomotic leak and lack of information on the natural history of the diverted rectal disease. It is probably best employed where the surgeon feels CD is more likely and where ileorectal anastomosis is feasible due to absence of significant anorectal disease.

Intraoperative Strategies

Q. What intraoperative steps during restorative proctocolectomy will help minimize the number of pouches made for Crohn's disease?

A. Assess the small bowel properly; inspect the resection specimen and collaborate with your pathologist.

Intraoperative macroscopic assessment may yield supportive or diagnostic information and should be done routinely during restorative proctocolectomy. The small bowel as well as the stomach and duodenum should be examined thoroughly. Features of fat-wrapping and serosal exudates with telangiectasia and bowel wall thickening with induration should be looked and felt for along the length of the small bowel, but particularly in the terminal ileum.

The colon should be opened in the operating room after resection and cleaned and inspected by the surgeon. At our institution, we will routinely examine the specimen together with our pathologist who attends at this point—before the rectal dissection is undertaken prior to pouch construction. This is done to minimize the risks of inadvertently constructing a pouch for CD. The pattern and distribution of the inflammatory changes are noted. Diffuse mucosal disease and left-sided predominance with rectal involvement support a diagnosis of UC.

Fissuring, bowel wall thickening, and transmural inflammation are changes strongly favoring CD. It must be remembered that discontinuous disease in the cecum or appendix and relative rectal sparing may be seen in genuine cases of UC. Any clearly atypical features occasionally found on opening the clean specimen will allow deferment of pouch construction until the colon has been thoroughly evaluated by multiple paraffin sections. These features of discontinuous disease may well become more common as UC is treated with topical agents and with newer drugs, possibly leading to a higher incidence of indeterminate colitis.

Some of the references for this chapter are included in other chapters on indeterminate colitis, on pouch pathology, and on UC and CD surgery. A complete 20-item bibliography is available at *lindseyilinz@yahoo.com*

Supplemental Reading

Davison AM, Dixon MF. The appendix as a "skip lesion" in ulcerative colitis. Histopathology 1990;16:93–5.

D'Haens G, Geboes K, Peeters M, et al. Patchy caecal inflammation associated with distal ulcerative colitis: a prospective endoscopic study. Am J Gastroenterol 1997;92:1275–9.

Edwards CM, George BD, Warren BF. Diversion colitis—new light through old windows. Histopathology 1999;34:1–5.

Grobler SP, Hosie KB, Thompson H, Keighley MRB. Outcome of restorative proctocolectomy when the diagnosis is suggestive of Crohn's disease. Gut 1993;34:1384–8.

Hyman NH, Fazio VW, Tuckson WB, Lavery IC. Consequences of ileal pouch-anal anastomosis for Crohn's colitis. Dis Colon Rectum 1991;34:653–7.

Lucarotti ME, Freeman BJC, Warren BF, Durdey P. Synchronous proctocolectomy and ileoanal pouch formation and the risk of Crohn's disease. Br J Surg 1995;82:755–6.

Panis Y, Poupard B, Nemeth J, et al. Ileal pouch/anal anastomosis for Crohn's disease. Lancet 1996;347:854–7.

Phillips RKS. Ileal pouch-anal anastomosis for Crohn's disease. Gut 1998;43:303–4.

Price AB. Overlap in the spectrum of non-specific inflammatory bowel disease—'colitis indeterminate.' J Clin Pathol 1978;31:567–77.

Sagar PM, Dozois RR, Wolff BG. Long-term results of ileal pouch-anal anastomosis in patients with Crohn's disease. Dis Colon Rectum 1996;39:893–8.

Sheehan AL, Warren BF, Gear MWL, Shepherd NA. Fat-wrapping in Crohn's disease: pathological basis and relevance to surgical practice. Br J Surg 1992;79:955–8.

Warren BF, Shepherd NA. The role of pathology in pelvic ileal reservoir surgery. Int J Colorectal Dis 1992;7:68–75.

Warren BF, Shepherd NA, Bartolo DCC, Bradfield JWB. Pathology of the defunctioned rectum in ulcerative colitis. Gut 1993;34:514–6.

Wells AD, McMillan I, Price AB, et al. Natural history of indeterminate colitis. Br J Surg 1991;78:179–81.

CHAPTER 52

GROWTH AND NUTRITIONAL PROBLEMS IN PEDIATRIC INFLAMMATORY BOWEL DISEASE

ERNEST G. SEIDMAN, MD, FRCPC

Inflammatory bowel disease (IBD) is recognized increasingly as a common diagnosis in the pediatric age group, accounting for approximately 25 percent of all patients with IBD. Virtually unknown prior to 1940, the annual incidence of pediatric Crohn's disease (CD) has increased sixfold over the past three decades. Inflammatory Bowel Disease is seen primarily in school-aged children, with CD outnumbering ulcerative colitis (UC) by approximately 4 to 1 in our population. A small but notable fraction of IBD cases are being diagnosed during infancy. As in adults, a wide variety of gastrointestinal manifestations and extra-intestinal complications are commonly encountered in children and adolescents with CD.

In view of the added metabolic requirements for growth, children are more likely to suffer from malnutrition and micronutrient deficiencies than adults. Furthermore, growth failure is a complication unique to the pediatric age group, which occurs in up to half of the cases of CD and in about 10 percent of those with UC. Although medications often achieve symptomatic relief, malnutrition and growth failure commonly persist, particularly in pediatric CD. The goal of completely suppressing disease activity and minimizing daily steroid use is detailed in the chapter on therapy of CD in children and adolescents.[*] Growth failure may be the presenting complaint, at times in the absence of gastrointestinal symptoms. The combination of short stature and delayed puberty is often more disturbing to the patient than all other symptoms. Thus, nutritional therapy represents a very important adjunctive to effective medical or surgical management strategies for many children, particularly when their disease is accompanied by growth failure. In this chapter, the extent of nutritional problems in pediatric IBD is reviewed, along with an evidence-based review of the role of nutritional therapy in IBD.

---

[*] Editor's Note: While this chapter focuses on nutrition and its effect on growth, the chapter on medical therapy in children and adolescents with CD presents a more thorough review of the importance of suppressing disease activity as well as focusing on nutrition. Some editorial additives also appear in the text. (TMB)

Nutritional Complications of Inflammatory Bowel Disease in Pediatric Patients

Impaired nutritional status often is an underestimated, if not overlooked, complication of IBD. This is particularly true for the pediatric age group, where the additional energy costs for growth are unlikely to be met. At the time of diagnosis, the majority of patients have lost weight, due mostly to poor intake. Hypoalbuminemia and negative nitrogen balance are more often due to a protein losing enteropathy than to inadequate protein intake. Common micronutrient deficiencies include iron, zinc, calcium, vitamins D, and B_{12} and folic acid.

Although several mechanisms can potentially contribute to malnutrition and micronutrient deficiencies, the most important factor is inadequate intake. This occurs because eating may exacerbate symptoms such as abdominal pain and diarrhea. Furthermore, active disease has a potent anorexic effect, due in part to an excess production of proinflammatory cytokines such as interleukin-1β or tumor necrosis factor-α. Malabsorption, resulting from diminished absorptive surface after resection or due to bacterial overgrowth, generally is far less important than the limited caloric intake. Malnutrition generally is more common in CD with proximal intestinal involvement, likely due to the more prominent pain after food ingestion in this subgroup. Chronically deficient energy and protein intake is of particular concern in children with IBD.

Slow Growth Velocity

Nearly half of pediatric CD patients present with growth failure, characterized by an abnormally slow growth velocity. This decreased growth velocity appears 1 or 2 years before any changes in weight gain velocity and before any intestinal symptoms in a significant portion of patients. There is evidence of growth-suppressing effects of some inflammatory cytokines, perhaps independent of nutrition. To distinguish secondary growth retardation caused by chronic IBD from constitutionally delayed growth or genetically short stature, repeated measurements of height gain over time are necessary, as well as

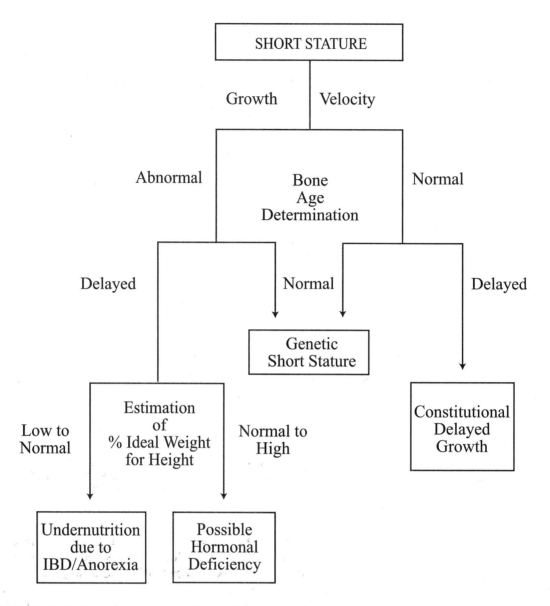

FIGURE 52–1. Evaluation of short stature in pediatric patients with IBD. Measurement of growth velocity (cm/yr) according to bone age or height age and estimation of the degree of acute malnutrition (% ideal weight for height) allow classification of patients according to etiology.

bone age determination and calculation of percent ideal weight for height. A practical approach to decipher the cause of short stature in the child with IBD is illustrated in Figure 52–1. As a rule of thumb, a height increase of less than 4 cm (1.5 inches) per year in a prepubertal patient should alert the physician. A major consequence of a prolonged reduction in growth velocity is permanent short stature, frequently seen in adults who had CD during childhood. More importantly, growth failure and delayed sexual maturation are often very debilitating symptoms for adolescent patients, potentially affecting their social interactions, school performance, and self-esteem.

Suppression of Disease Activity and Improving Nutrition

The dilemma in pediatric IBD is that adequate treatment of the inflammatory process and induction of remission with corticosteroids does not guarantee an improvement in growth. In contradistinction to nutritional therapy, steroids have potent proteolytic and osteolytic effects, resulting in a catabolic situation that inhibits bone growth. Thus, the management goal of IBD in the pediatric age group is to induce remission, minimize daily steroid use, and improve the energy-deficient and metabolic complications, allowing catch-up growth. It is

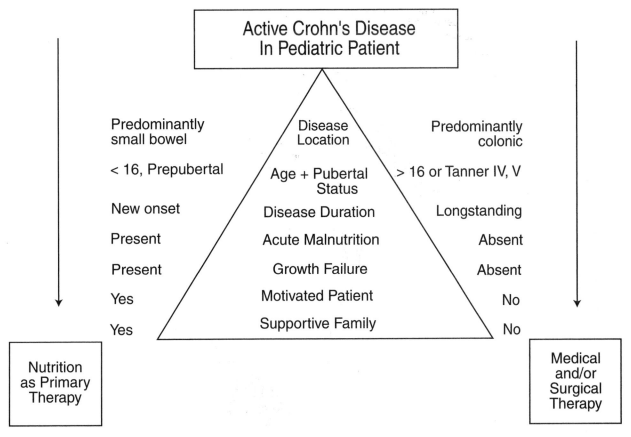

FIGURE 52–2. Factors that help determine the relative benefit of nutrition as primary therapy for active Crohn's disease in the pediatric age group.

critical for the physician to recognize that there is a limited period of time available for reversal of growth retardation in pubertal patients because of advancing bone maturation with eventual epiphyseal fusion.

Nutritional Therapy in Active Crohn's Disease

Enteral administration of elemental diets first was employed in CD in order to provide preoperative nutritional support. Several trials carried out over the last two decades have demonstrated that elemental diets effectively can induce remission in CD. In addition to controlling symptoms, inflammatory parameters and intestinal permeability improve with dietary treatment. A multicenter pediatric CD study using a semi-elemental diet showed that the remission rate of patients with new onset of disease was markedly higher (83%) compared to those with recurrently relapsing disease (50%). Enteral nutritional treatment is of therapeutic benefit in the pediatric age group to induce remission, even if its efficacy does not equal that of corticosteroids. The factors that have assisted us in the past in the decision to utilize

nutrition as primary therapy for active CD are summarized in Figure 52–2. Early immunomodulator use in pediatric patients may alter approaches in the future. There is a separate chapter on enteral nutrition and IBD.

In order to induce remission, we administered defined formula diets as the sole source of nutrition for 4 to 6 weeks, without concomitant corticosteroids. A potentially interesting but yet untested approach would be to combine diet therapy with low-dose steroids. Nutritional therapy has been used successfully in steroid-dependent and even steroid-resistant patients. Early use of immunomodulators has been shown to allow more rapid steroid tapering.

The choice of which type of formula should be administered is controversial. A multicenter trial comparing semi-elemental and polymeric formulas in a large number of pediatric patients is currently underway. In our experience, both elemental and semi-elemental diets definitely are effective in treating active CD. Although polymeric diets are less expensive, their efficacy in terms of induction of remission has not, in our opinion, been sufficiently proven to warrant their use outside of clinical trials at this time. Furthermore, despite their advantage in terms of better taste, compliance remains a problem with polymeric diets as well. This is due to the fact that defined formula diets are monotonous regardless of taste, requiring highly motivated patients. The formula to successful use of diet as primary therapy in CD is to have a medical team that is confident in this approach and supportive of the patient's and the family's needs. This involves a dedicated team that includes the attending physician, home care nurse, dietitian, and clinical psychologist. There is a separate chapter on use of elemental diets in IBD patients.

Important factors defining the potential for success using nutritional management in CD are summarized in Figure 52–2. These include disease duration and location. Nutritional therapy is, in our experience, less effective in patients with extensive colitis (whether CD or UC) or in those with upper gastrointestinal involvement. As noted above, the success rate of diets in treating longstanding CD is lower than in those newly diagnosed. Complications such as fistulae or abscesses may improve transiently with liquid formula diets. However, resolution of the problem is not often achieved, as fistulae generally reopen after a normal diet is reintroduced.

Diet for the Treatment of Growth Failure and Maintenance of Remission

Growth failure due to CD is the best-established indication for nutritional therapy. Using enteral diets on a cyclical basis, we first reported that height velocity increased to the point of achieving catch-up growth. Steroids, although more efficient in inducing remission, tend to impair linear growth. We and others have observed that the intermittent use of defined formulas as the sole source of nutrition for 1 of every 4 months on a cyclical basis decreased steroid requirements and reduced relapse rates, in addition to reversing growth failure.

The endocrine status in pediatric IBD patients is characterized by normal growth hormone secretion and somewhat low serum levels of insulin-like growth factor-I, due to impaired nutritional status. However, growth hormone, thyroxin, and cortisol status should be assessed in the rare cases that do not achieve improved growth despite disease activity suppression, adequate caloric intake, and weight gain.

Fish Oil Supplementation

A randomized and controlled trial in adults demonstrated that fish oil supplementation significantly reduced the relapse rate in patients considered to be at high risk for disease exacerbation (28% vs 69% for the fish oil-treated group vs. the placebo-treated controls, respectively; $p < .001$). Marine oils rich in omega-3 fatty acids act by competing in the substrate pool for the lipoxygenase pathway, reducing the production of pro-inflammatory eicosanoids such as leukotriene B4, while favoring the elaboration of leukotriene B5, a comparatively weak eicosanoid. The same approach, utilizing fish oil supplements, has been utilized successfully in UC. Controlled trials using fish oil in pediatric patients in order to maintain remission are lacking, as are any effects on growth.

Practical Issues on the Use of Nutritional Therapy

Diet therapy generally is instituted in one of three manners.[†] If the intent is to control disease activity, the formula (usually elemental or semi-elemental) is administered to the exclusion of other foods, for a 4- to 6-week period. The amount administered, either orally, via tube feeding, or both, is in the range of 50 to 70 kcal/kg ideal body weight per day. The volume can be increased to ensure satiety. Aside from the formula, patients are permitted some carbohydrates in the form of clear fluids and hard candies. Generally, formula not taken orally during the daytime is administered via nasogastric tube feeding, by constant infusion overnight. This program tends to interfere least with the child's daytime activities (school, social, etc.).

If, on the other hand, the primary indication is to correct growth velocity in the face of quiescent disease, the diet therapy (usually polymeric) can be administered nocturnally as a supplement to the patient's daytime intake. This supplementation is continued for at least 3 months per year, either continuously (1 month at a time) or intermittently (3 to 5 nights per week). Patients who do not tolerate nasogastric tube insertion may be candidates for gastrostomy tube placement.

Finally, if nutrition is to be employed to prevent relapses and enhance growth, the diet is administered to the exclusion of other food, as above, on an intermittent basis. Typically, the patient receives an elemental or semi-elemental formula for 4 weeks every 4-month period, for a total of three cycles over the course of a year.

The major advantage of nutritional management in CD is the avoidance of drug-related side effects. Disadvantages include low acceptability due to taste and the relatively high cost of diet therapy compared to most medications. A potential problem is early relapse (60 to 70%) within a year after the diet is stopped. As noted above, in order to maintain remission, we developed and validated a successful nutritional approach using elemental diets as sole-source nutrition on an intermittent basis.

Despite problems that potentially limit compliance, such as the questionable palatability and the monotony of these liquid diets, most adolescent patients are highly motivated and accept tube feedings. When administered

---

[2] Editor's Note: Increasing use of immunomodulator therapy including Remicade® (Centocor, Malvern, Pennsylvania), and of budesonide, a corticosteroid with less growth suppression will probably alter the practices of some pediatric gastroenterologists. (TMB)

nocturnally, adequate caloric intake is achieved while maintaining normal daily life. The advent of flavor packets has substantially decreased reliance on tube feedings in IBD, with significantly greater acceptance of these formulae taken orally.

Bone Mineral Density in Inflammatory Bowel Disease

As in adults, reduced bone mineral density (Z-score < −2) has been reported in about 30 percent of children and adolescents with IBD. As noted above, pediatric patients frequently have growth failure accompanied by significantly delayed bone age. In such cases, bone mineral density should be assessed on the basis of bone age, rather than chronological age. Bone density should be measured by dual energy x-ray absorptiometry (DEXA) routinely in children and adolescents with CD. Although patients with UC are at a lower risk of osteopenia, malnourished patients, those with growth failure, and those exposed to corticosteroids also merit screening. Appropriate use of vitamin D and calcium supplements should be ensured in all cases. In patients with persistent osteopenia, bisphosphonate therapy should be utilized. Bone mineral density measurement by DEXA should be repeated in order to document an adequate response. This topic is discussed further in other chapters on therapy in children concerning steroid use and osteopenia as well as osteoporosis. A supplemental reading list to this chapter is provided. Further information can be requested at *ernest.seidman@umontreal.ca*.

Supplemental Reading

Belli D, Seidman EG, Bouthillier L, et al. Chronic intermittent elemental diet improves growth failure in children with Crohn's disease. Gastroenterology 1988;94:603–10.

Griffiths AM, Nguyen P, Smith C, et al. Growth and clinical course of children with Crohn's disease. Gut 1993;34:939–43.

Griffiths AM, Ohlsson A, Sherman PM, et al. Meta-analysis of enteral nutrition as a primary treatment of active Crohn's disease. Gastroenterology 1995;108:1056–67.

Herzog D, Bishop N, Glorieux F, Seidman EG. Interpretation of bone mineral density values in pediatric Crohn's disease. Inflamm Bowel Dis 1998;4:261–7.

Herzog D, Bouthillier L, Deslandres C, Seidman E. The use of flavored defined formulas enhances the acceptability of nutrition as primary therapy in pediatric Crohn's disease. JPEN 2000; in press.

Hildebrand H, Karlberg J, Kristiansson B. Longitudinal growth in children and adolescents with inflammatory bowel disease. J Pediatr Gastroenterol Nutr 1994;18:65–73.

Hyams JS, Carey DE. Corticosteroids and growth. J Pediatr 1988;113:249–55.

Kanof ME, Lake AM, Bayless TM. Decreased height velocity in children and adolescents before the diagnosis of Crohn's disease. Gastroenterology 1988;95:1523–7.

Markowitz J, Grancher K, Rosa J, et al. Growth failure in pediatric inflammatory bowel disease. J Pediatr Gastroenterol Nutr 1994;18:165–73.

Papadopoulou A, Rawashdeh MO, Brown GA, et al. Remission following an elemental diet or prednisone in Crohn's disease. Acta Paediatr 1995;84:79–83.

Ruemmele F, Roy CC, Levy E, Seidman E. The role of nutrition in treating pediatric Crohn's disease in the new millennium. J Pediatr 2000;136:285–91.

Savage MO, Beattie RM, Camacho-Hubner C, et al. Growth in Crohn's disease. Acta Paediatr 1999;88(Suppl):89–92.

Seidman E, Bagnell P, Griffiths AM, et al. Canadian Collaborative Pediatric Crohn's Disease Study: growth failure and nutritional deficiencies in pediatric patients with active Crohn's disease. Gastroenterology 1991;100:249A.

Seidman EG, Jones A, Issenman R, et al. Relapse prevention/ growth enhancement in pediatric Crohn's disease: multicenter randomized controlled trial of intermittent enteral nutrition versus alternate day prednisone. J Pediatr Gastroenterol Nutr 1996;23:344A.

Seidman E. Nutritional therapy for Crohn's disease: lessons from the Ste.-Justine Hospital experience. Inflamm Bowel Dis 1997;3:49–53.

Semeao EJ, Jawad AF, Zemel BS, et al. Bone mineral density in children and young adults with Crohn's disease. Inflamm Bowel Dis 1999;5:161–6.

Whitington PF, Barnes HV, Bayless TM. Medical management of Crohn's disease in adolescence. Gastroenterology 1977; 72:1338–44.

CHAPTER 53

Dysplasia Surveillance Programs

Teresa A. Brentnall, MD

Does Surveillance Save Lives?

Several studies now show the benefits of endoscopic surveillance for neoplasia in ulcerative colitis (UC). The cancers that develop in patients under surveillance are detected at an earlier stage than those in patients who are not under surveillance. This earlier detection of cancer translates into improved 5-year survival rates–77 percent for those in surveillance versus 36 percent for those who are not. Do the benefits of surveillance outweigh the costs? Two decision analyses by Provenzale and colleagues suggest that *not only does surveillance increase life expectancy, but that it ultimately costs less than no surveillance.*[*]

The Dilemmas

The current standard of practice in all patients with extensive UC of 8 or more years duration is to perform life-long colonoscopic biopsy surveillance. Yet the optimal protocol for this surveillance has not been established. The lack of consensus on *which* patients warrant frequent colonoscopy is compounded by the divergent opinions regarding *what* constitutes adequate colonoscopic surveillance. A major problem in surveillance is the large surface area of the colon, which ranges from 0.5 to 1.0 square meters. Dysplasia may arise anywhere within this large area and frequently produces no endoscopically visible lesion.

Surveillance Protocol (Figure 53–1)

As indicated above, the current standard of practice is to perform life-long annual or biennial colonoscopic biopsy surveillance in patients with extensive colitis of 8 or more years' duration. Many physicians perform colonoscopy annually, taking an average of three to eight biopsies. The current guidelines from the World Health Organization (WHO) recommend annual to biennial colonoscopy with unspecified numbers of biopsies, taken from normal-appearing mucosa at 10- to12-cm intervals throughout the colon and extra biopsies taken from areas of mucosal irregularity. The American Gastroenterologic Association (AGA) has suggested a similar guideline; however, neither of these recommendations is based on a scientific data analysis. Our prospective studies have shown that in order to detect focal dysplasia in UC with 90 percent confidence, *33 colonoscopic biopsies must be examined histologically.* The acquisition of this many biopsies is both time and cost intensive; *however, once the patient's histologic diagnosis is established with confidence, it may be possible to extend the surveillance intervals.*

Our current protocol is to obtain biopsies at four quadrants every 10 cm from the cecum through the descending colon and at 5-cm intervals from the rectosigmoid, where cancer is most common. This provides an average of 44 biopsies per procedure. The biopsies are taken with jumbo biopsy forceps to provide a sample that is large enough to orient correctly and to minimize crush artifact.

The biopsies are oriented (straightened out from the forceps cup) and mounted flat on monofilament mesh prior to fixation. Four biopsies from each level are placed in a single fixative bottle (Hollande's gives the best nuclear detail) and labeled as to the location in the colon. After fixation, the four biopsies from each level are placed in a single paraffin block, serially sectioned and interpreted by an experienced gastrointestinal (GI) pathologist.

Patients who have mucosal irregularities, bumps, or polyps have the lesion sampled and, when possible, removed in its entirety for histologic evaluation. Samples from visible lesions are taken in addition to the usual number of surveillance biopsies and are placed in a separately labeled bottle of fixative. The location of the lesion is noted and described in the colonoscopy report.

The Importance of Interpretation by an Experienced Pathologist

The diagnosis of dysplasia in inflammatory bowel disease (IBD) is a subjective interpretation and requires an experienced pathologist for optimum accuracy. Because major clinical decisions rest on the histologic diagnosis, it is valuable to have the colonic biopsies evaluated by a pathologist who has expertise in the diagnosis of IBD and the associated neoplastic transformation. This caution is especially true when the diagnosis of dysplasia is made. For example, we recommend colectomy for high-grade

---

[*] Editor's Note: This chapter and the next both focus on surveillance strategies. Both authors have put a lot of thought into their recommendations, which are similar in some aspects but somewhat different in what they advise on low-grade dysplasia. This is such an important topic that we wanted several viewpoints. (TMB)

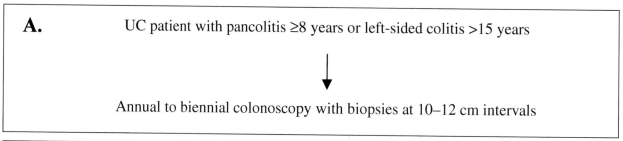

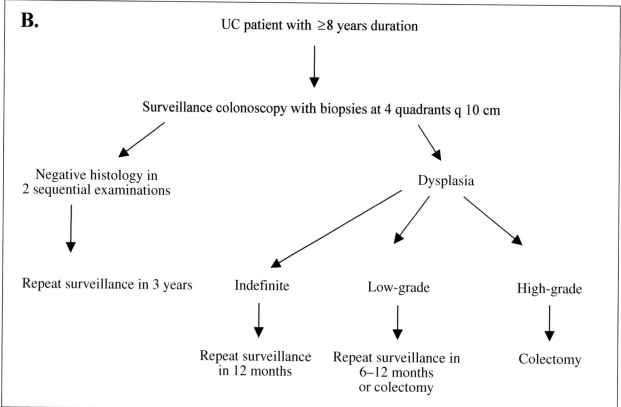

FIGURE 53–1. Surveillance strategies for IBD. Strategy A requires annual to biennial colonoscopy for the lifetime of the patient; Strategy B stratifies patients according to neoplastic risk.

dysplasia but usually not for low-grade dysplasia. Thus, unless the pathologist is experienced in the interpretation of dysplasia, a second opinion should be obtained on biopsies that will change clinical management.

Surveillance Intervals

According to WHO guidelines, if biopsies are classified as negative or indefinite for dysplasia, then surveillance colonoscopy should be repeated every 1 to 2 years. The current AGA guidelines suggest annual colonoscopy for IBD patients. *If the physician is taking only 8 to 10 biopsies per procedure, I think this is sage advice.* If, however, you perform a more thorough sampling of the colon, with more than 33 biopsies per procedure, the clinician and the patient can have confidence that dysplasia is less likely to have been missed. Our current recommendations are outlined in Table 53–1 and are based on the histologic

findings at colonoscopy, with the intervals longer for patients who are negative for dysplasia in two sequential examinations that are 1 to 2 years apart. This approach has several advantages: it costs less and it focuses the physician's time and effort on those patients who are most likely to progress to cancer.[†]

High-Risk Patients

Patients with UC and Crohn's colitis have an increased risk of colorectal cancer. Two chief factors determine which patients are at increased risk: disease *duration* of

---

[†] Editor's Note: We have tended to take "indefinite for dysplasia" somewhat more seriously and tend to repeat surveillance colonoscopy in 6 months, especially if the "indefinite" biopsy came from a mass or strictures. These "schedules" assume perfect compliance, foolproof scheduling, and an adequate cleansing preparation. Oh, that life was that perfect. (TMB)

TABLE 53–1. Time Intervals Between Surveillance Colonoscopies Assuming Adequate Sampling Has Been Achieved (see text)

Histology	Interval Between Colonoscopies
Negative for dysplasia × 2	3 years
Indefinite for dysplasia	1 year
Low-grade dysplasia	6–12 months or colectomy
High-grade dysplasia	Colectomy; for those who refuse colectomy then colonoscopy every 3–6 months

more than 8 years and disease *extent* proximal to the sigmoid colon. Primary sclerosing cholangitis (PSC) has been identified as a third factor; the risk of neoplasia approaches 50 percent after 25 years duration of UC in these patients. Patients with PSC have an 80 to 90 percent probability of having UC but *are often asymptomatic*, and the duration of UC may be difficult to determine. Therefore, PSC patients who have not been diagnosed with UC should have periodic flexible sigmoidoscopy with 5 to 10 biopsies to determine whether UC has developed. Patients with PSC found to have UC then should undergo surveillance colonoscopy as soon as they are diagnosed, rather than waiting for the usual 8-year duration prior to initiating surveillance. The reasons for this are because (1) duration of UC cannot be accurately determined in patients who may be asymptomatic and (2) these patients have the highest risk of developing neoplasia. The PSC patients with UC should have surveillance performed annually or biennially.

Management of Low-Grade Dysplasia

The optimal management of UC patients with low-grade dysplasia (LGD) is controversial. Some experts recommend colectomy, because a high probability of finding an occult cancer in the colectomy specimen from these patients has been reported. However, the retrospective studies upon which these recommendations are based used a variable number of biopsies (average 13 to 30 biopsies per 100 cm colon) obtained at inconsistent colonoscopic intervals varying from 1 month to 5 years. Thus, the finding of occult cancers in these studies is not surprising because insufficient numbers of biopsies were taken to make the correct histologic diagnosis.

While colectomy may be the least costly method for managing patients with LGD, many patients are reluctant to undergo this surgery. Patients who have had UC for 20 years, which is the average duration of disease prior to the development of dysplasia, often have minimal or no symptoms, and it can be difficult to convince them that a colectomy will benefit them. An informed discussion of the risks and benefits of colectomy for LGD requires an understanding of its natural history. Important questions about the biology of LGD include *Do all patients with*

LGD develop cancer? If so, over what time frame? Does LGD ever regress? Is high-grade dysplasia always an intermediate step between LGD and cancer? Can it be detected with confidence? Are there patient characteristics that predict who will progress to cancer?

We performed a prospective evaluation of the natural history of LGD in 18 patients with UC. The preliminary results suggest that only one-third of these patients with LGD will progress in the short term, and those who do progress usually do so within 18 months of the diagnosis of LGD. With our protocol of four quadrant biopsies every 10 cm and follow-up intervals occurring every 6 to 12 months, none of the 18 LGD patients developed cancer while under surveillance. Six patients who progressed in the study developed HGD and underwent colectomy; none had an unsuspected carcinoma in their colectomy specimen. Characteristics of those who were more likely to progress to HGD included (1) patients with three or more biopsies with LGD per colonoscopy and (2) *younger* patients. Two-thirds of LGD patients did not progress, but rather continue to have LGD or downgraded to indefinite or negative for dysplasia during an average follow-up of 3 years. Because of these data, we do not routinely recommend colectomy for UC patients with LGD, but rather discuss the risks and benefits of colectomy versus colonoscopic surveillance. Patients who choose surveillance should be followed endoscopically every 6 to 12 months for a lifetime or until multiple sites of LGD or a single site of HGD develops; then colectomy is strongly advised. If the patient chooses surveillance, he or she must agree (preferably in writing) to return for colonoscopy at intervals assigned by the GI physician. The endoscopist needs to take an adequate number of biopsies so that HGD or cancer will be detected. The protocol taking four quadrant biopsies every 10 cm from the cecum to the sigmoid and then every 5 cm thereafter until the rectum is recommended. Most UC patients have dysplasia located in the rectosigmoid, and it is helpful to note the location of the dysplasia in the chart (sigmoid, splenic flexure, etc.) so that additional biopsies can be taken from that area on follow-up colonoscopies. Biopsies revealing dysplasia or indefinite for dysplasia should be reviewed by a GI pathologist who has expertise in the diagnosis of IBD-associated neoplasia.

Management of Polyps

Part of the controversy regarding the management of polypoid lesions found in UC patients is embedded in the nomenclature associated with IBD neoplasia. Until recently, the finding of a dysplasia-associated lesion or mass (DALM) in the colon has been considered an indication for colectomy; however, the dilemma arises when trying to differentiate a sporadic adenoma (removed by polypectomy) from a DALM (requires colectomy). Many UC patients undergoing surveillance are in the age range

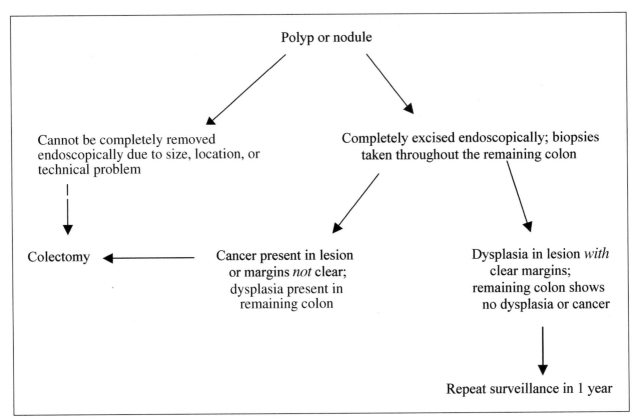

FIGURE 53–2. Management of polypoid lesions.

to have a 30 percent probability of sporadic adenoma. There are many approaches to the problem of polypoid lesions in the IBD patient. One approach is to perform *polypectomy* on lesions that arise in a field of normal colon (IBD-free) and a *colectomy* for dysplastic lesions that arise in a field of colitis. This approach is based on the concern that occult cancer is present, either in the lesion itself or elsewhere in the colon. The problem of this approach is that colectomies will be performed on many patients who would otherwise have a benign course.

An alternative approach is the performance of a complete *colonoscopic* resection of sessile and pedunculated polyps, regardless of whether they occur in IBD-affected colon or not, while at the same time taking sufficient numbers of biopsies to evaluate the remaining colon (Figure 53–2). If the biopsies of the lesion reveal invasive adenocarcinoma or if biopsies of the *flat* mucosa reveal dysplasia, then a colectomy is warranted. If histologic examination of the polyp reveals a completely resected dysplastic lesion, and if the remaining colon is dysplasia-free, then the patient should have a repeat surveillance colonoscopy in 1 year. (Two recent studies from Harvard and Mount Sinai Medical Centers used this paradigm. The studies involved 24 and 60 dysplastic polypoid lesions, respectively, from colitic sites.) A large number of the polypoid lesions were sessile. Approximately half of the patients had recurrent polyps on follow-up colonoscopy, often in the same location, which required

repeated polypectomy. However, the patients had a benign course: *no patients developed cancer and few patients developed flat dysplasia outside the polypoid lesion.*

We use this strategy for management of polypoid lesions and have found it to be successful (ie, patients have not developed cancer and have avoided colectomy), provided that the entire lesion is excised with clean margins, and the patient continues with annual surveillance.

Odds and Ends

A few important caveats are worth mentioning. Patients should have their colitis in remission prior to surveillance colonoscopy. It is difficult for the pathologist to interpret the subtleties of dysplasia when moderate to severe inflammation is present in the biopsy specimen. Therefore, every effort should be made to bring inflammation under control *prior* to surveillance colonoscopy. If the patient has active disease clearly evident at a scheduled surveillance colonoscopy, I postpone the procedure until I have it under control. If inflammation cannot be suppressed, the patient may be a candidate for a colectomy on the basis of intractable disease and an inability to monitor the mucosa histologically for dysplasia.

When in doubt about management or pathology, get a second opinion. Biopsies with dysplasia should be assessed by a pathologist with expertise in IBD. Barium enema should *not* be substituted for colonoscopy in IBD patients because dysplasia may not cause a visible defect.

Patients with ulcerative proctitis do not require surveillance because there appears to be no increased risk of colorectal cancer. Patients with Crohn's colitis have the same elevated neoplastic risk as those with UC and thus should be under similar surveillance protocols. There is a chapter on surveillance in patients with Crohn's colitis as well as another chapter on surveillance in IBD patients. References for supplemental reading have been edited to lessen duplication in these three chapters and the chapter on PSC (TMB)

Acknowledgment

I will be forever grateful to the late Dr. Rodger Haggitt for his sage advice and thoughtful comments regarding my work. The editors join Dr. Brentnall in mourning the untimely demise of Dr. Haggitt.

Supplemental Reading

Brentnall TA, Haggitt RC, Rabinovitch PS, et al. Risk and natural history of colonic neoplasia in patients with primary sclerosing cholangitis and ulcerative colitis. Gastroenterology 1996;110:331–8.

Choi PM, Nugent FW, Schoetz DJ, et al. Colonoscopic surveillance reduces mortality from colorectal cancer in ulcerative colitis. Gastroenterology 1993;105:418–24.

Ekbom A, Helmick C, Zack M, Adami H-O. Increased risk of large-bowel cancer in Crohn's disease with colonic involvement. Lancet 1990;336:357–9.

Ekbom A, Helmick C, Zack M, Adami H-O. Ulcerative colitis and colorectal cancer. A population-based study. N Engl J Med 1990;323:1228–33.

Engelsgjerd M, Farraye F, Odze R. Polyspectomy may be adequate treatment for adenoma-like dysplastic lesions in chronic ulcerative colitis. Gastroenterology 1999;117:1288–94.

Engelsgjerd M, Torres C, Farraye F, Odze D. Adenoma-like polypoid dysplasia in chronic ulcerative colitis: a follow-up study of 23 cases. Gastroenterology 1999;116:2100A.

Gurbuz AK, Giardiello FM, Bayless TM. Colorectal neoplasia in patients with ulcerative colitis and primary sclerosing cholangitis. Dis Colon Rectum 1995;38:37–41.

Nugent FW, Haggitt RC, Gilpin PA. Cancer surveillance in ulcerative colitis. Gastroenterology 1991;100:1241–8.

Provenzale D, Kowdley KV, Arora S, Wong JB. Prophylactic colectomy or surveillance for chronic ulcerative colitis? A decision analysis. Gastroenterology 1995;109:1188–96.

Provenzale D, Wong J, Onken J, Lipscomb J. Performing a cost-effectiveness analysis: surveillance of patients with ulcerative colitis. Am J Gastroenterol 1998;93:872–80.

Ransohoff DF. Colon cancer in ulcerative colitis. Gastroenterology 1988;94:1089–91.

Rubin CE, Haggitt, RC, Burmer GC, et al. DNA aneuploidy in colonic biopsies predicts future development of dysplasia in ulcerative colitis. Gastroenterology 1992;103:1611–20.

Rubin P, Friedman S, Harpas N, et al. Colonoscopic polypectomy in chronic colitis: conservative management after endoscopic resection of dysplastic polyps. Gastroenterology 1999;117:1295–300.

Winawer SJ, Fletcher RH, Miller L, et al. Colorectal cancer screening: clinical guidelines and rationale. Gastroenterology 1997;112:594–642.

Winawer SJ, St. John DJ, Bond JH, et al. Prevention of colorectal cancer: guidelines based on new data. Bull WHO 1995;73:7–10.

Woolrich AJ, DaSilva MD, Korelitz BI. Surveillance in the routine management of ulcerative colitis: the predictive value of low-grade dysplasia. Gastroenterology 1992;103:431–8.

CHAPTER 54

Cancer Prevention Strategies in Inflammatory Bowel Disease

Charles N. Bernstein, MD, FRCPC

Ulcerative colitis (UC) is associated with an increased risk of developing colorectal cancer (CRC). The risk of CRC is approximately 7 to 14 percent at 25 years of disease. Crohn's disease (CD) has a similar age-adjusted increased risk of developing CRC. The risks of developing CRC in UC correlate with increased disease duration and increased disease extent. Neoplasia (dysplasia, polyps, or cancer) usually is first evident after approximately 8 years of disease and is more likely to occur among patients with pancolitis than those with left-sided colitis. When cancer occurs in UC, it is more commonly found in the rectosigmoid. For CD, the increased risk is associated with disease duration and extent of "at risk mucosa" as well. Patients with limited cecal disease are at limited risk for developing CRC and isolated ileal disease does not appear to increase the risk of CRC.

There is some controversy as to whether patients who developed their disease at a younger age are at increased risk when followed over the same long duration as patients who developed their disease at an older age (ie, the difference between 20 years of disease in a 30 year old versus a 50 year old). Confounding this issue is that older patients may be in the age group who are at risk of developing sporadic CRC. Thus, it is simpler for the clinician to view all patients with longstanding UC or Crohn's colitis disease with equal concern. I am extrapolating much of what has been written regarding cancer surveillance and prevention in UC to CD.

Dysplasia

Neoplasia has a very different connotation than preneoplasia. Any grade of dysplasia is potentially worrisome because it can be associated with concurrent cancer, sometimes in an advanced stage.

The Inflammatory Bowel Disease Dysplasia Morphology Study Group (Riddell et al, 1983) scheme for assessing and grading dysplasia has been widely adopted. This includes low-grade, high-grade, and indefinite-for dysplasia. Low-grade dysplasia is of great concern because it can be associated with concurrent cancer at the time of surgery and has a high rate of ultimately progressing to high-grade dysplasia or frank cancer. Low-grade dysplasia was the highest grade of dysplasia identified in 50 percent of patients with CRC in UC in a series from St. Mark's

Hospital in the UK. Some studies that downplayed the premalignant significance of low-grade dysplasia have not had the study tissue reassessed by the pathologists. In other studies where this reassessment has been done much of what was originally judged as low grade was, when newly reviewed, not dysplasia at all. This led to a greater risk of progression to higher grades of neoplasia including cancer, from low grade. Although high-grade dysplasia is a more advanced neoplasm and is associated more often with cancer, low-grade dysplasia alone is sufficiently ominous to warrant colectomy.

Alteration of Cancer Risk

Chronic maintenance sulfasalazine therapy has been suggested as a factor in lower rates of CRC development in three different populations. In one UC cohort from Sweden with an increased risk for developing colorectal cancer, sulfasalazine use for at least 3 months was associated with a significantly decreased risk of developing CRC (relative risk, RR = 0.38 [95% CI, 0.20–0.69]). Significantly reduced rates of CRC also were reported in another group of patients from the UK with UC who used at least 1.2 g of 5-aminosalicylate per day compared to an age- and gender-matched population of UC patients who used less than this amount or none (RR = 0.19 [95% CI, 0.06–0.61]). Factors in this decreased risk may include less inflammation because of sulfasalazine use or simply more medical attention for those on chronic medications. Folic acid supplements have also been cited as a factor lowering cancer risk (RR = 0.72 [95% CI, 0.28 = 1.83]).

A concurrent diagnosis of primary sclerosing cholangitis (PSC) is widely agreed to be a risk factor for CRC development in IBD patients. Altering the bile salt milieu may alter repair and regeneration genes and/or factors in the colon. Since CRC in UC associated with PSC is more likely to be proximal to the splenic flexure, there may be a different cancer biology for PSC-associated CRC. As another possibility, those who are genetically programmed to develop PSC are similarly genetically programmed for their ulcerative colon mucosa to become cancerous.

Family history of sporadic CRC has been shown by groups in Rochester, Minnesota, and in Leicester, UK, to be a risk factor for cancer development among colitis patients.

Pitfalls of Dysplasia Surveillance

There are a number of pitfalls of dysplasia surveillance. First, the greatest barrier to effective surveillance is the huge area at risk, relative to the tiny fraction of tissue that is sampled to look for dysplasia. Second, there is no standard approach to the number of biopsies and the number of biopsy sites that are appropriate. Third, in 15 or 20 percent of patients, the neoplasia is diagnosed before the usual 8 years when surveillance programs are begun. Dysplasia or cancer was found in approximately 10 percent of cases who were undergoing their initial surveillance endoscopy. Dating the onset of disease may be difficult. In some patients, the diagnosis of UC is made after only 1 or 2 years of symptoms, yet the colon has the macroscopic and microscopic features of longstanding disease. This is especially true in patients with PSC or those diagnosed after age 40 (Fig. 54–1). Fourth, CRC presenting within 1 or 2 years of reportedly negative dysplasia surveillance examination has been described. Fifth, there are reports that in approximately 25 percent of patients with CRC in UC, no dysplasia could be found in the resection specimen. Finally, we are asking our pathology colleagues to differentiate dysplasia from inflammation when in fact expert pathologists have a relatively low concordance for making a diagnosis of low-grade or indefinite- for dysplasia.

Adenoma-like Masses versus Dysplasia-Associated Lesions or Masses

A major problem with dysplasia surveillance is searching for masses that may harbor dysplasia in colons that may have scattered fields of pseudopolyps. A dysplasia-associated lesion or mass (DALM) has typically mandated a colectomy because of the association with cancer in 40 percent of cases. However, all benign adenomas are by definition dysplastic lesions or masses. When they have been associated with adjacent flat dysplasia, this has boded poorly for the development of CRC. However, if the polyps are on a clear stalk and are proximal to the area of colitis or appear as adenoma-like masses (ALMs) (with characteristics of small benign lesions in non-colitis patients) within the colitis area, and a colectomy may not be necessary, then they are potentially resectable with polypectomy.

There are preliminary data on follow-up of 72 patients deemed to have ALMs with no synchronous flat dysplasia in chronic UC or Crohn's colitis from Boston and New York. All ALMs were removed and patients were followed for an average of 3 to 4 years with ongoing surveillance colonoscopies. None of these patients developed CRC. Until 5-year follow-up data are available, it is premature to assume that all presumed ALMs can be treated with polypectomy and not colectomy. A standard nomenclature that includes DALMs that are ominous and ALMs, which are not, is needed.

Benefits of Dysplasia Surveillance Colonoscopies

Being involved in cancer surveillance may provide the patient with some sense of control over an undetermined destiny. Data from the breast cancer literature suggest that younger women are more concerned about their breast cancer risk than older women. Since IBD is typically a disease of younger people who may also have heightened cancer concerns, this may lend support to their pursuing dysplasia surveillance. For many of these patients who are asymptomatic, a negative surveillance colonoscopy provides both emotional relief and satisfaction and an opportunity to be apprised of the activity status of their disease. Other less well-controlled studies have also shown improved cancer outcomes in surveilled patients compared to unmatched controls who were not studied[*]. Of patients who abandoned the dysplasia surveillance program at the St. Mark's Hospital, approximately 10 percent presented at a later time with CRC, of which 60 percent were fatal. Of the 344 patients remaining in surveillance, 5 percent developed cancers, of which only 12 percent were fatal. A recent case control study from the Karolinska Institute suggested that dysplasia surveillance will lead to the earlier diagnosis of cancers and result in less cancer-associated mortality. Based on the available literature, however, no definite improved outcome can be ascribed to the surveillance process.

A Suggested Approach

Simple clinical symptoms are rarely helpful to point to a diagnosis of colorectal cancer (Figure 54–2). As mentioned in the editor's note, if the symptoms are dissimilar enough from what would otherwise be typical UC then the cancer is likely far advanced and incurable.

Serum carcinoembryonic antigen screening is not helpful. Other potentially earlier colon mucosa markers are not likely to immediately impact on current clinical practice.

Patient Counseling

The patient with substantial Crohn's colitis or UC is informed of the increased risk of CRC. Surveillance is begun after 8 years of disease and patients with 20 years of disease are informed of the exponentially increasing

---

[*] Editor's Note: It is unlikely that a prospective control trial of surveillance versus no surveillance will be done. Our anecdotal experience was that 88 percent of 17 patients whose CRC was asymptomatic or was found as the result of a surveillance program or of prophylactic colectomy survived over 5 years. In contrast, only 18 percent of 22 patients who presented with colon cancer-related symptoms lived 5 years. These studies, although not perfectly controlled, should lead a prudent care giver to apply some type of prevention strategy, whether it be surveillance or prophylactic colectomy, to their patient with extensive colitis of over 8 years duration (Giandiello et al. Inflamm Bowel Dis 1996;2:30–5). (TMB)

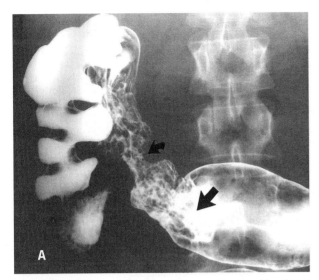

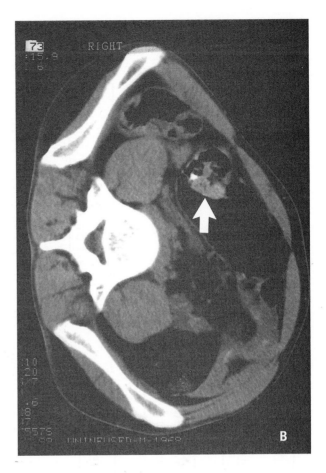

FIGURES 54–1a and 54–1b. A 30-year-old male with a 5-year history of Crohn's disease localized to his proximal transverse colon, who developed Dukes' stage B2 CRC (T4N0M0). *A*, Air contrast barium enema 5 years postdiagnosis at a time of increased clinical symptoms. The radiogram revealed a nodular pattern in the proximal transverse colon, with a segmental annular narrowing (*curved arrow*) at which a carcinoma could not be excluded. There is a large polypoid mass projecting into the lumen of the transverse colon (*arrow*). A colonoscopy revealed soft inflammatory-type pseudopolyps and a stricture through which a colonoscope could not pass. Biopsies distal to and through the stricture revealed nonspecific inflammation. *B*, Computed tomographic scan with air insufflation per anus, obtained with the patient in the left lateral position showing a broad-based lesion suggestive of a large pseudopolyp or a cancer (*arrow*). The patient then underwent segmental resection, which revealed a mucinous adenocarcinoma that extended to the serosal surface.

risk. The cancer risk should enter into the chronically active patient's algorithm for making decisions regarding surgery.

Finding a dysplastic lesion of any type in someone with chronic colitis-associated symptoms adds weight to the decision for colectomy. Because of recent reports of dysplasia or aneuploidy in ileoanal pouches and with a recent surgical trend to stapling and leaving a rectal cuff, patients should be informed of all possible outcomes of an ileoanal pouch, including the risk of neoplasia.

SURVEILLANCE TIMING

Multiple biopsies are obtained whenever a patient with Crohn's colitis or UC is colonoscopied because an occasional patient will present early in their course with neoplasia. Otherwise, dysplasia surveillance colonoscopies are begun after 8 years of disease. With two negative results from dysplasia surveillance colonoscopies within 1 year, the surveillance interval can be extended to 3 years until 20 years of disease. This suggestion is based on a low rate of dysplasia development after an initial negative surveillance endoscopy and a CRC rate of 0.5 to 1 percent/ year between 10 and 20 years of disease. At 20 years of disease, dysplasia surveillance is recommended annually.[†]

BIOPSY SITE AND NUMBER

At dysplasia surveillance colonoscopy, 4 large cup biopsies are taken from each zone. It has been estimated that 64 biopsies are required for a 95 percent probability of finding the highest grade of neoplasia in a colon containing dysplasia or cancer. However, 18 biopsies are required for a 95 percent certainty of finding either cancer or dysplasia in a patient who has cancer. Thirty biopsies is considered adequate to find at least some degree of dysplasia in 90 percent of patients. Biopsying every 10 cm is reliable only in a featureless colon, where intubation and withdrawal of the endoscope occurs without telescoping of the colon over the instrument. Biopsies are taken every 5 cm in the lower 20 cm. In patients with preserved landmarks, samples are taken at the cecum,

[†] Editor's Note: In my experience with over 50 patients with IBD and dysplasia or CRC, the frequency of surveillance needs to be individualized. Those with onset of IBD before age 20 have a shorter lag before dysplasia and cancer appear. Patients with pseudopolyps, active disease, or poor preps need to be studied more frequently. Patients who have indefinite- for dysplasia or an adenoma in an IBD area should be on a "worry list" and surveilled at least every 6 months. (TMB)

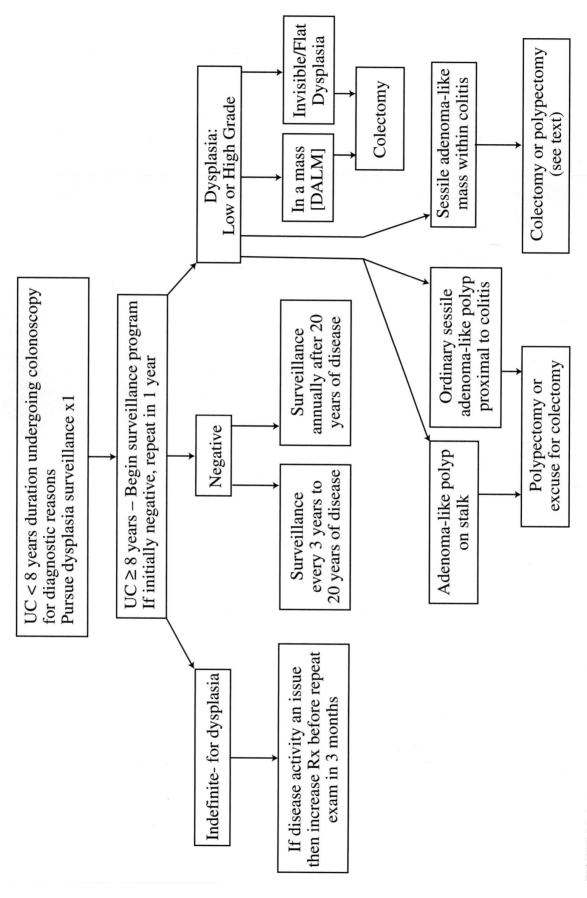

FIGURE 54–2. Approach to dysplasia surveillance colonoscopy.

ascending, proximal transverse, distal transverse, and descending colon segments. In the sigmoid and rectum, the commonest site of dysplasia, two sets of four biopsies are taken from each site. Additional biopsies are obtained from any suspicious-looking lesions anywhere in the colon. A pathologic diagnosis of low-grade dysplasia should be confirmed by another pathologist since definite low-grade and high-grade dysplasia are considered indications for colectomy in most patients.[‡]

ADENOMA-LIKE MASSES

A sessile or pedunculated polyp proximal to the extent of the colitis or a pedunculated polyp within the colitis zone is treated by polypectomy. Four quadrant biopsies are taken 1 to 2 cm away from that lesion to search for flat dysplasia. If there is no flat dysplasia, the patient is restudied in 1 year. The issue of colectomy is discussed with the patient on the basis that the mucosa is capable of neoplastic transformation. If a sessile, < 2 cm, smooth, and regular ALM within the colitis zone is removed, the choice of a colectomy versus repeat colonoscopy in 3 to 6 month, and annual surveillance thereafter is discussed with the patient. An ALM is found in a 30 year old who has many years of disease and many colonoscopies; the patient is urged to consider a colectomy. Alternatively, a 70 year old who is likely to form sporadic adenomas may choose further surveillance.

PRESENCE OF PSEUDOPOLYPS

If there are few typical pseudopolyps, then they should be biopsied. If there are multiple pseudopolyps, the endoscopist should search among them for lesions that are atypical from the rest, hard, or ulcerated, and these sites should be biopsied. These are difficult patients to follow.

Patients with UC who develop strictures identified by barium enema or colonoscopy should be considered to harbor a neoplasm until proven otherwise. The risk of malignancy is greatest if the strictures are proximal to the splenic flexure, if there is symptomatic large bowel obstruction, and if disease duration is over 20 years. There is a separate chapter on colonic strictures. If biopsies, CT scan, and endoscopic ultrasound do not convincingly exclude a cancer, or if it is impossible to traverse the stricture even with a narrower bore pediatric colonoscope, then a colectomy is recommended.

Markers as an Adjunct to Dysplasia Surveillance

Genetic testing of colon tissue, stool, or blood has not yet evolved to where cancer risk can be adequately assessed. Sialosyl TN, a mucin-associated carbohydrate, and sucrase-isomaltase, a mucosal disaccharidase, show some promise as complementary tests for defining dysplasia risk. Aneuploidy and p53 mutation may be earlier events than dysplasia and therefore their occurrence may alter one's surveillance approach. Currently, routine colonoscopy with multiple sampling for dysplasia assessment remains the single nonoperative cancer preventive approach for the typical clinician. Prophylactic colectomy is the other alternative. Preventing or removing CRC at an early stage in UC patients is as advantageous as diagnosing early CRC in the general population. The quest for early markers of neoplasia or even pre-neoplasia should continue.[§]

Supplemental Reading

Bernstein CN, Weinstein WM, Levine DS, Shanahan F. Physicians' perceptions of dysplasia and approaches to surveillance colonoscopy in ulcerative colitis. Am J Gastroenterol 1995;90:2106–14.

Choi PM, Nugent FW, Schoetz DJ, et al. Colonoscopic surveillance reduces mortality from colorectal cancer in ulcerative colitis. Gastroenterology 1993;105:418–24.

Connell WR, Lennard-Jones JE, Williams CB, et al. Factors affecting the outcome of endoscopic surveillance for cancer in ulcerative colitis. Gastroenterology 1994;107:934–44.

Engelsgjerd M, Torres C, Odze RD. Adenoma-like polypoid dysplasia in chronic ulcerative colitis: A follow-up study of 23 cases. Gastroenterology 2000; In press.

Gurbuz AK, Giardiello FM, Bayless TM. Colorectal neoplasia in patients with ulcerative colitis and primary sclerosing cholangitis. Dis Colon Rectum 1995;38:37–41.

Karlen P, Kornfeld D, Brostrom O, et al. Is colonoscopic surveillance reducing colorectal cancer mortality in ulcerative colitis? A population-based case control study. Gut 1998;42:715–20.

Lashner BA, Provencher KS, Seidner DL, et al. The effect of folic acid supplementation on the risk for cancer or dysplasia in ulcerative colitis. Gastroenterology 1997;112:29–32.

Lindberg B, Persson B, Veress B, et al. Twenty years' colonoscopic surveillance of patients with ulcerative colitis. Detection of dysplastic and malignant transformation. Scand J Gastroenterol 1996;31:1195–1204.

Riddell RH, Goldman H, Ransohoff DF, et al. Dysplasia in inflammatory bowel disease: standardized classification with provisional clinical applications. Hum Pathol 1983;14:931–68.

Rubin CE, Haggitt RC, Burmer GC, et al. DNA aneuploidy in colonic biopsies predicts future development of dysplasia in ulcerative colitis. Gastroenterology 1992;103:1611–20.

Rubin PH, Friedman S, Harpaz N, et al. Colonoscopic polypectomy in chronic colitis: are we removing adenomas or 'DALMs'? Gastroenterology 2000; In press.

Shetty K, Rybicki L, Brzezinski A, et al. The risk for cancer or dysplasia in ulcerative colitis patients with primary sclerosing cholangitis. Am J Gastroenterol 1999;94:1643–9.

[‡] Editor's Note: There are other chapters on dysplasia and cancer including surveillance in CD plus dysplasia in ileoanal pouch patients.

[§] Editor's Note: A requested chapter on this topic was not submitted by publication deadline. (TMB)

CHAPTER 55

Dysplasia Surveillance in Crohn's Disease

Peter H. Rubin, MD

Our knowledge of medicine, so black and white in internship and residency, so neatly condensed into mnemonics and lists, so suited for multiple-choice testing, has, like us, become progressively gray as we learn more. The more we study and experience patients, the more exceptions, amendments, and crossovers there are.

Cancer Risk in Crohn's Disease

A case in point is the traditional teaching that patients with chronic ulcerative colitis (UC) but not Crohn's disease (CD) are at increased risk for colorectal cancer. Many of us encountered or heard of the occasional case of colorectal cancer in CD. And ever since 1948 disturbing case reports have appeared, although no large series or prospective studies to match those in UC.

Studies from Europe, Scandinavia, and Australia, often population based, did not find an increase in cancer in CD. These studies, however, have been faulted for not dissecting the subpopulation at high risk (chronic, extensive colitis) from the larger cohort and for not taking into account the fact that much of their CD population had undergone segmental or total colonic resection because of intractable disease or stricturing.

Evidence has continued to accumulate suggesting that the risk of colorectal cancer indeed is elevated similarly in both UC and CD. Weedon and colleagues (1973) reported that colorectal cancer was more likely in Crohn's colitis than in the general population, with a standardized incidence ratio of 26.6. Gillen et al (1999), comparing the two inflammatory bowel diseases, found that the cumulative incidence of colorectal cancer in extensive, chronic UC and Crohn's colitis was similarly elevated.

Surveillance for Dysplasia and Cancer

A recent prospective study by Friedman and colleagues (1999) of colonoscopic screening and surveillance in a large outpatient cohort of 260 patients with Crohn's colitis of 8 or more years found dysplasia or cancer in 16 percent. Of the cases positive for dysplasia or cancer, 45 percent were found on screening and 55 percent on biennial surveillance exams. By life-table analysis, the probability of detecting dysplasia or cancer after a negative screening colonoscopy was 22 percent by the fourth surveillance examination. These rates are comparable to those reported in UC.

The preponderance of evidence to date, then, lends support to the prophecy by Sachar in 1983 that "when cases of ulcerative and Crohn's colitis of similar anatomical extent are followed for similar durations of time, the two diseases may ultimately prove to have similar increases in risk for colorectal cancer."

Although imperfect, our best tool for screening and surveying these patients is colonoscopy. As has been the practice with UC, these endoscopies probably should commence at 8 years of disease and be repeated every 1 or 2 years. Four-quadrant biopsies are taken every 10 cm throughout the colon and from any suspicious strictures or polyps, seeking dysplasia or cancer. A pediatric colonoscope is used to go through strictured areas.

But if we are now to extend the recommendations for UC and CD, there are a number of questions that arise specifically in screening and surveying patients with chronic Crohn's colitis:

Which Patients Should Have Screening and Surveillance Colonoscopies?

For UC, the profile is relatively straightforward: colitis greater than 8 or 10 years duration, and extensive colitis.[*] The risk is greatest for those with pancolitis, intermediate for left-sided colitis, and probably negligible for proctitis.

A similar profile is more problematic in Crohn's colitis. While patients with ileitis only or colitis limited to ileocecitis or a few scattered colonic aphthae do not appear to be at increased risk, cancers, sometimes multifocal, can arise in some patients with limited colonic CD. The most prominent of this group are those with chronic, severe, fistulous and perianal disease.

Therefore, it is my practice to screen and survey completely all patients with Crohn's colitis of 8 or more years duration who have any significant colonic involvement.[†] This includes all patients who have had previous segmental colonic resections.

[*†] Editor's Note: Dating the onset of colitis may be difficult in patients with coexistent, primary sclerosing cholangitis since the colitis is often mild and sometimes asymptomatic. Similarly, Crohn's colitis may not be detected for several years especially in patients first diagnosed after age 40. Therefore, surveillance should start soon after diagnosis in those types of IBD patients. (TMB)

Do Patients with Chronic Proctitis Need Screening and Surveillance?

While we probably would not regularly survey a patient with chronic ulcerative proctitis, the CD patient with chronic proctitis may be at greater risk. The relative risk of anal and rectal cancer in CD is elevated at least 10-fold over the general population. Anal neoplasms and cancers in fistulae arising in CD may be either squamous cell carcinomas or adenocarcinomas.

Some of these patients have had bypass surgery and the remaining distal colon unwisely may not be followed with surveillance endoscopy. Again, this emphasizes the importance of continued close follow-up of patients with Crohn's colitis after partial colon resection.

These patients may be difficult to study, however. Some have pain, induration, and stricturing. The neoplasms that arise here may be deep or submucosal and therefore not documented by superficial, tangential biopsy of the anal canal. To study these patients adequately, it may be necessary to resort to examination by rigid proctoscopy and by curetting fistulous tracts: both procedures often requiring anesthesia. Whether MRI or an endoscopic ultrasound will be useful in this area remains to be determined.

What is the Significance of Colonic Strictures?

In UC, stricturing that causes obstruction or prevents complete colonoscopy is considered an ominous feature, one for which colectomy is recommended. But in Crohn's colitis, inflammatory stricturing is more common and apt to be a consequence of the disease per se, rather than due to neoplasia.

Yamazaki and colleagues (1991) concluded that the risk of developing carcinoma in Crohn's colitis was greater in strictured than nonstrictured colons. But Friedman and colleagues (1999) found stricturing that precluded the passage of a conventional colonoscope in 25 percent of the 260 chronic Crohn's colitis patients they followed. In these cases, a pediatric caliber colonoscope significantly aided in achieving complete examination. In those patients in whom the thinner caliber endoscope could not traverse the stricture, a barium enema was performed to visualize the stricture and the rest of the colon. No dysplasia or carcinoma was found on follow-up of these patients with stricture.

Based on this data, there would appear to be justification for following asymptomatic strictures in Crohn's colitis with further endoscopic surveillance rather than surgery, presuming there is no dysplasia detected. A barium enema is obtained to study the nature of the stricture and the rest of the colon. Colonoscopy with a pediatric caliber endoscope is repeated at least yearly, with multiple biopsies taken within and through strictures as well as throughout the rest of the colon.

What Pathologic Findings Mandate Surgery?

In neither ulcerative nor Crohn's colitis has the progression from "indefinite" to "low-grade" to "high-grade" dysplasia to cancer been demonstrated. When "indefinite" dysplasia is found, it would seem prudent to repeat colonoscopy and biopsy within 6 months. Similarly, since the progression from low-grade to high-grade dysplasia and cancer is so uncertain, when only one focus of "low-grade" dysplasia is found. The author recommends complete colonoscopy be repeated within several months. Surgery is recommended for multifocal low-grade or any high-grade dysplasia, especially if it is detected in flat mucosa.

What if the Dysplasia is Found in Polypoid Mucosa?

Since 1981, the concept of "DALM" (dysplasia-associated lesion or mass) in UC has been held forth as a feature mandating colectomy. Recent studies by our group and others, however, have called this into question. On the basis of these studies, I suggest that when the dysplastic polypoid tissue is amenable to colonoscopic resection, that is what should be performed. In addition, multiple biopsies should be taken around the polypectomy sites and routinely throughout the colon, with follow-up examinations within several months to ensure complete removal of dysplastic mucosa. Surgery is reserved for those with dysplasia in flat mucosa or those with polypoid dysplasia that cannot be completely resected endoscopically. The approach to dysplastic polyps in CD has not been settled. But it seems reasonable to the author to follow the same approach in both UC and CD.[‡]

What Surgery Should be Performed?

For UC, the surgical decision is usually relatively straightforward: total colectomy, often with ileal pelvic reservoir if there is no dysplasia in the rectum (or even better, none in the entire colon). But in CD, the ileal pouch may not be an option due to the reluctance of surgeons to perform this procedure in known CD. Therefore, for lesions above the rectum, subtotal colectomy is the standard surgical procedure, and for rectal lesions, abdominoperineal resection with ileostomy or colostomy.

An exception to this may be the isolated dysplastic polyp that cannot be removed completely by endoscopic means. If there is no other dysplasia detectable and no other reason to do more extensive surgery, a simple segmental resection may suffice. After any of these surgical options, close follow-up endoscopic surveillance of remaining colon is mandatory.

[‡] Editor's Note: I'm afraid distinguishing a DALM in CD from a well-demarcated adenoma (as can occur proximal to a stricture) and from surrounding inflammatory nodules can be difficult. The author has the advantage of seeing many such patients, which increases his expertise; also patient compliance and scheduling snafus can compromise plans for every 6-month follow-up. (TMB)

Supplemental Reading

Bernstein D, Rogers A. Malignancy in Crohn's disease. Am J Gastroenterol 1996;91:434–40.

Friedman S, Rubin PH, Goldstein E, et al. The efficacy of a 10-year surveillance study in 260 chronic Crohn's colitis patients. Gastroenterology 1999;116:487A.

Gillen CD, Walmsley RS, Prior P, Andrews HA. Ulcerative colitis and Crohn's disease: a comparison of the colorectal cancer risk in extensive colitis. Gut 1994;35:1590–2.

Itzkowitz S. Inflammatory bowel disease and cancer. Gastroenterol Clin North Am 1997;26:136–9.

Ky A, Sohn N, Weinstein MD, Korelitz BI. Carcinoma arising in anorectal fistulas of Crohn's disease. Dis Colon Rectum 1998;41:992–6.

Nikias G, Eisner T, Katz S, et al. Crohn's disease and colorectal cancer: rectal cancer complicating long-standing active perianal disease. Am J Gastroenterol 1995;90:216–9.

Rubin PH, Friedman S, Harpaz N, et al. Colonoscopic polypectomy in chronic colitis: conservative management after endoscopic resection of dysplastic polyps. Gastroenterology 1999;117:1295–300.

Rubio CA, Befrits R. Colorectal adenocarcinoma in Crohn's disease. Dis Colon Rectum 1997;40:1072–8.

Weedon DD, Shorter RG, Ilstrup DM, et al. Crohn's disease and cancer. N Engl J Med 1973;289:1099–103.

Yamazaki Y, Riberio MB, Sachar DB, et al. Malignant colorectal strictures in Crohn's disease. Am J Gastroenterol 1991; 86:882–5.

CHAPTER 56

EXTRA-INTESTINAL MANIFESTATIONS

KIM L. ISAACS, MD, PHD

Inflammatory bowel disease (IBD) by definition affects the gastrointestinal tract, the colon in the case of ulcerative colitis (UC), and anywhere between the mouth and anus in Crohn's disease (CD). Both CD and UC are systemic diseases with extra-intestinal manifestations occurring in at least 25 to 40 percent of patients. If the secondary systemic effects of the disease and/or complications of therapy are also included, then almost 100 percent of patients will have "extra-intestinal manifestations." It is helpful to divide extra-intestinal manifestations into those that will improve with treatment of the underlying bowel disease and those that may progress despite successful therapy of bowel inflammation. A final category of extra-intestinal manifestations is those that are a direct pathophysiologic result of the disease process. These may respond to treatment of the disease process or replacement of nutrients affected by the disease process.

It is also useful to look at the organ system involved with the extra-intestinal manifestation since the treatment modalities within the organ system overlap. Treatment will be discussed and those processes that respond to therapy of underlying bowel disease will be identified (Table 56–1).

Bones and Joints

Peripheral Arthritis

Peripheral arthritis occurs in up to 25 percent of patients with IBD and is more common in patients with CD. There is a separate chapter on arthritis in IBD. Knees, ankles, wrists, and elbows are most commonly affected. The joint may have an effusion and is warm and tender. The effusion should be tapped to make sure that this is not a septic arthritis. Aggressive management of the bowel disease usually will result in improvement of the arthritis. The sulfapyridine component of sulfasalazine appears to have benefit in the therapy of enteropathic arthritis. Sulfasalazine is used preferentially in patients who are on a 5-aminosalicylic acid (5-ASA) compound and can tolerate sulfa products. In patients with mainly small bowel CD and arthritis, a combination of mesalamine (Pentasa®, Ferring-Shire Pharmaceuticals Inc., Florence, Kentucky) and sulfasalazine can be used. This allows for a

TABLE 56–1. Extra-intestinal Manifestations and Response to Treatment of Bowel Disease

Disease	Responds to Treatment of Underlying Bowel Disease
Bone and joint disease	
Axial arthritis: sacroiliitis, ankylosing spondylitis	No
Peripheral arthritis	Yes
Skin disease	
Pyoderma gangrenosum	No
Erythema nodosum	Yes
Ocular disease	
Episcleritis, scleritis	Yes
Uveitis	No
Hepatobiliary disease	
Sclerosing cholangitis	No

small bowel release of mesalamine for treatment of bowel inflammation and release of sulfapyridine from sulfasalazine in the large bowel for its therapeutic effects on arthritis. Systemic and injected corticosteroids also are beneficial in treating inflammatory arthritis but the use of systemic steroids should be limited, due to their adverse long-term effects on bone. Although nonsteroidal anti-inflammatory drugs (NSAIDs) are effective in the treatment of peripheral arthritis, they have been shown to increase bowel permeability in patients with IBD and may exacerbate bowel inflammation. I try to use local therapy with heat and acetaminophen for analgesia prior the use of nonsteroidals. If possible, NSAIDs should be avoided. Recently, cyclo-oxygenase 2 (COX-2) inhibitors such as rofecoxib (Vioxx®, Merck & Co., West Point, Pennsylvania) and celecoxib (Celebrex®, Searle and Pfizer, St. Louis, Missouri) have become available as anti-inflammatory agents. Inhibitors of COX-2 appear to cause less gastric ulceration than the nonselective COX-1 and COX-2 inhibitors. Although rofecoxib and celecoxib have a potential theoretic benefit over the nonselective NSAIDs such as ibuprofen, there are no data available on the effects of these drugs on the gastrointestinal tract in IBD. If an NSAID must be used, then consideration of COX-2 inhibitor is reasonable. Muscle relaxants such as diazepam or cyclobenzaprine hydrochloride also are a useful adjunct. Non-weight-bearing exercise such as swimming will help combat joint stiffness and may increase overall mobility. Surgical therapy of the underlying bowel disease also may lead to improvement of peripheral arthritis. Prompt improvement in joint complaints has occurred within days of Remicade® (Centocor Inc., Malvern, Pennsylvania) infusion in some patients with CD.

Axial Arthritis

This includes ankylosing spondylitis and sacroiliitis. Patients with ankylosing spondylitis typically have colitis and are human leukocyte antigen (HLA)-B27 positive. I do not routinely check HLA-B27 in patients presenting with ankylosing spondylitis as it does not change disease management. These patients often will need to use nonsteroidal drugs to control inflammatory symptoms. As with peripheral arthritis, sulfasalazine is the 5-ASA agent of choice. The arthritis can lead to bone fusion and marked skeletal limitations. Whereas analgesia is appropriate in patients with peripheral arthritis, both analgesia and anti-inflammatory activity may be needed in patients with axial arthritis to prevent the destructive effects of the joint inflammation. Selective COX-2 inhibitors theoretically may have an advantage in terms of decreased side effects in patients with IBD. Exercise and increasing mobility are very important for preventing disability from arthritis. In contrast to peripheral arthritis, resection of the inflamed bowel has no impact on the progression of axial arthritis. Anecdotal reports of improvement with Remicade have been received from patients.

Hypertrophic Osteoarthropathy

This entity consists of clubbing, periostosis, synovitis, and autonomic dysfunction and occurs more commonly in CD. Complaints of symptoms such as dull aching of feet, legs, spine, arms, and hands respond to nonsteroidals and treatment of the underlying bowel disease.

Osteoporosis and Osteomalacia

This may be due to prolonged steroid therapy, extensive small bowel inflammation, and/or extensive small bowel resection. Patients who have any of these potential complications should have a bone density study early in the course of their disease as a baseline. Some patients with CD already have diminished bone density at the time of diagnosis. Steroid avoidance or steroid sparing is indicated. Alternatives include 6-mercaptopurine (6-MP), azathioprine (AZA), and budesonide. Details of prevention and treatment of osteopenia and osteoporosis are in a separate chapter.

Skin

There are multiple skin diseases that have been described in conjunction with IBD. The most common lesions are erythema nodosum and pyoderma gangrenosum. Others include leukocytoclastic vasculitis and Sweet's syndrome.

There is a separate chapter on the therapy of skin diseases in IBD patients.

Erythema Nodosum

This is the most common skin manifestation of IBD occurring in up to 4 percent of patients with UC and 15 percent of patients with CD. It generally reflects the activity, though not necessarily the severity, of the bowel disease and should be treated by aggressive treatment of the bowel disease. Analgesia and bed rest may be required for very painful lesions. Occasionally hospitalization for intravenous (IV) steroid therapy is required to manage the erythema nodosum.

Pyoderma Gangrenosum

Pyoderma is a destructive cutaneous lesion that is seen in 1 to 5 percent of patients with UC. It runs a course that is independent of the bowel disease. These lesions can occur anywhere on the body but most commonly on the dorsum of the feet and the anterior tibial area. They start as pustular lesions that spread concentrically. This is followed by central ulceration. Biopsy can help to document the process but may be associated with poor healing and scarring. In clear-cut cases, I try not to biopsy these lesions. The initial therapy usually is high-dose steroids administered systemically. In a patient with a limited number of lesions, intralesional steroid therapy with triamcinolone may help resolve the inflammation. In patients in whom there is a relative contraindication to steroids or who have extensive pyoderma, I use cyclosporin A. There usually is a dramatic response to therapy. If a patient requires hospitalization for the pyoderma, cyclosporin A is initiated at 4 mg/kg/d in a continuous IV infusion for 3 to 7 days and then converted to oral cyclosporin A at twice the IV dose. The goal is to get the cyclosporin A level in the 200 to 300 ng/mL range. In patients who are not hospitalized, I start at 8 mg/kg/d in a divided oral dose. I continue this until all lesions are gone and then taper off the therapy over a 4-week period. Dapsone also is used. Local skin care including topical antibiotics also is important to help prevent secondary infection. Other thoughts on therapy are in the chapter on skin manifestations. Anecdotal reports of response to Remicade have been received by Centocor.

Cutaneous Crohn's Disease

Cutaneous CD also is referred to as metastatic Crohn's disease. Often it is under-recognized in cases that involve the perineal area. It is a granulomatous inflammatory process involving the skin. This entity usually responds to the same drug therapies, as does bowel inflammation, including steroids and immunosuppression. I also have used intralesional injection of triamcinolone in patients who have a limited number of lesions. It is important to define this entity in patients with perineal disease as it affects therapy. In perineal fistulous disease, I try to minimize steroid exposure and treat with antibiotics and immunosuppression, whereas with cutaneous CD, I will use both systemic and intralesional steroids as primary therapy, followed by immunosuppressive therapy. Patients with perineal lesions are examined under anesthesia with biopsy of the cutaneous lesions.[*]

Eye

Ocular manifestations associated with IBD have been reported in 1 to 11 percent of patients. The most commonly seen are anterior uveitis, iritis, scleritis, and episcleritis. Anterior uveitis and iritis are the most serious of the ocular manifestations. These patients present with photophobia, blurred vision, headache, and eye pain. With this presentation, I send the patient immediately to an opthalmologist for a good slit lamp examination. With this type of examination, disease in the anterior chamber can be identified by the presence of exudate in the chamber. Patients are treated with local steroid therapy and, in more severe cases, systemic steroid therapy. Cycloplegics such as cyclopentolate hydrochloride may be instilled into the eye to help with iridospasm. I also will patch the involved eye to help with the photophobia. Scleritis and episcleritis have less serious consequences. Patients present with burning eyes, watering, and itching. On physical examination, the conjunctiva appear red and inflamed. Patients usually will respond to treatment with steroid-containing eyedrops such as dexamethasone ophthalmic solution 0.1 percent. Initially, the dosage is two drops into the conjunctival sac of each eye every hour—gradually spreading this out to treatment every 4 hours as the patient responds. Scleritis and episcleritis usually will respond to treatment of the underlying bowel disease. Activity tends to parallel the activity of the bowel inflammation. Not all red eyes will respond to steroid therapy. A bacterial conjunctivitis should be recognized and eyedrops containing an antibiotic should be used. There is a combination eyedrop that contains neomycin and dexamethasone (Neo-Decadron®) that can be used if both conditions are suspected. Chapter 58 is devoted to ocular manifestations of IBD.

Hematology

Anemia

Anemia is common in most patients with IBD at some time during the course of their illness. This is discussed in detail in Chapter 69 on hematologic complications.

Iron Deficiency

For those patients who are iron deficient, ferrous sulfate (Fergon®), ferrous gluconate (Feosol®), and iron polysaccharide complex (Niferex®) are all available. The iron polysaccharide complex tends to be the most easily tolerated. Niferex-150® is given orally once or twice per day. This provides 150 mg to 300 mg of elemental iron daily. Patients who do not respond to or cannot tolerate oral iron are supplemented with IV iron. In patients who fail to respond to the IV iron supplementation and where erythropoietin response to anemia is suppressed, I treat again with IV iron and erythropoietin. Intravenous iron supplementation must be done cautiously as there is a 2 to 8 percent rate of side effects, with anaphylaxis as a rare but significant side effect. One protocol is to first calculate the iron deficit with the following formula: iron (mg) = (normal Hgb − patient Hgb × weight (kg) × (2.21 + 1,000). The patient is given methylprednisolone 20 mg IV and diphenhydramine 25 mg IV as a premedication and then a test dose of 25 mg is given IV. If the test dose is tolerated, the remaining iron is given IV over 3 hours.

Vitamin B$_{12}$ Deficiency

Patients who are B$_{12}$ deficient are given 1000 ug intramuscularly (IM) each week for 3 weeks and then 1000 µg IM each month. Vitamin B$_{12}$ now is available in a nasal preparation, Nascobal®, given as one spray into alternate nostrils each week. This is slightly less reliable than IM B$_{12}$, so after about 6 months of therapy, the vitamin B$_{12}$ level is checked to ensure adequate replacement.

Hypercoagulable States

The incidence of thrombosis in patients with IBD is 1.3 to 6.4 percent. Approximately two-thirds of patients will have active disease at the time of their thrombotic event. The etiology of thrombosis is multifactorial and may be related to thrombocytosis and an increase in acute-phase reactants during active inflammation. There has been an isolated report of hyperhomocysteinemia in patients with IBD. The role of this, in terms of excess thrombosis in IBD has not been proven; however, this state can be corrected with administration of folate, cobalamin, and pyridoxine. As testing for hyperhomocysteinemia becomes more prevalent, it will likely be added to the screening evaluation in IBD patients with thrombosis. I treat IBD patients with thrombosis in the same way as non-IBD patients with thrombosis, with anticoagulation as the mainstay of therapy. Although there is always a concern that anticoagulation will induce more bleeding in a patient with active bowel disease, it still must be done to prevent clot complications such as pulmonary embolus. There have been reports of primary treatment of UC with heparin. In those reports, there was not an increased incidence of life-threatening hemorrhage. An alternative to using Coumadin® as an outpatient is the use of low

---

[*] Editor's Note: Anecdotally, repeated Remicade infusions have been very helpful in four patients who did not respond to other immunomodulators. They are described in the next chapter, which is on cutaneous manifestations. (TMB)

molecular weight heparin (Lovenox®) subcutaneously. The major drawback is cost; however, in the event of a major bleed, its activity is diminished more quickly than that of Coumadin.

Other

Hepatobiliary Disease
Sclerosing cholangitis is seen in association with colitis and may progress independently of the bowel disease. It is covered thoroughly in a separate chapter.

Nephrolithiasis
Kidney stones have been reported in up to 19 percent of patients with IBD. Oxalate stones are most common in patients with small bowel CD and urate stones are most common in patients with an end-ileostomy. The management of oxylate stones is discussed in detail in a separate chapter.

Amyloidosis
Amyloidosis can be a complication of chronic inflammation. Deposition of amyloid may occur in the heart, skin, liver, and gastrointestinal tract; in the kidney, it may lead to renal failure. Symptoms depend on the site of deposition. In patients with secondary amyloidosis, the main goal is to decrease the bowel inflammation. Once amyloid has been deposited, decreasing bowel inflammation will not eliminate the deposits that already are present but may diminish further deposition. Colchicine has been used in the treatment of amyloidosis, and with a lack of other effective therapy, most patients are started on daily colchicine.

Pericarditis/Myocarditis
Pericarditis and myocarditis are not common extraintestinal manifestations of IBD, but they do occur—more commonly with UC than with CD. Review of a patient's medication is necessary in that this condition may occur as a side effect of 5-ASA medications. In severe cases with cardiac tamponade, drainage may be required. Patients are treated with salicylates or NSAIDs. It is possible that these agents may exacerbate underlying bowel disease. There are no data on the role of COX-2 inhibitors in the treatment of pericarditis.

Lungs
Four major categories of lung disease have been described in patients with IBD; however, the association often is not recognized. The categories include interstitial lung disease, airway disease, parenchymal nodules, and serositis. There is an allergic type of interstitial lung disease that has been described as an adverse effect of 5-ASA therapy and as in the case of pericarditis, a careful medication review must be performed. In patients who present with pulmonary disease, I will obtain baseline pulmonary function tests and have a bronchoscopy with biopsy/lavage performed. This will help define the category of lung disease and assist in therapeutic decisions. Lung disease often requires therapy with steroids. All 5-ASA products should be withdrawn. Methotrexate should not be used in treatment of the bowel disease, as it has been associated with irreversible pulmonary fibrosis and allergic pneumonitis.

Supplemental Reading
Cattaneao M, Vecchi M, Zighetti ML, et al. High prevalence of hyperhomocysteinemia in patients with inflammatory bowel disease: a pathogenic link with thromboembolic complications? Thromb Haemost 1998;80:542–5.

De Vos M, De Keyser F, Mielants H, et al. Review article: bone and joint diseases in inflammatory bowel disease. Aliment Pharmacol Ther 1998;12:397–404.

Faulds D, Goa KL, Benfield P. Cyclosporine: a review of its pharmacodynamic and pharmacokinetic properties and therapeutic use in immunoregulatory disorders. Drugs 1993;45:953–1040.

Fishbane SF, Ungureanu VD, Maesaka JK, et al. The safety of intravenous iron dextran in hemodialysis patients. Am J Kidney Dis 1996;28:529–34.

Gilmore JD, Hawkins PN, Pepys MB. Amyloidosis: a review of recent diagnostic and therapeutic developments. Br J Haematol 1997;99:245–56.

Greenstein AJ, Janowitz HD, Sachar DB. The extraintestinal complications of Crohn's disease and ulcerative colitis: a study of 700 patients. Medicine 1976;55:401–12.

Pardi DS, Tremaine WJ, Sandborn WJ, McCarthy JT. Renal and urologic complications of inflammatory bowel disease. Am J Gastroenterol 1998;93:504–14.

Schreiber S, Howaldt S, Schnoor M, et al. Recombinant erythropoietin for the treatment of anemia in inflammatory bowel disease. N Engl J Med 1996;334:619–23.

CHAPTER 57

CUTANEOUS MANIFESTATIONS OF INFLAMMATORY BOWEL DISEASE

HOSSEIN C. NOUSARI, MD, THOMAS T. PROVOST, MD, AND GRANT J. ANHALT, MD

Pyoderma Gangrenosum

Pyoderma gangrenosum is an idiopathic inflammatory skin disease manifested clinically by painful ulceration with characteristic purple to violaceous undermining borders. These ulcers most commonly present in an otherwise healthy patient as a single self-limited lesion of the lower extremities.

Chronic and multiple lesions, especially those that arise in areas other than lower extremities (such as the head and neck or upper extremities), are more commonly associated with an underlying systemic disease. The most common associated diseases fall into three groups: (1) inflammatory bowel disease (IBD), (2) hematologic disorders such as lymphoproliferative and myeloproliferative diseases, and (3) rheumatologic disorders such as connective tissue disease, vasculitides, and arthritides. When associated with IBD, the IBD may be asymptomatic, and the activity of the pyoderma gangrenosum does not directly parallel the activity of the underlying IBD. Similarly, pyoderma gangrenosum can develop in patients with occult or smoldering hematologic malignancies. In contrast, when associated with rheumatologic conditions, the disease almost always occurs in the context of overt and advanced rheumatologic disease.

The ulceration of pyoderma gangrenosum can be induced or extended by trauma. This phenomenon is called pathergy, and a similar finding also is seen in other neutrophilic dermatoses such as Behçet's syndrome and Sweet's syndrome. Periostomal ulceration in patients with IBD is not an uncommon presentation and may be difficult to distinguish from Crohn's disease (CD) of the skin.

Diagnosis

The diagnosis of pyoderma gangrenosum is a clinical diagnosis, for there are no histologic changes that are pathognomonic for the disease. It is important to obtain adequate skin biopsies for two purposes: (1) the histology should at least be compatible with the diagnosis and should include an intense neutrophilic infiltrate in the dermis and subcutaneous tissues without evidence of vasculitis or infection; and (2) the tissue must be submitted for bacterial, mycobacterial, and fungal stains and cultures to exclude a primary or superimposed infection.

The skin biopsy must include deep tissue from the borders of the ulcers.

Treatment

Although a significant number of pyoderma gangrenosum lesions may resolve spontaneously after many months, the debility from pain and the potential of a superimposed local and systemic infection in such a necrotic wound prompts the institution of early therapeutic intervention. The treatment of the pyoderma gangrenosum is based on immunosuppressive therapy. Corticosteroids are the first choice. Prednisone usually is initiated at a dose of 0.5 to 1 mg/kg/d, lean body weight. For rapidly evolving lesions, "pulse" steroid therapy can provide remarkably rapid pain relief and healing. This usually is given as intravenous methylprednisolone at a dose of 10 to 15 mg/kg/d for 3 consecutive days. This usually must be followed by oral corticosteroids to maintain improvement. A low threshold for early introduction of corticosteroid-sparing agents is encouraged. We and others have found that the most effective of these adjuvants are azathioprine (2 to 4 mg/kg/d), mycophenolate mofetil (30 to 35 mg/kg/d), cyclosporine (3.5 to 5 mg/kg/d; blood trough: 150 to 250 ng/mL), tacrolimus (150 to 200 µg/kg/d; blood trough: 10 to 20 ng/mL), cyclophosphamide (1.5 to 2.5 mg/kg/d), and chlorambucil.

Among these adjuvant drugs, the calcineurin inhibitors such as cyclosporine and tacrolimus are currently the most effective agents for IBD-associated pyoderma gangrenosum. For patients with debilitating lesions, these drugs should be introduced early in the course of therapy. A synergistic combination of these agents, for example, prednisone, cyclosporine, and mycophenolate mofetil, has proven to be a prudent and effective therapeutic modality for even the most refractory cases or for patients unable to tolerate full doses of these immunosuppressants in a single therapy. This combination can induce significant immunosuppression, so that one must be cautious when using all three drugs at full doses, and prophylaxis for *Pneumocystis carinii*, such as Bactrim DS® three times per week, should be added. The tapering of these corticosteroid-sparing agents should be performed slowly and based on clinical improvement of the skin disease.

In patients with more chronic disease, or in those who cannot tolerate the calcineurin inhibitors, azathioprine or mycophenolate mofetil can be used as steroid-sparing agents. These can be used individually in combination with prednisone, but because they have similar modes of action, they should not be used together, for no synergistic or additive effect will be gained. We have found that mycophenolate mofetil is not as reliably effective as azathioprine, but has a much lower incidence of side effects such as cytopenia, nausea, and hepatotoxicity.

Anti-inflammatory drugs such as dapsone or thalidomide have been reported to be effective in mild cases, when used in combination with prednisone. However, these agents should not be expected to be effective for more serious lesions, as they have rather modest anti-inflammatory actions. Topical tracrolimus has been proposed as a potential treatment for pyoderma gangrenosum. This approach has little promise, for the compound is very painful, and local absorption of the drug is not likely to be sufficient to inhibit significant lesions. As yet, there is no published evidence that anti-tumor necrosis factor therapy has a beneficial effect on pyoderma gangrenosum.

Because active lesions exhibit pathergy, aggressive surgical manipulation of these ulcers is contraindicated. However, careful débridement and even plastic reconstruction could be performed in patients who have received adequate medical treatment or who have controlled and limited disease.

Erythema Nodosum

Erythema nodosum (EN) is a reactive septal panniculitis characterized by extremely painful, nonulcerating erythematous nodules on pretibial areas. The vast majority of cases affect young women, and the triggering or underlying disease remains unknown. When a cause is identified, a preceding streptococcal infection is a common association. Other infections, sarcoidosis, drugs, rheumatologic disease, and IBD also can be associated with erythema nodosum. In contrast to pyoderma gangrenosum, the activity of erythema nodosum tends to reflect that of the associated intestinal disease.

Therapy

Erythema nodosum usually resolves spontaneously, and while waiting for resolution most cases will respond to nonsteroidal anti-inflammatory drugs. However, a small number of patients may require corticosteroid therapy (prednisone: 0.5 to 1 mg/kg/d) with or without the addition of a corticosteroid-sparing agent.

Differential Diagnosis

However, when patients have chronic and recurrent lesions that do not respond well to simple measures, or that exhibit any atypical clinical features such as ulceration or atypical locations, one must be careful to exclude other potential diseases that may mimic EN. These include other panniculitides secondary to lymphoproliferative disorders, infections, and vasculitis. Such lesions require large skin biopsies that include a significant amount of subcutaneous fat; these should be reviewed by a dermatopathologist with experience in the histologic features of these diseases, since obtaining a clear tissue diagnosis in panniculitis can be challenging.

Cutaneous Crohn's Disease

This is an unusual but potentially very debilitating complication of IBD. The most common presentation of cutaneous CD is perineal involvement secondary to enterocutaneous fistulae, and the clinical features of this presentation are draining sinuses, ulcerations, plaques, and nodules. The activity of the perineal disease tends to closely parallel that of the intestinal disease. However, the cutaneous diseases occasionally can occur in the presence of smoldering disease or may precede symptomatic gastrointestinal disease, particularly in children with genital lesions.

An unusual variant has been called metastatic cutaneous CD, and this is characterized by granulomatous cutaneous lesions distant from the perineum. These lesions most commonly present as ulcers, nodules, plaques on lower extremities, or ulcerated linear plaques involving intertriginous areas. Metastatic cutaneous CD usually follows a course independent from that of the intestinal disease activity. The treatment of cutaneous fistulae and perineal disease is similar to that for intestinal disease. The addition of metronidazole can be helpful.

The treatment of metastatic cutaneous CD often is challenging and requires combination immunosuppressive and anti-inflammatory therapy. Drug regimens that have been shown to be helpful include oral corticosteroids in combination with mycophenolate mofetil or azathioprine, cyclosporine, and thalidomide. In our experience, infliximab (Remicade®, Centocor, Malvern, Pennsylvania) (intravenously 5 mg/kg at weeks 0, 2, and 6) has provided dramatic improvement in several cases of even very refractory metastatic cutaneous disease. It is also reported to be very useful for the treatment of perineal lesions and enterocutaneous fistulae.[*]

Other Inflammatory Bowel Disease-Associated Cutaneous Disorders

Vasculitis

Vasculitis can complicate the course of IBD. In the vast majority of affected patients, the vasculitis is neutrophil-rich and affects only small superficial cutaneous blood

---

[*] Editor's Note: We share several patients with cutaneous Crohn's disease and continued infliximab infusions have been needed in all four such patients. (TMB)

vessels. It presents as palpable and nonpalpable purpura on the lower extremities. Whitish or porcelain-colored atrophic skin lesions that mimic Degos' disease also have been reported. Internal organ involvement is quite exceptional. Although cutaneous vasculitis can be the initial presentation of IBD, this complication usually presents in cases with active gastrointestinal symptoms.

Histologic and immunofluorescence examination of the skin is mandatory to confirm the diagnosis and to exclude immunoglobulin (Ig)A vasculitis (Henoch-Schönlein purpura) since the latter can present with a similar clinical picture (eg, diarrhea, gastrointestinal bleeding, arthritis, fever, and genital involvement). The association of medium-sized cutaneous vasculitis (such as polyarteritis nodosa) with IBD is controversial. Misdiagnosed IBD-associated EN could account for some cases of polyarteritis nodosa or vice versa. This reinforces the need for careful clinicopathologic correlation in the evaluation of these cases.

Corticosteroid therapy with or without adjuvant therapy and better control of the intestinal disease are usually effective therapeutic approaches.

Dermatosis-Arthritis Syndrome

Bowel-associated dermatosis-arthritis syndrome is characterized by fever, mild oligoarthritis, and a characteristic purpuric and pustular eruption that favors acral areas. Histologic examination of these lesions reveals dense neutrophilic dermal and subcutaneous infiltrates with or without full-blown vasculitis. This syndrome originally was described in patients with intestinal bypass surgery. However, several cases of this syndrome have been reported in association with IBD. A nonspecific pustular eruption observed in patients with IBD could be part of the spectrum of the bowel-associated dermatosis. The pathogenesis of this syndrome appears to be the presence of circulating immune complexes due to the bacterial overgrowth of intestinal flora. Antineutrophilic drugs like dapsone and antibiotics usually are effective therapies.

Sweet's Syndrome

Sweet's syndrome is another neutrophilic dermatosis that presents as painful urticarial plaques that favor the head, neck, and upper extremities. Most of the cases are idiopathic, but rheumatologic diseases, hematologic malignancies, drugs, and IBD are not uncommonly associated conditions. An atypical bullous variant of Sweet's syndrome generally is considered part of the spectrum of pyoderma gangrenosum. Corticosteroid, thalidomide, and dapsone therapy are usually effective.

Necrolytic Migratory Erythema

Necrolytic migratory erythema is an erythematous scaling eruption involving the perineum and periorificial areas associated with angular cheilitis and glossitis. The cutaneous eruption is similar, if not identical, to that observed in acrodermatitis enteropathica. The pathogenesis of this eruption is thought to be hypoaminoacidemia and zinc deficiency due to chronic diarrhea, and malabsorption secondary to glucagonoma. However, a pseudoglucagonoma syndrome with identical mucocutaneous features also has been observed in patients with IBD. Amino acid and zinc replacement along with better control of the intestinal disease usually are effective therapeutic interventions.

Other Inflammatory Bowel Disease-Associated Mucous Membrane Disorders

Aphthous stomatitis is the most common mucosal disease observed in patients with IBD. These oral ulcers usually present as painful grouped or scattered small superficial ulcerations on the buccal mucosae. These ulcers almost always appear in the setting of associated active IBD.

Orofacial granulomatosis presents with "cobble-stoned" mucosal plaques and granulomatous cheilitis. The histologic examination of these plaques reveals noncaseating granulomas. This could be classified as metastatic mucosal CD. Sarcoidosis should be carefully excluded in these patients.

Pyostomatitis vegetans is characterized by aseptic abscesses and spongy and friable erythematous plaques in the mouth. It is thought to represent a mucosal variant of pyoderma gangrenosum. Histologic and immunofluorescence studies should be performed to confirm the diagnosis and rule out a clinical variant of pemphigus called pemphigus vegetans.

Epidermolysis bullosa acquisita is an autoimmune mucocutaneous blistering disease that frequently heals with scarring. These patients have pathogenic autoantibodies against type VII collagen, a component of the basement membrane of stratified squamous epithelia. Localized mucosal epidermolysis bullosa acquisita including isolated esophageal involvement also can be observed in patients with IBD. This disease is treated with corticosteroids and immunosuppressive agents. Esophageal, laryngeal, conjunctival, or severe mucocutaneous disease should be treated with a combination of prednisone and cyclophosphamide.

Editor's Note

A complete 46-item reference list can be obtained at *gjanhalt@welch.jhu.edu*. We have included most of the references because of the rarity of some of these problems.

Supplemental Reading

Becuwe C, Delaporte E, Colombel JF, et al. Sweet's syndrome associated with Crohn's disease. Acta Derm Venereol 1989;69:444–5.

Cairns BA, Herbst CA, Sartor BR, et al. Periostomal pyoderma gangrenosum and inflammatory bowel disease. Arch Surg 1994;129:769–72.

Capella GL, Frigerio E, Fracchiolla C, Altomare G. The simultaneous treatment of inflammatory bowel disease and associated pyoderma gangrenosum with oral cyclosporin A. Scand J Gastroenterol 1999;34:220–1.

Castanet J, Lacour JP, Perrin C, et al. Cutaneous vasculitis with lesions mimicking Degos' disease and revealing Crohn's disease. Acta Derm Venereol 1995;75:408–9.

Corazza M, Ughi G, Spisani L, Virgili A. Metastatic ulcerative penile Crohn's disease. J Eur Acad Dermatol Venereol 1999;13:224–6.

Delaney TA, Clay CD, Randell PL. The bowel-associated dermatosis-arthritis syndrome. Australas J Dermatol 1989; 30:23–7.

D'inca R, Fagiuoli S, Sturniolo GC. Tacrolimus to treat pyoderma gangrenosum resistant to cyclosporine. Ann Intern Med 1998;128:783–4.

Dippel E, Rosenberger A, Zouboulis CC. Distant cutaneous manifestation of Crohn's disease presenting as a granulomatous erysipelas-like lesion. J Eur Acad Dermatol Venereol 1999;12:65–6.

Ferrer Rios T, Ramos Lora M, Pallares Manrique H, et al. Pyoderma gangrenosum with an atypical location and a rapid response to cyclosporin A. Gastroenterol Hepatol 1999;22:227–9.

Ficarra G, Cicchi P, Amorosi A, Piluso S. Oral Crohn's disease and pyostomatitis vegetans: an unusual association. Oral Surg Oral Med Oral Pathol 1993;75:220–4.

Gagoh OK, Qureshi RM, Hendrickse MT. Recurrent buccal space abscesses; a complication of Crohn's disease. Oral Surg Oral Med Oral Pathol Oral Radiol Endod 1999;88:33–6.

Gilson MR, Elston LC, Pruitt CA. Metastatic Crohn's disease: remission induced by mesalamine and prednisone. J Am Acad Dermatol 1999;41:476–9.

Grana Gil J, Alonso Aquirre P, Yebra Pimental MT, et al. Cutaneous polyarteritis nodosa and Crohn's disease. Clin Rheumatol 1991;10:196–200.

Kafity AA, Pellegrini AE, Fromkes JJ. Metastatic Crohn's disease: a rare cutaneous manifestation. J Clin Gastroenterol 1993;17:300–3.

Kay MH, Wyllie R. Cutaneous vasculitis as the initial manifestation of Crohn's disease in a pediatric patient. Am J Gastroenterol 1998;93:1014.

Levitt MD, Ritchie JK, Lennard-Jones JE, Phillips RK. Pyoderma gangrenosum in inflammatory bowel disease. Br J Surg 1991;78:676–8.

Marotta PJ, Reynolds RP. Metastatic Crohn's disease. Am J Gastroenterol 1996;91:373–5.

Matheson BK, Gilbertson EO, Eichenfield LF. Vesiculopustular eruption of Crohn's disease. Pediatr Dermatol 1996;13:127–30.

Mclelland J, Griffin SM. Metastatic Crohn's disease of the umbilicus. Clin Exp Dermatol 1996;21:318–9.

Nousari HC, Lynch W, Anhalt GJ, Petri M. The effectiveness of mycophenolate mofetil in refractory pyoderma gangrenosum. Arch Dermatol 1998;134:1509–11.

Nousari HC, Sragovich A, Kimyai-Asadi A, et al. Mycophenolate mofetil in autoimmune and inflammatory skin disorders. J Am Acad Dermatol 1999;40:265–8.

Ochonisky s, Bonvalet D, Caron C, et al. Granulomatous cheilitis with cutaneous extension in Crohn's disease. Regression with hydroxychloroquine. Ann Dermatol Venereol 1992;119:844–6.

Ploysangam T, Heubi JE, Eisen D, et al. Cutaneous Crohn's disease in children. J Am Acad Dermatol 1997;36:697–704.

Schattenkirchner S, Lemann M, Prost C, et al. Localized epidermolysis bullosa acquisita of the esophagus in a patient with Crohn's disease. Am J Gastroenterol 1996;91:1657–9.

Schlehaider UK, Suckow M, Rosenthal P, Kowalzick L. Cutaneous reactions in Crohn's disease. Vasculitis in various skin segments. Hutarzt 1997;48:328–31.

Sercki P, Janssen F, Vignon-Pennamen MD. Cutaneous manifestations of zinc deficiency in Crohn's disease. Ann Dermatol Venereol 1990;117:833–4.

Shelley ED, Shelley WB. Cyclosporine therapy for pyoderma gangrenosum associated with sclerosing cholangitis and ulcerative colitis. J Am Acad Dermatol 1988;18:1084–8.

Veloso FT, Carvalho J, Magro F. Immune-related systemic manifestations of inflammatory bowel disease. A prospective study of 792 patients. J Clin Gastroenterol 1996;23:29–34.

Von den Driesch P. Pyoderma gangrenosum: a report of 44 cases with follow-up. Br J Dermatol 1997;137:1000–5.

Waltz KM, Long D, Marks JG Jr, Billingsley EM. Sweet's syndrome and erythema nodosum: the simultaneous occurrence of 2 reactive dermatoses. Arch Dermatol 1999; 135:62–6.

Zlatanic J, Fleisher M, Sasson M, et al. Crohn's disease and acute leukocytoclastic vasculitis of skin. Am J Gastroenterol 1996;91:2410–3.

CHAPTER 58

Ocular Manifestations of Inflammatory Bowel Disease

Paul A. Latkany, MD, and Douglas A. Jabs, MD, MS

Crohn first reported the association of ulcerative colitis with ocular inflammation in 1925. Historically, inflammatory bowel disease–related ocular inflammation could result in blindness, although blindness is less likely today due to better treatments. Ocular inflammation in patients with inflammatory bowel disease (IBD) has a reported range of frequency from as low as 1.9 percent to as high as 13 percent of patients. Ulcerative colitis appears to be less likely to have associated ocular inflammation than does Crohn's disease. Although a large number of inflammatory conditions have been reported with IBD, including uveitis, episcleritis, scleritis, keratitis, conjunctivitis, retinitis, retinal vasculitis, choroiditis, optic neuritis, orbital myositis, and orbital pseudotumor, lesions that appear to be more clearly associated with IBD include anterior uveitis, scleritis, keratitis, and retinal vasculitis and/or posterior uveitis. Of these, anterior uveitis is the most common.

Anterior Uveitis

Anterior uveitis, also known as iritis or iridocyclitis, may be either acute or chronic, and both types are seen in patients with IBD. Acute anterior uveitis has a sudden onset with symptoms of pain, redness, and photophobia, whereas chronic anterior uveitis has an insidious onset with symptoms of blurred vision. Acute anterior uveitis may be episodic and recurrent but typically has periods of time with quiescent disease off treatment, whereas chronic anterior uveitis tends to recur whenever treatment is discontinued. Fifty percent of patients with acute anterior uveitis possess the tissue-type human leukocyte antigen (HLA)-B27, whereas chronic anterior uveitis has no known HLA association. Human leukocyte antigen-B27 is present in 8 percent of the Caucasian population and, even without concomitant IBD, is associated with the characteristic pattern of an alternating unilateral, acute, anterior uveitis. Inflammatory bowel disease–associated uveitis usually has a pattern similar to HLA-B27-associated uveitis. Patients with IBD and HLA-B27 have an incidence of uveitis higher than those with IBD alone and are more likely to have radiographic manifestations of spondylitis or sacroiliitis. The attacks of acute anterior uveitis in these patients do not parallel the activity of the IBD. Conversely, patients also may have, though less

frequently, a chronic anterior uveitis, the activity of which parallels that of the IBD, much in the same fashion as does enteropathic arthritis. Control of the underlying IBD activity will result in better control of the eye disease in these patients.

Scleritis

Episcleritis is a milder form of scleral disease with symptoms of irritation or discomfort, sectoral or nodular episcleral inflammation, and a low frequency of ocular complications and systemic disease associations. Scleritis is often (but not always) painful, may be diffuse, nodular, necrotizing, or even posterior, often has ocular complications, and is associated with systemic diseases in nearly one-half of the cases. Although either may be seen with IBD, scleritis is a more common association. Keratitis (inflammation of the cornea) may occur with or without scleritis. Keratitis may be infiltrative (interstitial keratitis) or ulcerative with a loss of epithelium and stroma (necrotizing keratitis, marginal corneal ulcer).

Accompanying Disorders

Patients with IBD may develop ocular problems incidental to the IBD or its treatment that are not directly related to the underlying immune-mediated process. Patients on chronic steroid therapy may develop *cataracts*. The incidence of cataract formation due to oral corticosteroids increases from 0 percent at doses less than 10 mg/d for a duration of less than 1 year to *86 percent for doses greater than 15 mg/d for a duration of over 4 years*. However, with modern cataract surgery, 95 percent of patients with uncomplicated cataracts will have a good surgical result (visual acuity 20/40 or better). *Glaucoma* is an uncommon but asymptomatic complication of oral corticosteroid therapy. Five percent of patients will have a substantial rise in intraocular pressure from *topical corticosteroids* (which appear *more likely* to raise the intraocular pressure than do oral corticosteroids). This rise is reversible with discontinuation of the steroids and treatable with anti-glaucoma eye drops if continued steroid therapy is needed. Since chronic glaucoma is asymptomatic until substantial permanent damage is done, an annual eye examination for patients on chronic steroid therapy is reasonable.

Patient Evaluation

Most patients with the serious ocular manifestations of IBD will be symptomatic, although the symptoms may need to be elicited. Any ocular symptoms should be evaluated by an ophthalmologist, as there are no symptoms that are specific for IBD-related eye disease, and the symptoms of several problems are similar. Acute problems often are manifested by pain, redness, photophobia, and sometimes blurred vision, whereas chronic problems may present with blurred vision. For example, chronic uveitis and cataracts could have similar presenting symptoms. Ophthalmologic examination including slit lamp examination and indirect ophthalmoscopy through a dilated pupil are needed to make a proper diagnosis.

As part of a workup for uveitis or scleritis, an internist or gastroenterologist might be asked to consult on a patient to rule out IBD as an associated disease. Although endoscopic evaluation is not usually warranted as part of a diagnostic workup of a patient with uveitis, attention should be paid to any signs or symptoms of IBD. We have not infrequently encountered patients in whom the symptoms of IBD were mild and the disease previously undiagnosed.

Treatment

The sooner therapy is instituted, the less likely patients with uveitis will develop long-term ocular complications. Typically, we treat patients with *anterior uveitis* with topical prednisolone acetate 1 percent every hour while awake, and once inflammation is controlled we begin to slowly taper the frequency of administration. We prefer aggressive treatment to control ocular inflammation and prevent ocular complications, such as adhesions between the iris and lens (posterior synechiae), cataract, glaucoma, and macular edema. A cycloplegic agent, such as atropine sulfate 1 percent or cyclopentolate 1 percent, is added to dilate the pupil to prevent posterior synechiae, which could lead to acute glaucoma, and to relieve pain secondary to spasm of the intraocular ciliary muscle. Nonsteroidal anti-inflammatory drugs (NSAIDs), either topical or oral, do *not* have a significant role in treatment of uveitis. Patients with acute anterior uveitis usually can have the steroid eye drops discontinued within 6 to 8 weeks of starting treatment, whereas those with chronic uveitis will require long-term, suppressive topical steroids (eg, one to four times daily).

Occasionally, patients with anterior uveitis will require supplemental treatment, either periocular corticosteroid injections or oral corticosteroids, due to the severity of the attack. For occasional patients with severe acute anterior uveitis, a short course of prednisone may help control the inflammation. Generally, we begin at a dosage of 1 mg/kg/d and taper it over 1 month. Occasionally, patients with chronic uveitis will require chronic low-dose prednisone ($\leq$10 mg/d) to control the uveitis.

Although *episcleritis* typically responds to treatment with mild topical corticosteroids (eg, fluorometholone four times daily), scleritis requires oral therapy. Anterior scleritis frequently responds to oral NSAIDs, and indomethacin appears to be particularly effective. For patients who do not respond to indomethacin, oral prednisone is necessary. For posterior scleritis, prednisone typically is needed, and for necrotizing scleritis, an immunosuppressive drug often is needed in addition to prednisone.

Keratitis with an intact corneal epithelium often responds to topical corticosteroids, whereas keratitis accompanied by loss of corneal epithelium and stroma (eg, marginal corneal ulcer, necrotizing keratitis) typically requires systemic corticosteroids. Patients with scleritis or keratitis requiring chronic oral corticosteroids may benefit from improved control of the IBD.

Other less frequent ocular manifestations of IBD may require urgent evaluation and aggressive systemic treatment. For instance, posterior uveitis, such as retinal vasculitis, typically requires oral corticosteroids. Topical corticosteroids do not penetrate well behind the lens and are not efficacious for posterior disease. We start our adult patients with posterior or symptomatic intermediate uveitis on prednisone at a dose of 1 mg/kg/d. We maintain our patients on this dose until the disease is quiet, but for no more than 4 weeks, before slowly tapering the steroids over a 2-month period while closely monitoring the activity of the ocular manifestation or inflammation. Steroid-sparing agents may be of benefit for patients who do not respond to high-dose oral prednisone, who require chronic steroid therapy at unacceptably high doses (prednisone >15 mg/d), or who develop steroid complications. However, these agents do not work quickly enough by themselves and therefore require concomitant prednisone therapy, at least initially, to control the acute ocular inflammation. Azathioprine, cyclosporine, and methotrexate each may be effective. We typically have not had to resort to the more potent but also more toxic alkylating agents (eg, cyclophosphamide or chlorambucil) for patients with IBD-associated severe uveitis. Colectomy for ulcerative colitis appears to decrease the incidence of ocular inflammation and has been associated with resolution of eye disease; however, ocular inflammation almost never should be the primary indication for colectomy as appropriate medical therapy usually controls the ocular inflammation.

Acknowledgment

The authors have no proprietary or financial interests in the subject matter or materials discussed in the manuscript.

Supplemental Reading

Billson FA, de Dombal FT, Watkinson G, Goliigher JC. Ocular complications of ulcerative colitis. Gut 1967;8:102–6.

Crohn BB. Ocular lesions complicating ulcerative colitis. Am J Sci 1925;169:260–7.

Edwards FC, Truelove SC. The course and prognosis of ulcerative colitis. Gut 1964;5:1–22.

Ellis PP, Gentry JH. Ocular complications of ulcerative colitis. Am J Ophthalmol 1964;58:779–85.

Greenstein AJ, Janoowitz HD, Sachar DB. The extra-intestinal complications of Crohn's disease and ulcerative colitis: a study of 700 patients. Medicine 1976;55:401–12.

Knox DL, Schachat AP, Mustonen E. Primary, secondary and coincidental ocular complications of Crohn's disease. Ophthalmology 1984;91:163–73.

Korelitz BBI, Coles RS. Uveitis (iritis) associated with ulcerative and granulomatous colitis. Gastroenterology 1967;52:78–82.

Lyons JL, Rosenbaum JT. Uveitis associated with inflammatory bowel disease compared with uveitis associated with spondyloarthropathy. Arch Ophthalmol 1997;115:61–4.

CHAPTER 59

ARTHRITIS ASSOCIATED WITH INFLAMMATORY BOWEL DISEASE

TIMOTHY R. ORCHARD, MA, MD, DM, MRCP

Arthritis is a relatively common complication of ulcerative colitis (UC) and Crohn's disease, affecting 10 to 20 percent of patients. It may predate the bowel disease and may be severe enough to warrant treatment in its own right, perhaps with nonsteroidal anti-inflammatory drugs (NSAIDs). This may, itself, exacerbate the underlying bowel disease. In this chapter, the different forms of arthritis associated with inflammatory bowel disease (IBD) are identified and their management discussed in terms of their prognosis, possible modes of treatment, and when expert help should be sought.

Natural History, Classification, and Diagnosis

The ability to predict and communicate the course of the disease to the patient is an important part of the management process in the arthritis of IBD. Several forms of joint disease are now recognized in IBD with differing natural histories, and these may require differing therapeutic approaches.

Axial Disease

SYMPTOMATIC DISEASE

Low back pain is a common complaint in both IBD and the general population. In IBD, it may represent inflammatory arthritis of the sacroiliac joints (sacroiliitis) or progressive ankylosing spondylitis (AS). Ankylosing spondylitis causes progressive ankylosis (fusion) of the vertebral facet joints. This progressive fusion leads to a characteristic "question mark" posture and may lead to respiratory embarrassment secondary to poor chest expansion and upper lobe pulmonary fibrosis. It is associated with peripheral arthritis in about 30 percent of cases. It has been suggested that the course of AS associated with IBD is less severe than idiopathic AS, but this is not universally accepted. In a patient presenting with back pain, it is therefore important to distinguish between mechanical low back pain and the inflammatory back pain associated with sacroiliitis and AS. The clinical features of inflammatory low back pain are an insidious onset over months, morning stiffness and exacerbation of pain by rest, and pain radiating into the buttocks (rather than central back pain). It tends to occur in patients under 40 years of age.

TABLE 59–1. Methods for Assessing Spinal Mobility

Test	Normal Values
Lumbar flexion (modified Schober test): mark the skin 5 cm below and 10 cm above the dimples of Venus. Ask the patient to flex forward fully and measure the distance between the two marks	The distance between the two marks should increase to ≥21 cm
Lateral flexion: from a vertical position the patient should slide each arm in turn down the leg. The distance moved by the fingertips should be measured and the mean calculated.	The fingertips should move ≥14 cm or to touch the joint line of the knee each side.
Chest expansion: measured in the 4th intercostal space	≥5 cm

Any decrease in the above not accounted for by preexisting conditions should be regarded as reflecting decreased spinal mobility and merits further investigation.

Mechanical back pain may be of sudden onset, is often central, and is better after rest, occurring generally in older patients. Plain radiographs of the sacroiliac joints are the conventional means of diagnosis, but x-ray changes occur only after several months and MRI scanning (with or without gadolinium enhancement) is more sensitive and avoids the necessity of a radiation dose.

If radiologic evidence of sacroiliitis is found, then a further assessment should be made to detect evidence of progressive axial disease. These should include the modified Schober test of lumbar flexion, lateral lumbar flexion, and chest expansion (see Table 59–1).

The most useful blood test in diagnosis is human leukocyte antigen (HLA)-B27 status. Although large studies of isolated sacroiliitis have not been performed, it appears that the prevalence of HLA-B27 in this group is significantly lower than in AS. A positive HLA-B27 result in an IBD patient with sacroiliitis is therefore a predictor of progression to AS. However, 20 to 50 percent of IBD-associated AS patients are HLA-B27 negative, so a negative result does not preclude the diagnosis, particularly in the presence of decreased spinal mobility. Patients with low back pain or decreased spinal mobility in the presence of sacroiliitis should be treated as having AS.

ASYMPTOMATIC DISEASE

Up to 20 percent of IBD patients may have asymptomatic sacroiliitis detectable by plain radiology, which may be diagnosed on the basis of routine abdominal x-rays. In many cases, there is no history of inflammatory back pain even on direct questioning.* If radiologic sacroiliitis is diagnosed a clinical assessment of spinal mobility should be undertaken along with HLA-B27 status. If there is evidence of decreased spinal mobility, the patient should be treated as having early AS.

Peripheral Arthritis

Peripheral joint pain is common in IBD, as it is in the general population, but in addition to nonspecific arthralgia, IBD patients may also suffer from an inflammatory arthritis. Arthralgia is often related to reducing doses of corticosteroids or starting immunosuppressants such as azathioprine. It normally settles with time and no further investigation is required.

The inflammatory arthritis has recently been characterized and falls into two main categories:

TYPE 1

Type 1 is a large joint pauciarticular arthritis that tends to occur with relapse of the IBD. It occurs in discrete episodes that may last for several weeks, but not normally for more than 12 weeks. Twenty-five to 40 percent of patients will have more than one episode of arthritis, and there is an increased risk of erythema nodosum and uveitis with this form of arthritis.

TYPE 2

Type 2 is a symmetric polyarthritis that may affect a wide range of joints. It runs a course independent of the IBD and is more persistent, lasting for a median of 3 years. It is associated with an increased risk of uveitis but not of erythema nodosum.

There is a degree of overlap between the two types, with 10 to 20 percent of oligoarthritis patients developing persistent symptoms. In cases of doubt, the association with disease activity is probably the most useful discriminator in terms of management. The two forms of arthritis are also associated with distinct immunogenetic identities. Type 1 is associated with HLA-B27, B35, and DR103 and type 2 is associated with HLA-B44. These tests are probably not helpful in the clinical setting at present, except that HLA-DR103 is present in 65 percent of patients who develop recurrent type 1 arthritis compared to 3 percent of the general population and may thus be a useful indicator of those at high risk of recurrent disease. Both forms of arthritis are rheumatoid factor negative and are not generally erosive or deforming. If there is evidence of erosive disease, then further investigation is required.

---

* Editor's Note: Scott et al reported that less than 10 percent of patients found to have sacroiliitis by CT scan were symptomatic. (TMB)

TABLE 59–2. Pharmacologic Treatments for Inflammatory Bowel Disease Arthritis

Drug	Uses
Sulphasalazine	5-ASA drug of choice in patients with arthritis. Most effective in peripheral arthritis, where it should be used early for maximal effect.
Analgesics	Paracetamol (acetaminophen) should be tried initially, but if it fails combinations with opioids should be used early. Constipation may be a problem.
Nonsteroidal anti-inflammatory drugs (NSAIDs)	These should be avoided where possible. They should never be used when there is active bowel disease. They may be used for persistent symptoms with AS or type 2 peripheral arthritis if the bowel disease is quiescent. They should be stopped if the bowel disease relapses. There is no rationale for choosing one NSAID over another at present.*
Steroids	Local: injection of steroid into an acutely inflamed joint is particularly effective in type 1 arthritis for symptom relief and early resolution of the inflammation. Oral: if used for the bowel disease, will improve type 1 arthritis and AS. Low-dose steroid may be used in resistant cases of AS or type 2 arthritis but should NOT be used for prolonged periods (>2 months).
Methotrexate	The immunosuppressant of choice in patients with resistant bowel and joint disease. May be useful in patients with AS or type 2 arthritis with persistent symptoms and quiescent bowel disease, where it may obviate the requirement for oral steroids.

* Editor's Note: The use of COX-2 inhibitor is also questioned later in the text. (TMB)

Diagnosis of IBD peripheral arthritis is largely based on clinical grounds, but other joint diseases should be excluded. For type 1 arthritis, the differential diagnosis includes gout and pseudogout, septic arthritis, and arthritis following genitourinary infections such as chlamydia and gonorrhea. These causes should be actively sought, particularly where there is no apparent relation to activity of the bowel disease. Serum urate and calcium should be checked routinely. Joint aspiration and examination should be performed in cases where there is any doubt. For type 2 arthritis, a rheumatoid factor and autoantibody screen should be performed to exclude seropositive rheumatic disease. Arthritis associated with IBD is very rarely erosive or deforming and is not associated with other manifestations of rheumatoid arthritis such as subcutaneous nodules. X-rays of the most severely affected joints should therefore be performed if symptoms are persistent to exclude erosive disease.

Management of Inflammatory Bowel Disease Arthropathies

General Considerations

The management of arthritis in IBD depends on the nature and duration of the arthritis, as discussed below. It involves alleviation of symptoms and preservation of function for the future, particularly in axial disease. Because of the relatively small number of patients involved, no controlled trials of treatment have been conducted, and most treatment modalities rely on general principles. Physical treatments (rest, range of movement exercises, and physiotherapy) are important components of management and should not be ignored. These may be enhanced by simple measures such as splinting affected joints and the use of assistive devices such as a walking stick.

ANALGESIA

This is a key element in management and is a potentially difficult area as nearly all analgesics have undesirable effects on the gut. A stepped approach should be used, starting with simple analgesia such as paracetamol (acetominophen) and then progressing to combinations of paracetamol and opioid analgesia such as co-dydramol (paracetamol 500 mg and Dihydrododeine 10 mg) and co-proxamol (paracetamol 325 mg and dextropropoxyphene hydrochloride 32.5 mg). In analgesics containing opioids, constipation may be a problem, particularly in patients with resistant distal colitis. Nonsteroidal anti-inflammatory drugs should be avoided if at all possible. They may cause enterocolitis in their own right and may trigger or exacerbate relapse of preexisting IBD. This may be associated with significant lower gastrointestinal bleeding. They should not be used at all in patients with active disease, and in these situations other therapies should be used depending on the circumstances (see below). The recent advent of cyclo-oxygenase-2 (COX-2) specific NSAIDs has raised the prospect of fewer unwanted gastrointestinal problems, particularly in the stomach. However, experiments in animals have demonstrated that the enterocolitis of NSAIDs is not primarily mediated by the cyclo-oxygenase pathway, and so it is likely that COX-2-specific NSAIDs will not improve the tolerability of these drugs in IBD patients and they should probably still be avoided if possible.

Axial Disease

Patients with AS should be managed in conjunction with a rheumatologist. Physical therapies are of particular importance, and all patients should take regular exercise to maintain the mobility of the spine. This may include swimming and spinal exercises with regular physiotherapy if necessary. These forms of exercise should also be recommended to patients with sacroiliitis associated with any form of low back pain or decreased spinal mobility. For patients with severely reduced spinal mobility or severe low back pain, injection of steroid into the sacroiliac joints may help, particularly in association with a period of intensive inpatient physiotherapy. The period of relief from sacroiliac injection alone may be brief.

DRUG TREATMENTS: ANALGESIA

Simple *analgesics* should be used if possible. Nonsteroidal anti-inflammatory drugs are the drugs of choice in idiopathic AS, and if there is active spinal disease in the absence of active IBD, then it is reasonable to use NSAIDs. However, they should be stopped if the IBD flares up. There is no rationale for using one NSAID rather than another in AS, and it remains to be seen whether the newer COX-2 inhibitors will have any advantage in this group of patients.

Sulfasalazine can be used for both the IBD and joint symptoms. It is most effective in patients with associated peripheral joint problems. Other 5-aminosalicyclic acid (5-ASA) drugs are not as effective as it is thought to be the sulfapyridine component that confers the articular effects rather than the 5-ASA.

If oral *steroids* are required for active disease, then they will also have a beneficial effect on the spinal disease. However, long-term steroid therapy for spinal disease alone should be avoided. This may be achieved by using *methotrexate*, which may be effective in both gut and spinal disease. In severe progressive disease unresponsive to the measures outlined above, radiotherapy remains a last resort; however, the increased risk of hematologic malignancy associated with this form of treatment has rendered it rarely used. A summary of drug treatments is shown in Table 59–2.

The most important part in the successful management of patients with AS and IBD is good communication between the patient, gastroenterologist, and rheumatologist to maximize the effectiveness of the available therapeutic options.[†]

Isolated sacroiliitis should be treated symptomatically with simple analgesia and regular exercise should be encouraged. However, further treatment should not be required in the absence of decreased spinal mobility or severe pain.

Peripheral Joint Disease

TYPE 1 ARTHRITIS

This is usually self-limiting, and so treatment is largely symptomatic. Resting the joint is important and use of a walking stick (cane) or splint to take pressure off the joint may lead to a significant improvement. Range of

---

[†] Editor's Note: The chapter "Lessons from Treatment of Rheumatoid Arthritis" focuses on parallels with Crohn's disease pathophysiology and treatment strategies. (TMB)

movement exercises should be performed to minimize any periarticular muscle atrophy and to prevent contractures. In severe cases, formal physiotherapy may be required to improve function.

Analgesia should be with simple analgesia, and as type 1 arthritis is usually associated with active bowel disease, NSAIDs should not be used. A good, but relatively seldom used, therapy is intra-articular injection of steroid. This may provide very effective symptom relief and may remove the requirement for other treatments. This may be done in the outpatient clinic, where a combination of local anesthetic such as lignocaine (lidocaine) and a steroid such as methylprednisolone may be injected into large joints such as the knee. If oral steroids are used to treat the active bowel disease, then these will normally treat the arthritis effectively. If not, an empirical change of 5-ASA drug to sulfasalazine may provide adequate symptom relief. If sulfasalazine fails, then a lower dose of oral steroid specifically for the joint disease may be effective (10 to 15 mg of prednisolone rather than 30 to 40 mg), but this should not be prolonged for more than a few weeks.[‡]

Long-term treatment is not usually required, although maintenance with sulfasalazine as the 5-ASA of choice may be appropriate, particularly in patients at risk of recurrent disease such as those who are HLA-DR103 positive. In the minority of patients with persistent problems, the treatment options are those of type 2 arthritis (see below).

TYPE 2 ARTHRITIS

These patients generally have persistent problems and may require long-term treatment. Again, as the disease is usually nonerosive and nondeforming, symptomatic relief is the major aim. Again, splinting of affected joints and rest are important components of management, but the persistent and polyarthritic nature of this condition makes this harder to achieve than in type 1 arthritis.

Simple analgesia should be tried initially. Nonsteroidal anti-inflammatory drugs should only be considered in patients with quiescent disease unresponsive to simple or combination analgesia such as co-dydramol, and if there is any evidence of an increase in the activity of the bowel disease they should be stopped immediately.

For patients with persisting problems, sulfasalazine or low-dose prednisolone (10 to 15 mg daily) may be used; however, prolonged courses of oral steroids should be avoided. In patients with active bowel disease, concurrent arthritis is a good indication for the use of methotrexate as the first-line immunosuppressant rather than azathioprine in order to treat both gut and joints. Rarely, methotrexate may be required for treatment of the joint disease alone. Patients who have evidence of erosive joint disease, a positive rheumatoid factor, or who do not respond to the measures outlined above should be managed jointly with a rheumatologist.

Summary

Arthritis is a relatively common complication of IBD. We now know more about arthritis in IBD and its natural history than previously and can tailor therapy to the pattern of joint disease. With the exception of AS the joint disease is largely non-deforming and non-progressive, and so can be managed symptomatically, although use of NSAID's should be avoided. Management involves judicious use of physical treatments in addition to the pharmacological treatments which are summarised in Table 2. Patients with AS or persistent or erosive peripheral joint disease should be referred to a rheumatologist.

Supplemental Reading

Bjarnason I, Zanelli G, Smith T, et al. Nonsteroidal anti-inflammatory drug induced intestinal inflammation in humans. Gastroenterology 1987;93:480–9.

De Vos M, Mielants H, De Keyser F, et al. Inflammatory arthropathy and inflammatory bowel disease. In: Rutgeerts P, ed. Advances in inflammatory bowel disease: Falk Symposium 106. London: Kluwer, 1999:280–8.

Orchard TR, Wordsworth BP, Jewell DP. Peripheral arthropathies in inflammatory bowel disease: their articular distribution and natural history. Gut 1998;42:387–91.

Scott WW Jr, Fishman EK, Kuhlman JE, et al. Computed tomography of the sacroiliac joints in Crohn's disease. Skeletal Radiol 1990;19:207–10.

Wright V, Watkinson G. The arthritis of ulcerative colitis. BMJ 1965;2:670–5.

Wright V, Watkinson G. Sacroiliitis and ulcerative colitis. BMJ 1965;2:675–80.

[‡] Editor's Note: Arthralgia associated with steroid withdrawal can be confusing and difficult to treat without small doses of NSAIDs or COX-2 inhibitors. (TMB)

CHAPTER 60

Lessons from Treatment of Rheumatoid Arthritis

Ulf Müller-Ladner, MD, and Jürgen Schölmerich, MD

Rheumatoid arthritis (RA) is a disease of very complex pathophysiology, combining genetic factors, alterations of cellular and humoral immune responses, potential involvement of infectious agents, and various mechanisms of tissue destruction. In addition, extra-articular organs can secondarily be affected. When compared to inflammatory bowel diseases (IBDs), remarkable similarities both in pathophysiologic mechanisms and in management of therapy exist, which may allow one to develop novel strategies for each of these disease entities derived from the knowledge of the counterpart.

The current paradigm regarding initiation and perpetuation of RA is that an inciting stimulus (eg, an infectious agent) initiates key mechanisms in a genetically susceptible host. Thereafter, subsequent pathways are activated by other stimuli—of which the most still remain to be determined—leading to intensive immune reactions and development of an aggressively growing synovial tissue and resulting in progressive destruction of the articular components. Inflammatory bowel diseases share a number of these mechanisms, forming a common basis for therapeutic approaches. Tables 60–1 and 60–2 illustrate the various pathophysiologic and therapeutic features that are found to be similar in IBD and RA.

Treatment Strategies

During the past years, both basic research and clinical studies revealed numerous novel aspects and approaches in all fields of RA therapy. The range of nonsteroidal anti-inflammatory drugs (NSAIDs) has been extended by the development of specific cyclo-oxygenase 2 (COX-2) inhibiting drugs and disease-modifying anti-rheumatoid drugs (DMARDs). Combination therapy has been proven to be both safe and effective. The inhibition of pyrimidine synthesis by leflunomide has been added to the spectrum of DMARDs, and targeting "biologic" molecules such as proinflammatory cytokines has generated a new class of drugs bearing the potential of steroid replacement in flares and providing a new component for long-term combination therapy.

TABLE 60–1. Similarities of Pathophysiologic Features of RA and IBD

Pathophysiologic Feature	Rheumatoid Arthritis	Inflammatory Bowel Diseases
Genetic factors	HLA DR4 (eg, HLA DRB1*40xx subtypes)	HLA DR2, DRB1*1502 (ulcerative colitis), HLA DQB1*0402, DRB1*1502 (Crohn's disease), HLA B27
Involvement of microorganisms	Unclassified (retro)viruses	Bacteria
Cellular infiltrates	Lymphocytes, macrophages, dendritic cells	Lymphocytes, macrophages, mast cells
Inflammatory mediators	Prostaglandins, cyclo-oxygenases, leukotrienes, nitric oxide	Prostaglandins, cyclo-oxygenases, leukotrienes, nitric oxide
Cytokines	IL-1, IL-6, TNF-α, and various others	IL-1, IL-6, TNF-α, and various others
Immune phenomena	Rheumatoid factor	Perinuclear cytoplasmic antibodies, anti-saccharomyces antibodies, anti-pancreas acini antibodies
Tissue destruction by disease components	Invading pannus	Fistula (CD)
Tissue destruction by vasculitis, fibrosis	MMPs, cysteine proteinases, possible secondary ankylosis	MMPs, possible intestinal stenosis
Extrafocal manifestations	Rheumatic nodules, serositides	Erythema nodosum, reactive arthritis

TABLE 60–2. Similarities of Response to Therapies in RA and IBD

Response to Established Therapies	Rheumatoid Arthritis	Inflammatory Bowel Diseases
Steroids	+	+
Immunosuppressants (combination therapy)	+ +	+ +
Cyclo-oxygenase inhibitors	+	–
Salicylates	(+) (Sulfasalazine)	+
Antibiotics	? (Minocycline)	(+) (Chinolones, imidazoles)

Early Disease-Modifying Anti-Rheumatoid Drug Therapy

Currently, most rheumatologists tend to use DMARDs much earlier in the course of the disease. *Methotrexate* (MTX) is the initial drug of choice for patients with at least moderate disease activity. Dosage ranges from 5 to 25 mg/week, complemented by an equivalent dose of folic acid 24 hours after MTX intake to minimize side effects. Improvement can be observed after 1 month; usually, the maximum is reached after 6 months. Using MTX monotherapy, complete remission is rare but as compared to other single-drug DMARD therapy, patient satisfaction is good, resulting in 30 percent of the patients still taking MTX after a period of 10 years. Application of gold is still an alternative, but tolerability is significantly better with MTX.

Combination Therapy

In addition, recent clinical trials have confirmed the efficacy and clinical advantage of the early use of DMARD combination therapy (including MTX) by improvement of the majority of standard disease variables (eg, the number of swollen and tender joints, duration of morning stiffness, and the erythrocyte sedimention rate). Among the patients receiving a DMARD combination therapy (MTX, sulfasalazine, hydroxychloroquine), 77 percent were reporting at least 50 percent improvement in disease parameters at 9 months until completion of the study after 24 months, whereas in the other groups (*sulfasalazine/hydroxychloroquine* and MTX monotherapy), only up to 40 percent of patients showed this extent of improvement after 24 months. Interestingly, combination of three DMARDs together with *steroids* resulted in remission in 36 of 97 patients after 2 years. In two other combination studies, significant improvement in swollen and tender joint count was achieved by combination DMARD therapy with MTX and cyclosporine A when compared to MTX monotherapy. Importantly, side effects were not significantly increased, supporting the use of DMARD combination therapy early in the course of the disease.

Leflunomide (Arava, Aventis Pharmaceuticals), is a novel immunomodulating molecule, which acts differently from other DMARDs. It is an inhibitor of tyrosinases and dihydroorotate dehydrogenase, with the latter being the key mechanism that is blocked in RA. Reduction of orotate synthesis by leflumomide leads to inhibition of pyrimidine synthesis and subsequently of DNA and RNA synthesis. Activation of T lymphocytes, in particular, which show an increased need for orotate, is downregulated following application of leflunomide, resulting in a reduction of joint swelling and pain comparable to other DMARDs such as sulfasalazine and MTX. At present, studies combining the effects of MTX (inhibition of purine synthesis) and leflunomide (inhibition of pyrimidine synthesis) are underway, most likely leading to new combination therapies for RA.

Lesson for the gastroenterologist

It is most likely that combinations of different immunosuppressive agents—proven to be safe and reliable in rheumatic diseases—might be beneficial for IBD. Subsequently, studies should be performed that not only evaluate the potential of combination therapy in long-term or "refractory" stages, but also in highly active early disease.

COX-2 INHIBITION: "THE" SOLUTION FOR NSAID SIDE EFFECTS?

The existence of two isoforms of COX, a key player in arachidonic acid metabolism, has been established. COX-1 is constitutively expressed in various tissues regulating physiologic pathways such as platelet function, gastric mucus synthesis, renal sodium balance, and vascular perfusion. Aside from constitutive synthesis, COX-2 is predominantly an inducible enzyme usually expressed following proinflammatory stimuli. It is also involved in regulation of pain and body temperature.

As the hitherto used NSAIDs are not selective for inhibition of one of the two isoforms, side effects such as induction of gastrointestinal ulcers (especially in combination with steroids) and inhibition of platelet aggregation are identical for all currently available NSAIDs. Thus, development of COX-2-specific inhibitors was a desirable goal for RA treatment, and following the semi-specific COX-2 inhibitor meloxicam, which could only be used for mild analgesia and antiphlogism, two highly specific COX-2 inhibitors, rofecoxib and celecoxib, are currently being introduced in clinical practice. Although trial data indicate that up to a fourfold analgesic effect can be achieved when compared to the maximum dosage of COX-1/-2 inhibitors, the most important benefit of specific COX-2 inhibitors might be the considerable reduction of gastrointestinal ulcers. On the other hand, long-term studies may reveal some problems inherent with inhibition of "physiologic" COX-2 mucosal repair functions seen in animal studies, which were further confirmed by key anti-inflammatory effects of COX-2 potentially operative in human intestinal mucosa. However, current clinical trial data in RA support the use of specific COX-2 inhibitors instead of COX-1/-2 inhibitors due to their advantages in increased reduction of pain and inflammation and less side effects.

Lesson for the gastroenterologist

Selective COX-2 inhibitors might resolve the problem of gastrointestinal ulcers during treatment of rheumatoid arthritis. In contrast, recent data indicate that COX-2 appears to be crucial for anti-inflammatory mechanisms in intestinal mucosa and COX-2 inhibitors most likely will not resolve the sequelae of currently used COX-1/-2 inhibitors in treatment of arthritic symptoms in IBD, which frequently aggravate intestinal inflammation or even trigger a flare.

Long-Term Disease-Modifying Anti-Rheumatoid Drug Treatment and Its Complications

Besides the potential decrease of clinical efficiency during long-term DMARD therapy, there are other complications that may force one to modify or alter the therapeutic regimen. The majority of side effects arise from the use of immunosuppressive and immunomodulatory drugs. In RA, these are corticosteroids, MTX, azathioprine, cyclosporine, sulfasalazine, gold, and hydroxychloroquine. Generally, side effects can be divided into three groups: (a) side effects that require termination of the use of this drug, (b) side effects that can be tolerated but must be monitored, and (c) side effects that are known to be temporary.

In long-term therapy, special attention has to be given to the use of steroids. Although few controlled studies exist that examine the cost/benefit value of these drugs, they are widely used, but side effects are constantly feared. However, there is ample clinical evidence for the effectiveness of steroids in rapid amelioration of the symptoms of RA and even for prevention of erosions especially in early RA. In addition to the control of flares and as part of a combination regimen, the main value for RA therapy—equivalent to IBD—may be the "bridging" in active disease before the effects of the DMARDs arise. Table 60–3 summarizes the side effects that have to be considered in long-term therapy in RA.

Lesson for the gastroenterologist

Side effects occurring during the use of immunomodulatory or immunosuppressive drugs do not necessarily imply the termination of the medication but instead an intensification of patient monitoring. Similar to rheumatic disease, short-term high-dose or long-term low-dose steroid should be considered part of the therapeutic armamentarium as a bridge to achievement of reevaluation and/or onset of active immunomodulatory therapy.

New Developments: The "Biologics"

A completely new class of antirheumatic drugs, the so-called "biologics," has been introduced into the therapeutic armamentarium. A number of different monoclonal antibodies and soluble cytokine receptors have been developed to inhibit the effects of proinflammatory cytokines. Among them, TNF-α–targeted substances have been shown to be the most promising. In RA synovium, TNF-α is produced by synovial fibroblasts, macrophages, and T cells. TNF-α stimulates the production of proinflammatory molecules such as interleukin-1, cyclo-oxygenases, and inducible nitric oxide and induces the expression of adhesion molecules such as VCAM-1 and ICAM-1. The latter are thought to be key players in RA pathophysiology, especially in the adhesion of the synovial lining layer to the adjacent cartilage and bone.

Inhibition of TNF-α has been achieved by two antibody-based "biologic" approaches: (a) soluble TNF-α (p55 and p75) receptors, etanercept (Enbrel®, Wyeth-Ayerst, Philadelphia, Pennsylvania) and lenercept, which "capture" circulating TNF-α, and (b) monoclonal murine-human and human antibodies against TNF-α, infliximab (Remicade®, Centocor, Malvern, Pennsylvania), and D2E7, which inactivate TNF-α by specific binding. Interestingly, infliximab also induces apoptosis in activated T cells in the mucosa. All anti–TNF-α biologics require subcutaneous or intravenous application, ranging from twice a week (etanercept, Enbrel) to one injection every 8 weeks (infliximab, Remicade). Current studies show a very rapid decrease in clinical and serologic inflammation parameters, and within days patients

TABLE 60–3. Side Effects of DMARDs in Long-Term RA Therapy and Their Clinical Consequences

Class of Side Effect/ Drug	Discontinuation Required	Continuous Monitoring/ Reduction of Dosage If Possible	Harmless, Frequently Temporary, Continue If Tolerated by the Patient
Corticosteroids	Gastrointestinal ulcers, severe infections	Osteoporosis, diabetes, myopathy, infections, psychotic reactions, cushingoid, osteopathy, cataract, positive tuberculine skin test, glaucoma	Sleep disorders
Methotrexate	Pneumonitis, severe cytopenia, liver cirrhosis, lymphomas	Moderate liver enzyme elevation, moderate cytopenia	Gastrointestinal discomfort
Azathioprine	Severe cytopenia, allergic reactions, lymphomas, pancreatitis	Moderate liver enzyme elevation	Gastrointestinal discomfort
Cyclosporine A	Progressive renal dysfunction, severe neuropathy, severe gingivitis and hypertrichosis, (lymphoma?)	Mild hypertension, mild gingivitis, and hypertrichosis	Mild neuropathy
Leflunomide	Persistent elevation of liver enzymes, allergic reactions	Reversible alopecia	Gastrointestinal discomfort
Sulfasalazine	Pancreatitis, cholestatic hepatitis, allergic (cutaneous) reactions, severe cytopenia, oligospermia	Mild elevation of liver enzymes, mild cytopenia	Gastrointestinal discomfort
Gold	Hypertension, progressive renal dysfunction, severe cytopenia, exanthema	Mild elevation of liver enzymes, mild cytopenia	Gastrointestinal discomfort
Hydroxychloroquine	Severe retinopathy, myopathy, severe cytopenia	Mild retinopathy, exanthema, mild cerebral dysfunction, mild cytopenia	Gastrointestinal discomfort

report amelioration of joint swelling and pain. There is also a rationale for combination of biologics with DMARDs. Infliximab in combination with MTX resulted in a higher number of patients reaching at least 50 percent reduction in clinical activity criteria than patients receiving either MTX or infliximab alone, and the addition of etanercept to MTX therapy in long-term RA treatment resulted in a significant reduction in the tender and swollen joint count.

However, at present, these potent drugs cannot be unrestrictedly recommended for first-line therapy, mainly due to a number of side effects and unanswered questions with long-term therapy. First, patients being considered for anti–TNF-α biologics should not show signs of active infection, as additional immunosuppression may be deleterious. Second, definite application schemes for anti–TNF-α biologics still need to be established. At the time of initiation of therapy, short-lasting soluble TNF-α receptors might be of advantage, whereas later the number of injections may be reduced by the use of anti–TNF-α antibodies. Third, a decrease in effectiveness might be due to development of neutralizing antibodies, especially when anti–TNF-α antibodies are used. Fourth, development of secondary malignancies due to reduced TNF-α activity needs to be monitored closely in long-term follow-up studies. Therefore, TNF-α–directed biologics should be currently used in patients with persistent active disease either in combination with DMARD therapy or to limit or replace the amount of steroids

usually needed to control a flare. Intensive follow-up should accompany these therapies, especially until the questions of whether anti–TNF-α therapies are also able to reduce joint destruction and/or lead to the development of malignancies and autoimmune diseases are sufficiently answered.

Lesson for the gastroenterologist

The development of novel drugs for long-term treatment and for acute flares of RA allows one to consider more intensive therapeutic regimens at an earlier stage of the disease in order to prevent joint destruction and avoid disability. These developments also resulted in replacement of the former therapeutic "pyramid" strategy, which implied an increase in drug dosage and number when increase in activity was noted, by modern "hit-early-and-hard" regimens to suppress inflammation and joint destruction early in the course of the disease. A modern therapeutic strategy for management of RA, which could be also be applied to IBD, is proposed in Table 60–4.

Future Outlook

Introduction of novel immunomodulatory drugs has greatly improved the therapeutic options in RA management in the past years, and combination of DMARDs with biologics may soon become the gold standard in all stages

TABLE 60–4. Current Therapeutic Strategies for Management of RA

Stage of RA	First-Line Therapy (Established)	Second-Line Therapy (Supported by Current Trials)
Presumably RA, criteria not fulfilled	NSAID	SAS + NSAID
Early RA, mild disease	MTX or SASP + NSAID	LEF + NSAID
Early RA, moderate to severe disease	MTX/SAS/HCQ + NSAID	MTX/BIO + NSAID
Long-term RA, mild disease	MTX or SASP + NSAID	LEF + NSAID
Long-term RA, moderate disease, stable	MTX/AZA/HCQ + NSAID	MTX/CyA + NSAID
Long-term RA, flares or progression to severe disease (not controllable with short-term increase in steroid dosage)	MTX/BIO + NSAID	LEF/BIO + NSAID

AZA = azathioprine, BIO = biologics, CyA = cyclosporine A, HCQ = hydroxychloroquine, LEF = leflunomide, MTX = methotrexate, NSAID = nonsteroidal anti-inflammatory drugs (COX-1/-2 inhibitors: diclofenac, ibuprofen, naproxen, and others; COX-2 inhibitors: rofecoxib, celecoxib), SASP = sulfasalazine.

of the disease. In addition, selective COX-2 inhibitors may also reduce the need for high doses of steroids in flares or long-term therapy. However, none of the drugs discussed above has yet proven to inhibit joint destruction completely or even delay it significantly for an extended period of time. Therefore, the outcome of studies examining matrix metalloproteinase inhibitors, due to their potential of inhibiting joint destruction directly at the "hot zone"—the areas of invasion of the aggressively growing synovium into the adjacent cartilage and bone—will be of utmost interest. Overexpression of the pleiotropic inhibitory cytokine IL-10 may also bear beneficial effects. In addition to preclinical data derived from animal models showing downregulation of proinflammatory cytokines, increase of metalloproteinase inhibitor TIMP-1, inhibition of MHC class II expression, and downregulation of adhesion molecule expression, the systemic administration of IL-10 in humans resulted in clinical improvement and reduction of proinflammatory cytokines (in IBD, the beneficial effects of IL-10 were not as obvious). Studies using gene therapy are underway to target key mechanisms at the molecular level, but clinical establishment will require considerable worldwide collaborative effort. Other approaches for curing RA and other immunomodulated diseases by bone marrow transplantation are being evaluated. An overview of some of the future therapeutic approaches for RA is shown in Table 60–5.

Supplemental Reading

Ajuebor MN, Wallace JL. Prostaglandins and nitric oxide: downregulators of intestinal inflammation. In: Rogler G, Kullmann F, Frick E, et al, eds. Cytokines and cell homeostasis in the gastrointestinal tract. London: Kluwer Academic, in press.

Alarcón GS, Tracy IC, Strand GM, et al. Survival and drug discontinuation analyses in a large cohort of methotrexate treated rheumatoid arthritis patients. Ann Rheum Dis 1995;54:708–12.

Jorgensen C, Gay S. Gene therapy in osteoarticular diseases: where are we? Immunol Today 1998;9:387–91.

Kirwan JR, Bálint G, Szebenyi B. Anniversary: 50 years of glucocorticoid treatment in rheumatoid arthritis. Rheumatology 1999;38:100–2.

Lewis EJ, Bishop J, Bottomley KMK, et al. Ro 32-3555, an orally active collagenase inhibitor, prevents cartilage breakdown in vitro and in vivo. Br J Pharmacol 1997;121:540–6.

Maini RN, Breedveld FC, Kalden JR, et al. Therapeutic efficacy of multiple intravenous infusions of anti-tumor necrosis factor alpha monoclonal antibody combined with low-dose weekly methotrexate in rheumatoid arthritis. Arthritis Rheum 1998;41:1552–63.

Martin DK, Singer PA. Bone marrow transplantation for rheumatoid arthritis: the costs for a cure. J Rheumatol 1999;26:1217–8.

Moreland LW, Baumgartner SW, Schiff MH, et al. Treatment of rheumatoid arthritis with a recombinant human tumor necrosis factor receptor (p75)-Fc fusion protein. N Engl J Med 1997;337:141–7.

Möttönen T, Hannonen P, Leirisalo-Repo M, et al. Comparison of combination therapy with single-drug therapy in early

TABLE 60–5. Future Therapeutic Strategies for RA Currently Being Investigated

Therapeutic Strategy	Target
Inhibitory cytokines	IL-10
Inhibition of matrix metalloproteinases	Oral collagenase inhibitors
Local overexpression of inhibitory and cartilage protective molecules	Gene therapy (IL-1Ra)
Anti-adhesion drugs	ICAM-1 antisense constructs

rheumatoid arthritis: a randomised trial. Lancet 1999;353:1568–73.

O'Dell JR, Haire CE, Erikson N, et al. Treatment of rheumatoid arthritis with methotrexate alone, sulfasalazine and hydroxychloroquine, or a combination of all three medications. N Engl J Med 1996;334:1287–91.

Rozman B, for the Leflunomide Investigators' Group. Clinical experience with leflunomide in rheumatoid arthritis. J Rheumatol 1998;25(Suppl 53):27–32.

Tugwell P, Pincus T, Yocum D, et al. Combination therapy with cyclosporine and methotrexate in severe rheumatoid arthritis. N Engl J Med 1995;333:137–41.

CHAPTER 61

Osteopenia and Osteoporosis: Prevention and Treatment

Jeffrey H. Lee, MD, and Jacqueline L. Wolf, MD

Twenty-eight million Americans have osteoporosis or a low bone mass that increases the risk of fracture. Osteoporosis is a major cause of hospitalization and disability in the elderly. Although less well recognized, in patients with inflammatory bowel disease (IBD), a decreased bone mass may be present. Reductions in bone mineral density (BMD) are termed osteopenia and osteoporosis. Osteoporosis is defined as 2.5 standard deviations (SDs) and osteopenia as 1 to 2.5 SDs below the mean peak bone mass.

According to some studies, greater lifetime calcium intake, adequate vitamin D, gender (male > female), and ethnicity (African American > Caucasians) positively affect bone density. Reduction in bone mass is affected by calcium absorption and factors causing high bone turnover. Bone loss occurs with age and is rapid following menopause and during corticosteroid therapy.

Bone consists of trabecular and cortical bone. The majority of osteoporosis-related fractures occur in the trabecular (less dense) bone found in vertebrae, ribs, the pelvis, and in the ends of long bones. However, fractures commonly occur in the femoral, neck, and long bones, sites that contain more cortical bone. Every year, more than 1.5 million Americans suffer from fractures related to osteoporosis. Cummings et al (1993), in a prospective study, showed that reduction of bone mass in the spine and hip by 1 SD compared with age-adjusted controls is associated with a 1.6- and 2.6-fold increased risk for hip fracture. The most important preventable cause of fractures is low bone mass. Thus, a low hip bone density is the most predictive of the risk of hip fracture.

Osteoporosis and Inflammatory Bowel Disease

Osteoporosis is present in 23 to 59 percent of patients with IBD, and bone loss occurs in both trabecular and cortical bone. Patients with IBD have not only the general risk factors for osteoporosis but also additional factors. Low weight and body mass index; poor calcium intake, owing to lactase deficiency; malnutrition; ileal resection; Ca and Mg malabsorption; sex hormone deficiency; reduced physical activity; smoking, in women; the presence of bone-resorptive cytokines (interleukin [IL]-6, IL-1, tumor necrosis factor [TNF]); and corticosteroid therapy all may contribute to the development of osteoporosis. In some studies, bone loss is higher in patients with Crohn's disease (CD) than ulcerative colitis (UC), but in others no difference has been observed between those with CD and those with UC. Gokhale et al (1998) found that low bone mineral density (BMD) occurs in children with IBD, especially pubertal and postpubertal girls, and more often in CD than in UC. It is important to realize that active disease, even before steroid use, is associated with excessive bone turnover and bone loss. Cumulative corticosteroid dose is an important predictor of low BMD.

Severe osteoporosis occurs in patients with primary sclerosing cholangitis, especially with longer duration of IBD and advanced liver disease. Ursodeoxycholic acid does not affect the rate of bone loss in primary sclerosing cholangitis.

Corticosteroids and Osteoporosis in Inflammatory Bowel Disease

Corticosteroids decrease net intestinal absorption of calcium, increase urinary phosphate and calcium loss by effects on the kidneys, increase the risk of kidney stones, suppress gonadal steroid production, and inhibit osteoblasts by inhibiting differentiation of osteoblast precursors and decreasing synthesis of osteoblast products, for example, osteocalcin. The most significant effect of corticosteroid use is on the trabecular bone. The reduction in bone mass of patients with IBD is, in part, attributed to the use of corticosteroids. Bone loss is dependent on both steroid dose and duration of therapy. With high-dose corticosteroids, bone loss may be rapid with rates of 5 to 15 percent per year and is most rapid in the first 6 to 12 months. Even low-dose corticosteroids may cause bone loss. Low-dose (< 10 mg/d) steroid therapy was associated with a reduced BMD in men and postmenopausal but not premenopausal women. The greatest decrease in bone density occurs in the first few months of therapy. Alternate-day corticosteroids in adolescent patients with IBD seem to prevent accelerated bone loss.

Rectal steroids do not significantly impair bone turnover in patients with IBD. Cyclosporine A causes time- and dose-dependent bone loss. Azathioprine (AZA) does not affect the bones.

Diagnostic Approach

Bone density measurement by dual-photon absorptiometry performed at both the hip and the spine is the best indicator of osteoporotic fracture risk. Further assessment of factors affecting bone health includes measurement of the serum 25-hydroxyvitamin D level, calcium, phosphorus, alkaline phosphatase (bone specific), osteocalcin, and intact parathyroid hormone (PTH) levels, urinary N-telopeptide (a measure of osteoclastic activity), and 24-hour urinary calcium. In steroid-treated men, testosterone measurements should be done because they often are low, and a decreased hormone level increases the risks of a reduction in bone density.

Prevention

The most important ways to prevent osteoporosis are to achieve the highest bone mass during young adulthood and to decrease the rate of subsequent bone loss. Preventive strategies include exercising (some weight-bearing exercise and walking 30 to 60 minutes three to four times a week), consuming an adequate amount of dietary calcium and vitamin D (400 to 800 IU), avoiding excess alcohol and smoking, and replacing sex steroids when they are deficient. Regular, moderate exercise can decrease the risk of falls and fractures and improve overall quality of life for subjects with osteoporosis. Daily dietary calcium requirements are listed in Table 61–1. Estrogen is recommended for postmenopausal women at high risk for osteoporosis without any contraindications.

Corticosteroid-treated patients should be placed on the lowest possible doses of steroids for the least possible time. Budesonide theoretically has fewer deleterious effects on bone turnover than the equivalent amount of prednisone; 9 mg of budesonide was statistically equivalent to 40 mg prednisone in producing remissions in patients with CD in the ileum and right colon. Alternatives such as AZA or 6-mercaptopurine (6-MP) should be considered in patients with IBD.

Treatment

Drugs used to treat osteoporosis can be grouped into two classes: antiresorptive drugs and drugs that increase bone mass. Antiresorptive drugs decrease the imbalance between bone resorption and formation, decrease the overall rate of bone turnover, or decrease both. The reduction in the resorption of trabecular plates that results from antiresorptive therapy stabilizes the bone structure and decreases the risk of fracture. Thus, antiresorptive drugs are well suited for the prevention of osteo-

TABLE 61–1. Daily Calcium Requirements

Patient	Required Calcium (mg)
Adult*	
Pregnant or lactating and > 19 yr	1300
19–50 yr	1000
51–70 yr	1200
Child†	
6 mo–1yr	400
1–3 yr	270
4–8 yr	500–800
9–18 yr	1,300

* Dietary Reference Intake (DRI) committee 1997: upper limit, 2500 mg; †DRI committee 1997: upper limit,

porosis and many are effective for the treatment of osteoporosis. They are the drugs most frequently used. Antiresorptive agents include calcium, hydrochlorothiazide, vitamin D, calcitriol (1,25-dihydroxyvitamin D), estrogen, estrogen receptor modulators, calcitonin, and bisphosphonates.

Drugs that increase bone mass increase bone formation more than bone resorption. These include sodium fluoride, PTH, and growth factors.

Antiresorptive Agents

CALCIUM

Supplemental calcium helps prevent bone loss in women with low baseline calcium intake, in older women and in women with osteoporosis. Calcium is bioavailable in milk. Calcium citrate is more bioavailable than calcium carbonate with fewer gastrointestinal (GI) side effects. A commonly recommended dosage of calcium citrate is 600 mg twice per day.

HYDROCHLOROTHIAZIDE

Low-dose hydrochlorothiazide therapy may correct hypercalciuria that is common in men with osteoporosis and in patients treated with glucocorticoids. Hydrochlorothiazide can lead to an increase in BMD. Hypercalciuria and nephrolithiasis occur commonly in corticosteroid-treated subjects and hyperoxaluria and calcium oxalate stones may develop in patients with malabsorption. In those patients with urinary calcium excretions > 300 mg/24 h, hydrochlorothiazide should be instituted to reduce the risk of nephrolithiasis formation and to improve calcium homeostasis. In those patients with hyperoxaluria, a low-oxalate diet should be followed.

VITAMIN D

Vitamin D is absorbed in the jejunum and ileum. For absorption, vitamin D requires bile acids, which undergo enterohepatic circulation. Therefore, patients with ileal resections are susceptible to vitamin D deficiency. Vitamin D is available in several preparations: oral vitamin D (intramuscularly in severe malabsorption), 25-hydroxyvitamin D (Calderol®, Organon, West Orange, New Jersey), 1,25-dihydroxyvitamin D (Rocaltrol®, Roche Labs, Nutley, New Jersey). Vitamin D commonly is a component of multivitamins (usually 400 IU) and calcium citrate and calcium carbonate tablets. Calcitriol, the active vitamin D metabolite (1,25-dihydroxyvitamin D), acts mainly by increasing calcium absorption but also may stimulate the function of osteoblasts. Calcitriol treatment improves calcium balance and decreases the rate of vertebral fracture. In some studies, but not all, it transiently increased bone mass. The "therapeutic window" between effective doses and those that induce hypercalcemia or hypercalciuria is relatively narrow. Calcitriol should be avoided in most cases because of the development of hypercalcemia in up to one-fourth of patients. When there is vitamin D deficiency (25-hydroxyvitamin D level less than 9 mg/mL), high doses of vitamin D preparations are necessary, and the patient is best monitored by a specialist in bone metabolism.

ESTROGENS

A third to half of all bone loss in women may be attributable to menopause. Estrogen therapy arrests bone loss in postmenopausal women. Long-term estrogen replacement therapy more than 6 years after menopause results in bone gain of about 3 to 5 percent over a period of about 12 months and, if continued, prevents a resumption of bone loss. If begun soon after menopause, estrogen therapy prevents the early phase of bone loss. In women with established osteoporosis, estrogen therapy still is effective. Raloxifene (an estrogen receptor modulator) is effective in preventing bone loss in postmenopausal women, although with less efficacy than estrogen. Women with a history of breast cancer or with a family history of breast cancer should find an alternative to estrogen for therapy.

CALCITONIN

Calcitonin acts directly on osteoclasts to inhibit bone resorption. It causes a gain in bone mass of about 4 to 5 percent over a period of 18 to 24 months when given parenterally at a daily dose of 100 IU. Calcitonin (Miocalcin®, Novartis Pharmaceuticals Corp., Greensboro, North Carolina) at a dose of 200 IU/d is available in the United States as an intranasal spray that is approved by the Food and Drug Administration (FDA) for the treatment of osteoporosis. It is sprayed into alternate nostrils on alternate days.

BISPHOSPHONATES

Bisphosphonates (etidronate, pamidronate, tiludronate, alendronate, and risedronate) are carbon-substituted analogues of pyrophosphate, an endogenous physiologic inhibitor of bone mineralization. Bisphosphonates inhibit

TABLE 61–2. Recommendations for Prevention and Treatment of Osteoporosis in Patients with Inflammatory Bowel Disease

Evaluation
   Dual-photon absorptiometry of hip and spine in all patients with IBD
      (1) At baseline
      (2) After 1 year in patients on glucocorticoids or with osteopenia or osteoporosis or after 1 to 2 years in patients with active IBD
   Serum 25-hydroxyvitamin D in all patients with malabsorption, malnutrition, or osteopenia/osteoporosis

Prophylaxis in all patients
   Calcium as outlined above
   Vitamin D (400–800 IU)
   Regular weight-bearing physical activity
   Elimination of smoking and excessive alcohol
   Testosterone replacement in deficient men
   Hormonal replacement in postmenopausal women unless contraindicated

Additional measures in patients on corticosteroids
   Calcium 1500 mg daily ingestion
   Maintainance of corticosteroids (or budesonide) at lowest possible level
   Measurement of 24-hour urinary calcium. If high and persistently elevated for 4 weeks, consider thiazide diuretics or other measures.
   If osteopenia, treat as osteoporosis if steroids are to be continued or if there are additional high factors, such as malabsorption or inactivity*

Established osteoporosis or vitamin D deficient
   Refer to a specialist in endocrinology or bone health for further treatment with bisphosphonate, calcitonin, or high doses of vitamin D

*Editor's Note: In the presence of osteopenia and continued corticosteroid use, there are those who recommend bisphosphonate therapy. I consider budesonide (6 mg/d) as steroid therapy and treat osteopenia hoping to prevent osteoporosis. Risedronate (Actonel) produces fewer upper gastrointestinal symptoms and fewer gastric and esophageal ulcers than alendronate (Fosamax) and may be useful in patients with IBD. Upper gastrointestinal symptoms with risedronate were no more frequent than with placebo. (TMB)

bone resorption by tightly binding to hydroxyapatite crystals. Both risedronate (Actonel®, Procter & Gamble, Cincinnati, Ohio), and alendronate (Fosamax®, Merck Research Laboratories, West Point, New Jersey) are potent bisphosphonates available in the United States and FDA approved for treatment and prevention of postmenopausal osteoporosis and treatment of glucocorticoid-induced osteoporosis. Risedronate also is approved for prevention of glucocorticoid-induced osteoporosis. Two 48-week, randomized, placebo-controlled studies of two dosages (5 and 10 mg/d) of alendronate in 477 men and women, 17 to 83 years of age, who were receiving glucocorticoid therapy, showed that alendronate produced a small increase in bone density in patients receiving glucocorticoid therapy. Risedronate (Actonel) (5 mg/d) was similarly protective. A trend toward fewer vertebral fractures was noted in study patients. Risedronate (Actonel), 5 mg, has been shown to prevent bone loss in the lumbar spine and femoral neck over a 12-month period in patients with rheumatoid arthritis and others not with IBD illness receiving an average of 20 mg/d of prednisone. It has been approved by the FDA for the treatment and prevention of glucocorticoid-induced osteoporosis.

Alendronate (Fosamax®) can cause esophagitis and esophageal ulcerations. It should be taken once a day on an empty stomach at least 30 minutes before breakfast with 8 ounces of water, and the person should remain upright after ingestion. Risedronate (Actonel®) is expected to cause less GI upset and should be useful in the IBD population. There were fewer gastric and esophageal ulcers among postmenopausal women taking 5 mg of risedronate than among those taking 10 mg of alendronate. Symptoms were similar to those seen in patients on placebo.

Summary

A summary of recommendations is given in Table 61–2.

References

Cummings SR, Black DM, Vogt TM, et al. Bone density at various sites for prediction of hip fractures. The study of Osteoporotic Fractures Research Group. Lancet 1993; 341:72–75.

Gokhale R, Favus MJ, Karrison T, et al. Bone mineral density assessment in children with inflammatory bowel disease. Gastroenterology 1998;114:902-11.

Supplemental Reading

Adams JS, Song CF, Kantorovich V. Rapid recovery of bone mass in hypercalciuric, osteoporotic men treated with hydrochlorothiazide. Ann Intern Med 1999;130:658–60.

Butler RC, Davie MW, Corsfold M, et al. Bone mineral content in patients with rheumatoid arthritis: relationship to low-dose steroid therapy. Br J Rheumatol 1991;30:86–90

Cohen S, Levy RM, Keller M, et al. Risedronate therapy prevents corticosteroid-induced bone loss: a twelve-month, multicenter, randomized, double-blind, placebo-controlled, parallel-group study. Arthritis Rheum 1999;42:2309–18.

Eastell R. Drug therapy: treatment of postmenopausal osteoporosis. N Engl J Med 1998;338:736–46.

Lanza FL, Hunt RH, Thompson ABR, et al. Endoscopy study comparing risedronate and alendronate in postmenopausal women [abstract]. Gastroenterology 2000;188.

LeBoff MS. Is prolonged use of corticosteroids safe in patients with Crohn's disease? Inflamm Bowel Dis 1999;3:169–73.

Pignot F, Roux C, Chaussade S, et al. Low bone mineral density in patients with inflammatory bowel disease. Dig Dis Sci 1992;37:1396–403.

Recker RR. Clinical review 41: current therapy for osteoporosis. J Clin Endocrinol Metab 1993;76;14–6.

Reid DM, Hughes RA, Laan RFJM, et al. Efficacy and safety of daily risedronate in the treatment of corticosteroid-induced osteoporosis in men and women: a randomized trial. J Bone Miner Res 2000;15:1006–13.

Riggs BL, Melton LJ III. The prevention and treatment of osteoporosis. N Engl J Med 1992;327:620–7.

Roux C, Abitol V, Chaussade S, et al. Bone loss in patients with inflammatory bowel disease: a prospective study. Osteoporos Int 1995;5:156–60.

Saag KG, Emkey R, Schnitzer TJ, et al. Alendronate for the prevention and treatment of glucocorticoid-induced osteoporosis. N Engl J Med 1998;339:292–9.

Schulte C, Dignass AU, Mann K, Goebell H. Bone loss in patients with inflammatory bowel disease is less than expected: a follow-up study. Scand J Gastroenterol 1999;34:696–702.

Silvennoinen JA, Karttunen TJ, Lehtola JK et al. A controlled study of bone mineral density in patients with inflammatory bowel disease. Gut 1995;37:71–6.

Valentine JF, Sninsky CA. Prevention and treatment of osteoporosis in patients with inflammatory bowel disease. Am J Gastroenterol 1999;94:878–83.

CHAPTER 62

ISCHEMIC NECROSIS OF BONE

THOMAS M. ZIZIC, MD, AND PETER A. HOLT, MD

Osteonecrosis (ON) and avascular necrosis of bone (AVN) are the commonly used terms for an entity that also is referred to as ischemic necrosis of bone, aseptic necrosis, and osteochondritis dissecans. Because the bone is truly avascular only in the end stage of the disease, the term ischemic necrosis of bone is preferred, emphasizing the period of ischemia that precedes actual bone death. Pathologically, it is characterized by death of cells in bone, resulting from an interruption of blood supply to bone.

Osteonecrosis afflicts between 10,000 to 20,000 new patients per year in the United States. Although patients can be affected at any age, the majority of patients develop the disease in the fourth decade of life. Since the disease does not affect longevity, there are several hundred thousand people living with the disease in the United States alone.

Osteonecrosis generally is divided into two major forms: post-traumatic and nontraumatic. Neither minor nor major trauma causes ON *unless* there has been a fracture or dislocation resulting in physical damage to the arterial circulation.

Disease Associations

There are a number of primary diseases that are associated with the development of ischemic bone changes, including hemoglobinopathies, Gaucher's disease, alcoholism, coagulopathies, decompression sickness, trauma, pancreatitis, systemic lupus erythematosus, and Crohn's disease. Diseases, such as inflammatory bowel disease (IBD), in which corticosteroids often are used in high doses and for prolonged periods pose an increased risk. Patients with IBD who present with ON may be younger than other patients with ischemic bone changes, and some have ON without having taken steroids.

Approximately 30 percent of patients have idiopathic osteonecrosis. Many of these patients may have subclinical coagulation abnormalities with thrombophilia or hypofibrinolysis. At Johns Hopkins, we recently evaluated 25 consecutive patients with nontraumatic ON and 22 (88%) were found to have one or more coagulation disorders as measured by thrombophilic factors, such as protein C, protein S, resistance to activated protein C, antiphospholipids, homocysteine, lupus, anticoagulant, or hypofibrinolytic factors, such as plasminogen activator

inhibitor, tissue plasminogen activator activity, and alpha lipoprotein. Occasionally, if plasma triglycerides are high, these can increase the risk of blood clotting, or affect how the body dissolves clots. Patients with coagulopathy-induced ON rarely have abnormalities in the routine coagulation tests (PTT or Bro-Time); consequently, they will be detected only if the above factors are tested (protein C, protein S, anticardiolipin etc.).

Sites of Involvement

Regardless of underlying disease or therapy, the hips most frequently are involved, followed by the knees and shoulders. More rarely, the scaphoid bone of the foot, the body of the talus (ankle), and the scaphoid bone of the hand are affected. There is a correlation between involvement of the talus with the diagnosis of IBD and the long-term administration of glucocorticoids. Multiple sites of bone involvement also correlate with the diagnosis of IBD or systemic lupus erythematosus, perhaps because both diseases often are treated with high doses of steroids for long periods.

Relation to Glucocorticoids

Glucocorticoids were first implicated in the development of ischemic necrosis of bone almost 30 years ago. In patients with systemic lupus erythematosus (SLE), the highest mean daily prednisone dose for a single month (Table 62–1) as well as the highest for 3, 6, and 12 months of consecutive therapy, is significantly higher in patients who develop ischemic necrosis of bone. The mean daily dose of prednisone was higher than 40 mg/d in 93 percent and higher than 25 mg/d in all patients who subsequently developed ischemic necrosis of bone. Thus, there

TABLE 62–1. Prednisone Dosage Parameters (SLE)

Parameter	Ischemic Necrosis of Bone	
	Present (28)	Absent (26)
Highest month (prednisone mg/day)	81.0* (25–220)	56.7 (5–190)
Total cumulative dose prednisone mg)	45,300 (2,970–124,215)	41,880 150–109,245)
Duration of steroid therapy (months)	64 (2–174)	91* (1–215)

*$p < .05$

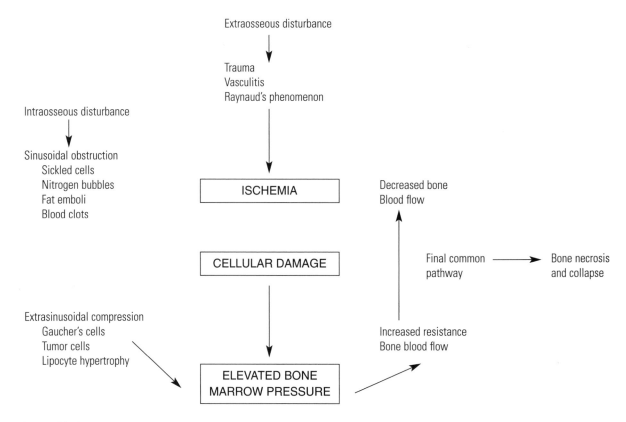

FIGURE 62–1. The etiology of ischemic necrosis of bone is multifactorial. There are a number of ways in which bone marrow pressure may be elevated directly (eg, lipocyte hypertrophy in steroid-treated patients) or via ischemia with resultant cellular damage and edema (eg, fatty emboli in alcoholids). The final common pathway appears to be elevated bone marrow pressure with increased resistance and decreased bone blood flow. The resultant ischemia and subsequent cellular damage with edema and eventual fibrosis cause a further increase in intraosseous pressure. If uninterrupted, this viscious amplification cycle eventuates in bone necrosis and collapse.

is a minimum threshold of approximately 25 mg of prednisone per day for more than a month for even the most susceptible patient to develop ON secondary to corticosteroids. This minimum threshold of dose and duration is required to alter fat metabolism sufficiently to produce ON. There is a statistically significant correlation between higher mean prednisone dose at all time intervals and increased number of bone sites involved. The total cumulative steroid dose was not significantly different in the patients who developed bone complications and those who did not. It should be noted that the minimum duration of corticosteroid therapy was more than 2 months. In a meta-analysis of more than 1,500 patients, Felson and Anderson (1987) found similar results. The vast majority of clinical studies clearly demonstrate that the higher the dose and the longer the duration of corticosteroids, the greater the number of patients who will develop osteo-necrosis. Patients with Crohn's disease and ON described by Vakil and Sparburg were younger and had a lower steroid exposure than the usual ON patient.

Pathogenesis

The vast majority of patients with corticosteroid-induced ischemic necrosis of bone become cushingnoid prior to the development of their bony complication. Just as enlarging fat cells can be seen to produce the moon-shaped face, intramedullary lipocytes enlarge by 69 percent. This lipocyte hypertrophy within the bone increases bone marrow pressure, producing progressive ischemia and eventual bone death.

The initial ischemic episode also can be produced by either *extraosseous or intraosseous circulatory disturbances* (Figure 62–1). Trauma such as a fracture or dislocation with severance of major vessels, vasculitis, or vasospasm (Raynaud's disease) can result in ischemia by interference with the extraosseous macrovasculature. Intraosseously, ischemia can occur through obstruction of the sinusoidal microcirculation by sickled erythrocytes in hemoglobinopathies, nitrogen bubbles in decompression sickness, fatty emboli in alcoholics or patients with pancreatitis, or by clots in patients with coagulation disorders. Compression of the microcirculation via elevation of intraosseus pressure can occur by *intramedullary lipocyte hypertrophy in steroid-treated patients* or by abnormal cells, such as metastatic tumor or Gaucher's cells filling the marrow space. It is the continued increase in bone marrow pressure compressing the microvasculature in the rigid osseous compartment in concert with weight-bearing that produces necrosis with eventual collapse, unless the cycle is interrupted early enough by a procedure such as core decompression.

Clinical Symptoms and Signs

In *femoral head necrosis*, the initial symptom is usually *pain in the groin* that intermittently radiates down the anteromedial thigh. It should be noted that there may be a delay of months to years between the onset of symptoms and the appearance of radiologic abnormalities. Most patients have "mechanical" pain induced by standing, walking, moving, or other mechanical stress but eased by rest. Another remarkable feature is that the *symptoms may begin suddenly* so that many patients remember the day and hour when they first felt a sudden, severe, and incapacitating pain. Approximately two-thirds have pain at rest and slightly more than one-third have pain at night, which may be associated with prolonged morning pain or stiffness. Involvement of the *knee* is similar to that of the hip except that limitations of motion, which eventually develop in two-thirds of patients with hip involvement, only occur in one-quarter of patients with knee involvement. Involvement of the *humeral head* may go undetected, because the shoulder is not a weight-bearing joint and symptoms may be transient or minimal. Generally, pain in the shoulder is *insidious* in onset, is made *worse by activity*, and *radiates to the deltoid tuberosity* of the humerus. The major complaint is pain on motion, but limitation of active motion also is seen early in the course. Collapse of the talus causes heel pain.

Imaging Techniques

There may be a delay between the onset of symptoms and the appearance of radiologic abnormalities ranging from several months to up to 5 years. Twenty percent of 310 ischemic bones found among the authors' study group were roentgenographically normal. Thus, the disease in these patients must be detected and diagnosed by other means. This is particularly important because these are the patients who will do best with treatment. *Early diagnosis before segmental collapse occurs is essential to effective treatment.*

Aggressive diagnostic evaluations should be done in patients in whom there is a *high index of suspicion of ON*. Patients with *unexplained hip pain* who have been taking *more than 25 mg/d of prednisone for more than 2 months*, patients who average *2 or more alcoholic drinks per day*, or patients with *coagulation disorders* are prime candidates. Additionally, the contralateral hip of patients who have unilateral symptoms should be carefully evaluated, since the prevalence of *bilaterality* has been reported to be between *50 and 80 percent*

Radiographic Evaluation

Good quality radiographs are the first step in the diagnosis of ON. If they are confirmative, it is not necessary to do magnetic resonance imaging (MRI). If one is attempting to assess the degree of collapse to help determine the best therapeutic option for that patient, then tomography or CT scans are generally superior to MRI for this purpose.

With respect to the hip, both *anteroposterior* and *frog-leg lateral radiographs* are necessary. Anteroposterior radiographs usually demonstrate the principal area of involvement. Because the anterior and posterior acetabular margins overlap the superior portion of the femoral head, subtle evidence of osteosclerotic or cystic changes in the subchondral regions may be missed. Consequently, it is imperative that good quality frog-leg lateral radiographs of the femoral head be performed.

Radionuclide Scanning Techniques

Radionuclide scans have definitive advantages over radiographs, since abnormalities evident on bone scans may precede radiologic changes by 2 to 18 months. In the earliest phase (days to weeks) following a vascular insult with subsequent development of ischemic necrosis, the involved area may appear "cold" on the scintiscan owing to absent blood supply in the avascular segment. Usually by the time a scan is obtained, weeks to months have gone by and revascularization and appositional new bone formation produce "hot" areas, because of increased uptake of radioisotope until repair is completed. False-negative qualitative scans are seen because, with bilateral involvement, there may be minimal but symmetric uptake on each side, so that both sides are interpreted as normal, and if uptake is asymmetric, the more severe side makes the less involved side look normal by comparison. Quantitative scintimetry detects about three-quarters of those patients with early (preradiologic) ischemic necrosis of bone. Three-phase radionuclide scanning may be even more helpful in detecting early ischemic necrosis of bone.

Increased uptake alone can be seen in reflex sympathetic dystrophy, infections, tumors, and transient migratory osteoporosis, as well as ON. A photopenic area, or "cold" spot, surrounded by an area of increased activity is highly suggestive of ON. Because a bone scan is a low-cost examination compared with MRI, it is generally the next step in evaluating a radiographically negative patient with suspected ON.

Magnetic Resonance Imaging

In high-risk patients with suggestive clinical symptoms and signs and normal radiographs and radionuclide scans, MRI is the next procedure used to evaluate those with possible ischemic necrosis of bone. Its major advantage is that it is a noninvasive study without radiation exposure. Its major disadvantage is its high cost, particularly if serial follow-up for multiple areas is required.

The earliest finding in ON is a single-density line (a low-intensity signal) on T^1-weighted images. Presumably, this represents a line of separation between normal and ischemic bone. On T^2-weighted images, a second, high-signal intensity line may be found within this line. This is the almost pathognomonic double-line sign and represents hypervascular granulation tissue. At times, even MRI does not detect very early ON. Koo and colleagues (1994) reported on 136 biopsy specimens that were consistent with ON; 10 had negative MRI.

Bone Marrow Pressure and Intraosseous Venography

Increased bone marrow pressure or decreased venous outflow is characteristic of ischemic necrosis of bone, irrespective of its radiologic stage. Among the authors' study group (Zizic et al, 1986), 223 (84%) patients with osteonecrotic bones had abnormal bone marrow pressure (baseline bone marrow pressure of 30 mm Hg or higher or an elevation of more than 10 mm Hg following the injection of 5 mL of saline as a stress test). The addition of intraosseous venography to the pressure studies increased detection capabilities, so that 94 percent of bones with radiologically or histologically proven ON were recognized. One of the important aspects of these hemodynamic studies is their predictive potential in patients with radiologically normal bones. Patients with unilateral ischemic necrosis of bone had bone marrow pressure measurements and intraosseous venograms performed on the asymptomatic and radiologically normal side. Thirty-six of 48 joints had increased bone marrow pressure and of these, 15 (42%) developed histologically or radiographically confirmed ischemic necrosis of bone. In none of the 12 bones with normal bone marrow pressure did ischemic necrosis of bone occur ($p = .005$) (Zizic et al, 1989).

Diagnosis

At times, the early diagnosis of ischemic necrosis of bone can be difficult. This is especially true in patients with IBD, since approximately 10 to 15 percent have arthritis involving, particularly, the large, lower extremity weight-bearing joints—the same areas most often affected by ischemic necrosis of bone. The key to diagnosis is in having a high index of suspicion in patients with appropriate clinical symptoms and signs who are at high risk for the development of ischemic bone changes. Diagnostic criteria for ON are presented in Table 62–2. The presence of any one of the four listed factors confirms the diagnosis of ON.

Treatment

If the bone disease is uninterrupted, the majority of patients have eventual destruction of the joints, because of the amplification loop with gradually progressive ischemia. Once the disease is roentgenographically evi-

TABLE 62–2. Diagnostic Criteria for Osteonecrosis

Test	Finding
Radiographs	Collapse of femoral head or Subchondral radiolucent line or Anterolateral sequestrium
Nuclear scans	Bone scan with "cold" spot surrounded by "hot" spot
Magnetic resonance imaging	Double band on T^2-weighted MRI
Bone biopsy	Empty lacunae involving multiple adjacent trabeculae

dent, it usually is progressive and eventually produces significant joint dysfunction. One of the major therapeutic challenges of ON in patients with IBD is that it generally affects young and otherwise physically active individuals. The excellent results of total joint replacement for other conditions in older patients have not been realizable in younger patients who are more active. Consequently, short of replacement arthroplasty, ways of salvaging ischemic bones continue to be explored.

Medical Management

Conservative or medical management consists primarily of nonload-bearing in an attempt to prevent collapse while repair is completed. Only about one-quarter of patients improve spontaneously and have a tolerable disability. Eventually, 90 percent of patients have some degree of collapse of the joint head, with the development of a progressive arthrosis. This is particularly true of the hip, where once radiologic changes occur, the patient almost always requires surgical intervention to have a reasonable chance to maintain acceptable hip joint function. However, conservative treatment of the shoulder is more successful. Almost half of the patients treated with intensive physical therapy, consisting of maintenance of motion through a vigorous program of pendulum exercises and a decrease in forces acting across the shoulder by avoidance of abduction, had excellent results, as measured by range of motion and the patient's success in returning to most normal activities.

Core Decompression Biopsy

Core decompression biopsy consists of inserting a hollow trephine up the neck and head of the femur. The rationale for this procedure is that by removing an 8- to 11-mm core of cancellous bone from the ischemic segment, there is a decrease in the intraosseous pressure (decompression), which reduces the forces compressing the sinusoidal microcirculation. This interrupts the amplification loop of the increased pressure that leads to the decreased bone blood flow that produces ischemia and edema and results in further increased pressure, decreased bone blood flow, and progressive ischemia (see Figure 62–1). By using a hollow trephine instead of a solid drill, a cylinder of bone is extracted that can be examined histologically to confirm the diagnosis in patients with preradiologic disease. It is likely that core biopsy and decompression stimulate the adjacent living bone and induce formation of new capillaries and progenitor cells as well as create avenues for revascularization and repopulation of the dead portions of the bone.

In a recent study from Johns Hopkins, the long-term results of core decompression were evaluated in 128 hips at an average of 11 years (range, 4 to 19 yr). On the basis of survival of the hip (no additional treatment required), a successful result was found in 22 (88%) of the 25 hips with stage I disease, 36 (71%) of the 51 hips with stage II disease, and 14 (27%) of the 52 hips with stage III disease. Survivorship analysis showed that 83 percent of patients would have a good result at 10 years. Since it is a simple procedure, with considerably less than an hour of intraoperative time, a short hospitalization, and significantly fewer requirements for postoperative nonweight-bearing than procedures such as bone grafting or osteotomy, it is a reasonable palliative procedure for stage III and IV disease. Additionally, since it does not interfere with any surgical procedures that may be needed subsequently, it should be included in the armamentarium for the management of ischemic necrosis of bone in young patients and in those who are poor surgical risks for more major procedures. Complications have been minimal; three fractures occurred through the core site, due to patient falls in the 6 weeks after surgery, and one patient developed a postoperative ipsilateral thrombophlebitis; no pulmonary embolus occurred and no infections or deaths have occurred.

Joint Replacement

Approximately 10 percent of total hip replacements are done in patients who have ON. The majority of studies demonstrate a higher rate of early failure compared to age-matched patients who have total hip replacements for other diagnoses. Consequently, the total societal cost is considerable; these patients are generally young, hold jobs, and have a life expectancy that makes additional operations probable. For these reasons, it is preferable to attempt to delay or eliminate the need for hip replacement by treating this condition with operative procedures that preserve the femoral head.

Total hip or knee replacements, although effective, are of greater risk than the more conservative procedures, such as core decompression. In one large series, the incidence of pulmonary embolism was almost 8 percent, with a 1.5 percent fatality rate. Other complications include infection, dislocation, and loosening of the prosthesis. The latter is particularly likely to occur in active patients under the age of 40 years, who have a 50-50 chance of having revision of their total joint replacement. Nevertheless, total hip replacement is the procedure of choice when there is multisystem disease, when patients are in poor general health, or for patients who are likely to require ≥ 25 mg of prednisone per day for prolonged periods of time.

Total shoulder replacement also has been reported to give excellent results in ischemic necrosis of bone of the humeral head. This is a more difficult procedure than total hip replacement, in which bone supplies stability or total knee replacement, in which the ligaments help provide some stability. Since the muscles are so critical for both stability and movement, optimal function requires as much skill in the reconstruction of rotator cuff and deltoid muscles as in the orientation and insertion of the implants.

References

Fairbank AC, Bhatia D, Jinnah RH, Hungerford DS. Long-term results of core decompression for ischemic necrosis of the femoral head. J Bone Joint Surg Br 1995;77:42–9.

Felson DT, Anderson JJ. A cross-study evaluation of association between steroid dose and bolus steroids and avascular necrosis of bone. Lancet 1987;1:902–6.

Koo KH, Kim RH, Ko KH, Cho SH. Changing pattern of bone marrow edema in early-stage osteonecrosis of the femoral head. A prospective study with repeated MR images. ARCO Proc 1994;5:50,.

Vakil N, Sparberg M. Steroid-related osteonecrosis in inflammatory bowel disease. Gastroenerology 1989;96:62–7.

Zizic TM, Lewis CG, Marcoux C, Hungerford DS. The predictive value of hemodynamic studies in preclinical ischemic necrosis of bone. J Rheumatol 1989;16:1559–64.

Zizic TM, Marcoux C, Hungerford DS, Stevens MB. The early diagnosis of necrosis of bone. Arthritis Rheum 1986; 29:1177–86.

Supplemental Reading

Conklin JJ, Alderson PO, Zizic TM, et al. Comparison of bone scan and radiograph sensitivity in detection of steroid-induced ischemic necrosis of bone. Radiology 1983;147:221–6.

Freeman HJ. Osteomyelitis and osteonecrosis in inflammatory bowel disease. Can J Gastroenterol 1997;11:601–6.

Shapiro SC, Rothstein FC, Newman AJ, et al. Multifocal osteonecrosis in adolescents with Crohn's disease: a complication of therapy? J Pediatr Gastroenterol Nutr 1985;4:502–6.

Zizic TM, Marcoux C, Hungerford DS, et al. Corticosteroid therapy associated with ischemic necrosis of bone in systemic lupus erythematosus. Am J Med 1985;79:596–604.

Zizic TM, Hungerford DS. Avascular necrosis of bone. In: Kelley WN, Harris ED, Ruddy S, Sledge CB, eds. Textbook of rheumatology. 2nd Ed. Philadelphia: WB Saunders, 1985:1689.

CHAPTER 63

Sclerosing Cholangitis

Young-Mee Lee, MD, and Marshall M. Kaplan, MD

Sclerosing cholangitis is a cholestatic liver disorder characterized by diffuse strictures of the bile ducts. The disorder may be primary (idiopathic) or secondary due to structural abnormalities of the bile ducts. Primary sclerosing cholangitis (PSC) is clinically indistinguishable from disorders that cause secondary sclerosing cholangitis. These include chronic bacterial cholangitis in patients with bile duct stricture or choledocholithiasis, ischemic bile duct damage due to treatment with floxuridine, infectious cholangiopathy associated with acquired immunodeficiency syndrome, prior biliary surgery, congenital biliary tree abnormalities, and bile duct neoplasms. In this chapter, we will review the relevant data on the management of PSC.

Primary sclerosing cholangitis is a chronic liver disorder of unknown etiology characterized by ongoing inflammation, obliteration, and fibrosis of both intrahepatic and extrahepatic bile ducts and the eventual development of biliary cirrhosis. Focal bile duct dilatation proximal to areas of stricturing produces a characteristic beaded appearance on cholangiography. There is a strong association of PSC and inflammatory bowel disease (IBD), particularly ulcerative colitis (UC). Approximately 4 percent of patients with IBD will either have or develop PSC. Primary sclerosing cholangitis can also occur in the absence of IBD. Until 1970, PSC was considered to be a medical curiosity. Fewer than 100 patients with PSC had been reported. However, the development of endoscopic retrograde cholangiography (ERCP) changed our perception of this disease. It is now recognized more frequently and, after chronic hepatitis C and alcoholic cirrhosis, is one of the common indications for liver transplantation.

The course of PSC is unpredictable but is usually progressive. It typically leads to cirrhosis, portal hypertension, and the need for liver transplantation. The disease may present in two forms: an acute one that is characterized by recurring episodes of fever, chills, right-upper-quadrant pain, jaundice, and dark urine and a more indolent one that is initially asymptomatic and recognized by abnormal liver function tests, typically an elevated alkaline phosphatase. Patients who are asymptomatic and have normal serum bilirubin levels at diagnosis survive longer than symptomatic patients but still have shortened survival compared to a healthy age- and sex-matched population. Median survival or referral for liver transplantation in asymptomatic patients is approximately 12 years.

Treatment Strategies

The treatment of PSC has been limited by uncertainty about its cause. As yet, no medical therapy has been proved effective. The medical management is divided into (1) management of symptoms and complications and (2) specific therapy of the underlying disease process. However, liver transplantation is the only effective treatment and is recommended for patients with end-stage disease who have symptomatic portal hypertension, liver failure, and recurrent or intractable bacterial cholangitis. There is a separate chapter on liver transplantation for PSC.

Management of Chronic Cholestasis and Complications

Many of the symptoms of PSC are similar to those of primary biliary cirrhosis. However, unique problems result from mechanical bile duct obstruction, including bacterial cholangitis, sepsis, and the formation of pigment stones within the obstructed bile ducts. In addition, patients with PSC are at risk of developing cholangiocarcinoma. This cancer may be very difficult to distinguish from the tight bile duct strictures typically seen in PSC.

Pruritus

One of the more bothersome symptoms is pruritus. Itching may be worse at night and in warm weather and may be exacerbated by a high dietary fat intake. The precise mechanism of pruritus remains unknown. Recent evidence suggests that pruritus may be mediated by opiodergic receptors rather than due to the retention of bile acids in skin. A variety of agents have been evaluated in the management of pruritus. *Cholestyramine*, a nonabsorbed resin, is effective in most patients as long as there is adequate bile flow. The usual dosage of cholestyramine is 4 g three times per day orally; however, it must be adjusted in individual patients. Cholestyramine may require 2 to 4 days before the itching remits. *Colestipol* hydrochloride, another ammonium resin, is as effective as cholestyramine and may be used in patients who cannot tolerate cholestyramine. *Antihistamines* are occasionally helpful in mild pruritus if given before bedtime. *Rifampin, naloxone, methyltestosterone, phenobarbital, ursodiol, S-adenosylmethionine, ondansetron, ultraviolet light,* and large-volume *plasmapheresis* have been used to control pruritus in some patients unresponsive to cholestyramine.

Steatorrhea and Vitamin Deficiency

Steatorrhea and malabsorption of fat-soluble vitamins may occur late in the course of PSC. Fat malabsorption in jaundiced patients is usually related to decreased secretion of conjugated bile acids into the small intestine. Other causes are pancreatic insufficiency and celiac disease, both of which may be associated with PSC. Vitamin A deficiency has been reported in up to 82 percent of patients with advanced PSC. Vitamin D and E deficiency occur in approximately 40 to 50 percent of patients with advanced PSC. Clinically important vitamin K deficiency rarely occurs unless the patient is chronically jaundiced and takes cholestyramine regularly. Fat-soluble vitamin level should be monitored and deficiencies treated with supplements.

Metabolic Bone Disease

As in primary biliary cirrhosis, the bone disease is due to osteoporosis rather than osteomalacia. The pathogenesis of osteoporosis in patients with PSC or other chronic cholestatic liver diseases is unknown. Osteoporosis is not related to vitamin D deficiency since the serum vitamin D concentration is often normal but may be related to osteoblast inhibitors in cholestatic serum. There is no proven medical treatment for osteoporosis. Therapies with 25-hydroxyvitamin D with calcium, ursodiol, and calcitonin have been suggested, but there are no controlled data. Patients with PSC are prone to develop fractures after liver transplantation due to immobilization and corticosteroid therapy.

Cholangitis

Bacterial cholangitis is typically associated with biliary procedures, bile duct stones or obstructing strictures. Antibiotics appear to have no role in slowing the progression of PSC but have been used to treat recurrent episodes of ascending cholangitis. Tetracycline was determined to be ineffective in one small study in PSC. *Ciprofloxacin* has been recommended for treatment and prophylaxis of bacterial cholangitis because of its high biliary tract penetration. Alternative agents are *amoxicillin* or *trimethoprim-sulfamethoxazole*. Anecdotal reports and our experience suggest that such drugs reduce the frequency and severity of bacterial cholangitis. Additional controlled trials are needed to test this hypothesis.

Dominant Biliary Strictures

Dominant strictures of the extrahepatic bile duct occur in 20 percent of patients with PSC. Several studies reported successful management with endoscopic balloon dilation or biliary stenting of the dominant strictures. We have also found endoscopic dilatation to be effective treatment in selected patients with dominant stricture and sudden worsening of bilirubin levels. In most of these patients, the stricture tended to recur within approximately 4 to 8 months so that *repeated ERCP with dilatations* was needed to keep liver function tests close to normal. The endoscopic treatment was associated with fewer episodes of cholangitis and improvement of cholangiographic appearance and biochemical tests. There are no randomized controlled trials evaluating the efficacy of endoscopic therapy, but there appears to be little risk and some potential benefit from this approach. The next chapter is devoted to stricture dilatations. Another approach to the dominant stricture, surgical dilatation or choledochojejunostomy, is rarely used now. Surgery carries the risk of postoperative infection and increases scarring in the portahepatis, potentially complicating future liver transplantation.

Cholangiocarcinoma

There is an increased incidence of cholangiocarcinoma in PSC, about 10 percent. Patients with longstanding chronic UC and cirrhosis are at highest risk. Early diagnosis of bile duct carcinoma is hampered by the lack of sensitive and specific serologic tumor markers as well as the insensitivity of biliary brush cytology. The serologic tumor markers have included CEA and CA-19-9. An unsuspected cholangiocarcinoma may be found after liver transplantation when the resected liver is examined in the pathology laboratory. Unfortunately, there is no reliable way to distinguish a dominant stricture from a cholangiocarcinoma, even after repeated imaging tests, endoscopic biopsies, and cytologic examination. Furthermore, treatment by resection, chemotherapy, and radiation has been discouraging, as have been the results with liver transplantation for clinically apparent tumors. Some experts have suggested earlier liver transplantation in patients with PSC before cholangiocarcinoma has a chance to develop.

Medical Therapy of Primary Sclerosing Cholangitis

A variety of immunosuppressive, anti-inflammatory, and antifibrotic agents have been used to treat PSC. However, no drug has been shown to improve its natural history. The evaluation of treatment has been limited by the unpredictable course of PSC and by the great variation in the severity of the disease at presentation. The course of PSC is indolent in most patients but may be rapidly progressive in some and associated with spontaneous exacerbations and remissions in others. Hence, even if a drug is effective, it will probably be years before its efficacy can be proven.

Corticosteroids and Azathioprine

Despite anecdotal reports of improvement with glucocorticoids and azathioprine in patients with PSC, there is little enthusiasm for their use. Approximately 75 to 90 percent of patients with PSC have chronic inflammatory bowel disease and were being treated with glucocorticoids and/or azathioprine or 6-mercaptopurine when PSC developed and progressed. Combination treatment with colchicine and glucocorticoids or either drug alone is not effective. In addition, glucocorticoids may accelerate the onset and progression of osteoporosis and increase spontaneous bone fractures. There is, however, one favorable report. In an uncontrolled trial, 10 patients with prefibrotic PSC had improvement in blood tests and liver histology. Four of these patients were well after 12 years and were still on low-dose prednisone (DR LaBrecque, personal communication).

D-penicillamine

Based on the observation of increased hepatic copper concentration in patients with PSC, D-penicillamine was evaluated in a double-blind prospective trial in 70 patients followed for 36 months. D-penicillamine produced the expected cupriuresis but had no beneficial effect on symptoms, biochemical tests, liver histology, disease progression, or survival. In addition, 21 percent of the patients developed major side effects from D-penicillamine. The toxicity and lack of efficacy have discouraged further use of D-penicillamine.

Colchicine

Eighty-four patients with PSC were randomized to receive either colchicine, 1 mg per day, or placebo in a double-blind study over 3 years. Liver biopsies were done at baseline and at 3 years. Patients were evaluated every 6 months. Colchicine had no beneficial effect on symptoms, biochemical tests of liver function, liver histology, or survival. Colchicine was clearly ineffective.

Cyclosporine

Cyclosporine was evaluated in a prospective, double-blind trial in 34 patients followed for 24 months. Twenty-two patients received cyclosporine while 12 patients received placebo. Cyclosporine doses were adjusted to keep trough blood levels between 80 and 100 ng/mL (HPLC whole blood) and averaged 3.1 mg/kg/day. Repeat liver biopsies were done in 30 patients. After 2 years of treatment, cyclosporine had no beneficial effect on pruritus, fatigue, biochemical tests of liver function, or survival free of liver transplantation. Nine of 10 patients (90 percent) on placebo showed histologic progression of disease compared to 11 of 20 (55 percent) on cyclosporine. The authors concluded that cyclosporine was not effective in the treatment of PSC.

Ursodeoxycholic Acid

Ursodeoxycholic acid (UDCA), a hydrophilic bile acid, has been widely used to treat PSC. Therapy with the drug leads to a two- to threefold increase in serum bile acid concentration. There is an increase in the biliary and urinary excretion of bile acids and an increase in bile flow. In vitro, UDCA stabilizes liver cell membranes exposed to toxic concentrations of the naturally occurring bile acid chenodeoxycholic acid.

Initially, several small studies reported improvements in symptoms and biochemical tests of liver function with UDCA. The long-term beneficial effects of UDCA on liver histology or cholangiographic appearance of the biliary tree was unclear since these trials were of relatively short duration and included few patients. A prospective, randomized, double-blind, placebo-controlled trial of 105 patients continued for 2 years confirmed earlier reports that UDCA (12 to 15 mg/kg bw/day) significantly improved some biochemical tests, primarily alkaline phosphatase and the aminotransferases. However, UDCA had no beneficial effect on time to treatment failure, which was defined as death, liver transplantation, progression to cirrhosis, histologic progression by two stages, sustained quadrupling of bilirubin, drug toxicity, or voluntary withdrawal. Furthermore, UDCA did not improve symptoms or liver histology. Although this study included a representative cross-section of patients with the disease, a large percentage of patients had histologically advanced disease at enrolment. The lack of clinical benefit may have been related to the advanced histologic stage of these patients. However, it is equally likely that UDCA alone may not be effective treatment in PSC. A longer, randomized trial of patients with earlier stages of the disease will be important in assessing the effectiveness of UDCA. Recently, Mitchell and associates reported results of a double-blind, placebo-controlled pilot study of higher dose (20 mg/kg) UDCA in PSC patients. Twenty-four patients were randomized for treatment with UDCA or placebo and were followed for 2 years. Ursodeoxycholic acid improved the alkaline phosphatase and the gamma-glutamyl transpeptidase levels, but the changes in the bilirubin and aspartate aminotransferase were not significantly different in the two groups. UDCA Ursodeoxycholic acid appear to have a beneficial effect on liver histology. Histologic inflammatory scores were unchanged or improved in 9 of 10 in the UDCA treatment group but worse in 5 of 9 in the placebo group. The histologic stage remained unchanged or improved in the treated group but progressed in the placebo group. Despite the higher dose of UDCA, it was well tolerated and had no significant side effects.

Methotrexate

Methotrexate has been evaluated at New England Medical Center during the past 20 years, based on favorable experiences with two patients treated in 1979 and 1980. These two men had dramatic symptomatic, biochemical, and histologic responses while receiving methotrexate. In an open-label study of 10 patients, none of whom had clinically advanced disease, all patients had improvement in serum alkaline phosphatase while on oral methotrexate, approximately 0.25 mg/kg/week. Symptoms of right-upper-quadrant pain, fever, chills, itching, and recurrent jaundice improved in the six patients who had these symptoms. Histology improved in six of nine patients and was unchanged in three. Patients with advanced disease, that is, cirrhosis and portal hypertension, did not respond to methotrexate, UDCA, or the combination of these two. The addition of antibiotics to these two drugs did not help in these patients with advanced disease.

In a double-blind, controlled trial of 24 patients, there was no therapeutic benefit for patients receiving methotrexate compared to those on placebo. Twelve patients received methotrexate, 15 mg/week, and 12 placebo. Each patient was followed for 2 years. The only statistically significant change was a decrease in the serum alkaline phosphatase in the patients receiving methotrexate. Half of the 24 patients in the study already had cirrhosis when enrolled, including 7 of the 12 patients receiving methotrexate. Patients with cirrhosis probably have medically irreversible PSC. There was no toxicity from methotrexate. There is still no firm evidence that methotrexate by itself favorably alters the natural history of PSC, but studies using it with ursodiol and antibiotics are in progress.

Pentoxifylline

Tumor necrosis factor (TNF) has been postulated to have a role in the hepatic injury in PSC. Pentoxifylline prevents the production of TNF. In a pilot study of 20 patients, pentoxifylline was not beneficial in improvement of symptoms or liver function tests in patients with PSC.

Tacrolimus

Tacrolimus (FK 506) is a macrolide antibiotic that has been used to prevent rejection in transplant recipients. Tacrolimus was evaluated in an open-label trial of 10 patients who were followed for 1 year. After 1 year, the median serum bilirubin fell by 75 percent, the alkaline phosphatase by 70 percent, and aminotransferases by 83 percent. The dose was that that kept trough levels of Tacrolimus between 0.6 and 1.0 ng/mL. No toxicity was reported. There were no data on liver histology or cholangiography. The short duration and uncontrolled nature of the study did not allow Tacrolimus to be evaluated meaningfully as treatment for PSC.

Conclusion

Primary sclerosing cholangitis remains an elusive, difficult-to-treat disease. Progress in treating this disease will be slow until the cause is better understood. In the future, patients in the early stages should be included in prospective trials. New treatment strategies employing combinations of drugs such as UDCA, methotrexate, antibiotics, and other immunomodulatory drugs appear to be the most promising approach to treatment at this time.*

Supplemental Reading

Broome U, Linberg G, Lofberg R. Primary sclerosing cholangitis in ulcerative colitis: a risk factor for the development of dysplasia and DNA aneuploidy? Gastroenterology 1992;102:1877–80.

Chapman RW. Role of immune factors in the pathogenesis of primary sclerosing cholangitis. Semin Liver Dis 1991;11:1–4.

D'Haens GR, Lashner BA, Hanauer SB. Pericholangitis and sclerosing cholangitis are risk factors for dysplasia and cancer in ulcerative colitis. Am J Gastroenterol 1993;88:1174–8.

Fausa O, Schrumpf E, Elgjo K. Relationship of inflammatory bowel disease and primary sclerosing cholangitis. Semin Liver Dis 1991;11:31–9.

Kaplan MM. Medical approaches to primary sclerosing cholangitis. Semin Liver Dis 1991;11:56–63.

Knox TA, Kaplan MM. A double-blind controlled trial of oral-pulse methotrexate therapy in the treatment of primary sclerosing cholangitis. Gastroenterology 1994;106:494–9.

Lindor KD, The Mayo PSC-UDCA Study Group: ursodiol for primary sclerosing cholangitis. N Engl J Med 1997;336;691–5.

Ludwig J. Small-duct primary sclerosing cholangitis. Semin Liver Dis 1991;11:11–7.

Mitchell S, Bansi D, Hunt N, et al. High dose ursodeoxycholic acid (UDCA) in primary sclerosing cholangitis: results after 2 years of randomized double-blind placebo-controlled trial (abstract). Gastroenterology;1997;112:A1335.

Wiesner RH. Current concepts in primary sclerosing cholangitis. Mayo Clin Proc 1994;69:969–82.

---

* Editor's Note: The course of the colitis, usually UC but sometimes Crohn's disease, is independent of the PSC. No one is seemingly advocating colectomy for PSC anymore. However, the colitis in PSC patients seems to be milder than the usual UC, often going unrecognized until the PSC is diagnosed. They are seemingly at very high risk for colonic neoplasia. The chapters on colonic dysplasia and colon cancer surveillance point out that in some series, half of the UC patients with PSC had developed either dysplasia or colon cancer by 28 years. The PSC patient should enter a colonoscopic surveillance program as soon as an IBD diagnosis is made. (TMB)

CHAPTER 64

STRICTURE MANAGEMENT IN PRIMARY SCLEROSING CHOLANGITIS

ANTHONY N. KALLOO, MD, FACP

The major biliary complication of inflammatory bowel disease (IBD) is a stricturing disease of the biliary tree, namely, primary sclerosing cholangitis (PSC). The mainstay of treatment of PSC is liver transplantation with survival rates of greater than 80 percent at 5 years. Therefore, the use of other palliative therapeutic modalities such as endoscopic, nontransplant surgical or radiologic interventions should be evaluated in the context of the efficacy of liver transplantation. Furthermore, the concern of underlying cholangiocarcinoma should always be a priority when evaluating and treating these strictures. The indications, technique, and results of endoscopic intervention for biliary strictures in patients with PSC will be discussed.

Diagnostic Modalities

Endoscopic Retrograde Cholangiopancreatography

Although endoscopic retrograde cholangiopancreatography (ERCP) may be performed in patients with PSC to confirm the diagnosis, endoscopic intervention should not be a routine procedure if the patient is asymptomatic. This holds true even if significant strictures are seen at initial diagnostic ERCP. Of concern is the observation that an underlying cholangiocarcinoma may also have a similar presentation. If there is a suspicion of underlying cholangiocarcinoma, then endoscopic evaluation with biopsies and brush cytology may be helpful. In general, the yield of endoscopic biopsies and brush cytology is poor. The use of image cytometry may be a useful diagnostic technique for distinguishing benign from malignant disease. K-ras mutation analysis and oncoprotein p-53 immunocytochemistry are shown to offer no additional diagnostic benefit. The best results are obtained with a combination of biopsy and brush cytology with a sensitivity of about 80 percent using this approach.

Magnetic Resonance Imaging

Magnetic resonance imaging (MRI) is an evolving technique that is able to provide much useful information for patients with PSC, especially with the advent of MR cholangiography. Magnetic resonance imaging (MRI) may detect bile duct thickening, stenosis, dilatation, and abnormalities of liver parenchyma. Periportal lymphadenopathy and liver masses may also be detected. Magnetic resonance imaging can provide information on the biliary tree in areas not visualized by ERCP because of high-grade obstruction.

Endoscopic Interventions

The major indications for endoscopic interventions are worsening jaundice or pruritus or bouts of acute cholangitis. Cholangiographic features of PSC that favor a good endoscopic outcome include the presence of dominant extrahepatic stricture(s) with relative sparing of the intrahepatic ducts. Severe intrahepatic disease or significant stenoses of the left and right hepatic ducts are features that suggest a poor outcome of endoscopic therapy.

The use of prophylactic antibiotics is recommended simply because there may be areas in the biliary tree that may not drain after the injection of contrast through strictured areas. Once a satisfactory cholangiogram is obtained, the first step in endoscopic therapy is endoscopic sphincterotomy. This is performed not only to facilitate passage of endoscopic accessories but to direct therapy at the sphincter itself, which may be sclerotic as part of the diffuse inflammatory process and also may be responsible in part for bile outflow obstruction. The second step is to gain access across the strictures. This is easily accomplished with hydrophilic guide wires. Loading the wire into a balloon catheter may be helpful to aid placement of the wire since the inflated balloon will prevent retrograde movement of the wire and allow for different directing angles for wire manipulation. Once the wire is in place across the stricture, then a dilating balloon is placed across the stricture and inflated to approximately 150 psi. In very tight strictures, slippage of the balloon may occur during inflation and therefore it may be necessary to apply manual tension to the dilating balloon catheter during inflation. Our practice is to keep the balloon inflated for 60 seconds at each station. Then the balloon is deflated and withdrawn to the next narrow segment so that there is overlap in the dilating stations. The stricture is then dilated from proximal to distal to achieve a diameter comparable to the nonstrictured portion of the duct.

The use of biliary stents in the treatment of PSC generally has been unsatisfactory. This is because early stent occlusion is a problem, presumably as a result of the low bile flow rates in these patients. However, stents may be a useful alternative in patients who have strictures that are unresponsive to dilation. Other endoscopic options that have been tried without success are saline lavage of the biliary tree and infusion of steroids in the ducts.

Outcome of Endoscopic Therapy

There are only a few trials that have examined the role of endoscopic intervention. in PSC. Even in patients with endoscopically favorable cholangiographic features, once there is established cirrhosis, then endoscopic therapy is unlikely to be helpful. This is also true of the nontransplant surgical, percutaneous, and medical approaches in cirrhotic patients. In this group of patients, liver transplantation remains the treatment of choice. There is now a growing trend for earlier liver transplantation in patients with PSC, making long-term follow-up trials of endoscopic therapy difficult to perform. In general, one can expect a response rate of approximately 70 to 75 percent with endoscopic therapy in patients with ideal cholangiographic features (dominant stricture with minimal intrahepatic structuring) for 2 to 3 years if no cirrhosis is present.

Supplemental Reading

Cotton PB, Nickl N. Endoscopic and radiologic approaches to primary sclerosing cholangitis. Semin Liver Dis 1991;11:40–8.

Deviere J. Therapeutic endoscopy and primary sclerosing cholangitis. Endoscopy 1996;28:576–7.

Ito K, Mitchell DG, Outwater EK, Blasbalg R. Primary sclerosing cholangitis: MR imaging features. AJR Am J Roentgenol 1999;172:1527–33.

Johnson GK, Geenen JE, Venue RP, et al. Endoscopic treatment of biliary tract strictures in sclerosing cholangitis: a larger series and recommendation for treatment. Gastrointest Endosc 1991;37:38–43.

Kalloo AN. Primary sclerosing cholangitis: an overview. In: Cameron JL; ed. Current surgical therapy. 5th Ed. Mosby 1995:375–7.

Lee JG, Schutz SM, England RE, et al. Endoscopic therapy of primary sclerosing cholangitis. Hepatology 1995;21:661–7.

Lemmer ER, Bornman PC. Endoscopic dilatation of dominant strictures in primary sclerosing cholangitis. HPB Surg 1998;11:68–70.

Ponsioen CY, Vrouenraets SM, van Milligan de Wit AW, et al. Value of brush cytology for dominant strictures in primary sclerosing cholangitis. Endoscopy 1999;31:305–9.

Van Milligen de Wit AW, Van Bracht J, Rauws EAJ, et al. Endoscopic stent therapy for dominant extrahepatic bile duct strictures in primary sclerosing cholangitis. Gastrointest Endosc 1996;44:293–9.

Van Milligen de Wit AW, Rauws EA, van Bracht J, et al. Lack of complications following short-term stent therapy for extrahepatic bile duct strictures in primary sclerosing cholangitis. Gastrointest Endosc 1997;45:344–7.

Wagner S, Gebel M, Meier P, et al. Endoscopic management of biliary tract strictures in primary sclerosing cholangitis. Endoscopy 1996;28:546–51.

CHAPTER 65

Liver Transplantation for Primary Sclerosing Cholangitis

Paul J. Thuluvath, MD, FRCP, Henkie Tan, MD, PhD, Sateesh Nair, MD, and Andrew Klein, MD

Primary Sclerosing Cholangitis

Primary sclerosing cholangitis (PSC) is a chronic, usually progressive liver disease characterized by cholangiographic appearance of intrahepatic or extrahepatic duct stricturing and dilatation ("beaded" appearance). Perinuclear antineutrophil cytoplasmic antibodies (pANCA) are commonly seen, but pANCA titers do not appear to correlate with clinical activity or histology. Moreover, pANCA persists after liver transplantation and does not appear to be related to recurrence of PSC. Human leukocyte antigen (HLA)-DR4 may be associated with an accelerated disease progression.

Prevalence

The prevalence of PSC in the United States is approximately 1 to 6 cases per 100,000 population. The disease is seen predominantly in males (M:F—7:1) in their late thirties. A majority of patients (about 70%) have inflammatory bowel disease (IBD), ulcerative colitis (UC) being more common than Crohn's disease (9:1). It is estimated that about 5 percent of patients with UC may develop PSC sometime in their lifetime. There is no correlation between the severity of IBD and the occurrence of PSC. On many occasions, the diagnosis of IBD is made after the diagnosis of PSC. It has been suggested that patients with PSC may have a less symptomatic form of IBD. Colectomy does not influence the natural history of PSC, and PSC may appear several years after colectomy. In patients with both PSC and UC, there appears to be a fivefold increase in risk of colon cancer compared to patients with UC without PSC.

Presentation

Currently, many patients are diagnosed during evaluation of abnormal liver enzymes noted on routine blood tests. Elevated alkaline phosphatase or gamma-glutamyl transferase (GGT) is the most common abnormality found in these patients. About 10 to 15 percent patients with PSC present with symptoms of cholangitis that may or may not be bacterial in nature. However, it may be prudent to treat them with broad-spectrum antibiotics if they have leukocytosis and sustained fever. In advanced stages, patients present with jaundice, pruritus, and fatigue. It is not uncommon to find patients with transient jaundice even in early stages, which may be due to bile plugs, stones, or dominant strictures. Ascites, hypoalbuminemia, coagulopathy, weight loss, encephalopathy, and variceal bleeding are seen only in very advanced stages.

Diagnosis

The diagnosis of PSC is based on cholangiographic appearance, and endoscopic retrograde cholangiography (ERC) remains the investigation of choice. The "beaded" appearance is generally seen in both intrahepatic and extrahepatic ducts, but in a small proportion (10%) of patients, the disease may be limited to intrahepatic ducts. It is very uncommon to see patients with extrahepatic disease without intrahepatic lesions. One has to be very cautious before making a diagnosis of PSC on the basis of extrahepatic duct structuring alone. It has been suggested that some patients with histologic features of PSC may have a normal cholangiogram since the lesion is limited to small ducts and therefore cholangiographic changes may be difficult to appreciate. Ischemic strictures may mimic PSC on cholangiogram and histology and are often indistinguishable from PSC. Arteriogram may be necessary in doubtful cases. The liver biopsy is not essential nor is it generally useful in making a diagnosis of PSC, since the classic periductal fibrosis ("onion skin" appearance) is rarely seen on needle biopsies. The histology, however, is helpful for staging and also to exclude other diseases like sarcoidosis.

Prognosis

The median survival is 9 to 12 years from the time of diagnosis. In patients without cirrhosis, the 5-year survival is around 70 percent. Cirrhosis, jaundice, ascites, encephalopathy, and variceal bleeding are poor prognostic indicators. It has been suggested that the presence of symptoms at the time of diagnosis may indicate shorter survival, but this has not been confirmed in all studies.

The present UNOS[*] allocation system for liver transplantation gives priority to patients with more advanced liver disease based on the Child-Turcotte-Pugh (CTP)

---

[*] United Network for Organ Sharing.

scoring system. Since CTP score is predominantly based on hepatocellular synthetic function, patients with cholestatic liver disease, with relatively well-compensated synthetic function, may have to wait longer to receive a liver transplant. As in all liver diseases, the morbidity, mortality, and cost of liver transplantation increase with worsening liver disease. Despite the limitation imposed by the current UNOS allocation system, accurate methods of estimating survival in PSC are important in the decision-making process regarding an individual's candidacy for liver transplantation. Moreover, the increasing acceptance of living donor transplantation (or xenotransplantation in the future) may make it possible to transplant patients with PSC in a more timely fashion.

Prognostic Models

Various prognostic models have been proposed in PSC. These models are useful for epidemiologic studies and clinical trials but are of only limited benefit when applied to an individual patient. However, the criteria derived from these studies can be used as a guide to decide the need for liver transplantation. The prognostic model developed by Dickson and colleagues (1992), based on 426 patients from five international centers, identified four poor prognostic variables: *serum bilirubin level*, *age*, *histologic stage*, and *splenomegaly*. Using these variables, patients were stratified into *low-*, *moderate-*, and *severe-risk* categories by a Cox regression model with 5-year survivals of 91 percent, 55 percent, and 16 percent, respectively. It has been shown that patients with a low Mayo risk score (< 4.4) undergoing liver transplantation had a better survival than those with a higher (> 5.3) Mayo risk score. Unfortunately, none of these predictors could identify patients at risk for developing cholangiocarcinoma. Based on a retrospective study of 94 patients, it has been suggested that high-grade intrahepatic strictures might indicate early jaundice and a shorter survival. This observation merits further examination in a prospective manner.

Diagnosis of Cholangiocarcinoma in Primary Sclerosing Cholangitis

Cholangiocarcinoma is an unpredictable complication of PSC and is seen in about 10 to 15 percent of patients with PSC. In one series, the cumulative incidence of cholangiocarcinoma was found to be 13 percent at 5 years and 31 percent at 10 years after onset of PSC. Prevalence of cholangiocarcinoma was found to be as high as 42 percent in an autopsy series.

The diagnosis of cholangiocarcinoma is extremely difficult in the presence of PSC. This is highlighted by the fact that a significant number of unsuspected carcinomas are found in the explants of patients undergoing transplantation, despite rigorous pretransplant investigations, which failed to identify a malignancy. Rapid worsening of liver function tests in a stable patient, weight loss, abdom-

inal pain, and anorexia should alert the clinician to a possible cholangiocarcinoma. Endoscopic retrograde cholangiography is a useful diagnostic tool to obtain brushings from the dominant strictures and to obtain bile for cytology. The diagnostic yield can be increased significantly by obtaining bile from the duct proximal to the dominant stricture, which is a rich source of exfoliated malignant cells. Bile can be obtained proximal to tight strictures these days without much difficulty using glidewire-guided catheters.

Tumor markers like carcinoembroyonic antigen (CEA) and carbohydrate antigen 19-9 (CA 19-9) are of limited value to make the diagnosis, because these glycoproteins are nonspecifically increased in the presence of biliary obstruction or liver disease. The sensitivity of these tumor markers is around 50 to 60 percent with a specificity of 80 to 90 percent. A study from Kings College, London, suggested that the specificity could be improved significantly by a combination of CEA and CA 19-9. An index was derived by this group using a formula CA 19-9 + (CEA × 40). By imposing an upper limit of 400 units (> 400 units + abnormal), they could increase the specificity of the index to 100 percent. However, the sensitivity of the index was only 66 percent. Positron emission tomography with [18^F] fluoro-2-deoxy-D-glucose is a relatively new noninvasive imaging study that looks promising in the detection of small cholangiocarcinomas and may have potential in the decision whether to accept a PSC patient on a waiting list for liver transplantation.

Older age, longer duration of IBD, and smoking behavior are associated with an increased risk of cholangiocarcinoma in patients with PSC. Tumors arise most commonly around the common hepatic duct or its bifurcation, and rapid progression of the disease is not uncommon.

Management—Medical, Endoscopic and Surgical

There is no consistently effective medical therapy for PSC. There is a chapter on medical therapy. A variety of drugs, including corticosteroids (both oral and intrabiliary), penicillamine, colchicines, methotrexate, azathioprine, and cyclosporine, have been used, but there is no convincing evidence that any of these agents are effective. These drugs should not be used alone or in combination until they are found to be of benefit in randomized, controlled trials. The exception to this group is ursodeoxycholic acid. This drug is relatively nontoxic and is well tolerated by patients. The current data suggest that this drug improves liver function tests and some of the symptoms. There is as yet no convincing evidence that ursodeoxycholic acid improves the histology, the survival, or the need for liver transplantation. Because ursodeoxycholic acid is relatively free of side effects, it is recommended for both symptomatic and asymptomatic PSC patients until there is evidence to the contrary.

In noncirrhotic patients with localized disease such as dominant strictures of common bile duct, common hepatic duct, and right or left hepatic duct, endoscopic treatment is preferable to surgery. The dominant strictures can be progressively dilated with balloon dilators followed by stenting if necessary. Since the natural history of PSC is variable, the uncontrolled reports of success with any form of treatment need to be considered with caution. Although it is technically possible to dilate intrahepatic strictures, it is important to assess the potential complications associated with repeated manipulation of a diseased biliary tree. Bacterial colonization is very common after endoscopic or transhepatic manipulation of bile ducts, and it is not uncommon to see low-grade sepsis after such an intervention in a patient with PSC. Rarely, this may make the patient unsuitable for liver transplantation. Aggressive dilatation or manipulation of intrahepatic ducts, even in the absence of cirrhosis, needs to be discouraged.

The role of biliary surgery in PSC has diminished with the growing success of liver transplantation. Biliary surgery, including transhepatic stents, does not alter the natural history of the disease and may indeed make liver transplantation more difficult. Previous biliary surgery is associated with a significantly longer operation time, greater intraoperative blood loss, and a higher incidence of post-transplant biliary complications; however, previous biliary surgery had no effect on patient survival after transplantation. Nevertheless, biliary surgery in patients with PSC should be minimized and reserved for selected noncirrhotic patients, who have marked cholestasis or recurrent cholangitis caused by a dominant extrahepatic or biliar stricture not amenable to endoscopic or percutaneous dilatation. In general, the outcome of biliary surgery or colectomy is poor in the presence of cirrhosis. Arguably, the only indication for nontransplant, operative management in the cirrhotic PSC patient is the suspicion of a cholangiocarcinoma.

Liver Transplantation

Liver transplantation is the treatment of choice for patients with advanced PSC. Liver transplantation for a patient with sclerosing cholangitis was first reported in 1976 from the University of Colorado. In 1998, 4,450 of 13,835 patients on the waiting list in the United States received a liver transplant. Currently, 9 percent of patients undergoing liver transplantation in the United States have a preoperative diagnosis of PSC.

Selection and timing of liver transplantation in PSC is difficult. The prognostic model developed by Dickson et al (1992) can be used as a general guide, but it is not always helpful in an individual patient. As a rough guide, patients with cirrhosis should be evaluated for liver transplantation. Other indications include persistent jaundice, extreme fatigue, ascites, encephalopathy, or variceal bleeding. Unlike other liver diseases, it is preferable to transplant patients with PSC early in the

clinical course due to the significant risk of cholangiocarcinoma, for which there is no proven therapy. The average life expectancy in a patient with PSC and cholangiocarcinoma is approximately 5 months, and this should be constantly borne in mind.

The contraindications to transplantation are (1) patients with known cholangiocarcinoma, (2) patients with debilitating systemic disease that would preclude an extensive operation, (3) active alcohol use in the previous 6 months by a patient with a diagnosis of alcohol abuse or dependence, (4) active illicit drug use in the previous 6 months by a patient with a diagnosis of substance abuse, and (5) extrahepatic malignancy other than skin cancer.

Survival After Liver Transplantation

The survival after liver transplantation for PSC is 75 to 90 percent at 5 years. These survival rates are comparable to those achieved for other transplant indications such as primary biliary cirrhosis (Table 65–1). The survival rate is significantly higher than could be expected, based on the Mayo model. In a study from France, the actuarial patient survival of 5 years after liver transplantation was 89 percent, which was significantly higher than 31 percent that could be expected from prognostic models.

Transplantation in Patients with Cholangiocarcinoma

The prognosis for patients with PSC and cholangiocarcinoma with or without liver transplantation is very poor, with a reported survival shorter than 1 year from the time of diagnosis in most patients. The main reason for the shorter survival is the high recurrence of cancer during the first 6 months post-transplantation.

In a recent study, patients with incidental, microscopic cholangiocarcinoma without regional lymph node involvement were found to have a long-term survival similar to those PSC patients without cholangiocarcinoma after liver transplantation. The survival of 47 patients with cholangiocarcinoma (27 patients with hilar cholangiocarcinoma [Klatskin tumor] and 20 unresectable, peripheral cholangiocarcinoma) who had orthotopic liver transplantation (OLT) at the University of Pittsburgh was also reported recently. In patients with hilar tumor, the surgical margins were positive for malignant cells in 22 percent of patients. The 1-, 3-, and 5-year survival rates were 59.3 percent, 36.2 percent, and 36.2 percent, respectively, with a perioperative mortality of 22.2 percent. There was no 5-year survival in patients with lymph node involvement. In the 20 patients with unresectable peripheral cholangiocarcinoma who underwent liver transplantation, the 1-, 3-, and 5-year survival rates were 70 percent, 29 percent, and 18 percent, respectively. In multivariate analysis, positive margins, multiple tumors, and lymph node involvement were independently shown to be associated with poor prognosis. Similarly, in the Australian registry, Sheil (1995) reported a 5-year survival of 22 percent in the eight

TABLE 65–1. Patient Graft Survival Results of Liver Transplantation for Primary Schlerosing Cholangitis (%)

	1 year	2 year	5 year	10 year
Mayo Clinic and University of Pittsburgh (n = 216)				
Patient	85	80	75	
Mayo Clinic (n = 150)				
Patient	93.7	92.7	86.4	69.8
Graft	83.4	83.4	79.4	60.5
UCLA (n = 127)				
Patient	90	86	85	
Graft	82	77	72	
UCSF (n = 37)				
Patient	96.9	91.6	87.9	
Graft	83.1	74.2	65.2	
Villejuif, France (n = 51)				
Patient	89	89	89	
Graft	82	65	65	

patients who underwent liver transplantation for cholangiocarcinoma.

Preliminary results from small ongoing studies in patients with PSC and cholangiocarcinoma suggest that preoperative radiation and chemotherapy may be associated with a prolonged disease-free survival. However, in another study, in 17 patients with cholangiocarcinoma who had adjuvant radiochemotherapy 8 weeks after liver transplantation, the overall 1-year patient survival was 53 percent with a disease-free 3-year survival of only 13 percent. Since PSC patients with known cholangiocarcinoma are expected to have a poor prognosis, these patients should not be considered for transplantation outside clinical trials. However, the intraoperative identification of intrahepatic cholangiocarcinoma in the absence of lymph node spread is not considered to be a contraindication to proceeding with the liver transplantaiton.

Recurrence of Primary Sclerosing Cholangitis After Liver Transplantation

The diagnosis of recurrent PSC after OLT is difficult since many other complications, such as hepatic artery thrombosis, preservation-related ischemia, cytomegalovirus infection, chronic ductopenic rejection, and ABO, incompatibility, can cause nonanastomotic biliary strictures mimicking recurrent PSC.

Several studies have reported a higher incidence of biliary strictures after liver transplantation in patients with PSC when compared to all other conditions requiring liver transplantation. In a retrospective 10-year study of 643 liver transplant recipients, including 100 liver transplants for PSC, Sheng and associates (1996) noted a higher frequency of intrahepatic (27% [30/112] vs 13% [75/575], $p < .0001$) and nonanastomotic extrahepatic strictures (6% [7/112] vs 2% [10/575], $p = .008$). However, there was no difference in the incidence of anastomotic strictures in the two groups, both of which underwent choledochojejunostomy. In a later study by the same group, 32 liver grafts of patients with PSC and strictures were compared to 32 control grafts (non-PSC) matched for the location, length, and number of strictures and duct dilatation. The control group was matched with the PSC group for the type of biliary anastomosis (choledochojejunostomy), presence of strictures, and the time interval between liver transplantation and stricture diagnosis. The study concluded that mural irregularity and diverticulum-like outpouchings (suggestive of recurrent PSC) and an overall appearance resembling PSC occurred more frequently in PSC transplants than in transplants for other diseases.

Although several studies have shown a higher incidence of strictures suggestive of recurrent PSC, this diagnosis cannot be confirmed by cholangiographic features alone. Hence, definite evidence of recurrent PSC requires characteristic cholangiographic features, histologic evidence, and absence of any other known cause of biliary stricture after liver transplantation. In a retrospective study of 24 patients who developed nonanastomotic biliary strictures after non–PSC-related liver transplantation, antecedent liver biopsies and failed grafts were analyzed to determine the pattern of histologic injury and identify potential contributing factors in their pathogenesis. Twenty-three patients had features consistent with sclerosing cholangitis, with a combination of periductal fibrosis and features of large duct obstruction, whereas the remaining patient had ischemic-type lesions without periductal fibrosis. Numerous associated factors may explain the pathogenesis of these strictures: ABO incompatibility (10 patients), hepatic artery thrombosis (12 patients), focal arterial intimal hyperplasia (3 patients), chronic ductopenic arteriopathic rejection (3 patients), and/or preservation-related ischemia (4 patients). Thus, most patients with features of secondary sclerosing cholangitis after non-PSC liver transplantation had evidence of potential etiology.

In order to compare whether characteristic histologic lesions of PSCs (fibro-obliterative lesions and fibrous cholangitis) occurred more frequently in liver allografts from patients with PSC than other similarly matched controls, Harrison et al (1994) reviewed all histologic material in a 3-year period from a series of 207 liver transplants. Of 22 patients receiving liver transplant for PSC, 7 (32%) patients had biopsy results showing features of biliary obstruction, 6 (27%) showing fibrosing cholangitis and 3 (14%) showing classic fibro-obliterative lesions. These findings compared with 3 (14%), 1 (5%), and 0 patients, respectively, among 22 non-PSC controls who underwent

Roux-en-Y surgery, and 19 (10%), 4 (2%), and 0 patients, respectively, among 185 controls without PSC who underwent choledochocholedochostomy. They concluded that, although some of these lesions could represent a secondary sclerosing cholangitis, the frequency and characteristic nature of these lesions suggest that PSC rarely recurs in the liver allografts.

In a recent report, Gross et al (1997) reported a single center's 12-year experience with 127 liver transplants for PSC. Recurrent sclerosing cholangitis developed in 11 (8.6%) patients. The 5-year patient survival of this group was 90 percent, but there was a trend toward lower graft survival (52%) in patients who had recurrent disease. Although the lower graft survival was not statistically significant, this may suggest that a significant number of patients who develop recurrent PSC may require re-transplantation. In another study, Jeyarajah et al (1998) reported their experience in 100 patients who had OLT for PSC. Eighteen (15.7%) patients developed recurrent PSC and 115 (13%) patients developed chronic rejection. The 5-year graft survival was 65 percent in those who developed recurrent disease, 33 percent in those who had chronic rejection, and 76 percent in the remainder; re-transplantation rates were 28 percent, 47 percent, and 8.5 percent, respectively. Histopathologic analysis revealed that recurrent disease and chronic rejection shared many common features and were indistinguishable on histology. A cost analysis has not been performed in patients who develop recurrent disease, but it is probable that these patients use more resources. Recently, Graziadel et al (1999) reported cholangiographic evidence of nonanastomotic biliary strictures in 24 of 120 (20%) patients transplanted for PSC. This study may have overestimated recurrence of PSC because hepatic Doppler ultrasonography, not angiography, was used to exclude hepatic artery occlusion of stenosis. In our experience, Doppler ultrasonography underestimates hepatic artery stenosis in post-transplant patients, and we believe that hepatic angiography should be the gold standard to rule out hepatic artery stenosis or occlusion.

We had one patient with the unequivocal evidence of recurrence of PSC-like biliary strictures in two consecutive liver allografts (Figures 65–1, 65–2). This patient did not have any contributing factors such as ischemia or infection. The diagnosis was confirmed on both explants. From our own observations and the reports from other centers, it appears that recurrent PSC is a distinct entity seen in 5 to 10 percent of patients. Patients with PSC also seem to have a higher incidence of chronic ductopenic rejection and nonanastomotic biliary strictures compared to patients with primary biliary cirrhosis or other liver diseases.

Post-Orthotopic Liver Transplantation Follow-Up of Ulcerative Colitis

The association of PSC and UC appears to increase the risk of carcinoma of the colon about fivefold compared to

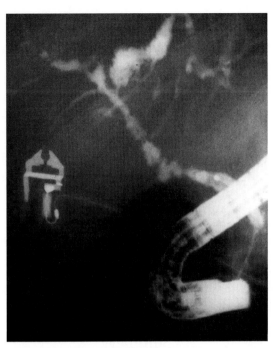

FIGURE 65–1. Endoscopic retrograde cholangiogram after the first liver transplantation showing diffuse mucosal abnormalities of intra- and extrahepatic ducts with stricturing and dilatation consistent with the diagnosis of sclerosing cholangitis.

UC patients without PSC. In a prospective study using multivariate analysis, Brentnall and colleagues (1996) found a significant increase in the development of dysplasia, up to 9 years of follow-up, in patients with UC and PSC (45%) compared with carefully matched controls with UC alone (16%). Details of colorectal neoplasia risk in PSC/UC patients are given in the chapter on dysplasia surveillance in IBD. At our own institution, 50 percent of patients had colonic neoplasia of some type after 28 years (actuarial table).

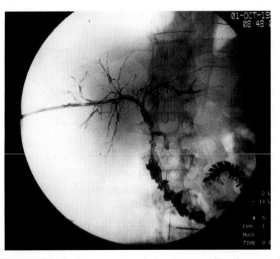

FIGURE 65–2. Percutaneous cholangiogram after the second transplantation showing diffuse intrahepatic strictures. A percutaneously placed stent is in place to bypass the dominant strictures in the extrahepatic ducts and at the choledochojejunal anastomosis.

The incidence of colorectal cancer after liver transplantation in patients with PSC and UC is estimated to be 1.25 percent per person per year and the cumulative incidence of colorectal dysplasia is about 15 percent at 5 years after liver transplantation. Therefore, the colon should be screened for early cancer before and after transplantation, at least on a yearly basis. In general, the presence of UC after liver transplantation is not thought to pose a significant medical problem. Most patients with symptoms of active colitis improved post-transplantation, perhaps due to the fact that these patients were receiving immunosuppressive medications. However, some patients with quiescent IBD have had an exacerbation of the IBD post-OLT despite immunosuppression use (Paptheodoridis et al. Gut 1998;43:639–44). Neuberger and colleagues (1999), using the Cox regression model, found that UC was associated with increased post-transplant survival, whereas Crohn's disease was associated with decreased post-transplant survival.

Summary

Primary sclerosing cholangitis is a chronic, progressive, cholestatic disease with a median survival of 10 years from the time of diagnosis. There is currently no effective medical therapy. Dominant, symptomatic strictures can be managed endoscopically. Reconstructive biliary surgery has no role in the management of PSC. Liver transplantation is the treatment of choice. Five-year survival after liver transplantation is approximately 80 to 90 percent. Actuarial patient survival after liver transplantation is significantly better than the survival rate of patients treated with nontransplantation biliary surgery or the predicted survival from prognostic models. Ten to 15 percent of patients with PSC develop cholangiocarcinoma, which is difficult to diagnose and rarely curable; however, in patients with small incidental cholangiocarcinomas, recognized only at liver exploration (in the absence of lymph node spread), the prognosis is more encouraging. It is recommended that patients with PSC are transplanted earlier than patients with other liver diseases. The high risk and poor prognosis for cholangiocarcinoma in longstanding PSC are an argument in favor of performing liver transplantation in an earlier phase of the disease. Colonoscopic surveillance for dysplasia is essential. Due to space limitation, all of the references prepared for this chapter could not be included. For a complete reference list, the reader is referred to pjthuluv@welch.jhu.edu. A number of references are included with other chapters in this text.

Supplemental Reading

Abu-Elmagd KM, Malinchoc M, Dickson R, et al. Efficacy of hepatic transplantation in patients with primary sclerosing cholangitis. Surg Gynecol Obstet 1993;177:335–44.

Angulo P, Lindo KD. Primary sclerosing cholangitis. Hepatology 1999;30:25–32.

Boberg KM, Lundin KE, Schrumpf E. Etiology and pathogenesis in primary sclerosing cholangitis [review]. Scand J Gastroenterol Suppl 1994;204:47–58.

Broome U, Olsson R, Loof L, et al. Natural history and prognostic factors in 305 Swedish patients with primary sclerosing cholangitis. Gut 1996;38:610–5.

Casavilla FA, Marsh JW, Iwatsuki S, et al. Hepatic resection and transplantation for peripheral cholangiocarcinoma. J Am Coll Surg 1997;185:429–36.

Dickson ER, Murtaugh PA, Wiesner RH, et al. Primary sclerosing cholangitis: refinement and validation of survival models. Gastroenterology 1992;103:1893–901.

Gores GJ, Steers JL, Burch PA, et al. Prolonged, disease-free survival following orthotopic liver transplantation (OLT) for cholangiocarcinoma. Transplantation 1999;67:S235.

Goss JA, Shackleton CR, Farmer DG, et al. Orthotopic liver transplantation for primary sclerosing cholangitis: a 12-year single center experience. Ann Surg 1997;225:472–83.

Graziadei IW, Wiesner RII, Batts P, et al. Recurrence of primary sclerosing cholangitis following liver transplantation. Hepatology 1999;29:1050–6.

Graziadei IW, Wiesner RII, Marotta PJ, et al. Long-term results of patients undergoing liver transplantation for primary sclerosing cholangitis. Hepatology 1999;30:1121–7.

Jeyarajah DR, Klintmalm GD. Is liver transplantation indicated for cholangiocarcinoma? J Hepatol Bil Panc Surg 1998; 5:48–51.

Jeyarajah DR, Netto GJ, Lee SP, et al. Recurrent primary sclerosing cholangitis after orthotopic liver transplantation. Transplantation 1998;66:1300–6.

Keiding S, Hansen SB, Rasmussen HH, et al. Detection of cholangiocarcinoma in primary sclerosing cholangitis by positron emission tomography. Hepatology 1998;28:700–6.

Lindor KD. Ursodiol for primary sclerosing cholangitis. Mayo Primary Sclerosing Cholangitis-Ursodeoxycholic Acid Study Group. N Engl J Med 1997;336:91–5.

Narumi S, Roberts JP, Emond JC, et al. Liver transplantation for sclerosing cholangitis. Hepatology 1995;22:451–7.

Nashan B, Schlitt HJ, Tusch G, et a. Biliary malignancies in primary sclerosing cholangitis: timing for liver transplantation. Hepatology 1996;23:1105–11.

Neuberger J, Gunson B, Komolmit P, et al. Pretransplant prediction of prognosis after liver transplantation in primary sclerosing cholangitis using a Cox regression model. Hepatology 1999;29:1375–9.

Seaberg EC, Belle SH, Beringer KC, et al. Liver transplantation in the United States from 1987–1998: updated results from the Pitt-UNOS liver transplant registry. In: Cecka JM, Terasaki PI, eds. Clinical transplants 1998. Los Angeles: UCLA Tissue Typing Laboratory, 1999:17–37.

Sheng R, Campbell WI, Zajko AB, Baron RL. Cholangiographic features of biliary strictures after liver transplantation for primary sclerosing cholangitis: evidence of recurrent disease. AJR Am J Roentgenol 1996;166:1109–13.

Shetty K, Ribicki I, Carey WD. The Child-Pugh classification as a prognostic indicator for survival in primary sclerosing cholangitis. Hepatology 1997;25:1049–53.

Voigt M, Schmidt W, LaBracque D, et al. Successful treatment of early stage cholangiocarcinoma in patients with PSC using combined liver transplantation, pancreaticoduodenectomy and brachytherapy. Transplantation 1999;67:5579A.

CHAPTER 66

CHOLANGIOCARCINOMA IN THE INFLAMMATORY BOWEL DISEASE PATIENT

BENEDICT M. DEVEREAUX, MB, BS, FRACP, STUART SHERMAN, MD, AND GLEN A. LEHMAN, MD

Cholangiocarcinoma (CC) is the most dreaded complication of primary sclerosing cholangitis (PSC) due to its overall poor prognosis and limited prospects for curative treatment. In the general population, CCs are rare tumors but occur in 5 to 15 percent of patients with PSC. Despite this frequency, there are limited publications on CC complicating PSC. Caution must therefore be exercised in the interpretation of data on CC if it has not been derived in the setting of PSC. Cholangiocarcinomas are mucin-producing adenocarcinomas that are slow growing and locally invasive, migrating along the nerves and nerve sheaths and invading adjacent vascular structures. The hepatic parenchyma can be infiltrated and lymph node metastases occur in approximately one-third of cases, but distant metastases are infrequent. Two-thirds of CC develop proximal to the junction of the cystic duct and common hepatic duct. The sclerosing type of CC is usually located in the hilar region. The papillary and nodular types are predominantly distal.

Cholangiocarcinomas are commonly grouped according to location: intrahepatic, perihilar, and extrahepatic tumors. This classification is useful as each category correlates with a distinct anatomic distribution and necessitates a different surgical resection. Cholangiocarcinomas associated with PSC classically involves the extrahepatic and hilar biliary tree with secondary extension into the intrahepatic bile ducts and liver parenchyma. Intrahepatic cholangiocarcinoma or cholangiocellular carcinoma (CCC) arises from the peripheral, small, intrahepatic bile ducts. It has a significantly weaker association with IBD and PSC, reported to be in the range of 0 to 7 percent, but is associated with hepatolithiasis and liver fluke infestation (eg, *Clinorchis sinensis*).

The occurrence of CC represents a devastating development in the course of PSC as the prognosis is very poor, with a median survival of 5 months. Orthotopic liver transplantation (OLT) has been very disappointing in the treatment of PSC complicated by CC due to the very high incidence of tumor recurrence in the donor liver. The literature reports a 1-year survival rate after OLT of only 30 percent and a 5-year survival approaching zero. The challenge, therefore, is to more precisely time definitive

treatment of PSC with OLT, before the development of CC, or diagnose CC at a sufficiently early, preinvasive stage so that curative resection can be achieved. The chapter on liver transplantation in PSC addresses these issues.

Risk Factors

The major risk factor for CC development is chronicity of PSC. This duration of disease is somewhat difficult to prove, as the precise date of onset of PSC is often uncertain. Most CC patients have already developed cirrhosis and have longstanding ulcerative colitis. In our own recent multicenter, case-controlled study, alcohol consumption was significantly associated with the development of CC in patients with PSC, conferring a three times increased risk.

Diagnosis

Screening

Ideally, stable PSC patients could undergo serologic, radiographic, or other noninvasive testing to detect early CC. Limited data reveal that the use of serum tumor markers and transcutaneous ultrasound have to date failed in this quest. No studies have been reported assessing the role of routine endoscopic retrograde cholangiopancreatography (ERCP) screening of PSC patients for the development of CC. Positron emission tomography (PET) using fluoro 2-2-deoxy-D-glucose reportedly has been able to detect small, potentially treatable CCs. Its use for screening PSC patients awaits testing.

Typical Clinical Presentation

The most frequent symptom of CC is jaundice, which is reported to occur in 90 to 98 percent of cases. Other common symptoms include weight loss, abdominal pain, and fever. The serum liver chemistries indicate biliary obstruction but do not differentiate benign from malignant processes.

Serum Tumor Markers

Measurement of serum tumor markers has been of some but limited value in differentiating benign strictures of

PSC from CC. Carbohydrate antigen (CA) 19-9 (a mucin-type glycoprotein) has been most widely used. Serum CA19-9 was elevated in 60 to 89 percent of patients with CC, but, unfortunately, moderate elevations can also be seen in PSC patients with cirrhosis and cholangitis without a tumor. An index combining serum CA19-9 and carcinoembryonic antigen (CEA) concentrations (CA19-9 + CEA × 40 > 400) reportedly afforded an accuracy of 86 percent in detecting CC in the PSC patient. Recent limited data reveal CA19-9 alone to be as sensitive as combined analysis of CA19-9 and CEA for CC detection. Our current practice is to monitor serum CA19-9 concentration at 6-month intervals. Goytos et al (1998) in a prospective study reported that a high level of the cytokine interleukin (IL)-6, which acts to promote the acute inflammatory response, was present in patients with a variety of liver malignancies, especially cholangiocarcinoma (sensitivity 100%, specificity 91.4%). In addition, its level correlated with tumor burden both pre- and postresection. This may represent a valuable, future marker for the development of CC. Further confirmatory studies are required.

Noninvasive Imaging Techniques

TRANSABDOMINAL ULTRASOUND

Transabdominal ultrasound's utility, in the assessment of CC, is limited to detection of biliary dilatation as it fails to identify a tumor mass in the majority of cases.

COMPUTED TOMOGRAPHY

Over an 11-year period, a variety of computed tomography (CT) scanning techniques detected possible tumor in 83 percent of patients with CC and definite or probable tumor in 74 percent in a series of 30 patients with PSC. Computed tomography was particularly valuable for showing intrahepatic tumor and therefore complemented cholangiography; cholangiography was insensitive for the detection of intrahepatic tumor but surpassed CT for detection of extrahepatic duct lesions. Importantly, this and other series conclude that the detection of enlarged lymph nodes on CT scan is not predictive of the development of carcinoma in the PSC patient. Quad-phase spiral CT scanners will be available in the near future. These may afford greater sensitivity than the current dual-phase CT scanners in the detection of CC in PSC patients.

MAGNETIC RESONANCE IMAGING

Magnetic resonance imaging (MRI) adds little to CT scan in the detection of CC. It may afford greatest benefit when CT and other modalities are equivocal or contraindicated due to iodine allergy.

MAGNETIC RESONANCE CHOLANGIOPANCREATOGRAPHY

Magnetic resonance imaging (MRCP) acquires a noninvasive cholangiogram without the need for ionizing radiation or intravenous contrast. It is effective in the detection of an obstructing biliary lesion but its specific application in the setting of PSC and differentiating benign from malignant dominant biliary strictures requires further investigation.

Invasive Imaging Techniques

ENDOSCOPIC ULTRASOUND

Endoscopic ultrasound (EUS) is of value mainly in evaluating the extrahepatic bile ducts. Nodular tumors are seen as masses but sclerosing tumors appear as nonspecific thickening. Fine-needle aspiration (FNA) is required for diagnosis. Its sensitivity in detecting invasion through the wall of the bile duct has been reported to be 78 percent with a specificity of 100 percent. Accurate N staging requires FNA. The use of intraductal ultrasound probes to differentiate benign from malignant strictures has, to date, been disappointing.

PERCUTANEOUS TRANSHEPATIC CHOLANGIOGRAPHY

Percutaneous transhepatic cholangiography (PTC) affords excellent images of the biliary tree, if the ducts can be entered. Tissue samples can also be obtained by FNA or intraductal sampling. The gold standard for the nonoperative detection of CC remains histologic assessment of cholangiographically guided tissue samples. However, PTC is not always possible in the PSC patient due to lack of dilatation of the intrahepatic ducts. Ducts with even high-grade obstruction downstream may fail to dilate due to hepatic fibrosis or cirrhosis.

ENDOSCOPIC RETROGRADE CHOLANGIOPANCREATOGRAPHY

The most useful nonoperative technique for the diagnosis of CC is endoscopic retrograde cholangiopancreatography (ERCP). The key benefit is the ability to define the presence and location of dominant strictures, obtain tissue specimens for diagnosis, and relieve obstruction during a single procedure, which does not traverse the peritoneal cavity.

DOMINANT STRICTURE EVALUATION

A dominant stricture is a tight stricture that occurs in the extrahepatic biliary tree or hilum resulting in cholestasis (in the absence of high-grade diffuse intrahepatic disease). The prevalence of these strictures in PSC is estimated to be approximately 20 to 30 percent. Approximately 90 percent can be traversed via ERCP, whereas the remainder require PTC assistance. Obtaining a tissue specimen from the strictured region of bile duct can be achieved percutaneously or at ERCP using a brush, FNA biopsy, intraductal forceps biopsy, or cytologic examination of aspirated bile.

BRUSH CYTOLOGY

The sensitivity of brush cytology for cancer detection, if present, is approximately 60 percent. This figure was not improved by the addition of K-ras and p53 analysis despite reports of an increase in mutations in these markers in PSC patients with CC compared with PSC patients without CC. The specificity and negative predictive value were reported to be 89 percent and 89 percent, respectively. Simultaneous application of FNA, endobiliary forceps biopsy, and exfoliative bile cytology testing will increase overall sensitivity to 70 to 75 percent. Whether the sensitivity of bile duct brushings is improved following dilation of dominant strictures is currently under investigation. Acquisition of multiple brush samples may afford greater sensitivity than a single brush sample.

Staging

The resectability rates for CC depend on the location of the lesion and careful staging to detect advanced local or metastatic disease that precludes resection. Complete preoperative assessment of resectability may require hepatic arteriography, portal venography, and/or EUS in addition to the standard imaging techniques discussed above.

Treatment

The options for curative therapy are very limited in the context of PSC because CC is frequently at an advanced stage at the time of diagnosis, and there is potential for multifocal involvement of the biliary tree. The focus of treatment following the detection of CC in the PSC patient is usually palliation.

Surgical

Surgical resection represents the only curative treatment strategy for CC. Resection of CC is *precluded* in the presence of cirrhosis; bilateral intrahepatic bile duct spread or multifocal disease on cholangiography; involvement of the main trunk of the portal vein; bilateral involvement of hepatic arterial or portal venous branches or both; and a combination of unilateral hepatic arterial involvement with cholangiographic evidence of extensive contralateral ductal spread. The most reproducible independent predictor of survival, following resection, is microscopically clear resection margins. The histologic subtype of the lesion, nutritional status, and postoperative sepsis may also impact on the outcome. Only rare CCs qualify for resection with curative intent. Palliative resection or surgical bypass is unwarranted in view of less invasive alternatives.

Chemoradiotherapy

Postoperative chemotherapy or radiotherapy has been universally disappointing in its lack of impact on the natural history of CC. Similarly, brachytherapy using iridium wires has not resulted in a significant survival benefit and is not widely undertaken. McMasters et al (1997), however, report that neoadjuvant chemoradiotherapy using 5-fluorouracil as a radiosensitizer was associated with a high rate of pathologic complete response as defined by no viable tumor detectable on histologic examination of the surgical specimen. Of nine patients to receive preoperative chemoradiation, all experienced a response, and in 3 (33%) this was a complete pathologic response. This represents a promising future development in the treatment of CC as it may increase the proportion of patients who can undergo resection with clear resection margins. Palliative use of chemotherapy or radiation therapy is of little value and generally not recommended.

Endoscopic

The aim of endoscopic intervention in the management of CC is to resolve cholestasis and bacterial cholangitis if present with resulting improved quality of life. Endoscopic therapy is technically successful in approximately 85 percent of cases in experienced centers. Failed cases are those with very tight, tortuous strictures and obstruction of multiple hilar branches.

Dominant biliary strictures can be dilated with either a graduated dilating catheter or preferably a balloon (typically 4 to 8 mm). The risk of perforation is small (approximately 1%), but care must be exercised so as not to dilate the stricture to a diameter greater than the smallest adjacent bile duct.

Endoscopic stent placement can use either plastic or expandable metal endoprostheses. Plastic 10 French stents typically remain patent for 3 to 4 months. Metal stents are superior in their duration of patency and may result in a lower incidence of cholangitis. In the event of metal stent occlusion, from tumor ingrowth, patency can be restored by inserting a plastic or second metal stent within the existing stent. It is essential to *confirm* the malignant and unresectable nature of a stricture prior to placement of an expandable metal stent as it usually cannot be removed and may hinder surgical intervention if undertaken.

Photodynamic Therapy

Photodynamic therapy (PDT) of nonresectable has been reported in small series to be effective in reducing the serum bilirubin and improving the quality of life. Photodynamic therapy may represent an additional treatment strategy, pending confirmation of this benefit in future studies.

Interventional Radiology

Biliary decompression is not always endoscopically achievable, and hilar strictures, in particular, can represent a challenge to the endoscopist. For endoscopically impassable strictures, the percutaneous route is usually effective. Percutaneous transhepatic cholangiography and percutaneous stent placement is facilitated by dilated intrahepatic ducts. Initial decompression of the biliary tree can be followed by internal/external drain placement and subsequent internalization of the drain once effective biliary drainage has been confirmed. Metal stents can be

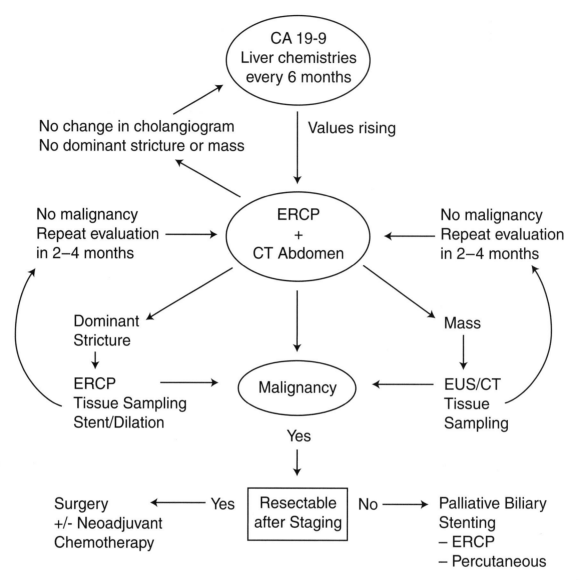

FIGURE 66–1. Management algorithm for patients with primary sclerosing cholangitis.

delivered percutaneously without endoscopic assistance. Occasionally, it is necessary to combine endoscopic and interventional radiologic efforts in a "rendezvous" procedure. A guidewire is inserted percutaneously through the stricture and subsequently snared in the duodenum and brought out through the endoscope.

Complications

Cholangitis

Biliary tract infection is a common complication in patients with PSC and CC. The reported overall infection rate during the course of biliary tract cancer is 50 to 60 percent, and it is the main cause of death in 25 percent of cases. The risk of infection is greater following instrumentation of the biliary tree at ERCP; therefore, the use of pre-procedure antibiotics is essential. We also

advocate a post-procedure 7-day course of antibiotics, particularly if there is injection of contrast into a segment of the biliary tree with poor drainage. The fluoroquinolones (eg, ciprofloxacin and levofloxacin) achieve excellent biliary concentration and are our antibiotics of choice. Should recurrent (greater than two episodes) or persistent cholangitis occur in the absence of stent dysfunction, then continuous administration of antibacterial prophylaxis is reasonable. Trimethoprim-sulfamethoxazole, augmentin, and ciprofloxacin are effective agents and can be cycled at monthly intervals.

Prognosis

It is important to decipher the literature carefully so as to differentiate between the prognosis of de novo CC and that complicating PSC. Nakeeb et al (1996) reported an actuarial survival of 17 percent in a series of 294 patients with CC who underwent resection. Of these, only 5 percent of patients, however, had PSC. Iwatsuki et al (1998) report 1- and 5-year survival rates of 60 percent and 25 percent, respectively, for patients undergoing OLT for hilar cholangiocarcinoma. In this series, only 34 percent of patients had PSC. These results are in stark contrast to the very poor prognosis for CC complicating PSC. The 5-year survival following OLT for PSC complicated by CC is essentially zero. This disparity could be explained by the multifocal nature of CC in advanced PSC and the presence of micrometastases in regional lymph nodes. The outlook for CC complicating PSC is grim, with a median survival of 5 months. See Figure 66–1 for recommended management.

Conclusion

Cholangiocarcinoma is a dreaded complication of PSC due to its poor prognosis and limited treatment options. Its detection in the setting of PSC necessitates a high index of clinical suspicion in addition to serial assessments of serum biliary biochemistry and possible imaging with CT scan of the abdomen and ERCP with tissue sampling of dominant strictures. Early detection of potentially curable CC remains the challenge, and no proven technique exists. Serum IL-6 concentration and PET scanning may prove to be helpful in this regard. The only definitive treatment is surgical resection as the prognosis following OLT remains unacceptably poor. Neoadjuvant therapy with chemoradiation may offer some benefit in reducing tumor bulk and increasing the proportion of patients suitable for curative resection. Palliative therapy aims to relieve the symptoms of biliary obstruction and optimize quality of life. Endoscopic stricture dilation and biliary stent placement is possible in the majority of patients and highly successful in effecting biliary decompression. A multidisciplinary approach optimizes the treatment strategy in the management of patients with CC.

Supplemental Reading

Campbell WL, Ferris JV, Holbert BL, et al. Biliary tract carcinoma complicating primary sclerosing cholangitis: evaluation with CT, cholangiography, US, and MR imaging. Radiology 1998;207:41–50.

Goytos JS, Brumfield AM, Frezza E, et al. Marked elevation of serum interleukin-6 in patients with cholangiocarcinoma. Ann Surg 1998;227:398–404.

Iwatsuki S, Todo S, Marsh JW, et al. Treatment of hilar cholangiocarcinoma (Klatskin tumors) with hepatic resection or transplantation. J Am Coll Surg 1998;187:358–64.

McMasters KM, Tuttle TM, Leach SD, et al. Neoadjuvant chemoradiation for extrahepatic cholangiocarcinoma. Am J Surg 1997;74:605–9.

Nakeeb A, Pitt HA, Sohn TA, et al. Cholangiocarcinoma. A spectrum of intrahepatic, perihilar and distal tumors. Ann Surg 1996;224 :463–75.

Peters RA, Williams SGJ, Lombard M, et al. The management of high-grade hilar strictures by endoscopic insertion of self-expanding metal endoprostheses. Endoscopy 1996;28:10–6.

Ponsioen, et al. Value of brush cytology for dominant strictures in primary sclerosing cholangitis. Endoscopy 1999;31:305–9.

Ramage JK, Donaghy A, Farrant JM, et al. Serum tumor markers for the diagnosis of cholangiocarcinoma in primary sclerosing cholangitis. Gastroenterology 1995;108:865–9.

Rogers SA, Podolsky DK. Predicting cholangiocarcinoma in patients with primary sclerosing cholangitis: an analysis of serological marker CA19-9. Hepatology 1994;19:543–5.

Vauthey JN, Blumgart LH. Recent advances in the management of cholangiocarcinomas. Semin Liver Dis 1994;14:109–14.

CHAPTER 67

GALLSTONE MANAGEMENT IN INFLAMMATORY BOWEL DISEASE

KONSTANTINOS N. LAZARIDIS, MD, AND KEITH D. LINDOR, MD

The association between inflammatory bowel disease (IBD) and hepatobiliary disorders has been well established. Both Crohn's disease (CD) and chronic ulcerative colitis (UC) can affect the liver and biliary system. Indeed, hepatobiliary involvement in patients with IBD varies from the asymptomatic state to the development of symptomatic complications related to chronic liver injury. The spectrum of hepatobiliary associations in IBD is outlined in Table 67–1. Of all of those conditions, gallstones represent one of the most frequently encountered clinical hepatobiliary problems in patients with IBD especially those with Crohn's disease.

In this chapter, we present an overview of the management of gallbladder stones and biliary sludge in patients with IBD. A summary of the epidemiology and pathogenesis of gallstones and biliary sludge in these patients is provided to guide therapeutic decision-making, which should aim not only to address symptomatic stones but also to prevent their development.

Epidemiology and Pathogenesis of Gallstones in Inflammatory Bowel Disease

Multiple investigations have shown a greater prevalence of cholelithiasis in patients with CD compared to the general population. Two recent independent retrospective studies from England and Sweden have reported the prevalence of gallstones to be 28 percent and 26 percent, respectively, in patients with CD. Lapidus et al demonstrated a 1.8 relative risk of developing cholelithiasis in CD patients compared to a control population. A case-control study by Lorusso et al (1990) also revealed an increased relative risk of gallstones in patients with CD (odds ratio: 3.6).

Gallstone formation is considered to be multifactorial. Indeed, cholesterol supersaturation, nucleation of cholesterol crystals, hypersecretion of gallbladder mucus, and gallbladder motility are important factors that participate in the formation of gallstones. However, the pathogenesis of cholelithiasis in CD remains obscure. In Western societies, cholesterol stones account for almost 90 percent of gallstones, with pigment stones making up the rest. Knowing the type of stones present in CD may help to elucidate the mechanism of gallstone formation in these

TABLE 67–1. Hepatobiliary Manifestations of Inflammatory Bowel Disease

Hepatic	Biliary Tract
Amyloidosis	Cholelithiasis
Abscess	Pericholangitis
Cirrhosis	Primary sclerosing cholangitis
Fibrosis	Cholangiocarcinoma
Hemosiderosis	
Hepatitis	
Hepatic vascular abnormalities	
Sarcoidosis	
Steatosis	

patients. Nevertheless, studies using stone analysis in patients with CD are lacking. It was thought that cholesterol stones represent the majority of gallstones in CD patients; however, data suggest that pigment stones may also exist in these patients. Moreover, it has been demonstrated that gallbladder bile from patients with CD involving the ileum has high bilirubin concentration compared to a group of patients with Crohn's colitis or chronic UC. This observation suggests the enterohepatic circulation of bilirubin, which represents an additional risk factor for pigment stone formation. Another contributing factor in gallstone formation is cholesterol crystal precipitation or nucleation. Evidence indicates an increased nucleation time in bile from patients with CD compared to those with a history of UC. Studies on the secretion of gallbladder mucus in IBD are limited.

The effect of CD on gallbladder motility remains controversial. In patients with CD, some investigators have shown gallbladder hypokinesia while others have reported no abnormalities in gallbladder emptying. Despite the debate on the possible direct effect of CD on gallbladder motility, one must realize that many of these patients receive total parenteral nutrition (TPN) for long periods of time as therapeutic management, which can also be associated with gallbladder hypomotility.

It has been postulated that the increased prevalence of cholelithiasis in CD patients may be related to bile acid malabsorption because of a diseased or surgically resected terminal ileum. It was felt that decreased ileal absorption of bile acids produces supersaturation of cholesterol in bile and the subsequent development of cholesterol stones. However, studies have shown that intestinal loss of

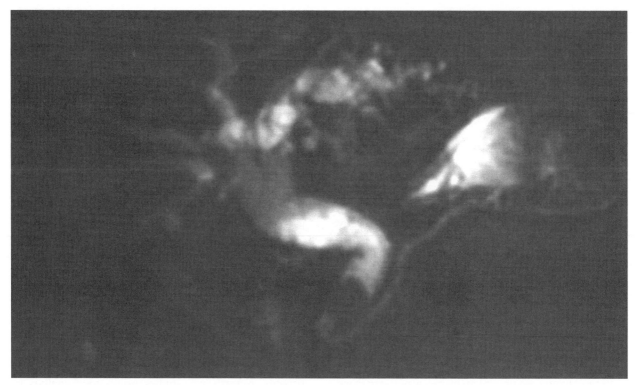

Figure 67–1. Magnetic resonance cholangiopancreatography shows choledocholithiasis in a patient with inflammatory bowel disease. (Courtesy of D. C. Johnson, MD, Department of Radiology, Mayo Clinic, Rochester, Minnesota).

bile acids increases their *de novo* hepatic synthesis. Moreover, patients with CD produce bile that is less saturated with cholesterol compared to bile from patients with cholelithiasis in the general population. Indeed, Hutchinson et al reported that in patients with CD, neither the site of disease nor previous intestinal resection were predisposing factors for development of cholelithiasis. Nevertheless, in the same study, previous surgery (laparotomy) alone was an independent risk factor for development of gallstones and the risk was correlated with the number of laparotomies. More recently, Lapidus et al. using a defined cohort of patients with CD, have shown that only the number of previous intestinal resections was an independent risk factor for cholelithiasis, not the localization of disease or type of surgery. Therefore, it is reasonable to assume that perioperative factors inducing gallbladder hypomotility such as protracted fasting and use of TPN may predispose a patient to gallstone formation rather than ileal dysfunction or intestinal resection.

The prevalence of biliary sludge and gallstones in patients with CD receiving TPN has been reported to be approximately 40 percent. Biliary sludge represents a combination of particulate substances and bile that forms in the gallbladder when solutes in bile precipitate. In patients with no history of hepatobiliary disease, sludge develops in 6 percent after 3 weeks and in 100 percent after 6 weeks of TPN. Biliary sludge usually persists during TPN and may resolve after its discontinuation.

Diagnosis of sludge is achieved by abdominal or endoscopic ultrasound with sensitivity of about 55 percent and 96 percent, respectively. In cases of suspected biliary sludge, extensive evaluation may be needed to prove its presence. The "gold standard" test for diagnosis is the presence of cholesterol crystals on bile microscopy. Biliary sludge may cause complications including acute cholecystitis, acute pancreatitis, and biliary colic. In patients with CD, gallbladder sludge may represent a predisposing factor for cholelithiasis.

In patients with chronic UC, cholelithiasis is less frequent compared to Crohn's disease. Lorusso et al have reported an increased risk of gallstones in patients with chronic UC (odds ratio: 2.5). Inflammatory bowel disease, more commonly chronic UC than CD, may coexist with primary sclerosing cholangitis (PSC). Cholelithiasis and choledocholithiasis occur in approximately 30 percent of patients with PSC. In these patients, chronic cholestasis predisposes to formation of cholesterol gallstones, with bile stasis and bacterial cholangitis inducing the development of pigment stones. If patients with PSC who have intact gallbladders are surveyed by ultrasonography, gallstones will be found in about 25 percent. Because most of these patients are young men, this high incidence of gallstone disease probably denotes an increased frequency of cholelithiasis in PSC. Choledocholithiasis can cause bacterial cholangitis as a complication of PSC. Diagnosis can be extremely difficult in these patients, since bacterial cholangitis may develop in the absence of biliary stones. A cholangiogram to exclude choledocholithiasis superimposed on PSC should be considered, particularly in patients who have not had biliary surgery and who have recently experienced the onset or recurrent episodes of bacterial cholangitis. The advent of magnetic resonance cholangiopancreatography (MRCP) has provided an effective and nonradioactive modality for detection of choledocholithiasis with a sensitivity between 75 and 95 percent. (Figure 67–1)

Treatment of Gallstones in Inflammatory Bowel Disease

In patients with IBD and gallbladder and/or biliary stones or sludge, the therapeutic approach should be individualized depending on the clinical presentation and underlying status of primary disease.

Patients with CD and symptomatic cholelithiasis or complications related to gallbladder stones such as acute pancreatitis and biliary colic should have elective cholecystectomy. In CD patients with a prior history of intestinal resections, open cholecystectomy is preferred over the laparoscopic approach.* Alternative surgical approaches in high-risk patients include surgical cholecystostomy, percutaneous cholecystostomy, and percutaneous cholecystolithotomy. Surgical cholecystostomy is used in emergent conditions to accomplish gallbladder decompression via an open tube cholecystostomy. Today, a safer and more frequently used procedure is the percutaneous cholecystostomy, which is carried out using ultrasound or fluoroscopic guidance. It provides decompression and drainage of the gallbladder. When performed by experienced individuals, percutaneous cholecystostomy has lower morbidity and mortality compared to surgical cholecystostomy. Finally, percutaneous cholecystolithotomy represents a combination of percutaneous cholecystostomy and direct endoscopic lithotomy and requires advanced expertise and technology. It is indicated in patients with insoluble gallstones. Potential complications of all of these alternative surgical approaches include abscess formation, sepsis, intractable bleeding, and intraperitoneal bile leakage.

Pharmacologic dissolution of cholesterol gallstones is reserved for patients with high surgical risk. The two natural bile acids that have been used for dissolution of radiolucent cholesterol stones include ursodeoxycholic acid (ursodiol) and chenodeoxycholic acid (chenodiol).

---

* Editor's Note: Some therapeutic questions: Symptomatic gallstones and a long asymptomatic ileal stricture? Do both laparascopically and laparascopically assisted (see separate chapter)? Laparoscopic cholecystectomy and separate open ileal resections? Asymptomatic stones and a long symptomatic ileal resection? Many surgeons would take out the gall bladder. They would think that cholecystectomy is almost inevitable. One down side, cholereic diarrhea with a low ileal resection and cholecystectomy. (TMB)

Candidates for pharmacologic dissolution treatment should have radiolucent stones and a patent cystic duct. In the general population, the overall success rate for dissolution of gallbladder stones up to 20 mm in diameter is between 30 and 50 percent. Therapeutic doses of ursodiol and chenodiol are 8 to 10 mg/kg and 13 to 15 mg/kg, respectively. In a meta-analysis of randomized studies using ursodiol > 7 mg/kg or > 500 mg daily for 6 months, the dissolution rate was 37 percent. Following complete dissolution of stones, continuation of ursodiol therapy is recommended for 3 additional months. An absent or minimal decrease in stone diameter after 6 to 12 months of therapy with ursodiol represents a poor prognostic sign. Recurrence of gallstones following complete dissolution ranges between 50 and 70 percent over a period of 11 years.

Maintenance low-dose ursodiol (300 mg/d) decreases the reappearance rate of gallstones by approximately 50 percent compared to an untreated group over a period of 9 years. Data regarding the effects of ursodiol as treatment for patients with gallstones and IBD are not available but the results are likely to be poor, given the risk of pigment stones being present.

Additional nonsurgical approaches include gallstone contact dissolution with methyl-tert-butyl-ether (MTBE) and extracorporeal shock wave lithotripsy (ESWL). However, both MTBE and ESWL are considered experimental in the United States. Methyl-tert-butyl-ether is a contact solvent that works by dissolving cholesterol stones in the gallbladder; it is infused via either percutaneous transhepatic cholecystostomy or retrograde nasobiliary tubing. Successful dissolution has been reported to be 95 to 100 percent over 2 to 3 days but is followed by a high rate of new gallstone formation. Extracorporeal shock wave lithotripsy depends on the generation of acoustic shock waves that are transmitted to the body and facilitate the breakage of stones at the interface of substances with varying acoustic impedance. Gallstones should be less than 3 cm in diameter. Continuous oral bile acid dissolution therapy for 1 to 2 years is required following gallstone fragmentation to accomplish complete clearance of gallbladder stones.

In patients with IBD and biliary sludge, the therapeutic approach depends on the presence of symptoms or complications such as episodes of acute cholecystitis, acute pancreatitis, or biliary colic. Asymptomatic sludge need not be monitored regularly; however, precipitating factors or conditions including prolonged fasting, TPN, and use of ceftriaxone or octreotide must be avoided. Patients with symptomatic sludge or complications should have cholecystectomy. In poor surgical candidates, alternative interventions include oral agents for bile acid dissolution and percutaneous cholecystostomy.

In patients with chronic UC associated with PSC, symptomatic cholelithiasis or its complications require cholecystectomy. In these patients, the presence of chole-docholithiasis obligates evaluation for biliary strictures. This can be achieved by either ERCP or percutaneous transhepatic cholangiography and perhaps MRCP. Dominant strictures should be dilated and biliary stones should be lavaged or extracted. Recurrence of choledo-cholithiasis can be a therapeutic challenge and requires a multispecialty approach. There are separate chapters on PSC and on dilating strictures in PSC.

More studies are needed to better define the patho-genesis and natural history of gallstones in IBD prior to implementing more effective treatments. In addition, attention should be given to secondary prevention of stones in these patients. For example, in patients with CD, prophylactic use of ursodiol or cholecystokinin during TPN may prevent gallstone formation.

Editor's Note

The next edition will have a chapter by a surgeon as to the need for and timing of cholecystectomy in patients with Crohn's disease. The chapters on small bowel surgery in Crohn's disease address some of the issues. (TMB)

Supplemental Reading

Barish MA, Soto JA, Yucel KE. Magnetic resonance cholangio-pancreatography of the biliary ducts: techniques, clinical applications, and limitations. Top in Magn Reson Imaging 1996;8:302–11.

Brink MA, Slors JFM, Keulemans YCA, et al. Enterohepatic cycling of bilirubin: a putative mechanism for pigment gall-stone formation in ileal Crohn's disease. Gastroenterology 1999;116:1420–7.

Damiao AOMC, Sipahi AM, Vezozzo DP, et al. Gallbladder hypokinesia in Crohn's disease. Digestion 1997;58:458–63.

Hutchinson R, Tyrrell PNM, Kumar D, et al. Pathogenesis of gallstones in Crohn's disease: an alternative explanation. Gut 1994;35:94–7.

Ko CW, Sekijima JH, Lee SP. Biliary sludge. Ann Intern Med 1999;130:301–11.

Lapidus A, Bangstad M, Astrom M, et al. The prevalence of gallstone disease in a defined cohort of patients with Crohn's disease. Am J Gastroenterol 1999;94:1261–6.

Lorusso D, Leo S, Mossa A, et al. Cholelithiasis in inflammatory bowel disease: a case-control study. Dis Colon Rectum 1990;33:791–4.

Rubin RA, Kowalski TE, Khandelwal M, et al. Ursodiol for hepatobiliary disorders. Ann Intern Med 1994;121:207–18.

CHAPTER 68

Urologic Complications

David Y. Chan, MD, and H. Ballentine Carter, MD

A significant percentage of patients (4 to 23%) with inflammatory bowel disease (IBD) will develop complications involving the genitourinary tract. These urologic complications are sequelae of the metabolic derangements associated with IBD, the chronic underlying disease process, and its treatment. The most pervasive problems include renal calculi, enterovesical fistulae, ureteral obstruction, infertility, and iatrogenic ureteral injury. These complications can be insidiously asymptomatic and often are obscured by concomitant bowel symptoms. Consequently, integration of urologic evaluation as a part of IBD assessment can help prevent urologic complications.

Urinary Tract Calculi

It has been estimated that between 1 and 25 percent of patients with IBD will develop urinary tract calculi, a rate 10 to 100 times greater than that of the general hospital population. This risk is higher in patients with Crohn's disease (CD) than with ulcerative colitis (UC) and in patients with ileostomies.

In general, if the patient with IBD has a functional colon, most urinary calculi in these patients are composed of calcium oxalate, primarily due to increased oxalate absorption in the colon, while patients with ileostomy diversions with no functional colon tend to present with uric acid stones, primarily due to dehydration and acidosis. The etiology of nephrolithiasis is multifactorial. Dehydration, oliguria, obstruction, urinary tract infection, acidic urine, steroid use (which increases intestinal calcium absorption), prolonged bed rest (which increases calcium mobilization), and increased fecal sodium loss from persistent diarrhea (which results in dehydration) all can predispose and contribute to stone formation. Typically, these patients present with dysuria, abdominal or flank pain, and microscopic hematuria.

Calcium Oxalate Stones

The pathophysiology of calcium oxalate stone formation is related to disturbances in the permeability of the colonic mucosa. Intestinal transport of oxalate is increased by the secondary influences of bile salts and fatty acids. Intestinal fat malabsorption, characteristic of ileal disease, can exaggerate calcium-soap formation,

sequestering free calcium from complexing with intestinal oxalate, thereby indirectly increasing the enteric oxalate pool for absorption in the colon. Exposure of colonic mucosa to bile salts, which is increased in IBD, increases oxalate absorption in the colon. Other factors, such as excessive fluid loss from the gastrointestinal tract leading to reduced urinary output, hypomagnesuria from poor intestinal magnesium absorption, hypocitruria due to hypokalemia, and metabolic acidosis, may predispose patients to stone formation. Magnesium and citrate are potent urinary inhibitors of stone formation. Thus, low urinary levels predispose these patients to stone formation. There is a chapter on hyperoxaluria and nephrolithiasis.

Uric Acid Stones

Uric acid stones in IBD are primarily a consequence of dehydration and acidic urine secondary to metabolic acidosis. Uric acid has a pKa of 5.5. Consequently, low urinary pH precipitates the formation of uric acid crystals that can form uric acid stones or serve as nidus for calcium stone formation.

Prevention of New Stone Formation

The fundamental management of calcium oxalate and uric acid stones includes maintaining good hydration and high urinary output. Urinary measurements of citrate, oxalate, and uric acid can help guide therapy. Although some patients with calcium oxalate stones may benefit from magnesium replacement, most patients do not tolerate the diarrhea that accompanies magnesium supplementation. Simple dietary oxalate restriction can be useful in some patients with malabsorption. The mainstay of treatment is correction of metabolic acidosis, aciduria, and hypocitraturia with potassium citrate. The details of dietary and medication management of oxylate stones are given in the chapter on hyperoxylurea.

For patients with uric acid stones, serum and urinary uric acid levels are valuable. Patients with mild to moderate hyperuricosuria associated with hypocitruria will benefit from potassium citrate. However, patients with severe hyperuricosuria or hyperuricemia will require treatement with allopurinol 300 mg each day. Sodium bicarbonate, 650 mg three times each day, can be used to alkalinize urine to maintain an optimal pH near 7.0. However, if the patient also has hypercalciuria, potassium citrate may be a better choice as an alkalinizing agent since the increased sodium load from sodium bicarbonate will increase sodium delivery to the proximal tubule and can increase urinary calcium. Over-alkalinization can be detrimental as alkaline solution can precipitate apatite stones. Patients should be instructed to test the urine with pH paper to maintain pH in the proper range. At times, patients with ileostomy and excessive fluid losses from chronic diarrhea can be extremely difficult to manage and may require additional antidiarrheal medications. In some patients, increased sodium and potassium intake may also increase diarrhea. In these patients, the medication dosage must be individualized to avoid unwanted gastrointestinal side effects. In select cases, these patients may need nighttime alkalinization with carbonic anhydrase inhibitors.

Treatment of Existing Stones

Symptomatic patients with nephrolithiasis can be managed with minimally invasive techniques such as extracorporeal shock wave lithotripsy or endoscopic techniques. With the development of percutaneous and ureteroscopic approaches, open surgery rarely is indicated today for the treatment of urinary tract stones. Complete obstruction, especially when associated with urinary tract infections or fever, demands immediate decompression with either a ureteral stent or nephrostomy tube.

Enterovesical Fistula Formation

Although internal fistulae are common in CD (24 to 32%), fistulae between the gastrointestinal tract and the urinary tract are less common (1 to 8%), but do pose a significant management problem. These patients generally present with prominent, irritative urinary tract symptoms, such as dysuria, frequency, and suprapubic discomfort. Classic symptoms also include pneumaturia and fecaluria with frequent urinary tract infections.

The majority of enterovesical fistulae are seen in patients with CD and involve the terminal ileum and bladder dome. Colovesical fistulae also can occur but usually are noted in patients with UC or diverticulitis. When suspected clinically, the diagnosis of enterovesical fistulae is confirmed with computed tomography (CT) scan and cystoscopy. The details of CT localization of enterovesical fistulae are in the chapter on use of CT in IBD patients.

Diagnosis

Computed tomographic scan without intravenous contrast should be the initial diagnostic study before any other manipulation that can potentially introduce air into the bladder, resulting in a false-positive result, since air in the bladder that has not been instrumented is diagnostic of a fistula. Other studies such as plain abdominal films, intravenous pyelography, cystography, and barium enema tend to have a low yield. The typical CT scan findings reveal air in the bladder with focal apposition of the bladder and bowel and bladder and bowel wall thickening. Cross-sectional imaging is useful for ruling out abscess formation, for extrinsic pathology, and for planning a surgical approach to the disease process. Cystoscopy usually demonstrates an erythematous inflamed area on the anterior or posterior bladder wall, but the fistulous tract may not be evident.

Management

Spontaneous closure of enterovesical fistulae is rare. The most effective management is surgical intervention. The preferred operation is a single-stage procedure with surgical resection of the diseased bowel, closure of the bladder fistula, and, if possible, interposition of omentum between bowel and bladder. A Foley catheter is placed to ensure adequate bladder drainage while healing takes place. Patients with colonic obstruction, sepsis, extensive inflammation, complex fistulae, poor nutritional status, or frank abscess may require staged procedures for management. A gravity cystogram should be performed postoperatively prior to a voiding trial to exclude a bladder leak. Immunosuppressive agents, such as 6-mercaptopurine and methotrexate, have been described as possible medical therapy for ileovesical or colovesical fistulae, but are less successful in the long-term than surgery. The role of immunomodulator therapy is described in several chapters in this text. Whether anti–tumor necrosis factor therapy will play any predictable role is yet to be described.

Ureteral Obstruction

Ureteral obstruction in IBD usually is not caused by stone disease. Retroperitoneal inflammation and retroperitoneal fibrosis are responsible for most cases of ureteral obstruction. Noncalculous ureteral obstruction is detected incidentally in 5 to 15 percent of patients with IBD undergoing intravenous pyelogram for various other indications. In CD, retroperitoneal inflammation with periureteral fibrosis is usually the source of obstruction. Right-sided obstruction predominates in over 70 percent of these cases associated with ileal or ileocecal disease. Stent placement to prevent iatrogenic ureteral injury is discussed in a later section. In UC, the distribution of obstruction is more uniform, and iatrogenic surgical complications or colon cancer are more often the causes of obstruction.

Patients with noncalculous ureteral obstruction often are asymptomatic. When symptoms are present, they are nonspecific and suggest bladder irritability. Despite the absence of symptoms in these patients, ureteral obstruction is not benign, and upper tract pathology may

CHAPTER 69

Hematologic Problems in Inflammatory Bowel Disease

Henry Cymorek, MD, and Joel B. Levine, MD

The hematologic abnormalities encountered in the management of inflammatory bowel disease (IBD) are varied and range from overt and occult gastrointestinal bleeding to an increased risk for thromboembolic complications. Blood disorders are prevalent: anemia is present in more than 50 percent of patients, and a decreased serum iron level is found in over one-third. Iron loss, defective iron transport, insufficient erythropoietin production, and even inhibition of marrow colony formation all have been described. Much of the pathophysiology associated with these abnormalities now is seen as either a direct or derivative consequence of the inflammatory cell responses that characterize these disorders. Effective clinical management arises from recognizing these relationships and adapting our overall advances in inflammation and immune modulation to these specific clinical settings.

Gastrointestinal Bleeding

Although it is rare, occurring in less than 5 percent of patients, massive hemorrhage may occur in ulcerative colitis (UC) or in Crohn's disease (CD) where it may be secondary to deep submucosal ulcers or filiform polyps. As with other intestinal blood loss, restoration of volume is essential though recent data suggest that, unless the patient is unstable, central line monitoring may not be needed and may be associated with an increased risk of thrombotic catheter occlusion. In addition, nutritional- or antibiotic-mediated decreases in clotting factors also may be present, amplifying the amount of blood loss.

Iron Deficiency Anemia

Chronic blood loss may lead to iron deficiency anemia. In the face of sustained iron depletion, ineffective erythropoiesis may occur when transferrin saturation is below 10 percent, and many iron-dependent tissue enzymes decrease in functional activity. Ferrous sulfate (300 mg tablets providing 60 mg of elemental iron) remains in therapeutic fashion. Although the recommended dosage is 120 to 180 mg of elemental iron per day, even a single tablet exceeds daily intestinal absorptive capacity. Gastrointestinal distress due to oral iron is reducible if the initial dose, given with or during meals, is gradually increased from one tablet per day. A longer duration of therapy, extending to 4 months, is preferable to high doses over a short duration. In ordinary circumstances, parenteral iron is no more effective than ferrous sulfate in correcting iron deficiency. If ferrous sulfate proves intolerable at any dose, carbonyl iron powder is available and has milder though similar side effects.

When iron loss exceeds the efficiency of oral iron therapy, or if the patient does not respond, parenteral iron may be used. Colloidal suspensions, especially iron dextran (Imferon® 50 mg elemental iron/mL) may be given intramuscularly (IM) or intravenously (IV) but are inconvenient, painful, and carry a small but real risk of anaphylactic reaction. This adverse response is not dose-dependent nor can it be excluded by a history of previously tolerated test injections. Although most of the chelated iron exists as microspherules of ferrous oxide cloaked with dextran, small amounts of iron leak from their polysaccharide shells. Since there is no physiologic mechanism to excrete excess iron, doses should be carefully calculated (gm FE = normal Hb–patients Hb, in g/100 mL × 0.255) and judiciously given (2 mL IV or 5 mL IM), with 6 to 10 5 mL injections usually required. A formula for IV use is given in Chapter 56.

The severity of anemia in IBD patients may be related to disease activity and correlated to levels of specific cytokines, such as interleukin (IL)-6 and monocyte-derived IL-1β. These cytokines may impair both the production and the stimulatory effect of **erythropoietin** on the proliferation and maturation of erythroid precursors. Affected patients may exhibit an incomplete response with concentrations of erythropoietin inadequate for the degree of anemia. Patients refractory to conventional courses of iron and vitamins may significantly increase their hemoglobin levels in response to a combination of oral iron and **recombinant erythropoietin** (150 units kg *sc* twice a week). Although there may be an increase in the magnitude response when IV iron is supplemented with erythropoietin, it is important to emphasize that, in light of the cost of this supplemental therapy, 75 percent of IBD patients may still respond adequately to 8 weeks of IV iron saccharate. Erythropoietin may, however, be especially effective in proven nonresponders.

Interpretation of Hypochromic Anemia

Hypochromic anemias need careful resolution. Although a primary disorder of heme synthesis (sideroblastic anemia) may be encountered, the more common challenge is to distinguish true iron deficiency from disorders of iron—erythroblast transport, poorly termed "the anemia of chronic disease." Isolated measurements of the serum iron level may be misleading, since hypoferritinemia may appear despite abundant stores of iron. Variations in the serum iron levels may, in part, reflect the levels of circulating IL-1 and a decreased iron may thus be a reflection of increased disease activity. As a clinical guideline, serum iron concentrations below 70 mg/dL, serum transferrin greater than 350 mg/dL, and a percent saturation of less than 16 percent are statistically valid predictors for true iron deficiency.

The serum ferritin level in many clinical circumstances accurately reflects the adequacy of iron stores. Bone marrow iron is absent when serum ferritin is less than 10 ng/dL. Ferritin release from polysomes appears contingent upon the incorporation of iron into ribosomal-associated apoferritin. In uncomplicated cases of iron deficiency, ferritin release (synthesis) decreases as available iron declines. When responding as a liver-synthesized acute-phase reactant, the serum ferritin value (reflecting both ferritin and iron-poor apoferritin) increases as part of the adaptive response to active inflammation. Impairment of iron transport to the erythroblast also is present and may be a consequence of an increased number of macrophage-associated transferrin and lactoferrin receptors expressed in response to the inflammatory stimulus. Increased IL-1 production also has been implicated in the release of granulocyte lactoferrin and inhibition of bone marrow colony formation.

In summary, although gastrointestinal bleeding has center stage in IBD, hematologic abnormalities may reflect the impact of the inflammatory process on hematopoiesis and iron metabolism. The interpretation of specific hematologic measurements (serum iron level) and the amount of available carrier protein (transferrin and ferritin [apoferritin]), the expression of receptors (lactoferrin, transferrin) that influence the transfer of serum iron from the macrophage, and even the degree of marrow responsiveness all may be consequences of ongoing, even subclinical, inflammation.

Alterations in Blood Coagulation

Clinical and laboratory studies have suggested that blood coagulation is activated in patients with either CD or UC. Molecular activation of coagulation is crucial to the full expression of the inflammatory response and clotting activation is well studied in IBD. Activated blood coagulation, evidenced by increases in thrombin activated clotting factors, products of fibrin formation and fibrinolysis (fibrinopeptide A [FPA]), thrombin-antithrombin complex, fragments 1 + 2 and d-dimers, is well validated. Conversely, thrombin can, in turn, influence inflammation by stimulating adhesion molecules for leukocytes and endothelial cell surface leukocyte rolling. Some measurements of clotting activation may reflect, therefore, inflammation; for example, monocyte activation is well correlated with plasma levels of FPA. Serial levels of FPA may measure the true state of subclinical inflammation and even predict the appearance of a clinical recurrence. Of potential clinical value is the rapid decline of fibrinogen and fibrin degradation products in patients who achieve remission with corticosteroid therapy. Residual elevations of markers of activated clotting may identify patients with partial remission or who are at risk for relapse. Plasma concentrations of markers of activated coagulation may deserve further study as useful measures of disease activity in IBD.

Thromboembolic Complications

Accelerated clotting also may add real risk to patients with IBD. Thromboembolic complications are reported to occur in 12 to 39 percent of patients with IBD and may be associated with an increased mortality rate. Reports of cerebral vascular, mesenteric, and pulmonary vessel occlusion in young people are not infrequent. Risk of mortality increases in patients with their first thrombotic episode and there is a 20 percent risk for recurrent thrombosis. Those who clot once frequently will clot again (multiple episodes occur in 12 percent of patients), often involving unusual sites. Though the early case reports limited the thrombosis risk to active colitis, there is a 70 percent association with clinical inactivity. This may be due to ongoing release of proinflammatory cell products and platelet activation.

In recent years, there is evidence that activated clotting may be a pathogenic factor and not just a secondary response to inflammation. The thrombotic tendency in IBD is only infrequently reported to be causally related to abnormal amounts of protein C or cofactor protein S, decreased antithrombin III, or the antiphospholipid antibody syndrome. Using a three-dimensional latex injected model of CD pathology, investigators have suggested that a primary granulomatous vasculitis, perhaps triggered by retained measles virus genome, may be the initiating event in the disease. Finally, and receiving strong interest, is the accumulating evidence for a predisposing endothelial injury or a genetic defect in factor V Leiden that would reduce natural antithrombotic defenses and create a susceptible environment for any of the myriad coagulation-triggering events mentioned earlier. Conversely, reduction in the ability to clot (hemophilia) appears beneficial and is associated with fewer cases of IBD than would be predicted.

Heparin Use in IBD

In concert with this and similar observations, there has been increasing interest in the therapeutic role for heparin. Heparin's effect on inflammation is well studied. It may inhibit selectin-mediated leukocyte tethering and rolling, leukocyte cell adhesion with ligands, and leukocyte integrin upregulation. Of special interest in IBD are recent abstracts suggesting heparin-associated decreases in IL-6 and tumor necrosis factor alpha in both UC and CD.

A prospective trial of unfractionated heparin in UC, given by continuous infusion to prolong the partial thromboplastin time (PTT) to greater than 60 seconds, has been reported. Although remission was achieved in as many as 50 percent of cases, massive colonic bleeding has been reported to occur as late as day 11 of a 2-week infusion. These studies, using heparin as therapy, differ in the degree of clinical activity that may respond and to the extent of improvement in endoscopic/histologic versus clinical activity index measurements. There are conflicting reports on the effect of heparin in CD. Of particular interest, however, is the reporting that extra-intestinal manifestations of IBD, for example, peripheral arthritis and pyoderma gangrenosum, resolved during the course of heparin therapy.

It is likely that the physiologic basis for heparin therapy is sound but the heterogeneity of IBD (both UC and CD) patients tempers the predictability of a response for a given patient. This is of practical importance as the use of heparin may add significant risk to a subset of active colitis patients. The chapter on novel manipulations of inflammatory mediator pathways has more information on heparin use in UC.

Hemolysis

Hemolysis presents in a small but significant number of cases of IBD. Heinz body anemia does occur and competitive inhibition of folate transport was known to develop when sulfasalazine was more commonly used in IBD therapy. Sulfasalazine is also associated with idiosyncratic leukopenia, even to the extent of agranulocytosis, thrombocytopenia, sulfhemoglobinemia, and methemoglobinema. Slow acetylation may be a risk factor for these complications but acetylation status is not routinely clinically tested. Warm antibody hemolytic anemias, mainly immunoglobulin G in type, occur in IBD, usually is association with UC. When hemolysis occurs in the setting of blood loss anemia or the anemia of chronic disease, its impact may be amplified.

Supplemental Reading

Folwaczny C, Wiebecke B, Loeschke K. Unfractionated heparin in the therapy of patients with highly active inflammatory bowel disease. Am J Gastroenterol 1999;94:1551–9.

Gasche C, Dejaco C, Waldhoer T, et al. Intravenous iron and erythropoietin for anemia associated with Crohn's disease. A randomized, controlled trial. Ann Intern Med 1997;126:782–7.

Jackson L, O'Gorman P, O'Connell J, et al. Thrombosis in inflammatory bowel disease: clinical setting, procoagulant profile and factor V Leiden. QJM 1997;90:183–93.

Levine J. Activated coagulation and inflammatory bowel disease: noise or music? Inflamm Bowel Dis 1996;2:313–4.

CHAPTER 70

Pancreatitis in Inflammatory Bowel Disease

Sonia Friedman, MD, and Peter A. Banks, MD

There is a higher incidence and prevalence of pancreatitis in patients with inflammatory bowel disease (IBD) than in the general population. The pancreatitis can be acute or chronic, or subclinical or overt, and has many causes. The most common cause is medications used to treat IBD, especially azathioprine and 6-mercaptopurine (6-MP). Other causes of pancreatitis include duodenal involvement from Crohn's disease (CD), gallstones, and primary sclerosing cholangitis (PSC). Pancreatitis also can be caused by high serum concentrations of triglycerides during total parenteral nutritional (TPN) therapy for CD, and may also be a primary extra-intestinal manifestation of IBD.

Incidence

The incidence and prevalence of pancreatitis in IBD patients differs depending on the way it is measured. In a large Danish population study, the nationwide standardized incidence ratio (observed cases/expected cases) of the first case of acute pancreatitis was 4.3 percent in Crohn's patients and 2.1 percent in ulcerative colitis (UC) patients. Other studies have estimated incidences of 1.2 to 1.5 percent, about 250 times normal.

The incidence and prevalence is much higher, however, when one includes subclinical disease. The first evidence of a significant association between pancreatic lesions and IBD was from a postmortem study almost 50 years ago. Pathologic examination revealed 14 percent gross and 53 percent histologic interstitial pancreatic lesions in UC patients. The same laboratory found mild to moderate pancreatic fibrosis at necropsy in 15 of 39 patients with CD. Remarkably, no patient had previous clinical evidence of pancreatic disease.[*]

Several studies have documented abnormal pancreatic function and structure in IBD patients without clinical evidence of pancreatic disease. In one cross-sectional study, 4 percent of 237 IBD patients had an abnormal secretin test of pancreatic function, and 8 percent of these patients had ductal abnormalities as imaged by endoscopic retrograde cholangiopancreatography (ERCP). In another study, 143 CD patients and 115 control subjects were given a Lundh test meal to study pancreatic function. As a group, CD patients had significantly decreased activity of both amylase and lipase in duodenal aspirates. The lowest enzyme levels were found in patients with the most extensive CD.

Other studies have documented increases in pancreatic enzymes in the serum of IBD patients. In a recent cross-sectional study that measured the serum pancreatic enzymes in 237 IBD patients, the authors found hyperamylasemia in 11 percent (17% CD and 9% UC) and hyperlipasemia in 7 percent (9% CD and 7% UC) of the total study group. High levels were associated with extensive colonic disease and severe histologic activity. Eight percent of the IBD patients with increased pancreatic enzymes had clinical pancreatitis. Elevation of serum pancreatic enzymes among IBD patients may be caused by pancreatic inflammation or possibly by increased gut permeability of intraluminal enzymes with enzyme leakage into the bloodstream.

Etiology and Diagnosis

Although it is unclear why so many IBD patients have subclinical pancreatic abnormalities, the causes of clinical pancreatitis are better defined.

Drug-Induced Pancreatitis

Drugs used to treat IBD are the most common cause of acute pancreatitis (Table 70–1). 6-Mercaptopurine and azathioprine cause acute pancreatitis in 3 to 5 percent of IBD patients. The pancreatitis is unrelated to the dosage of medication, typically occurs within the first 3 to 4 weeks of initiating therapy, and disappears when the drug is discontinued. Patients who are rechallenged, even

TABLE 70–1. IBD Drugs Associated with Acute Pancreatitis

Drugs Definitely Associated	Drugs Probably Associated
6-Mercaptopurine	Metronidazole
Azathioprine	Corticosteroids
5-ASA compounds	
Sulfasalazine	

5-ASA = 5-aminosalicylic acid.

[*] Editor's Note: Perhaps, malnutrition, a cause of pancreatitis, may have been present in at least some of those patients who died with IBD. However, this should not detract from the important new data linking CD and pancreatitis that are in this chapter. (TMB)

with as little as one-eighth of the original dose, develop recurrent pancreatitis as severe as the initial pancreatitis, usually within 24 hours. This reaction appears to be a form of hypersensitivity. Patients allergic to 6-MP or azathioprine who are rechallenged with the other agent react similarly. Acute pancreatitis caused by sulfasalazine is rare, occurs with rechallenge, and is caused by both the sulfapyridine and the 5-aminosalicylic acid (ASA) part of the molecule. It is also a complication of olsalazine and mesalamine. Acute pancreatitis occurs mainly with very high-dose steroids (500 mg to 1 g of Solu-Medrol per day) as used to treat optic neuritis or central nervous system vasculitis and recurs with rechallenge.

Duodenal Crohn's Disease

About half of the cases of clinical pancreatitis other than drug-induced cases are reported to occur from duodenal CD. Crohn's disease of the duodenum occurs in only 2 percent of patients. Pancreatitis may be caused by direct fistulization from the duodenum into the pancreatic duct, by direct ampullary involvement with stenosis, or by duodenal strictures causing reflux of duodenal contents into the pancreatic duct and probably activation of pancreatic enzymes.

The complication of pancreatitis in duodenal CD may be more common than expected. In 10 patients with duodenal CD at the Mayo Clinic, 3 had clinical pancreatitis. Two of these cases were documented by surgical exploration. Other case reports confirm the presence of clinical pancreatitis in this setting, documented by surgical exploration, ERCP, or barium studies demonstrating reflux into the pancreatic duct in association with clinical symptoms and pancreatic enzyme elevations.

Since duodenal CD presents with abdominal pain, it can be difficult to diagnose a concurrent pancreatitis. If pancreatitis is suspected, one should obtain pancreatic enzymes and an abdominal computed tomographic (CT) scan. An upper gastrointestinal series is the best study to both diagnose duodenal CD and demonstrate a fistula or reflux into the pancreatic duct.

Biliary Tract Disease

Both cholelithiasis and PSC are associated with acute pancreatitis in IBD patients. Cholelithiasis is more common in Crohn's patients than in the general population and is due to alterations in the bile salt pool secondary to ileal dysfunction or resection. There is a chapter on cholelithiasis in IBD patients. Pancreatic ductal changes are associated with sclerosing cholangitis, probably due to autoimmune and genetic mechanisms. There is an increased frequency of human leukocyte antigen (HLA)-B8 and -DR2 in patients with UC and PSC and familial occurrence of UC and PSC. In a study from Norway, of 151 patients with UC, 7 had PSC; 4 of these had ductal changes on ERCP consistent with chronic pancreatitis, and 1 had clinical

symptoms. In a more recent study of IBD-associated pancreatitis, 58 percent of UC patients and 12.5 percent of CD patients had bile duct involvement.

Total Parenteral Nutrition-Induced

A rare cause of acute pancreatitis in Crohn's patients is hypertriglyceridemia due to lipid emulsions in TPN. In several case reports, fat emulsions in TPN preparations have caused acute pancreatitis that can recur following rechallenge. Fatty acids can then be given with oral preparations and TPN used without lipids.

Idiopathic or Autoimmune

In one-third to one-half of cases, no cause can be found, and the pancreatitis is likely a primary extra-intestinal manifestation of IBD and due to autoimmune mechanisms. The pancreas can be a primary site of granulomatous inflammation in CD. This entity recently was described in a patient with gastric and duodenal CD and common bile duct obstruction due to a pancreatic mass. Upon surgical exploration, the pancreas contained granulomas.

The fact that CD can present in the pancreas is not so surprising when one looks at the studies of autoantibodies directed against the pancreas. In a study of 273 patients with IBD, 31 percent of CD patients and 4 percent of UC patients had serum antibodies against pancreatic acinar cells or pancreatic autoantibodies (PABs). The UC patients had very low titer PABs and none were found in patients with various chronic inflammatory diseases and healthy controls. Pancreatic autoantibodies persisted for extended periods of time and did not correlate with disease activity, extra-intestinal manifestations, or anti-inflammatory drugs. Seven of the CD patients had a history of pancreatic disease and four had PABs. Thus, PABs might be a serologic marker for CD and, in particular, CD-associated pancreatitis.

Current studies described further differences in the manifestations of pancreatic disease in UC and CD patients. The clinical and morphologic features were studied in 8 cases of idiopathic chronic pancreatitis in IBD patients and an additional 20 from the literature. Ulcerative colitis patients were more likely to have common bile duct involvement with painless jaundice and weight loss. In contrast, CD patients were more likely to have calcifications of the parenchyma, disease involving the main pancreatic duct and the side branches, and abdominal pain.

Two different immunologic mechanisms may account for these two types of chronic pancreatitis in IBD. Pancreatic autoantibodies can be divided into two different subgroups. Those classified as subtype I are of the immunoglobulin (Ig)G1 and IgG2 subclasses. They are directed to the pancreatic duct and acini and have diffuse "droplike" immunofluorescence of acinar cells. The type I autoantibodies, seen mostly in CD, are thought to cause ductal inflammation with stricture, ductal hypertension, decreased water and electrolyte secretion with the resultant protein plug and pancreatic stone formation, and severe abdominal pain—similar to the pathophysiology seen in CD patients and alcoholic patients with chronic pancreatitis.

Conversely, PABs classified as subtype II are of the IgG1 subclass only and have a "speckled" immunofluorescence pattern of acinar cells. The type II autoantibodies, seen in both CD and UC, are directed to the acinar cells and result in decreased pancreatic enzyme secretion, maldigestion, and weight loss—similar to the pathophysiology observed in UC patients and patients with nonalcoholic idiopathic chronic pancreatitis.

In contrast to perinuclear cytoplasmic antibody, which is seen in 15 to 20 percent of first-degree relatives of UC patients and may signify a genetic predisposition to disease, PABs were found only in 2.5 percent of first-degree relatives of CD patients, and most had anamnestic data compatible with IBD. Thus, rather than having a genetic inheritance pattern, PABs are likely either produced from intestinal antigens or antigens that cross the intestinal barrier during active inflammation in IBD. At the present time, there is only a rare clinical need to document PABs. A diagnosis of idiopathic IBD-associated pancreatitis is made when other etiologies are excluded.

Management

Treatment for the pancreatitis depends on the cause. For asymptomatic patients with pancreatic enzyme elevations on routine blood tests, no diagnostic tests or treatment are necessary. However, in an IBD patient with epigastric or back pain, pancreatic and liver enzymes should be checked and an abdominal ultrasound and CT performed. For patients in whom the pancreatitis is likely due to 6-MP (or azathioprine), the drug should be stopped and the patient should not be rechallenged. When it is not clear whether 6-MP (or azathioprine) caused the pancreatitis, the drug should also be stopped; however, if 6-MP (or azathioprine) is deemed essential in the management of IBD, it is reasonable to reinstitute the medication with the patient's informed consent, starting with one-quarter of the original dose. For pancreatitis induced by hypertriglyceridemia from TPN, lipid emulsions should be removed and the infusion restarted.

If there is duodenal thickening on CT scan or evidence of duodenal CD on esophagogastroduodenoscopy, an upper gastrointestinal series should be performed to rule out extensive duodenal/ampullary CD with reflux of barium into the pancreatic duct and/or a duodenal-pancreatic fistula. If there is no duodenal CD; if an abdominal ultrasound is negative for gallstones, sludge, or biliary dilation; and if there is no offending medication, alcohol abuse, or use of TPN, then magnetic resonance cholan-

giopancreatography should be performed to rule out common bile duct stones and PSC. If a patient has had two or more episodes of acute pancreatitis and the above studies are negative, an ERCP should be performed to visualize the pancreatic and bile ducts and to aspirate bile for cholesterol crystals. If all of the above studies are negative, the patient likely has idiopathic (autoimmune) IBD-related pancreatitis. Pancreatic autoantibodies then might be helpful in a research setting as evidence for primary pancreatic autoimmune disease.

Treatment

Treatment is different for each cause. For drug-induced pancreatitis, discontinuation of the drug should improve the pancreatitis. For TPN-induced pancreatitis, oral medium-chain triglycerides should be substituted for the lipid emulsion. For pancreatitis that has developed from gallstones, the usual treatment is laparoscopic cholecystectomy. Common bile duct stones can be retrieved endoscopically following ERCP.

If the pancreatitis has developed from duodenal CD, the optimal management is unclear. If the CD is inflammatory, suppression of the inflammation with Pentasa® (Ferring-Shire Pharmaceuticals, Florence, Kentucky), omeprazole, corticosteroids, and/or immunosuppressives is the therapeutic approach. Remicade® (Centocor, Inc., Malvern, Pennsylvania) may prove effective for refractory cases. For patients who do not improve with medical management, surgical options are a gastrojejunostomy or a Whipple procedure. For patients with narrow duodenal strictures that appear to cause reflux of luminal contents into the pancreatic duct, endoscopic duodenal dilation may be possible. For patients with duodenal fistulas to the pancreatic duct, antibiotics, immunomodulatory agents such as 6-MP or azathioprine, and Remicade for refractory cases should be given. Corticosteroids are not recommended in fistulous CD. A gastrojejunostomy may be necessary to divert bowel contents away from a duodenal-pancreatic fistula. A Whipple procedure can be offered as a last resort.[†]

The most interesting therapy is that for idiopathic pancreatitis. Since the pancreatitis is presumed to be due to antibodies that are either produced from intestinal antigens or antigens that cross the intestinal barrier during active inflammation, treating the CD may be effective in the acute episode and in preventing additional episodes. Several papers have shown remission of idiopathic IBD-associated pancreatitis with treatment directed against the gut, that is, corticosteroids, 6-MP, or surgical resection of the inflamed intestine.

[†] Editor's Note: In one patient with a duodenal-pancreatic duct fistula and recurrent pancreatitis despite a gastrojejunostomy, Dr. Paul Thuluvath obliterated the fistulae with an injection of scleroscent. There have been no further episodes of pancreatitis. (TMB)

Conclusion

Pancreatitis occurs in as many as 1.5 percent of cases of IBD, about 250 times more than in the general population. Subclinical disease as measured by pancreatic enzymes, tests of pancreatic function, ERCP, or surgical pathology is common but is of little clinical significance. Inflammatory bowel disease–associated pancreatitis can be drug or TPN induced, due to biliary complications of IBD or duodenal CD, or idiopathic. Pancreatic autoantibodies are common in IBD and differ in CD and UC patients, most likely defining two different types of pancreatic disease. Treatment depends on the etiology of the pancreatitis. If the pancreatis is idiopathic, one should treat the gut disease.

Supplemental Reading

Barthet M, Hatier P, Bernard JP, et al. Chronic pancreatitis and inflammatory bowel disease: true or coincidental association. Am J Gastroenterol 1999;94:2141–8.

Borkje B, Vetvik K, Odegaard S, et al. Chronic pancreatitis in patients with sclerosing cholangitis and ulcerative colitis. Scand J Gastroenterol 1985;20:539–42.

Eland IA, van Puijenbroek EP, Sturkenboom MJCM, et al. Drug-associated acute pancreatitis: twenty-one years of spontaneous reporting in the Netherlands. Am J Gastroenterol 1999;94:2417–22.

Heikius B, Niemela MD, Lehtola J, et al. Elevated pancreatic enzymes in inflammatory bowel disease are associated with extensive disease. Am J Gastroenterol 1999;94:1062–9.

Lashner BA, Kirsner JB, Hanauer SB. Acute pancreatitis associated with high-concentration lipid emulsion during total parenteral nutrition therapy for Crohn's disease. Gastroenterology 1986;90:1039–41.

Legge DA, Hoffman HN, Carlson HC. Pancreatitis as a complication of regional enteritis of the duodenum. Gastroenterology 1971;61:834–7.

Meyers S, Greenspan J, Greenstein A, et al. Pancreatitis coincident with Crohn's ileocolitis: report of a case and review of the literature. Dis Colon Rectum 1987;30:119–22.

Present DH. 6-Mercaptopurine and other immunosuppressive agents in the treatment of Crohn's disease and ulcerative colitis. Gastroenterol Clin North Am 1989;1:57–71.

Rasmussen HH, Fonager K, Sorensen HT, et al. Risk of acute pancreatitis in patients with chronic inflammatory bowel disease. Scand J Gastroenterol 1999;349:199–201.

Seibold F, Mork H, Tanza S, et al. Pancreatic autoantibodies in Crohn's disease: a family study. Gut 1997;40:481–4.

CHAPTER 71

CROHN'S DISEASE: THERAPEUTIC IMPLICATIONS OF DISEASE SUBTYPES

LLOYD R. SUTHERLAND, MDCM, MSc, FRCPC, FACP

Clinicians and their patients are interested in either the identification of subgroups or the development of classification systems that would guide particular therapeutic interventions. This concept of "responsive" subgroups can also be expanded to examine the converse, namely, the selection of medications that are more likely to be effective in a particular "unresponsive" patient population. The development of a classification system that would assist in decision-making regarding the choice of therapy would be helpful to all concerned. This is an important issue, as one of the major trends in the therapy of Crohn's disease is the increasing acceptance of a role for immunomodulators earlier on in the management of disease compared to past practices. If one could identify, in advance, which patients were at greater risk of severe disease, then clinicians might feel more comfortable offering aggressive therapy to their patients.

Another force for classification of Crohn's disease is the availability of the new biologic therapeutic interventions (of which infliximab is only the first). Identification of subgroups of patients more likely to respond will make these costly medications more cost effective.

This chapter will summarize what is currently known in terms of disease subgroups and speculate as to how that might influence therapeutic management. It should be acknowledged that the first successful classification of inflammatory bowel disease (IBD) was the separation of colonic disease into three categories: Crohn's disease, ulcerative colitis, and indeterminate colitis. The usefulness of this separation can be demonstrated when one considers the approach to a patient prior to colectomy. Physicians and surgeons speak positively about the possibility of a "cure" following a colectomy for ulcerative colitis, but that is not appropriate when the patient has a colectomy for Crohn's disease. The chapters on indeterminate colitis describe the dilemma when considering an ileal pouch-anal anastomosis.

Classification Systems

A classification system is defined as a system in which assignment to predesignated classes can be based on perceived common characteristics. The characteristics of a satisfactory classification system include (1) naturalness, (2) exhaustiveness, (3) usefulness, (4) simplicity, and (5) constructability. Naturalness refers to the quality that the classes correspond to the nature of the thing being classified. Exhaustiveness requires that every individual be placed into only one category. Classifications, to be helpful and accepted by the practice community, need to be both useful and relevant. They need to be simple. They should also be so well described that anyone can look at the data and arrive at the same classification structure (constructability).

Classification systems, however, pose a variety of problems. Often the clinician is never sure how aggressive to be in determining which group the patient should enter. For example, let's assume that disease location is important. Is it appropriate to distinguish Crohn's disease of the large intestine from ileal-colonic Crohn's disease? Should every patient have a colonoscopy at the time of the initial diagnostic workup to determine whether there is any ileal involvement? Another potential controversy is whether one should be simply satisfied with demonstrating macroscopic disease or whether it is important to define the disease microscopically as well.

Grouping Based on Medication Response

The aminosalicylates can be classified by their release formulation. Sulfasalazine, olsalazine, and balsalazine all require bacterial action to break the azo bond and release the 5-aminosalicylic acid. Theoretically, patients with Crohn's disease affecting only the small bowel or cecal area are less well served by medications that require bacterial action. Conversely, the microsphere formulation begins to release mesalamine in the proximal small intestine, suggesting that it may be particularly effective in small bowel disease.

Steroid Responsiveness

Another possible grouping based on medication might be the response to corticosteroids. Munkholm and colleagues (1994) described the prognosis in a group of patients with Crohn's disease receiving their first course of corticosteroids. Three patient groups were identified based on their response to the steroid therapy: steroid responders (44%), steroid dependent (36%), and steroid resistant (20%). If their definitions were accepted, and if it was shown that patients remained within their initial category, then most IBD patients could be characterized in this fashion. Ideally, this would stream patients into two groups based on their response to a course of corticosteroids. The resistant/dependent patients might be offered immunomodulators earlier in the disease course compared to the responders; giving azathioprine at the outset of therapy could allow more rapid tapering of prednisone and lead to a prolonged remission.

Disease Duration

In terms of Crohn's disease, various authors have commented that the disease can often be separated into two groups: an aggressive form and a more indolent form. As a clinician, I would be more aggressive in introducing immunomodulators early in the treatment of a patient who reported frequent episodes of disease activity in the past 2 years compared to a patient with only two disease flares in the past 10 years. This phenomenon may also be seen in ulcerative colitis, with some patients having a flare every 2 to 3 years, whereas others appear to be chronically active and require surgery or immunomodulators.

Activity Indices

A variety of activity indices have been developed in IBD and are described in the first chapter of this text. For the most part, they were developed as tools to be used in randomized, controlled trials of therapy. The most cited index for ulcerative colitis would be the Truelove-Witts Index. The index characterizes patients into three categories (mild, moderate, and severe) based on stool frequency, fever, rectal bleeding, tachycardia, anemia, and erythrocyte sedimentation rate. Although the index is commonly cited as an inclusion criterion for patient entry into randomized controlled trials of therapy, it has little relevance to the day-to-day management of patients.

The Crohn's Disease Activity Index (CDAI) is the most cited index for Crohn's disease patients. Developed for the National Cooperative Crohn's Study, it incorporates several elements that are delineated in the opening chapter. Since it requires a 7-day diary collection for the calculation of the index, it has little clinical relevance in the day-to-day management of patients' disease activity. However, it has served as a standard by which various trials can be examined and compared to one another. A CDAI of less than 150 implies that the patient is in remission. There continues to be debate as to what the minimal clinically significant change in disease activity should be to justify the term "response." Some clinicians require a 100-point drop in the CDAI, whereas others require a 50- to 70-point drop in the CDAI.

Clinical Pattern

The clinical pattern as described by the Cleveland Clinic group suggests that disease location is an important predictor of disease activity in patients with Crohn's disease.

Patients with colonic disease, for example, have lower recurrence rates following surgery than patients who have ileal or ileocecal involvement. This classification has not been assessed for its therapeutic implications and may suffer some of the problems associated with any tertiary referral center, that is, a lack of generalizability to the general patient population. However, there is general agreement that surgery for fistulization, abscesses, and obstruction is more frequent in patients with ileitis or ileocolitis than with colitis alone.

Disease Behavior

The Mount Sinai group and others have popularized the concept of disease behavior as having implications for disease recurrence. The indications for surgery in patients who underwent resection were divided into two groups: perforating and nonperforating indications. For the most part, patients who have a perforating classification as their initial indication for a first operation will have that as the indication for their second operation as well. Conversely, those who have nonperforating indications for their first surgery will often have nonperforating indications for their second surgery. Patients with perforating disease tend to have more rapid recurrence and again might be candidates for more aggressive maintenance therapy. This is discussed in the chapter on fistulizing disease.

Other Potential Variables

Familial Aspects

Potential classifying variables in the future might include a better understanding of the familial aspects of the disease. Many centers have reported that within families the disease tends to behave in a similar manner between siblings or sometimes from parents to siblings. If there is a family history of severe disease, then an argument could be made to introduce immunomodulators earlier on in the disease course. Genetic markers have been identified suggesting that some patients are at greater risk of having more extensive disease, and, thus, one might decide to be more aggressive in selection of therapy as compared to a patient who does not have these markers.

Age at Onset

Extremes of age may also have therapeutic implications. The best example of this would probably be the willingness of prepubertal children with Crohn's disease to accept nutritional therapy rather than corticosteroids because they are worried about the cosmetic effects of corticosteroids and are reluctant to take them. The promise that the young patient will go through puberty provided that the enteral feed is consumed is a powerful incentive!

Smoking

Smoking status could be used to classify patients. Crohn's disease patients who smoke may be a subgroup that requires more aggressive therapy. There is increasing evidence that smokers have more refractory disease, are more apt to require the use of immunomodulators, and have an increased risk for surgery.

Functional Status Classification

In this era of interest in outcomes research, it is conceivable that in the future a functional status classification system will be incorporated, somewhat analogous to the various functional classifications available in cardiology for patients with angina or congestive heart failure. One could imagine a hypothetical IBD functional index. *IBD Stage I* would cover patients who report full activities of daily living, are employed, and demonstrate little evidence of the social costs of the disease. *IBD Stage III* patients would include those who are confined to home, unemployed, and requiring constant social support. *IBD Stage II* would be intermediate. In the argument for the use of the new biologic therapies, the return to a higher functional status might be one of the most compelling reasons to approve their funding.

Multiple Variable Systems

There have been two attempts to provide classification systems incorporating more than one variable. The Roma 91 classification incorporated four variables: disease location (six subgroups), extent of disease (two subgroups), primary behavior (three subgroups), and operative history (two subgroups). This classification provided 72 subgroups, which probably limited its clinical relevance. A more recent attempt, the Vienna Classification, offers three classifying variables: location (terminal ileum, colon, ileocolonic, and upper gastrointestinal), age (<40 years, >40 years), and behavior (nonstricturing, nonpenetrating, stricturing, penetrating). This, at least, offers the opportunity for simplicity with only 24 cells. Whether the classification will have therapeutic implications remains to be determined in the future.

Conclusion

The classification systems referred to in this chapter assume that Crohn's disease has a single etiology and that, thus, it is possible to classify various parts of the disease. An alternate hypothesis would be that the gut has a limited capacity to respond to a variety of etiologic insults. If reality is Crohn's syndrome rather than Crohn's disease, many of the suggested classifications would be invalid.

Although it may be important to develop subgroups for therapeutic interventions, the question begs an additional question as to whether we have effective therapies available at this time. For example, although the aminosalicylates have been shown to be effective in maintaining remission in ulcerative colitis, their efficacy in the management of patients with Crohn's disease is coming increasingly under question. Until we have new effective therapeutic options available to offer our patients with Crohn's disease, the development of classification systems may be premature.[*]

Reference

Munkholm P, Langholz E, Davidsen M, Binder V. Frequency of glucocorticoid resistance and dependency in Crohn's disease. Gut 1994;35:360–2.

Supplemental Reading

Cosnes J, Carbonnel F, Beaugerie L, et al. Effects of cigarette smoking on the long-term course of Crohn's disease. Gastroenterology 1996;110:424–31.

Farmer RG, Brown CH. Emerging concepts of proctosigmoiditis. Dis Colon Rectum 1972;15:142–6.

Farmer RG, Hawk WA, Turnbull RB Jr. Clinical patterns in Crohn's disease: a statistical study of 615 cases. Gastroenterology 1975;68:627–35.

Gasche C, Scholmerich J, Brynskov J, et al. A simple classification of Crohn's disease. Inflamm Bowel Dis 2000;1:8–15.

Greenstein AJ, Lachman P, Sachar DB, et al. Perforating and non-perforating indications for repeated operations in Crohn's disease: evidence for two clinical forms. Gut 1988;29:588–92.

Last JM. A dictionary of epidemiology. 2nd Ed. Oxford: Oxford University Press, 1988:115–6.

Sachar DB, Andrews HA, Farmer RG, et al. Proposed classification of patient subgroups in Crohn's disease. Gastroenterology 1992;5:141–54.

---

[*] Editor's Note: Perhaps I am less objective than the author or perhaps more optimistic, but I believe our therapeutic decision-making has improved as more agents and subgrouping of patients have become more widely used. In the next chapter, the expectations with various medications are discussed. (TMB)

CHAPTER 72

Therapeutic Expectations of Medical Management of Crohn's Disease

THEODORE M. BAYLESS, MD, AND MICHAEL F. PICCO, MD, PhD

The experienced clinician bases his or her therapeutic expectations, and those of the patient, on, first, the assessment of the patient in terms of that individual's place in the heterogeneity of Crohn's disease, and, second, on the reputation of a particular medication or combination of medications. A useful checklist for determining expectations would include (1) patient individuality; (2) subgroups leading to the clinical heterogeneity of Crohn's disease; (3) goals of therapy; (4) medication characteristics; (5) an individual's therapeutic management history, including adverse events; and (6) surgical history. The therapeutic implications of the various disease subtypes are discussed in the preceding chapter. A detailed outline of items that influence therapeutic expectations is presented in Table 72–1. Some of the views in this chapter are anecdotal and experience based but are not necessarily evidence based.

Patient Individuality

Age at Onset

Age at onset influences the patient's clinical manifestations or phenotype. Those whose illness began in childhood or adolescence (less than age 20 yr) are more likely than older-onset patients to have a positive family history; jejunoileitis and other small bowel disease; and fistulae, abscesses, and obstruction, the complications that commonly accompany small bowel disease. In contrast, patients whose illness started later in adult life less commonly have a positive family history. Perhaps their disease is more influenced by environmental rather than genetic factors. They usually have colonic disease, which is inflammatory in nature, and are less likely to need surgery for fistulae or obstruction. Smoking at the time of diagnosis seemingly decreases the age of diagnosis in CD.

Coexistent Irritable Bowel Syndrome

There is an overlap of irritable bowel syndrome (IBS) and inflammatory bowel disease (IBD) in at least 20 or 30 percent of patients referred to a tertiary care center. Recognizing the coexistence of these two chronic conditions that both tend to run in families is extremely helpful in patient education and patient management. Coexistent IBS symptoms make evaluation of therapeutic

results, by both the patient and the doctor, difficult. This subject is discussed in two separate chapters and in the chapter on postresection diarrhea.

Extrinsic Aggravating Factors

Continued smoking correlates with more small bowel disease, more disease activity, more need for immunomodulators, more fistulizing complications, and more postresection recurrences. Urging patients to stop smoking might improve the results of therapy. Just a few tablets of nonsteroidal anti-inflammatory drugs (NSAIDs) have been incriminated in exacerbations of ulcerative colitis and, perhaps, of Crohn's disease. Intake of dietary secretoagogues, such as caffeine, lactose (in the lactose intolerant person), or fat (in the patient with steatorrhea or coexistent IBS), can contribute to diarrhea, bloating, or abdominal cramps and interfere with the patient's response to therapy. Gassy food ingestion, including carbonated beverages, lactose, fructose (fruits), sorbitol (dietetic gums), and excessive fiber also can cause distressing complaints of abdominal distension and discomfort, further confusing evaluation.

Personality and Psychological Profile

An old truism in gastroenterology allows that "it isn't what the patient eats, it's what eats the patient." Each patient and each family bring their own unique situations to the doctor, who also has his or her individual traits and characteristics, and these multiplex factors influence the response to therapy and resultant quality of life. Patients with Crohn's disease may have to endure chronic pain, and medication abuse can further cloud evaluation of the patient's symptoms. Since narcotics can increase colonic spasm, creating a vicious cycle of pain, analgesic use, increased spasm and distension, and then more pain, trying to avoid narcotic use can simplify long-term patient care. There are two chapters on chronic pain management.

Clinical Heterogeneity

There are therapeutic implications of the various disease subtypes in Crohn's disease. These are discussed in detail in the preceding chapter that reviews the various classification systems, including disease duration; activity index; clinical pattern (jejunoileitis, ileitis, ileocolitis, and colitis); disease behavior (inflammatory, fistulizing, or

TABLE 72–1. Factors That Influence Results of Medical Management of Crohn's Disease

Patient Individualtiy
  Demographics
    Age at onset (diagnosis)
    Growth and development status
    Family history of IBD or sporadic case
    Extrinsic aggravating factors: smoking history, NSAIDs

  Constitutional
    Coexistent irritable bowel syndrome
    Medication adverse event profile

  Psychosocial
    Quality of life
    Underlying psychological and psychiatric profile
    Patient and family responses to illness (and to stress)
    Personal history of compliance with medication instructions
    Medication abuse tendency
    Insurance and financial resources

  Knowledge, attitude, and practices
    Understanding of the illness and of the medications

Heterogeneity of Crohn's Disease
  Disease site ("natural history" or potential outcome)
    Gastroduodenal
    Jejunoileitis
    Distal ileitis
    Ileocolitis
    Colitis
    Perianal disease

  Disease behavior subtype (differences in transmural aggressiveness)
    Inflammatory
      Extent (limited disease that is not transmurally aggressive, more easily suppressed)
      Severity (mild–moderate; severe)
      Tendency to relapse after medical therapy or after resection
      Chronic, less suppressible course, approximately 15 to 20%
      Usually suppressible with immunomodulator therapy
      Prophylactic medications may lessen postresection recurrence

    Fisulizing or Perforating
      Transmural aggressiveness usually manifested in first 2 to 4 years
      Distal ileum is usual site; occasional perforation in left colon
      Postresection recurrences may be of similar nature
      One-third may be suppressible with immunomodulator therapy
      Over half transiently suppressible with anti-TNF therapy

    Stenosing
      More common in small bowel; does occur in colon
      Clinical manifestations of obstruction usually 7 to 10 yr after onset or previous resection
      May develop fistula or perforation secondary to obstruction
      Seemingly not preventable with current medications

Course of inflammation
  Acute intermittent
  Chronic, incompletely responsive

Occurrence of intestinal complications
  Fistulae
  Abscess; perforation
  Fixed obstruction
  Carcinoma

Goals of Therapy
  Clinical remission (CDAI < 150)
  Laboratory remission
  Continuous disease suppression (eg, prepubescent adolescents)
  Mucosal healing
  Combination therapy
  Responding to symptomatic recurrences with flexible medication alterations
  Maintenance of clinical remission without deviation in therapy (eg, rigid clinical trial)
  Quality of life

Medication Characteristics
  5-ASA
  Corticosteroids; budesonide
  Antibiotics
  Bowel rest
  Immunomodulators; azathioprine or 6-MP; methotrexate; cyclosporine
  Cytokine or anticytokine strategies: infliximab (Remicade); IL-10

Individual Therapeutic History
  Individual patient pharmacogenetics (influences dose, response, duration of response)
    Azathioprine or 6-MP
    Steroid resistance
    5-ASA intracellular metabolism

  Prior Therapy
    Patient's previous response to medications
    Adequacy of dosage and duration
    Requirement for steroids or immunomodulators

  Mechanism of Remission
    Spontaneous
    Steroids
    Immunomodulator
    Surgical

  Surgical History
    Indication for surgery
    Extent of resection; residual gross disease
    Rate of recurrence postresection
    Endoscopic; clinical; re-resection
    Response to postresection prophylactic medications and dosage

IBD = inflammatory bowel disease; NSAID = nonsteroidal anti-inflammatory drug; TNF = tumor necrosis factor; CDAI = Crohn's Disease Activity Index; 5-ASA = 5-aminosalicylic acid; 6-MP = 6-mercaptopurine; IL = interleukin.

perforating, and stricturing); combinations of pattern and behavior; grouping based on medication prescribed and therapeutic response (eg, steroids, immunomodulators); need for surgery; and postresection recurrences. Each of these can be considered in one's assessment of therapeutic expectations.

Clinical Pattern

Jejunoileitis

Patients with jejunoileitis usually are diagnosed in teenage years and their early twenties. It is rare to see a patient over 30 years of age with a new diagnosis of jejunoileitis. Their course usually is an indolent one of exacerbations, remissions, and later surgery for obstruction. A few respond dramatically to steroids, but most require long-term disease suppression, including mesalamine (Pentasa®, Ferring-Shire Pharmaceuticals, Florence, Kentucky) and azathioprine (Imuran®, Glaxo Wellcome Inc., Research Triangle Park, North Carolina). One expects to use long-term immunomodulation in this subgroup, and discontinuing therapy has been difficult.

The chapters on jejunoileitis point out the importance of conserving small bowel by judicious use of strictureplasties and short resections. Although most of the reports on strictureplasty do not discuss postoperative medications, long-term use of azathioprine (AZA) or 6-mercaptopurine (6-MP) seems to be necessary to limit the need for further resection in these patients who are vulnerable to excessive removal of small intestine. The authors have noted symptomatic restricturing of some strictureplasty sites more frequently than some surgical articles imply. Several patients with active jejunoileitis have had dramatic responses when Remicade® (Centocor Inc., Malvern, Pennsylvania) was added to their long-term azathioprine (Imuran®, Glaxo-Wellcome Inc., Research Triangle Park, North Carolina) therapy. How long Remicade will have to be continued is not known.

Ileitis and Ileocolitis

Patients with ileitis and those with ileocolitis comprise at least two-thirds of the patients with Crohn's disease. The majority lead an indolent course for at least 4 years, with infrequent relapses and a prolonged period that is free of relapses if they continue on maintenance therapy, especially immunomodulators. Of those with mild-to-moderate ileitis, about 30 to 40 percent respond to large doses of Asacol (Procter & Gamble, Cincinnati, Ohio) (3.6 to 4.8 g/d) or Pentasa (3 to 4 g/d). Adding metronidazole or Cipro (Bayer, West Haven, Connecticut) is seemingly helpful in achieving a remission in some, minimizing the need for adrenocortical steroids, and managing mild symptomatic recurrences in others.

Patients with more severe disease or with systemic symptoms are given prednisone, usually orally. At least 50 to 60 percent of those without complications go into a clinical remission on 40 to 60 mg/d. From day one, efforts should be made to minimize steroid side effects and adrenal suppression by starting with a divided dose for 1 to 2 weeks and then switching to an all-in-the-morning dose. Prednisone as a single agent is not recommended. Mesalamine and antibiotics are continued and prednisone is tapered weekly, to an alternate-day routine from 30 mg/d. Topical rectal therapy is used if there is rectal symptomatology. Proton pump inhibitors are added if there is gastroduodenal disease and beclomethasone (obtained from compounding pharmacies) has been used for upper gastrointestinal disease as a form of steroid

sparing. Discontinuing prednisone therapy invariably leads to a relapse if that was the only therapy or if acute-phase reactants, such as the erythrocyte sedimentation rate or mucosal lymphocyte tumor necrosis factor (TNF) content, are elevated even in the asymptomatic patient. There is an excellent chapter on biologic markers of disease activity that provides some useful clinical parameters for assessing response to therapy.

Ileocolonic-released budesonide (Entocort CIR®, Astra Draco, AB, Lund, Sweden), 6 mg/d, which causes less steroid side effects and less adrenal suppression, can be used to allow more rapid prednisone tapering or can be used at a dose of 9 mg in the morning, for 6 to 8 weeks, as the primary corticosteroid. The responses with active disease are statistically similar to those achieved with 40 mg of prednisone, with a 50 percent remission rate with 9 mg/d. The remission rate with prednisone was 60 percent, and there is a more rapid fall in the Crohn's Disease Activity Index (CDAI). After 6 to 8 weeks, the dosage of budesonide is lowered to 6 mg per day. There is a separate chapter on budesonide that provides more details on its use. About a fourth of the patients on a maintenance dosage of 6 mg/d may have mild steroid side effects, including sleeplessness, bruising, or acne. There is adrenal suppression at this dosage, and presumably, some increased bone turnover.

Because of the excellent results with AZA or 6-MP, these medications are discussed with the patient at the initial visit. Patients are told that immunomodulators are the recommended treatment for extensive disease, transmurally aggressive disease (about 25% of patients), steroid dependence, or steroid resistance. With a 1.0 to 1.5 mg/kg dose for 6-MP and 1.5 to 2.0 mg/kg dose for AZA, a 70 percent response rate is expected after an average 12-week lag. Less than 10 percent of patients respond to placebo. At a dosage of 2.0 to 2.5 mg/kg, perhaps monitored with 6-thioguanine (6-TG) levels, the response rate theoretically may be higher, and the lag may be shortened to about 8 weeks, but at the potential risk of increased adverse events. There is a separate chapter describing the details of 6-MP metabolism and the use of 6-TG levels in monitoring AZA and 6-MP therapy.

In the future, it may be possible to measure an individual patient's level of thiopurine methyltransferase (TPMT) activity. Because of a genetic polymorphism, negligible activity is present in 0.3 percent and low levels in 11 percent of the population. These low levels of TPMT activity have been associated with increased cytotoxicity by allowing 6-MP metabolism to be shunted toward excessive production of 6-TG nucleotides. One would prefer to use a lower dose, such as 1 or perhaps 1.5 mg/kg, in those with present but low levels of TPMT activity. In contrast, 10 percent of individuals have elevated TPMT activity and are rapid metabolizers of 6-MP. Whether this influences therapeutic responses in IBD is not known, but in the treatment of leukemia, patients with high TPMT activity are at increased risk of relapse even though they are on a presumably therapeutic dosage of AZA. In a recent report, patients with "high-normal or high" TPMT levels were given 2 mg/kg of AZA. Only 20 percent went into remission compared to the 60 to 70 percent response rates in other unselected population series, perhaps owing, at least in part, to presumably accelerated 6-MP metabolism.

Five percent of patients are expected to be allergic to AZA or 6-MP and to develop a rash, fever, or flu-like illness in the first 3 weeks; at 1.0 to 1.5 mg/kg, 2 percent develop pancreatitis. Leukopenia and infectious complications are rare. A higher rate of adverse events is expected at 2.0 to 2.5 mg/kg. At present, about two-thirds of 500 patients being followed are on immunomodulators. Levels of 6-TG are monitored when the dosage of AZA or 6-MP is being increased in incompletely responsive patients or when there is any question about therapeutic efficacy or compliance. Levels of 6-TG also are useful in determining that a prophylactic dosage of AZA is actually therapeutic.

AGGRESSIVE COURSE

The tendency in patients with a chronic unresponsive form of Crohn's disease is to administer prolonged steroid and immunomodulator therapy in an attempt to suppress disease activity. Increasingly, physicians are using immunomodulator therapy earlier in the course of this aggressive form of Crohn's disease

Approximately half of the patients who are unresponsive to AZA (1 to 1.5 mg/kg) respond to methotrexate given as 25 mg/wk, intramuscularly. The period to response (about 8 weeks) and the adverse events (especially allergic pneumonitis and hepatotoxicity) are described in a separate chapter. Maintenance therapy with 15 mg/wk given intramuscularly or subcutaneously has been effective in over half of the responders, but the therapeutic response seems to diminish at 9 to 12 months. Reportedly, returning to a 25 mg/wk/m per week dose is helpful in some patients who relapse on 15 mg/wk/m (N Engl J Med 2000;342:1627–32). Since therapy often is limited to a year or less, hepatic fibrosis (hopefully predicted by a rise in alkaline phosphatase) is not as common as when methotrexate was given daily in the treatment of psoriasis.

Cyclosporine use in Crohn's disease is discussed in a separate chapter. The best responses have been achieved in Crohn's disease of the colon and pyoderma gangrenosum. Patients are maintained on AZA at a dosage that achieves therapeutic levels of 6-TG.

The role of infliximab (Remicade) is evolving. As described in several chapters in this text, rapid improvement in intestinal inflammation occurred in about two-thirds of the 125 patients in the clinical trials. Over a third

went into remission. Since Remicade received Food and Drug Administration (FDA) approval, over 30,000 patients have received at least one infusion. The anecdotal reports from many centers as well as the authors' experience has been similar to that of the trials. At least 60 percent of patients with active ileitis or colitis experience a rapid response with an infusion of 5 mg/kg. Those with systemic symptoms and extra-intestinal manifestations note improvement in days. Sedimentation rates and C-reactive protein (CRP) levels fall in days. Improvement at 2 weeks is impressive in many patients. In the trials, less than a third of those nonresponsive to 5 mg/kg responded to 10 mg/kg. Four patients with Crohn's disease of the skin or "metastatic" Crohn's disease at our institution have responded favorably to Remicade infusions. This is discussed in the chapter on cutaneous manifestations of IBD.

Despite the sometimes dramatic responses to the first infusion, relapses begin to appear at 8 to 12 weeks after a single infusion. Rutgeerts and Baert (1998) reported that four additional infusions of 10 mg/kg prolonged the responses in 70 percent of the responders during a 32-week trial. However, the data in their report suggest that after the therapy was stopped at 32 weeks, relapses were occurring by 48 weeks. Because concomitant methotrexate therapy seemed to prolong the responses to repeated Remicade infusions in rheumatoid arthritis (see the chapter on lessons from rheumatoid arthritis), many physicians are hoping that long-term AZA or methotrexate administration will prolong responses in Crohn's disease. No known published data exist on this approach. The current questions include how long one should continue Remicade infusions and whether adverse events will increase with time. The trial of Remicade and methotrexate in rheumatoid arthritis is planned to go on for 2 years. Reportedly, a 2-year trial is planned for Crohn's disease. Fortunately, a number of centers are documenting their experience, and this could be helpful in the absence of controlled trials; some of those observations are mentioned in this book. The manufacturers are planning a registry of patients receiving Remicade, which will provide more data.

COMPLICATIONS

Fistulizing or perforating complications may occur in about 20 percent of patients with ileitis or ileocolitis, leading to surgery in the first 4 years. Postresection recurrences commonly are also of a fistulizing or perforating nature and occur early, often in the next 4 years. Although there is no trial showing that immunomodulators prevent recurrences in a series of patients undergoing ileocolonic resection for transmurally aggressive fistulizing or perforating disease, some practitioners do prescribe AZA postoperatively for patients with IBD who can tolerate that medication. A clinical trial in this particular group is needed. Guidelines for the use of Remicade for fistulizing complications are evolving in the absence of long-term controlled trials.

Imaging and endoscopic techniques can, at times, help identify these individuals by demonstrating deep ulcerations, fissuring, or fistulae. The chapter on computed tomography discusses some of these "complications." In the future, biologic markers, such as high interleukin-6 (IL-6) levels or alleles of the gene encoding for TNF-alpha, may facilitate identification of those at highest risk of running an aggressive course or not responding to the usual doses of a particular agent. Azathioprine will probably remain the treatment of choice for patients with deep ulcerations or fissuring as well as for the patient with involvement of a number of loops of ileum. The current trend is to start immunomodulators earlier in the course and not to wait for a prolonged period on steroids (steroid dependence) or lack of response to steroids (steroid resistance). There are two trials, one in adolescents (Markowitz) and one in adults (Ewe, references in other chapters), that have demonstrated that use of AZA or 6-MP at the onset of steroid therapy in unselected patients allowed more rapid tapering of steroids. Presumably one would then continue the immunomodulator as maintenance therapy. A multicenter trial of early use of AZA is being conducted in Boston. Although it rarely is mentioned in articles, many experienced gastroenterologists continue treatment with mesalamine along with AZA or 6-MP. The use of AZA, 6-MP, methotrexate, cyclosporine, and Remicade for fistulizing disease is discussed in other chapters.

Relapse-Free Maintenance

Remission maintenance has been the watchword of ulcerative colitis therapy for decades. Recently, attention has become focused on maintenance therapy in Crohn's disease. During treatment of 60 prepubescent adolescents in the 1960s and 1970s in an open-label setting, it became clear that both continuous disease activity suppression (including laboratory evidences of activity) and avoidance of daily steroids was necessary for sustained growth. Adequate nutrition was an additional factor, but disease suppression seemed essential. This approach seemingly lessened morbidity and avoided relapses, hospitalizations, and surgeries.

That experience of caring for growing teenagers suggests that the goals of therapy in all patients with Crohn's disease should include long-term control of disease activity. Ideally this could be accomplished without the adverse effects of prolonged daily prednisone therapy. In a series using combination therapy, two-thirds of adults with Crohn's disease who had not undergone resection could be kept relapse-free for 4 years. They were maintained on combination medical therapy, including alternate-day steroids, 5-aminosalicylic acid (5-ASA)

compounds, and immunomodulators (in a third). Importantly, a flexible dosing schedule allowed minor changes in doses or the addition of antibiotics at the time of mild symptomatic recurrences. The majority of patients with colitis needed AZA or 6-MP.

Some patients with mild-to-moderate uncomplicated ileitis and ileocolitis, who do not require steroids or immunomodulators, can be kept in a clinical and laboratory remission on Asacol (3.6 or 4.8 gm/d) or Pentasa (3 to 4 gm/d) and perhaps metronidazole (250 mg three times/d) or Cipro (500 mg twice/d). Some require budesonide (6 mg/d) to remain in remission. Often this is necessary while waiting 2 or 3 months for AZA to become effective. Before the availability of budesonide, 20 mg of prednisone on an alternate-day basis could be used if needed. All of the patients on budesonide (or formerly on alternate-day steroids) are on supplemental calcium and weight-bearing exercise. If bone density measurements (done in almost all patients) reveal osteopenia and steroids are to be continued, alendronate (Fosamax®, Merck, West Point, New Jersey) or nasal calcitonin (Miacalcin, Novartis Pharmaceutical Corp., East Hanover, New Jersey) is added, sometimes involving consultation with an endocrinologist. Risedronate (Actonel®, Procter & Gamble, Cincinnati, Ohio), a new compound effective in lessening corticosteroid-induced bone demineralization, may cause less upper gastrointestinal side effects than alendronate. If osteoporosis is present, the budesonide (or alternate-day steroids) is discontinued and AZA is continued or substituted. Patients who clearly require steroids to go into remission usually do not stay in remission on mesalamine, except perhaps in high doses. Most require addition of intermittent budesonide or, more often, AZA. Those who do not respond until AZA or 6-MP is instituted invariably need an immunomodulator to maintain the remission. Presumably, long-term immunosuppression also is needed with Remicade therapy, because of the high relapse rate.

Fibrostenotic Disease

Small bowel obstruction as a result of muscular hypertrophy and fibrosis, occurs in about half of the patients with ileitis and seemingly takes 7 years to develop after a previous resection for obstruction. Patients with partial obstruction usually describe a change in their symptomatology with right lower quadrant or periumbilical pain, worse after meals, often accompanied by borborygmi. Most have lost some weight because they have altered their diet to lessen discomfort. In a group of 60 childhood- or adolescent-onset patients, the start of the clinically recognizable phase of their Crohn's disease could be dated to a change in growth velocity in over 80 percent of the patients. Using this as the onset of disease, there was an average lag of 9.1 years before ileal resection was needed for fixed small bowel obstruction. Interestingly,

Dr. Greenstein, the lead author of the Mt. Sinai study report describing recapitulation of the same indication for surgery (perforating or nonperforating) in the majority of the over 350 patients in their series (Greenstein), stated that the lag between first and second operations, both for obstruction, also was 9.1 years. Presumably, there are inflammatory cytokines that stimulate muscle hypertrophy and fibrosis, and these are not inhibited by the currently used anti-inflammatory medications. There is as yet no evidence that AZA or 6-MP prevents fibrostenotic disease either primarily or after resection. In terms of infliximab (Remicade), there are a few reports of worsening intestinal obstruction in patients with stenotic areas prior to infusion therapy. At this early stage in the use of Remicade, fixed stenotic areas with proximal dilatation would not seem to be a favorable indication for its use.

Crohn's Colitis

A subgroup of patients with Crohn's colitis comprises 20 to 30 percent of most series, and among patients with the onset of Crohn's disease after age 40, over 80 percent have colonic involvement. The disease process is inflammatory in the vast majority, and the goal of therapy is suppression of disease activity and, if possible, maintenance of remission. Asacol (4.8 g/d) and AZA is the maintenance regimen for most of the authors' patients. Some also are on Cipro or metronidazole, especially if there is concomitant perianal disease. Over 90 percent of patients will continue in remission as long as the AZA is continued. There are data that suggest that after 4 years in remission, one can slowly taper AZA, perhaps by 25 mg every 4 to 6 months. If colonoscopy shows mucosal healing, AZA may be tapered, but the mesalamine or sulfasalazine should be continued. Other patients, including those in a French study (Bouhnik et al, referred to in Chapter 75), have been able to stop the immunomodulators abruptly after 4 years without relapse. Unfortunately, several patients have developed an abscess or free perforation when AZA or 6-MP or methotrexate immunomodulation was withdrawn after only 6 to 12 months of remission. The issue of duration of immunomodulator use is discussed in the chapter on unanswered clinical questions in Crohn's disease.

Most patients in an early series who did not respond to AZA or 6-MP had colitis. Currently, some can be expected to improve on higher doses of these medications, perhaps monitored by measuring 6-MP metabolite levels. About 40 to 50 percent respond to intramuscular methotrexate; some respond to intravenous cyclosporine and then require long-term AZA. Infliximab (Remicade) has led to a rapid but short-lived response, even with temporary mucosal healing, in about 60 percent of patients in the trials of this new medication. Whether adding AZA or methotrexate will prolong the response in some patients is not proven. How long one could and should safely continue Remicade also is not yet known.

Colonoscopic Surveillance

All patients with Crohn's colitis should be entered into a colonoscopic surveillance program for dysplasia and colon cancer. There is an excellent chapter in this text that describes such a program with a 16 percent neoplasia yield. In that chapter, the opinion is expressed that 6-MP use lessened cancer risk among the subjects, presumably by suppressing active inflammation. However, immunomodulator therapy may allow some colons to be salvaged that would ordinarily have been removed surgically; these severely damaged organs presumably are at increased risk of cancer development. This is speculation, but it motivates practitioners to insist on surveillance colonoscopies in all patients with Crohn's colitis and especially those who have severe and extensive disease.

Reference

Rutgeerts P, Baert F. Immunosuppressive drugs in the treatment of Crohn's disease. Eur J Surg 1998;164:911–5.

Supplemental Reading

Bayless TM, Bayless JA, O'Brien JO, et al. Crohn's disease: long-term disease activity suppression with multiple drug therapy. Gastroenterology 1991;100:A196.

Bayless TM, Tokayer AZ, Polito JM II, et al. Crohn's disease: concordance for site and clinical type in affected family members: potential hereditary influences. Gastroenterology 1996;111:573–9.

Cohen S, Levy RM, Keller M, et al. Risedronate therapy prevents corticosteroid-induced bone loss. Arthritis Rheum 1999;42:2309–18.

Cuffari C, Theoret Y, Latour S, et al. 6-Mercaptopurine metabolism in Crohn's disease: correlation with efficacy and toxicity. Gut 1996;39:401–6.

Greenstein, AJ, Lachman P, Sachar DB, et al. Perforating and non-perforating indications for repeated operations in Crohn's disease: evidence for two clinical forms. Gut 1988;29:588–92.

Hamedani R, Feldman RD, Feagan BG. Drug development in inflammatory bowel disease: budesonide, a model of targeted therapy. Aliment Pharmacol Ther 1997;11(Suppl 3):98–107.

O'Brien JJ, Bayless TM, Bayless JA. Use of azathioprine or 6-mercaptopurine in the treatment of Crohn's disease. Gastroenterology 1991;101:39–46.

Stein RB, Hanauer SB. Medical therapy for inflammatory bowel disease. Gastroenterol Clin North Am 1999;28:297–321.

Vandeputte L, Haens G, Baert F, Rutgeerts P. Methotrexate in refractory Crohn's disease. Inflamm Bowel Dis 1999;5:11–5.

Whitington PF, Barnes HV, Bayless TM. Medical management of Crohn's disease in adolescence. Gastroenterology 1977;72:1338–44.

CHAPTER 73

SEQUENTIAL AND COMBINATION THERAPY FOR SMALL BOWEL DISEASE

GEERT D'HAENS, MD, PhD

Inflammation of at least part of the small intestine occurs in the majority of patients with Crohn's disease. Approximately 40 percent of Crohn's disease patients have an ileocolonic location of their disease (right colon and distal ileum) and 30 percent have small bowel disease alone. This chapter is focused on the specific management of small bowel Crohn's disease and its complications.

Management of Small Bowel Crohn's Disease: Key Issues

When dealing with patients with small bowel Crohn's disease, a number of important issues need to be addressed: How extensive is the involvement? What are the metabolic consequences? Is there inflammation of other parts of the gastrointestinal tract? Are there any active extraintestinal manifestations? Most importantly, *what causes the patient's symptoms*: inflammation and/or obstruction or other complications such as abscess formation or fistulization to other organs? The answers to these questions will allow the clinician to select the most appropriate therapy. Indeed, there is no "standard therapy" for small bowel Crohn's disease: the clinical presentation will determine the management. Furthermore, the management of any type of Crohn's disease consists of two consecutive steps: the *induction* of remission, that is, the control of acute symptoms, and the *maintenance* of remission, that is, the prevention of further relapses.

Induction of Remission (Table 73–1)

Patients with severe small bowel inflammation need effective anti-inflammatory therapy. Two types of approaches can be taken: (1) the classic, sequential "*step-up*" therapy in which a stronger agent is added to the ongoing treatment until the symptoms can be controlled with this *combination* therapy or (2) the alternative "*top-down*" approach, in which the patient is treated with the most potent therapeutic agent first. Controlled trials are currently comparing both strategies. Sequential and combination therapy as it is routinely being done at most centers will be the focus of discussion.

Mild small bowel inflammation can be treated with mesalamine in doses of at least 4 g per day. Pentasa® (Ferring-Shire Pharmaceuticals, Florence, Kentucky), a

sustained-release formulation of mesalamine, is the most useful agent for small bowel involvement proximally to the terminal ileum. For the most common "terminal ileitis," other pH- or time-dependent mesalamine release preparations such as Asacol® (Procter & Gamble Pharmaceuticals, Cincinnati, Ohio) can also be used. In patients with symptomatic spondylarthropathy, sulfasalazine, the only agent shown to be effective for this particular problem, can be considered. In the absence of joint symptoms or in patients with inflammation proximal to the distal ileum, sulfasalazine use is not appropriate. Patients who are intolerant to mesalamine/sulfasalazine can be treated with antibiotics such as quinolones or metronidazole, often with comparable short-term success rates. The *combination* of mesalamine and antibiotics such as quinolones or metronidazole can lead to rapid symptomatic improvement, in particular if peri-intestinal inflammation (periviseritis) is present.[*]

Moderate to severe small bowel disease, in particular in the presence of extra-intestinal manifestations, often requires *corticosteroid therapy*. Oral corticosteroids were used successfully in the National and the European Cooperative Crohn's Disease Study. In the National Cooperative Crohn's Disease Study, remission was achieved with prednisone 0.25 to 0.75 mg/kg/d in 60 percent of the patients and in the European Cooperative Crohn's Disease Study (ECCDS), 80 percent of patients had a remission after 100 days. (There was no additional benefit from sulfasalazine in either of these trials.) French investigators have even used higher doses of glucocorticosteroids (prednisolone metasulphobenzoate 1 mg/kg/d), with remission rates as high as 92 percent. These high doses and the side effects they cause have never been compared to more "conventional" doses. I generally start glucocorticosteroids in a dose of 32 mg of methylprednisolone or 40 mg of prednisone. This dose needs to be continued for a number of weeks (2 to 3 weeks) until symptomatic improvement has been achieved. After this, the dose can slowly be tapered by 4 to 5 mg/wk, depending on clinical parameters. One should

---

[*] Editor's Note: Perhaps this is a manifestation of transmural disease. One might even consider immunomodulators at this point. (TMB)

TABLE 73–1. Sequential Therapy of Small Bowel Crohn's Disease

	Mild Attack	Moderate Attack	Severe Attack
Terminal ileitis	Mesalamine Budesonide	Budesonide (Methyl)predniso(lo)ne (antibiotics) Azathioprine	(Methyl)predniso(lo)ne ± antibiotics Azathioprine Infliximab
Proximal ileitis/ jejunoileitis	Mesalamine (Pentasa®) Antibiotics	(Methyl)predniso(lo)ne Antibiotics Azathioprine	(Methyl)predniso(lo)ne ± antibiotics Azathioprine Infliximab

aim at *clinical* improvement; it is of no use to perform endoscopy or radiology to assess healing of lesions. A common mistake is to start corticosteroid therapy at too low a dose, with only partial improvement and need for longer therapy duration and a progressive increase of the dose as a consequence. With this type of approach, it will take longer before the patient becomes free of symptoms and the cumulative corticosteroid dose will be higher. Some clinicians combine corticosteroids and mesalamine for the treatment of an acute attack. The French Consortium GETAID demonstrated that the addition of mesalamine permits an easier corticosteroid taper. Another approach is to start mesalamine (3 to 4 g/d) during the corticosteroid taper, for instance, when a dose of 16 mg methylprednisolone has been reached.[†] Azathioprine is effective in over 70 percent of patients with active small bowel disease that is "steroid dependent" or unresponsive. This is discussed in detail in other chapters and under maintenance.

For an acute attack of terminal ileitis, topical corticosteroids such as budesonide are more potent than mesalamine, have less side effects than prednisone, and should be considered as a first-line treatment. Ileocolonic-released budesonide ileal release tablets (Entocort CIR®, Astra Draco AB, Lund, Sweden) are generally safe and induce improvement of symptoms within the first 2 weeks. In a randomized double-blind trial comparing the efficacy and safety of budesonide CIR, 9 mg/d in a single dose before breakfast, with prednisolone 40 mg/d for 2 weeks (with taper thereafter) for the treatment of active ileocolonic Crohn's disease, remission rates at 10 weeks were not significantly different (53 vs 66%). Although the drop in the Crohn's Disease Activity Index was significantly greater with prednisolone than with budesonide, the incidence of steroid side effects was higher in the prednisolone group. A similar budesonide preparation, Budenofalk® (Falk Pharma, Freiburg, Germany), has been equally effective for terminal ileitis and possibly also for Crohn's colitis.

[†] Editor's Note: Steroid sparing from the onset is a reasonable goal so that immediate institution of combination therapy with mesalamine and antibiotics and early use of immunomodulators could be considered. Budesonide is discussed in a subsequent paragraph. (TMB)

COMPLICATIONS

If an inflammatory mass is present, in particular if the patient runs a fever, intra-abdominal abscesses should be ruled out by means of ultrasound or computed tomography (CT) scan. An abscess is not always an indication for immediate surgery, but if corticosteroid therapy is to be given, antibiotic coverage is mandatory. In the ECCDS (prior to the availability of CT or ultrasound), three patients with a palpable mass died of septic complications during treatment with 6-methylprednisolone. Abscesses that can be reached percutaneously should be drained if technically possible.

SYSTEMIC GLUCOCORTICOSTEROIDS AND POSSIBLE ALTERNATIVES

Patients presenting with severe inflammation, those with important extra-intestinal manifestations, and those with proximal small bowel disease will need systemic corticosteroid therapy or, alternatively, anti-tumor necrosis factor (TNF) antibody therapy with infliximab (Remicade®, Centocor, Malvern Pennsylvania). A few patients with complicated proximal small bowel Crohn's disease have been successfully treated with FK 506® (Tacrolimus®, Fujisawa, Japan), an immunomodulatory drug with a much better intestinal absorption than cyclosporine.

The *intravenous* use of corticosteroids has not been studied in a controlled fashion, but it is generally accepted as the next therapeutic step when oral steroids fail. Approximately 75 percent of patients will have a remission with intravenous corticosteroids in a dose comparable to methylprednisolone 40 to 60 mg/d in continuous infusion.

BOWEL REST

A few trials have studied the effect of exclusive parenteral or enteral nutrition ("bowel rest") on active Crohn's disease. The problem with this approach is that, although it can be effective to relieve symptoms, relapse was often observed as soon as normal food intake was resumed. Personally, I only use nutritional therapy in patients with intestinal obstruction (total parenteral nutrition) or

---

[‡] Editor's Note: Another approach is to use bowel rest while immunomodulator therapy such as azathioprine is being introduced. (TMB)

TABLE 73–2. Maintenance Therapy of Small Bowel Crohn's Disease

Following Mild Attack	Following Moderate/Severe Attack
Mesalamine	Azathioprine/6-mercaptopurine
	Exceptional: budesonide, low-dose corticosteroids, repeated infusions of infliximab, MTX, FK 506, cyclosporine

MTX = methotrexate; FK 506 = Tacrolimus

malnutrition (enteral or parenteral nutrition), in particular if surgical intervention is to be performed.‡

An attractive alternative to both oral and intravenous corticosteroids or a rescue therapy if they fail to induce improvement is antibody therapy against TNF (infliximab [Remicade]). A single IV dose of infliximab 5 mg/kg improves symptoms in 82 percent of the patients regardless of the location of the inflammation. An additional benefit of infliximab is the mucosal healing, reduction of the length of the inflamed bowel segment, and favorable short-term side-effect profile. As more information on remission maintenance and more long-term safety data become available, this biologic drug may be considered as first-line "induction" therapy in some patients with extensive or transmurally aggressive disease.

Maintenance of Remission (Table 73–2)

Few drugs have a well-proven maintenance benefit in Crohn's disease. A large number of studies including meta-analyses have demonstrated the limited impact of mesalamine on the prevention of relapses. This therapy is usually advocated for maintenance purposes in patients with a mild or moderate disease course. The most effective maintenance drugs for more severe Crohn's disease are undoubtedly azathioprine and 6-mercaptopurine, which successfully prevent relapses in up to 75 percent of patients. In patients with postoperative recurrent ileitis in the neoterminal ileum, we have demonstrated healing of the inflamed mucosa with azathioprine. Patients with extensive jejunitis or jejunoileitis need azathioprine/6-mercaptopurine therapy early on, since the disease course is often severe and complicated. The development of stenoses and strictures is considered by some as a complication of immunomodulatory therapy for Crohn's disease. As discussed in another chapter, these can be managed endoscopically (balloon dilatation of ileocolonic anastomosis) or surgically. We have the impression that surgical resections can be limited after prior use of immunomodulators.

Most studies do not support the use of maintenance corticosteroids and they are considered unacceptable by most authors. Only in patients intolerant to azathioprine/6-mercaptopurine, in those who are refractory to this type of therapy and who cannot be managed surgically, would I use the lowest possible dose of corticosteroids, possibly on an alternate-day scheduled basis. In case of terminal ileitis, a switch to budesonide CIR 6 or even 3 mg/d can be attempted and is probably safer in the long run. There is a chapter on budesonide use in small bowel and right colon Crohn's disease and in collagenous colitis.

Patients with extensive small bowel disease who suffer frequent relapses in spite of first-line immunomodulation are a particular challenge to the gastroenterologist. Malabsorption is a problem in many patients. Cyclosporine is sometimes effective in chronically ill patients and the onset of action is rapid. However, relapse occurs rapidly after stopping cyclosporine. Valuable alternative options are FK 506 or weekly injections of methotrexate, 25 mg/week. Patients who improve with infliximab therapy but suffer relapse after a short period of time can benefit from repeated administration of infliximab. With the latter therapy, however, we are still faced with a degree of uncertainty about long-term safety, and the cost of this drug is considerable. There is a separate chapter on anti-TNF strategies.

Management of Complications

Patients with small bowel Crohn's disease may present with purely obstructive symptoms, that is, with postprandial bowel cramps without any other abdominal pain indicating inflammation. It is a challenge to the clinician to determine and localize the stenosis causing these symptoms, most frequently by means of small bowel follow-through studies or enteroclysis. A short stenosis of an ileocolonic anastomosis can be dilated endoscopically, whereas stenoses higher up in the small bowel need to be resected or treated with strictureplasties. These interventions are very rewarding, since the patient almost immediately becomes free of symptoms. Intestinal obstruction accompanying severe inflammation, however, is not a good indication for surgery, since postoperative recurrence often appears quickly in this situation. Hence, patients with an inflammatory stenosis should first be treated medically.

Patients with intra-abdominal abscesses should also undergo careful radiologic investigation in order to localize the abscess and possibly to drain it percutaneously. Surgical intervention is usually inevitable. There is a chapter on fistulizing Crohn's disease.

Another common complication of small bowel Crohn's disease is malnutrition, with electrolyte and mineral deficiencies. These can be substituted orally or parenterally as necessary. Iron deficiency can be treated with intravenous iron supplements and, in refractory cases, with recombinant erythropoietin. Details are provided in chapters on nutrition and on hematologic complications.

Editor's Note

Similar to ulcerative colitis, potent immune suppressants such as cyclosporine and Tacrolimus provide rapid improvement in CD symptoms and decreased fistula drainage. However, neither provides maintenance benefits at tolerable doses. With the advent of infliximab, we rarely need to revert to this class of agents. Mycophenolate mofetil may be a reasonable substitute for azathioprine/6-mercaptopurine maintenance therapies, but additional trials and clinical experience are needed. The recent data regarding long-term methotrexate, 15 mg/wk for methotrexate responders, also afford an alternative sequential approach to maintenance therapy (SBH)

Supplemental Reading

Caesar I, Gross V, Roth M, et al. Treatment of active and postactive ileal and colonic Crohn's disease with oral pH-modified-release budesonide. Hepatogastroenterology 1997;44:445–51.

Colombel JF, Lémann M, Cassagnou M, et al. A controlled trial comparing ciprofloxacin with mesalazine for the treatment of active Crohn's disease. Gastroenterology 1997;113.A.

D'Haens G, Geboes K, Ponette E, et al. Healing of severe recurrent ileitis with azathioprine therapy in patients with Crohn's disease. Gastroenterology 1997;112:1475–81.

Modigliani R, Colombel JF, Dupas JL, et al. GETAID: mesalamine in Crohn's disease with steroid-induced remission: effect on steroid withdrawal and remission maintenance. Gastroenterology 1996;110:688–93.

Present DH, Korelitz BI, Wisch N, et al. Treatment of Crohn's disease with 6-mercaptopurine. A long-term randomized double-blind study. N Engl J Med 1980;302:981–7.

Rutgeerts P, D'Haens G, van Deventer SJH, et al and the Crohn's Disease cA2 Study Group. Retreatment with anti-TNF-α chimeric antibody (cA2) effectively maintains cA2-induced remission in Crohn's disease. Gastroenterology 1999;117:761–9.

Rutgeerts P, Lofberg R, Malchow H, et al. A comparison of budesonide with prednisolone for active Crohn's disease. N Engl J Med 1994;331:842–5.

Sandborn WJ. Preliminary report on the use of oral Tacrolimus (FK 506) in the treatment of complicated proximal small bowel and fistulizing Crohn's disease. Am J Gastroenterol 1997;92:876–9.

Sutherland LR, Martin F, Bailey RJ, et al. and the Canadian Mesalamine for Remission Study Group. A randomized, placebo-controlled, double-blind trial of mesalamine in the maintenance of remission of Crohn's disease. Gastroenterology 1997;112:1069–77.

Targan SR, Hanauer SB, van Deventer SJH, et al. for the Crohn's Disease cA2 Study Group. A short-term study of chimeric monoclonal antibody cA2 to tumor necrosis factor α for Crohn's disease. N Engl J Med 1997;337:1029–35.

Thomsen OO, Cortot A, Jewell D, et al. A comparison of budesonide and mesalamine for active Crohn's disease. N Engl J Med 1998;339:370–4.

CHAPTER 74

Oral 5-Aminosalicylic Acid Medications in Crohn's Disease

Cosimo Prantera, MD, and Maria Lia Scribano, MD

Imagine a man in a wood, four centuries before Christ. He chews a willow leaf while he looks for wood to burn. Slowly a mild toothache improves and this sets the man to thinking. He is Hippocrates of Cos, a Greek, the most famous physician of his time, and thinking is his business. Another few trials perhaps—on his patients, on his friends—and the pain-killing property of willow bark and leaf is discovered.

Many years after Hippocrates, in the middle of the 18th century, the clergyman Edward Stone in England found that willow bark could lower fever. At the end of the 19th century, Felix Hoffman added acetic acid to salicylic acid for improving gastric tolerability. Aminosalicylic acid (ASA) was born.

Pharmacokinetics of 5-Aminosalicylic Acid

After oral administration, a considerable amount of 5-ASA is excreted unabsorbed with the feces. The absorbed fraction is rapidly acetylated to acetyl-5-ASA (ac-5-ASA) in the gastrointestinal wall and in the liver, and, contrary to that of sulfasalazine (SASP), this process is independent of the patient's acetylator phenotype. Excretion occurs in urine and in bile, predominantly in the acetylated form. Plasma levels of 5-ASA are very low, whereas those of ac-5-ASA are higher because of a slower elimination. About half of the absorbed 5-ASA is bound to the plasma proteins compared with 80 percent of ac-5-ASA. The half-life of 5-ASA is between 40 and 90 minutes, depending on the dose administered, whereas that of ac-5-ASA is at least 6 hours.

Because it is orally ingested, 5-ASA is rapidly absorbed in the stomach and in the proximal portions of the small intestine. Several methods have been used to prevent this absorption by the upper gastrointestinal tract and to ensure the release of the active drug in the distal ileum and in the colon, the most common sites of inflammation. In delayed-release preparations, such as Asacol® (Procter & Gamble Pharmaceuticals, Cincinnati, Ohio), Salofalk® (Axcan Phama Inc., Minneapolis, Minnesota), and Claversal, 5-ASA is coated with acrylic-based resins that dissolve at specific intraluminal pH values, liberating the active drug in different tracts of the small bowel and

colon (Table 74–1). A new formulation of mesalamine (Asacol microgranular) consists of 5-ASA contained in microgranules coated with Eudragit S. With this delivery system the drug is released mainly in the terminal ileum. In a slow-release preparation (Pentasa®, Ferring-Shire Pharmaceuticals, Florence, Kentucky), 5-ASA is contained in microgranules coated with a semipermeable and gastroresistant membrane of ethylcellulose. These tablets disintegrate in the stomach and liberate the microgranules that deliver the 5-ASA gradually and continuously throughout the small and large intestines. Finally, in azo-bond compounds, colonic bacterial reductase either liberates two 5-ASA molecules (olsalazine) or splits off 5-ASA from an inert carrier (balsalazide and ipsalazide), as it does with SASP, thus releasing the active substance in the colon.

Treatment of Acute Flares of Crohn's Disease

5-Aminosalicylic acid (mesalamine-mesalazine) was first employed in the treatment of Crohn's disease (CD) active phase at the beginning of the 1980s, based on important information acquired in preceding years. Sulfasalazine (Salazopyrine or Azulfidine®, Pharmacia and Upjohn Inc., Peapack, New Jersey), a chemical compound of 5-ASA and sulfapyridine (SP), was shown to be superior to placebo in treating CD acute flares, and better results were obtained with high doses of this drug. Side effects were mainly connected with SP, the probable clinically inactive carrier of 5-ASA. This led to the elaboration of products made up exclusively from 5-ASA. Different 5-ASA compounds were prepared with different delivery systems and, consequently, with different sites of release (see Table 74–1).

Controlled trials have been carried out employing 5-ASAs with different delivery systems. The studies showed a therapeutic advantage over placebo but undoubtedly inferior to steroids (Table 74–2).

An important study on mesalamine involved 310 patients on different doses of Pentasa (1, 2, or 4 g/d) compared to placebo. The lower doses were ineffective, but 43 percent of the patients treated with 4 g were in remission (Crohn's Disease Activity Index [CDAI] ≤150) at 16 weeks in comparison with 18 percent on placebo. In a

TABLE 74–1. Properties of Oral 5-Aminosalicylic Acid (5-ASA) Preparations

Product	Preparation	Solubility	Site of Release
Asacol	Mesalamine coated with Eudragit S	pH >7	Distal ileum-colon
Asacol microgranular	Mesalamine encapsulated in microgranules coated with Eudragit S	pH >7	Distal ileum-right colon
Claversal, Mesasal, Salofalk	Mesalamine coated with Eudragit L	pH >6	Jejunum-ileum-colon
Rowasa	Mesalamine coated with Eudragit L 100	pH >6	Jejunum-ileum-colon
Enterasin	Mesalamine encapsulated in microgranules coated with Eudragit S	pH = 7	Distal ileum-colon
Pentasa	Mesalamine encapsulated in ethylcellulose microgranules	Time released	Jejunum-ileum-colon
Dipentum	Olsalazine (5-ASA + 5-ASA)*	Colonic bacteria	Colon
Colazide	Balsalazide (4-aminobenzoyl-β-alanine + 5-ASA)*	Colonic bacteria	Colon
—	Ipsalazide (4-aminobenzoyl-β-glycine + 5-ASA)*	Colonic bacteria	Colon
—	4-ASA (PAS) (enteric coated with Eudragit S and L)	pH = 6.8	Colon

*Olsalazine, balsalazide, and ipsalazide deliver the 5-ASA in the colon after splitting of the azo-bond by colonic bacterial reductase.

pooled analysis of 542 patients in two trials by the same group, 4 g of mesalamine was significantly better than placebo. In another study, 4.5 g/d of mesalamine (Salofalk) showed no difference from 6-methylprednisolone 48 mg/d in inducing remission in 34 patients with ileocolonic involvement.

A randomized controlled trial published in 1999 was a multicenter Italian study with two formulations of mesalamine. Ninety-four patients with CD localized to the terminal ileum and with mild to moderate activity (CDAI between 180 and 350) were randomly assigned to receive mesalamine tablets (Asacol) 4 g, 6-methylprednisolone 40 mg, and a new formulation of mesalamine (Asacol microgranular) 4 g for 12 weeks. The last formulation of 5-ASA differed from the tablets by containing in a gelatine capsule 400 mg of mesalamine microgranules coated with Eudragit S. This preparation had been shown to deliver microgranules in the terminal ileum, overcoming the problem of eventual drug loss. The best results at 12 weeks were obtained with this formulation: 79 percent of remission in this group in comparison with 61 percent of remission on steroid and 60% with the mesalamine tablets. Considering the mild to moderate activity of the trial patients, the low rate of success in the group on steroid was caused by the withdrawal of five patients on account of steroid side effects. Given the small sample size, a possible type II error should be considered.

TABLE 74–2. Controlled Trials on Efficacy of 5-Aminosalicylic Acid (5-ASA) in Active Crohn's Disease

Author	Year	Active Drug	Dose of 5-ASA (g/d)	Number of of Patients	Period	Control	Therapeutic Advantage 5-ASA (%)
Maier et al	1985	Salofalk	1.5	30	8 wk	SASP	+ 7
Saverymuttu et al	1986	Pentasa	1.5	12	10 d	Placebo	**+ 50**
Rasmussen et al	1987	Pentasa	1.5	67	16 wk	Placebo	+ 10
Mahida and Jewell	1990	Pentasa	1.5	40	6 wk	Placebo	+ 5
Scholmerich et al	1990	Claversal	2.0	62	24 wk	Steroid	**− 39**
Maier et al	1990	Salofalk	3.0	50	12 wk	Steroid + SASP	− 5.5
Martin et al	1990	Salofalk	3.0	50	12 wk	Steroid	+ 1
Singleton et al	1993	Pentasa	4.0	310	16 wk	Placebo	**+ 25**
			2.0				+ 6
			1.0				+ 5
Singleton et al	1994	Pentasa	4.0	232	16 wk	Placebo	NS
			2.0				
Tremaine et al	1994	Asacol	3.2	38	16 wk	Placebo	**+ 23**
Gross et al	1995	Salofalk	4.5	34	8 wk	Steroid	− 16.3
Wright et al	1995	Dipentum	2.0	91	4 mo	Placebo	**− 32**
Prantera et al	1999	Asacol	4.0	94	12 wk	Steroid	− 1
		Asacol microgranular	4.0				+ 18
Thomsen et al	1998	Budesonide	4.0	182	16 wk	Pentasa	**− 26**
Colombel et al	1999	Ciprofloxacin	4.0	40	6 wk	Pentasa	− 1

Therapeutic advantage is the difference between the response rate of 5-ASA minus the control group response. Bold type indicates a statistically significant therapeutic advantage; SASP = sulfasalazine; NS = not significant, figures not given.

TABLE 74–3. Controlled Trials on Efficacy of 5-Aminosalicylic Acid (5-ASA) for Remission Maintenance in Crohn's Disease

Author	Year	Active Drug	Dose (g/day)	Number of of Patients	Period (months)	Control	Therapeutic Advantage (%)
Wellman et al	1988	Salofalk	1.5	67	12	Placebo	+ 12
IMSG	1990	Mesasal/Claversal	1.5	206	12	Placebo	**+ 13.8**
Bondesen et al	1991	Pentasa	3.0	202	12	Placebo	0.0
Prantera et al	1992	Asacol	2.4	125	12	Placebo	**+ 21**
Brignola et al	1992	Pentasa	2.0	44	4	Placebo	+ 6.7
Gendre et al	1993	Pentasa	2.0	161	24	Placebo	**+ 16**
Arber et al	1995	Rafassal	1.0	59	12	Placebo	**+ 28**
Thomson et al	1995	Mesasal/Claversal	3.0	286	12	Placebo	NS
Modigliani et al	1996	Pentasa	4.0	129	12	Placebo	+ 4
Sutherland et al	1997	5-ASA	3.0	293	12	Placebo	**+ 11.4**
de Franchis et al	1997	Claversal	3.0	117	12	Placebo	− 6.1

Bold type indicates a statistically significant therapeutic advantage; NS = not significant, figures not given.

5-Aminosalicylic Acid Compared to Other Agents

In one study, 9 mg/d budesonide, a new steroid with a topical anti-inflammatory and lower systemic activity than conventional steroids, was compared with Pentasa 4 g/d in 182 patients with flare-up of CD affecting the terminal ileum and/or the right colon. The remission rates after 16 weeks were lower in the mesalamine group (36%) than in the budesonide group (62%). It was speculated that the 36 percent remission rate was not dissimilar from that obtainable with placebo in mild to moderate active CD (Thomsen et al).

A study of ciprofloxacin, an antibiotic that had been shown, in combination with metronidazole, to be effective in the treatment of active CD, has verified the efficacy of this drug comparing 1 g/d of ciprofloxacin with Pentasa 4 g/d. Forty patients with different Crohn's location were enrolled. Similar rates of success were obtained with these two treatments: exactly 56 percent of patients on ciprofloxacin and 55 percent of those on mesalamine were in remission at 6 weeks.

Maintenance in Crohn's Disease

Maintenance is the most important goal in CD. Although many drugs can be successfully used for inducing remis-

sion of an acute phase, maintenance with the same drugs often fails or is discontinued because of side effects. Given the high safety profile of 5-ASAs, these agents have been evaluated for maintaining remission of CD. A large number of trials have been published on this topic, unfortunately with contradictory results (Tables 74–3, 74–4).

In order to clarify this dispute, three meta-analyses have analyzed the results of all of the studies on 5-ASA employed in CD maintenance.

The first meta-analysis (1994) analyzed eight randomized trials, two of which were studies on recurrence prevention, namely, the prevention of the appearance of endoscopic lesions or of symptoms after surgery. The other six trials concerned the prevention of symptoms relapse after a medically induced remission. Mesalamine significantly reduced the relapse frequency in CD patients with inactive disease. A second meta-analysis (1994) also favored the treatment of mesalamine for relapse prevention. A therapeutic benefit existed for mesalamine but not for SASP. A third meta-analysis (1997) included 15 randomized trials, including 2,097 patients, and concluded that mesalamine significantly decreased the symptomatic relapse of CD. However, *treatment of 16 patients was necessary for preventing one relapse.* The effectiveness of mesalamine was statistically significant in the prevention of recurrence in the surgically induced remission

TABLE 74–4. Controlled Trials on Efficacy of 5-Aminosalicylic Acid (5-ASA) in the Prevention of Clinical (C) and Endoscopic (E) Recurrence after Surgery of Crohn's Disease

Author	Year	Active Drug	Dose (g/d)	Number of of Patients	Period (months)	Control	C/E	Therapeutic Advantage (%)
Fiasse et al	1991	Claversal	1.5	37	12	Placebo	C	− 19
Caprilli et al	1994	Asacol	2.4	110	24	NT	E	**+ 24**
Brignola et al	1995	Pentasa	3.0	87	12	Placebo	E	**+ 32**
McLeod et al	1995	Salofalk	3.0	163	36	Placebo	C	**+ 19**
Florent et al	1996	Claversal	3.0	126	3	Placebo	E	+ 13
Lochs et al	1997	Pentasa	4.0	318	18	Placebo	C	+7

NT = no treatment; bold type indicates a statistically significant therapeutic advantage.

TABLE 74–5. Side Effects Caused by 5-Aminosalicylic Acid

Organ System	Side Effects
Gastroenterologic	Diarrhea
	Abdominal pain
	Nausea
	Vomiting
	Dyspepsia
	Pancreatitis
Nephrologic	Nephrotic syndrome
	Interstitial nephritis
Hepatic	Hepatotoxicity
Hematologic	Mild neutropenia
Pulmonary	Interstitial pneumonitis
	Bronchospasm
Cardiologic	Peri- or myocarditis
Dermatologic	Skin rash
	Lichen planus
	Kawasaki-like syndrome
Rheumatologic	Lupus-like syndrome
Neurologic	Peripheral neuropathy
Miscellaneous	Headache
	Fever
	Chest pain
	Hair loss

group ($p = .0028$) but not in the group with medically induced remission. The effectiveness of treatment was increased in patients with Crohn's ileitis and in patients with prolonged remission duration. We must take into account, however, that all of the meta-analyses, and especially those that show a marginal benefit of the active treatment, can be exposed to a publication bias, namely, the tendency for negative trials with a small sample size to remain unpublished. This criticism may be especially valid in the case of mesalamine because the majority of the positive studies included few patients; hence, an indefinite number of negative studies, with a similarly small sample size, may have slipped through the net. After this last meta-analysis, a trial on Pentasa prophylaxis of postoperative CD was published as an abstract. Four grams of mesalamine tended to decrease the recurrence rate at 18 months in comparison with placebo. The difference between placebo and active drug, in the entire population of 318 patients of the study, was not statistically significant, but the subgroup analysis showed a significant difference in favor of the treatment when the disease was in the small bowel ($p = .020$) and no difference when the colon was involved.

5-Aminosalicylic Acid Side Effects

5-Aminosalicylic acids were first introduced into clinical practice to overcome the side effects of SASP. The main side effects of 5-ASA are reported in Table 74–5. The use of higher doses of these drugs, however, could change their

safety profile in the future. Currently, 5-ASA drugs are very well tolerated, but from 10 to 20 percent of patients intolerant to SASP show the same side effects with 5-ASA. Many side effects are not severe but are the cause of treatment interruption because of their characteristics. Diarrhea and abdominal pain, with an incidence of 4 to 6 percent, are troublesome effects in patients who often have these symptoms because of active disease. Diarrhea is particularly frequent with olsalazine. Side effects, probably caused by absorption of drug in the small bowel, are reported with mesalamines, which are in part delivered in this site. Pancreatitis and renal toxicity are fortunately rare but worrying. In the Singleton Pentasa study, the most frequent side effect, which affected 7.3 percent of the patients, was gastric intolerance to the drug. The safety profile of mesalamine has been evaluated in a large prospective long-term study involving nearly 3,000 American patients. They received different doses ranging from 0.4 g to 7.2 g/d of mesalamine (Asacol) coated with Eudragit S for up to 5.2 years. Only 8.8percent of patients discontinued treatment because of adverse events. The nine most common adverse events were abdominal pain, diarrhea, headache, bloody stools, nausea, flatulence, pain, flu-like syndrome, and asthenia. In 0.2 percent of this cohort of patients, an alteration of renal function tests was reported. 5-Aminosalicylic acid seems to be safe in pregnancy. A study from Canada on 19 pregnancies and a subsequent study on 165 Canadian women have shown that mesalamine does not represent a teratogenic risk in humans in the doses normally employed. Nevertheless, the mean birth weight of the babies born on mesalamine therapy was about 200 g lower than that of the control babies. An increase in preterm delivery rate was also reported. It was suggested that these findings could also be attributed to relapses and greater disease activity of the mothers who experienced these adverse events.

Conclusion

The conclusion of the analysis of all of these studies both in acute flare and in maintenance has to be drawn bearing in mind several caveats. The first caveat concerns the difference in dosage of 5-ASA employed in the studies, varying from 1.5 g to 4.5 g. Second, the inclusion in the maintenance trials of patients with surgically induced remission together with patients who were in remission because of medical therapy has introduced an important selection bias. In fact, induced medical remission is fairly often not concomitant with a complete healing of lesions, as opposed to surgery, where all of the diseased intestine is nearly always removed. The consequence, then, is that the time of relapse is different in the two situations, maintenance of clinical remission usually lasting longer after surgery.

Another difference among the trials is that some of them have included only patients in whom the remission was homogeneously induced, whereas others have enrolled patients already in remission. The different drugs employed for inducing remission of the acute phase could influence the subsequent relapse rate, inasmuch as they may favor the inclusion of patients with different disease severity. For example, steroids, which have a greater therapeutic efficacy in the acute setting, could provide patients for the maintenance study who have a more severe disease and are more prone to an early relapse.

Another possible source of error is the different bioavailability of the 5-ASAs because of the eventual fecal loss of the drug, following the accelerated transit or an extensive bowel resection. In spite of these criticisms, the results of all of these studies permit us to draw some important conclusions:

• 5-Aminosalicylic acids should work better when the site of disease coincides with the site of their splitting; their efficacy in other parts of the intestine is uncertain. A recent study confirms that the mean value of mucosal mesalamine concentration was lower in patients with recurrent disease after surgery, in comparison with those without recurrence.
• The delivery system of the 5-ASA should permit a homogeneous splitting in the area of inflammation and, because of their local action, 5-ASA should be more effective when the disease is localized in the superficial layer of the gut.

5-Aminosalicylic acid should be reserved for patients with mild to moderate disease and/or with long remission duration, because these groups should include patients with more superficial lesions. Patients with fistulizing disease should be generally unresponsive to 5-ASA and for recurrence prevention in patients with inactive disease because of surgery. 5-Aminosalicylic acid with pH or mechanically dependent delivery should be used for patients with mild to moderately active disease, localized in the ileum or in the right side of the colon. Doses of 4.8 g or more, if tolerated, should be administered in an acute setting. Doses of 4 g would be advisable in maintenance. Whether the 5-ASAs with an azo-bond (olsalazine-balsalazide) could be effective in the left-sided Crohn's colitis, where they are split, should be evaluated in the near future.

Editor's Note

As described in other chapters, combination therapy, including mesalamine in the higher doses and in an appropriate release form, is being used in mild to moderate disease and for some degree of steroid sparing along with azathioprine or 6-mercaptopurine.

Only a portion of the 78-reference bibliography could be reproduced. A complete copy can be obtained upon request to the author at prantera@tinit. A number of the references appear in other chapters. (TMB)

Supplemental Reading

Agnholt J, Sorensen HT, Rasmussen SN, et al. Cardiac hypersensitivity to 5-aminosalicylic acid [letter]. Lancet 1989;1:1135.

Alstead EM, Wilson AG McT, Farthing MJG. Lichen planus and mesalazine. J Clin Gastroenterol 1991;13:335–7.

Camma' C, Giunta M, Rosselli M, Cottone M. Mesalamine in the maintenance treatment of Crohn's disease: a meta-analysis adjusted for confounding variables. Gastroenterology 1997;113:1465–73.

Deltenre P, Berson A, Marcellin P, et al. Mesalazine (5-aminosalicylic acid) induced chronic hepatitis. Gut 1999;44:886–8.

Dent MT, Ganapathy S, Holdsworth CD, Channer KC. Mesalazine induced lupus-like syndrome. BMJ 1992;305:159.

Frieri G, Pimpo MT, Andreoli A, et al. Prevention of postoperative recurrence of Crohn's disease requires adequate mucosal concentration of mesalazine. Aliment Pharmacol Ther 1999;13:577–82.

Hanauer SB, Verst-Brasch C, Regalli G. Renal safety of long-term mesalamine therapy in inflammatory bowel disease (IBD). Gastroenterology 1997;112:A991.

Messori A, Brignola C, Trallori G, et al. Effectiveness of 5-aminosalicylic acid for maintaining remission in patients with Crohn's disease: a meta-analysis. Am J Gastroenterol 1994;89:692–8.

Novis BH, Korzeta Z, Chen P, Bernheim J. Nephrotic syndrome after treatment with 5-aminosalicylic acid. BMJ 1988;1:1442.

Popoola J, Muller AF, Pollock L, et al. Late onset interstitial nephritis associated with mesalazine treatment. BMJ 1998;317:795–7.

Prantera C, Cottone M, Pallone F, et al. Mesalamine in the treatment of mild to moderate active Crohn's ileitis: results of a randomized, multicenter trial. Gastroenterology 1999;116:521–6.

Prantera C, Pallone F, Brunetti G, et al. Oral 5-aminosalicylic acid (Asacol) in the maintenance treatment of Crohn's disease. Gastroenterology 1992;103:363–8.

Prantera C, Scribano ML, Berto E. Treatment of active Crohn's disease with salazopyrine and derivatives of aminosalicylic acid (5-ASA). In: Prantera C, Korelitz BI, eds. Crohn's disease. New York: Marcel Dekker, 1996:233–51.

Rao SS, Cann PA, Holdsworth CD. Clinical experience of the tolerance of mesalazine and olsalazine in patients intolerant to sulphasalazine. Scand J Gastroenterol 1987;22:332–6.

Reinoso MA, Schroeder KW, Pisani RJ. Lung disease associated with orally administered mesalazine for ulcerative colitis. Chest 1992;101:1469–71.

Sachedina B, Saibil F, Cohen LB, Whittey J. Acute pancreatitis due to 5-aminosalicylate. Ann Intern Med 1989;110:490–2.

Singleton JW, Hanauer SB, Gitnick GL, et al. Mesalamine capsules for the treatment of active Crohn's disease: results of a 16-week trial. Gastroenterology 1993;104:1293–301.

Singleton JW. Second trial of mesalamine therapy in the treatment of active Crohn's disease. Gastroenterology 1994;107:632–3.

Thomsen OO, Cortot A, Jewell D, et al. A comparison of budesonide and mesalazine for active Crohn's disease. N Engl J Med 1998;339:370–4.

Waanders H, Thompson J. Kawasaki-like syndrome after treatment with mesalazine. Am J Gastroenterol 1991;86:219–21.

Woodward DK. Peripheral neuropathy and mesalazine [letter]. BMJ 1989;299:1224.

CHAPTER 75

CLINICAL QUESTIONS IN CROHN'S DISEASE NOT ANSWERED BY CONTROLLED TRIALS

RICHARD J. FARRELL, MD, MRCPI, AND Z. MYRON FALCHUK, MD

Despite advances in our understanding of Crohn's disease and the development of novel medical therapies for inflammatory bowel disease (IBD), the treatment of patients with Crohn's disease remains ever challenging. Because of the diversity of responses to the same therapeutic approach in different patients with Crohn's disease, there are a number of important areas for which definitive data are not yet available, current clinical opinions are divergent, and management controversies exist. The heterogeneous nature of clinical presentations of Crohn's disease can overwhelm the clinician managing these patients whose disease is often refractory to standard anti-inflammatory therapy. Such is the explosion in the armamentarium of medical therapies for Crohn's disease that long-term or controlled trial data on many of these newer agents are not available. In this chapter, we attempt to address several therapeutic questions about Crohn's disease management that currently remain contentious or for which there are insufficient data in the literature to mandate management decisions.

How long should patients with Crohn's disease be treated with azathioprine or 6-mercaptopurine?

There are no good data on how long to maintain patients on azathioprine (AZA) or 6-mercaptopurine (6-MP) who are in remission. Toxicity does not seem to be in proportion to duration of therapy. The most influential factor in stopping 6-MP therapy is its failure. This usually takes a full year to determine, and certainly at least 6 months of maintenance therapy before failure of therapy can be assumed with confidence. The chapter on measurement of 6-MP metabolites addresses the issue of optimizing azathioprine or 6-MP dosage and avoiding toxicity. Bouhnik and colleagues (1996) performed a long-term follow-up study of Crohn's disease patients treated with AZA or 6-MP for more than 6 months who were in prolonged clinical remission (over 6 months without steroids). They found that after 4 years of remission on these drugs, the risk of relapse appeared to be similar, whether the therapy

was maintained or stopped, and concluded that given the potential risks of long-term immunosuppressive therapy, the usefulness of maintaining AZA or 6-MP in patients who have been in remission for more than 4 years is questionable. Consequently, several authors have adopted this 4-year limit for maintenance immunomodulator therapy. However, there is also preliminary evidence that the longer the duration of therapy, the longer the remission lasts after the drug is stopped. We also do not know the adequacy of the maintenance doses in 6TG levels in those who relapsed on continuous therapy in the French study.

Current Practice

Our own practice follows the old dictum "if it ain't broke, don't fix it." In other words, decisions are made on an individual patient basis, and if patients are tolerating their maintenance immunomodulator therapy and their monthly blood profiles are stable, we recommend that they be kept on the treatment at dosages of 1.5 to 2.5 mg/kg/d of AZA or 1 to 1.5 mg/kg/d of 6-MP. For patients who are tolerating therapy but who are particularly worried about long-term effects, our practice is not to stop therapy but rather encourage the patient to reduce the dose to 1.5 mg/kg/d of AZA or 1 mg/kg/d of 6-MP. One advantage of this approach is the mildness of the recurrence compared with what occurs when the drug is stopped and the greater likelihood of response when the dose is increased again. In patients who are in remission and are tolerating maintenance 5-aminosalicyclic acid (5-ASA)/sulfasalazine and immunomodulator therapy, our own practice is to encourage the patients to maintain the combination therapy. Although future trials are needed to assess if 5-ASA/sulfasalazine therapy can be successfully withdrawn in these circumstances, we feel that the different modes of action of these agents combined with their topical and systemic sites of action may help to prolong remission compared to immunomodulator therapy alone. There are also preliminary data supporting a potential role for colorectal cancer protective effects of long-term 5-ASA therapies in ulcerative colitis patients, possibly mediated through COX-2 inhibition, which, in theory, may benefit patients with longstanding extensive Crohn's colitis.

How safe is azathioprine or 6-mercaptopurine therapy?

Although the potential side effects related to long-term use of immunomodulator therapy are of particular concern, the reported side effects in long-term studies are reassuringly low, in the range of 10 to 15 percent. Over half of the reported side effects are infections, the frequency of which is not unlike what can be expected in a background control population. Approximately 3 percent of patients experience pancreatitis that is usually reversible, 2 percent significant bone marrow depression, and 2 percent allergic reactions. Although it is suspected that long-term treatment with AZA or 6-MP increases the risk for various neoplasms including lymphoma and colorectal cancer in IBD patients, it is worth remembering that as many cases of lymphoma in IBD patients were reported in the literature prior to the introduction of immunomodulator therapy as have been reported since then. A study by Connell and colleagues in London failed to find any increased risk of either colorectal cancer or non-Hodgkin's lymphoma in 755 IBD patients treated with 2 mg/kg of AZA for a median of 12.5 months after a median follow-up of 9 years.

In those patients who have had successful treatment with immunomodulators, the most common priority in stopping the drug is the desire for pregnancy. Although 5-ASA and sulfasalazine can be used safely in pregnancy, there is a general reluctance to consider AZA/6-MP in young patients who are considering starting a family. Unfortunately, there are very few data specific to AZA/6-MP safety during pregnancy in IBD patients. Data from Alstead and colleagues (1990) suggests that AZA can be used in patients with refractory Crohn's disease who wish to become pregnant. Furthermore, the renal transplant experience with these drugs is very reassuring. In many cases, if it was not for AZA/6-MP therapy, often in much higher doses than used in IBD, hundreds of post-transplant patients would not have had successful pregnancies. There are two chapters on IBD and pregnancy that address the issue of immunomodulators' use in pregnancy.

Although AZA and 6-MP are therapeutically similar and have similar toxicity profiles, a number of cases have been reported where patients who discontinued AZA therapy because of poor response or toxicity either responded to 6-MP or had no recurrence of side effects when treated with 6-MP. However, if a patient experiences pancreatitis or significant bone marrow depression on AZA therapy, it is likely that he/she will experience the same side effects with 6-MP therapy, whereas, if the main reason for discontinuing AZA therapy is gastrointestinal intolerance, myalgia, or rash, it is possible that he/she may not experience these side effects on 6-MP. In our institution, we have had experience with a few patients with steroid-dependent Crohn's disease who responded to 6-MP but not AZA. Thus, it may be worth considering consecutive treatment with both agents in particularly refractory cases.

Does any "prophylactic" medication prevent recurrent ileal stenosis, and what do you routinely recommend for patients postileal resection for Crohn's disease?

A major frustrating feature in the surgical management of Crohn's disease is the high recurrence rate, which may lead to reoperation. Postoperative recurrence of lesions is endoscopically present in 70 to 90 percent of cases within 1 year after surgery and is already present in as many as 75 percent of cases after 3 months. This has made the prevention of recurrence after resection one of the main goals in the treatment of Crohn's disease. Yet, the role of prophylactic therapy following resection remains a controversial issue. Despite a number of controlled trials assessing several medical therapies over the last 20 years, the data on preventing recurrence of Crohn's disease, although promising, are difficult to interpret. Multiple definitions of what constitutes a recurrence, that is, endoscopic, radiologic, clinical, or surgical recurrence, accounts for much of the confusion in interpreting these studies. Additionally, several trials' study groups were poorly stratified and not homogeneous with respect to pretrial clinical characteristics such as small and large bowel disease, smoking, and presence of fistulizing disease. There is a chapter on efforts to lessen postoperative recurrence in Crohn's disease.

Two large randomized clinical trials failed to demonstrate a clinically important effect of medical therapy with sulfasalazine (2 to 3 g/d) in preventing recurrence of ileal Crohn's disease. Some authors have suggested that the full therapeutic dosage of 3 to 4 g/d is required to maintain remissions. Since sulfasalazine theoretically requires intestinal bacterial action to release its active 5-ASA moiety, it is likely that this protective effect is due to admixture of ileal and colonic contents in the area of the neoterminal ileum, the site of the majority of Crohn's disease recurrences. Meta-analysis of the 5-ASA data demonstrates that, interestingly, the greatest prevention of recurrence is in patients with colitis or ileocolitis, with less effect observed in patients with only small bowel disease. Three to four grams of sulfasalazine is not an unreasonable first-line "prophylactic" agent in a patient who has had a colo-colonic anastomosis.

Although data on various 5-ASA preparations in preventing small bowel recurrence are more favorable, the efficacy is modest, showing a 10 to 24 percent therapeutic advantage compared to placebo at 12 months. One randomized open trial showed that 2.4 g/d of 5-ASA (Asacol®, Procter & Gamble Pharmaceuticals, Cincinnati, Ohio) was effective in preventing endoscopic recurrence in patients who had undergone resection for Crohn's ileitis. At 24 months, the cumulative proportion of recurrence was 0.52 in the 5-ASA group compared to 0.85 in the control group. The results of this study, however, must be interpreted in light of the absence of a placebo-controlled group and the fact that the endoscopists were aware of which patients were assigned 5-ASA therapy. Another 1-year placebo-controlled trial of 3 g/d of 5-ASA (Pentasa®, Ferring-Shire Pharmaceuticals, Florence, Kentucky) concluded that 5-ASA was effective in reducing the grade of endoscopic activity of disease recurrence, but only a small difference concerning clinical relapse was observed. Although it is intuitive that the longer patients stay on 5-ASA maintenance therapy, the stronger the prophylactic effect, a recent large multicenter study demonstrated a therapeutic advantage with 3 g/d of 5-ASA (Salofalk®, Axcan Pharma Inc., Minneapolis, Minnesota) over placebo of only 19 percent at 3 years. As mentioned, there is a separate chapter on postoperative prophylaxis and a chapter on 5-ASA.

Current Practice

Recent work by D'Haens and colleagues has shown that the initiation of recurrence in Crohn's disease occurs almost immediately, within days of a healthy bowel being reconnected. Thus, patients who tolerated 5-ASA/sulfasalazine therapies prior to their bowel resection should be encouraged to stay on maintenance therapy in the perioperative as well as postoperative periods. We currently recommend oral 5-ASA 3 to 4 g/d for patients who have a moderate risk of recurrence—in other words, all patients who have had small or large bowel Crohn's disease resected. Their position as first-line "prophylaxis" agents is based on their good cost-benefit relation between side effects and efficacy. Although higher doses probably could increase the therapeutic advantage, it would be at the risk of a higher percentage of side effects. Our strategy in minimizing recurrence in the moderately at-risk patient is to inform all patients about the risk of smoking and establish the optimal dosage of 5-ASA for each patient, while aiming for the 3 to 4 g/d dosage range, all the while ensuring

---

* Editor's Note: The important question about preventing recurrent ileal stenosis is not addressed by these authors. This would have to be a 7- to 10-year study. None of our current medications have the property of inhibiting muscle hypertrophy or fibrosis. This would best be studied in a group undergoing resection for ileal stenosis since at least 40 percent could be predicted to undergo a second resection for a nonperforating obstruction 7 to 10 years later. (TMB)

that they stay on their maintenance medication and understand that recurrence is always a risk and surgical resection never a cure for their disease.*

Is it possible to predict patients at higher risk of recurrence? What about prophylaxis in patients with more aggressive disease such as fistulizing ileitis?

Unfortunately, it remains difficult to identify those patients who are destined for symptomatic recurrence. Factors that have been shown to increase a patient's risk of relapse and recurrence include a young age at diagnosis, multiple resections, extensive disease, short onset between symptoms and surgery, the presence of perforating or fistulizing disease, and concurrent cigarette smoking. In patients with aggressive Crohn's disease with a higher risk of recurrence, the modest therapeutic advantages offered by 5-ASA maintenance therapy clearly may not be enough to minimize disease recurrence. In such circumstances, the options of immunomodulator agents, AZA/6-MP or antibiotic therapy, should be considered.

Immunomodulator Therapy

6-Mercaptopurine, which is cleaved off the AZA molecule, appears to be the active moiety of this compound. The two drugs seem to have identical therapeutic effects but at different dosages. The molecular weight of AZA is almost twice that of 6-MP; hence, the dose of 6-MP represents about 50 percent of the dose of AZA needed to produce comparable therapeutic and toxic effects. What typically happens in practice, however, is that both drugs are given at a starting dose of 50 mg/d, which is probably too low a dose for AZA. The upper limit of relative safety of AZA is approximately 2.5 to 3 mg/kg/d, corresponding to 1.5 mg/kg/d of 6-MP. Only a couple of small studies assessing the benefits of immunomodulator therapy in preventing Crohn's disease recurrence have been published. In a recent multicenter controlled study by Korelitz and colleagues (1998) with a 2-year follow-up, 6-MP (50 mg/d) was found to be superior to 5-ASA (3 g/d) and placebo in preventing clinical (53% vs 61% vs 70%), endoscopic (68% vs 80% vs 90%), and radiologic (68% vs 82% vs 85%) postoperative recurrence of Crohn's disease. Although the therapeutic advantage with 6-MP was modest, future controlled studies of the long-term effects of AZA/6-MP on recurrence prevention are forthcoming, and it is likely that their beneficial effects, using higher maintenance doses, will be better established.

Antibiotics

There is good evidence to support the hypothesis that bacteria in the gut lumen play an important role in the pathogenesis of Crohn's disease, including disease recurrence. The importance of fecal stream and reflux of colonic contents in determining the pattern of ileal recurrence after ileocolectomy for Crohn's disease has been demonstrated by several groups after side-to-side ileocolonic anastomosis. The excluded blind end of ileum was seemingly protected from the recurrence seen at the site of end-to-end anastomoses. Infusion of intestinal luminal contents into excluded ileum in patients with Crohn's disease who had undergone a curative ileocolonic resection with ileocolonic anastomosis and temporary protective proximal loop ileostomy induced focal infiltration of inflammatory cells in the lamina propria in the excluded neoterminal ileum proximal to the ileocolonic anastomosis within a matter of days. Antibiotics for the prevention of recurrence of Crohn's disease following surgical resection have yielded encouraging results. Rutgeerts and colleagues (1995) found that metronidazole therapy (20 mg/kg/d) for 3 months decreased the severity of early recurrence of Crohn's disease in the neoterminal ileum and significantly reduced the clinical recurrence rate at 1 year (4% vs 25%). However, the side-effect profile of metronidazole, particularly the occurrence of paresthesias resulting from peripheral neuropathy with doses over 1 g, has limited long-term use. Reductions in disease recurrence were not seen beyond 1 year. Because of potential teratogenic effects, metronidazole is absolutely contraindicated in the first trimester of pregnancy, and we do not use it in women of child-bearing age who are not using adequate birth control methods or who are planning a family.

Current Practice

Although the combination of metronidazole plus ciprofloxacin or metronidazole plus 5-ASA for the prevention of Crohn's disease postresection is in need of future study, we are attempting to maintain postoperative remission in numerous patients with these combination regimens. Our current practice in patients who are at high risk of disease recurrence, including those patients who have experienced a recurrence on 3 to 4 g/d of 5-ASA therapy, is to recommend careful discussion of the benefits and side effects of both AZA/6-MP as well as short-term antibiotic regimens. We usually start AZA or 6-MP at a dose of 50 mg/d. If tolerated and weekly blood counts do not drop precipitously, the dose is increased by 25-mg increments every month, to reach a maximum of 2.5 mg/kg/d of AZA or 1.5 mg/kg/d of 6-MP.[†] After the first month of treatment, blood counts are usually checked monthly for the duration of the therapy. In selected patients who have active perirectal disease, Crohn's colitis, or a recent history of abscess or fistula, or patients who become intolerant of AZA/6-MP therapy or are reluctant to commence treatment, we

usually recommend metronidazole therapy alone or in combination with ciprofloxacin or both antibiotics as part of an alternating regimen. Because of its aerobic coverage, ciprofloxacin may be superior to metronidazole therapy in patients with predominantly small bowel disease and absence of perianal symptoms. Metronidazole is commenced at a dose of 10 mg/kg/d, increased to a maximum of 20 mg/kg/d after 1 month, and continued for a total of 3 months.[‡] Ciprofloxacin is started at a dose of 250 mg bid for 2 weeks and increased to a maximum of 500 mg bid thereafter. We have found a 3-month postoperative course of antibiotics a particularly useful short-term option in high-risk patients who have to wait 3 to 6 months for AZA/6-MP to take effect; we then discontinue the antibiotics as we increase the immunomodulator dosage.

Is there any role for maintenance therapy with alternate-day prednisone or budesonide to prevent disease recurrence?

The relatively high effectiveness of long-term alternate-day prednisone treatment (20 to 25 mg alternate days) and the low rate of side effects reported make it a valid option for selected patients with Crohn's disease, such as young patients in whom AZA/6-MP is not indicated because of intolerance. However, in practice, we do not prescribe prednisone solely for the maintenance of Crohn's disease patients or indeed with the intention of preventing disease recurrence, and we would always consider a trial of mesalamine, immunomodulator therapy, or antibiotics first in patients with steroid-dependent disease. Although the development of topically acting corticosteroids (budesonide) promises a maintenance steroid with minimal systemic toxicity, results from a recent multicenter, double-blind, randomized trial by Hellers and colleagues (1999) showed that although oral budesonide 6 mg/d reduced the recurrence rate in patients who had undergone surgery for disease activity, the differences at 3 and 12 months were not significant, and, more importantly, budesonide offered no benefit in preventing endoscopic recurrence after surgery for ileal/ileocecal fibrostenotic Crohn's disease. Consequently, given the concerns of long-term "minimal" steroid toxicity, while acknowledging that we have had some success with budesonide (9 mg/d) in maintaining remission in steroid-dependent patients, we do not recommend long-term budesonide therapy as a means of preventing disease recurrence. There is a chapter on use of topically active corticosteroids with a focus on budesonide in this text. Use for maintaining remission is discussed.

[†] Editor's Note: Use of 6-MP metabolite levels could be helpful in this type of dose schedule in which there are no symptoms to follow. This approach is discussed in a chapter in this text. (TMB)

[‡] Editor's Note: With metronidazole doses over 1 g/d for 8 weeks, most patients will develop neuropathy. The 10 mg/1 kg dose was effective in the Belgian Study. (TMB)

What is the experience with infliximab in clinical practice? Is there any role for infliximab in combination with immunomodulator therapy?

The emergence of infliximab, a cytokine-directed biologic therapy, represents a significant advancement in our understanding of the pathophysiology and treatment of Crohn's disease. Clinical efficacy of infliximab in patients with intractable Crohn's disease has been conclusively shown in several acute studies, and a long-term study (multiple infusions) suggests benefit for maintenance of the effect in patients with severe disease. In patients with fistulous disease, infliximab has demonstrated rapid onset of fistulae closure (usually within 2 weeks) with lasting median benefit of action (exceeding 3 months). However, although the chimeric monoclonal antibody is well tolerated in the short term, and serious adverse events are infrequent, its potential long-term toxicities remain uncertain. The appropriate patient populations need to be defined; its use as sequential or concomitant treatment with conventional therapy, particularly immunomodulator therapy, and its ability to "reset" the mucosal immune system remain areas of continued investigation.

Current Practice

To date, we have had experience in treating over 130 patients with almost 250 infliximab infusions (5 mg/kg). Therapy was successful in approximately two-thirds of patients who received infliximab for either active disease or symptomatic perianal fistulae, with the more active the disease, the more dramatic the response, prompting successful inpatient trials in a handful of patients with fulminant Crohn's disease. Most patients who responded did so within 2 weeks of receiving their infusion, whereas the mean duration of response was 10 weeks, underscoring the short-term role of this expensive therapy. In practice, those patients with active disease who tolerate and respond to their first infliximab infusion tend to have a subsequent infusion only when their disease relapses. Unfortunately, some patients have developed serum sickness-like reaction when there was a 2-year lag between infusions. There are anecdotal reports of similar reactions after a 6-month lag. Regarding those patients with active disease who fail to respond to but tolerate the first infusion, we generally reschedule a second infusion, given the current data demonstrating a 15 percent subsequent response rate among first-time nonresponders. Our clinical experience also supports this policy in that patients with active disease who fail to respond to two infusions should probably not receive further infusions. Our preliminary experience among patients who received infliximab as a steroid-sparing therapy demonstrated an ability to discontinue steroids in 40 percent of patients following one to two infusions. Whether successive infusions become the mainstay of therapy for steroid-dependent Crohn's disease patients who are intolerant of immunomodulator therapy remains to be defined in prospective studies. Whereas most patients tolerated the infusions, 7 percent of patients experienced significant adverse events; several patients who had received multiple infusions had to have infusions aborted because of allergic-type reactions. Patients who were receiving concomitant prednisone appeared to have higher infection rates, which accounted for almost one-third of late adverse events. Placing a seton drain before treating a patient with a perianal fistula may lessen the risk of abscess formation. Infliximab appeared to be responsible for converting partial to complete bowel obstruction in one patient, prompting us to be more vigilant in ruling out narrow fibrostenotic disease prior to contemplating infliximab therapy.

Given the limited data and concerns regarding long-term toxicity of infliximab, particularly regarding the development of lupus syndromes and lymphoma, and the fact that the long-term safety profile of immunomodulator therapy is better documented, we are reluctant to consider infliximab therapy in patients with steroid-dependent or refractory Crohn's disease who have not had a trial of AZA/6-MP. However, in patients with particularly aggressive and active Crohn's disease, we currently use infliximab as a bridge to long-term immunomodulator therapy, in a similar fashion to intravenous cyclosporine in severe steroid refractory ulcerative colitis. In practice, once we are confident that a patient with aggressive, active disease has no significant intra-abdominal abscess or fibrostenotic disease, he/she receives infliximab and is then commenced on AZA/6-MP therapy. In this situation, infliximab serves as a useful short-term bridge in aggressive steroid-dependent Crohn's disease while waiting for AZA/6-MP therapy to take effect. While we await future clinical trials on the efficacy of this "two-punch" regimen, preliminary data on combination therapy with infliximab and methotrexate in aggressive rheumatoid arthritis show considerable promise for this approach.

What do you recommend regarding colonoscopic surveillance in Crohn's disease?

The issue of dysplasia surveillance in Crohn's disease is addressed in more detail in a separate chapter but deserves comment here because of the limited data available to support colonoscopic surveillance recommendations. Whereas one study by Weedon and colleagues (1973) reported a significantly high risk of colorectal cancer (standardized incidence ratio = 26.6), admittedly in a cohort of patients with extensive Crohn's colitis who were older than the general population, several studies have failed to demonstrate as large a magnitude of risk of colorectal cancer associated with Crohn's colitis with standardized incidence ratios ranging between 1.0 and 4.3. This relative lack of risk of colorectal cancer has made the development of firm surveillance recommendations for patients with Crohn's colitis more difficult. At present, there is no indication that patients with Crohn's disease limited to the small bowel area are at an increased risk of colorectal cancer.

However, there is growing evidence that the biology of colorectal cancer is similar in Crohn's disease and ulcerative colitis, with patients having longstanding, extensive colitis being at greatest risk for colorectal cancer. Gillen and colleagues (1994) demonstrated similar cumulative incidence of colorectal cancer in patients with extensive Crohn's colitis and patients with extensive ulcerative colitis (8% at 22 years in Crohn's disease and 7% at 20 years in ulcerative colitis). Although less attention has been addressed toward reducing the risk of colorectal cancer in patients with Crohn's disease, it is important to bear in mind that many patients with Crohn's colitis will have undergone resections of the involved portion of the colon, thus reducing their overall cancer risk. Our own practice is to enroll patients who have longstanding Crohn's colitis (>8 years duration) who have extensive disease, which would include patients who have patchy colonic involvement extending beyond the sigmoid colon, in a cancer surveillance program with colonoscopy performed at least every 2 years with multiple biopsy specimens taken every 10 cm. Patients with Crohn's disease confined to the small bowel probably have the same colorectal cancer risk as the general population, and, as such, colorectal cancer screening recommendations that apply to the general population based on patient age, family history of colorectal cancer, and previous history of cancer or adenomatous polyps are more important in these circumstances. Finally, it is worth noting that a considerable number of Crohn's colitis patients are only diagnosed with Crohn's disease several years after the onset of their initial gastrointestinal symptoms, which, in many cases, may be falsely ascribed to irritable bowel syndrome or acute self-limiting colitis. Therefore, the time of onset of symptoms rather than the time of diagnosis becomes an important consideration in calculating when to initiate colonoscopic cancer surveillance so as not to underestimate their duration of disease. In our experience, patients referred with newly diagnosed Crohn's disease whose initial symptoms stretch as far back as childhood or the early teen years should always have a colonoscopy when their disease is inactive to assess the extent of their disease and rule out colonic dysplasia.

References

Bouhnik Y, Lemann M, Mary JY, et al. Long-term follow-up of patients with Crohn's disease treated with azathioprine or 6-mercaptopurine. Lancet 1996;347:215–9.

Connell WR, Kamm MA, Dickson M, et al. Long-term neoplasia risk after azathioprine treatment in inflammatory bowel disease. Lancet 1994;343:1249–52.

D'Haens GR, Geboes K, Peeters M, et al. Early lesions of recurrent Crohn's disease caused by infusion of intestinal contents in excluded ileum. Gastroenterology 1998;114:262–7.

Gillen CD, Andrews HA, Prior P, et al. Crohn's disease and colorectal cancer. Gut 1994;35:651–5.

Hellers G, Cortot A, Jewell D, et al. Oral budesonide for prevention of postsurgical recurrence in Crohn's disease. The IOIBD Budesonide Study Group. Gastroenterology 1999;116:294–300.

Korelitz B, Hanauer S, Rutgeerts P, et al. Post-operative prophylaxis with 6MP, 5-ASA or placebo in Crohn's disease: a 2-year multicenter trial. Gastroenterology 1998;114: A1011.

Rutgeerts P, Hiele M, Gebbos K, et al. Controlled trial of metronidazole treatment for prevention of Crohn's recurrence after ileal resection. Gastroenterology 1995;108:1617–21.

Weedon DD, Shorter RG, Ilstrup DM, et al. Crohn's disease and cancer. N Engl J Med 1973;289:1099–103.

Supplemental Reading

Alstead EM, Ritchie JK, Lennard-Jones JE, et al. Safety of azathioprine in pregnancy in inflammatory bowel disease. Gastroenterology 1990;90:443–6.

Farrell RJ, Ladhavia P, Shah S, et al. Clinical experience with infliximab in 100 Crohn's disease patients. Am J Gastroenterol 1999;94:2642A.

Lewis JD, Deren JJ, Lichtenstein GR. Cancer risk in patients with inflammatory bowel disease. Gastroenterol Clin North Am 1999;28:459–77.

Michetti P, Peppercorn MA. Medical therapy of specific clinical presentations. Gastroenterol Clin North Am 1999;28:353–70.

CHAPTER 76

ANTIBIOTICS AS THERAPEUTIC AGENTS IN CROHN'S DISEASE

R. BALFOUR SARTOR, MD

The use of antibiotics as primary or adjunctive therapeutic agents in Crohn's disease remains controversial due to a paucity of definitive, rigorously designed controlled trials. However, these agents are widely used by experienced clinicians who, on empirical grounds, are convinced of their efficacy in certain clinical situations as an adjunct to or as an alternative to corticosteroids. Although their utility as primary therapeutic agents remains contentious, antibiotics are clearly indicated in conjunction with surgical or percutaneous drainage of abscesses for the frequent septic complications of Crohn's disease (Table 76–1). This chapter will briefly review the rationale for the use of antibiotics in intestinal inflammation; summarize the major clinical trials investigating their use as primary therapeutic agents in Crohn's disease and prevention of postoperative recurrence of disease; relate the personal experience of the author; and suggest future clinical trials to establish more definitively the optimal use of single or combination antimicrobial agents in primary, adjunctive, or preventive protocols.

Experimental Models

Rationale of Antibiotic Therapy in Intestinal Inflammation

Antibiotics have several potential activities that could decrease intestinal and systematic inflammation (Table 76–2). Results in induced and genetically engineered rodent models demonstrate compellingly that normal resident luminal bacteria provide the constant stimulus for genetically susceptible hosts to develop chronic, immune-mediated intestinal inflammation and associated extra-intestinal manifestations. At least 10 different

TABLE 76–1. Complications of Crohn's Disease Requiring Antibiotics

Intra-abdominal or perirectal abscess

Perianal fistula and chronic fissure

Intra-abdominal inflammatory mass

Enterovesical fistula

Small bowel bacterial overgrowth

Secondary infection (*Clostridium difficile*, parasites, enteric pathogens)

Postoperative infection

TABLE 76–2. Mechanisms of Antibiotic Responses in Intestinal Inflammation

Decrease overall concentrations of luminal bacteria

Selectively eliminate certain enteric bacterial subsets

Diminish tissue invasion and microabscesses

Decrease bacterial translocation and systemic dissemination of bacterial constituents

models in rats, mice, and guinea pigs fail to exhibit colitis and enterocolitis in the absence of viable luminal enteric bacteria. Moreover, colitis occurs within 1 to 4 weeks of colonizing sterile (germ-free) rodents with normal flora, and, conversely, experimental disease is attenuated with antibiotics. In these experimental models, metronidazole and regimens that eliminate *Bacteroides* species are superior in prevention protocols to agents with predominantly aerobic spectra, but combinations of broad-spectrum antibiotics are the only means to reverse established disease. Chronic use of broad-spectrum antibiotics does not change the total luminal bacterial concentrations, although they do alter the composition by eliminating *Bacteroides* species and decrease the numbers of adherent and/or translocating bacteria. Of considerable clinical relevance, not all resident flora have equal capacities to induce inflammation, since anaerobic bacteria and *Bacteroides* species preferentially induce colitis in HLA B_{27}/β_2 microglobulin transgenic rats, and *Lactobacillus* and *Bifidobacterium* species provide protection in several experimental models. These results suggest that selective *elimination* of certain subsets of the complex enteric bacterial population has therapeutic possibilities, perhaps in conjunction with *enhancement* of protective subpopulations by *probiotic* or *prebiotic* approaches.

Clinical Observations

These results in experimental models complement clinical observations in Crohn's disease. Concentrations of certain anaerobic bacteria, including *Bacteroides* species, as well as serum antibodies to anaerobic coccobacilli and a broad panel of enteric commensals, are increased in patients with Crohn's disease, and fecal concentrations of *Bacteroides* correlate with clinical responses to metronidazole. Enteric bacteria translocate in areas of fistulae and fissure ulcers, whereas systemic uptake of inflammatory bacterial products such as endotoxin (lipopolysaccharide) correlates with disease activity and response to treatment. Finally, Crohn's disease tends not to recur in bypassed distal ileal segments, but inflammation is evident within a week of re-infusion of ileostomy contents into the bypassed ileum, and disease recurs soon after restoration of bowel continuity, suggesting that luminal components induce intestinal inflammation. These results support the concept that certain subsets of the normal resident bacterial flora provide the stimulus for chronic, relapsing intestinal inflammation and provide an attractive rationale for therapeutic approaches that broadly suppress luminal bacteria or selectively inhibit subsets responsible for disease induction.

Clinical Trials

Although broad-spectrum and sequentially rotated antibiotics (ampicillin, tetracycline, sulphamethoxazole, or trimethoprim/sulphamethoxazole) have been used by experienced clinicians and have been reported to achieve symptomatic improvement in 93 percent of patients, with radiographic improvement in 57 percent in a 6-month uncontrolled trial, these agents have never been subjected to an adequate multicenter, controlled trial.

Metronidazole

Metronidazole has been the most thoroughly studied antibiotic used in Crohn's disease, but the numbers of patients investigated are relatively low and protocols have varied, so that results are somewhat inconsistent. Ursing et al (1982) demonstrated that metronidazole 800 mg/day was equal to sulfasalazine in a 16-week trial, with improvement occurring in 57 percent of unselected patients and 25 percent of patients entering remission. These results were not significantly different from the group treated with sulfasalazine (55% improvement, 40% remission), although serum orosomucoid, an acute-phase reactant that reflects the inflammatory response, was significantly lower with metronidazole therapy. In the larger North American Cooperative Study comparing metronidazole 10 and 20 mg/kg/d to placebo, a dose-dependent significant decrease in the Crohn's Disease Activity Index (CDAI) was noted at the end of the 16-week trial (-67, 10 mg/kg; -97, 20 mg/kg; 1, placebo), although the rates of remission were not different with metronidazole therapy (36%, 10 mg/kg; 27%, 20 mg/kg; 25% placebo), and only 53 percent of patients completed the trial. In both the Scandinavian and North American studies, patients with colonic involvement (colitis and ileocolitis) had the best response, with no improvement noted with isolated ileal disease. In addition, no peripheral neuropathy was reported in either study. Together, these studies support the use of metronidazole for active colonic Crohn's disease.

Rutgeerts et al (1995 and 1999) have reported that metronidazole and related nitromidazol compounds have promise in preventing postoperative recurrence of ileal Crohn's disease. Patients who were treated with metronidazole 20 mg/kg/d for 3 months beginning immediately after ileal resection had significantly fewer severe endoscopic lesions at 3 months (13% vs 43% placebo, $p = .02$) and decreased clinical recurrence at 1 year (4% vs 25%, $p = .04$), with a trend toward decreased clinical recurrence for the remainder of the 3-year observation period (30% vs 50% relapse at 3 years, NS). Similar improvement was noted in a preliminary 1-year administration of ornidazole (1 g/d). Severe endoscopic lesions were noted in 41 percent of ornidazole-treated patients at 3 months versus 74 percent of placebo controls ($p < .02$) and in 62 percent versus 94 percent at 1 year ($p = .059$). Unfortunately, these trials, particularly the metronidazole study, are conceptually flawed by treating patients with a life-long propensity to relapse with a short course of antibiotics. It is quite surprising that a trend toward clinical improvement persisted for 3 years in the 3-month metronidazole study.*

Ciprofloxacin

Recent data support the use of ciprofloxacin, either alone or in combination with metronidazole. Colombel et al (1999) prospectively evaluated ciprofloxacin 500 mg bid versus mesalamine 2 gm bid for 6 weeks and showed no difference in rate of remission (56% vs 55%, NS) or overall improvement (73% vs 60%, respectively, NS). Only one patient taking ciprofloxacin withdrew because of side effects, and the failure rate was 17 percent ciprofloxacin versus 36 percent placebo. In a recent preliminary placebo-controlled study, Arnold et al (1999) found that 6-month administration of ciprofloxacin (500 mg bid) resulted in a significantly lower CDAI (122 vs 205 placebo group, $p < .001$) at the end of the study. Prantera et al (1996) compared ciprofloxacin (500 mg bid) plus metronidazole (250 mg qid) versus methylprednisolone 0.7 to 1.0 mg/kg/d for 12 weeks; 45.5 percent of the antibiotic group and 63 percent of the corticosteroid group ($p = $ NS) entered a clinical remission but 27 percent of the antibiotic group versus 11 percent of steroid-treated patients were classified as treatment failures. In an open-label study of ciprofloxacin (500 mg bid) plus metronidazole (250 mg tid), Greenbloom et al (1998) demonstrated that 68 percent of patients entered remission after 10 weeks of therapy, with superior results in those patients with colonic involvement, concurrent steroid therapy, and no prior surgical resection.

Clarithromycin

In preliminary studies, *clarithromycin*, either alone or in combination with broad-spectrum antibiotics or with

---

* Editor's Note: In terms of antibiotic therapy of intestinal diseases, after treating patients with tropical sprue with tetracycline for 6 months, improvement in jejunal structure and function continued over the ensuing months (Guerra et al, Ann Intern Med 1964). (TMB)

antimycobacterial agents, appears promising. In a double-blind crossover study, Graham et al (1995) reported that five of seven patients treated with clarithromycin 500 mg bid for 3 months entered a clinical remission versus one of eight placebo controls; these patients remained in remission during the 1-year follow-up. However, only one of seven patients treated with clarithromycin in the crossover phase went into remission. In two additional open-label experiences, 58 to 78 percent of patients improved. Thirty *Helicobacter pylori*-positive patients with Crohn's disease treated with omeprazole, clarithromycin 500 mg bid, and amoxicillin 1 g bid had a mean drop in CDAI from 310 to 133, with results comparable to prednisolone controls. Finally, Gui and colleagues (1997) reported in an uncontrolled trial that 52 patients treated with clarithromycin 250 mg bid (42 patients) or *azithromycin* 500 mg daily for 4 days/week plus *rifabutin* 450 mg daily for a mean of 18 months had significant improvement in disease activity and inflammatory markers, with 82.5 percent of patients achieving remission at some point during the trial, and 69 percent of those patients who achieved remission remained clinically quiescent after 24 months. Twelve percent of patients were intolerant of these medications. This study was designed to test the hypothesis that treatment of *Mycobacterium paratuberculosis* would cure Crohn's disease, but this aspect is difficult to interpret because the antibiotics chosen have broad antimicrobial activities. The results of most antimycobacterial trials with traditional triple antibiotic regimens have been negative.[*]

Author's Experience

In my experience, antibiotics are effective in many patients with active Crohn's disease involving the colon (colitis and ileocolitis), especially when an inflammatory mass or fistula is present (Table 76–3). I rarely use antibiotics alone, instead adding these agents to 5-aminosalicylic acid (5-ASA), steroids, or immunosuppressive drugs. In my experience, many patients unresponsive to 5-ASA alone or with partial responses to steroids respond to the addition of antibiotics. Although 6-mercaptopurine (6-MP)/azathioprine is the first-line approach to steroid-dependent patients, the addition of antibiotics for 3 months can accelerate clinical responses and steroid reduction and provide adjunctive benefit to those patients not responding optimally to immunosuppressive agents.

Choice of antibiotics, dosing, and duration of therapy are critical determinants for successful outcomes, in addition to selection of appropriate candidates for treatment. I usually begin with *metronidazole*, 10 mg/kg/d in

TABLE 76–3. Suggested Clinical Situations for Antibiotics in Crohn's Disease

Active Crohn's colitis or ileocolitis

Postoperative disease recurrence

Inflammatory mass with sinus tracks

Small bowel bacterial overgrowth from partial obstruction or internal fistulae

Perianal fistulae

Enterovesical fistula

divided doses (usually 250 mg tid) for primary colonic Crohn's disease and 20 mg/kg/d for perianal disease, implementing therapy slowly with one pill after a meal the first day and increasing by one pill per day until the target dose is reached over several days. Slow onset of therapy diminishes the frequent (20%) dose-dependent nausea, anorexia, and metallic taste experienced with metronidazole. The most important long-term side effect is peripheral neuropathy, which is rare (< 5%) with 10 mg/kg/d, but frequent when higher doses (20 mg/kg/d) are used for greater than 6 months. A toxic interaction with alcohol is rare (< 5%), but patients should be warned of this possibility.

If metronidazole is not tolerated or is not effective within 1 month of use, my next choice is *ciprofloxacin* 500 mg bid, which is well tolerated but expensive and more frequently leads to *Candida* overgrowth. If neither of these medications is effective or tolerated, *tetracycline* (500 mg tid) or *clarithromycin* (500 mg bid) provides an effective alternative, although the former is much less costly. If antibiotics are used as primary treatment of Crohn's disease, they must be viewed as *long-term therapeutic agents*, with minimum use of 1 month and preferred duration of therapy of 3 months. The most frequent mistake I see with the use of antibiotics is short-term administration (7- to 10-day course), which is doomed to failure similar to the results obtained by pulse therapy with corticosteroids. In complex or refractory perianal fistulae unresponsive to single antibiotics, I will frequently *combine* metronidazole and ciprofloxacin while immunosuppressive drugs are initiated. Chronic, relapsing fistulae may respond to *rotating* antibiotics as bacterial resistance develops. Complex patients may require prolonged (several years) antibiotic use, which is safe as long as peripheral neuropathy secondary to metronidazole is carefully monitored.

Metronidazole offers an alternative as a potential means to prevent recurrence of disease in patients undergoing bowel resection who cannot afford or who are unwilling to take 16 mesalamine pills per day on a long-term basis, who refuse to consider 6-MP or azathioprine because of perceived or demonstrated toxicities, or who have had an early recurrence of disease despite mesalamine or immunosuppressive prophylaxis with previous surgery. In these patients, I use a combination of

---

[*] Editor's Note: Although gastroenterologists are generally skeptical of the association between *Mycobacteria paratuberculosis* and Crohn's disease, the cattle industry in Pennsylvania, Australia, and New Zealand have decided to make their herds free of Johne's disease, which is caused by that organism. (TMB)

mesalamine 1 g and metronidazole 250 mg bid, which is a reasonably easily remembered and less expensive approach, but for which there is no published experience in preventing disease relapse.

Conclusions and Future Directions

There is irrefutable evidence in rodent models that chronic intestinal inflammation is a consequence of an overly aggressive cellular immune response to a subset of normal resident luminal bacteria. Abundant clinical evidence in Crohn's disease supports this hypothesis, providing a firm rationale for the therapeutic use of antibiotics in this disorder. Although most clinical trials demonstrate positive effects of metronidazole, ciprofloxacin, and clarithromycin in patients with colonic Crohn's disease, no single study is definitive, and the majority are underpowered, are open labeled, have serious design flaws, or compare antibiotics to 5-ASA compounds, which themselves have questionable activity as primary therapeutic agents.

Thus, although antibiotics should continue to be used in appropriately selected patients with active disease or septic complications, it is imperative that clinical investigators design appropriate multicenter control trials to determine optimal regimens and clinical indications for the use of antibiotics in Crohn's disease. Results in animal models suggest that broad-spectrum combination protocols (imipenem/vancomycin or metronidazole/neomycin) will be superior to single agents, whereas insights into pathophysiology of disease mechanisms suggest that optimal long-term responses will result from combining antibiotics, which eliminate the constant antigenic drive activating antigen presenting cells and T lymphocytes with medications that suppress cell-mediated immune responses and restore barrier function. It is likely that antibiotics will synergistically interact not only with other medications that have different mechanisms of action but also will synergize with *probiotic* and *prebiotic* agents to alter the composition of the luminal microflora on a long-term basis. Several clinical situations seem particularly promising: active Crohn's colitis (in combination with traditional medication), perianal fistulae (with and without 6-MP/azathioprine or anti-TNF-α antibodies), and long-term prevention of postoperative relapse (in combination with 6-MP or mesalamine).

References

Arnold G, Patel H, Becker KG, Boyd H. Ciprofloxacin in active Crohn's disease: preliminary report of a 6 month randomized placebo controlled study [abstract]. Gastroenterology 1999;116:G2898.

Colombel JF, Lemann M, Cassagnou M, et al. A controlled trial comparing ciprofloxacin with mesalazine for the treatment of active Crohn's disease. Groupe d'Etudes Therapeutiques des Affections Inflammatoires Digestives (GETAID). Am J Gastroenterol 1999;94:674–8.

Graham DY, Al-Assi M, Robinson M. Prolonged remission in Crohn's disease following therapy for *Mycobacterium paratuberculosis* infection [abstract]. Gastroenterology 1995;108:A826.

Greenbloom SL, Steinhart AH, Greenberg GR. Combination ciprofloxacin and metronidazole for active Crohn's disease. Can J Gastroenterol 1998;12:53–6.

Gui GP, Thomas PR, Tizard ML, et al. Two-year-outcomes analysis of Crohn's disease treated with rifabutin and macrolide antibiotics. J Antimicrob Chemother 1997;39:393–400.

Prantera C, Zannoni F, Scribano ML, et al. An antibiotic regimen for the treatment of active Crohn's disease: a randomized, controlled clinical trial of metronidazole plus ciprofloxacin. Am J Gastroenterol 1996;91:328–32.

Rutgeerts P, Hiele M, Geboes K, et al. Controlled trial of metronidazole treatment for prevention of Crohn's recurrence after ileal resection. Gastroenterology 1995;108:1617–21.

Rutgeerts PJ, D'Haens G, Baert F, et al. Nitromidazol antibiotics are efficacious for prophylaxis of postoperative recurrence of Crohn's disease: a placebo controlled trial [abstract]. Gastroenterology 1999;116:G3506.

Ursing B, Alm T, Barany F, et al. A comparative study of metronidazole and sulfasalazine for active Crohn's disease: the cooperative Crohn's disease study in Sweden. II. Result. Gastroenterology 1982;83:550–62.

Supplemental Reading

D'Haens GR, Geboes K, Peeters M, et al. Early lesions of recurrent Crohn's disease caused by infusion of intestinal contents in excluded ileum. Gastroenterology 1998;114:262–7.

Feagan BG. Antibiotics are not effective therapy for Crohn's disease (time to remove the rose-coloured glasses). Inflamm Bowel Dis 1997;3:314–7.

Mantzaris GJ, Petraki K, Archavlis E, et al. Short-term remission of Crohn's disease after treatment of *H. pylori* infection [abstract]. Gastroenterology 1999;116:G337.

Moss AA, Carbone JV, Kressel HY. Radiologic and clinical assessment of broad-spectrum antibiotic therapy in Crohn's disease. AJR Am J Roentgenol 1978;131:787–90.

Peppercorn MA. Antibiotics are effective therapy for Crohn's disease. Inflamm Bowel Dis 1997;3:318–9.

Sartor RB. Microbial factors in the pathogenesis of Crohn's disease, ulcerative colitis and experimental intestinal inflammation. In: Kirsner JB and Hanauer S, eds. Inflammatory bowel disease. 5th Ed. Philadelphia: WB Saunders, 1999:153–78.

Sutherland L, Singleton J, Sessions J, et al. Double blind, placebo controlled trial of metronidazole in Crohn's disease. Gut 1991;32:1071–5.

Thomas GA, Swift GL, Green JT, et al. Controlled trial of antituberculous chemotherapy in Crohn's disease: a five year follow up study. Gut 1998;42:497–500.

CHAPTER 77

Appropriate Use of Corticosteroids in Inflammatory Bowel Disease

Francisco A. Sylvester, MD, and Jeffrey S. Hyams, MD

Glucocorticoids are a mainstay for the treatment of severe inflammatory bowel disease (IBD). The efficacy of corticosteroids to induce remission in both Crohn's disease and ulcerative colitis has been well established in large randomized controlled trials. At times, a focus on adverse events has diminished the recognition of the usefulness of corticosteroids. The aim of this chapter is to suggest approaches for the appropriate use of corticosteroids, including corticosteroid-sparing strategies, in patients with IBD.

Mode of Action

Glucocorticoids act at multiple levels in the immune system (Table 77–1) (Cato and Wade, 1996; Didonato et al, 1996). Upon entering the cell by passive diffusion, they bind to a cytoplasmic receptor. The hormone-receptor complex then translocates to the nucleus, where it binds to DNA sequences called glucocorticoid-responsive elements (GRE). Binding to the GRE results in either repression or activation of transcription of specific genes. Glucocorticoids can also modulate transcription by interfering with the activity of certain transcription factors, such as activator protein-1 (AP-1) and nuclear factor (NF)-κB. These transcription factors are involved in the expression of key elements of the inflammatory cascade, such as cytokines and metalloproteinases. By interfering with these factors, glucocorticoids can inhibit cytokine and metalloproteinase gene expression. Glucocorticoids also have effects on mast cells, lymphoid cells, macrophages, endothelial cells, and fibroblasts that augment their anti-inflammatory activity. Glucocorticoids inhibit the expression of adhesion molecules that direct the traffic of circulating immunocompetent cells to the site of inflammation. They also inhibit the production of lipid mediators derived from the breakdown of cell membranes and the release of arachidonic acid by phospholipase A2. This effect is mediated by the glucocorticoid-dependent increase in synthesis of lipocortin-1, an inhibitor of phospholipase A2. Glucocorticoids also directly inhibit the expression of cyclo-oxygenase 2, which is responsible for prostaglandin synthesis.

Corticosteroids used in the treatment of IBD are prednisone, prednisolone, methylprednisolone, and budesonide. Prednisone and prednisolone have comparable glucocorticoid potency, whereas methylprednisolone is slightly more potent. All three have minimal mineralocorticoid activity. Prednisone is preferentially used in North America, prednisolone in the United Kingdom, and methylprednisolone in Europe. Budesonide, a topically active steroid that is rapidly metabolized by the liver, is available in Canada, Europe, and Scandinavia.

Strategies for the Use of Corticosteroid Therapy

Use Corticosteroids When Indicated

Corticosteroids are associated with significant side effects because of the ubiquitous nature of their receptors (Table 77–2) (Frauman, 1996). In IBD, their use should be restricted to severe, active disease, to induce remission (Stein, 1999). Simple dosing principles can decrease the

TABLE 77–1. Mechanisms of Action of Corticosteroids

Mechanism	Effect
Molecular mechanisms	
Binding to GRE in DNA and to transcription factors (AP-1, CREB, NF-κB)	Downregulate expression of proinflammatory factors
Gene regulation (transcriptional and post-transcriptional)	
Anti-inflammatory and immunosuppressive effects	
On neutrophils, monocytes-macrophages, eosinophils, mast cells	Decreased myelopoiesis, decreased adhesion to endothelial cells, decreased cytokines synthesis
On endothelial cells	Decreased vascular permeability, decreased adhesion-molecule synthesis
On fibroblasts	Decreased collagen synthesis
On prostaglandin synthesis	Inhibition of phospholipase AZ synthesis, activation of enzyme inhibitors (lipocortin-1), inhibition of cyclo-oxygenase 2 expression
Stabilization of lysosomal membranes	
Decreased cell-mediated immunity	
T lymphocytes	Transient reduction of circulating cells, increased apoptosis, inhibition of T-cell activation
B cells	Decreased antibody formation

GRE = glucocorticoid-responsive elements; AP-1 = activator protein-1; CREB = cyclic adenosine monophosphate-responsive element binding protein; NF = nuclear factor.

TABLE 77–2. Adverse Effects of Corticosteroids

Immediate onset in majority of patients

Sleep disturbances	Increased appetite	Dyspepsia, heartburn
Mood changes	Fluid retention	Acne
Fatigue	Cushingoid facies	

Aggravating presumed predisposition

Hypertension	Gastric, duodenal ulcers
Hyperglycemia, diabetes	Psychoses

Effects of long-term use

Osteopenia, osteoporosis	Skin striae
Stunting of growth	Central redistribution of fat
Myalgia, myopathy	Headaches, seizures

Perhaps idiosyncratic but dose dependent
  Avascular necrosis
  Cataracts

possibility of serious side effects. For example, corticosteroids should be given as a single morning dose to coincide with the natural circadian rhythm of endogenous corticosteroids. This strategy also takes advantage of the principle that tissue effects of corticosteroids outlast drug concentrations in serum. Therefore, a single daily dose of a corticosteroid will be as therapeutically efficacious as if it is given in divided doses, and will cause fewer side effects and less suppression of the hypothalamic-pituitary-adrenal axis.

There is no clinical evidence that corticosteroids have benefit in the maintenance of remission of IBD. To induce remission, oral doses over 1 mg/kg (maximum 40 to 60 mg/d) of prednisone do not offer additional benefit and increase the possibility of side effects. This high-dose course should be continued for 2 to 6 weeks, followed by gradual tapering. In patients with severe ulcerative colitis or Crohn's disease who do not respond to oral therapy, intravenous steroid therapy and parenteral nutrition ("bowel rest") may be needed. Parenteral glucocorticoids may be administered as hydrocortisone 300 mg/d or methylprednisolone 40 to 60 mg/d. Intravenous adrenocorticotropic hormone (ACTH) was found in one study to be efficacious in severe ulcerative colitis, particularly in patients who had not received prior courses of corticosteroids; currently, such patients rarely are encountered in hospitals. Adrenocorticotropic hormone stimulates adrenal production of a mixture of corticosteroids in pharmacologic concentrations. Importantly, the prolonged use of ACTH is associated with a risk of adrenal hemorrhage.

Topical Therapy

Topical corticosteroids are available for the induction of remission of distal active colitis. The standard steroid formulations include hydrocortisone hemisuccinate or acetate and prednisolone 21-phosphate. These are not effective in maintenance therapy; they are absorbed from the rectum and prolonged administration is associated

with systemic side effects (Marshall and Irvine, 1997). Newer agents are being developed that have high topical activity and lower systemic bioavailability after rectal administration.

Ideally, corticosteroids should be tapered as quickly as possible once clinical remission has been attained. Tapering by 5 mg weekly is a common approach. Some patients may benefit from slower reductions (eg, decreasing the dose by 5 mg every other day each week, or by 5 mg every other week). The use of alternate-day therapy decreases side effects and should be considered in patients who are steroid-dependent or have chronic active disease. This approach is particularly advantageous in children, because it helps to prevent the stunting associated with corticosteroid use and causes fewer side effects in general (Hyams et al, 1988). Steroid-sparing strategies should be considered from the beginning of therapy.

Corticosteroids should not be used for mild-to-moderate disease. Several agents are available to treat patients who do not have severe symptoms. These include both oral and topical agents. Some of these drugs have steroid-sparing effects. Following is an outline of these agents; for a more extensive discussion, refer to the appropriate chapters in this book.

Corticosteroid-Sparing Strategies

NUTRITION

Diet factors may be of crucial importance for the development of IBD, and elemental diets and total parenteral nutrition are effective in inducing remission in Crohn's disease. Nutritional therapy is probably less efficacious than corticosteroids in the induction of remission in Crohn's disease, but should be considered first-line therapy in children with impaired linear growth, or in those patients who relapse frequently or have chronic active disease.

Fish oil, containing a large amount of omega-3 fatty acids, recently has proved efficacious in a controlled trial for prevention of relapse in Crohn's disease. Active IBD does not respond to fish oil, probably owing to its late onset of action.

BUDESONIDE

The "perfect" steroid would have high topical glucocorticoid potency, low systemic bioavailability, rapid first-pass metabolism in the intestine or liver, and rapid excretion. Although none of the currently available agents fully meet these criteria, budesonide comes close. Budesonide has potent topical activity, and therefore has been used for both oral and intrarectal administration. The main advantage of budesonide is its significant "first-pass effect" in the liver after intestinal absorption. The liver rapidly degrades budesonide into inactive metabolites, so that only 9 to 12 percent of an oral dose is available systemically. This property limits its systemic bioavailability and, therefore, its toxicity. Clinical trials have documented that budesonide causes less systemic side effects than prednisolone.

Oral budesonide has been studied mainly in patients with Crohn's disease. Several randomized controlled trials have shown that oral budesonide is slightly less effective at inducing remission than prednisone. However, budesonide is more effective than 5-aminosalicylic acid (5-ASA) in active Crohn's disease (Thomsen et al, 1998). The optimal dose appears to be 9 mg/d. Data in ulcerative colitis are limited but encouraging (Feagan, 1996).

Budesonide comes in two forms. Entocort® (Astra Draco, AB, Lund, Sweden) releases the drug more proximally and is suitable for the treatment of ileal and right ileocolonic disease. Entocort has been used in most randomized trials. Budenofalk® (Falk Pharma, Freiburg, Germany) releases more budesonide in the colon and might be more suitable to treat colonic disease, although data are lacking. For intrarectal administration, topical budesonide seems to be as effective as other topical corticosteroids. Budesonide is not yet approved for use in the United States. Other chapters discuss topically active corticosteroids.

Budesonide at a dose of 3 to 6 g was shown to be efficacious, compared to a placebo, in a randomized trial in maintaining remission short term, but its benefit dissipated after 1 year (Greenberg et al, 1996).

AMINOSALICYLATES

Sulfasalazine and its 5-ASA derivatives are efficacious in the treatment of active mild-to-moderate Crohn's colitis and ulcerative colitis and should be used in preference to conventional corticosteroids to induce remission in this clinical situation. Both oral sulfasalazine and its 5-ASA derivatives are efficacious in maintaining remission in patients with ulcerative colitis. Corticosteroids are not used for maintenance. In the postsurgical setting, mesalamine may be of value for preventing recurrence after intestinal resection for Crohn's disease (Modigliani, 1996), but the role of maintenance therapy in relapse-prone patients is less evident. Topical 5-ASA is effective in maintaining remission of distal ulcerative colitis.

ANTIBIOTICS

Antibiotics probably act by a combination of antimicrobial and immunologic effects on the inflamed gastrointestinal mucosa and can be used for steroid sparing. In a large randomized trial, metronidazole was as effective as sulfasalazine for mild-to-moderately active Crohn's colitis. Clinical experience has shown that metronidazole also is useful in perianal Crohn's disease and ileal reservoir pouchitis after colectomy for ulcerative colitis. Ciprofloxacin has steroid-sparing properties and has been used in patients with active Crohn's disease and perianal disease. Other chapters discuss antibiotic usage in Crohn's disease and ulcerative colitis.

AZATHIOPRINE AND 6-MERCAPTOPURINE

Azathioprine (AZA), a prodrug of 6-mercaptopurine (6-MP), is cheaper and equally efficacious. Recently there has been an emerging interest in the earlier use of these immunomodulators in IBD.

Azathioprine and 6-MP are established adjuvant drug therapy in patients with Crohn's disease who are corticosteroid-dependent or relapse-prone, particularly those with extensive ileal or colonic involvement and those with persistent perianal disease, including fistulae. Both medications have a corticosteroid-sparing effect, allowing dose reduction or complete weaning from corticosteroids in many patients. In the authors' opinion, the use of AZA or 6-MP needs to be considered early in the course of the disease, perhaps if a patient needs two consecutive courses of oral corticosteroids for chronic active disease. Their use in ulcerative colitis has been more limited, but remission is expected in 70 percent of patients with chronic unresponsive disease. In patients with ulcerative colitis, it is important to weigh the risks of prolonged immunosuppression with the possibility of performing curative surgery.

METHOTREXATE

Methotrexate (MTX) appears to be useful in Crohn's disease for patients who do not tolerate or respond to AZA or 6-MP. In a multicenter study comparing the efficacy of MTX, 25 mg once weekly, with placebo in 141 patients with chronic active steroid-dependent Crohn's disease, patients treated with MTX were more likely to be able to discontinue prednisone and to go into clinical remission than those given the placebo (39% vs 19%, $p = .03$). A significant reduction in the dose of prednisone also was noted. The placebo effect in this trial was modest. There are risks of allergic pneumonitis, bone marrow suppression, and long-term liver toxicity. In ulcerative colitis, MTX has not yet been proven effective in clinical trials.

CYCLOSPORINE

Cyclosporine has been used in severe ulcerative colitis, with the goal of avoiding or postponing colectomy and in fistulizing Crohn's disease. The initial enthusiasm for cyclosporine use has been dampened by subsequent negative long-term follow-up from the initial studies, and the occurrence of several deaths among patients treated for steroid-resistant, severe attacks of ulcerative colitis. Use of cyclosporine in patients with IBD can be associated with significant toxicity, including renal insufficiency, septic complications, and opportunistic infections (eg, *Pneumocystis carinii* and cytomegalovirus [CMV]).

ANTI-TUMOR NECROSIS FACTOR-ALPHA

Remicade® (Centocor Inc., Malvern, Pennsylvania) is a chimeric IgG1 monoclonal antibody directed against tumor necrosis factor-alpha (TNF-α) that is discussed in separate chapters. Intravenous Remicade has been useful in patients with refractory Crohn's disease and in severe perianal disease. Four repeated treatments of Remicade maintained clinical response for 8 weeks after the last infusion in 70 percent of patients. There are anecdotal reports of prolonged steroid sparing with repeated dosing, often with the addition of azathioprine. Use of Remicade needs to be balanced against the possibility of side effects, including malignancy and the appearance of antibodies against the agent, and its cost. To date, there is only limited, anecdotal experience of the use of Remicade in ulcerative colitis. This new era of molecularly engineered recombinant therapies likely will yield therapies that will lessen dependence on corticosteroids for those with more severe IBD.

Editor's Note

To lessen overlap with other chapters, some of the references in the bibliography have been omitted. A complete bibliography can be reqested at *jhyams@ccmckids.org*. (TMB)

References

Cato ACB, Wade E. Molecular mechanisms of anti-inflammatory action of glucocorticoids. Bioessays 1996;18:371–8.

Didonato JA, Saatcioglu F, Karin M. Molecular mechanisms of immunosuppression and anti-inflammatory activities by glucocorticoids. Am J Respir Crit Care Med 1996;154:S11–5.

Feagan BG. Oral budesonide therapy for ulcerative colitis: a topical tale. Gastroenterology 1996;110:2000–17.

Frauman AG. An overview of the adverse reactions to adrenal corticosteroids. Adverse Drug React Toxicol Rev 1996; 15:203–6.

Greenberg GR, Feagan BG, Martin F, et al. Oral budesonide as maintenance treatment for Crohn's disease: a placebo-controlled, dose-ranging study. Gastroenterology 1996;110:45–51.

Hyams JS, Moore RE, Leichtner AM, et al. Relationship of type I procollagen to corticosteroid therapy with inflammatory bowel disease. J Pediatr 1988;112:893–8.

Marshall JK, Irvine EJ. Rectal corticosteroids versus alternative treatments in ulcerative colitis: a meta-analysis. Gut 1997;40:775–81.

Modigliani R. Mesalamine in Crohn's disease with steroid-induced remission: effect of steroid withdrawal and remission maintenance. Gastroenterology 1996;110:688–93.

Stein RB, Hanauer SB. Medical therapy for inflammatory bowel disease. Gastroenterol Clin North Am 1999;28:297–321.

Thomsen OO, Cortot A, Jewell D, et al. A comparison of budesonide and mesalamine for active Crohn's disease. N Engl J Med 1998;339:370–4.

Supplemental Reading

Bar-Meir S, Chowers Y, Lavy A, et al. Budesonide versus prednisone in the treatment of active Crohn's disease. Gastroenterology 1998;115:835–40.

Campieri M, Ferguson A, Persson T, et al. Oral budesonide is as effective as oral prednisolone in active Crohn's disease. Gut 1997;41:209–14.

Greenberg GR, Feagan GB, Martin F, et al. Oral budesonide for active Crohn's disease. Canadian Inflammatory Bowel Disease Study Group. N Engl J Med 1994;331:836–41.

CHAPTER 78

TOPICALLY ACTIVE STEROID PREPARATIONS

ROBERT LÖFBERG, MD, PhD

Glucocorticosteroids (GCS) remain the mainstay of primary medical treatment for induction of remission in moderate and severe attacks of Crohn's disease (CD). The anti-inflammatory effects of GCS in active CD are unsurpassed by any other type of drug. However, drawbacks with conventional GCS include problems with a wide array of side effects and the risk for steroid dependency in a substantial proportion of patients who initially respond favorably to the treatment. Elimination of, or at least a substantial reduction of, unwanted short- and long-term systemic side effects would make GCS an even more important anti-inflammatory modality for the treatment of CD.

Efforts in developing superior steroids for inflammatory bowel disease (IBD) aim at obtaining increased and selective topical action, with no, or only limited, systemic impact (Löfberg, 1998). The original cortisone and its derivative, prednisone, are prodrugs with a low affinity for the GCS receptor. Prednisolone and 6-methylprednisolone have a better separation between glucocorticoid and mineral corticoid activity. The introduction of lipophilic substituents on the GCS skeleton has given betamethasone and the developed agent **beclomethasone diproprionate** enhanced efficacy and a high rate of hepatic biotransformation. Beclomethasone diproprionate was the first of the topically acting steroids to be evaluated in CD. Using an acid-resistant capsule, this compound was delivered intact to the small bowel, and although no large trials have been performed, beclomethasone still is used in North America and elsewhere, in extempore-type preparations for active CD, and other upper gastrointestinal inflammatory states, including graft-versus-host disease. This type of galenic formulation showed that a topically acting GCS could be delivered locally in the gut, exert its action, and then undergo extensive biotransformation during the first passage through the liver.

Budesonide is another improved, new generation GCS, primarily developed for use in asthma. It has a high topical potency with great affinity for the GCS receptor and a high first-pass metabolism in the liver (via the cytochrome P450 CYP3A4 enzymes) to metabolites with much less GCS activity. Hence, budesonide has low systemic impact when it is administered to the bowel.

Because of a relatively high water solubility, budesonide is readily dissolved and, thus, more readily transported to the bowel wall. Lipophilic properties ensure a high tissue uptake, resulting in high concentrations and high activity in the target tissues (eg, gut mucosa) when the drug is applied topically (Löfberg, 1998).

Budesonide has been extensively evaluated for several IBD conditions, and has been proven effective in enema form for active distal ulcerative colitis and proctitis. With a beneficial efficacy versus side-effect ratio, it also has emerged as a valuable peroral alternative to conventional GCS in mild-to-moderately active CD localized to the terminal ileum or proximal colon, and is now considered to be one of the first-line options for active CD (Lowry and Sandborn, 1999).

Oral Budesonide Preparations

Oral capsule preparations of budesonide recently have been approved in Europe, Israel, and Canada for treatment of active CD. The first and most extensively documented preparation for ileal and ileocolonic disease is a time- and pH-dependent, controlled ileal-release formulation (Entocort®, Astra Draco, AB, Lund, Sweden) with 5-mm-sized enteric-coated (Eudragit L100-55) pellets with a rate-limiting polymer containing the active drug. This targeted type of release delivers around 70 percent of budesonide to the distal ileum, cecum, and ascending colon (Löfberg, 1998). An acid-resistant resin, similar to that used in several slow-release 5-aminosalicylic acid (ASA) preparations (Eudragit L; dissolving above a pH ca. 6.0), is used for the ca. 400 pellets in the other oral capsule formulation of budesonide (Budenofalk®, Falk Pharma, Freiburg, Germany) (Gross et al, 1996). The latter formulation delivers somewhat more of the active drug to the colon.

Dosing

The optimal dose of oral budesonide for induction of remission in active CD is 9 mg/d. The results from both controlled studies and clinical practice support a practical once-daily dosing, which increases compliance (Rutgeerts et al, 1994; Campieri et al, 1997; Thomsen et al, 1998). Giving the daily dose at one time makes sense also from a theoretic standpoint. Owing to formation of intracellular conjugates, budesonide seems to remain within the mucosa for longer than prednisolone, for example; thus, the time-frame for interaction with the intracellular GCS receptor may be increased.

It is apparent in clinical practice that some patients may need, and also tolerate, higher doses than 9 mg daily, although this has not been unequivocally documented in formal trials. Some patients are experiencing neither any GCS-related side effects nor suppression of plasma cortisol levels when treated with doses of 12 mg or even 15 mg of budesonide daily. If such doses are required to control symptoms in active CD but are not causing side effects, they may be acceptable, at least for a limited period in selected patients. The dose is subsequently reduced after 2 to 4 weeks of initial treatment, down to the standard dose of 9 mg/d.

Conversely, some patients may be more sensitive to the actions of budesonide than others, and in those, the low systemic availability may still lead to problematic side effects when the standard 9-mg dose is administered, such as easy bruising and subcutaneous bleeding. Those patients may need dose adjustment downward to 6 mg and sometimes even 3 mg/d in the active phase.

In the vast majority of patients with a mild-to-moderate flare of ileal or proximal colonic CD, a clear and prompt symptomatic response is seen during the first few weeks of budesonide therapy. If the patient has not responded to some extent after 8 weeks of treatment, there is rarely any benefit to continuing. However, in those patients who achieved a significant response or remission at 8 weeks, further improvement of symptoms may be seen during an additional 8 weeks of continuous treatment (Thomsen et al, 1998). Therefore, up to 4 months of acute therapy seems to be a reasonable treatment period with the standard 9-mg dose, provided no troublesome side effects arise. Maintenance therapy is discussed in later paragraphs.

Budesonide versus Standard Steroid Regimens

An 8-week course with oral budesonide, 9 mg daily, has been proven statistically to be as efficacious and at least as rapid for acute therapy in patients with active ileal or ileocecal CD as a standard GCS regimen (ie, 40 mg/d of prednisolone, with gradual tapering over 8 to 10 weeks (Gross et al, 1996; Rutgeerts et al, 1994; Campieri et al, 1997). The symptomatic Crohn's Disease Activity Index (CDAI) fall was somewhat faster with prednisolone, but not significantly so. In large, randomized, controlled trials, altogether comprising more than a thousand patients, symptomatic remission rates with a 9-mg dose of budesonide have ranged from 51 to 69 percent. Importantly, budesonide has been found to induce significantly less suppression of endogenous cortisol levels than prednisolone and also to be associated with a decreased frequency and intensity of GCS-related side effects. As up to

60 percent of patients treated with standard prednisone or prednisolone regimens may experience GCS-associated side effects, with acne, moon-face, mood swings, and insomnia being some of the most common, an improvement in the adverse-event profile of GCS used in IBD is of great clinical value. However, even if the overall GCS-related side-effect profile appears to be significantly more benign with budesonide in comparison with conventional GCS therapy, the impact on the patients' perceived quality of life has not been found to be better, at least not in the short-term perspective. A decrease in certain GCS side effects, such as cosmetic ones, may have the greatest importance in younger age groups, after more prolonged use or at a second or third treatment.

When complications, such as an abdominal mass, fistula, or abscess, are present in active CD, GCS should be given with caution and preferably with antibiotic coverage. The chance of a septic, and in rare cases even fatal, complication should not be underestimated when conventional GCS is used, but seems to be less likely with budesonide.

Another advantage with budesonide is that tapering after a course for active disease does not seem to be necessary when therapy is to be terminated. To avoid the risk for iatrogenic long-term suppression of endogenous cortisol production, the dose of prednisolone or prednisone normally is decreased gradually over 1 to 3 months, depending on the level of the starting dose. Budesonide, however, usually conveys no, or only limited, impact on the hypothalamic-pituitary-adrenal (HPA) axis and may be continued at an optimal therapeutic level throughout the active disease phase and then abruptly discontinued (Thomsen et al, 1998). If one is in doubt as to whether there may be significant suppression or not, following prolonged treatment with 9 mg or more of budesonide per day, a normal morning plasma-cortisol sample indicates a low risk for clinically significant suppression and, thus, may aid the decision-making in terms of tapering.

The systemic bioavailability of the oral Entocort preparation is only around 10 percent in adults, and even less in children (6%). This makes the drug a more attractive GCS option for pediatric CD. Moreover, the risk for certain interactions is lower (eg, increased plasma concentrations of GCS in women using oral contraceptives and prednisolone are not seen with budesonide therapy).

Even though the oral budesonide preparations are associated with substantially fewer side effects and less impact on endogenous cortisol production, they still seem to have the same impact on some extra-intestinal manifestations, such as arthralgia, compared with a standard regimen with conventional GCS. This observation indicates a primary, topical effect on the target organ (ie, the terminal ileum or ascending colon) when IBD is treated with budesonide, resulting in secondary beneficial effects in other organs or tissues that have been influenced by the disease process in the bowel. The hypothesis that the action of budesonide is predominantly topical also is supported by the fact that commonly observed hematologic or clinical chemistry abnormalities during conventional GCS use, such as increased white blood cell count or hypokalemia), rarely are seen with budesonide therapy.

Budesonide versus Mesalazine in Active Crohn's Disease

In a study of patients with mild-to-moderately active ileal or ileocecal CD, oral controlled ilealocolonic-released budesonide (Entocort, 9 mg/d) recently has been shown to be significantly superior to treatment with a dose of 4 g of oral, sustained slow-release 5-ASA (Pentasa®, Ferring-Shire Pharmaceuticals, Florence, Kentucky) for induction of symptomatic remission (Thomsen et al, 1998). The maximal remission rate was strikingly higher (69% vs 45%) and the mean CDAI score was significantly more improved in the budesonide group during the 16-week study (Figure 78–1). The response to budesonide therapy was found to be more rapid and more profound. Not surprisingly, quality of life, as assessed by the psychological general well-being (PGWB) index, also was significantly improved among budesonide-treated patients. Furthermore, since 5-ASA treatment was associated with more withdrawal symptoms and more severe adverse events (Thomsen et al, 1998), the case for budesonide as a first-line option for flares in CD is strengthened.

Colonic Targeting

There still are no commercially available preparations of oral budesonide optimized for delivery throughout the

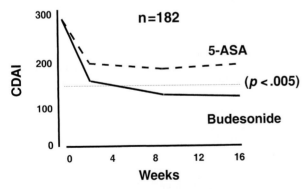

FIGURE 78–1. Mean Crohn's Disease Activity Index (CDAI) scores during a 16-week study showing the efficacy of oral budesonide in a controlled ilealocolonic-released preparation (Entocort®, 9 mg/d) versus oral slow-release mesalazine (Pentasa®, 4 g/d) in patients with active disease localized in the terminal ileum or proximal colon. The dotted line indicates the level of symptomatic remission (CDAI 150 pts). (Adapted from Thomsen OO, Cortot A, Jewell D, et al. A comparison of budesonide and mesalamine for active Crohn's disease. International Budesonide-Mesalamine Study Group. N Engl J Med 1998;339:370–4.)

large bowel, although a preliminary controlled colonic-release preparation has shown promising results in a trial with patients having left-sided and extensive ulcerative colitis (Löfberg et al, 1996). Currently, to treat cases of extensive colonic CD, a combination of oral ileal-release therapy with the preparation used for ileocecal CD ($\geq$ 9 mg/d) together with the 2-mg enema envisaged for distal ulcerative colitis (Entocort) at bedtime may be tried. The enema has limited systemic bioavailability, and thus, the total systemic load of GCS is kept low. This combination of budesonide preparations may cover a substantial part, if not all, of a diseased colon. Albeit somewhat cumbersome for the individual patient, the oral-rectal combination still may offer advantages over other therapeutic options in active colonic or colorectal CD.

Only anecdotal reports support the use of the budesonide enema for isolated rectal and distal colonic CD, but this may be a valuable alternative to conventional hydrocortisone and prednisolone formulations (foams, enemas). Those may in fact have substantial impact on endogenous cortisol production, particularly if used for prolonged periods, and may then also cause GCS-associated side effects, which are highly unlikely when the budesonide enema is used. The Entocort enema preparation comes in a package containing the 2 mg of drug and the 100-mL water enema separately, making the volume of the enema easily adjustable by the patient. For CD patients having difficulties retaining the full 100-mL enema, the 50-mL enema with double budesonide concentration may be a better preparation.

Combination Therapy

In the clinical setting, for ileal, ileocolonic, or pure colonic CD, budesonide seems to be particularly versatile in combination with other drugs, including metronidazole, ciprofloxacin, mesalamine, and sulfasalazine, for treatment of IBD. Combination therapy may allow lower doses of these drugs to be prescribed. Controlled trials evaluating different combinations with budesonide are in progress, but similar strategies are already in clinical use at many centers. For example, a reduction of the daily dose of metronidazole when used in combination with budesonide (an often used combination) may be of great importance for the patient, as tolerance for the metronidazole is enhanced if the daily dose is kept at no more than 800 mg. This increases safety (no risk for neuropathy) and improves overall, long-term compliance. At least one large ongoing study is addressing the usefulness of budesonide with ciprofloxacin, another popular combination.

A regimen of oral budesonide and an immunomodulator, such as azathioprine or 6-mercaptopurine (6-MP), may be another useful option. Budesonide is effective initially (with low risk for short-term adverse events), whereas an immunomodulator achieves its maximal efficacy after a 2- to 3-month course of therapy, and at that point, there is a low risk of long-term side effects if the patient tolerates the drug. Budesonide and azathioprine also are likely to have synergistic effects that may be of benefit in more severe cases, or may lead to a reduction in daily doses of both drugs while still maintaining the same level of efficacy in mild-to-moderate disease. Using this concept, it is possible to reduce the daily dose of azathioprine to 50 to 75 mg and of budesonide to 3 to 6 mg daily or every other day and still keep patients with ileocolonic CD in long-term symptomatic and endoscopic remission. Similar experience has been noted by others, for example, after balloon dilatation of colonic strictures.

Maintenance Therapy

Glucocorticosteroids generally are not thought to have relapse prevention properties in IBD, although certain patient subgroups may benefit from prolonged treatment. In practice, a patient attaining symptomatic remission in ileocolonic CD after budesonide therapy may experience a significant prolongation of the subsequent period in remission, possibly several months, by using oral budesonide as maintenance treatment in a dose of 6 mg/d (Löfberg, 1998). However, lower daily doses of budesonide do not seem to be of benefit in the long-term management of CD. Furthermore, if one continues the 6-mg dose, there is little benefit compared with placebo remaining after 1 year of treatment. On the other hand, certain patients may experience longer periods of remission when an adaptive dose regimen is used. Using the 6-mg dose of budesonide as the baseline, the dose may be raised temporarily, for example, to 9 mg/d, when the first symptoms of a potential relapse are encountered. Such long-term, flexible dosing seems to work in selected cases and is now being evaluated in appropriate randomized trials.

Budesonide seems to be particularly useful in patients experiencing difficulties in the weaning phase of conventional GCS (prednisolone or prednisone) therapy. In these patients, 6 mg/d of controlled ilealocolonic-released budesonide may be succesfully introduced as a substitute to maintain remission in almost 70 percent of the cases, but without the GCS-related side-effect profile (Cortot et al, 1999).

Hellers et al (1999) demonstrated that the overall risk of having an endoscopic recurrence at the site of an anastomosis following resective surgery for ileal or ileo-colonic CD was not altered if treatment with 6 mg/d of budesonide was initiated directly after the operation and then maintained for 12 months. However, the risk for recurrence may be decreased in a subgroup of patients undergoing surgical resection predominantly for inflammatory activity rather than for fibrostenotic disease. The chapter on efforts to lessen postresection recurrences discusses the high rate of recurrence in patients resected for active disease.

Long-Term Safety of Budesonide

Abundant data from several large studies with oral budesonide indicate a benign toxicity profile. At an oral dose of 6 mg/d, the side-effect profile is similar to that of a placebo, and the reported risk for sustained adrenal-gland suppression is low.

Still, a slight impairment of the HPA axis probably is not the major concern in the long-term perspective. Instead the impact on bone metabolism, risk for cataract formation, and other potential metabolic side effects during prolonged use of budesonide at 6 mg/d need to be further elucidated. Several studies already indicate advantages of budesonide compared to conventional GCS in this respect, at least in the short-term perspective. One study failed to show any impact during a 10-week course of 9 mg/d of controlled ilealocolonic-released budesonide on osteocalin, a sensitive marker of bone formation, whereas methylprednisolone caused marked suppression (D'Haens et al, 1998). In a comprehensive safety survey, the use of budesonide was associated with a 0.9 percent risk of clinical fractures in comparison with 1.1% risk for patients treated with placebo (Østergaard-Thomsen, 1996).

In the long-term perspective, budesonide may become one of the preferred drugs for certain high-risk groups, to minimize the risk for deleterious GCS-associated side effects, including growth retardation in children with CD and fractures in elderly CD patients having osteoporosis. Studies in children are being conducted, and the long-term effect on bone mineralization as well as the risk for fractures will be assessed in longitudinal studies incorporating sensitive osteodensitometry assessment. Enhanced topical GCS with even higher potency and improved delivery systems, to the proximal colon in particular, are likely developments for the future.

References

Campieri M, Ferguson A, Doe W, et al. Oral budesonide is as effective as prednisolone in active Crohn's disease. Gut 1997;41:209–14.

Cortot A, Colombel JF, Huriez C, et al. Budesonide controlled ileal-release (CIR) capsules in prednisolone-dependent patients with Crohn's disease. Gastroenterology 1999;116:A692.

D'Haens G, Verstraete A, Cheyns K, et al. Bone turnover during short-term therapy with methylprednisolone or budesonide in Crohn's disease. Aliment Pharmacol Ther 1998;12:419–24.

Gross V, Andus T, Caesar I, et al. Oral pH-modified release budesonide versus 6-methylprednisolone in active Crohn's disease. Eur J Gastroenterol Hepatol 1996;8:905–9.

Hellers G, Cortot A, Jewell DP, et al. Oral budesonide in post-surgical recurrence prevention of Crohn's disease: a placebo controlled multi-center study. Gastroenterology 1999;116:294–300.

Löfberg R. New data on inflammatory bowel disease treatment with topical steroids. Res Clin For 1998;20:179–86.

Löfberg R, Danielsson Å, Suhr O, et al. Oral budesonide versus prednisolone in patients with active extensive and left-sided ulcerative colitis. Gastroenterology 1996;110:1713–8.

Lowry PW, Sandborn WJ. A comparison of budesonide and mesalamine for active Crohn's disease. Gastroenterology 1999;116:1263–4.

Østergaard-Thomsen O. Safety overview of budesonide in inflammatory bowel disease. Res Clin For 1996;18:91–100.

Rutgeerts P, Löfberg R, Malchow H, et al. A comparison of budesonide with prednisolone for active Crohn's disease. N Engl J Med 1994;331:842–5.

Thomsen OO, Cortot A, Jewell D, et al. A comparison of budesonide and mesalamine for active Crohn's disease. International Budesonide-Mesalamine Study Group. N Engl J Med 1998;339:370–4.

CHAPTER 79

AZATHIOPRINE AND 6-MERCAPTOPURINE USE IN CROHN'S DISEASE

RAMONA O. RAJAPAKSE, MD, AND BURTON I. KORELITZ, MD

Since the first description of regional ileitis by Crohn, Ginzburg, and Oppenheimer in 1932, much research has been performed in an attempt to elucidate the etiology of the disease and to find a lasting therapy. The concept of autoimmune diseases was introduced in the 1960s, and the early days of transplant surgery began. Hitchings and Elion used azathioprine to prevent rejection of organ transplants, and the concept of using immunosuppressive drugs to treat any disease perceived to be due to an autoimmune process evolved.

Following reports of success with the use of 6-mercaptopurine (6-MP) and azathioprine in the treatment of Crohn's disease and ulcerative colitis, a 2-year placebo-controlled, double-blind, crossover study of 6-MP in the treatment of refractory Crohn's disease was undertaken (Present et al, 1980). The major findings of this study were as follows: (1) over a 1-year period, there was a 67 percent improvement in the 6-MP group in comparison to a placebo group; (2) steroids were eliminated in 55 percent of patients, and the dose was reduced in another 20 percent; (3) fistulae closed in one-third of patients within 3 months and improved in another one-third; (4) toxicity was minimal; and (5) it was shown that the drug was slow acting, with a mean response time of 3.1 months.

Other early observations included (1) 6-MP appeared to be more effective in Crohn's colitis and ileocolitis than when only the small bowel was involved, (2) the response once accomplished was maintained over a 1-year period, and (3) when 6-MP was reintroduced after relapse, the mean time to response was more rapid than the first response. Subsequent studies have confirmed that 6-MP, used over a long term, maintains remission, closes fistulae, prevents the recurrence of extra-intestinal manifestations, such as arthritis, erythema nodosum, and pyoderma gangrenosum, after steroids are eliminated, and prevents the recurrence of Crohn's disease proximally after resection.

Pharmacokinetics

Azathioprine and 6-MP are biochemically classified as thiopurines; 6-MP was the first of the two used to treat disease, specifically as an antileukemic agent for childhood leukemias. Shortly thereafter, it was recognized that it possessed immunosuppressive properties. Azathioprine was initially conceived as a masked form of 6-MP that might yield higher tissue concentrations of the latter at requisite sites. It is a 6-substituted purine that is rapidly cleaved in vivo to 6-MP.

The immunosuppressive properties of azathioprine and 6-MP probably are mediated via their interference with protein synthesis and nucleic acid metabolism as well as by their cytotoxic effects on lymphoid cells. The transformation of 6-MP into active metabolites occurs along the competing routes catalyzed by thiopurine methyltransferase (TPMT) and hypoxanthine phosphoribosyltransferase (HPRT), giving rise to 6-methyl-mercaptopurine (6-MMP), 6-methyl-thioinosine 5′-monophosphate (6-Me-tIMP), and 6-thioguanine (6-TG) nucleotides, respectively.

When to Initiate Therapy

Early hesitance to use 6-MP or azathioprine in the treatment of Crohn's disease was due mostly to the fear of toxicity. As a result, treatment was delayed until some manifestations of the disease no longer offered hope of response to nonoperative therapy.

The question arises whether more goals would be achieved if 6-MP were started earlier in the course of disease, when complications are less severe. Intestinal inflammation and strictures secondary to cellular infiltrate and edema are more likely to respond than the more fibrotic phase of longstanding disease. Once the diagnosis of Crohn's disease is made and the manifestations are mild, therapy should be initiated with one of the oral 5-aminosalicylic acid (ASA) products that are most effective in colitis, moderately effective in ileocolitis, and least effective in small bowel disease. For patients with more advanced disease, corticosteroids should be used, either orally or intravenously, depending on the severity of the illness, to bring the disease into remission. If the steroids cannot be eliminated without recurrent flares of disease, 6-MP should be introduced either alone or with concurrent steroids, to bring the disease into control. The current trend is toward starting 6-MP sooner after the diagnosis of Crohn's disease is made, especially in children and adolescents in whom the disease is more virulent, and in older patients when the response to 5-ASA products is not rapid.

If the dominant manifestation is a perirectal fistula, a trial of metronidazole can be instituted, with 6-MP used only if this fails. For all other fistulae, 6-MP should be initiated early in therapy as it has an overall efficacy of 64 percent for healing. For perirectal abscesses, drainage or a modified Parks' procedure followed by the introduction of 6-MP would be appropriate.

6-Mercaptopurine has seemingly prevented recurrent attacks of small bowel obstruction in 45 percent of patients; this result is less gratifying than when the indication is primarily inflammation or abscesses. The response is more favorable when the stricture is caused by inflammation than when fibrosis is the cause. Therapy should be instituted earlier rather than later. In contrast, 83 percent of colonic strictures respond to 6-MP, although the possibility of carcinoma, when the stricture cannot be adequately biopsied, may tip the balance in favor of surgery in these patients. It is probable that colonic strictures respond better because the wider lumen is less likely to cause obstruction.

Abdominal masses in Crohn's disease usually are attributable to matted loops of bowel with or without fistulization. Nonsurgical elimination of an abdominal mass, using steroids, antibiotics, and then 6-MP, has been successful in 50 percent of cases.

Recurrent ileitis in the ileostomy and stomal abscesses, Crohn's disease of the stomach and duodenum, and extra-intestinal manifestations (eg, erythema nodosum, pyoderma gangrenosum, and arthritis) also have been treated effectively with 6-MP.

In addition, patients should be offered the opportunity to start 6-MP after surgery to prevent proximal recurrence and progression of disease. The prophylactic value of 50 mg of 6-MP postoperatively was shown in a preliminary study comparing 6-MP, 5-ASA, and a placebo (Korelitz et al, 1998).

Comparison of 6-Mercaptopurine and Azathioprine

The authors favor 6-MP over azathioprine, having had more experience with it. Theoretically, 6-MP has advantages over azathioprine in that it is a more active product and its potency compared to that of azathioprine is approximately 2:1. Azathioprine has been tried in patients who are intolerant of 6-MP for any number of reasons, including leukopenia, hepatitis, pancreatitis, and failed attempts at desensitization to 6-MP for other allergies.

Dosage and Monitoring

Initially, the starting dose of 6-MP used in the double-blind study was 1.5 mg/kg (Present et al, 1980). Currently, the starting dose is 50 mg/d independent of weight. Complete blood counts are monitored weekly for the first 3 weeks. If the patient is doing well, the dose can be continued at 50 mg/d and the time between blood counts

extended to 2 weeks and later 3 weeks. The longest period permitted between blood counts has been 8 weeks. However, if clinical judgment warrants an increase in dosage, the time between blood counts again is reduced to once weekly for 3 weeks. It should be noted that, because leukopenia has been noted as late as 88 months after starting therapy, blood counts should be checked regularly for the duration of therapy.

The dose may be increased in increments of 25 mg, prescribed as alternating 50 mg on one day with 50 mg twice daily on the next day (for a 75-mg/d dosage), 50 mg twice daily, and in a few cases 100 mg on one day alternating with 150 mg on the next. Occasionally patients may not tolerate the 50-mg/d dose, in which case it may be given twice or 3 times weekly, or the tablet may be halved.

Even though azathioprine is considered to have half the potency of 6-MP and, therefore, usually requires double the dose of 6-MP, we feel patients should be started at a dose of 50 mg, which can be increased, depending on the clinical situation. Monitoring is as for 6-MP.

Recently attempts have been made to study 6-MP metabolism in patients with inflammatory bowel disease (IBD), correlating dose responsiveness with outcome and toxicity. An apparent genetic polymorphism has been observed in TPMT activity, with negligible activity noted in 0.3 percent and low activities in 11 percent of subjects. Low TPMT activity has been associated with increased toxicity and early response, by allowing 6-MP metabolism to be shunted toward the excessive production of 6-TG nucleotides. There are commercially available tests for TPMT genotyping and for the measurement of 6-MP metabolites. The clinical usefulness of these tests is discussed in other chapters. With careful hematologic monitoring as outlined above, the majority of 6-MP-related toxicities can be identified early and managed effectively. In many patients, 6-MP is initiated while the patient is on steroids, which blunts the severity of leukopenia and other forms of toxicity.

Duration of Therapy

How long should the drug be continued? This is a question that is often posed by the patient, and is one that can only be resolved by discussion between the physician and the patient. The factors that need to be taken into consideration are the duration and severity of disease, patient anxiety, and the desire for pregnancy. In general terms, it should be continued indefinitely, because cessation of therapy may cause recurrence of disease in about 75 percent of cases. The progressive efficacy of the drug, with prolonged therapy, is impressive. It may reassure patients to know that some have been on the drug for more than 20 years without ill effects. It should be noted that 6-MP is effective even when it is reintroduced after a period off medication, and in fact, the time to response is shorter for the second course of therapy than for the first. A retrospective study by Bouhnik et al (1996) suggests that, after

4 years of effective therapy, 6-MP may be discontinued with little risk of relapse. Although this is not the widely accepted view and requires further prospective controlled trials, patients who have major concerns regarding long-term therapy should be encouraged to continue therapy for at least 4 years.

Toxicity

Original data on toxicity of 6-MP in IBD had been compiled for 396 patients, including follow-up information in 356, seen by Drs. Korelitz and Present in their private practices. The mean follow-up time was 60 months. Currently, additional data are available on allergic reactions, malignant neoplasms, herpes zoster, and other infections during therapy with 6-MP.

Pancreatitis

This type of toxicity, allergic reaction, occurs in 3.3 percent of patients, usually within 32 days of starting the drug. Patients may present with abdominal pain, nausea, vomiting, and elevated amylase. All of these symptoms disappear quickly upon discontinuation of the drug. Rechallenge results in recurrence of pancreatitis, and most attempts to desensitize patients have been unsuccessful. A bout of pancreatitis has served as a contraindication for future use, but if clinically warranted, a cautious trial of azathioprine in small desensitization doses has been attempted in a limited number of these patients.

Leukopenia

Leukopenia (white blood cell count [WBC]) < 4000) was noted at some time in most patients treated with 6-MP, but clinically significant bone marrow depression occurred in 2% and was reversed when the drug was discontinued. In this study, most cases occurred in the early days of 6-MP use. Currently, with careful monitoring, this problem is rarely encountered. If the WBC decreases during therapy, the dose of 6-MP should be decreased or it should be stopped altogether, depending on the clinical situation. In almost all cases, therapy can be continued at lower doses given either daily or once or twice weekly. In a study of 21 patients who developed leukopenia while taking 6-MP, there appeared to be a preferential suppression of neutrophils. Other agents used for IBD, such as prednisone and 5-ASA products, also preferentially affect the neutrophils. Clinical relapse of IBD is characterized by an influx of neutrophils into the intestinal wall. These migrated cells produce oxygen-reactive molecules and release lysosomal enzymes when they come into contact with chemoattractants. These products produce nonspecific tissue injury and probably play an important role in the inflammation of the gastrointestinal tract. It is possible that 6-MP may modulate this effect through the induction of leukopenia, thus explaining the more profound and durable response to therapy noted in patients who develop leukopenia. This is an area that requires further investigation. Leukopenia as

a marker for adequacy of dosing is discussed in the next chapter. 6TG levels are apparently more important.

Allergic Reactions

Allergic reactions, such as fever, rash, and joint pain, have been reported to occur in 2 to 5 percent of all patients. In a recent analysis of 591 patients receiving 6-MP for IBD, followed up for 28 years, there were 16 allergic reactions (3%). These symptoms usually appeared early and disappeared when the drug was stopped. Fever was the most common symptom, followed by joint pains and severe back pain. A minority developed a sepsis-like syndrome, uremia, sinusitis, neck swelling, red nodular palms, blepharitis, and pneumonitis. The allergic symptoms lasted an average of 5 days. Nausea is common during the first month of 6-MP use but eventually disappears with continued use.

Hepatitis, possibly on an allergic basis, is seen less often and is the only allergic form of toxicity that may occur late in the course of treatment. About half do not again develop hepatitis with rechallenge, and still others can be successfully desensitized with either azathioprine or 6-MP, starting with small doses as with other allergic manifestations.

Infections

The authors have seen two or three patients with cytomegalovirus infection (associated with bone marrow depression), one with a liver abscess, and 15 patients with pneumonia in the course of treatment; all responded to antibiotic therapy, including those in whom the 6-MP was not stopped. Herpes zoster has been seen in 20 patients and resolved in all, half of them having continued 6-MP therapy. A recent review of 550 patients with IBD treated with 6-MP and followed over a 25-year period revealed 12 cases of shingles (herpes zoster), an incidence similar to that described in a previous review. It appears that the risk of developing shingles during 6-MP therapy is slightly higher than for the general IBD population. We have temporarily lowered or discontinued 6-MP therapy, but this may not be necessary. Acyclovir should be instituted upon diagnosis, although its effectiveness in this group of patients has not been established. If the disease severity requires it, the 6-MP can be restarted after the shingles subsides.

Neoplasms

Neoplasms occur more frequently in patients with IBD whether or not they have received immunosuppressive therapy; this is particularly true for those with Crohn's disease. Many neoplasms noted in patients who have taken 6-MP occur within the limits expected statistically in the population at large. These neoplasms have included melanoma (n = 1), carcinoma of the lung (n = 3), and carcinoma of the rectum or colon (n = 1). The one tumor believed to have a probable association with immunosuppressive therapy was a histiocytic lymphoma of the brain in a male patient with a 35-year history of Crohn's disease, who had earlier used 6-MP for less than a year. The probable association is based on the relatively high incidence of this tumor in transplant patients who have received high doses of immunosuppressive medications. A more recent analysis of 550 patients with IBD treated with 6-MP and followed for a mean of 17 years revealed 25 malignancies. The cancers encountered included colon, breast, lung, testicle, cervix, ovary, non-Hodgkin's lymphoma, and leukemia. These neoplasms were not believed to be attributable to the 6-MP. However, the suspicion of a relation between 6-MP and leukemia or lymphoma still exists, although it remains unproven. Consideration must tentatively be given to possible acceleration by the 6-MP of a neoplasm to which the patient might be predisposed. We have raised the question whether prolonged leukopenia may predispose to neoplasia.

Death

There have been six deaths in this series of patients, but in only one patient (with histiocytic lymphoma of the brain) could the death in any way be attributed to 6-MP. A review of 1,000 patients with Crohn's disease hospitalized during a 15-year period revealed 25 deaths. Of these, at least 72 percent, and perhaps more, were related to the Crohn's disease and its complications. This underlines the importance of early and aggressive medical therapy to prevent the development of complications and postpone or eliminate the need for surgery, especially in patients with onset at a young age and virulent disease.

Pregnancy Concerns

There is no clear consensus regarding the safety of these medications in terms of pregnancy outcomes when taken by male or female patients. The transplant literature and data from Present et al's group at the Mount Sinai Hospital suggest that they can safely be used in pregnancy. However, the present study found a slightly increased incidence of abnormal amniocenteses, requiring therapeutic abortions, in females who took the drug prior to conception, and an increased incidence of pregnancy complications when the fathers took 6-MP within 3 months of conception. The numbers in these studies are too small to make definitive recommendations. However, until larger studies are performed and reported, it is the authors' practice to discontinue 6-MP, if feasible, from 1 to 3 months prior to planned conception.

The Future

The future for the treatment of IBD ultimately lies in elucidating its etiology. Until such time, the best hope of therapy is in the form of better, more focused, and less toxic immunosuppressive agents. The main drawback to therapy with 6-MP and azathioprine is the long time to response. Perhaps the use of intravenous preparations or higher doses may bring about a faster response. Thiopurine methyltransferase genotyping and measurement of 6-MP metabolites may then become useful to predict toxicity and monitor dosing. With the more widespread use of antitumor necrosis factor (anti-TNF), the role of 6-MP will be redefined. Early experience with anti-TNF suggests that 6-MP and azathioprine maintain priority for maintenance after the initial improvement. Whether intravenous steroids or anti-TNF will lead to a more rapid or more complete initial response has yet to be determined.

Editor's Note

This chapter is the essence of our book. A perceptive "student" of Crohn's disease and of immunomodulator use has refined his experience into useful ideas on the use of an important group of therapeutic agents. Information on other views on dosing, metabolite levels, and leukopenia appears in the next chapter. It would be difficult to be the "complete" IBD doctor without knowledge of how to safely use azathioprine and 6-MP. (TMB)

References

Korelitz BI, Hanauer S, Rutgeerts P, et al. Post-operative prophylaxis with 6-MP, 5-ASA, or placebo in Crohn's disease: a 2-year multicenter trial. Gastroenterology 1998;114:A4141.

Present DH, Korelitz BI, Wisch N, et al. Treatment of Crohn's disease with 6-mercaptopurine. A long-term randomized double-blind study. N Engl J Med 1980;302:981–7.

Supplemental Reading

Bouhnik Y, Lemann M, Mary J-Y, et al. Long-term follow-up of patients with Crohn's disease treated with azathioprine or 6-mercaptopurine. Lancet 1996;347:215–9.

Cuffari C, Theoret Y, Latour S, Seidman G. 6-Mercaptopurine metabolism in Crohn's disease: correlation with efficacy and toxicity. Gut 1996;39:401–6.

Korelitz BI, Adler DJ, Mendelsohn RA, Sacknoff AL. Long-term experience with 6-mercaptopurine in the treatment of Crohn's disease. Am J Gastroenterol 1993;88:1198–205.

Korelitz BI, Fuller SR, Warman JI, et al. Shingles during the course of treatment with 6-mercaptopurine for inflammatory bowel disease. Am J Gastroenterol 1999;94:424–6.

Korelitz BI, Mirsky FJ, Fleisher MR, et al. Malignant neoplasms subsequent to treatment of inflammatory bowel disease with 6-mercaptopurine. Am J Gastroenterol 1999;94:3248–53.

Korelitz BI, Present DH. Favorable effect of 6-mercaptopurine on fistulae of Crohn's disease. Dig Dis Sci 1985;30:58–64.

Present DH, Meltzer SJ, Krumholz MP, et al. Management of inflammatory bowel disease: short- and long-term toxicity. Ann Intern Med 1989;111:641–9.

Rajapakse RO, Korelitz BI, Zlatanic J, et al. Outcome of pregnancies when fathers are treated with 6-mercaptopurine for inflammatory bowel disease. Am J Gastroenterol 2000;5:684–8.

CHAPTER 80

Azathioprine Metabolism in Inflammatory Bowel Disease: Correlation with Efficacy and Toxicity

Carmen Cuffari, MD

6-Mercaptopurine (6-MP) and its parent compound azathioprine (AZA) are purine analogues that interfere with nucleic acid metabolism and cell proliferation. In active Crohn's disease, when combined with corticosteroids, azathioprine induces remission faster, more frequently, and with a lower cumulative steroid dose than prednisone alone. Furthermore, AZA and 6-MP have been shown to eliminate the need for corticosteroids in about 75 percent of patients, with a median response time of 12 to 16 weeks, and they have proven efficacy in maintaining long-term remission.

Pearson's meta-analysis of several well-controlled clinical trials in patients with Crohn's disease has affirmed that the clinical response to azathioprine therapy largely is dependent on the duration of therapy. Indeed, patients who were weaned from prednisone before azathioprine could achieve its effect did not have a favorable clinical response to therapy. In most patients, treatment required at least 4 months of combination therapy. However, 30 percent of patients do not respond favorably to the usually administered doses (1 to 2 mg/kg).

Most physicians measure drug efficacy either by an improvement in clinical symptoms and quality of life or by the ability to maintain remission while weaning off corticosteroid therapy. Practitioners tend to rely on their clinical judgment and experience in determining the dose of azathioprine to be used in treating patients with inflammatory bowel disease (IBD). Some start with 50 or 75 mg per day regardless of weight and then increase by 25-mg increments. It is not uncommon for the daily dose to be less than 1.5 mg/kg of AZA. Colonna and co-workers (1994) noted that in 51 patients with moderate to severe Crohn's disease on long-term 6-MP therapy (1 to 1.5 mg/kg), clinical responsiveness correlated well with drug-induced leukopenia (< 5,000). A true distinction between immunosuppression and 6-MP-induced cytotoxicity has yet to be defined in IBD.

The wide dose range of azathioprine currently used in clinical practice would suggest that a safe and established therapeutic dose has not yet been established. As a consequence, clinicians must always remain aware of potential adverse effects, including allergic reactions, hepatitis, pancreatitis, bone marrow suppression, and lymphoma, while attempting to achieve a therapeutic response.

The high-performance liquid chromatography (HPLC) measurement of erythrocyte 6-MP metabolites has become a useful clinical tool for adjusting AZA/6-MP doses to maximize clinical efficiency while avoiding adverse events, including leukopenia, and also for monitoring patient compliance. Ongoing studies have developed the concept of a "therapeutic window" of efficacy and toxicity based on the measure of erythrocyte 6-MP metabolite levels. This technology allows physicians to tailor 6-MP therapy to suit a patient's individual needs, as is done when prescribing anticonvulsant and antimicrobial drugs.

Pharmacology of 6-Mercaptopurine

The immunosuppressive properties of 6-MP and azathioprine most likely are mediated through their interference with protein synthesis and nucleic acid metabolism in the sequence that follows antigen stimulation, as well as by their cytotoxic effects on lymphoid cells. Since 6-MP and azathioprine by themselves are inactive, they must be transformed intracellularly into ribonucleotides, which function as purine antagonists. These antimetabolites then are incorporated into deoxyribonucleic acid (DNA), causing DNA breakage and interference with DNA and protein interactions involved in DNA replication.

6-Mercaptopurine undergoes rapid and extensive catabolic oxidation to 6-thiouric acid in the intestinal mucosa and liver by the enzyme xanthine oxidase (Figure 80–1). The bioavailability of 6-MP ranges from 5 to 37 percent. In comparison, the intestinal absorption of azathioprine is somewhat better than that of 6-MP. Once absorbed into the circulation, azathioprine is rapidly converted to 6-MP and S-methyl-4-nitro-5-thioimidazole on exposure to sulfhydryl-containing compounds in the plasma and tissues. Twelve percent of azathioprine is excreted in the form of S-methyl-4-nitro-5-thioimidazole. This reaction has been shown to occur nonenzymatically. Beyond this metabolic step, in vivo studies in both animals and man have shown that azathioprine metabolism is identical to

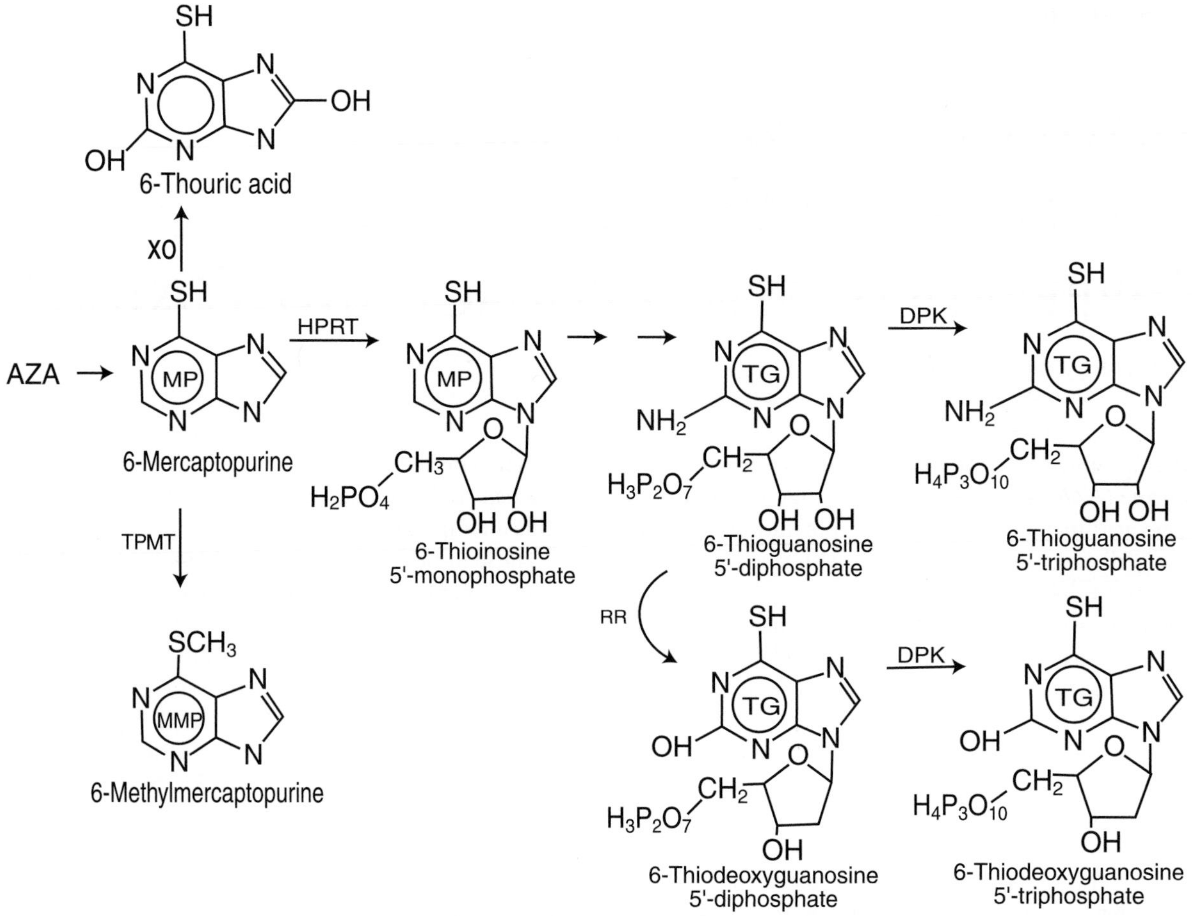

FIGURE 80–1. Azathioprine (AZA) metabolism: AZA is rapidly converted to 6-MP by a nonenzymatic process in the plasma. The metabolism of 6-MP occurs along the competing pathways catalyzed by thiopurine methyltransferase (TPMT), xanthine oxidase (XO), and hypoxanthine phosphoribosyltransferase (HPRT). The di- and triphosphates are formed by their respective mono- and diphosphate kinases (DPKs). 6-Thioguanosine nucleotides are then metabolized to 6-thiodeoxyguanosine nucleotides and incorporated into RNA and DNA.

that of 6-MP. It is also important to note that azathioprine is 55 percent of 6-MP by molecular weight. All of these factors may contribute to the conversion factor of 2.08 when converting a dose of 6-MP to azathioprine.

The plasma half-life of 6-MP is short, ranging from 1 to 2 hours partially because of the rapid absorption of 6-MP into erythrocytes and organ tissues. The anabolic transformation of 6-MP into its active metabolites occurs intracellularly along the competing routes catalyzed by thiopurine methyltransferase (TPMT) and hypoxanthine phosphoribosyltransferase (HPRT), giving rise to 6-methylmercaptopurine (6-MMP), 6-methyl-thioinosine 5′-monophosphate (6-Me-tIMP), and 6-thioguanine nucleotides (6-TG), respectively (see Figure 80–1). The 6-**TG nucleotides** are thought to be lymphocytotoxic and beneficial in the treatment of patients with leukemia. Indeed, low erythrocyte 6-TG levels have been associated with a low 6-MP dose and with an increased risk of a disease relapse. In patients with IBD, there is a correlation between 6-TG levels and the therapeutic response.

An apparent **genetic polymorphism** has been observed in **TPMT activity**. Negligible activity has been noted in 0.3 percent, and low levels in 11 percent of individuals. Indeed, low TPMT activity has been associated with increased cytotoxicity, by allowing 6-MP metabolism to be shunted toward the excessive production of 6-TG nucleotides. Irreversible bone marrow suppression occurred in a patient with acute lymphoblastic leukemia and absent TPMT activity on long-term 6-MP therapy. This patient had markedly elevated erythrocyte 6-TG levels despite a reduced maintenance dose of 6-MP. One would not administer large intravenous doses to patients with low TPMT levels.

Genetic polymorphism in TPMT activity also affects the extent of 6-MMP production. Ten percent of patients are considered rapid metabolizers, with elevated TPMT activity levels. In these patients, 6-MP metabolism is shunted away from 6-TG production and into the formation of 6-MMP. Patients with high TPMT activity are considered to be at an increased risk for disease relapse.

Furthermore, these patients potentially may remain refractory to therapy despite a presumed therapeutic drug dosing regimen. High levels of 6-MMP have been associated in some patients with hepatic toxicity.

Although the lymphocytotoxic properties of 6-MP are thought to be mediated by its active 6-TG metabolites, recent data on a human lymphoblastic T-cell line have suggested a putative role for methylated metabolites. In vitro studies with Malt F4 lymphoma cells have shown that the inhibition of de novo purine synthesis by 6-MetIMP was crucial in achieving 6-MP-induced toxicity. These studies would suggest that both methylated and nonmethylated 6-MP metabolites may be critical in the treatment of leukemia.

Azathioprine Metabolism in IBD: 6-Thioguanine Levels

In patients with IBD, HPLC measurement of erythrocyte 6-MP metabolites showed a strong inverse correlation between 6-TG levels and disease activity (Cuffari et al, 1996). Although a wide range of erythrocyte 6-TG levels was associated with clinical responsiveness to therapy, patients with 6-TG levels > 250 pmol/8×10^8 red blood cells (RBCs) were uniformly asymptomatic. A lack of clinical response was associated with low erythrocte 6-TG metabolite levels. Neither drug dose nor the level of 6-MP-induced leukopenia correlated with responsiveness to therapy. This was the first study to support the immunosuppressive role of 6-MP based on the production of its 6-TG metabolites. Noncompliance was suspected in several patients in view of low erythrocyte 6-TG levels, and was subsequently confirmed by the patients. Several anecdotal cases support the usefulness of 6-MP monitoring in verifying patient compliance.

To date, 93 pediatric patients with IBD have had their erythrocyte 6-MP metabolite levels monitored and those who maintained 6-TG levels > 230 pmol/8×10^8 RBCs usually were in remission. In 82 adult patients on long-term azathioprine therapy (> 3 mo), an erythrocyte 6-TG level > 250 pmol/8×10^8 RBCs was more often associated with clinical remission.

High erythrocyte 6-MMP rather than high 6-TG levels were associated with 6-MP-induced complications, including pancreatitis (4 cases), hepatitis (1 case), and bone marrow suppression (2 cases). Most of the patients in the studies by Cuffari et al (1996) and Dubinsky et al (2000) were taking either sulfasalazine or related 5-aminosalicylic acid (5-ASA) compounds at the time of the study.

Like 6-MP, 5-ASA must be metabolized by N-acetyltransferase (NAT-1) into its active N-acetyl 5-ASA metabolite, and there are variant NAT-1 alleles present within the population that may potentially affect 5-ASA metabolism. Patients with the variant NAT-1 allele do not convert 5-ASA effectively into its active N-acetyl 5-ASA metabolite. Since 5-ASA has been shown to interfere with TPMT activity in vitro, patients with the variant NAT-1 allele may be predisposed to 6-MP-induced cytotoxicity. Proujansky and colleagues (1999) have shown that inherent differences in 5-ASA metabolism may predict complications to 6-MP therapy. Patients with the NAT-1 variant allele were at a significantly increased risk for 6-MP-related cytotoxicity, including pancreatitis. In contrast, patients who were identified as carriers (heterozygotes) of TPMT-deficient allele responded favorably to 6-MP therapy, but were at an increased risk for developing hepatitis. This study would suggest that combined TPMT genotyping and the measure of NAT-1 enzyme activity may help identify those patients susceptible to 6-MP-related toxicity. Further studies are required to determine whether the putative influences of the NAT-1 variant allele on 5-ASA metabolism can be correlated with alterations in erythrocyte metabolite levels.

Thiopurine Methyltransferase Activity

Genetic polymorphism in TPMT activity can be qualitatively measured by genotype testing. This is useful in identifying patients at risk for 6-MP-related toxicity. Eleven percent of the population are heterozygous carriers of the TPMT-deficient allele, and are potentially at risk for hepatotoxicity. Homozygous patients with absent TPMT activity are at added risk of severe, irreversible bone marrow suppression if given large amounts of AZA or 6-MP. Patients with Crohn's disease and a "mutant" TPMT allele incur significant azathioprine-induced leukopenia and were compelled to discontinue treatment, whereas patients with the wild-type allele achieve a good clinical response, and without side effects. Theoretically, one could interpret these findings as suggesting that all patients with the heterozygote allele are at an increased risk for drug toxicity and should not receive AZA or 6-MP. However, this would exclude 11 percent of the population who could potentially benefit from carefully monitored low-dose AZA therapy.

Clinical Implications

The genetic polymorphism in TPMT activity observed in the general population also may influence patient responsiveness to therapy and delay in clinical response times. Ten percent of the population are considered rapid catabolizers of 6-MP and in theory would require larger than standard doses of 6-MP to achieve a therapeutic drug benefit.

Patients with TPMT enzyme activity levels known to be over 5.0 U/mL RBCs (normal activity) could theoretically be challenged with a higher dose of 6-MP at the onset of therapy without increased risk of drug toxicity. Some patients treated with higher doses of AZA (2 mg/kg) at the start of therapy have had significantly shortened clinical response times and have maintained remission more effectively. Conversely, patients with low TPMT enzyme activity levels (< 5 U/mL RBCs) could have their AZA dose tailored carefully, through serial measurements of erythrocyte 6-MP metabolite levels, while avoiding untoward cytotoxicity.

Dose Adjustments

The "tailoring" of 6-MP therapy based on an individual patient's needs was studied prospectively in a group of 10 pediatric patients with active Crohn's disease on standard 6-MP therapy (0.8 to 1.2 mg/kg/d) for at least 3-month durations, but with subtherapeutic erythrocyte 6-TG levels (< 250 pmol/8 × 10^8 RBCs). Noncompliance was identified in four patients by very low 6-TG levels. Median erythrocyte 6-TG levels were 55 (range, 0 to 148) pmol/8 × 10^8 RBCs. Prospective studies in adults are validating the therapeutic efficacy of a median erythrocyte 6-TG level of 250 pmol/8 × 10^8 RBCs. Dose adjustments of 25 mg monitored with 6-TG levels have been associated with clinical response in over two-thirds of patients who were incompletely responsive and had 6-TG levels below 250 pmol/8 × 10^8 RBCs. This was accomplished without producing leukopenia.

Intravenous Therapy

Intravenous forms of AZA therapy were studied by Sandborn et al (1995) in an attempt to establish a role for this drug in the treatment of severe active Crohn's disease. Patients with TPMT activity less than 5 U/mL/blood ("non-metabolizers") were considered at risk for AZA-induced cytotoxicity and were excluded. Patients with normal activity received an intravenous AZA infusion (50 mg/hr × 36 hr) followed by daily oral AZA (100 mg) therapy. The erythrocyte 6-TG levels obtained at the end of the intravenous infusion were equivalent to those seen after several weeks of continuous daily oral AZA therapy. Clinical improvement was noted at 4 weeks. However, a subsequent double-blind study in a population of patients with high-normal TPMT activity levels, comparing intravenous AZA with high-dose oral AZA (2 mg/kg) therapy, showed no added benefit. Remission rate (only 20%) was equal at 8 weeks. Importantly, patients who received high-dose oral AZA therapy achieved therapeutic erythrocyte 6-TG metabolite levels after just 2 weeks. A therapeutic benefit of bolus AZA therapy in IBD has not been proven.

Generic versus Nongeneric

In general, pediatric gastroenterologists tend to prescribe 6-MP, whereas, in adult medicine, AZA is preferred. Comparison of 6-MP metabolite levels in adult and pediatric patients with IBD show that pediatric patients achieve higher metabolite levels (Cuffari et al, 1996). This difference in 6-MP metabolite levels correlates with patient responsiveness to therapy. Initially, the difference was thought to be either attributable to an observational bias or perhaps due to altered drug metabolism. However, ongoing studies have now suggested that there may exist differences in drug bioavailability when comparing generic and nongeneric forms of AZA, based on the measurement of erythrocyte 6-TG levels.

Conclusion

Measurement by HPLC of erythrocyte 6-MP metabolites can be useful in treating patients with IBD. As done with anticonvulsant and antimicrobial drugs, patients on 6-MP therapy can be closely monitored to achieve a desired therapeutic effect based on the measurement of erythrocyte 6-TG levels. Furthermore, drug dosage can be carefully tailored based on the inherent differences in 6-MP metabolism. Theoretically, it is now possible to achieve a favorable clinical response in patients with IBD, while avoiding excessive 6-MP-induced toxicity.

Editor's Note

A complete list of 34 articles suggested for supplemental reading can be obtained from Dr. Cuffari at *ccuffari@jhmi.edu* (TMB)

References

Colonna T, Korelitz BI. The role of leukopenia in 6-mercaptopurine-induced remission of refractory Crohn's disease. Am J Gastroenterol 1994;89:362–6.

Cuffari C, Theoret Y, LaHaie R, et al. 6-Mercaptopurine (6-MP) metabolite levels in adult and pediatric IBD: correlation with drug efficacy. Gastroenterology 1996;110:A890.

Cuffari C, Theoret Y, Latour S, Seidman G. 6-Mercaptopurine metabolism in Crohn's disease: correlation with efficacy and toxicity. Gut 1996;39:401–6.

Dubinsky MC, Lamothe S, Yang HY, et al. Pharmacogenomics and metabolite measurement for 6-mercaptopurine therapy in inflammatory bowel disease. Gastroenterology 2000; 118:705–13.

Proujansky R, Maxwell M, Johnson J, et al. Molecular genotyping predicts complications of 6-mercaptopurine therapy in childhood IBD. Gastroenterology 1999;116:A800.

Sandborn WJ, Van Os EC, Zins BJ, et al. An intravenous loading dose of azathioprine decreases the time to response in patients with Crohn's disease. Gastroenterology 1995;109:1808–17.

Supplemental Reading

Black AJ, McLeod HL, Capell HA, et al. Thiopurine methyltransferase genotype predicts therapy-limiting severe toxicity from azathioprine. Ann Intern Med 1998;129:716–8.

Bostrum B, Erdman G. Cellular pharmacology of 6-mercaptopurine in acute lymphoblastic leukemia. Am J Pediatr Hematol Oncol 1993;15:80–6.

Cuffari C, Picco M, Hunt S, et al. Azathioprine metabolite levels predict clinical responsiveness to therapy in IBD. Gastroenterology 1999;116:A694.

Cuffari C, Sharma S. 6-Mercaptopurine metabolites tailored to achieve clinical responsiveness in pediatric IBD. Gastroenterology 1999;116:A694.

Lennard L. The clinical pharmacology of 6-mercaptopurine in acute lymphoblastic leukemia. Eur J Clin Pharmacol 1992; 43:329–39.

Lennard L, Lilleyman JS. Variable mercaptopurine metabolism and treatment outcome in childhood lymphoblastic leukemia. J Clin Oncol 1989;7:1816–23.

Lennard L, Rees CA, Lilleyman JS, Maddocks JL. Childhood leukemia: a relationship between intracellular 6-mercaptopurine metabolites and neutropenia. Br J Clin Pharmacol 1983;16:359–63.

O'Brien JJ, Bayless TM, Bayless JA. Use of azathioprine or 6-mercaptopurine in the treatment of Crohn's disease. Gastroenterology 1991;101:39–46.

Pearson DC, May GR, Fick GH, et al. Azathioprine and 6-mercaptopurine in Crohn's disease: a meta-analysis. Ann Intern Med 1995;122:132–42.

Sandborn WJ, Tremaine WJ, Wolf DC, et al. Lack of effect of intravenous administration on time to respond to azathioprine for steroid-treated Crohn's disease. Gastroenterology 1999;117:527–35.

Szumlanski C, Weinshilboum RN. Sulphasalazine inhibition of thiopurine methyltransferase: possible mechanism of interaction with 6-mercaptopurine. Br J Clin Pharmacol 1995;39:456–9.

Van Os EC, Zins BJ, Sandborn WJ, et al. Azathioprine pharmacokinetics after intravenous, oral, delayed-release oral, and rectal foam administration. Gut 1996;39:63–8.

CHAPTER 81

METHOTREXATE IN INFLAMMATORY BOWEL DISEASE

BRIAN GORDON FEAGAN, MD, AND PRASANNA KUMARANAYAKE, MD

Despite many recent advances, some notable deficiencies exist in the medical management of patients with inflammatory bowel disease (IBD). Although glucocorticoids are highly effective for the induction of remission in both ulcerative colitis and Crohn's disease, the chronic use of these drugs is associated with a high incidence of adverse events. Therefore, a need exists to identify treatment alternatives for patients who are refractory to glucocorticoid therapy. In other chronic inflammatory diseases, such as psoriasis and rheumatoid arthritis (RA), methotrexate is an effective and safe treatment for corticosteroid-dependent patients (Klippel and Decker, 1985; Willkens et al, 1995). Thus, it was logical that methotrexate should be evaluated as a therapy for inflammatory bowel disease.

The development of methotrexate as a treatment for leukemia was based on knowledge of the activity and three-dimensional structure of the enzyme dihydrofolate reductase. The synthesis of methotrexate as a competitive antagonist of folic acid is one of the earliest examples of the construction of a "designer drug." Inhibition of dihydrofolate reductase by high-dose methotrexate interferes with DNA synthesis, which ultimately results in cell death. During an initial experience with methotrexate in oncology, it was serendipitously recognized that some leukemic children who had concomitant psoriasis and RA showed improvement of these conditions. This observation led to the evaluation of low-dose (5 to 25 mg/wk) methotrexate as a treatment for autoimmune diseases. Over the past decade, clinical trials have shown that methotrexate has an emerging role for the treatment of Crohn's disease.

Pharmacology

Methotrexate can be administered by the oral, subcutaneous, intramuscular, or intravenous routes (Jundt et al, 1993). Although the drug is highly bioavailable at doses of 15 mg or less, absorption may be erratic with higher oral doses (Hillson and Furst, 1997).

Following absorption, methotrexate is concentrated in the liver, kidneys, and synovium with a steady-state volume of distribution of approximately 1 L/kg. The parent molecule is transported into cells by an energy-dependent process. In the liver the enzyme hepatic aldehyde converts methotrexate to the major metabolite, 7-hydroxymethotrexate. Drug excretion is by the kidneys (glomerular filtration); both tubular secretion and re-absorption occur. Other organic acids, such as aminosalicylic (ASA), and some nonsteroidal anti-inflammatory drugs may interfere with renal tubular secretion and increase serum methotrexate levels. Therefore, patients with chronic renal failure may be at an increased risk of toxicity. However, therapeutic drug monitoring of methotrexate has not been shown to be useful in patients with RA (Bannwarth et al, 1996).

Although the mechanism of the anti-inflammatory effect of methotrexate is poorly understood, it is not likely through the inhibition of dihydrofolate reductase, since folate supplementation does not reduce clinical efficacy (Morgan et al, 1994). In vitro, a number of immunosuppressive properties have been demonstrated. They include suppression of proinflammatory molecules, a decrease in cytotoxic T-cell function, and reduction in neutrophil activity (Cronstein et al, 1993).

Toxicity

Low-dose methotrexate first was established as an effective treatment for severe psoriasis in the early 1960s. However, an unacceptably high incidence of hepatic toxicity was noted. For example, among 104 patients with psoriasis treated daily for a mean duration of 3.38 years with standard doses of 20 to 25 mg/wk, 23.1 percent of individuals showed significant pathologic changes (cirrhosis or active hepatitis) on liver biopsy (Malatjalian et al, 1996). Subsequent pharmacokinetic investigations demonstrated that daily drug administration results in high hepatic polyglutamic folic acid and methotrexate concentrations. Since methotrexate is a folate analogue, the drug accumulates in the liver and causes toxicity. However, methotrexate does not accumulate if sufficient time is allowed between doses for the drug to be excreted by the kidney (Lewis and Schiff, 1988). This awareness of the pharmacokinetics of methotrexate led to the development of once-weekly dosing schedules and a significant reduction in the incidence of hepatic toxicity. The rate of methotrexate-induced hepatic toxicity also may relate to the underlying disease state, as the incidence of this complication is higher in psoriasis and lower in RA. This may reflect differences among populations in the prevalence of known risk factors (alcohol use, diabetes mellitus, and obesity) for methotrexate toxicity. Only limited data are available to assess the potential risk of methotrexate-associated hepatic fibrosis in IBD but the risk does not appear to be high.

Other important adverse effects of methotrexate include nausea, bone marrow suppression, and hypersensitivity pneumonitis (Feagan et al, 1995; Al-Awadhi et al, 1993; Searles and McKendry, 1987). Methotrexate must not be given to women of childbearing potential owing to the risk of teratogenicity (Kozlowski et al, 1990).

Methotrexate as Therapy for IBD

Crohn's Disease

The majority of patients who are treated with a course of conventional glucocorticoid therapy become either steroid dependent (36%) or steroid resistant (20%). Only a minority (44%) of patients experience a durable treatment response to glucocorticoid therapy.

Patients who require chronic steroid therapy are appropriate candidates for immunosuppressive drug therapy. The purine antimetabolites, 6-mercaptopurine (6-MP) and azathioprine, are effective in the majority of, but not all, patients both for induction of remission and for maintenance therapy in Crohn's disease. Approximately 30% of patients are unresponsive to low-to-moderate doses of azathioprine. Also, the onset of action of azathioprine is relatively slow (3 to 6 mo), and in some studies less than half of patients who receive maintenance therapy with the purine antimetabolites remain free of a relapse longer than 1 year. Although these agents are relatively well tolerated as chronic therapy, serious toxicity can occur; therefore, alternative medical treatments are desirable.

Kozarek and colleagues (1989) pioneered the use of methotrexate for the treatment of IBD. In their initial open-label series with 21 patients (14 with Crohn's disease, 7 with ulcerative colitis) with chronically active disease, methotrexate was administered intramuscularly at a dose of 25 mg once weekly, with conversion to a maintenance dose of 15 mg orally in patients who responded to therapy. Two-thirds of patients had improvement in symptoms and a steroid-sparing effect also was documented. Colonoscopic improvement was demonstrated in one-third of the patients with Crohn's disease but not in the patients with ulcerative colitis.

REMISSION INDUCTION

Four randomized, double-blind, placebo-controlled trials of methotrexate in chronic active, steroid-dependent Crohn's disease have been reported. In the North American Crohn's Study Group (NACSG) study, 141 patients with chronically active steroid-dependent disease

received 25 mg of intramuscular methotrexate weekly or a placebo (Feagan et al, 1995). Following 16 weeks of treatment, 39.4 percent of methotrexate-treated patients were in remission without prednisone compared with 19.1 percent in the placebo arm ($p = .025$). Beneficial effects of methotrexate treatment were seen for disease activity, quality of life, and prednisone use. The effect of treatment was greatest in those patients who had required more than 20 mg/d of prednisone to control their symptoms. Although withdrawal from therapy for adverse events occurred more frequently in the methotrexate group (17% vs 2%), the majority related to the occurrence of asymptomatic elevations of hepatic enzymes.

In another trial, there was no significant difference in remission rate at 9 months between a lower oral dose of methotrexate (12.5 mg/wk), 6-MP (50 mg/d) and placebo in 84 patients with chronically active steroid-dependent disease (Oren et al, 1997). Patients also were allowed treatment with 5-ASA. Remission was defined as a Harvey-Bradshaw score of < 4 without steroid use at the end of 9 months. The methotrexate-treated patients had a significant improvement in general well-being and reduction in abdominal pain relative to the other two groups.

In another trial, oral methotrexate (15 to 22.5 mg/wk) was compared to placebo in 33 patients with Crohn's disease who were treated for 1 year (Arora et al, 1999). Fewer methotrexate-treated patients experienced disease-related exacerbations (46% vs 80%), but this difference was not statistically significant. However, a trend toward an increased number of side effects in the methotrexate-treated patients (33% vs 0%) was observed.

MAINTENANCE THERAPY

As further confirmation of the Kozarek report, a placebo-controlled maintenance study in 76 patients showed that low-dose methotrexate (15 mg/wk) is effective as a maintenance therapy over 40 weeks in patients with quiescent disease (Feagan et al, 1999). Prior to the trial, the patients had chronically active steroid-dependent disease and had been successfully treated with a methotrexate-induction regimen (16 to 24 wk of 25 mg/wk by intramuscular [IM] injection). At the end of the 40-week study, 26 patients (65%) were in remission in the methotrexate group, compared with 14 patients (38.9%) in the placebo group ($p = .015$). Methotrexate-treated patients were less likely to require prednisone (27.5% vs 58.3%) and had lower disease activity. Over half of the patients who relapsed were successfully retreated with the induction regimen of methotrexate (25 mg/wk) and were free of prednisone and in remission in the placebo group at the end of the trial. One possible explanation for the relatively high rate of remission in the placebo group is the possibility that the induction regimen of methotrexate, which patients had received prior to randomization, resulted in healing of mucosal ulceration and a durable clinical response.

Although there were no serious adverse events associated with methotrexate therapy in this 40-week maintenance study, the participants were selected for tolerance of methotrexate in the induction study.

Clinical Implications

The largest studies support the efficacy of methotrexate both in active disease and for maintenance therapy in previously steroid-dependent patients. Methotrexate given intramuscularly at a relatively high dose (25 mg/wk) in conjunction with prednisone was an effective remission induction therapy. Fifteen milligrams of methotrexate intramuscularly was effective for maintenance therapy.

In contrast, oral methotrexate dose of 12.5 mg was not consistently beneficial for induction of remission whereas a beneficial response was suggested when a higher oral dose was administered (15.0 to 22.5 mg/wk). Collectively, these data may mean that the dose-response curve for methotrexate therapy in Crohn's disease is shifted to the right in comparison to that in rheumatoid arthritis, where methotrexate doses as low as 7.5 mg/wk are effective. If drug doses greater than 15 mg/wk are required for efficacy, then oral administration may be suboptimal, owing to incomplete drug absorption from the gastrointestinal tract. Since intramuscular injection is inconvenient and relatively costly, one solution to this problem is the use of subcutaneous administration of the drug. This approach has been used in RA with good results (Bannwarth et al, 1996). Patients can easily be taught to self-inject the drug subcutaneously.

Important questions remain regarding the potential clinical applications of methotrexate in Crohn's disease. An initial uncontrolled experience suggests that methotrexate is effective for fistula treatment in patients who have been refractory to therapy with purine antimetabolites (Mahadevan et al, 1997). There is also anecdotal experience that methotrexate is effective for some extra-intestinal manifestations including arthralgias and arthritis, erythema nodosum, and pyoderma gangrenosum.

Ulcerative Colitis

Although no large randomized controlled trials have evaluated the use of the purine antimetabolites in patients with chronically active ulcerative colitis, Hawthorne and colleagues (1992) have performed a withdrawal study that evaluated the efficacy of azathioprine in 79 patients who entered remission after receiving azathioprine therapy. Patients who were assigned to withdraw from azathioprine had a greater rate of relapse at 1 year compared to those who remained on drug therapy (59% vs 35%, $p = .04$).

In the only randomized, double-blind, placebo-controlled 9-month trial of methotrexate in chronic active ulcerative colitis, oral methotrexate (12.5 mg/wk) was not better than placebo in 67 patients who had received steroids or immunosuppressive drugs for at least 4 of the 12 preceding months (Oren et al, 1996).

Although Kozarek's pilot study suggested a 40 percent response rate in ulcerative colitis, currently, no reliable data from controlled trials exist to support the use of methotrexate as a therapy for ulcerative colitis.

Future Directions

Over the past decade, methotrexate has emerged as a new therapy for chronically active Crohn's disease. In RA, use of methotrexate has superseded azathioprine because of its superior efficacy and long-term tolerability.

In the absence of reliable comparative data, clinicians must decide whether methotrexate or a purine antimetabolite is the preferred induction treatment for unresponsive Crohn's disease. Extensive long-term experience exists with the purine antimetabolites, whereas the risk of liver disease from methotrexate remains an issue. However, the risk of significant hepatic toxicity in RA is low, and surveillance liver biopsy is no longer recommended. In the absence of biopsy data from patients with Crohn's disease, the American Rheumatism Association guidelines regarding surveillance for hepatic toxicity should be followed (Kremer et al, 1994).

The development of infliximab as a new therapy for patients with refractory Crohn's disease should focus additional attention on the use of methotrexate as an alternative to the purine antimetabolites. In patients with RA concomitant treatment with methotrexate has been shown to enhance the response to infliximab therapy. Furthermore, patients who are receiving methotrexate are less likely to develop human anti-chimeric antibodies (Maini et al, 1998). These antibodies, which may block the beneficial action of infliximab or cause adverse effects, are a significant limitation to the long-term use of this form of treatment. Thus, a strong rationale exists to consider combination therapy with these agents in Crohn's disease.

Controlled trials to compare the relative efficacy and safety of azathioprine and methotrexate in therapy-resistant patients are warranted. The use of both drugs in combination with infliximab should be explored.

Editor's Note

A copy of the complete bibliography supplied by the authors can be requested at *feagan@lctrg.com*. (TMB)

References

Al-Awadhi A, Dale P, McKendry R. Pancytopenia associated with low-dose methotrexate therapy: a regional survey. J Rheumatol 1993;20:1121–5.

Arora S, Katkoc W, Cooley J, et al. Methotrexate in Crohn's disease: results of a randomized double-blind, placebo-controlled trial. Hepatogastroenterology 1999;46:1724–9.

Bannwarth B, Pehourcq F, Schaeverbeke T, Dehais J. Clinical pharmacokinetics of low-dose pulse methotrexate in rheumatoid arthritis. Clin Pharmacokinet 1996;30:194–210.

Cronstein BN, Naime D, Ostad E. The anti-inflammatory mechanism of methotrexate. J Clin Invest 1993;92:2675–82.

Feagan BG, McDonald J, Hopkins M, et al. A randomized controlled trial of methotrexate (MTX) as a maintenance therapy for chronically active Crohn's disease (CD). N Engl J Med 2000:342 (May).

Feagan BG, Rochon J, Fedorak RN, et al. Methotrexate for the treatment of Crohn's disease. N Engl J Med 1995;332:292–7.

Hawthorne AB, Logan RFA, Hawkey CJ, et al. Randomized controlled trial of azathioprine withdrawal in ulcerative colitis. BMJ 1992;305:20–2.

Hillson JL, Furst DE. Pharmacology and pharmacokinetics of methotrexate in rheumatic disease. Practical issues in treatment and design. Rheum Dis Clin North Am 1997;23:757–78.

Jundt JW, Bowne BA, Fiocco GP, et al. A comparison of low dose methotrexate bioavailability: oral solution, oral tablet, subcutaneous, and intramuscular dosing. J Rheumatol 1993;20:1845–9.

Klippel JH, Decker JL. Methotrexate in rheumatoid arthritis. N Engl J Med 1985;312:853–4.

Kozarek RA, Patterson DJ, Gelfand MD, et al. Methotrexate induces clinical and histologic remission in patients with refractory inflammatory bowel disease. Ann Intern Med 1989;110:353–6.

Kozlowski RD, Steinbrunner JV, MacKenzie AH, et al. Outcome of first-trimester exposure to low-dose methotrexate in eight patients with rheumatic disease. Am J Med 1990;88:589–92.

Kremer JM, Alarcon GS, Lightfoot RW, et al. Methotrexate for rheumatoid arthritis. Suggested guidelines for monitoring liver toxicity. Arthritis Rheum 1994;37:316–28.

Lewis JH, Schiff EAC. Methotrexate-induced chronic liver injury: guidelines for detection and prevention. Am J Gastroenterol 1988;83:1337–45.

Mahadevan U, Mario JF, Present DH. The place for methotrexate in the treatment of refractory Crohn's disease. Gastroenterology 1997;113:A1031.

Maini RN, Breedveld FC, Kalden JR, et al. Therapeutic efficacy of multiple intravenous infusion of anti-tumor necrosis factor alpha monoclonal antibody combined with low-dose weekly methotrexate in rheumatoid arthritis. Arthritis Rheum 1998;1:1552–63.

Malatjalian DA, Ross JB, Williams CN, et al. Methotrexate hepatotoxicity in psoriatics: report of 104 patients from Nova Scotia, with analysis of risks from obesity, diabetes, and alcohol consumption during long-term follow-up. Can J Gastroenterol 1996;10:369–75.

Morgan SL, Baggott JE, Vaughn WH, et al. Supplementation with folic acid during methotrexate therapy for rheumatoid arthritis. Ann Intern Med 1994;121:833–41.

Oren R, Arber N, Odes S, et al. Methotrexate in chronic active ulcerative colitis: a double-blind, randomized, Israeli multicenter trial. Gastroenterology 1996;110:1416–21.

Oren R, Moshkowitz M, Odes S, et al. Methotrexate in chronic active Crohn's disease: a double-blind, randomized, Israeli multicenter trial. Am J Gastroenterol 1997;92:2203–9.

Searles G, McKendry RJ. Methotrexate pneumonitis in rheumatoid arthritis: potential risk factors: four case reports and a review of the literature. J Rheumatol 1987;14:1164–71.

Willkens RF, Sharp JT, Stablein D, et al. Comparison of azathioprine, methotrexate, and the combination of the two in the treatment of rheumatoid arthritis. A forty-eight-week controlled clinical trial with radiologic outcome assessment. Arthritis Rheum 1995;38:1799–806.

Supplemental Reading

Black RL, O'Brien WM, Van Scott EJ, et al. Methotrexate therapy in psoriatic arthritis: double-blind study on 21 patients. JAMA 1964;189:743–7.

Feagan BG, Rochon J, Fedorak RN, et al. Methotrexate for the treatment of Crohn's disease. N Engl J Med 1995;332:292–7.

Goodman LS, Gilman A. The pharmacologic basis of therapeutics. New York: McGraw-Hill, 1996.

Hall PD, Jenner MA, Ahern MJ. Hepatotoxicity in a rat model caused by orally administered methotrexate. Hepatology 1991;14:906–10.

Korelitz BI, Present DH. Methotrexate for Crohn's disease. N Engl J Med 1995;333:600–1.

Munkholm P, Langholz E, Davidsen M, Binder V. Frequency of glucocorticoid resistance and dependency in Crohn's disease. Gut 1994;35:360–2.

Weinblatt ME, Coblyn JS, Fox DA. Efficacy of low-dose methotrexate in rheumatoid arthritis. N Engl J Med 1985;312:818–22.

Weinstein GD, Jeffes E, McCullough JL. Cytotoxic and immunologic effects of methotrexate in psoriasis. J Invest Dermatol 1990;95:49S–52S.

CHAPTER 82

Cyclosporine in Crohn's Disease

Mary Lawrence Harris, MD

Patients with Crohn's disease refractory to mesalamine, oral and topical products, and corticosteroids are candidates for immunomodulator therapy. Cyclosporine (CYSA), extracted from the soil fungus *Tolypocladium inflatum*, has been proposed as an alternative or adjunct to antimetabolite therapy, such as 6-mercaptopurine (6-MP) or azathioprine (AZA), for refractory disease. Cyclosporine inhibits cellular immunity by interrupting the production of interleukin-1 (IL-1) and two receptors by helper T lymphocytes. Cyclosporine does not alter the function of granulocytes, monocytes, or macrophages but does alter B-cell function, by inhibiting the production of B-cell activating factors and interferon-gamma by helper T cells. Whereas 6-MP and AZA have a prolonged time of onset of action and pose risks of bone marrow suppression, pancreatitis, or malignancy, intravenous cyclosporine provides a rapid onset of response, usually in less than 7 days. Cyclosporine is a mainstay of immunosuppressive therapy in organ transplantation and also has been used with success in various autoimmune diseases.

Both controlled and uncontrolled data suggest that high-dose cyclosporine is beneficial in some patients with chronically active Crohn's disease and can also be potentially useful in fistulizing Crohn's disease. Some patients respond to intravenously administered cyclosporine (4 mg/kg) and maintain their clinical response during divided dose oral therapy for 3 months. However, the majority of patients relapse when oral cyclosporine is discontinued; therefore, concomitant use of other immunomodulator agents is common practice. Oral high-dose (7.5 mg/kg) therapy reputedly also is effective initially in some patients. Cyclosporine use for perianal disease, enteric fistulae, unresponsive colitis, and pyoderma gangrenosum is discussed in other chapters.

Pharmacokinetics

Cyclosporine is a lipophilic, hydrophobic, cyclic undecapeptide that inhibits T-helper lymphocyte production of interleukin-2 (IL-2) and interferon-gamma (INF-γ) with additional effects on production of cytokines. By inhibiting the production of interleukins-2, -3, -4, and -5 as well as tumor necrosis factor-alpha and -beta (TNF-α and -β), T-cell and B-cell functions are altered. However, it is not known which of these cyclosporine-induced effects on humoral or cellular immunity accounts for a therapeutic action in Crohn's disease. In intravenous solution, cyclosporine must be stabilized with alcohol and polyoxyethylated castor oil and, in oral solutions, with alcohol and olive oil. Cyclosporine is maximally absorbed at approximately 4 hours after an orally administered dose. Bioavailability varies greatly, with a range of 12 to 35 percent. Cyclosporine absorption from the small intestine also varies with motility and length of small bowel and, thus, is a function of contact time. Disease activity that compromises mucosal integrity can impair absorption of cyclosporine in the gastroduodenal and small bowel. The presence of biliary diversion can result in cyclosporine malabsorption but microemulsion formulations have improved bioavailability not dependent on the presence of bile. Intravenous doses of cyclosporine ranging from 2 to 4 mg/kg/d which are equivalent to oral divided doses up to 8 mg to 16/kg/d, have been tested in Crohn's disease.

Clinical trials evaluating intravenous cyclosporine include a continuous intravenous infusion over 24 hours, starting at a dose of 4 mg/kg/d. However, some studies have evaluated intravenous infusion over 4 hours to facilitate obtaining true 12-hour trough levels in whole blood concentrations. Trough concentrations of cyclosporine are measured by high-performance liquid chromatography (HPLC) or monoclonal radioimmunoassay (RIA). A therapeutic window of approximately 150 to 300 mg/mL has been established for these assays in organ transplantation. In addition to cyclosporine trough levels, the serum creatinine, electrolytes, and complete blood counts should be determined daily during intravenous administration and every week during oral cyclosporine administration. There are no complaints of nausea and headache with 4 hour infusions than with 24-hour infusions.

Data from Clinical Trials

Three large, controlled trials of oral low-dose cyclosporine (5 mg/kg/d) for treatment of chronically active Crohn's disease did not show beneficial treatment affect (Feagan et al, 1994; Jewell et al, 1994; Stange et al, 1995). Brynskov evaluated 71 patients with active Crohn's disease using a higher oral dose of cyclosporine (7.6 mg/d). There was an initial benefit from this oral protocol; however, response did not persist when cyclosporine was discontinued.

Absorption was the rate-limiting factor in this study. There have been numerous uncontrolled trials of intravenous cyclosporine and oral cyclosporine for inflammatory bowel disease (IBD) as well as for fistulizing Crohn's disease that do suggest efficacy. Definition of response can be defined as resolution of diarrhea and abdominal pain, with partial response noted as a decrease in stool frequency and abdominal pain as compared to the clinical baseline prior to cyclosporine treatment. In patients with fistulizing Crohn's disease, reduction in the size of fistulae and drainage and discomfort were compared with complete response, defined as closure of the fistulae and lack of drainage. Egan et al (1998), at the Mayo Clinic, published a study evaluating intravenous cyclosporine in the treatment of refractory inflammatory and fistulizing Crohn's disease. Most patients who responded to intravenous cyclosporine maintained a response when converted to oral cyclosporine.

It has been postulated that when patients are converted to oral therapy that a concomitant immunosuppressant drug (eg, AZA) should be instituted to provide a bridge when the cyclosporine therapy is discontinued. The role of concomitant antibiotics, metronidazole, or ciprofloxacin has not been firmly established but they often are prescribed. There were no significant differences between responders and nonresponders in the mean whole blood or intestinal tissue cyclosporine concentration in patients with Crohn's disease treated with cyclosporine (8 mg/kg/d) (Sandborn, 1996).

The use of cyclosporine for Crohn's disease remains controversial and will need to be compared with other induction therapies, such as Remicade® (Centocor Inc., Malvern, Pennsylvania). Newer forms of cyclosporine, such as Neoral (Novartis Pharmaceuticals Corp., Basel, Switzerland), are better absorbed and make feasible high-dose oral therapy.

Toxicity

The most common adverse effects of cyclosporine include headaches, tremor, paresthesias, hypertension, infection, gingival hyperplasia, and hypertrichosis. The most severe adverse events include nephrotoxicity, increase in serum creatinine greater than 30 percent above baseline, and central nervous system (CNS) toxicity. The reported incidence of malignant lymphoma is 0.3 percent in the transplant literature.

The potential for permanent renal damage is the greatest concern associated with cyclosporine treatment. It has been reported that glomerular filtration rate may be reduced by one-third in 20 percent of patients undergoing long-term cyclosporine treatment for IBD and other autoimmune diseases. If cyclosporine therapy is terminated, renal function usually returns to normal within 1 to 2 weeks. However, irreversible histologic nephropathy has been described. Hepatic toxicity in patients treated with cyclosporine is predominantly one of cholestasis rather than elevation of aminotransferases. Patients with serum cholesterol levels less than 120 mg/dL should not receive cyclosporine, to avoid CNS toxicity, most commonly demonstrated by seizures. Because of the risk of *Pneumocystis carinii* pneumonia, prophylaxis with trimethoprim-sulfamethoxazole (double strength, 3 times/wk) is recommended for patients who also receive high-dose steroids and AZA.

Conclusion

The use of high-dose cyclosporine in Crohn's disease is equivocal with an average response of 67 percent and a need for long-term suppression with AZA or 6-MP. Cyclosporine-associated nephrotoxicity, opportunistic infections, and possible oncogenesis suggest caution and the need for future controlled trials to evaluate its efficacy for Crohn's disease. Perhaps the best application for cyclosporine administration is use as a rapidly active agent for persistently active disease or fistulae that can serve as bridges to other immunosuppressive agents for maintenance of disease remission and fistula closure. The use of cyclosporine is put into perspective with other therapies in other chapters in this text. The section on perianal disease compares cyclosporine and Remicade therapy for that indication. Cyclosporine use in pyoderma gangrenosum is discussed in a separate chapter.

References

Egan LJ, Sandborn WJ, Tremaine WJ. Clinical outcome following treatment of refractory inflammatory and fistulizing Crohn's disease with intravenous cyclosporine. Gastroenterology 1998;93:442–8.

Feagan BG, McDonald JWD, Rochon J, et al. Low-dose cyclosporine for the treatment of Crohn's disease. N Engl J Med 1994;330:1846–51.

Jewell DP, Lennard-Jones JE, Cyclosporin Study Group of Great Britain and Ireland. Oral cyclosporin for chronic active Crohn's disease. A multicentre controlled trial. Eur J Gastroenterol Hepatol 1994;6:499–505.

Sandborn WJ. A review of immune modifier therapy for inflammatory bowel disease: azathioprine, 6-mercaptopurine, cyclosporine, and methotrexate. Am J Gastroenterol 1996;91:423–33.

Sandborn WJ, Tremaine WJ, Sawson GM. Clinical response does not correlate with intestinal or blood cyclosporine concentrations in patients with Crohn's disease treated with high-dose oral cyclosporine. Am J Gastroenterol 1996; 91:37–43.

Stange EF, Modigliani R, Penna AS, et al. European trial of cyclosporine in chronic active Crohn's disease: a 12-month study. Gastroenterology 1995;109:774–82.

Supplemental Reading

Sandborn WJ. Cyclosporine therapy for inflammatory bowel disease: definitive answers and remaining questions. Gastroenterology 1995;109:1001–3.

Sandborn WJ, Tremaine WJ. Cyclosporine treatment of inflammatory bowel disease. Mayo Clin Proc 1992;67:981–90.

Anticytokine Therapy in Crohn's Disease

Loren C. Karp, MA, and Stephan R. Targan, MD

Research into the immunopathogenetic processes of inflammatory bowel disease (IBD) has resulted in the identification of a variety of inflammatory mediators, including cytokines, which are elevated in the mucosa of patients with Crohn's disease (CD). The current trend in treatment development is the manipulation of these mediators to render anti-inflammatory effects more specific than are provided by the traditional therapeutic options. Recent developments have centered on selective inhibition of expression or activity of these mediators of inflammation. Most progress has been made in the compounds that downregulate or completely inhibit the effect of tumor necrosis factor-alpha (TNF-α). Remicade® (Centocor Inc., Malvern, Pennsylvania) and Enbrel® (Wyeth-Ayerst Laboratories, Philadelphia, Pennsylvania), both of which recently received FDA approval for use in CD and juvenile rheumatoid arthritis, respectively, are anti-TNF-α preparations with different mechanisms of action. Another promising agent with potent anti-TNF properties is thalidomide. Thalidomide and a range of its analogues are under investigation at present. It is recommended that these agents, however effective, not be used as first-line therapy. This chapter provides guidelines for the use of anticytokine therapy for patients with CD and summarizes the clinical experience to date with TNF blockade.

Cytokines and Mucosal Inflammation

Normal mucosa is in a state of perpetually orchestrated inflammation, characterized by an intricate balance of immune mediators, in response to various antigenic stimuli in a genetically regulated environment. Failure of normal regulatory mechanisms, and perhaps persistent antigen presence, may inhibit downregulation of inflammation. Inflammatory bowel disease pathogenesis may be the result of an abnormal immune response to a common antigen, or may represent a failure to suppress the "normal" immune response. T-helper (Th1) cells and macrophages produce proinflammatory cytokines, including interleukin (IL)-1, IL-6, IL-8, IL-12, TNF-α, and interferon-gamma (IFN-γ), all of which incite inflammation. Production of Th1-type cytokines is stimulated by TNF-α, particularly in the mucosa.

It is feasible that the therapeutic effect of cytokines in the regulation of inflammation may be to reset the immune response to a normal level of balanced Th1 and Th2 cytokine secretion. The regulatory properties of cytokines may persist beyond the point that the therapeutic cytokine can be measured in the case of cytokine therapy, or the absence thereof detected, as with the use of anticytokines. Therefore, alteration of the basic mechanism of inflammation can result in long-term regulation.

Based on these hypotheses, new compounds designed to block the effect of, or eliminate, TNF-α have been developed and are now being used to treat patients with CD. The newness of these treatments and the presence of several potentially dangerous side effects are considerations in selecting patients for treatment and in the approach to patient management.

Anticytokine Therapy in the Management of Patients with Inflammatory Bowel Disease

Currently, it is difficult to advocate the use of any of the anticytokine preparations as a first-line treatment for CD. As previously mentioned, the undefined side-effect potential of these agents suggests that they are best reserved for steroid-resistant or steroid-dependent patients and those not responding to optimized therapy with 6-mercaptopurine (6-MP) or azathioprine (AZA). Furthermore, Remicade and thalidomide are not good choices for prevention of postoperative occurrence; 6-MP and AZA are preferred in those instances, with an anticytokine therapy remaining available in the event of severe flares. With these cautions, there are many patients and clinical situations in which these treatments are appropriate and beneficial.

In contemplating the use of anticytokine therapy for the patient with medically resistant disease, one must consider both the acute and chronic treatment plans. The physician must assess whether these agents are best employed as a bridge to long-term treatment with 6-MP or AZA or whether the patient will require treatments repeated once or at specified intervals. Concomitant treatment with 6-MP or AZA has been shown to prolong the effectiveness of anticytokine therapy and reduce the likelihood that the patient will develop human anti-chimeric antibodies (HACA). Furthermore, judicious use of anticytokine modalities, particularly Remicade, can obviate concerns about attenuation of effect.

Recent clinical trials, in which patients were treated successfully with intravenous infusions of anti-TNF-α, highlight the importance of TNF-α in the inflammatory process of the majority of patients with Crohn's disease. Approximately two-thirds of patients responded to treatment, as measured by changes in the Crohn's Disease Activity Index (CDAI) or closure of fistulae. Differences among types of mucosal inflammation may account for the disparity in response among the studied populations. Parallel laboratory investigations show that enhanced levels of Th1-type cytokines were found in pretreatment mucosal samples from the group of responsive patients.

Because TNF plays a central role in the inflammation present in inflammatory bowel disease, other anti-TNF therapies have been developed and are in the early stages of investigation. These include recombinant TNF receptors (designed to bind TNF and prevent its subsequent effects) and the humanized immunoglobulin (Ig)G$_4$ antibody CDP571, which demonstrated promising results in a short-term (2-wk) efficacy trial conducted in 31 patients with Crohn's disease (Stack et al, 1997); however, long-term efficacy and safety have not yet been established.

Remicade

Clinical Trial Data

In a multicenter, double-blind, placebo-controlled 12-week trial of Remicade in medically resistant, moderate-to-severe Crohn's disease, 81 percent of patients treated with a single infusion of 5 mg/kg of Remicade were significantly improved compared to the placebo group at the end of 4 weeks (Targan et al, 1997). In the same trial, 64 percent of patients treated with 5 to 20 mg/kg of anti-TNF-α also demonstrated significant clinical improvement at week 4; 33 percent of trial participants achieved remission (CDAI < 150).

In another study, endoscopic and histologic effects of treatment with Remicade were assessed (D'Haens et al, 1999). At 4 weeks after treatment, patients underwent ileocolonoscopy with biopsies. Using the Crohn's Disease Endoscopic Index of Severity (CDEIS), investigators noted a significant improvement in patients treated with Remicade. No endoscopic improvement was seen in patients receiving placebo. Histologically, samples from patients who received Remicade showed elimination of inflammatory infiltrate, but the same response was not seen in placebo-treated patients.

Multiple infusions of Remicade were studied in 73 patients who initially responded to a single Remicade infusion (Rutgeerts et al, 1999). These patients received four infusions of Remicade at a dose of 10 mg/kg or placebo, at 8-week intervals starting at 12 weeks following the initial infusion. At the end of 44 weeks, 66 percent of patients were able to maintain a clinical response to Remicade, and 51 percent were able to be maintained in remission, compared to 35 percent and 21 percent, respectively, of patients treated with placebo after only one infusion. There also was an additional increase in the number of patients who achieved remission over the 12- to 44-week treatment period. These encouraging results support the use of multiple infusions to maintain and sometimes improve disease response and remission following initial treatment with Remicade.

Remicade also has been studied for the treatment of fistulae in a 14-week trial of 94 patients with active, fistulizing Crohn's disease (Present et al, 1999). Patients were administered three infusions at 5 mg/kg or 10 mg/kg, or placebo. These were given at 0, 2, and 6 weeks. Sixty-eight percent and 56 percent of Remicade-treated fistulae were 50 percent closed, respectively, versus only 26 percent of those treated with placebo. A statistically significant 55 percent and 38 percent of fistulae treated with 5 mg/kg or 10 mg/kg, respectively, completely resolved by the end of the study. A fistula was considered closed if no drainage could be expressed over a 1-month period. Improvement in fistulae often was observed within 2 weeks of treatment and lasted a median of at least 3 months. These results show that Remicade may be a rapid and effective treatment for fistulizing Crohn's disease and a promising alternative for those who do not respond to standard therapy. Placement of a seton drain prior to Remicade and then removing it after the 2-week infusion may lessen the occurrence of abscesses at the site of fistula closure.

As previously mentioned, an interesting feature of treatment with Remicade is the potential for a long duration of response even after cessation of therapy. In one trial, responses were shown as long as 1 year after a single initial dose (Stack et al, 1997). In a study of the extended response to Remicade, it was found that relapse occurred later in patients who received higher doses of the medication and in those treated concomitantly with AZA (D'Haens et al, 1999). Furthermore, patients treated with multiple infusions had longer remissions than those treated with a single infusion, particularly in the presence of 6-MP or AZA.

More recently, data have come to the fore about the potential for delayed hypersensitivity reactions among patients treated with Remicade. In contrast to the simpler infusion reaction, which can be managed in most patients without discontinuation of treatment, the delayed hypersensitivity reaction requires immediate cessation of the drug. In one study, as many as 25 percent of patients, most of whom had received their first infusion 2 years earlier, experienced serum sickness characterized by myalgia,

polyarthralgia, fever, pruritis, urticaria, facial edema, or dysphagia. Since Remicade has become more widely available, the incidence of such delayed hypersensitivity reactions is much lower, less than 19 percent. A lag period between infusions is apparently one factor.

Clinical Management

Remicade is indicated (FDA approved) in steroid-dependent or steroid-resistant patients who have not responded to optimized use of 6-MP or AZA. This anti-TNF-α antibody also is effective in patients with chronic fistulous disease that is unresponsive to antibiotic therapy or 6-MP or AZA.

Standard inflammatory parameters should be assessed at baseline: complete blood count (CBC) with differential, erythrocyte sedimentation rate (ESR), C-reactive protein (CRP), and platelets. Remicade, 5 mg/kg, is delivered in a 2-hour infusion. Administration in a closely observed infusion center or similar environment is strongly recommended. Approximately 3 percent of patients develop an infusion reaction. The great majority of such reactions can be successfully treated with concomitant medication. Patients should be monitored for flushing, chest tightness, and panic symptoms. In the presence of any of these occurrences, the infusion should be slowed or stopped and intravenous Benadryl (Warner-Lambert, Morris Plains, New Jersey) or acetaminophen should be administered. However, if blood pressure drops, and urticaria or other anaphalyctoid symptoms develop, the infusion should be stopped immediately and not restarted. It is important to query patients for potential exposure to mice or other murine-derived compounds. Such prior sensitization can intensify infusion reactions. Steroid prophylaxis and simultaneous Benadryl administration will generally permit a successful Remicade infusion in these patients.

After a patient has been infused, he or she should be advised to report any rashes, joint pain, fever, wheezing, or urticaria and to be in contact with the physician in 7 to 10 days. In the patient with bowel strictures, uneven healing may result in complete obstruction and may require hospitalization. To avoid such outcomes, patients with fixed strictures or strictures with fistulae behind them should not be treated with Remicade. Fistulae should be treated beforehand and then 6-MP at 1.5 mg/kg (or AZA at 2.5 mg/kg) can be instituted in patients that are homozygous for high thiopurine methyltransferase (TPMT) activity.

Patients should return for follow-up in 2 to 4 weeks and inflammatory parameter reassessment. Retreatment with Remicade at 8 weeks or other therapy should be based on the laboratory parameters rather than delayed until a clinical manifestation of a flare. Steroids should be stable until 2 weeks after infusion and should be tapered at the standard intervals. The goal is to maintain the patient in remission with 6-MP or AZA. Optimal dosing of 6-MP and AZA can be defined by the use of metabolite testing. Red blood cell levels of 6-thioguanine (6-TG) and 6-methylmercaptopurine (6-MMP) can be used as a guide in monitoring clinical response, adjusting dosage, and steroid weaning. This is discussed in a separate chapter.

In nonresponding patients, determination of whether to re-infuse can theoretically be assisted with the use of serologic markers. In general, CD patients who are perinuclear antineutrophil cytoplasmic antibodies (pANCA)-positive seemed to respond poorly to Remicade. Re-infusion with 10 mg/kg may be of therapeutic benefit.

Thalidomide

Clinical Trial Data

Thalidomide appears to have beneficial anti-inflammatory and immunomodulatory effects for a wide variety of severe conditions, including erythema nodosum leprosum (for which thalidomide is FDA approved), rheumatoid arthritis, and Behçet's syndrome (Gutiérrez-Rodriguez et al, 1989; Hamuryudan et al, 1998). Thalidomide downregulates TNF-α production and inhibits production of IL-12, an important immunoregulatory cytokine critical to the development of cellular immune responses. (Blockage of IL-12 by anti-IL-12 antibody therapy has been shown to ameliorate mucosal inflammation in an animal model of colitis.) This inhibition of TNF-α production resulting in reduction of the elevated levels of TNF-α makes thalidomide of potential therapeutic importance in any disease state in which high TNF-α levels cause primary problems or secondary complications. In a study of 12 patients who received 50 or 100 mg of thalidomide, Vasiliauskas and colleagues (1999) found that disease activity decreased consistently in all patients during weeks 1 to 4: 58 percent response, 17 percent remission. Clinical improvement was generally maintained despite steroid taper during weeks 5 to 12. All patients were able to reduce steroids by 50 percent or more; 44 percent discontinued steroids entirely. In weeks 5 to 12, 70 percent of patients responded and 20 percent achieved remission. Side effects were mild and mostly transient, with the most common being drowsiness, peripheral neuropathy, edema, and dermatitis. Ehrenpreis and colleagues (1999), in a study of 22 patients with a different formulation of thalidomide (200 or 300 mg at bedtime), found that each of the 14 patients who completed 12 weeks of therapy responded: 9 achieved clinical remission (3 luminal, 6 fistula patients).

Clinical Management

Thalidomide is manufactured by more than one pharmaceutical company and the compound varies in terms of strength and effectiveness. Thalidomide has well-known, severe teratogenic effects; thus, prescribing the agent for women requires special vigilance. Celgene Corporation (Warren, New Jersey) has devised the System for Thalidomide Education and Prescribing Safety (STEPS). Participation in STEPS by prescribing physicians and treated patients is mandatory. This program is designed to ensure that there is no risk of pregnancy in treated women and to keep participants safe and aware of the risks and benefits of thalidomide. Thalidomide manufactured by Celgene Corporation is prescribed at 50 mg/kg and given as one oral dose in the evenings.

Drowsiness and neuropathy are the two most frequently noted adverse effects of thalidomide. In most cases, the nighttime administration overcomes the sedative effects of thalidomide. It is important to query the patient specifically about neuropathy to establish a baseline and to note changes. Neuropathies can be nonspecific and patients often need to be cued to report symptoms. Furthermore, since Flagyl® (Searle, Skokie, Illinois) is also known to cause neuropathy, it is necessary to differentiate which agent is responsible. Electromyography detects evidence of neuropathy prior to the appearance of clinical symptoms. Neuropathy is more common with the higher doses used for graft-versus-host disease. Thalidomide can be steroid sparing in most patients that respond to treatment. After 3 to 4 weeks of thalidomide therapy, steroids can be tapered in the standard fashion. For patients not responding to treatment with 50 mg/kg of thalidomide, the dose can be moved as high as 100 mg/kg. If there is no response by 8 weeks, the treatment should be terminated. Until controlled studies of thalidomide are completed, it is recommended that this agent be used only within the context of a clinical trial.

Future of Anticytokines in the Treatment of Inflammatory Bowel Disease

Cytokine and anticytokines show great promise for the treatment of IBD. Anti-TNF-α and IL-10 have been demonstrated to be beneficial, albeit for varying percentages of the affected populations. Data from laboratory investigations performed in parallel with the clinical trials indicate that it may be possible to determine which patients will respond to a particular treatment modality. Furthermore, the magnitude and duration of the response may be predictable as well. Currently, a panel of tests to detect the presence of specific serum immune markers associated with ulcerative colitis and Crohn's disease is being evaluated for their usefulness in this regard.

Although the evidence for the use of cytokines and anticytokines individually is encouraging, perhaps their greatest potential will be realized in combination or sequential administration. Additional laboratory and clinical investigations will help to define the appropriate combinations and the patients most likely to respond to

TABLE 83–1. Potential Sequences and Combinations for Future Cytokine and Anticytokine Therapy of IBD

Modality	Sequential/Combination	Modality
Anti-TNF-α	$\rightarrow$	6-MP
Anti-TNF-α	$\rightarrow$	Anti-IL-12, anti-IL-18
Anti-TNF-α	$\rightarrow$	Antigen manipulation
Anti-TNF-α	+	IL-10
Anti-TNF-α	+	Downregulatory cells/ TR3 (IL-10)

Antisense-cytokine specific
Induction of antigen-specific regulatory cells

TNF = tumor necrosis factor; 6-MP = 6-mercaptopurine; IL = interleukin.

the therapy. Table 83–1 presents potential cytokine–anticytokine combinations that, based on their effects on the immune system, may prove to be highly beneficial.

The use of antibodies to proinflammatory cytokines may be to reset the immunoregulator functions of the gut, whereas another, less potent immunomodulator can then be used to maintain it. Alternatively, based on a cytokine profile of an individual patient, a combination of cytokines–anticytokines may be indicated. Once antigen culprits have been further identified, disease may be brought under control by cytokines–anticytokines and then maintained by antigen manipulation. Alternatively, an agent such as anti-TNF-α can be used to downregulate Th1 function and then another agent employed for its potent anti-inflammatory effects.

Serologic markers in combination with genetic and immunologic profiles allow specific characterization of patients and implicate certain therapeutic interventions. For example, a patient who is shown to produce high-level IFN-γ or TNF-α is most likely to respond to anti-TNF-α. As more characteristics are defined, the available therapeutic armamentarium will increase.

References

D'Haens GR, Aerden I, van Hogezand R, et al. Duration of response following cessation of infliximab therapy for active or fistulizing Crohn's disease. Gastroenterology 1999;116:A696.

D'Haens G, van Deventer S, van Hogezand R, et al. Endoscopic and histological healing with infliximab anti-tumor necrosis factor antibodies in Crohn's disease. Gastroenterology 1999;116:1029–34.

Ehrenpreis ED, Kane SV, Cohen LB, et al. Thalidomide therapy for patients with refractory Crohn's disease: an open-label trial. Gastroenterology 1999;177:1271–7.

Gutiérrez-Rodriguez O, Starusta-Bacal P, Gutiérrez-Montes O. Treatment of refractory rheumatoid arthritis: the thalidomide experience. J Rheumatol 1989;16:158–63.

Hamuryudan V, Mat C, Saip S, et al. Thalidomide in the treatment of the mucocutaneous lesions of the Behçet syndrome: a randomized, double-blind, placebo-controlled trial. Ann Intern Med 1998;128:443–50.

Present DH, Rutgeerts P, Targan S, et al. Infliximab for the treatment of fistulas in patients with Crohn's disease. N Engl J Med 1999;340:1398–405.

Rutgeerts P, D'Haens G, Targan S, et al. Efficacy and safety of retreatment with anti-tumor necrosis factor antibody (infliximab) to maintain remission in Crohn's disease. Gastroenterology 1999;117:761–9.

Stack WA, Mann S, Roy AJ, et al. Randomised controlled trial of CDP571 antibody to tumour necrosis factor-alpha in Crohn's disease. Lancet 1997;349:521–4.

Targan SR, Hanauer SB, van Deventer SJ, et al. A short-term study of chimeric monoclonal antibody cA2 to tumor necrosis factor-alpha for Crohn's disease. Crohn's Disease cA2 Study Group. N Engl J Med 1997;337:1029–35.

Vasiliauskas EA, Kam LY, Abreu MT, et al. An open-label, step-wise dose-escalating pilot study of low-dose thalidomide in chronically active, steroid-dependent Crohn's disease. Gastroenterology 1999;117:1278–87.

CHAPTER 84

PERIANAL FISTULA

DANIEL H. PRESENT, MD

Perianal Fistula

Clinical Classification of Perianal Crohn's Disease

Depending on the clinical classification, anywhere from 20 to 80 percent of Crohn's patients suffer at some point in their course from perianal complications. Fistula is not the only abnormality seen in the perianal area. Large and swollen areas around the anal orifice that initially appear to be hemorrhoids are related to Crohn's disease and are known vernacular as "elephant ears." The patients' chief complaints are those of difficulty in keeping the area clean and disfigurement. Anecdotally, surgical removal could lead to persistent ulcerations. I do have one patient who, against my advice, had them surgically removed and did well.

In the differential diagnosis of a perianal fistula that presents without any evidence of bowel involvement, one should also consider the diagnosis of actinomycosis, tuberculosis, or trauma. There is a separate chapter on perianal disease in Crohn's disease written by a colorectal surgeon.

Fissures

Patients may also suffer from fissures, which tend to involve the squamous lining of the anal canal. They are similar to fissures seen in patients who do not have Crohn's disease. They are usually very painful; however, in Crohn's patients, they can be painless. Fissures tend to be in the midline and when they extend laterally, Crohn's disease becomes a likely diagnosis.

Perineal Skin Changes

Other findings on physical examination include a redness and thickened skin completely surrounding the perianal area. Hemorrhoids and skin tags are also observed, but they may be difficult to distinguish when there are extensive perianal complications, and there should be a careful search for ulcerations as well as discharge of pus secondary to fistula.

Vulvar Fistula

It is not unusual to have a female patient present with what was thought to be a Bartholin's abscess. This will be incised by the gynecologist with the anticipation of healing; however, persistence of drainage may then ensue, and it subsequently becomes clear that this is a fistula arising from the anal canal.

Rectovaginal Fistula

The diagnosis of a small rectovaginal fistula is suspected only when the patient volunteers or is asked if there has been the passage of air or fecal material from the vagina. It is also very difficult to identify the site of the fistula when the patient is examined by the gynecologist or the gastroenterologist. A rectovaginal fistula is usually quite small and arises from the distal portion of the rectovaginal septum. Rectovaginal fistula can occur in Crohn's disease, in ulcerative colitis, or after a gynecologic or obstetric complication. There is an excellent chapter on surgical management of rectovaginal or anovaginal fistula.

Surgical Evaluation

With the variety of perianal disease, a colorectal surgeon should be involved early in the course, initially for evaluation as well as for his/her knowledge of the anatomy around the anal area, and subsequently for therapy. When there appear to be multiple complex lesions, the surgeon will usually perform an examination under anesthesia. This is a valuable diagnostic and therapeutic procedure, in that abscesses can be drained or setons placed to facilitate healing.

An MRI can help delineate the course of fistula, but there are no large prospective studies comparing MRIs with examination under anesthesia. Transanal sonography is often limited by significant rectal scarring. Fistulograms also have not been helpful in the majority of cases. At this point, I consider examination under anesthesia as the best diagnostic and potentially therapeutic modality.

Clinical Course in Perianal Fistula

Fifteen or 20 percent of patients have perianal fistula as their initial presentation of inflammatory bowel disease (IBD). In the past, the patient was often referred to the surgeon, who, without realizing that the patient had Crohn's disease, attempted a repair. Fortunately, a high percentage of patients would heal; however, some patients went on to experience persistent drainage and lack of healing. Obviously, it is important that Crohn's disease be considered before an attempt is made to surgically cure a perianal fistula, especially in a young person. The literature on the clinical course is quite variable. The long-term course of fistula in some patients is relatively benign and the fistula heals or becomes asymptomatic if followed for long enough periods of time. At the other extreme, some patients require proctectomy in order to obtain healing.

Clinical Variables

There appear to be multiple variables that may influence whether the course is benign or aggressive. If the rectum is actively involved with Crohn's disease, the prognosis tends to be poor. Patients with transsphincteric fistula appear to have a better outcome than those patients with ischiorectal fistula. Likewise, the best prognosis occurs with subcutaneous fistula.

Although a proximal diversion can be helpful, this improvement is often temporary and usually not associated with complete healing. I strongly advise against diversion until all medical therapy has been used and has failed. Under these circumstances, I often advise proctectomy rather than diversion alone.*

Initial surgical therapy should be directed at the control of symptoms such as pain. This is accomplished by drainage, with the clear understanding that a fistula might develop at the site of the incision. Before repair of the fistula is attempted, medical therapy should be instituted, since surgical repairs can be associated with some incontinence. There is a very balanced discussion of the role of surgery for perianal fistula in the surgical section of this book.

Medical Management

There are only two controlled trials that have randomized for fistula healing, and these include one paper using 6-mercaptopurine (6-MP) and another more recent paper using infliximab.

5-Aminosalicylic Acid

Sulfasalazine or 5-aminosalicylic acid (5-ASA) does not play any major role in the management of perianal fistula aside from helping suppress coexistent intestinal disease. Actually, many patients have developed fistula while taking adequate doses of oral 5-ASA. I continue 5-ASA drugs if the patient develops a fistula but only in terms of the management of the active bowel disease.

Corticosteroids

Neither the National Cooperative Crohn's Disease Study nor the European Cooperative Crohn's Disease Study randomized patients with fistulization. It has been my personal experience that steroids retard the healing of both perianal and enteroenteric fistula because of the frequent development of abscess formation. In a recent study of 6-MP in patients with enterovesical fistula, those on steroids were much more difficult to heal. Often the fistula did not close until steroids were discontinued. Budesonide has not been evaluated in patients with fistula but would not be expected to play a role in the management of fistula aside from suppressing ileocolonic disease activity.

Metronidazole

Metronidazole as treatment for perianal fistula has been evaluated in several uncontrolled studies. These are described in detail in the chapters on antibiotic use in Crohn's disease and on fistulizing Crohn's disease. In the paper by Bernstein, complete fistula healing occurred in about half of the 21 patients who were maintained on therapy. Five others showed advanced healing but dosage reduction was associated with reactivation of fistula activity. Only one-fourth of the patients could discontinue the drug without worsening. Paresthesias occurred in 50 percent of patients, with a mean of about 6 months after initiation of therapy. Although some patients took metronidazole for as long as 3 years, reduction of the dose or stopping the drug usually resulted in exacerbation of disease. Several smaller uncontrolled studies have confirmed the initial data, and in one small study, better healing was observed with metronidazole as compared to surgery. No long-term data are available.

I initiate metronidazole as 1 to 1.5 g daily for 2 to 4 weeks and then lower the dose to 750 mg daily for maintenance. The generic preparation of metronidazole causes many more side effects than the brand form (Flagyl®, Searle, Skokie, Illinois), which is coated, and I routinely use the latter preparation.† Long-term maintenance without peripheral neuropathy can be obtained when using even lower doses, 250 to 750 mg daily for maintenance. It has been my experience that when patients go on and off metronidazole they become less responsive, and if the drug is to be used with fistula, I try to maintain low dosages for long periods of time. The "Antabuse effect" is seen in only 1 to 2 percent of patients taking metronidazole and I therefore allow my patients to drink, although I advise a trial dose of alcohol at home rather than risk the embarrassment of the nausea and vomiting that can occur in a social setting.‡ A controlled trial is needed to look at long-term efficacy of low-dose metronidazole in the management of fistula.

---

* Editors Note: As Remicade® (Centocor, Inc., Malvern, Pennsylvania), which is described in this chapter, has appeared, some young people opt for a diverting ostomy, hoping that a new medication will help to avoid a proctectomy. (TMB)

† Editor's Note: The 375-mg Flagyl® is acceptable to some HMOs because there is no generic preparation at that strength. (TMB)

‡ Editor's Note: I advise patients to take 250 mg metronidazole at breakfast and at lunch, and then skip the dinner dose if they wish to have wine or beer with dining. One patient remarked, "that if I'm not so drunk I can't find the pills, I'll take the third one at bedtime." (TMB)

Ciprofloxacin

There have been several studies evaluating ciprofloxacin in the treatment of active Crohn's disease. Colombel reported 1 g daily to be equivalent to 4 g of mesalamine; however, once again, patients were not randomized for fistula. In a small uncontrolled study of 10 patients with fistulae, 70 percent responded to 1 to 1.5 g of ciprofloxacin for 3 months. When fistula recurred, they once again responded to repeat initiation of ciprofloxacin. It is difficult to be certain of the value of this agent; however, in practice, the vast majority of patients are managed with a combination of metronidazole and ciprofloxacin. Some patients who are not responding to 500 mg of ciprofloxacin twice per day subsequently respond to 750 mg twice daily. A small subset of patients with fistula do maintain a response with long-term ciprofloxacin, but once again a controlled trial for chronic perianal fistula is warranted.

6-Mercaptopurine/Azathioprine

The first controlled trial to evaluate for fistula response was a randomized, double-blind 2-year study of 6-MP versus placebo in unresponsive Crohn's disease. Clinical response and steroid sparing were observed in over two-thirds of patients. In terms of fistula, 9 of 29, or 31 percent of patients. closed their fistulae, compared to 1 of 17 patients (6%) on placebo who closed fistulae. In addition, some healing was seen in 7 of 29 patients (24%) with 6-MP as compared to 3 of 17 (18%) with placebo. Korelitz and Present (1985) reported more data on their patients with complete closure using 6-MP in 39 percent of patients, partial response in 26 percent, and no response in 35 percent. Mean time to response was 3.1 months, and by 4 months, 77 percent of patients had responded. At 8 months, all of those who were going to respond had done so. In looking at the long-term data of the 13 patients who each had fistula that closed within 1 year, all 13 remained closed. After an additional year, 6 of the 13 patients who remained on the drug long term continued to show closure, whereas of the 7 patients who stopped the drug, only 2 fistulae remained closed and 5 reopened. Of the 5 that reopened, 3 patients were once again placed back on 6-MP with closure. We observed not only closure of perianal fistula but also closure of internal fistula. These data have been confirmed in other series, such as that of O'Brien and Bayless, in which 85 percent of individuals with any type of fistula showed improvement, but it was most effective in perianal fistula, where 75 percent responded. All 8 patients with a single perianal fistula had complete healing.

6-Mercaptopurine is effective both in closing and maintaining closure of perianal fistula without evidence of superinfections or development of neoplasia in these patients. I therefore recommend that no matter which medication is used to induce a response with fistula, that 6-MP/azathioprine (AZA) is the appropriate maintenance drug for long-term use.

Methotrexate

There has been one controlled trial showing the steroid-sparing effect of methotrexate as compared to placebo, and there have been several uncontrolled trials using methotrexate intramuscularly or subcutaneously in the treatment of active Crohn's disease. Data on fistulization are limited to one uncontrolled study by Muhadevan et al (1997) in 33 patients. Clinical remission was seen in 62% of patients. Fistula closed in 4 of 16 (25%) and improved in another 5 of 16 (31%). The overall response was 56 percent; however, relapse was frequently observed, even when the drug was continued in a dose of 20 to 25 mg intramuscularly weekly. It would therefore appear that methotrexate is temporarily effective in the treatment of fistula but is probably best used only when patients have failed or have been intolerant of 6-MP/AZA.

Cyclosporine

Cyclosporine is a rapidly acting and potent immunosuppressive agent in which uncontrolled trials showed efficacy in patients with active chronic Crohn's disease. On occasion during these studies, fistulae were seen to improve and heal. An initial placebo-controlled trial showed efficacy in the management of Crohn's disease using a mean dosage of 7.6 mg/kg daily. Three subsequent controlled trials used lower doses (5 mg/kg/d) and showed no response. The healing of fistula was not reported in these studies. There have been several uncontrolled reports in the treatment of fistula using intravenous cyclosporine in a dose of 4 mg/kg daily. This is comparable to a dose of 9 to 10 mg daily of oral cyclosporine. Hanauer et al (1993) evaluated 5 patients with a total of 12 fistulae and complete resolution of drainage was observed in 10 of the 12. Response was quite rapid within days. However, relapse was noted as the dose was lowered. In a larger study of 16 patients with active fistula, 10 had perirectal disease, 4 had enterocutaneous fistula, and 2 had rectovaginal fistula. Fourteen of the 16 patients (88%) responded acutely, and there was complete closure in 7 (44%). Subsequently, 5 patients (36%) relapsed; however, 9 (64%) maintained their improvement. Chronic steroids were discontinued in 75 percent of patients.

Cyclosporine is a dramatically effective drug for inducing fistula response and closure but maintenance therapy is needed. The drug does have significant toxicity (9%) when administered in higher doses. The patient is sent home on an oral dose of 6 to 8 mg/kg daily and the dose gradually reduced to between 5 and 6 mg/kg daily. Since cyclosporine is not effective when the doses are reduced to below this level, we introduce 6-MP/AZA for maintenance. Cyclosporine is continued for between 6 and 12 months, allowing for the 6-MP/AZA to take effect. Because of potential toxicity, we advise caution in the administration of cyclosporine with measurement of renal function and whole-blood monoclonal cyclosporine concentrations.

Infliximab

Tumor necrosis factor-alpha has been shown to be a pivotal mediator of the inflammatory response in patients with Crohn's disease. A chimeric monoclonal antibody has shown efficacy and safety in the treatment of chronically active Crohn's disease. During the preliminary trials, it became evident that the drug could also positively affect perianal fistulization. Twelve centers in the United States and Europe participated in a randomized, double-blind, placebo-controlled trial in 94 patients with single or multiple draining fistulae. They received three infusions, comparing 5 mg/kg of infliximab versus 10 mg/kg versus placebo, at weeks 0, 2, and 6. Thirty-five percent were receiving steroids, 40 percent 6-MP/AZA, 55 percent aminosalicylic acid, and 30 percent antibiotics.

The primary endpoint of this study was that of a 50 percent or greater reduction in the number of draining fistulae for two consecutive evaluations (a time period of 1 month). Fistulae were considered closed if they were no longer draining despite gentle finger compression. A secondary endpoint was closure of all fistulae for at least two consecutive visits. A perianal activity index (PDAI) in which five simple elements were graded on a 5-point scale was also recorded.

At 5 mg/kg, the primary endpoint was achieved in 62 percent of infliximab-treated patients as compared to 26 percent of placebo patients ($p = .002$). Complete closure of fistula was demonstrated in 46 percent of patients as compared to 13 percent with placebo ($p = .001$). The 5 mg/kg dose was the most effective and closed 55 percent of all fistulae. Most had closed before the third infusion (scheduled at 6 weeks). One could consider the final 6-week dose as maintenance therapy. In terms of responses, there were no differences as regards duration or extent of disease, prior surgery, number of fistulae, concomitant activity, or medication use.

These findings represent the first controlled trial that demonstrates a statistically significant therapeutic benefit of any agent in the treatment of perianal fistula. Since the controlled trial, I have observed complete closure in 39 percent of 38 open-label patients and partial closure in another 39 percent.[§]

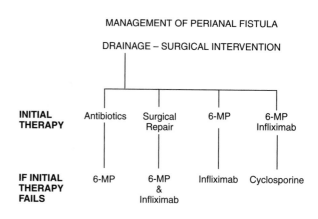

FIGURE 84–1. Outline of management therapy preferred by the author. 6-MP = 6-mercaptopurine.

Other Therapies

Other agents used in the treatment of the perianal fistula of Crohn's disease include hyperbaric oxygenation, total parenteral nutrition, and combinations of antimycobacterial agents. Thus far, data are limited and no prospective controlled trials have been reported.

Unanswered Questions

Since we have data on only 94 patients in one controlled trial and 1 year of experience of open-label infliximab, it is difficult to be certain exactly how to use it in combination with other agents. Will other immunomodulators prolong the response? Also, there are no good data regarding the closing of rectovaginal fistula. We cannot predict which patients will respond, and we are uncertain as to whether infliximab should be a first-line therapy or reserved for patients who do not respond to other therapies. Most importantly, we do not know how often infliximab will be required to maintain closure once it has been induced. Finally, with this new agent, we have no data on long-term toxicity.

Personal Management Preferences

My preferred management choices are outlined in Figure 84–1. Pain should be promptly relieved by abscess drainage. If there is a complex fistula, the surgeon should perform the examination under anesthesia. If setons are needed, they are placed through the fistula tract and tied loosely to maintain the patency of the fistula without cutting through the sphincters. The setons can be removed later after medical therapy is initiated. With infliximab, this has usually been if there was improvement with the first two infusions.

Most patients are placed on metronidazole (1 to 1.5 g daily) or ciprofloxacin and metronidazole. Patients are then observed for protracted periods on metronidazole 500 mg/d to see if the fistula will remain healed. If metronidazole is withdrawn, the majority of patients relapse.

[§] Editor's Note: Relapses after drainage had stopped during infliximab (Remicade) use are a concern to patients and physicians. Improvement continues in some patients given additional infusions at 8-week intervals. Whether 6-MP/AZA or methotrexate will help sustain the response to infliximab is not known. As the author states, there are a lot of unanswered questions. Additional trials are underway and the results are needed. (TMB)

An alternative approach would be antibiotics plus 6-MP. The mean time to respond to this drug at 1 to 1.5 mg/kg would be approximately 3 months, and 6-MP can be used as a long-term agent to maintain improvement.

If the patient has had a prior fistula and a second one develops, I always initiate 6-MP at that time. One could also argue that 6-MP should be withheld only if antibiotics are effective. A potential alternative would be use of infliximab initially with antibiotics and then the adding of 6-MP.

If the combination of 6-MP/AZA and infliximab is unsuccessful, the patient is admitted for intravenous cyclosporine. 6-Mercaptopurine is added or continued as a maintenance agent.

If cyclosporine is ineffective, surgical diversion and/or resection is considered. Unhealed perianal wounds or fistula may require medical therapy after surgery.

The chapters on surgical approaches to perianal and perineal disease and on rectovaginal fistula provide additional useful information.

References

Hanauer SB, Smith MB. Rapid closure of Crohn's disease fistulas with continuous cyclosporin A. Am J Gastroenterol 1993; 88:646–9.

Korelitz BI, Present DH. The favorable effects of 6-mercaptopurine in the fistula of Crohn's disease. Dig Dis Sci 1985;30:58–64.

Muhadevan U, Marion J, Present DH. The place for methotrexate in the treatment of refractory Crohn's disease. Gastroenterology 1997;112:A1031.

Supplemental Reading

Brandt LJ, Bernstein LH, Boley SJ, et al. Flagyl therapy for perineal Crohn's disease. A follow-up study. Gastroenterology 1982;83:383–7.

Present DH, Korelitz BI, Wisch N, et al. Treatment of Crohn's disease with 6-mercaptopurine in a long term, randomized, double blind study. N Engl J Med 1983;2:981–7.

Present DH, Lichtiger S. Efficacy of cyclosporine in treatment of fistula of Crohn's disease. Dig Dis Sci 1994;39:374–80.

Present DH, Rutgeerts P, Targan S, et al. Infliximab for the treatment of fistulas in patients with Crohn's disease. N Engl J Med 1999;340:1398–405.

OPTIONS IN MANAGING ENTERAL FISTULAE IN INFLAMMATORY BOWEL DISEASE

CHARLES O. ELSON, MD, AND NUZHAT IQBAL, MD

Over the past few years the understanding of the pathogenesis of inflammatory bowel disease has improved and so have the treatment options (Elson, 1996). However, fistulae associated with Crohn's disease still present a difficult therapeutic problem.

Differential Diagnoses of Enteral Fistulae

Fistulae usually result from penetration of the inflammatory process from a segment of Crohn's disease into adjacent tissue. Most but not all fistulae occurring in patients with Crohn's disease are attributable to the Crohn's disease. Fistulae occurring within 7 to 10 days after gastrointestinal surgery most likely are related to anastomotic failure. There is a chapter on management of postoperative fistulae. Causes of fistulae other than Crohn's disease and surgery include diverticular disease, radiation, malignancy, ischemia, peptic ulcer disease, and pancreatitis. However, excluding postoperative complications, the most common cause of enteral fistulae in the Western world is Crohn's disease.

Types of Fistulae in Crohn's Disease

Intestinal fistulae are classified as internal, external, or mixed. Internal fistulae (in which a fistulous connection exists between two segments of bowel or between a segment of intestine and another hollow viscus), are relatively uncommon compared with external fistula, in which a direct communication exists between the intestine and the skin of the abdominal wall or the vagina.

External fistulae are further classified as low-output (≤ 200 mL/day) or high-output fistulae (> 500 mL/day). Mixed fistulae are more complex and involve both internal and external communications, often through an abscess cavity. Small bowel fistulae are usually high output, whereas colon fistulae more often are low output. Enterocutaneous and perirectal fistulae are a cause of local pain, drainage, and considerable inconvenience; their medical and surgical care is covered in detail in another chapter.

Internal fistulae commonly arise from the terminal ileum and include enteroenteric and enterogenitourinary fistulae. Ileoileal and ileosigmoid fistulae are most common and are often discovered incidentally on radiographs because they are asymptomatic and usually do not compromise the nutritional status of the patient. Ileojejunal fistulae are uncommon and can result in malabsorption and incapacitating diarrhea, owing to bypass or bacterial overgrowth in a long segment of small intestine. Enterovesical fistulae occur in 2 to 5 percent of patients. These present as urinary tract infections with symptoms of dysuria, pneumaturia, or fecaluria. These are twice as likely to occur in men as in women. There is a separate chapter on surgical management of enterovesical fistulae. Cologastric and coloduodenal fistulae are uncommon; patients present with abdominal pain, diarrhea, and weight loss. Fecal vomiting is pathognomonic but infrequent. Unusual fistulae include esophagopleural and duodenopancreatic duct fistulae (Newman et al, 1987).

Diagnosis

Barium contrast radiography is the main diagnostic modality for fistulae detection. Endoscopy can be used to identify the diseased segment of bowel giving rise to the fistula; however, the endoscopist often is unable to find the intestinal orifice of the fistula. Computed tomography (CT), ultrasound, and magnetic resonance imaging (MRI) each can have a role in the definition of abscesses and fistulae. The best choice among these modalities depends on the local expertise and availability.

Treatment

Although the natural history of a Crohn's disease fistula often parallels the activity of underlying bowel disease, fistulae rarely close spontaneously and do not respond to sulfasalazine or steroids. Many clinicians believe that steroids have the detrimental effect of impairing the response to local sepsis, but this never has been established in a systematic study. Surgery often is required. However, because of the high recurrence rate, surgery is reserved for the patients who fail to respond to medical therapy or who have obstruction or an associated abscess. Fistulae can occur proximal to a stricture, an eventuality that should be considered relative to the timing of surgery. Control of the associated inflammatory component by medical therapy and bowel rest may allow for a

TABLE 85–1. Types of Fistula and Management Options

Types of Fistula	Therapy
Enteroenteric	Observation; 6-MP or AZA
Enterocutaneous	Spontaneous remission; TNF-α mab; 6-MP or AZA; IV cyclosporine; surgery followed by postoperative bowel rest, fluid, and nutritional support
Enterovesical	Antibiotics; 6-MP or AZA; surgery
Rectovaginal	Metronidazole; 6-MP or AZA; TNF-α mab; IV cyclosporine; surgery
Perianal	Metronidazole; 6-MP or AZA; TNF-α mab; IV cyclosporine; surgery

AZA = azathioprine; TNF-α mab = tumor necrosis factor-alpha monoclonal antibody; 6-MP = 6-mercaptopurine; IV = intravenous.

smaller resection and fewer postoperative complications. It also is important to control any underlying infection and optimize nutrition prior to surgery. As previously stated, the more proximal the fistula, the higher the output and thus the greater the nutrition loss as a result of decreased absorptive capacity.

Types of fistulae and their respective therapies are presented in Table 85–1.

Bowel Rest

Total parenteral nutrition (TPN) improves nutrition and temporarily decreases the volume of flow through a fistula. However, the role of TPN and bowel rest in the management of fistulae is a topic of debate. In one study, bowel rest and TPN resulted in spontaneous closure of fistulae in 63 percent of patients (Ostro et al, 1985); however, another study demonstrated no response to TPN and bowel rest (Schraut and Block, 1984). Fistulae arising from nondiseased bowel at the site of surgical anastomosis usually respond to antibiotic treatment to control infection, local wound care, drainage of any existing abscess, and TPN, which may lead to closure of up to 90 percent of these fistulae within 4 to 6 weeks. Fistulae arising from diseased bowel are much less likely to respond to TPN and conservative management alone.

Octreotide

Recently, octreotide, a somatostatin analogue with a long half-life, has been used to treat high output small bowel fistulae with favorable results in some patients. One study reported a 77 percent spontaneous closure rate in postoperative fistulae within a week of using TPN and octreotide, whereas a similar response took 4 to 6 weeks with TPN alone (Nubiola et al, 1989).

Specific Medical Therapy

Medical management of fistulae in Crohn's disease includes the use of antibiotics; immunomodulating agents including azathioprine, 6-mercaptopurine (6-MP), and cyclosporine; and anti-TNF-alpha antibody (Remicade®, Centocor Inc., Malvern, Pennsylvania). Most of the data

on the use of immunosuppressive agents relate to perianal fistulous disease but we are making an unproven assumption in this chapter that the response of enteral fistulae would be similar. This important assumption should be clear to the reader. Few data exist on internal fistulae, largely because of patient differences in the degree of underlying obstruction and remaining diseased bowel.

METRONIDAZOLE

Metronidazole was first used in the treatment of Crohn's disease in 1975, and since then several studies have suggested a beneficial role, especially in patients with perianal disease (Brandt et al, 1982). There also are documented instances of resolution of internal fistulae occurring during metronidazole therapy (see the chapter on fistulizing Crohn's disease). In one controlled study, 8 patients with perianal fistulae related to Crohn's disease were treated with high-dose (20 mg/kg) metronidazole therapy and benefit was noted in half at 10 weeks (Jakobovits and Schuster, 1984). Two of the patients had both perianal and enteroenteric fistulae.

Complete but temporary resolution of symptoms occurred in half the patients; however, all patients experienced significant (at times irreversible) peripheral neuropathy and metallic taste. The dose of metronidazole used was as high as the patients could tolerate, usually above 1000 mg/d. The treatment was long term, often more than 6 months, and most patients appeared to have an exacerbation of disease upon discontinuation. The associated side effects and long treatment time limit the usefulness of high-dose metronidazole as a therapeutic option for fistulae.

When using metronidazole for Crohn's disease fistulae one should probably limit the dose to ≤ 1000 mg/d and question the patient about peripheral neuropathy.

Ciprofloxacin has shown benefit in Crohn's disease, and it can be used together with or in rotation with metronidazole. Studies of effectiveness and duration of therapy are needed. There are anecdotal reports of improvement in perianal disease with decreased drainage but not closure of fistulae.

AZATHIOPRINE OR 6-MERCAPTOPURINE

Therapy with 6-MP, an active metabolite of azathioprine, has been beneficial in some patients during the period of immunomodulation (Korelitz and Present, 1985). In one large anecdotal series, the fistulae that responded best to 6-MP included rectovaginal (83%), ileorectal and ileosigmoid (80%), ileocutaneous (56%), and ileovesical (50%). Perirectal complications were the most difficult to heal with 6-MP. Response usually paralleled improvement in underlying bowel disease. The dose used in the study was 1.5 mg/kg of 6-MP, and the time for initial response to treatment was 3.1 months. The dose was adjusted downward if necessary to keep the white blood cell (WBC) count above 4,500 m^3. This was accomplished by weekly blood counts until stabilization of values was achieved and then by monthly follow-up. Leukopenia was dose dependent and reversible upon stopping the drug. The most common type of toxicity clearly related to 6-MP was pancreatitis with an incidence of 3 percent. It occurred usually within 30 days of taking the drug and, although symptoms improved upon stopping the drug, rechallenge resulted in recurrence. Allergic reactions such as fever, rash, and joint pain were noted in 2 percent of patients, usually in the first 3 weeks, and were reversed upon stopping 6-MP. Infections also were noted in 1.8 percent of patients.

Azathioprine has been reported to be similarly beneficial. The dose required is 1.5 to 3.0 mg/kg/d, and is titered to the response of the individual patient. If there is no response to these agents after 6 months, despite a biologic effect manifested by a drop in the WBC count to low-normal range, the treatment should be considered a failure and another agent should be prescribed. Use of 6-MP metabolite levels may help with dose titration, as described in a separate chapter. In patients with aggressive fistulous disease and a partial response, 6-MP or azathioprine can be maintained as useful adjunctive therapy to surgery. There is some evidence that giving azathioprine intravenously (2 mg/kg) may shorten the lag before onset of decreased disease activity from 8 weeks to 4 weeks.

METHOTREXATE

Methotrexate has shown efficacy in about half of the patients treated, but its effect on fistula healing has not been evaluated in any controlled studies. In one uncontrolled study, 33 patients were treated with intramuscular methotrexate; 16 had fistula (site not stated), and of these, 4 had complete healing with treatment. However, relapse was frequent, especially when the dose was lowered or switched to oral methotrexate (Muhadevan et al, 1997). The beneficial effects of methotrexate on active Crohn's disease at 15 mg/wk last less than a year in most patients.

CYCLOSPORINE

The slow onset of action of azathioprine or 6-MP in patients with inflammatory bowel disease has led to trials of more potent immunosuppressive drugs, such as cyclosporine. Uncontrolled studies in small number of patients have suggested that high-dose intravenous cyclosporine (4 mg/kg/d, as a constant infusion) may be of benefit as a bridge to other therapies in patients with active inflammatory and fistulizing Crohn's disease (Hanauer and Smith, 1993). Continuous intravenous infusion (4 mg/kg/d) has proven effective, whereas low-dose oral regimens have not. In one study, 9 of 18 patients had complex fistulizing disease, and the types of fistulae were perineal, enterocutaneous, or enterovaginal (Egan et al, 1998). Seven of these nine patients had partial response to high-dose intravenous cyclosporine, defined as reduction in size, drainage, and discomfort. Five of the responders maintained their response while receiving oral cyclosporine but relapsed within a month of stopping the drug.

Primary side effects of cyclosporine include decreased glomerular filtration, interstitial nephritis, and hypertension. Other complications included neurotoxic effects, seizures (especially in patients with low serum cholesterol), and opportunistic infections. Cyclosporine usually is reserved for the treatment of severe refractory disease when surgery is not appropriate, or as a bridge to other therapies with a slower onset of effect. There is a chapter on the use of cyclosporine in Crohn's disease.

TUMOR NECROSIS FACTOR-ALPHA MONOCLONAL ANTIBODY

One of the major breakthroughs in treatment of fistulizing Crohn's disease is the use of infliximab (Remicade), a human chimeric tumor necrosis factor-alpha (TNF-α) monoclonal antibody. There are several chapters on this new class of agents. Infliximab resulted in complete healing in about one-half of patients in a double-blind placebo-controlled study of 94 patients with draining fistulae (mainly perianal) related to Crohn's disease (Present et al, 1999). The effect of treatment became evident rapidly and lasted for about 3 months. There is a chapter on perianal fistulae and infliximab use. The most commonly reported side effects are headache and upper respiratory tract infection. Delayed-type hypersensitivity reactions have been reported when there was a 6- to 24-month lag between infusions, but this is rare. Acute infusion reactions were noted especially in patients with positive human anti-chimeric antibody. Concomitant immunosuppression is strongly recommended to prevent this reaction and to perhaps lengthen the duration of response. The use of infliximab is recommended for short-term treatment of enterocutaneous fistulae and as a bridge to maintenance therapy with azathioprine or 6-MP for patients who have not already failed this therapy. Others are using methotrexate with infliximab as was studied in a 2-year trial in patients with rheumatoid arthritis. There is a chapter comparing Crohn's disease to rheumatoid arthritis in terms of therapy.

Specific Management Issues

Rectovaginal Fistulae

Rectovaginal fistulae present a difficult therapeutic problem and are most common with severe colonic disease. There is an excellent chapter in the surgical section of this book. The authors' approach is to initiate immunosuppressive therapy to control active bowel disease and induce remission. Partial and complete healing of rectovaginal fistulae have been demonstrated with 6-MP. Also, there may be transient symptomatic improvement when metronidazole or ciprofloxacin is added to the immunosuppressive regimen. Patients with refractory symptoms ultimately require surgical management, but the success of surgery depends on aggressive preoperative management of inflammation. Details are provided in the aforementioned chapter on surgical management of retrovaginal fistulae. The traditional approach has consisted of surgical fecal diversion and often proctocolectomy. In some patients, primary repair has been attempted once the inflammation is under control, by advancement of an anorectal flap of mucosa, submucosa, and muscle, which obliterates the fistula. Other approaches include excision of ulcerated fibrous tissue and closure of the rectal mucosa with or without a rectal advancement flap. Antibiotics and immunosuppressive therapy are continued in the postoperative period to maintain remission. Fecal diversion and fistula repair at the time of disease remission is recommended in difficult cases of a high rectovaginal fistula or if control of inflammation is difficult to achieve. The role of infliximab and the duration of therapy are yet to be determined.

Gastrocolic and Duodenocolic Fistulae

Frequently, gastrocolic and duodenocolic fistulae do not respond to medical therapy, and surgical management is necessary in symptomatic cases. Most cases can be managed by excision of the diseased section of bowel and simple closure of the duodenum or stomach, but sometimes partial gastric resection is necessary. Side-to-side duodenojejunal anastomosis and a two-stage procedure involving diversion of the fecal stream followed by resection and primary closure of the duodenum are procedures usually employed in surgical treatment of these fistulae. There is a chapter on the surgery of gastroduodenal Crohn's disease.

Enterovesicular Fistulae

Enterovesicular fistulae can be managed with antibiotics, bowel rest, and immunosuppressive agents to induce remission. Surgery is considered if the patient has an obstructed segment of bowel or is unresponsive to medical therapy and continues to have symptoms and complications. Surgical management consists of resection of diseased bowel, excision of the fistula, and partial bladder resection with or without temporary diversion of the fecal stream. This subject is discussed in detail in several other chapters.

References

Brandt LJ, Bernstein LH, Boley SJ, Frank MS. Metronidazole therapy for perineal Crohn's disease: a follow-up study. Gastroenterology 1982;83:383–7.

Egan LJ, Sandborn WJ, Tremaine WJ. Clinical outcome following treatment of refractory inflammatory and fistulizing Crohn's disease with intravenous cyclosporine. Am J Gastroenterol 1998;93:442–8.

Elson CO. The basis of current and future therapy for inflammatory bowel disease. Am J Med 1996;100:656–62.

Hanauer SB, Smith MB. Rapid closure of Crohn's disease fistulas with continuous intravenous cyclosporin A [see comments]. Am J Gastroenterol 1993;88:646–9.

Jakobovits J, Schuster MM. Metronidazole therapy for Crohn's disease and associated fistulae. Am J Gastroenterol 1984;79:533–40.

Korelitz BI, Present DH. Favorable effects of 6-mercaptopurine on fistulae of Crohn's disease. Dig Dis Sci 1985;30:58–64.

Muhadevan U, Marion J, Present DH. The place of methotrexate in the treatment of refractory Crohn's disease. Gastroenterology 1997;112:A1031.

Newman LH, Wellinger JR, Present DH, Aufses AH Jr. Crohn's disease of the duodenum associated with pancreatitis: a case report and review of the literature. Mt Sinai J Med 1987;54:429–32.

Nubiola P, Badia JM, Martinez-Rodenas F, et al. Treatment of 27 postoperative enterocutaneous fistulas with the long half-life somatostatin analogue SMS 201-995. Ann Surg 1989;210:56–8. Erratum Ann Surg 1990;211:246.

Ostro MJ, Greenberg IR, Jeejeebhoy KN. Total parenteral nutrition and complete bowel rest in the management of Crohn's disease. JPEN J Parenter Enteral Nutr 1985;9:280–7.

Present DH, Rutgeerts P, Targan S, et al. Infliximab for the treatment of fistulas in patients with Crohn's disease. N Engl J Med 1999;340:1398–405.

Schraut W, Block G. Enterovesical fistula complicating Crohn's ileocolitis. Am J Gastroenterol 1984;79:186–90.

CHAPTER 86

Bowel Rest and Parenteral Nutrition

Rosemarie L. Fisher, MD

The basis of the use of bowel rest in patients with Crohn's disease has its origin in several theories. Along the path for the search for the etiology of Crohn's disease there have been multiple times when the possibility of an intraluminal antigen, be it bacterial, viral, food related, or other, has been seriously considered. With this consideration, it only made sense that the idea of "putting the bowel to rest" might add to our therapeutic armamentarium. Take away the antigenic stimulus, and one might stop the progression or exacerbation of the disease process. Surely, if one removes gluten from the diet of a patient with celiac disease, the disease goes into remission. So, if Crohn's disease is caused by some dietary or intraluminal antigen, does it not make sense to try to remove it? However, as the antigen is unknown, one would have to stop giving anything by mouth, thus putting the bowel to rest. Second, it has been considered that any nutrients delivered to the intestinal tract do, as part of normal physiology, stimulate various gastrointestinal hormones, increase gastrointestinal secretions, increase gastrointestinal motility, and change mucosal permeability. If we stop this increased activity, would it not have a positive effect on the course of the disease? In a disease where we are still searching for an etiology, all therapeutic options surely must still be considered. Last, the old home remedy of "if it hurts when you move it, don't move it" has given the above two considerations more power.*

What is an obvious problem to this approach, however, is that unless the patient receives some form of parenteral nutrition while putting the bowel to rest, malnutrition is either going to occur or worsen. In addition, as we have progressed in our understanding of the role of nutrition in the maintenance of the gastrointestinal mucosa and the role of various nutrients in cellular functions, it has become less clear that putting the bowel to rest will result in any benefit to the patient or alter the course of their disease.

Is there evidence, however, that bowel rest is helpful in any patients with Crohn's disease, and is there any evidence that, in fact, it may be harmful to this patient group? What follows will attempt to delineate the evidence for and against the use of bowel rest and my approach to the use of bowel rest in patients with Crohn's disease. However, one must ask, what is the definition of "bowel rest?" Is it actually "nothing by mouth" or may it include the use of elemental diets, which, in the view of some clinicians, is equivalent to bowel rest? In addition, one must consider the use of bowel rest in both the short-term (acute disease) and long-term, or home, total parenteral nutrition (TPN) in these patients.

Physiologic Effects of Bowel Rest

Although the above theories about the benefits of bowel rest all seem quite reasonable, we have data from in vitro and in vivo studies as well as postoperative studies demonstrating that excluding nutrients from the lumen of the intestine will result in mucosal atrophy and may result in further malabsorption and perhaps even bacterial translocation. One must be very careful to distinguish what role malnutrition itself plays in mucosal atrophy, as opposed to the absence of luminal nutrients and the accompanying hormonal stimuli. Early studies compared the effects of bowel rest with what was effectively starvation. We know from studies in developing countries that severe malnutrition will result in intestinal mucosal changes. When one compares rats fed intravenously to those fed orally, there is a decrease in mucosal weight, mucosal protein content, and mucosal enzyme content in those fed intravenously. In vivo, patients with short-bowel syndrome who are fed orally postoperatively, as opposed to being maintained on TPN, even though a well-nourished state is maintained, have a more rapid and higher rate of adaptive changes in the remaining small bowel. More recently, several studies have challenged the importance of intraluminal nutrients in the maintenance of mucosal function. Resection of the distal bowel in rats has been shown to result in hyperplasia of the more proximal bowel. Enteral amino acids given alone were not incorporated into the proliferative zone of the intestinal crypt unless intravenous amino acids were administered as well. A recent study by Reynolds et al (1997) random-

---

* Editor's Note: A third consideration is that bowel rest alters the luminal contents by starving the lower intestinal tract bacteria. Systemic endotoxin disappears from the blood stream within days of instituting complete bowel rest. As described in the chapter on antibiotic use in Crohn's disease, the gut flora is thought to play a role in the pathogenesis of Crohn's disease. Most of the genetically engineered experimental colitides in mice do not occur in germ-free animals. (TMB)

ized 67 patients undergoing major gastrointestinal surgery to either TPN or TEN and fed them for 7 days postoperatively. They found no clinical benefit in either systemic parameters or intestinal permeability parameters that were measured.

With these somewhat contradictory statements of the effect of bowel rest on the normal or postoperative gut, the physician must also consider the possibility that the increased mucosal permeability that is seen in patients with Crohn's disease may be the chicken, not the egg, or the cart, not the horse. Is there an underlying primary mucosal permeability disorder that allows the penetration of various antigenic stimuli, or is it the presence of a luminal stimulus that causes the increased permeability? In the first scenario, bowel rest might increase the permeability, causing further systemic problems, whereas in the second scenario, the removal of the stimulus should lead to an improvement in pathology and systemic abnormalities.

We know from several studies that there is an increased mucosal permeability in patients with Crohn's disease. It has been suggested from studies by Hollander et al (1986, 1988) that the increased permeability may be primary in nature. They found increased permeability in patients with inactive Crohn's disease and in two-thirds of healthy relatives of Crohn's disease patients. Teahon et al (1992), on the other hand, showed that there was no real difference between first-degree relatives of patients with Crohn's disease and healthy controls. It has also been shown, however, that first-degree relatives have an exaggerated increase in permeability after treatment with agents that increase permeability.

If it is correct that the increased permeability is primary, and if it is correct that lack of luminal nutrients leads to further abnormalities in gut mucosal function and permeability, then putting the gut to rest may only result in further injury locally and systemically. However, as the primary abnormality is unknown, perhaps the only way in which to evaluate the role of bowel rest in the treatment of Crohn's disease is to look at the clinical trials in patients. In order to do this, one must also attempt to separate the possible roles and benefits of providing the bowel rest:

1. Is this meant to be primary therapy for active disease without the addition of other medications?
2. Is this meant to be adjunctive therapy for active disease while giving drugs in addition?
3. Are elemental diets considered to be equivalent to bowel rest in the above populations?
4. Is this meant to treat the complications of the disease such as fistulae?
5. Is this meant to treat intractable disease or gut failure secondary to short bowel syndrome?
6. Does the trial showing a benefit of growth hormone injections and a high-protein diet say bowel rest is the wrong road? (N Engl J Med May 2000)

Clinical Experience

Total Parenteral Nutrition and Nothing by Mouth as Primary Therapy

The available data on the use of TPN and bowel rest for the primary treatment of Crohn's disease are extremely difficult to summarize to reach some conclusions. Many of the studies are retrospective and uncontrolled as to the extent and location of the disease process and the presence of complications of the disease. In addition, the numbers of patients have been small, and the criteria for remission have not been consistent. Overall, it is seen, however, that approximately 64 percent (40 to 90%) of patients with Crohn's disease will enter some form of remission after 3 to 6 weeks of TPN and taking nothing by mouth (NPO). The subsequent relapse rate was noted to be between 28 and 85 percent after 1 year and 40 and 62 percent at 2 years after therapy. A recent retrospective review again showed similar results, but specifically in patients with Crohn's colitis. However, only 12 patients were included in this study: 11 of 12 improved significantly, with only 1 patient requiring surgery. There was, however, no control group and no group that was treated with prednisone (or other medications) as opposed to TPN.

A prospective but noncontrolled trial examined the effect of TPN, bowel rest, and no medications in patients who had been judged to be refractory to medical therapy. Thirty patients were kept NPO and on TPN for 3 months. At the end of this period, 25 patients avoided surgery, but there was a cumulative recurrence rate of 60 percent over 2 years and 85 percent after 4 years. This recurrence rate is four times higher than the recurrence rate after surgery at that same institution. This prompted the authors to state that TPN is not as beneficial as surgery in this group of medically unresponsive patients.

A multicenter, prospective, controlled trial published by Greenberg et al (1988) presents the best data regarding the use of TPN and bowel rest. Patients with active Crohn's disease unresponsive to medical therapy were randomized to receive either TPN and nothing by mouth, a defined polymeric tube feeding, or a standard oral diet supplemented by partial parenteral nutrition. There was no difference in either the remission rate, the avoidance of surgery, or symptomatic improvement among any of the three groups.[†] There was thus no advantage in the use of bowel rest as opposed to good nutritional support. This study by Greenberg et al raised the entire question of whether the response of patients with Crohn's disease to TPN and NPO was not as much secondary to the use of bowel rest but to the supply of adequate nutrients and energy.

[†] Editor's Note: A problem with that study was that the conclusions were drawn at a year, which was many, many months after the actual therapeutic maneuvers. (TMB)

Total Parenteral Nutrition and Nothing by Mouth as Adjunctive Therapy

The use of TPN as adjunctive therapy to standard drug therapy cannot be questioned if the patient is unable to take nutrients in adequate supply to maintain their energy needs and protein stores. This may be seen in cases where there is either bowel obstruction secondary to chronic scarring or acute inflammation. This may also be appropriate in the patient who enters the hospital with an acute exacerbation and no obstruction but severe malnutrition and an inability to tolerate oral nutrients or tube feedings.

Use of Elemental Diets as a Substitute for Bowel Rest

The use of an elemental diet was proposed for the same reasons that the use of bowel rest was initially proposed: less antigenic stimulation to the intestine, with only free amino acids, glucose, and short-chain fatty acids, as opposed to whole proteins, glucose polymers, and long-chain or mixed long- and short-chain triglycerides. In addition, as elemental diets were presumed to be more completely absorbed in the proximal intestine, there would be less volume delivered to the distal bowel, thus allowing patients with near total obstruction to tolerate oral or enteral supplements.‡

The studies showing superiority of an elemental diet when compared to steroid therapy in patients with acute exacerbations of Crohn's disease, not on other medical therapy, are reviewed in detail in the chapter on elemental diets. A meta-analysis showed no difference between the use of an elemental versus a polymeric diet. Another meta-analysis showed the inferiority of diet therapy to steroids and no advantage for elemental versus nonelemental diets.

If one does, however, consider that there might be certain groups of patients where steroid therapy may not be desired—such as in children and patients with complications of steroid therapy (ie, diabetes)—then enteral nutrition may be considered as primary therapy. Whether an elemental formula is preferred is not totally clear in my mind. Elemental and semi-elemental diets for the most part are largely unpalatable, and I have not been able to find more than two patients over my career who have been able to tolerate an elemental diet. Using this therapy would thus necessitate tube feeding in the majority of patients with its own set of complications. The two chapters on nutrition and growth cover the topic of elemental diets as primary therapy in detail.

Bowel Rest as Therapy for Fistulous Disease

Information is now available that bowel rest and TPN, and in some cases the addition of octreotide, will result in the closure of non-Crohn's disease–related enterocutaneous fistulae in some patients, with high rates of long-term closure in patients who are postoperative. However, this does not appear to be the case for patients with fistulae secondary to Crohn's disease. An initial review cited an overall closure rate of 38 percent but a much lower maintenance of closure after the reinstitution of oral nutrition. A study from Japan treated 22 fistulae with either bowel rest and TPN or enteral alimentation. None of the internal fistulae closed and 42 percent of the external fistulae closed. The reopening rate after nutritional therapy was 88.9 percent, as compared to 53.8 percent in those patients requiring surgery. There have also been case reports showing that fistulae have developed in patients on TPN and total bowel rest. Prior to the approval of Remicade® (Centocor Inc., Malvern, Pennsylvania), it appeared that surgery, when possible, was still the preferred method of therapy in patients with Crohn's disease with enteroenteric fistulae. Whether Remicade preoperatively and even postoperatively will change our approach is not known. There is a separate chapter on enteric fistulae by a surgeon. However, in those patients where immunomodulator therapy is not successful and surgery is not possible, long-term bowel rest and immunomodulators and home TPN may be the only therapeutic maneuver possible to maintain nutritional health.

Home Total Parenteral Nutrition in Crohn's Disease

The scenario then where bowel rest and home TPN in patients with Crohn's disease is in fact shown to be very effective is in that group of patients with multiple strictures, fistulae, or complications of medical therapy who are not surgical candidates. Several databases from around the world provide the opportunity to follow up these patients. The present availability of small bowel transplantation in non-Crohn's disease patients with short-bowel syndrome, as discussed in a separate chapter, makes patients with Crohn's disease one of the larger groups maintained on home TPN.

In the United States, the OLEY Registry collected data from 217 nutritional support programs between 1985 and 1992 on more than 4,000 patients. In examining survival, complication rates, etc., Howard and Hassan (1998) reviewed 562 patients with Crohn's disease. Mean age of the patients was 36 ($\pm$ 17 years SD), with a 1-year survival of 96 percent. At 1 year, 70 percent had resumed full oral nutrition and 25 percent continued on home therapy. Sixty percent (60%) had established complete rehabilitation, defined as the ability to sustain normal age-related activities. Another 38 percent reached partial rehabilitation status at 1 year or a partial return to these activities. The complication rate per year (those that resulted in readmission to the hospital) was 0.9 related to the TPN and 1.1 for non-TPN causes.§ A recent review of the data of the group on home TPN followed up at the Mayo

---

‡ Editor's Note: Once again, the fecal flora is altered by elemental diets, thus, its use as a preoperative prep in the past. (TMB)

§ Editor's Note: The role of concomitant medical therapy in this improvement is not clear. (TMB)

Clinic showed that 22.2 percent of their 225 patients had IBD and short-bowel syndrome. The mean age at the time of institution of therapy was 37 years, compared to 51 years for the entire group. The median duration of TPN in the Crohn's disease patients was 62.2 months, compared to all other groups (median duration 5.1 to 19.7 months). The patients with IBD had a better survival when compared to all other diagnostic groups—92% at 5 years.

The use of bowel rest and TPN in these patients is not a question. Here it is not in truth a form of therapy of Crohn's disease but the only form of nutritional support in this group of patients with true gut failure. The fact, however, that such a large portion of these patients can return to full oral intake further emphasizes the importance of good nutritional status in the management of patients with Crohn's disease and their disease progression. Perhaps we should not be focusing so much on bowel rest but whether the provision of specific nutrients to the gut (ie, glutamine, short-chain fatty acids, nucleotides, etc.) in order to improve the nutritional status of the patients would be more productive and beneficial to our patients. These aspects are discussed in the chapters on the short-bowel syndrome. A recent report in *The New England Journal of Medicine* on human growth hormone injections and a high-protein diet is of interest.

References

Greenberg GR, Fleming CR, Jeejeebhoy KN, et al. Controlled trial of bowel rest and nutritional support in the management of Crohn's disease. Gut 1988;29:1309–15.

Hollander D. Crohn's disease—a permeability disorder of the tight junction? Gut 1988;29:1621–4.

Hollander D, Vadheim CM, Brettholz E, et al. Increased intestinal epithelial permeability in patients with Crohn's disease and their relatives: a possible etiologic factor. Ann Intern Med 1986;105:883–5.

Howard L, Hassan N. Home parenteral nutrition. 25 years later. Gastroenterol Clin North Am 1998;27:481–512.

Reynolds JV, Kanwar S, Welsh FK, et al. 1997 Harry M. Vars Research Award. Does the route of feeding modify gut barrier function and clinical outcome in patients after major upper gastrointestinal surgery? J Parenter Enteral Nutr 1997;21:196–201.

Teahon K, Smethurst P, Levi AJ, et al. Intestinal permeability in patients with Crohn's disease and their first degree relatives. Gut 1992;33:320–3.

Supplemental Reading

Buchman AL, Moukarzel AA, Ament ME, et al. Effects of total parenteral nutrition on intestinal morphology and function in humans. Transplant Proc 1994;26:1457.

Buchman AL, Moukarzel AA, Ament ME, et al. Parenteral nutrition leads to a decrease in intestinal mucosal thickness and an increase in intestinal permeability in man. Gastroenterology 1993;104:612.

Dieleman LA, Heizer WD. Nutritional issues in inflammatory bowel disease. Gastroenterol Clin North Am 1998;27:435–51.

Fernendez-Banares F, Cabre E, EsteveoComas M, et al. How effective is enteral nutrition in inducing clinical remission in active Crohn's disease? A meta-analysis of the randomized clinical trials. J Parenter Enteral Nutr 1995;19:356–63.

Griffiths AM, Ohlsson A, Sherman PM, et al. Meta-analysis of enteral nutrition as a primary treatment of active Crohn's disease. Gastroenterology 1995;108:1056–67.

Guedon C, Schmitz J, Lerebours E, et al. Decreased brush border hydrolase activities without gross morphologic changes in human intestinal mucosa after prolonged total parenteral nutrition of adults. Gastroenterology 1986;90:373–8.

Hernandez G, Velasco N, Wainstein C, et al. Gut mucosal atrophy after a short enteral fasting period in critically ill patients. J Crit Care 1999;14:73–7.

Hilsden RJ, Meddings JB, Sutherland LR. Intestinal permeability changes in response to acetylsalicylic acid in relatives of patients with Crohn's disease. Gastroenterology 1996;110:1395–403.

Inoue Y, Espat NJ, Frohnapple DJ, et al. Effect of total parenteral nutrition on amino acid and glucose transport by the human small intestine. Ann Surg 1993;217:604–12.

Johnson LR. Regulation of gastrointestinal mucosal growth. Physiol Rev 1988;68:456–502.

Muller JM, Keller HW, Erasmi H, et al. Total parenteral nutrition as the sole therapy in Crohn's disease—a prospective study. Br J Surg 1983;70:40–3.

O'Morain C, Segal AW, Levi AJ. Elemental diets as primary treatment of acute Crohn's disease: a controlled trial. BMJ 1984;288:1859–62.

Parks RW, Rowlands BJ, Gardiner KR. Preoperative total parenteral nutrition is not associated with mucosal atrophy or bacterial translocation in humans. Br J Surg 1996;83:713.

Scolapio JS, Fleming CR, Kelley DG, et al. Survival of home parenteral nutrition-treated patients: 20 years experience at the Mayo Clinic. Mayo Clin Proc 1999;74:217–22.

Sedman PC, Macfie J, Palmer MD, et al. Preoperative total parenteral nutrition is not associated with mucosal atrophy or bacterial translocation in humans. Br J Surg 1995;82:1663–7.

Sedman PC, Macfie J, Sagar P, et al. The prevalence of gut translocation in humans. Gastroenterology 1995;107:643–9.

Seo M, Okada M, Yao T, et al. The role of total parenteral nutrition in the management of patients with acute attacks of inflammatory bowel disease. J Clin Gastroenterol 1999;29:270–5.

Stokes MA, Irving MH. How do patients with Crohn's disease fare on home parenteral nutrition? Dis Colon Rectum 1988;31:454–8.

Van der Hulst RRW, van Kreel BK, von Meyenfeldt MF, et al. Glutamine and the preservation of gut integrity. Lancet 1993;341:1363–5.

Winborn WB, Seeling LL Jr, Nakayama H, et al. Hyperplasia of gastric glands after small bowel resection in the rat. Gastroenterology 1982;66:384.

Wright HK, Poskitt T, Cleveland JC. The effect of total colectomy on morphology and absorptive capacity of the ileum in the rat. J Surg Res 1969;9:301–4.

Yamazaki Y, Fukushima T, Sugita A, et al. The medical, nutritional and surgical treatment of fistulae in Crohn's disease. Jpn J Surg 1990;20:376–83.

CHAPTER 87

Enteral Nutrition and Dietary Management

ANNE M. GRIFFITHS, MD, FRCP(C)

Many patients with Crohn's disease feel that their condition is caused by or in need of a particular diet. Discussion of diet with patients should differentiate two issues: (1) Can diet influence the frequency and severity of symptoms such as diarrhea or abdominal cramps? and (2) Can diet actually modify intestinal inflammation, that is, treat exacerbations or maintain disease quiescence? In consideration of the first question, what is eaten will affect stool pattern in patients with Crohn's disease, just as in healthy individuals. Furthermore, foods that are high in residue may precipitate abdominal cramps in the presence of a stenotic ileum. However, neither of these occurrences should be construed as signifying a worsening of intestinal inflammation. The response to the second question encompasses the role of nutrition in the primary treatment of Crohn's disease. This chapter focuses on enteral nutrition, that is, administration of formulated food, as anti-inflammatory therapy. Adult gastroenterologists in North America have frequently been skeptical of the efficacy of enteral nutrition as primary therapy, whereas their pediatric colleagues often consider the conventional regimens too difficult to implement or too demanding for their young patients to accept. In Europe, however, liquid diet therapy is more commonly employed among adult patients and, in several pediatric centers, constitutes the first line of treatment for active Crohn's disease (Walker-Smith, 1996). The earlier chapter on growth and nutrition in pediatric patients also discussed elemental diets in detail.

Enteral Nutrition as Primary Therapy of Acute Disease

Evidence of Efficacy

Primary therapeutic efficacy was established in a small controlled trial in adults, comparing an elemental formula with conventional corticosteroids (O'Morain et al, 1984). However, in most trials, more patients achieve clinical remission with steroids than with enteral nutrition (Lochs et al, 1991). There is a table of these trials in the earlier chapter on growth and nutrition. Examining the data in meta-analytic fashion, the pooled odds ratio for likelihood of clinical response to enteral nutrition using elemental, semi-elemental, or polymeric formulae versus corticosteroids is 0.35 (95% CI = 0.23 to 0.53) (Griffiths et al, 1995). The multiple trials are in agreement: overall, there is a treatment benefit to corticosteroids. Furthermore, poor compliance, although a factor, does not constitute the major reason for the lower response rates to enteral nutrition, as evident from a secondary meta-analysis excluding dropouts for apparent intolerance.

Comparison of observed response rates to exclusive liquid diet therapy with usual placebo response rates in the controlled clinical trial setting suggests that enteral nutrition is of therapeutic benefit, even if efficacy does not equal that of corticosteroid treatment. Moreover, a reduction in gastrointestinal protein loss, a decrease in intestinal permeability, and a reduction in fecal excretion of indium-labeled leukocytes have been demonstrated, suggesting a direct effect on intestinal inflammation (Teahon et al, 1991). The mode of action of enteral nutrition as primary treatment of active Crohn's disease remains conjectural. Hypotheses have included alteration in intestinal microbial flora, elimination of dietary antigen uptake, diminution of intestinal synthesis of inflammatory mediators via reduction of dietary fat, overall nutritional repletion, or provision of vital micronutrients to the diseased bowel (Fernandez-Banares et al, 1994).

Factors Influencing Effectiveness of Enteral Nutrition

Anatomic Localization of Disease

The site of intestinal inflammation may influence the likelihood of response to nutritional therapy in that Crohn's colitis responds less well to enteral feeding than does ileocolitis or isolated small bowel disease. Nevertheless, excellent clinical response rates of 67 percent and 73 percent to elemental and polymeric formulae, respectively, were observed in the comparative trial of Rigaud and co-workers (1991), even though two-thirds of the adult patients receiving the nutritional treatment had disease confined to the colon. Teahon et al (1990) reported that relapse occurred earlier and more frequently among patients with colonic inflammation versus isolated small intestinal disease, but initial response rates were similar. Others note that Crohn's colitis is less likely to respond to

TABLE 87–1. Formula Composition and Outcomes in Trials of Elemental versus Nonelemental Liquid Diet Therapy

Study	Number of Patients Treated	Percentage Achieving Remission	Protein Source	Percentage of Total Calories as Fat
Raouf et al, 1991				
Elemental	13	69	Amino acids	16.4
Nonelemental	11	73	Intact milk	Not stated
Rigaud et al, 1991				
Elemental	15	67	Amino acids	0.8
Nonelemental	15	73	Intact milk protein and egg or milk protein*	27.0 or* 36.0
Park et al, 1991				
Elemental	7	29	Amino acids	11.0
Nonelemental	7	71	Whole whey	27.0
Royall et al, 1994				
Elemental	19	84	Amino acids	3.0
Nonelemental	21	71	Oligopeptides	33.0 (10.0 LCT + 23.0 MCT)
Middleton et al, 1991				
Elemental	11	73	Amino acids	16.4
Nonelemental	15	73	Oligopeptides	24.0

*Two polymeric formulae used; LCT = long-chain triglyceride; MCT = medium-chain triglyceride.

enteral nutrition (Wilschanski et al, 1996). This is perhaps not surprising, in that colonic Crohn's disease was relatively refractory even to corticosteroid therapy in the National Collaborative Crohn's Disease Study and the European Cooperative Crohn's Disease Study. Moreover, administration of liquid diets often is associated, at least initially, with a decrease in stool consistency and an increase in stool frequency, which may be intolerable to patients with colitis and more baseline diarrhea. Liquid diet therapy may provide nutritional support, but the author does not recommend it as single therapy to promote healing of Crohn's colitis.

Formula Composition

Both the protein and the fat content of liquid diets have been hypothesized to influence efficacy. Results from directly comparative trials do not support the proposed benefit of elemental formulae (Table 87–1). The pooled odds ratio for likelihood of attainment of remission using an elemental versus nonelemental formula was 0.87 (95% CI = 0.41 to 1.83) (Griffiths et al, 1995). However, the number of patients included in the total sample would preclude detection of a difference in response rate even as large as 30 percent. Furthermore, the elemental and "nonelemental" formulae used in these studies were not consistently disparate. All elemental formulae contained amino acids as their protein source, but the nonelemental formulae contained either oligopeptides (also of low antigenicity) or intact proteins. Similarly, the percentage of total calories derived from fat varied greatly. Both a low total fat content and a low ratio of n-6 to n-3 polyunsaturated fatty acids have been hypothesized to be necessary for reduction of intestinal inflammation (Fernandez-Banares et al, 1994). Too few data exist to establish definitively whether either decreased antigenicity related to the

protein content or an immunomodulatory or anti-inflammatory effect related to low fat content is important in reduction of intestinal inflammation. The hypothesis that diets low in n-6 fatty acids, precursors for arachidonate-derived eicosanoid synthesis, are more efficacious is continuing to be explored in the comparative trial setting.

Meanwhile the practicing gastroenterologist must choose a formula based on the available data. Polymeric formulae are certainly more palatable, but given the limited published experience with their efficacy, in pediatric practice the more tried-and-true low-fat elemental or semi-elemental formulae are preferred, recognizing that nasogastric infusion is required.

Importance of Bowel Rest

When employed in the treatment of active Crohn's disease, enteral nutrition is generally combined with bowel rest. However, in an oft-quoted randomized trial of adjunctive nutritional treatments, Greenberg et al (1988) observed that partial parenteral nutrition plus an ad libitum oral diet was as effective in inducing clinical remission as either elemental liquid diets administered by nasogastric tube or total parenteral nutrition and complete bowel rest. However, this study was conducted among patients hospitalized because of activity of their disease despite high-dose steroid therapy, so that the continuing co-intervention with steroids may have influenced the result. Also, they looked at long-term results a year later and without added medical therapy.

When treating active Crohn's disease with enteral nutrition, initially clear fluids by mouth are the only other allowed food source. Although such exclusivity of enteral nutrition is not proven to be essential, a stomach full of other food will certainly compromise tolerance of a nasogastric infusion and thereby jeopardize the success of the regimen. Once the patient is comfortable with the enteral feeding and the activity of disease is lessened, the stringency of the bowel rest can be modified.

Compliance

Poor compliance with orally administered enteral nutrition compromises effectiveness. Twenty-one percent of patients randomized to nutritional therapy in comparative trials versus corticosteroids did not complete the study because of intolerance to formulated food (Griffiths et al, 1995). Studies wherein patients first attempted to drink the formula had a higher rate of nonacceptance (34% of patients) than those wherein administration of formula was exclusively via nasogastric infusion from the outset (8% of patients intolerant).

In the nutritional treatment of exacerbations of Crohn's disease it is preferable to administer formulated food via nocturnal nasogastric infusion; children who are unwell and anorexic are not able to ingest the required amounts orally. Almost all young patients initially resist the suggestion of nasogastric tube feeding. Encouragement from members of the medical, nursing, and dietetic team involved with the child's management is important in ensuring success. With such input, children quickly become adept at swallowing the silastic catheter, infusing the formula overnight in the home setting, and removing it each morning to allow normal daytime activities. In post-treatment surveys, 45 percent of children and adolescents reported a preference for enteral nutrition versus corticosteroid treatment, with which they had had prior experience, whereas 27 percent favored the drug treatment (Wilschanski et al, 1996).

Maintenance of Remission with Enteral Nutrition

One of the limitations of liquid diet therapy has been the observed tendency for symptoms to recur promptly following its cessation. In most studies, 60 to 70 percent of patients experience a relapse within 12 months of stopping enteral nutrition and resuming a normal diet. Relapse is, of course, common following cessation of steroids in drug-induced remission as well.[*] Three different nutritional strategies have been employed after attainment of remission through use of exclusive enteral nutrition.

Cyclic Enteral Nutrition

A regimen of exclusive enteral nutrition and avoidance of regular food 1 month of 4 has been suggested to provide beneficial effects on disease activity and growth (Bellet al,

1998). In a subsequent Canadian pediatric randomized multicenter trial, this regimen was compared with low-dose alternate-day prednisone given to maintain remission. Nine (47%) of 19 patients treated with alternate-day prednisone and 12 (67%) of 18 treated with cyclic enteral nutrition remained in continuous clinical remission during the 18-month study period ($p = .32$) (Seidman et al, 1996). Although time to first relapse and number of clinical relapses were not significantly different, patients receiving the nutritional therapy achieved greater gains in height.

Supplementary Enteral Nutrition

As an alternate nutritional strategy, continuation of nocturnal nasogastric feeding four to five times weekly as supplement to an unrestricted ad libitum daytime diet also was associated with prolonged disease quiescence and improved growth in a historic cohort study (Wilshanski et al, 1996). These findings, although yet to be confirmed in prospective randomized fashion, suggest that administration of formulated food is useful in diminishing the activity of Crohn's disease even when dietary restrictions are not imposed. This remains the favored approach of the author; in the long-term, allowing normal food at times when family and friends are eating is particularly important in achieving compliance.

Specific Foods Exclusion Diet

Adult gastroenterologists in the United Kingdom have employed a type of elimination diet to maintain remission achieved with exclusive enteral nutrition. Patients are advised to introduce one food at a time in a specified sequence. If symptoms develop, that food becomes one to be avoided. A prolongation of clinical remission was reported. This study is discussed in the chapter on nutritional consultation and guidance.

Growth Impairment as Indication for Enteral Nutrition

Inflammatory disease occurring during early adolescence is likely to have a major impact on nutritional status and growth because of the rapid accumulation of lean body mass that normally occurs at this time. Boys are more vulnerable to disturbances in growth than girls because their growth spurt comes at a later stage of normal pubertal development and is ultimately longer and greater. Impairment of linear growth is common prior to disease recognition as well as during the subsequent years, and height at maturity is often compromised (Griffiths et al, 1993). Height velocity is the most sensitive parameter by which to recognize growth delay. Normal height velocity is an important marker of control of disease activity and success of any therapy.

---

[*] Editor's Note: If the trend toward using immunomodulator therapy in young patients continues, one might expect less need for prolonged enteral nutrition. (TMB)

Role of Active Disease

Several interrelated factors contribute to growth impairment in children with Crohn's disease. Most emphasis formerly was placed on the importance of chronic undernutrition as the primary cause of growth retardation, but a simple nutritional hypothesis does not explain all of the observations related to growth patterns among children with inflammatory bowel disease (IBD). A direct growth-retarding effect of chronic inflammation is now recognized. Inflammatory mediators secreted from the inflamed gut may interfere with growth-plate kinetics and thereby suppress linear growth (DeBenedetti et al, 1997). Daily corticosteroid use may inhibit growth, but often it is difficult to separate the relative contributions of disease activity from corticosteroid usage in the pathogenesis of slow linear growth in pediatric Crohn's disease.

Reduction of Inflammation and Provision of Nutrition

Children with Crohn's disease need special approaches to therapy because of their need to grow. **Reduction of intestinal inflammation and provision of adequate nutrition are of paramount importance**. Among growth-impaired young patients, liquid dietary supplements recommended for oral administration generally are not accepted or at best displace ingested calories from regular food without increasing total caloric intake. Nasogastric tube feeding of liquid diets can provide optimal macro- and micronutrients and appears to ameliorate intestinal inflammation, all of which should facilitate growth. Children with extensive small intestinal disease and growth impairment respond well to enteral nutrition alone. Those with severe colonic inflammation are best treated with immunomodulatory steroid-sparing drugs (eg, azathioprine), but adjunctive enteral nutrition also may be required if growth continues to be delayed despite pharmacologic optimization of anti-inflammatory therapy.

When more than 6 months of enteral nutrition is contemplated, insertion of a gastrostomy tube makes administration easier. This procedure appears to be uncomplicated in Crohn's disease patients; one patient in a pediatric series had a persistent gastrocutaneous fistula when the gastrostomy tube was removed, but surgical closure proved successful (Israel and Hassall, 1995).

Other Dietary Management

The success of enteral nutrition in ameliorating Crohn's disease stands apart from the apparent lack of benefit of other dietary measures. Controlled studies have not supported a role for a low-residue diet nor for a high-fiber–low-refined sugar diet in the maintenance of remission in Crohn's disease. Lactase deficiency and lactose intolerance may coexist with IBD, but are in general no more common than would be expected in an age- and ethnically matched control population. A major problem with dietary modifications is that they frequently result in a less appetizing diet that discourages optimal caloric intake. Imposition of dietary restrictions can result in a major source of conflict between children and their parents. Except in specific circumstances (eg, a low-residue diet to reduce obstructive symptoms in the setting of small intestinal stricture), the most important advice is to consume a diet liberal in protein, with calories sufficient to maintain or restore weight, or to support growth in children and adolescents.

The ability of pharmacologic amounts of certain nutrients, such as n-3 polyunsaturated fatty acids found in marine oils, to modulate proinflammatory cytokine synthesis is intriguing. However, the specific fish-oil preparation that has been most efficacious in the clinical trial setting is unique in its design for ileal release and is not currently obtainable.

Editor's Note

References on this topic are also included in the supplemental reading lists of the related chapters on nutrition and diet.

References

Belli DC, Seidman E, Bouthillier L, et al. Chronic intermittent elemental diet improves growth failure in children with Crohn's disease. Gastroenterology 1988;94:603–10.

DeBenedetti F, Alonzi T, Moretta A, et al. Interleukin-6 causes growth impairment in transgenic mice through a decrease in insulin-growth factor I. J Clin Invest 1997;99:643–50.

Fernandez-Banares F, Cabre E, Gonzalez-Huix F, Gassull MA. Enteral nutrition as primary therapy in Crohn's disease. Gut 1994;35:S55–9.

Greenberg GR, Fleming CR, Jeejeebhoy KN, et al. Controlled trial of bowel rest and nutritional support in the management of Crohn's disease. Gut 1988;29:1309–15.

Griffiths AM, Nguyen P, Smith C, et al. Growth and clinical course of children with Crohn's disease. Gut 1993;34:939–43.

Griffiths AM, Ohlsson A, Sherman P, Sutherland LR. Meta-analysis of enteral nutrition as primary treatment of active Crohn's disease. Gastroenterology 1995;108:1056–67.

Israel DM, Hassall E. Prolonged use of gastrostomy for enteral hyperalimentation in children with Crohn's disease. Am J Gastroenterol 1995;90:1084–8.

Lochs H, Steinhardt HJ, Klaus-Ventz B, et al. Comparison of enteral nutrition and drug treatment in active Crohn's disease. Results of the European Cooperative Crohn's Disease Study IV. Gastroenterology 1991;101:881–8.

O'Morain C, Segal AW, Levi AJ. Elemental diet as primary treatment of acute Crohn's disease. BMJ 1984;288:1859–62.

Rigaud D, Cosnes J, Le Quintrec Y, et al. Controlled trial comparing two types of enteral nutrition in treatment of active Crohn's disease. Gut 1991;32:1492–7.

Seidman E, Jones A, Issenman R, Griffiths AM. Cyclical exclusive enteral nutrition versus alternate-day prednisone in maintaining remission of pediatric Crohn's disease. J Pediatr Gastroenterol Nutr 1996;23:344.

Teahon K, Bjarnason I, Levi AJ. Elemental diets in the management of Crohn's disease: a ten year review. Gut 1990; 31:1133–7.

Teahon K, Smethurst P, Pearson M, et al. The effect of elemental diet on permeability and inflammation in Crohn's disease. Gastroenterology 1991;101:84–7.

Walker-Smith JA. Management of growth failure in Crohn's disease. Arch Dis Child 1996;75:351–4.

Wilschanski M, Sherman P, Pencharz P, et al. Supplementary enteral nutrition maintains remission in paediatric Crohn's disease. Gut 1996;38:543–8.

Supplemental Reading

Belluzzi A, Brignola C, Campieri M, et al. Effect of an enteric coated fish-oil preparation on relapses in Crohn's disease. N Engl J Med 1996;334:1557–61.

Malchow H, Steinhardt HJ, Lorenz-Meyer H, et al. European Cooperative Crohn's Disease Study III. Scand J Gastroenterol 1990;25:235–44.

Riordan AM, Hunter JO, Cowan RE, et al. Treatment of active Crohn's disease by exclusion diet: East Anglian multicentre controlled trial. Lancet 1993;343:1131–4.

Vointk AJ, Echave V, Feller JH, et al. Experience with elemental diet in the treatment of acute Crohn's disease. Arch Surg 1973;107:329–33.

CHAPTER 88

CROHN'S DISEASE IN CHILDREN AND ADOLESCENTS

RANJANA GOKHALE, MD, AND BARBARA S. KIRSCHNER, MD

Crohn's disease (CD) and ulcerative colitis (UC) increasingly are being recognized as important causes of chronic gastrointestinal disease in children and adolescents. An increased incidence of CD has been observed in recent years. Barton et al (1989) reported a threefold rise in newly diagnosed CD in children in Scotland between 1968 and 1983 (6.6 to 22.9/100,000), followed by a further increase between 1984 and 1986 to 29/100,000. Similar increases in CD in children have been reported from Wales, Sweden, and Canada.

Comparison of patients diagnosed with CD before age 20 years with those over 40 years shows higher frequencies of small bowel disease, strictures (46% vs 29%), and surgery (71% vs 55%) in the younger group. Children and adolescents with CD have unique presentations, extra-intestinal manifestations, and therapeutic considerations. Whereas the focus of therapy is reduction of disease activity and symptoms, management of the special nutritional, extra-intestinal, and emotional features of inflammatory bowel disease (IBD) in children requires attention as well. Thus, gastroenterologists managing children with CD may be faced with patients with more refractory disease than in their adult patients.

Diagnostic Studies

The importance of excluding enteric pathogens before confirming the diagnosis of CD cannot be overemphasized. Stool specimens are sent for analysis to rule out *Salmonella*, *Shigella*, *Campylobacter*, *Aeromonas*, *Plesiomonas*, *Yersinia*, and *Clostridium difficile*, and, when clinically indicated, *Escherichia coli* 0157:H7, *Giardia lamblia*, *Entamoeba histolytica*, and *Histoplasma*. When infection precedes IBD, intestinal symptoms either fail to resolve or recur within days to weeks.

In the absence of enteric infections, hematologic screening tests, endoscopy with biopsy, and radiography are conducted to confirm the diagnosis. New diagnostic tools include perinuclear antineutrophil cytoplasmic antibodies (pANCA) and anti-*Saccharomyces cerevisiae* antibodies (ASCA): pANCA is detected in 66 to 83 percent of children with UC and 14 to 19 percent with CD (Proujansky et al, 1993; Hoffenberg et al, 1997), and ASCA in children with CD is reported to have 44 to 54 percent sensitivity and 89 to 97 percent specificity

(Ruemmele et al, 1998). Endoscopy in children requires adequate sedation using either conscious sedation (usually midazolam combined with Demerol or fentanyl) or deeper sedation with propofol generally administered by an anesthesiologist. The latter approach is easier for children and younger adolescents and shortens procedure time. However anesthesiology arrangements reduce flexibility in timing the procedure. Bowel preparation for children having colonoscopy is achieved using a clear liquid diet for 1 to 2 days, followed by oral Fleet Phospho-Soda in an age-appropriate dose (1 to 2 ounces repeated in 2 doses). Fleet PhosphoSoda is better tolerated with comparable cleansing to high-volume balanced polyethylene glycol electrolyte lavage. However, aphthous ulcers have been reported with this preparation (TMB).

Approach to a Child with Crohn's Disease

Medical approach to treating children with CD varies depending on the severity of symptoms, areas and extent of intestinal involvement, and associated extra-intestinal manifestations. Goals in managing pediatric patients include reducing gastrointestinal symptoms, optimizing nutritional status (linear growth, weight gain, and dietary intake), alleviating extra-intestinal symptoms (arthralgia and arthritis, malaise, dermatologic lesions, etc.), and paying attention to the impact of the disease on social activities and school attendance.[*]

Drug Therapy

Table 88–1 summarizes drug dosages used for treating children with CD.

Corticosteroids

Corticosteroid medications are effective in decreasing disease activity in children with CD. Daily prednisone or its equivalent is given until symptoms subside (generally 4 to 8 wk); the dosage is gradually lowered by 2.5 to

---

[*] Editor's Note: In order to optimize growth before and during puberty, we have added another therapeutic goal: complete suppression of clinical and laboratory evidence of inflammation, including sedimentation rate, albumin, and iron levels. As discussed, avoiding prolonged daily prednisone use is essential if growth is to be maximized. (Gastroenterology 1977;72:1338–44.) (TMB)

TABLE 88–1. Drug Dosages for Treating Children with Crohn's Disease

Agent	Dosage
Corticosteroids	1.0–2.0 mg/kg/d prednisone equivalent IV or PO in 1–2 doses/d Maximum 60 mg/d
Sulfasalazine	Initial dose: 25–50 mg/kg/d in divided doses Can be increased to 75 mg/kg/d Maximum 4 g/d
Mesalamine	30–60 mg/kg/d Maximum 4.8 g/d
Metronidazole	10–20 mg/kg/d
Azathioprine	1.5–2.0 mg/kg/d
6-Mercaptopurine	1.0–1.5 mg/kg/d
Methotrexate	10–20 mg/m^2/wk

5.0 mg every 1 to 2 weeks. To avoid growth suppression from daily use of corticosteroids, an alternate-day administration may be efficacious. Linear growth usually is normal with alternate-day corticosteroids, if disease activity is relatively quiescent and dietary intake is adequate. Growth hormone secretion in children receiving alternate-day corticosteroids is similar to that in normal children (Sadeghi-Nejad and Senior, 1969). Adverse cosmetic effects of glucocorticoid therapy (round facies, acne) usually regress after 1 to 2 months of alternate-day treatment.

Once clinical remission is achieved, attempts are made to discontinue corticosteroids. However, children often have a recurrence of clinical symptoms when the dose is lowered below a threshold level. Under these circumstances, alternate-day or low-dose corticosteroids (≤ 5 mg/d) reduces disease activity in patients whose course is characterized by low-grade, chronically active disease. In many children, multiple drugs are used concurrently in an attempt to reduce the need for corticosteroids. Even 5 mg of prednisone on the low-dose day of an alternate-day dosing taper has the potential to delay growth.

Budesonide, a potent steroid that undergoes extensive first-pass hepatic metabolism, may be useful in pediatric patients with CD. There are no published studies of the efficacy of budesonide in children. The long-term effects of budesonide on bone turnover in pediatric patients undergoing linear growth remains to be studied.

Sulfasalazine and 5-Aminosalicylic Acid

Sulfasalazine and mesalamine (5-ASA) may reduce disease activity and steroid dosage. Unlike the newer 5-ASA preparations, sulfasalazine can be prepared as a liquid and thus is useful in young children. Headaches are the most common side effects and can sometimes be averted by starting at a lower dose and gradually increasing the dose as tolerated. Other signs of intolerance include hemolytic anemia and pruritic dermatitis.

5-Aminosalicylic acid preparations are effective and are frequently accompanied by fewer side effects. In a review of 153 pediatric patients who received mesalamine, D'Agata (1996) noted that the average dose for both active disease and maintenance over a 10-year period increased from 36 to 43 mg/kg/d. The most common cause for withdrawal from mesalamine therapy was exacerbation of diarrhea.

Antibiotics

METRONIDAZOLE

Perianal disease is common in pediatric patients with CD and is manifest by skin tags (35%), fissures (51%), fistulae (15%), and perirectal abscesses (13%). Clinical experience has shown that these perineal complications often improve with metronidazole. Rarely, a child may develop sensory peripheral neuropathy; complete resolution or improvement is noted after discontinuation of therapy.

CIPROFLOXACIN

Ciprofloxacin has been advocated for adults with perianal CD. The occurrence of impaired cartilage growth in experimental animals has produced hesitancy to use this antibiotic for long-term therapy in children. However, a recent analysis of children with cystic fibrosis on long-term ciprofloxacin did not demonstrate radiographic evidence of cartilage damage.

Immunomodulatory Agents

6-MERCAPTOPURINE AND AZATHIOPRINE

Azathioprine (AZA) and 6-mercaptopurine (6-MP) increasingly are being used in children with CD. Indications include steroid dependency, medical intractability (particularly in the absence of focally resectable disease), and steroid toxicity. These drugs permit significant reduction in corticosteroid requirement in 70 to 87 percent of children. They are prescribed for children with extensive disease, particularly those with previous intestinal resection, or those who are steroid dependent (≥ 5 mg/d) or have gastroduodenal and perirectal disease, especially fistulous refractory disease. The recommended dosages are 1.0 to 1.5 mg/kg/d for 6-MP and 1.5 to 2.0 mg/kg/d for azathioprine. Hematologic toxicity (leukopenia, anemia, thrombocytopenia) is monitored on a regular basis. Toxicity to 6-MP or AZA is infrequent (Kirschner, 1998). The most common adverse reactions are elevated alanine transaminase (ALT) or aspartate aminotransferase (AST) (13.7%), and leukopenia, defined as white blood cell (WBC) count less than 4,000 (10.5%). These side effects revert to normal with reduction in AZA or 6-MP dose. Four children reportedly developed acute pancreatitis: three within the first 4 weeks of therapy, the fourth after

22 months. All side effects resolved with discontinuation of the drug, but three children required hospitalization and intravenous fluids. Blood levels of the 6-MP metabolite, 6-thioguanine (> 225 pmol per 8 × 103 erythrocytes), are reported to correlate with disease remission, whereas high levels of 6-methylmercaptopurine (6-MMP) (>6,000 pmol) can be associated with hepatic toxicity. There is a chapter on the use of 6-thioguanine levels to monitor therapy.

Because a high rate of relapse occurs when these drugs are discontinued in adults, the authors attempt to taper the dose after 12 to 24 months and follow clinical activity, acute-phase reactants, and the blood counts in establishing an individual child's maintenance dose. Parents are frequently concerned about the risk of malignancy with these drugs. The data indicate that the risk of induction of malignancy is no greater in adult patients with CD than for the general population. This can be reassuring information for parents.

METHOTREXATE

Preliminary experience in children with CD suggests that methotrexate may improve clinical status and provide steroid sparing in those with refractory disease. The authors found that subcutaneous methotrexate (MTX) (12.5 to 25.0 mg/wk) for 24 to 64 months reduced corticosteroid requirement (mean dosage, 25 to 6 mg/d) in steroid-dependent children with CD. Liver biopsy was normal in the child with the highest cumulative dose (4.83 g). Subsequently, Mack et al (1998) described 14 children with CD who had failed (n = 11) or were hypersensitive (n = 3) to 6-MP. All received subcutaneous MTX (10 to 25 mg/wk depending on body weight). Improvement was seen in 64 percent of children within 4 weeks, including 55 percent who had failed to respond to 6-MP. Nausea and headache resulted in withdrawal from therapy of 2 of the 14 children (14%).

CYCLOSPORINE AND TACROLIMUS

Cyclosporine may be beneficial in selected children with CD, such as those with refractory perianal disease. The authors have used cyclosporine in four highly selected growth-impaired patients with severe extensive CD, who were steroid dependent and unresponsive to AZA or 6-MP, an elemental diet, or home total parenteral nutrition (TPN). A reduction in corticosteroid dose led to improved growth in all four patients, including one who also experienced closure of multiple perineal fistulae. Mahdi et al (1996) used intravenous cyclosporine (4 mg/kg/d in two divided doses) in 10 children with severe refractory active Crohn's colitis. There was a 70 percent response rate, although 30 percent relapsed within 2 to 6 months. Thus, 40 percent responded and remained in remission 3 to 22 months after cyclosporine therapy was discontinued. In that series, children refractory to 6-MP

did not respond to cyclosporine. Further studies are needed to determine the range of response in children with CD. A limited study of Tacrolimus in six children with severe colitis demonstrated improvement to the point of discharge in five patients and maintenance of remission with 6-MP in three of the six patients.

THALIDOMIDE

Published experience in the pediatric age range with thalidomide is limited. Thalidomide was beneficial in a 13-year-old with severe oral ulceration due to CD (Weinstein et al, 1999). Within 1 week, improvement was observed, with complete healing noted after 1 month. The effect is thought to result from inhibition of tumor necrosis factor-alpha (TNF-α) production by monocytes.

Biologic Therapy: Anti-Tumor Necrosis Factor Antibody

Chronic inflammation in CD can be attributed in part to increased production of inflammatory cytokines, especially TNF. The amount of TNF is found to be increased both in histologically normal and in inflamed mucosa in CD. Baldassano et al (1999) reported the safety and efficacy of a single infusion of TNF at the end of 4 weeks after infusion. Five of 12 children with treatment-resistant CD achieved remission after a single infusion of 1, 5, or 10 mg/kg of infliximab. Hadigan et al studied the effects of a single TNF infusion given to 21 patients with CD. At weeks 4 and 8, respectively, clinical response was achieved in 65 percent and 90 percent, and 25 percent and 38 percent were in remission. None of the children experienced adverse reactions and none developed antibodies to TNF. However, there are no published data on long-term safety, dosing, and efficacy in children.

Monitoring Response to Medical Therapy

Pediatric rating systems include the Lloyd-Still-Green Clinical Score and the Pediatric Crohn's Disease Activity Index (PCDAI). Each study found good correlation between the relatively complex clinical scores and simpler subjective ratings. Recently the PCDAI has been shown to correlate more closely with Physician Global Assessment and laboratory indices than the CDAI when used in pediatric patients. Laboratory studies, including ESR, are used to monitor therapy. Endoscopy is used for diagnosis and for evaluating unresponsive patients.

Nutritional Intervention

Nutritional deficiencies are common in children with IBD. Lack of calorie intake, whether from dietary insufficiency or malabsorption, alters weight gain, body composition, linear growth, and endocrine function. Specific nutrient complications include iron, folate and cyanocobalamin deficiencies, which may cause anemia; hypoalbuminemia; zinc deficiency; osteoporosis; and osteomalacia. Malabsorption based on fecal fat, d-xylose, or cyanocobalamin absorption does not account for the nutritional deficits found in most growth-impaired children. Children reduce dietary intake below that recommended for age as a means of decreasing postprandial symptoms. A variety of enteral and parenteral methods to enhance caloric intake lead to reversal of growth failure.

Nutritional Support

Some pediatric gastroenterologists use nutritional intervention to control disease activity, prevent deficiencies and provide restitution, and reverse growth failure. Whether steroids or elemental or polymeric formulas are more effective in reducing disease activity and promoting prolonged remission and long-term normalization of growth is discussed in two chapters on elemental diet. Presumably immunomodulator use will change some of these practice patterns in the future. Continuous nasogastric infusion at night is effective when dietary intake is suboptimal, although up to one-third of children may be unwilling or unable to tolerate the nightly passage of a nasogastric tube. Gastrostomy feedings can be an effective alternative. This approach is more effective in newly diagnosed children with ileal disease than in children with longstanding disease or extensive gastroduodenal or colonic disease. As discussed in two of the chapters, administering an elemental formula for 1 month of 4 enhances weight gain and growth in some adolescents with CD. Nutritional recommendations for caloric and protein intake should at least meet the recommended daily allowance (RDA) for age. Caloric needs for undernourished children at the onset of therapy usually are higher than for healthy children, since most patients have lost weight. Recently, it was shown that children with CD fail to downregulate their resting energy expenditure (REE) in response to weight loss, which might further contribute to malnutrition. Recommendations for protein intake are similar to those for healthy children. Because excess enteric protein loss also is common, protein status (albumin, prealbumin, arm muscle circumference) should be followed.

Mineral Deficiencies

Several mineral deficits are observed in children with IBD. Of these, **iron deficiency anemia** is the commonest and usually is accompanied by microcytosis and low ferritin levels, although ferritin may be normal since it is an acute-phase reactant. Intravenous iron dextran complex may be beneficial in children with chronic anemia resistant to oral iron. Test doses are mandatory to identify hypersensitivity reactions and avoid anaphylaxis. **Recombinant human erythropoietin** (EPO) has been used in children with low endogenous EPO production. Hemoglobin levels normalize within 6 weeks. **Zinc deficiency** may contribute to the growth failure and delayed sexual maturation. Plasma zinc levels are lower in growth-impaired than in normally growing teenagers with CD. Very low alkaline phosphatase may be a clue to zinc deficiency. Mineral losses of calcium, magnesium, or phosphorus also may occur.

Bone Mineralization

Osteopenia or reduced bone mineral mass is an important potential complication of pediatric CD. Contributing factors include nutritional status, circulating cytokines, total cumulative corticosteroids, sex hormone levels, pubertal status, and the level of physical activity. In a series of 95 children with IBD, significant differences in bone mineral density were noted between pediatric patients with CD and those with UC, despite similar total cumulative corticosteroid doses in the two groups (Gokhale et al, 1998). The Z-scores for boys and girls with CD were −0.55 and −0.88 versus +0.06 and −0.34 for those with UC. Therapies that reduce the risk of osteopenia, such as alternate-day steroids, aminosalicylates, and immunomodulatory drugs, should be used in children. In view of the importance of bone calcium accretion during adolescence, adequate **calcium** and **vitamin D intakes** are essential. Commercially available chocolate or strawberry flavored chewable calcium preparations may be particularly useful in children and adolescents with CD.

Emotional Needs

Most children with CD have not experienced serious health problems prior to the diagnosis of IBD. They are frequently unprepared for the invasive and painful diagnostic studies. Sensitivity on the part of physicians is required. Care must be taken that pediatric patients are reassured that their comfort and concerns are being addressed. There are two chapters on the pediatric patient, family, and doctor interactions. Adjusting to IBD is an evolving process for children and their families; fluctuations in mood and medication compliance occur as disease activity varies. Relapses and extra-intestinal symptoms, such as malaise, joint pain, delayed growth and sexual maturation, combined with the cosmetic side effects of corticosteroids, interference with social activities, and absenteeism from school, converge to reinforce feelings of being different and isolated from their peers.

Psychiatric studies have shown that anxiety, depression, and low self-esteem are present with increased frequency in children with IBD. Quality-of-life questionnaires reveal several areas of difficulty, including lack of energy to engage in sports, problems with long trips because of unavailable toilet facilities, and inability to remain overnight at friends' houses. Parents were concerned about side effects of medications, their children's behavior, their own absence from work, and their children's future.

Since only a minority of pediatric patients have a family history of IBD, most children and their parents are unfamiliar with these disorders. Parents may inappropriately restrict their child's activities; this needs to be addressed by the treating physician. In view of the length of time children spend in school, teachers have an especially important role in the life of children with IBD. Special consideration may be necessary with regard to gymnastic activities and bathroom privileges.

Surgical Intervention

The indications for surgery in children with CD include medical intractability, suspected perforation or abscess, intestinal obstruction, and hemorrhage. A special circumstance in children is the potential of surgery for reversing growth failure especially when there is a localized area of resectable disease. This is optimally performed before the onset of puberty.

References

Baldassano R, Vasiliauskis E, Braegger CP, et al. A multicenter study of infliximab (anti TNF-α antibody) in the treatment of children with active Crohn's disease. Gastroenterology 1999;116:A665.

Barton JR, Gillon S, Ferguson A. Incidence of inflammatory bowel disease in Scottish children between 1968 and 1983; marginal fall in ulcerative colitis, three-fold rise in Crohn's disease. Gut 1989;30:618–22.

D'Agata ID. Mesalamine in pediatric inflammatory bowel disease: a 10-year experience. Inflamm Bowel Dis 1996; 2:229–35.

Gokhale R, Favus MJ, Karrison T, et al. Bone mineral density assessment in children with inflammatory bowel disease. Gastroenterology 1998;114:902–11.

Hadigan C, Baldassano R, Braegger CP, et al. Pharmacokinetics of infliximab (anti-TNF-α) in children with Crohn's disease: a multicenter trial. J Pediatr Gastroenterol Nutr

Hoffenberg EJ, Fidanza S, Logan L. New serologic tests for inflammatory bowel disease in children. J Pediatr Gastroenterol Nutr 1997;25:450.

Kirschner BS. Safety of azathioprine and 6-mercaptopurine in pediatric patients with inflammatory bowel disease. Gastroenterology 1998;115:813–21.

Mack DR, Young R, Kaufman SS, et al. Methotrexate in patients with Crohn's disease after 6-mercaptopurine. J Pediatr 1998;132:830–5.

Mahdi G, Israel DM, Hassall E. Cyclosporine and 6-mercaptopurine for active, refractory Crohn's colitis in children. Am J Gastroenterol 1996;91:1355–9.

Proujansky R, Fawcett PT, Gibney KM, et al. Examination of anti-neutrophil cytoplasmic antibodies in childhood inflammatory bowel disease. J Pediatr Gastroenterol Nutr 1993;17:193–7.

Ruemmele FM, Targan S, Levy G, et al. Diagnostic accuracy of serological assays in pediatric inflammatory bowel disease. Gastroenterology 1998;115:822–9.

Sadeghi-Nejad A, Senior B. Adrenal function, growth, and insulin in patients treated with corticoids on alternate days. Pediatrics 1969;43:277–83.

Weinstein TA, Sciubba JJ, Levine J. Thalidomide for the treatment of oral aphthous ulcers in Crohn's disease. J Pediatr Gastroenterol Nutr 1999;28:214–6.

CHAPTER 89

GASTRODUODENAL CROHN'S DISEASE

ROBERT BURAKOFF, MD

Involvement of the stomach or duodenum in Crohn's disease occurs in 0.5 to 13 percent of patients with ileocolonic disease. However, these statistics are rather misleading if one defines the meaning of gastroduodenal Crohn's disease in terms of histologic, radiologic, or endoscopic signs. For treatment purposes, obviously, only clinically significant Crohn's disease should be considered, and this is uncommon, representing 2 to 4 percent of all patients with Crohn's disease. These patients present with symptoms from erosive gastritis, gastroparesis, duodenal strictures, and fistulas. Signs of upper gastrointestinal (GI) Crohn's disease can be observed on double-contrast radiographs in 20 to 40 percent of patients with established lower tract Crohn's disease. A histologic diagnosis of gastroduodenal Crohn's disease (focally enhanced gastritis) has been reported to occur in 76 percent of *Helicobacter pylori*–negative patients with Crohn's disease. For practical purposes, the most appropriate definition of gastroduodenal Crohn's disease should relate to clinical symptoms and how these symptoms impact on the management of the disease.

Presenting Symptoms

Patients with gastroduodenal Crohn's disease often present with symptoms indistinguishable from those of peptic ulcer or drug therapy including 5-aminosalicylic acid (5-ASA) drugs, prednisone, and 6-mercaptopurine (6-MP) or azathioprine. These symptoms include postprandial pain and nausea and may progress to more continuous pain associated with nausea and vomiting, indicating the presence of gastric outlet obstruction secondary to gastroduodenal stricture formation.

Less commonly, gastroduodenal Crohn's disease has been associated with upper GI bleeding and with gastrocolic fistulae resulting in feculent vomiting, diarrhea, and weight loss. Upper GI tract fistulae usually arise from the ileum or the colon. Rare cases of pancreatitis and malignant degeneration in gastroduodenal Crohn's disease have been reported.

Radiology Findings

In a recent study of 55 patients with Crohn's disease, there was radiologic evidence of gastroduodenal disease in 42 percent (Zalev and Prokipchuk, 1992). Five patients

TABLE 89–1. Common Endoscopic Findings in Gastroduodenal Crohn's Disease

Notching of Kerckring's folds	Ulcerations
Erythema	Cobblestoning
Friability	Thickened folds
Erosions	Narrowing

had gastroduodenitis and 18 duodenitis. Only 13 percent of the patients with duodenitis had strictures. Radiologic features included nodularity and "cobblestoning" of the antrum as well as narrowing of the antrum, and, at times, poor gastric emptying. In the duodenum, the most common findings included ulcerations, mucosal (cobblestoning) nodularity, thickening of the folds, and gastroduodenal narrowing. Less common are intramural fissures comparable to those observed in small bowel disease. Gastrocolic fistulae are best diagnosed by a barium enema.

Endoscopic Findings

There are multiple nonspecific abnormalities noted with endoscopy in patients with gastroduodenal Crohn's disease (Table 89–1). The two most helpful observations in diagnosing gastroduodenal Crohn's disease are the absence of duodenal ulceration and the presence of "notching" of Kerckring's folds in the duodenum in a patient with upper GI symptoms. In two studies comprising 74 patients with Crohn's disease with or without upper GI symptoms, approximately 75 percent of the patients had endoscopic abnormalities, including mucosal edema, erosions, nodular lesions, thickened folds, and gastroduodenal narrowing. If ulcerations were present, they usually were longitudinal or serpiginous (Weterman, 1990). In a recent Japanese endoscopic study in patients with Crohn's disease, the presence of bamboo joint-like erosions and furrows on the lesser curvature of the gastric body and cardia was observed in 22 of 41 patients. Histologically, these endoscopic findings were significantly correlated with stromal edema and granulomas (Yokota et al, 1997).

Histologic Abnormalities and *Helicobacter pylori*

Granulomas are present in antral and duodenal biopsies in only 7 percent of patients if the mucosa appears normal. However, if endoscopic abnormalities are present, then the yield increases to approximately 30 percent. Histologically, the majority of patients have nonspecific acute and chronic inflammation. Two histologic observations that may be more specific for Crohn's disease have been made: (1) increased numbers of **macrophages** were observed by immunostaining in noninflamed gastroduodenal mucosa in patients with Crohn's disease compared to normal controls and patients with ulcerative colitis (Yao et al, 1996); (2) "**focally enhanced gastritis**" was noted on gastric biopsy in the absence of *H. pylori*. Focally enhanced gastritis was characterized by a focal infiltration of CD3+ lymphocytes, CD68R+ histiocytes, and granulocytes. Focally enhanced gastritis was found in 72 percent of patients and only in 0.8 percent of controls. There was no association between these histologic findings and clinical symptoms (Oberhuber et al, 1997).

Special staining techniques may significantly increase the ability of physicians to definitively diagnose Crohn's disease. The prevalence of *H. pylori* (30%) is not increased in Crohn's disease, but with persistent upper GI symptoms in a patient with Crohn's disease, upper endoscopy should be performed to rule out the presence of *H. pylori*. Of course, if *H. pylori* is present, then appropriate and complete therapy for eradication should be instituted to eliminate confusion regarding the upper GI symptoms.

Differential Diagnosis

The majority of endoscopic findings in Crohn's disease are nonspecific. In addition to *H. pylori*, the differential diagnosis includes peptic disease, eosinophilic gastroenteritis, sarcoidosis, Zollinger-Ellison syndrome, lymphoma, and adenocarcinoma. Therefore, multiple biopsies should be taken in any area of endoscopic abnormality.

Management of Gastroduodenal Crohn's Disease

Medical Therapy

Most patients with Crohn's disease do not need specific medical management of their gastroduodenal Crohn's disease. Treatment of the Crohn's disease should be based on the severity of the patient's overall symptoms with 5-ASA drugs, immunomodulatory therapy (6-MP or azathioprine), antibiotics, and judicious use of corticosteroids as indicated. Unfortunately, no controlled prospective study data exist on the use of any of the drugs cited for the primary treatment of gastroduodenal Crohn's disease. Endoscopy is the first diagnostic step to determine if an ulceration is present and whether it is secondary to Crohn's or *H. pylori*. The majority of patients with nonobstructing duodenal Crohn's disease without ulceration respond to corticosteroid therapy and in the largest studies to date, 42 of 46 patients treated with corticosteroids had a good-to-excellent result with a median follow-up of 10 years (Nugent and Roy, 1989). However, before using corticosteroids for chronically isolated gastroduodenal Crohn's disease, *H. pylori* should be ruled out and patients should be treated with adequate doses of proton-pump inhibitor and mesalamine (Pentasa®, Ferring-Shire Pharmaceuticals, Florence, Kentucky). There are now several case reports of duodenal ulcers secondary to Crohn's disease healing with proton-pump inhibitors.

Before using corticosteroids, effort should be made to ensure that the patient's upper GI symptoms are not due to nonsteroidal anti-inflammatory drugs (NSAIDs) or to medical therapy for Crohn's disease. Intermittent or persistent upper GI discomfort or nausea can occur with sulfasalazine, 5-ASA, 6-MP, or azathioprine, as well as from metronidazole. Before using corticosteroids, one should attempt to decrease or even temporarily withdraw the primary drug therapy for Crohn's disease to determine if one of these medications is the offending agent.

The topically active corticosteroid, beclomethasone, which is rapidly metabolized and has fewer side effects than prednisone, has been used with Pentasa and omeprazole in some patients. Azathioprine also reportedly is helpful. There are no published data on Remicade® (Centocor Inc., Malvern, Pennsylvania) usage for gastroduodenal Crohn's disease.

Endoscopic Balloon Dilatation

For patients with gastroduodenal strictures, the development of endoscopic balloon dilatation has been a major advance that has resulted in the avoidance of surgery for some patients with obstruction of the antrum and gastroparesis secondary to stricture formation. Patients with gastroduodenal strictures, especially short strictures, are good candidates for balloon dilatation. Adequate and, at times, intermittent dilatation must be undertaken to provide long-term symptomatic relief. With a rigiflex balloon (8 mm) or microvasive balloons (10 to 20 mm), progressive dilatation is most successful in achieving symptomatic relief. The risk of perforation is approximately 1 to 2 percent.

Surgical Therapy

Surgery for gastroduodenal Crohn's disease usually is reserved for patients with clinically significant gastric outlet obstruction. Rarely is surgery necessary because of continued upper GI bleeding. There is a chapter from the Lahey Clinic on this subject.

References

Nugent FW, Roy MA. Duodenal Crohn's disease: an analysis of 89 cases. Am J Gastroenterol 1989;84:249–54.

Oberhuber G, Puspok A, Oesterreicher C, et al. Focally enhanced gastritis: a frequent type of gastritis in patients with Crohn's disease. Gastroenterology 1997;112:698–706.

Weterman IJ. Oral, esophageal, and gastroduodenal Crohn's disease. In: Allan RN, Keighly MRB, Alexander-Williams J, Hawkins C, eds. Inflammatory bowel diseases. New York: Churchill Livingstone, 1990:319–27.

Yao K, Iwashita A, Yao T, et al. Increased numbers of macrophages in noninflamed gastroduodenal mucosa on patients with Crohn's disease. Dig Dis Sci 1996;41:2260–7.

Yokota K, Saito Y, Einami K, et al. A bamboo joint-like appearance of the gastric body and cardia: possible association with Crohn's disease. Gastrointest Endosc 1997;46:268–72.

Zalev AH, Prokipchuk EJ. Crohn's disease of the proximal small intestine: radiologic findings in 55 patients. Can Assoc Radiol J 1992;43:170–8.

Supplemental Reading

Inca R, Sturniolo G, Cassaro M, et al. Prevalence of upper gastrointestinal lesions and *Helicobacter pylori* infections in Crohn's disease. Dig Dis Sci 1998;43:988–92.

Matsui T, Hatakeyama S, Ikeda K, et al. Long-term endoscopic balloon dilation in obstructive gastroduodenal Crohn's disease. Endoscopy 1997;29:640–5.

Wagtmans MJ, van Hogezand RA, Griffioen G, et al. Crohn's disease of the upper gastrointestinal tract. Neth J Med 1997;50:S2–S7.

CHAPTER 90

CROHN'S JEJUNOILEITIS

C. NOEL WILLIAMS, MRCS, LRCP, FRCP(C), FACP

Involvement of the jejunum is one of the more unusual manifestations of Crohn's disease. The exact frequency is unknown, but about one patient per year presents to major centers, that is, centers with more than 1,000 patients with Crohn's disease attending their clinics. The incidence is highest in young patients. The importance of jejunoileitis is the associated high morbidity and frequent need for surgical management with the potential for creating intestinal insufficiency.*

Diagnosis

Patients with jejunoileitis tend to present at a younger age than those with distal ileal Crohn's disease. The predominant symptoms are periumbilical, colicky abdominal pain, in association with weight loss and diarrhea. Fever and growth retardation are not uncommon. Most patients require eventual surgical management, and some require two or more operations. Long-term follow-up of patients suggests that the disease tends to become less active with time, so that decreasing morbidity and conserving intestine, by strictureplasty, is essential.

There often is coexistent disease, either distal ileal disease, colon disease, or disease affecting the duodenum. In the largest radiologic study published, all 55 patients had presented before the age of 30 years: 14 had jejunitis alone, 18 jejunoileitis, 18 jejunitis and duodenitis, and 5 jejunitis and gastroduodenitis. Nineteen patients had previously undergone ileocecal resection. The terminal ileum was not affected in 11 of the 36 patients who had not undergone ileocecal resection. In contrast to ileal disease, the coincident presence of fistulae is uncommon. The symptom presentation is predominantly that of obstructive or subacute obstruction. Duodenal involvement is invariably a skip lesion in patients with disease of the terminal ileum. The diagnosis of proximal enteric Crohn's disease depends on the presence of one or more characteristic lesions in the jejunum or terminal ileum, perhaps associated with a duodenal or jejunal abnormality. Radiologic evidence of mucosal ulceration is seen in 88 percent of the patients with disease of the terminal ileum; it is less common in the jejunum (53%) and proximal ileum (57%). Sinuses are more common than fistulae. Proximal enteric

fistulae were seen in only 4 of 55 patients. By far the commonest radiologic appearance was that of strictures, occurring in up to 70 percent of the patients with jejunitis. These were uncommon in the duodenum and less common than in the distal ileum. Gadolinium-enhanced MRI, PET scanning, and labeled leukocyte studies are potentially more sensitive studies of small bowel mucosal inflammation and will play a greater role in the future.

Differential Diagnosis

In patients with multiple jejunal ulcerations, specific causes include drug reactions (potassium chloride, aspirin, nonsteroidal anti-inflammatory drugs [NSAIDs]), vasculitis, ischemia, rare infections (tuberculosis and syphilis), Zollinger-Ellison syndrome, rarely, celiac disease (gluten-responsive enteropathy), and small bowel neoplasia, especially lymphoma.

Nongranulomatous Ulcerative Jejunoileitis

In patients who present with colicky abdominal pain and diarrhea, especially with steatorrhea and weight loss, sometimes with fever, radiography may demonstrate an ulcerated appearance in the jejunum. Usually these patients are older, in their forties and fifties. The absence of other sites of involvement and a negative family history for inflammatory bowel disease (IBD) point to the need for a small bowel biopsy. There may be total or subtotal villous atrophy, and often no response to gluten restriction. No granulomas are seen. Immune deficiencies (hypoglobulinemia) may be present. This condition in patients without a primary diagnosis has been labeled "nongranulomatous ulcerative jejunoileitis." Prednisone may be of benefit. A high risk of lymphoma often requires full-thickness biopsy to establish the correct diagnosis. These patients often do poorly, with bleeding, obstruction, or perforation of their ulcers, sometimes while receiving prednisone. There is a separate chapter on this unusual syndrome.†

---

* Editor's Note: In my clinic 8% of 530 consecutive patients had jejunal involvement. (TMB)

† Editor's Note: I receive approximately six referrals over 2 years of patients with unexplained jejunal ulcers: one may have Crohn's jejunitis; one may have lymphoma (rarely, angiocentric lymphoma); one may be taking NSAIDs or potassium; one may have an unusual ileal or ulcerative jejunitis; one may be vasculitic; and one may have some unexplained presumed infectious process. (TMB)

TABLE 90–1. Medical Therapy of Crohn's Jejunoileitis

5-Aminosalicylic acid	Pentasa
Oral mesalamine suspension	Salofalk oral suspension
Corticosteroid	Prednisone
IV Methylprednisolone	Beclomethasone
Immunosuppressant	Imuran
Inflammatory mediators	
Chimeric antibody to TNF-α	Remicade
Total parenteral nutrition (TPN)	
Enteral nutrition	
Rarely, home TPN	

IV = intravenous; TNF-α = tumor necrosis factor-alpha.

Management

5-Aminosalicylic Acid

Management of Crohn's jejunoileitis is difficult and often challenging. Of the originally introduced agents, sulfasalazine is an unsuitable medication for use in jejunal disease because its action depends on bacterial cleavage in the colon. Of the newer 5-aminosalicylic acid (5-ASA) preparations, the microencapsulated granules of Pentasa® (Ferring-Shire Pharmaceuticals Inc., Florence, Kentucky), with release starting in the duodenum, are of benefit (Table 90–1). Four grams per day is used to both induce and maintain remission. Few reports exist on Pentasa use with jejunoleitis.

Mesalamine suspension (enema) 4 g/d has been used successfully as oral therapy in this group of patients. A normal bioavailability improved after several weeks of therapy, with control of symptoms.

Corticosteroids

Corticosteroids are absorbed proximally, act throughout the gut, and are of benefit. Prednisone frequently is used in these patients because of the site of the disease and is successful treatment in at least half of the patients. A rapid decrease of the inflammatory response narrowing the lumen, which is the cause of the colicky pain, results in amelioration of the symptoms. The newer, focally released preparation with fewer side effects, ilealocolonic released budesonide (Entocort CIR®, Astra Draco, AB, Lund, Sweden) capsules, are unsuitable for proximal small bowel disease because the medication is absorbed in the distal ileum and undergoes major first-pass metabolism in the liver. Beclomethasone, another topically active and rapidly metabolized agent (or steroid), is given as a solution and is reportedly helpful in upper gastrointestinal (GI) tract Crohn's disease. Intravenous methylprednisolone is the drug of choice for patients requiring hospitalization because of uncontrolled symptoms.

Immunomodulators

In those patients unresponsive to prednisone, immunomodulation (most commonly with Imuran [Glaxo Wellcome Inc., Research Triangle Park, North Carolina] or 6-mercaptopurine) can be used. The drawback of this medication is the time for induction of remission, up to 3 months, although high-dose initial oral therapy may shorten this delay. Unfortunately, relapse is common when Imuran is discontinued; therefore, it should be used for 3 or 4 years, anticipating that the disease "burns out" with time. Imuran is not believed to promote stricture formation.

The introduction of Remicade® (Centocor Inc., Malvern, Pennsylvania), an antibody directed against the major inflammatory mediator, tumor necrosis factor-alpha (TNF-α), is a major advance in the management of Crohn's disease resistant to prednisone and Imuran. To date, there have been no reports of Remicade use in patients with jejunoileitis. However, from a pharmacologic viewpoint, this should work well and may be of advantage in the future.

Bowel Rest

Patients with jejunoileitis may present with significant malnutrition. Intravenous hyperalimentation is used to replenish nutrition. When tolerated, enteral nutrition is also useful in this situation.

Strictureplasty

The major surgical advance in managing these patients is bowel conservation by the introduction of **stricture-plasty**. Multiple strictureplasties have been performed, saving the bowel from being resected and preventing manifestations of the short-bowel syndrome. Patients with evidence of subacute obstruction whose symptoms cannot be medically controlled should be referred for surgical assessment. Innovative, **isoperistaltic, side-to-side strictureplasty** also can be used in selected situations to conserve bowel. **Bypass operations** of major affected areas are no longer performed now that strictureplasty is available. The chapter on strictureplasty provides details on results as well as a discussion of the risk of malignancy in strictures where continued immunomodulation may be necessary.

Short-Bowel Syndrome

In the past, many patients underwent multiple resections because of active disease, and a new syndrome, the short-bowel syndrome, followed. In such cases, the complications of renal stones; gallstones; vitamin B_{12}, folate, or iron deficiency anemia; and malnutrition become the focus of management. The consequences of steatorrhea and diarrhea may require supplements of calcium, magnesium, and fat-soluble vitamins A, D, E, and K. Enteral nutrition is of benefit for controlling the symptoms and promoting the well-being of these patients. Ursodeoxycholic acid is useful to prevent gallstone formation following ileal resection. High doses (15 to 20 mg/kg/d) may help reduce diarrhea by improving fat malabsorption. Renal oxalate stones can be addressed by increasing calcium in the diet and increasing fluid intake to 3 to 4 L/d. In the past, occasionally a patient with short-bowel syndrome would require home hyperalimentation, but, fortunately, this is now rarely necessary. Chapters on the short-bowel syndrome, gallstones in IBD patients, and oxaluria provide details on management.

Editor's Note

Jejunoileitis is a curse of young patients, perhaps genetically modulated, which has the potential for shortening lives if management is not well conceived and executed. In the past, three of my young patients with major problems due to jejunoileitis and its therapy died suddenly and unexpectedly. Fortunately, management of jejunoileitis has improved. (TMB)

Supplemental Reading

Baer AN, Bayless TM, Yardley JH. Intestinal ulceration and malabsorption syndromes. Gastroenterology 1980;79:754–65.

Bodzin JH. Home hyperalimentation for inflammatory bowel disease. Nutr Clin Pract 1992;7:70–3.

Dehn PC, Kettlewel MG, Mortensen NJ, et al. Ten years' experience of strictureplasty for obstructive Crohn's disease. Br J Surg 1989;76:339–41.

Fazio VW, Galandiuk S. Strictureplasty in diffuse Crohn's jejunoileitis. Dis Colon Rectum 1985;28:512–8.

Fazio VW, Tjandra JJ, Lavery IC, et al. Long-term follow-up of strictureplasty in Crohn's disease. Dis Colon Rectum 1993;36:355–61.

Michelassi F. Side-to-side isoperistaltic strictureplasty for multiple Crohn's strictures. Dis Colon Rectum 1996;39:345–9.

Saxon A, Stevens RH, Ashman RF, Parker NH. Dual immune defects in nongranulomatous ulcerative jejunoileitis with hypogammaglobulinemia. Clin Immun Immunopathol 1977;2:272–9.

Tan WC, Allen RN. Diffuse jejunoileitis of Crohn's disease. Gut 1993;34:1374–8.

Touze I, Gower-Rousseau C, Grandbastien B, et al. Diffuse jejunoileitis of Crohn's disease: a separate form of the disease? Gastroenterol Clin Biol 1999;23:307–11.

Williams CN. Pharmacokinetics of 5-aminosalicylic acid enteral suspension in patients with Crohn's disease and in normal volunteers. Can J Gastroenterol 1990;4:458–62.

Zalev AH, Prokipchuk EJ. Crohn's disease of the proximal small intestine. Radiological findings in 55 patients. Can Assoc Radiol J 1992;43:170–8.

CHAPTER 91

MEDICAL THERAPY OF CROHN'S COLITIS

E. JAN IRVINE, MD, MSC, FRCPC, AND FOROUGH FARROKHYAR, PHD

It was first recognized in the 1960s that Crohn's disease could involve just the large bowel. This observation, together with the increased diagnostic accuracy afforded by colonoscopy, likely contributed to the apparent increase in the incidence of Crohn's disease in the 1970s. Approximately 25 percent (range, 21 to 31%) of new cases have Crohn's colitis, and an additional 40 percent have both small and large bowel involvement (Harper et al, 1987). Indeed, descriptions of the demographics of patients enrolled in most clinical trials reveal a similar distribution. However, most trials have insufficient power to adequately address drug efficacy by site of disease, and even meta-analyses rarely are able to determine efficacy by site of disease, owing to the heterogeneity of the diseased populations.

The treatment goals for patients with Crohn's disease, irrespective of the sites involved, are to reduce symptoms, induce and maintain remission, improve health-related quality of life (HRQOL), and stimulate mucosal healing. Specific management also is based on patient preferences and the use of the most cost-effective strategies. Selection of treatment for Crohn's colitis is based on several important features of the disease, including the disease site (whether colitis alone or both small and large bowel), extent, severity, presence of complications or extra-intestinal manifestations, prior response to specific drugs, and perhaps disease behavior (inflammatory, fistulizing, stenotic). However, patient characteristics also are extremely important. Adverse effects of treatment; the patient's personality; the presence of anxiety or depression, which may reduce compliance; and the presence of comorbid conditions, which is more prevalent in older patients, also impact upon both the selection of and response to different therapies. Rectal and perianal disease (anal tags, fissures, anal canal ulcers, fistulae) occur in up to 35 percent of patients with Crohn's disease, is associated more frequently with colonic than with small bowel disease, and can help distinguish Crohn's disease from ulcerative colitis. Distal disease, involving the rectum or sigmoid colon, occurs more frequently in elderly patients and may be difficult to distinguish from ischemic colitis or the segmental colitis of diverticulitis (Carr and Schofield, 1982). This aspect is discussed in a chapter on colitis in the elderly. Segmental disease occurs when only

TABLE 91–1. Crohn's Disease Activity Index (CDAI) Scores, Symptoms, and Clinical Impression of Disease Severity

Characteristic	Mild to Moderate	Severe
CDAI	151–450	>450
Stool frequency	3 or less/d	6 or more/d
Blood in stool	Small amount, macroscopic	Obvious
Pus in stool	Small amount	Obvious
Pain	Occasional or mild	Continuous or severe
Systemic symptoms	Minor fever or weight loss	Fever, anemia, weight loss >6 kg

one or two colonic segments are affected or there are extensive "skip areas." Strictures may also occur. Extensive disease requires involvement of most of the large bowel. First-line drug recommendations are based on administering the drug to the site of maximum inflammation. Most of the commonly used drugs for Crohn's disease can be given intravenously, rectally (as a suppository, foam, or enema), or as a tablet (fixed or delayed release).

Crohn's Disease Activity Index

The Crohn's Disease Activity Index (CDAI) is used in clinical trials to assess disease severity but, although well validated, is not used in clinical practice. The CDAI measures eight variables, including stool frequency and consistency, abdominal pain, well-being, weight, hematocrit, use of antidiarrheal agents, and the presence of extra-intestinal problems associated with Crohn's disease. The presence of an abdominal mass appears to be highly predictive of the need for ileocecal resection. The score range (0 to >750) is used to classify disease as in remission (CDAI < 150), mild to moderate (CDAI 151–450), and severe (CDAI > 450). Table 91–1 lists typical symptoms of patients by disease severity. Patients with a CDAI > 450 generally are hospitalized.

Management of Crohn's Colitis

Medical treatment can be classified as supportive or specific. General measures include treatment of dehydration, anemia, nutritional or vitamin deficiencies, and the use of antidiarrheal agents, such as loperamide, or analgesics

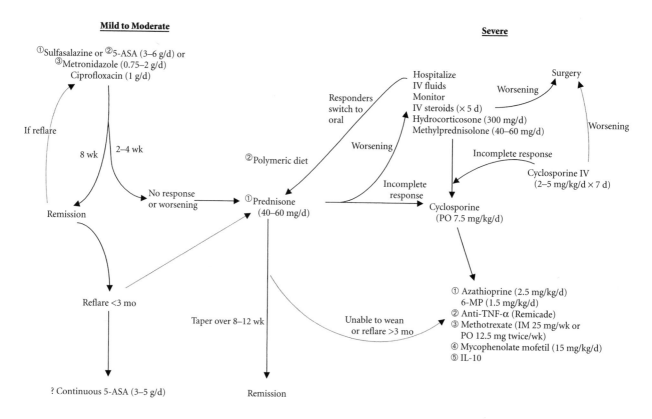

FIGURE 91–1. Suggested therapies for acute Crohn's colitis. ① – ⑤ = order of preference; 5-ASA = 5-aminosalicyclic acid.

when needed. Patients are encouraged to reduce fiber and caffeine intake if they have substantial diarrhea. Testing for lactose intolerance also may be appropriate. Specific measures are directed at the management of inflammation and halting the disease process. More potent drugs are needed in subjects whose disease has been flaring for an extended period without treatment or who respond poorly to initial treatment. Patients are encouraged to optimize their nutritional status, get adequate rest, and minimize stress. Those who smoke are strongly urged to discontinue, as continued smoking is a predictive factor of a poorer disease outcome. For general discussion purposes, it is assumed that patients may have either ileocolitis or colitis. When treatment differs for each of these sites, it is specified accordingly.

Acute Crohn's Colitis

MILD AND MODERATE DISEASE

Suggested guidelines for the treatment of active Crohn's colitis are shown in Figure 91–1. Newly diagnosed patients, who have mild or moderate colitis or ileocolitis, or those who have previously responded to these drugs, should be treated with sulfasalazine or a 5-aminosalicylic acid (5-ASA) in doses of 3 to 6 g/d for at least 8 weeks. Results of the National Cooperative Crohn's Disease Study (NCCDS), a multicenter, double-blind, placebo-controlled trial,

supported oral doses of 3 to 5 g/d sulfasalazine for colonic Crohn's disease. Higher doses usually are needed to control Crohn's disease compared to ulcerative colitis. Some patients may be slower to respond, and in those patients it is worth continuing treatment for up to 16 weeks. In subjects who are allergic to sulfa or who experience significant dose-related side effects of sulfasalazine, such as headache or nausea, other mesalamine compounds should be tried, based on tolerability, site of maximal inflammation, and availability. For colonic disease only, Asacol® (Procter & Gamble Pharmaceuticals, Cincinnati, Ohio) or balsalazide should be considered, whereas Asacol, Pentasa® (Ferring-Shire Pharmaceuticals Inc., Florence, Kentucky), Salofalk® (Axcan Pharma Inc., Minneapolis, Minnesota), Mesasal® (SmithKline Beecham, Philadelphia, Pennsylvania), Quintasa® (Ferring-Shire Pharmaceuticals Inc.), or Rowasa® (Solvay Pharmaceuticals Inc., Marietta, Georgia) are preferred if the small bowel is also involved. For male patients wishing to plan a family, 5-ASAs are preferred over sulfasalazine, because they do not affect sperm count or motility. When cost is an important consideration, there are considerable cost savings if patients can tolerate oral sulfasalazine, as it is cheaper than the mesalamine compounds. Mesalamine or sulfasalazine given in combination with oral steroids may or may not be more effective for acute colitis than steroids alone, but seem to work more rapidly in some patients.

Rectal preparations should be considered for patients with distal involvement, although some may refuse to use topical therapy. Rectal therapies are generally well tolerated and because of the limited absorption, even steroid adverse effects are minimal. If disease is limited to the rectum (distal 15 cm), 5-ASA suppositories (1.0 to 1.5 g/d) for 4 weeks or longer are needed. For more extensive disease, enemas are more likely to be efficacious because the larger volume (60 to 100 mL) is delivered more proximally and, therefore, is in contact with more of the inflamed mucosa. Patients should continue therapy for at least 2 weeks after symptoms disappear. Compliance is better if dosing is less frequent, making larger dosing units preferable. Steroid suppositories (hydrocortisone 10 to 40 mg), foams, or enemas can be used as an alternative to rectal 5-ASA but may be less effective. Combining oral and rectal preparations also is useful and may improve efficacy. These recommendations are based on observations, as most clinical trial data concerning rectal therapy come from ulcerative colitis.

For patients who do not respond or are allergic to 5-ASA, or those with moderately severe disease, corticosteroids given as 40 to 60 mg/d of prednisone or prednisolone in a single morning dose is suggested. A lower dose, such as 30 to 40 mg/d, should be considered for milder disease or if patients experience adverse effects, particularly hyperphagia, worsening diabetes, difficulty sleeping, or mood swings. Seventy-eight percent of patients in the NCCDS responded to steroids given similarly. Patients should continue this dose for 1 to 2 weeks, and then taper gradually, by approximately 5 mg/wk until the drug can be discontinued or symptoms worsen. If patients are unable to completely discontinue steroids without deterioration, or have been maintained on steroids for over 3 months, even at a relatively low dose, they should be tried on an immunosuppressive drug to permit steroid weaning. In the NCCDS, among patients who were already taking steroids at the time of flare, there was no benefit in switching to sulfasalazine or 5-ASA. Most practitioners use maximum doses of 5-ASA in patients with Crohn's colitis who require steroids; some also prescribe metronidazole or ciprofloxacin at the same time.

In controlled studies, antibiotics, particularly metronidazole, given orally at a dose of 750 mg to 2g/d, were useful only in milder disease. In the Cooperative Crohn's Disease Study in Sweden (CCDSS), a double-blind, randomized, crossover trial, metronidazole was most useful in mild Crohn's colitis that had failed to respond to 5-ASA (Ursing et al, 1982). Ciprofloxacin is also effective at a dose of 1g/d and can be combined with metronidazole for mild to moderate ileal or colonic Crohn's disease (Colombel et al, 1999). As with all treatment regimens, only a subgroup of patients will respond. In practice, some physicians add metronidazole or ciprofloxacin or both to the treatment regimen of incompletely responsive patients. This might be while awaiting the onset of immunomodulator therapy. There is a separate chapter on antibiotic use in Crohn's disease. Patients who receive more than 1 g/d of metronidazole for longer than 8 weeks are at high risk of developing peripheral neuropathy.

Corticosteroids are the first-line therapy for moderate or severe Crohn's colitis. Most clinicians test the stool for *Clostridium difficile* toxin prior to steroid treatment, because a small number of patients have a superimposed infection, making them appear refractory to treatment. In the NCCDS, prednisone, 0.5 mg/kg and 0.75 mg/kg, was used for mild and moderate disease, respectively, and was superior to placebo for inducing remission, irrespective of disease distribution. For patients with ileal or ileocecal Crohn's disease who experience serious adverse effects, the topically acting corticosteroid, budesonide, has been shown to be effective in several trials in a controlled ileal-release formulation at a recommended dose of 9 mg/d (single dose) or 4.5 mg twice daily (bid) for 8 weeks. Frequency of side effects is similar to that of placebo. However, a dosage form that provides colonic delivery is not widely available and has not been conclusively effective for extensive colitis in preliminary testing. As described in the chapter on topically active corticosteroids, ileocolonic-released budesonide (Entocort CIR®, Draco, AB, Lund, Sweden) can be helpful when tapering prednisone in patients with extensive colonic disease.

Nutritional therapy with polymeric oral or enteral feeding may be useful in some patients with Crohn's disease, particularly those with small bowel disease who refuse to take corticosteroids, children in whom use of corticosteroids is contraindicated because of the growth retardation factor, or in those who have malnutrition. Enteral feeding does not appear to be superior to corticosteroids, and polymeric diets are as efficacious as elemental or oligomeric protein diets. There are two chapters on enteral feeding. If enteral feeding is used, intake of regular food should be limited during the 4 to 6 weeks of treatment necessary. Nutritional therapy is worthwhile considering, perhaps even in patients with colonic disease. Poor palatability, high cost, and inconclusive results in patients with colonic disease preclude widespread use of such regimens. Bowel rest and total parenteral nutrition (TPN) until the onset of action of immunomodulators is discussed in a separate chapter.

The use of immunosuppressive agents such as azathioprine (AZA) (2.5 mg/kg/d) or 6-mercaptopurine (6-MP) (1.5 mg/kg/d) appears to be beneficial in meta-analysis for acute Crohn's disease even as a first-line therapy (Pearson et al, 1995). These drugs may be useful in milder disease, in patients who refuse to use corticosteroids, or, alternatively, in combination with standard-dose corticosteroids. Patients may then continue maintenance therapy after steroid withdrawal. For patients who have more severe disease, they are less useful as monotherapy because of the relatively long interval until maximum benefit (3 to 4 mo). A bridging therapy, such as cyclosporine in large doses, or perhaps Remicade® (Centocor Inc., Malvern, Pennsylvania), may need to be considered.

Severe Disease

Patients with severe Crohn's disease who have not responded to oral steroids in doses of up to 60 mg/d, or combination therapies, require hospitalization and initiation of intravenous steroids, using a regimen similar to that used for fulminant ulcerative colitis (hydrocortisone 300 mg/d or methylprednisolone 60 mg/d). Correction of dehydration and nutritional deficiencies, careful monitoring of blood counts, electrolytes, albumin, and inflammatory markers, as well as watching for complications, such as toxic megacolon or perforation, are important. Treatment of sepsis or impending perforation with broad-spectrum antibiotics may be necessary. Enteral or parenteral nutrition or supplementation may be considered for patients with significant malnutrition or those with extensive or fistulizing disease. Observational evidence suggests that the addition of intravenous cyclosporine in patients with fulminant Crohn's colitis (2 to 5 mg/kg/d), given as continuous therapy, may avoid colectomy for some patients. This is usually started, as for ulcerative colitis, after 5 to 7 days, if steroids alone have not resulted in substantial improvement. Careful monitoring of renal function and blood levels and anticipation of serious opportunistic infections, such as *Pneumocystis carinii* or cytomegalovirus, are mandatory. Treatment can be continued for 7 to 10 days and responders often show dramatic clinical improvement and a rapid decrease in inflammatory markers, such as erythrocyte sedimentation rate or C-reactive protein. Subjects may then be switched to oral therapy before discharge. Patients who fail to respond to this regimen should undergo urgent subtotal colectomy Patients who avoid colectomy, should receive gradual tapering of their prednisone, maintenance for up to 2 months with oral cyclosporine, and gradual crossover from cyclosporine to an antimetabolite in standard doses. Again, opportunistic infection must be anticipated and Bactrim DS given thrice weekly as prophylaxis is employed by some groups. Appropriate monitoring is needed (blood levels, renal function), and long-term outcome may still result in subsequent surgery. Remicade is being used in some patients with severe disease.

Refractory Disease and Steroid-Dependent Disease

Immunomodulators

Immunosuppressive drugs, such as AZA, 6-MP, cyclosporine, methotrexate, and new biologic, may be valuable in refractory disease (steroid-resistant) or steroid-dependent disease by increasing remission rate, reducing steroid requirement, or aiding avoidance of surgery. Patients who have responded to and tolerate AZA after withdrawal of drug have relapse rates approximately twice those of patients who continue therapy (Pearson et al, 1995). This benefit seems to last for up to 5 years. Although relatively rare, life-threatening toxicity, such as bone marrow suppression and sepsis, remains an ongoing risk, irrespective of treatment duration. Recently, mycophenolate mofetil (15 mg/kg/d) plus prednisolone was shown to work more quickly and with less toxicity than AZA (2.5 mg/kg) with prednisolone (50 mg), particularly in patients with more severe chronic active Crohn's disease (Neurath et al, 1999).

Cyclosporine and Methotrexate

Results of one trial support the use of a relatively high dose of oral cyclosporine (7.6 mg/kg/d) in patients with steroid-resistant Crohn's disease (Brynskov et al, 1989). Adverse effects, particularly renal compromise and hypertension, must be carefully monitored. Methotrexate given by intramuscular injection at a dose of 25 mg/wk for 16 weeks also was superior to placebo in patients with chronically active Crohn's disease, irrespective of disease site, but only in the subgroup that required prednisone more than 20 mg/d in the previous 3 months (Feagan et al, 1995). Oral methotrexate also is somewhat useful when given orally, in the absence of intestinal malabsorption, although data supporting this strategy are observational. Frequent monitoring of blood counts and liver function is needed. The possibility of allergic pneumonitis must be discussed with patients beforehand. Unexplained shortness of breath or cough necessitates immediate pulmonary-function assessment to rule out a restrictive defect. The drug should be discontinued if this occurs.

Biologic Therapies

For patients with moderate disease that flares despite ongoing treatment with 5-ASA, steroids, or AZA, a single intravenous infusion of chimeric monoclonal antibody to tumor necrosis factor-alpha (TNF-α) (Remicade) can be considered at a dose of 5 mg/kg. Significantly higher remission and decreased disease activity was noted in actively treated patients (all doses combined). Adverse effects include risk of infection, possible serum sickness in some subjects if a prolonged interval occurs between infusions, and lymphoma, which has been reported in several cases. The high cost of this treatment will likely limit its use. There is a separate chapter on biologic anti-inflammatory therapy.

Another study with similar entry criteria suggested significant benefit from daily intravenous recombinant human interleukin (IL)-10, given for 1 week at various doses (0.5, 1, 5, 10, and 25 μg/kg body weight) in active steroid-resistant Crohn's disease. Although no dose-

TABLE 91–2. Indications for Surgery in Patients with Crohn's Colitis

Problem	Recommended Surgery
Fulminant disease, unresponsive to treatment (perforation, megacolon)	Subtotal colectomy, ileostomy
Refractory disease, steroid dependent	Subtotal colectomy, ileostomy
Segmental disease	Segmental resection
Stricture	Balloon dilatation, resection
Intra-abdominal fistula or abscess	Drainage, subsequent resection
Simple perianal disease	Fistulotomy, drainage of abscess or seton insertion
Complex perianal disease	Defunctioning ileostomy (temporary or permanent)

response effect was noted, 81 percent of IL-10-treated patients experienced a clinical response compared to 46 percent of a placebo group. Flu-like symptoms were the commonest side effects (van Deventer et al, 1997). The cost of the biologic agents, need for careful monitoring, and limited availability may restrict their use.

Maintenance of Remission

The role of 5-ASA as maintenance therapy in Crohn's disease is controversial. No strong evidence exists except for patients with surgically induced remission. Soft evidence suggests a benefit in ileitis, a possible benefit in colitis, and little benefit from sulfasalazine. Doses required are 3 to 5 g/d, and although long term-use of 5-ASA is safe, there is considerable cost associated with indefinite use (Belluzzi et al, 1996; Messori et al, 1993). Ongoing treatment with AZA and 6-MP is supported by steroid sparing and a reduced relapse rate. Methotrexate at acute therapy doses (25 mg/wk) as well as a lower dose (15 mg/wk) is supported by observational data. Preliminary evidence suggests that an enteric-coated fish-oil preparation may be beneficial in some patients for prevention of relapse, but this is not yet widely available and confirmatory studies are needed. Indications for surgery are listed in Table 91–2.

Editor's Note

Remicade information and references are given in other chapters.

References

Belluzzi A, Brignola C, Campieri M, et al. Effect of an enteric-coated fish-oil preparation on relapses in Crohn's disease. N Engl J Med 1996;334:1557–60.

Brynskov J, Freund L, Rassmussen SN, et al. A placebo-controlled double-blind randomized trial of cyclosporine therapy in active Crohn's disease. N Engl J Med 1989; 321:845–50.

Carr N, Schofield PF. Inflammatory bowel disease in the older patient. Br J Surg 1982;69:223–5.

Colombel JF, Lemann M, Cassagnou M, et al. A controlled trial comparing ciprofloxacin with mesalazine for the treatment of active Crohn's disease. Am J Gastroenterol 1999;94:674–8.

Feagan BG, Rochon J, Fedorak RN, et al. Methotrexate for the treatment of Crohn's disease. N Engl J Med 1995;332:292–7.

Harper PH, Fazio VW, Lavery IC, et al. The long-term outcome in Crohn's disease. Dis Colon Rectum 1987;30:174–9.

Messori A, Brignola C, Trallori G, et al. Effectiveness of 5-aminosalicylic acid for maintaining remission in patients with Crohn's disease: a meta-analysis. Am J Gastroenterol 1993;89:692–8.

Neurath MF, Wanitschke R, Peters M, et al. Randomised trial of mycophenolate mofetil versus azathioprine for treatment of chronic active Crohn's disease. Gut 1999;44:625–8.

Pearson DC, May GR, Fick GH, Sutherland LR. Azathioprine and 6-mercaptopurine in Crohn's disease: a meta-analysis. Ann Intern Med 1995;122:132–42.

Ursing BO, Alm T, Barany F, et al. A comparative study of metronidazole and sulfasalazine for active Crohn's disease study in Sweden. II. Result. Gastroenterology 1982;83:550–62.

van Deventer SJ, Elson CO, Fedorak RN. Multiple doses of intravenous interleukin-10 in steroid-refractory Crohn's disease. N Engl J Med 1997;113:383–9.

CHAPTER 92

Fistulizing and Perforating Crohn's Disease

Gary R. Lichtenstein, MD

The transmural nature of Crohn's disease predisposes to the formation of fistulae. The presence of fistulae indicates the penetration of the inflammatory response into adjacent organs, tissue, or skin. Fistulae have been categorized as either **internal** if they terminate into adjacent organs (eg, enterovesicular, ileocolic) or into the nearby mesentery and **external** if they terminate on the surface of the body (eg, enterocutaneous, perianal).

External fistulae occur most commonly in the form of enterocutaneous or perianal fistulae and frequently are associated with the presence of local pain, drainage, and possible abscess formation. Internal fistulae may be major, such as a gastrocolic fistula, which has the potential to cause short-gut syndrome by bypassing the majority of the digestive tract, or minor, such as ileocecal or ileoileal fistulae, which commonly are asymptomatic.

The incidence of intestinal fistulae complicating the course of Crohn's disease varies from as low as 17 percent to as high as 85 percent. The treatment for fistulae is dependent upon location and symptoms complicating their course. Perianal fistulae may be painful and associated with abscess formation, requiring surgical drainage or even proctectomy. At the other end of the spectrum, patients may have internal fistulae, such as ileoileal or ileocecal fistulae, that are asymptomatic and require no intervention.*

Medical Therapy of Fistulous Crohn's Disease

There have been few studies of medications specifically for treatment of fistulous disease. Corticosteroids have not been demonstrated to have efficacy in the treatment of fistulous Crohn's disease and in one report there was a suggestion that the use of corticosteroids increased the need for surgery. Also, in controlled trials of Crohn's disease some deaths occurred among patients with fistula-related abdominal masses who took concurrent corticosteroids in the era before computed tomography (CT) and sonography.

Antibiotics

Ciprofloxacin and Metronidazole

There have been no controlled trials specifically designed to evaluate the efficacy of antibiotics in the treatment of fistulous Crohn's disease; rather, these medications have been used empirically with success.

Ciprofloxacin, a fluoroquinolone antibiotic has a broad spectrum of coverage including gram-negative aerobic organisms. In two uncontrolled trials, reports indicated improvement in physician and patient global assessments in 12 of 13 patients using 1,000 to 1,500 g daily of ciprofloxacin for 3 to 12 months in severe perineal Crohn's disease (Turunen et al, 1989). In one of these reports, perianal pain diminished in four of five patients with active perianal disease after they received ciprofloxacin therapy for 4 days to 5 weeks. One patient with a rectovaginal fistula had partial closure.

Combination therapy with ciprofloxacin and metronidazole has been based on the rationale that metronidazole has antimicrobial activity against anaerobic bacteria and ciprofloxacin is efficacious against gram-negative organisms. After 12 weeks of therapy with metronidazole (500 to 1,500 mg/d) and ciprofloxacin (1,000 to 1,500 mg/d), there was improvement in 9 of 14 patients with complex fistulae (one rectovaginal) and healing in 3 patients. After cessation of medication, repeat administration was needed in 9 of 14 patients.

There also are uncontrolled trials of metronidazole for chronic fistulous perineal Crohn's disease. A clinical response was seen in 20 of 21 patients given 20 mg/kg of metronidazole daily with complete "healing" in 10 (56%) of 18 if the medication was maintained. Symptomatic improvement occurred in 90 percent within 2 weeks, and the remaining 10 percent noted improvement within 6 to 8 weeks. In another report, four of eight patients had fistula closure while on high-dose metronidazole. There was a symptomatic recurrence in over three-fourths of 30 patients within 4 months of ceasing use of metronidazole. Metronidazole must be used continuously to be effective. Adverse effects related to medication use

---

* Editor's Note: The thesis of this chapter is that patients with fistulizing or perforating disease may have inherently more transmurally aggressive disease. As a group, they require surgery earlier and more often, and they may benefit from earlier use of immunomodulator therapy. (TMB)

included paresthesia, which usually but not always is reversible, dyspepsia, a metallic taste, and an "Antabuse effect" (limiting the ability to ingest ethanol).[†]

Immunomodulators

6-MERCAPTOPURINE AND AZATHIOPRINE

Immunomodulatory medications are the most effective medical treatment for fistulous Crohn's disease, but relapses occur when the immunomodulation is discontinued. There are separate chapters on immunomodulators and on perianal fistulae. In the only controlled trial of 6-mercaptopurine (6-MP) (1.5 mg/kg) on fistulae in Crohn's disease, complete fistula closure was seen in 9 of 29 patients (31%) compared to 1 of 17 (6%) in the placebo arm. There was a partial response in seven patients (24%) who received 6-MP compared to three patients (18%) who received a placebo. The overall response rate was 55 percent for those patients who received 6-MP. These same patients plus five others were later reported to have a 39 percent complete closure rate with another 26 percent demonstrating improvement. Twenty-four patients had a single fistula and 10 had multiple fistulae, including perirectal, abdominal wall, rectovaginal, vulvar, and enteroenteric fistulae. The mean time to response was 3.1 months with 77 percent of patients responding at 4 months, and 100 percent of patients who responded did so by 8 months. Continuous therapy was needed to maintain fistula closure. Six patients remained on 6-MP with continued fistula closure, whereas in five of seven who discontinued medication the fistulae reopened. With reinstitution of 6-MP, the fistulae reclosed. In an uncontrolled trial from Baltimore, 26 patients (35 fistulae) experienced complete closure of all fistulae noted in 31 percent of patients; 54 percent had partial healing.

There are uncontrolled reports of 6-MP or azathioprine (AZA) being effective for the closure of a few gastrocolic and about half of enterovesicular fistulae. In a recent review of the world's literature there were 27 gastrocolic fistulae reported, with 24 individuals being treated surgically. There were three patients who were treated with 6-MP or AZA, all of whom responded. Enterovesicular fistulas in 18 (58%) of 31 patients reportedly closed with 6-MP and AZA therapy; 12 patients (39%) maintained their response.[‡]

METHOTREXATE

Methotrexate has been demonstrated to be efficacious for induction of remission in active Crohn's disease. The response time was 4 to 8 weeks, more rapid than with 6-MP or AZA therapy. Intramuscular methotrexate was reportedly transiently helpful in 9 (56%) of 16 patients with fistulae; closure was achieved in 4 and improvement in 5. When the dose was lowered or converted to oral medication, relapses occurred.

CYCLOSPORIN A

An important feature of intravenous cyclosporin A (CyA) use is the rapidity with which clinical efficacy is observed, often within 1 to 2 weeks. When CyA was administered intravenously at a dose of 4 mg/kg in a continuous fashion, 14 of 16 patients with fistulous disease responded acutely. There was complete closure in seven patients and moderate improvement in seven. The mean time to response was 7.4 days, and 9 of 10 patients who failed 6-MP or AZA therapy responded to CyA. A 1998 review cited a 90 percent response rate to intravenous CyA in the 39 patients reported in the literature. Relapse after cessation of oral therapy was significant (82%). (Patients were given oral therapy for a finite time after being converted from intravenous to oral therapy with CyA.) These uncontrolled data suggest that intravenous CyA is efficacious for fistulizing Crohn's disease as a rapidly acting bridge to maintenance therapy with AZA, 6-MP, or, perhaps, methotrexate.

INFLIXIMAB

There are several chapters on the biologic agent infliximab in this text. A statistically significant efficacy for infliximab (Remicade®, Centocor Inc., Malvern, Pennsylvania) treatment of fistulous Crohn's disease has been demonstrated in a randomized, multicenter, double-blind, placebo-controlled trial. In this study, which is described in detail in the chapter on perianal fistulae, 94 adults with draining abdominal or perianal fistulae that had been present for at least 3 months were given either placebo (31 patients), 5 mg/kg of infliximab (31 patients), or 10 mg/kg of infliximab (32 patients) intravenously at weeks 0, 2, and 6.

Sixty-eight percent of patients who received infliximab at a dose of 5 mg/kg and 56 percent who received infliximab at 10 mg/kg experienced closure of at least half of their fistulae compared to 26 percent of the patients in the placebo group ($p = .002$ and $p = .02$, respectively). Fifty-five percent of the patients receiving 5 mg/kg and 38 percent receiving 10 mg/kg had closure of all fistulae compared with 13 percent who received placebo ($p = .001$ and $p = .04$, respectively). The median length of time for fistula closure was approximately 3 months.[§]

[†] Editor's Note: If the metronidazole dose is less than 1 g/d, few patients develop neuropathy. At dosages of 1,500 to 2,000 mg, many patients will complain of neuropathic symptoms, especially in the feet. (TMB)

[‡] Editor's Note: If the enterovesicular fistula is the result of intestinal obstruction, surgical resection may be the most effective long-term option. (TMB)

[§] Editor's Note: Men seemingly respond better than women. There were no data on success with rectovaginal fistulae. Only half of the patients had received 6-MP or AZA therapy before the trial. Reportedly the relapse rate after several months was high; thus, again, long-term immunomodulator therapy presumably will be needed. (TMB)

Other modalities and agents have been used for the treatment of fistulous Crohn's disease, including hyperbaric oxygen. The use of a temporary fecal diversion (such as occurs with a temporary diverting ileostomy) also has been successful; however, fistula recurrence is common upon takedown of the ileostomy or colostomy. Proctectomy for individuals with severe perirectal disease has been used, but perineal healing may be slow. Preliminary data are emerging regarding the use of fibrin glue, and mycophenolate mofetil and Tacrolimus have been used in preliminary uncontrolled studies with some short-term success.

Medical and Surgical Therapy

The collaboration of the gastroenterologist and the colorectal surgeon for examination under anesthesia, drainage of abscesses, and placement of setons is critical. There is a separate chapter on surgical approaches. Avoidance of muscle-cutting procedures and control of the infectious process are important goals. When simple fistulae are present, surgery (without a significant risk for incontinence and without the potential risk of immunosuppressive therapy) is appropriate. There are chapters on management of enteral and of postoperative fistulae.

Postoperative Recurrence of Crohn's Disease

It still remains exceptionally difficult to accurately predict the course of disease in an individual patient with fistulous disease. At least 70 percent of patients with Crohn's disease require surgery during their disease course and anywhere from 33 to 82 percent will require reoperation for their disease. In an attempt to better categorize the disease course a patient may follow, several patterns of Crohn's disease and its recurrence postoperatively have been described.

Indolent versus Aggressive Disease

In 1971 (De Dombal et al), two distinct populations of individuals were described among 169 patients: the first, those who had preoperative illness, often colonic disease, for less than 12 months and presented with postsurgical recurrence within 2 years (early), and the other, those with preoperative history longer than 14 months who presented with recurrence after 5 to 10 years (late). Two forms of Crohn's disease were delineated: an aggressive form that requires surgery soon after diagnosis and a more benign or indolent form, not associated with late surgery and that recurred less often and later after resection.

This concept of having two forms of Crohn's disease, one aggressive and one indolent, has been confirmed by other groups. Sachar and colleagues (1983) at Mount Sinai Hospital in New York reported that the risk of recurrence postoperatively in patients with symptoms for

less than 10 years was 65 percent, twice that of patients who had symptoms for more than 10 years (23%).

Two patterns of endoscopic recurrence also have been described: early recurrence, with severe lesions in the ileum proximal to the ileocolic anastamosis, and late recurrence, with less severe lesions. The severe lesions were large serpiginous ulcerations. There is a chapter by Rutgeerts on postoperative recurrences in this text.

Perforating versus Nonperforating Types

Greenstein and colleagues (1988) at Mount Sinai Hospital in New York reinforced this subtyping in a review of surgical indications for initial and subsequent operations in 770 patients with Crohn's disease undergoing intestinal resection. They observed that disease occurred in two different clinical patterns, independent of anatomic distribution. The relatively aggressive "perforating" type, which forms fistulae and abscesses (eg, acute free perforations, subacute perforation with abscess formation, and chronic perforation with internal fistulization), was present in 375 patients at the initial surgery. The more indolent "nonperforating" type, which was associated with obstruction, intractability, hemorrhage, and toxic dilatation, was present in 395 patients at the initial surgery. These types tended to retain their identities between repeated operations, and they influenced the rapidity with which reoperation was performed. Among 292 patients (38%) who underwent second operations for recurrent Crohn's disease, the indications for the second operation were closely dependent upon the indication for primary resection. Operations for perforating indications were followed by reoperation nearly three times as often and in half the time interval compared to operations for nonperforating indications whether going from first to second operation (perforating, 4.7 yr vs nonperforating, 8.8 yr) or from second to third operation (perforating, 2.3 yr vs nonperforating, 5.2 yr).[//]

Subsequent studies have not all agreed about the importance of surgical indication in predicting early postoperative recurrence. A Swiss study of 56 patients confirmed that a perforating indication for initial surgery was the main factor associated with early postoperative recurrence. Studies from the Cleveland Clinic and a small prospective study from Mount Sinai did not confirm the concept. Recently, our group at the University of Pennsylvania published the largest study, to date, to address the issue of predictors of early postoperative recurrence of Crohn's disease since the original two studies conducted at Mount Sinai Hospital and a subsequent one at the Cleveland Clinic. We used multivariable analysis to more accurately determine the independent role of surgical

---

[//] Editor's Note: Greenstein and colleagues later suggested that there are cytokine and molecular differences that may explain the aggressive and indolent forms of Crohn's disease. (TMB)

indication in predicting earlier recurrence. We found that a perforating indication and a longer preoperative duration of disease were independent predictors of an earlier recurrence of Crohn's disease after initial resection. In addition, a longer preoperative duration showed a borderline association with earlier recurrence after second resection. Finally, the type of indication for the initial resection strongly predicted a similar indication for subsequent resection. This suggests that the essential character of Crohn's disease in a patient is already firmly determined at the time of first resection regardless of future interventions. Despite advances in the understanding of Crohn's disease, it remains exceptionally difficult to accurately predict the course of the disease in an individual patient. In terms of medical therapy it may be appropriate to place those patients who are of the perforating phenotype on aggressive medical therapy, such as AZA or 6-MP preoperatively or following resection. The role of Remicade is being determined.

Specific Fistulae

ENTEROVESICULAR FISTULAE

Enterovesicular fistulae are discussed in a separate chapter, and the issue of medical versus surgical therapy is debated.

RECTOVAGINAL FISTULAE

The vagina may be a site of involvement by Crohn's disease, with reports of prevalence ranging from 3.5 percent to 23 percent among patients with Crohn's disease. When rectal pain occurs in conjunction with the fistulae, there is frequently an undrained or partially drained intermuscular abscess; an attempt should be made to drain it. Feculent vaginal drainage is problematic, and correction of the underlying problem should be pursued. Therapy can be by surgery alone or in combination with medication. There is a separate chapter on the surgical options.

Medical therapy has been somewhat helpful in a minority of patients, and preliminary evidence has shown some promise for use of fibrin glue; however, results for complex fistulae in patients with Crohn's disease have been disappointing. In a 1985 report assessing efficacy of 6-MP in the treatment of fistulizing Crohn's disease, two of six patients experienced closure of rectovaginal fistulae and one of two with vulvar fistulae improved. Intravenous cyclosporine led to a rapid but often temporary improvement in five patients who had a total of 12 fistulae (5 enterovaginal, 3 perianal, 3 enterocutaneous, 1 enterovesical). Complete resolution of drainage occurred in

10 of the 12 fistulae with initial response after a mean of 3.6 days, and complete cessation of drainage after a mean of 7.9 days. Relapse occurred in two perianal fistulae and in two enterovaginal fistulae. In another report of a 2-week course of intravenous cyclosporine (4 mg/kg) with subsequent continued oral conversion, 4 of 10 patients with perirectal disease and 1 of 2 with rectovaginal fistula experienced fistula closure after 2 weeks of therapy. After a mean follow-up of 1 year, 7 of 10 patients with perineal disease continued their oral cyclosporine; about half had improved and half had fistula closure. Both individuals who had rectovaginal fistulae had recurrence, and one required surgery. No controlled trial with the endpoint of fistula closure has been conducted to assess enterovesicular fistulae or enterovaginal fistulae. There was no mention of enterovaginal fistulae in the report on infliximab (Remicade) by Present et al in *The New England Journal of Medicine* (1999).

References

De Dombal FT, Burton I, Goligher JC. Recurrence of Crohn's disease after primary excisional surgery. Gut 1971;12:519–27.

Greenstein AJ, Lachman P, Sachar DB, et al. Perforating and nonperforating indications for repeated operations in Crohn's disease: evidence for two clinical forms. Gut 1988;29:588–92.

Present DH, Rutgeerts P, Targan S, et al. Infliximab for the treatment of fistulas in patients with Crohn's disease. N Engl J Med 1999;340:1398–405.

Sachar DB, Wolfson DM, Greenstein AJ, et al. Risk factors for postoperative recurrence of Crohn's disease. Gastroenterology 1983;85:917–21.

Turunen U, Farkkila M, Seppala K. Long-term treatment of perianal or fistulous Crohn's disease with ciprofloxacin. Scand J Gastroenterol 1989;24:144.

Supplemental Reading

Hanauer SB, Smith MB. Rapid closure of Crohn's disease fistulas with continuous intravenous cyclosporin A. Am J Gastroenterol 1993;88:646–9.

Jakobovits J, Schuster M. Metronidazole therapy for Crohn's disease and associated fistulae. Am J Gastroenterol 1984;79:533–40.

Korelitz BI, Present DH. Favorable effect of 6-mercaptopurine on fistulae of Crohn's disease. Dig Dis Sci 1985;30:58–64.

Lautenbach E, Berlin JE, Lichtenstein GR. Risk factors for early postoperative recurrence of Crohn's disease. Gastroenterology 1998;115:259–67.

McDonald PJ, Fazio VW, Farmer RG, et al. Perforating and nonperforating Crohn's disease: an unpredictable guide to recurrence after surgery. Dis Colon Rectum 1989;32:117–20.

Crohn's Disease of the Anal and Perianal Area

As in the emerging therapies for the treatment of intestinal conditions, there is now renewed hope that many of the manifestations of Crohn's disease in the anal area can be treated with continence-sparing operations combined with newer and more effective medications. Although the reported frequency of anal Crohn's varies widely in the literature, it probably occurs to some degree in over half of patients with Crohn's disease, and perhaps more commonly in patients with large intestinal Crohn's disease. Patients with anal Crohn's disease usually are symptomatic, and occasionally symptoms can be disabling, especially when there is the added problem of loose consistency of the stools. Nonetheless, with the proper management of anal Crohn's disease, the vast majority of patients will not require a permanent stoma.

Management Strategies

Patients need a multifaceted approach to the treatment of anal Crohn's disease. Stool consistency needs to be optimized, and certain types of anal manifestations need not be treated. There is no need to surgically treat large tags or hemorrhoids in these patients. Excisional therapy for such problems can lead to serious scarring, infection, and poor healing. A common scenario is the patient who has moderate to severe symptoms who undergoes a painful office examination, precluding thorough evaluation. These patients need to be examined under anesthesia, with a thorough evaluation and drainage of any abscess present, placement of a drain, and gentle dilatation of any narrowing. Then the patient, surgeon, and gastroenterologist can proceed with a medical plan that may include antibiotic therapy, immunosuppresives, and, currently, anti-tumor necrosis factor treatment for maximization of healing of the area.

When fistulae are present, depending on the severity and location, operative intervention has a high probability of helping the patient. Low asymptomatic fistulae do not require treatment; low symptomatic fistulae can be treated by fistulotomy, if there is no major inflammation in the area, including the rectum (Williams et al, 1991). Complex fistulae with major sphincter involvement or multiple tracks require maximization of medical management, and then consideration of some type of palliative drainage procedure or an advancement flap operation. The latter should be considered only when there is reasonably controlled disease elsewhere and minimal to mild rectal disease. Advancement flap operations in Crohn's disease, with appropriate medical management and patience (meaning willingness to consider repeating the flap procedure or diversion and repeating of the procedure when it first fails), can lead to healing of

the fistula in as high as 60 or 70 percent of patients (Hull and Fazio, 1997). With newer medical therapies and the use of new intraoperative techniques, such as fibrin glue tissue adhesives, it may be possible to achieve even higher success rates in patients with complex anal Crohn's disease, in the near future. The authors generally do not "give up" on consideration of a continence-sparing approach for patients with anal Crohn's disease unless the sphincters are severely compromised and the rectum itself also is refractory to medical therapy, or if the patient is quite elderly and it is more reasonable to ask the patient to live with a permanent stoma.

References

Allan A, Andrews MB, Hilton CJ, et al. Segmental colonic resection is an appropriate operation for short skip lesions due to Crohn's disease of the colon. World J Surg 1989;13:611–6.

Cooke WT, Mallas E, Prior P, et al. Crohn's disease: course, treatment, and long-term prognosis. QJM 1980;49:363–84.

Cooper JC, Jones D, Williams NS. Outcome of colectomy and ileorectal anastomosis in Crohn's disease. Ann R Coll Surg Engl 1986;68:279–82.

Farmer RG, Hawk WA, Turnbull RB. Indications for surgery in Crohn's disease: analysis of 500 cases. Gastroenterology 1976;71:245–50.

Fazio VW, Marchetti F, Church J, et al. Effects of resection margins on the recurrence of Crohn's disease in the small bowel: a randomized controlled trial. Ann Surg 1996;224:563–73.

Harper PH, Fazio VW, Lavery IC, et al. The long-term outcome in Crohn's disease. Dis Colon Rectum 1987;30:174–9.

Hull TL, Fazio VW. Surgical approaches to low anovaginal fistula in Crohn's disease. Am J Surg 1997;173:95–8.

Longo WE, Oakley JR, Lavery IC, et al. Outcome of ileorectal anastomosis for Crohn's colitis. Dis Colon Rectum 1992;35:1066–71.

Milsom JW, Boehm B, Hammerhofer KA, et al. A prospective randomized trial comparing laparoscopic versus conventional techniques in ileal Crohn's disease. Presented at the Annual Meeting of the American Society of Colon and Rectal Surgeons, Washington DC, May 4, 1999.

Ozuner G, Fazio VW, Lavery IC, et al. How safe is strictureplasty in the management of Crohn's disease? Am J Surg 1996;171:57–61.

Ozuner G, Fazio VW, Lavery IC, et al. Reoperative rates for Crohn's disease following strictureplasty: long-term analysis. Dis Colon Rectum 1996;39:1–5.

Williams JG, Rothenberger DA, Nemer FD, et al. Fistula-in-ano in Crohn's disease: results of aggressive surgical treatment. Dis Colon Rectum 1991;34:378–84.

Supplemental Reading

Heilberg R, Hulten L, Rosengren C, et al. The recurrence rate after primary excisional surgery for Crohn's disease. Acta Chir Scand 1980;146:435–49.

Lock MR, Farmer RG, Fazio VW, et al. Recurrence and reoperation for Crohn's disease. N Engl J Med 1981;304:1586–90.

CHAPTER 94

INDICATIONS AND PROCEDURES FOR SURGERY OF SMALL BOWEL CROHN'S DISEASE

ADRIAN J. GREENSTEIN, MD, FACS, FRCS

Crohn's disease is a panenteric nonspecific granulomatous inflammatory disease. Because of the tendency to recurrence following resection, patients with Crohn's disease are generally managed by medical therapy. Most respond to dietary or drug therapy. Surgical treatment for small bowel disease is advised for those who develop complications.

Indications for Surgery

Indications for surgery may be classified as **perforating, nonperforating,** or **inflammatory** (Greenstein et al, 1988). Perforating indications include free perforation, abscess, and fistula. Nonperforating indications include intestinal obstruction, medical intractability, and severe hemorrhage. Inflammatory disease, especially extensive jejunoileitis with weight loss and malnutrition, is generally considered a contraindication to surgical intervention unless strictures develop and strictureplasty or resection is required. Postoperative prophylactic medical therapy is helpful, especially in patients with inflammatory disease as the indication for resection.

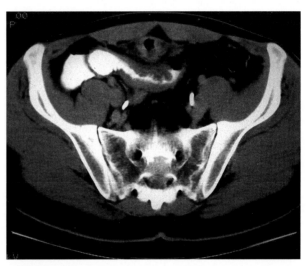

FIGURE 94–2. Computed tomographic scan with contrast demonstrating an irregularly narrowed small bowel loop with thickened bowel wall producing chronic progressive intestinal obstruction.

Nonperforating Indications

INTESTINAL OBSTRUCTION

Approximately half of the patients with distal ileal disease require surgery for intestinal obstruction (Figures 94–1 and 94–2). For the first episode of major obstruction, simple nonoperative measures, such as tube decompression and intravenous fluid support, suffice. Virtually all patients respond to such measures, but recurrent attacks are usual and constitute an inescapable indication for operative intervention, particularly in longstanding disease.[*]

MEDICAL INTRACTABILITY

Failure of medical management is most frequently an indication for surgical intervention in Crohn's disease involving the colon, but less commonly in small bowel disease. Surgery is required for failure of medical therapy with persistent and progressive symptoms, such as malnutrition, growth retardation, fever, and toxemia; steroid complications, such as osteoporosis, osteonecrosis, or

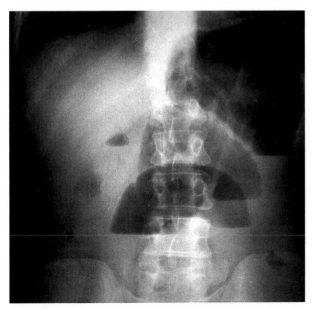

FIGURE 94–1. Flat plate of the abdomen showing an obstructed loop of small bowel.

---

[*] Editor's Note: In a series of 60 cases of childhood- or teenage-onset ileal disease, 30 underwent resection for obstruction at an average of 9.1 years after onset of disease. (TMB)

psychosis; and inability to use drugs, such as sulfasalazine, other 5-aminosalicylic acid (5-ASA) derivatives, and 6-mercaptopurine (6-MP), owing to side effects. In these patients, planned elective segmental resection with reconstruction of intestinal continuity is carried out.

HEMORRHAGE

Massive or recurrent hemorrhage, with or without severe anemia due to deep ulcerations, occasionally is an indication for surgical intervention.

Perforating Indications

Perforating complications may be subdivided into three groups, depending upon the rapidity of perforation, and adherence to surrounding structures: acute free perforation, subacute perforation with abscess formation, and chronic fistula formation. The latter is usually amenable to elective surgery, but free perforation and intra-abdominal or retroperitoneal abscess usually require urgent surgery.

ACUTE FREE PERFORATION

Acute free perforation into the greater peritoneal cavity is an uncommon complication of Crohn's disease and requires immediate laparotomy.

INTRA-ABDOMINAL AND RETROPERITONEAL ABSCESS

Intra-abdominal abscess results from perforation of the fissure ulcers of Crohn's disease into the perienteric areas. These abscesses are common and occur in approximately 20 percent of patients with regional enteritis. Presenting features include high spiking fevers, night sweats and chills, tachycardia, and elevated white blood cell count. However, the classic clinical picture may be obscured or attenuated by administration of steroids in high dosage. Most abscesses (53%) develop in the right lower quadrant of the abdomen and arise from the terminal ileum (Greenstein et al, 1985). Retroperitoneal abscesses may result in hydronephrosis, hydroureter, and fixed flexion of the thigh.

FISTULAE

Fistulae in Crohn's disease may be internal or external, with an incidence of approximately 33 percent and 15 percent, respectively. Internal fistulae are multiple in approximately one-third of patients. The most common, enteroenteric fistulae (Broe et al, 1982), seldom are symptomatic, and rarely require operation. Ileocolic fistulae are the most frequently occurring enteroenteric fistulae and the majority of these are ileosigmoid (Figure 94–3).

Enterovesical fistulae are found in approximately 6 percent of patients with Crohn's disease (Greenstein et al, 1984). The majority (approximately 60%) are ileovesical, with 15 percent colovesical and 15 percent ileocolovesical. Male patients outnumber female because of the anatomic

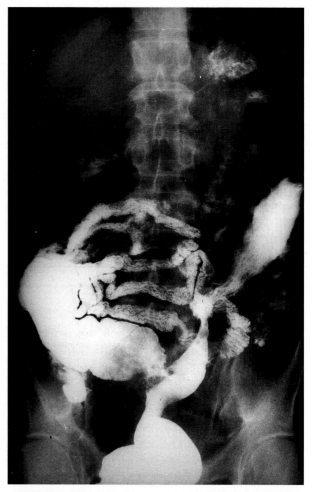

FIGURE 94–3. Two ileosigmoid fistulae in ileocolitis in a 52-year-old man with a 20-year history of ileocolitis, which required simultaneous ileocolic and sigmoid resection with reanastomosis and temporary diverting ileostomy.

location of the uterus in the female. The classic presenting symptoms are pneumaturia, dysuria, and fecaluria. Surgery almost always is required sooner or later, especially if obstruction of the bowel is present.

Enteric fistulae communicating with the renal pelvis, ureter, and urethra are rare and reportable cases.

Spontaneous external abdominal fistulae are rare. Only one of our five cases originated in the ileum (four colocutaneous, one ileocutaneous).

Ileocutaneous fistulae generally appear through the site of a postoperative scar. The author noted that peri-ileostomy fistulae, a particularly complex form of external fistula, occurred in 15 percent of patients. There is a separate chapter on postoperative fistula management.

Surgical Management

Preoperative Management

Surgery for Crohn's disease usually is reserved for patients who develop complications. Over 90 percent of patients who eventually require surgery have been treated with steroids, sometimes with sulfasalazine (Azulfidine®, Pharmacia and Upjohn Inc., Peapack, New Jersey), mesalamine (Asacol® [Procter & Gamble Pharmaceuticals, Cincinnati, Ohio] or Pentasa® [Ferring-Shire Pharmaceuticals Inc., Florence, Kentucky]), and in recent years with 6-MP or azathioprine (AZA; Imuran®, Glaxo Wellcome, Research Triangle Park, North Carolina). Steroids result in Cushing's syndrome, with fluid retention, hypotension, edema of skin and tissues, and friability and thinning of the integument, and impaired wound healing. Side effects of 6-MP and AZA include pancreatitis and bone marrow depression. These side effects, as well as anemia, leukopenia, and fluid and electrolyte imbalance, should be taken into account in the preoperative preparation. Preoperative and perioperative needs may include total parenteral nutrition (TPN) for malnutrition, intravenous fluids for metabolic abnormalities, blood transfusion for severe anemia, and Neupogen® (Amgen Inc., Thousand Oaks, California) for leukopenia.

The patient should be prepared carefully for surgery, both psychologically and physically. Complications, outcomes, and any long-term sequelae should be fully discussed prior to surgery.

Clear liquids should be given for 1 to 2 days preoperatively (longer in cases with obstruction) and polyethylene glycol, mannitol, or Fleet Phospho-soda (unless there is obstruction) the day prior to surgery. Preoperative antibiotics should include oral neomycin and erythromycin, 1 g each, at 2, 6, and 10 pm on the day prior to surgery and intravenous Kefzol and metronidazole on call to the operating room. High-colonic enemas with tap water until clear are recommended. In selected cases, such as patients confined to bed for long periods and those with severe edema owing to steroid medication, anticoagulants, such as perioperative intravenous or subcutaneous heparin, should be considered and compression stockings or venodynes used.

Surgery: Emergency versus Elective

Surgical operations for Crohn's disease may be subdivided into emergency and elective procedures. Emergency surgery is carried out soon after stabilization of the patient and is associated with a relatively high mortality rate. When elective procedures are planned carefully, with endoscopic and imaging studies repeated and the patient and bowel well prepared, mortality should be low. Laparoscopy has been advocated for selected elective cases, and trials are now in progress. There is a separate chapter on laparoscopically assisted bowel resection.

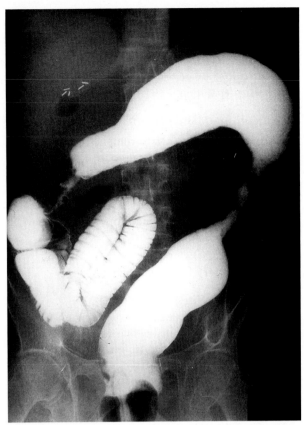

FIGURE 94–4. Two strictures in a 30-year-old woman following previous ileocolic resection. This required an extended secondary ileocolic resection with ileosigmoidostomy.

Surgery for Obstructing Disease

SIMPLE OBSTRUCTION

Ileocolic resection with ileotransverse colostomy was the earliest procedure used for intestinal obstruction (Figure 94–4). More recently, limited ileocecal or ileocolic resection with ileoascending colostomy has become the procedure of choice. These patients may be ideal candidates for laparoscopically assisted resection.

A particular form of obstruction in which an even more limited surgical procedure has been recommended is obstruction with multiple small bowel strictures, usually involving the jejunum, and associated with malabsorption. Strictureplasty, similar to a Heineke-Mikulicz pyloroplasty, may be of value in selected patients with short bowel, and in universal jejunoileitis with multiple areas of saccular dilatation alternating with areas of stricture (Lee and Papaioannou, 1982). Strictures always should be opened and biopsies taken of suspicious areas to rule out carcinoma. There is a separate chapter on techniques and results with strictureplasty.

CLOSED-LOOP OBSTRUCTION

Emergency surgery may be required in cases with closed-loop obstruction. In these patients, only limited preparation is possible. Inability to mechanically empty the bowel may make diversionary ileostomy necessary. Patients with incomplete obstruction, gas-filled loops, and fluid levels usually respond to nasogastric suction and then can be treated electively, perhaps after formal bowel rest preparation.

MASSIVE HEMORRHAGE

Massive hemorrhage is a rare complication in Crohn's disease. True massive hemorrhage occurs in 1 to 2 percent of patients. Ideally, the site will be known preoperatively. Following resection, the specimen should be examined immediately for a bleeding site. If no obvious bleeding site is found, intraoperative endoscopy should be carried out for an occult source.

Surgery for Perforating Disease

INTERNAL FISTULAE

Patients with fistulae usually can have complete bowel preparation and be operated upon electively.

Ileocecal and ileoileal fistulae rarely require surgery, because they bypass only a small segment of bowel and cause few symptoms. Surgery is necessary only for associated abscess with sepsis. An ileocolic or ileal resection with reanastomosis is the procedure of choice.

Ileosigmoid fistulae are the most common enteroenteric type of fistula, occurring in approximately 10 percent of patients. They are the most challenging, surgically, of the internal fistulae (see Figure 94–3). There is considerable debate as to whether ileocolic resection should be carried out with simultaneous sigmoid resection (Fazio et al, 1977), or whether simple closure of the sigmoid colon is adequate. Preoperative colonoscopy is essential and complete bowel preparation leaves various options open. If colonic disease demonstrated by colonoscopy is minimal, simple closure should suffice. If there is segmental colonic disease, especially with a stricture, or multiple fistulae, simultaneous ileocolic and sigmoid resection en bloc with two separate anastomoses is advisable. A concomitant proximal diverting loop is seldom necessary with the CEEA stapler currently available. For universal or extensive colonic disease, subtotal colectomy or proctocolectomy may be necessary.

Ileovesical fistulae are common, occurring in about 6.5 percent of patients with Crohn's disease coming to surgery. They are complicated in half of the patients by sepsis, which may be relieved by rupture into the bladder or may require surgical drainage.

The optimal surgical treatment for ileovesical fistulae consists of separation of the bowel from bladder, resection of the diseased segment of bowel with reanastomosis, and closure of the bladder with interrupted sutures. The most important aspect is leaving the urinary catheter in for a week. Among 38 patients treated in this manner, no recurrent bladder fistulae occurred (Greenstein et al, 1984).

Colojejunal fistulae are relatively uncommon and may originate in either colon (approximately two-thirds) or jejunum (one-third). These may be single or multiple and may be associated with localized or diffuse or discontinuous jejunal disease. Resection of the diseased bowel, proximal, distal, or both, cures the problem.

EXTERNAL FISTULAE

Patients with rare spontaneous fistulae that originate in the colon require ileocolic or colonic resection.

Most external fistulae follow previous surgical intervention, and most require surgical therapy. External fistulae usually develop immediately following surgery as a result of an anastomotic leak, or later in the postoperative course, as recurrent disease. The former often is a high-volume fistula and may heal with total intravenous hyperalimentation, but may require reexploration and proximal diversion to deal with septic complications. Reanastomosis may be carried out at a later date when the inflammatory process has resolved. Late fistulae may develop spontaneously or following incision and drainage of an intra-abdominal abscess; elective surgical treatment is recommended. Resection of the fistulous tract and area of recurrent ileitis with immediate reanastomosis should be carried out for perianastomotic recurrence. For peri-ileostomy fistulae, resection of the ileostomy, fistulous tract, and diseased bowel, with reconstruction of the ileostomy, with or without transposition, is the preferred surgical therapy.

FREE PERFORATION

The cornerstone of treatment of free perforation of the small bowel into the general peritoneal cavity is immediate laparotomy and proximal diversion with delayed reconstruction of intestinal continuity, or primary reanastomosis (Greenstein et al, 1987). Laparoscopic drainage with resection has been suggested by some but open laparotomy remains the procedure of choice.

INTRA-ABDOMINAL ABSCESS

Intra-abdominal abscesses may occur in any quadrant of the abdomen, but most frequently occur in the right lower quadrant, originating in the ileocecal region of the bowel. Pelvic abscesses are frequently encountered, usually arising from terminal ileum.

The safest treatment, especially for the enteroparietal form, consists of immediate incision or percutaneous drainage. Following resolution of the toxemia, a postoperative enterocutaneous fistula commonly forms. When recovery is complete, and steroid dosage is reduced as much as possible, a planned elective resection should be carried out. Deep intraloop or intramesenteric abscesses require drainage and resection, usually with defunctioning ileostomy to divert the intestinal contents.

Although percutaneous drainage of intra-abdominal abscess has been advocated in recent years, its value in Crohn's disease where thickened loops of bowel may be punctured is still to be proven. Percutaneous drainage as an initial procedure has been somewhat successful. Percutaneous drainage may be attempted in the critically ill patient with a deep abscess as a temporizing procedure to limit mortality. However, superficial abscesses usually should be opened surgically to evacuate the debris and necrotic tissue found within these abscesses.

Cancer and Crohn's Disease

Small bowel cancers are usually found in a strictured area of Crohn's disease. The surgical therapy of malignancy takes precedence over that of the Crohn's disease, because the primary objective is cure of the cancer. Surgery for cancer should be carried out with adequate resection of lymph nodes. Cure is relatively rare in small bowel cancer despite radical surgery.

Conclusion

Surgical intervention in Crohn's disease is one of the most challenging problems in clinical medicine. The decision to operate should be made by surgeon and gastroenterologist together. Surgical intervention, when made at an appropriate time following failure of medical therapy, can lead to a better quality of life, reduce morbidity, and minimize mortality in this chronic intestinal affliction.

Editor's Note

This detailed and very specific chapter illustrates the importance of considering the various subgroups of Crohn's disease as separate situations, each requiring different philosophies of management. The frequency of recurrence and the use of prophylactic medications postoperatively are discussed in another chapter. (TMB)

References

Fazio VW, Wilk I, Turnbull RB Jr. The dilemma of Crohn's disease: ileosigmoidal fistula complicating Crohn's disease. Dis Colon Rectum 1977;20:381–6.

Greenstein AJ, Lachman P, Sachar DB, et al. Perforating and nonperforating indications for repeated operations in Crohn's disease: evidence for two clinical forms. Gut 1988;29:588–92.

Greenstein AJ, Sachar DB, Tzakis A, et al. The course of enterovesical fistulae in Crohn's disease. Am J Surg 1984; 147:788–92.

Greenstein AJ, Sachar DB, Greenstein RJ, et al. Intra-abdominal abscess in Crohn's (ileo)colitis. Am J Surg 1985;143:727–37.

Greenstein AJ, Sachar DB, Lachman P, et al. Spontaneous free perforated abscess in 30 patients with Crohn's disease. Ann Surg 1987;205:72–6.

Lee EC, Papaioannou N. Minimal surgery for chronic obstruction in patients with extensive or universal Crohn's disease. Ann R Coll Surg Engl 1982;64:229–33.

Supplemental Reading

Broe PJ, Bayless TM, Cameron JL. Crohn's disease: are enteroenteral fistulas an indication for surgery? Surgery 1982;91:249–53.

Greenstein AJ, Meyers S, Dicker A, Aufses AH Jr. Peri-ileostomy fistulae in Crohn's disease. Ann Surg 1983;197:199–201.

CHAPTER 95

PERIOPERATIVE NUTRITION SUPPORT

MICHAEL D. SITRIN, MD

Nutritional therapy has become an integral part of the treatment of patients with inflammatory bowel disease (IBD). It must be appreciated, however, that nutritional treatments are used for various purposes in these patients, such as reversal of nutritional deficits due to IBD, primary treatment of the inflammatory disorder, or prevention of complications associated with IBD surgery. The goals of nutritional therapy should clearly be established at the outset, as these will determine the most appropriate type and duration of treatment. In this chapter, issues related primarily to nutrition and surgical management of IBD will be discussed. Other chapters in this book explore nutrition as primary therapy, the approach to specific nutritional complications, the special nutritional considerations of children with IBD and the short-bowel syndrome.

Perioperative Nutrition Support

One of the most common questions regarding nutritional management of IBD concerns perioperative nutrition support for the patient undergoing elective surgery. In the past, many IBD patients would receive a course of preoperative total parenteral nutrition (TPN) prior to elective surgery on the assumption that this would decrease postoperative complications and permit excellent bowel preparation for the procedure. Relatively scant data from controlled clinical trials are available on the impact of preoperative TPN specifically on IBD surgery. Collins et al reported that TPN decreased postoperative complications in patients undergoing proctocolectomy or proctectomy.

Recent studies of perioperative nutrition support in general, however, have raised some important issues regarding this approach. A large cooperative multicenter trial conducted in Veterans' Administration (VA) hospitals has explored the role of perioperative nutrition support in patients undergoing major elective abdominal or thoracic operations. Overall, patients who received a 7- to 15-day period of preoperative TPN support did not have fewer postoperative complications than those who did not receive nutrition therapy, and, in fact, had significantly more postoperative infections.

Nutritional Assessment

Further analysis of these data was performed by stratifying the patients according to their nutritional status. A Subjective Global Assessment that uses data from the history and bedside physical examination and a Nutrition Risk Index that considers body weight and serum albumin were used. Both techniques have been extensively validated as predictors of postoperative morbidity and mortality. Patients with severe malnutrition who received preoperative TPN had significantly fewer noninfectious complications and no increase in postoperative infections compared to those who did not receive nutrition support. In contrast, patients with borderline or mild malnutrition who received preoperative TPN had more postoperative infections than those who did not receive intravenous feedings and were not protected from noninfectious complications such as anastomotic leaks, respiratory failure, cardiac complications, wound dehiscences, etc. The higher postoperative infection rate in those receiving TPN was not explained by catheter-related infections, but was due mainly to more episodes of pneumonia and empyema.

Risks of Excessive Hyperalimentation

This VA cooperative study has been criticized by some who note that many of the patients treated with TPN received excessive intravenous energy intakes, putting them at higher risk for hyperglycemia, which can interfere with neutrophil function and predispose them to infection. Others have claimed that use of intravenous lipid emulsions to provide a substantial portion of the energy intake promoted infections. Nevertheless, other analyses of perioperative TPN also have quite consistently demonstrated an increase in postoperative infections in mild to moderately malnourished patients who received TPN.

Importance of Nutritional Risk Assessment

These observations emphasize the importance of performing a nutritional assessment of patients with IBD prior to surgery. Various assessment techniques and tools can be used, each with their own advantages and disadvantages. Although the causes of increased infection risk in TPN are at present controversial and uncertain, current data support the use of preoperative TPN only in patients with substantial protein-calorie malnutrition.

Optimal Duration of Nutritional Repletion

The optimal duration of TPN prior to elective surgery also is often debated. Faced with a severely cachectic patient with complex IBD, the surgeon often is tempted to request prolonged, weeks to months, of parenteral nutrition prior to operating on these high-risk individuals. Christie and Hill (1990) have studied the physiologic effects of nutritional repletion of patients with IBD awaiting surgical treatment. They observed rapid improvements in the function of respiratory and other muscles and increased levels of serum proteins *within 1 week* after initiation of TPN. These occurred at a time before significant changes in body composition could be demonstrated, and subsequent further improvements in physiologic function and repletion of body cell mass progressed very slowly. It is likely that the rapid gain of physiologic function following parenteral nutrition reflected enhanced cellular metabolism.

In general, a 5- to 14-day period of preoperative TPN prior to surgery can be justified for patients with severe malnutrition, but a longer duration has not been proven to be beneficial and would significantly increase medical costs. A recent analysis of the literature of perioperative TPN has found that preoperative TPN in malnourished patients decreased the complication rate, but TPN initiated *only* during the *postoperative period* was associated with a higher complication rate than was observed in untreated controls.

Effect of Preoperative Total Parenteral Nutrition on Operability

Using a case-control methodology, Lashner et al reported that Crohn's disease (CD) patients who received short-term preoperative TPN had somewhat smaller resections than matched patients who were not nutritionally treated prior to surgery. This important observation needs to be confirmed before recommending preoperative TPN as an approach to limiting the amount of bowel resection.* It must be emphasized that urgently needed surgery when complications of IBD such as abscess, perforation, or high-grade obstruction are suspected should not be delayed in the hope of improving the patient's nutritional status.

Enteral Nutrition

Controlled clinical trials have not been performed specifically comparing preoperative TPN with enteral nutri-

---

* Editor's Note: As a complementary aspect to this issue, Talamini and his colleagues report in the chapter on laparoscopically assisted bowel resection on the significance of preoperative weight loss. Weight loss was a predictor of having to convert a laparoscopic procedure to an open and more extensive operation. There is a message there. (TMB)

tional support of patients with IBD. Patients with ulcerative colitis (UC) and CD often tolerate tube feedings very well, and enteral nutrition support can provide both effective nutritional repletion and excellent bowel preparation in these patients. Furthermore, enteral nutrition support may avoid the postoperative infectious complications associated with current TPN regimens in those with mild to moderate malnutrition. Gonzalez-Huix et al (1993) compared enteral versus parenteral nutrition as adjunctive therapy in patients with acute UC treated with corticosteroids. Remission rate and need for colectomy were similar in both groups. In those who required colectomy, postoperative infections were more common with parenteral nutrition. Complications of nutrition support occurred more frequently in the parenteral nutrition patients. These considerations suggest that, when possible, tube feeding should be the first choice for preoperative nutritional rehabilitation.

The possible benefits of combining perioperative nutrition support with growth hormone as a means of more effectively promoting nitrogen balance and of repleting lean body mass of patients with inflammatory bowel disease is currently being investigated. Growth hormone and a high-protein diet is also being studied as treatment for active CD.

Fistulae

Gastrointestinal fistulae are among the most difficult complications in patients with CD. There are two chapters on enteric fistulae and their management. Patients with fistulae are often very malnourished, due to the severity of the IBD, loss of nutrients through the fistula track secretions, and predisposition for small bowel bacterial overgrowth and malabsorption. Several groups have examined the effect of TPN and bowel rest on fistula healing in CD. Some have reported high rates of healing whereas others found that fistulae rarely closed and stayed healed after TPN. These disparate results largely can be explained by recognizing that there are different types of fistulae in patients with CD. Postoperative fistulae occur due to anastomotic leaks or leaks at the site of drainage tubes, and generally are not associated with active IBD. These types of fistulae have high healing rates and generally close with 30 days or less of TPN and bowel rest. In contrast, enterocutaneous and enteroenteric fistulae due to CD per se generally originate from areas of active disease proximal to a site of obstruction, and perianal fistulae usually occur in the context of active rectal CD. These types of fistulae have poorer response to TPN and bowel rest. Although they frequently will close temporarily, they commonly reopen once oral food intake resumes. Overall, long-term closure of these fistulae occurs in less than 30 percent of patients, and surgical treatment usually is needed. Because of the high prevalence of severe malnutrition in patients with fistulae, nutritional therapy may play an important adjunctive role prior to corrective surgery. The chapters on surgical approaches and on Remicade® (Centocor Inc., Malvern, Pennsylvania) with enteric fistulae provide additional information.

Enteral nutrition support also has been successfully used to manage fistulae in CD, although the reported series are small and controlled comparisons with TPN have not been performed. Elemental formulas are nearly completely absorbed in the proximal small bowel, and generally are well-tolerated in patients with fistulae from the more distal intestine. In addition, fistulae from the stomach, duodenum, or proximal jejunum often can be bypassed by placing a feeding tube distal to the origin of the fistula, and tube feedings generally will not increase fistula output. Enteral nutrition support has been reported to improve perianal fistulae, but healing often is not complete.

Fistula track secretions often contain large amounts of certain micronutrients, such as zinc and vitamin C, that are important for wound healing. This has prompted some to recommend additional supplementation of these nutrients, although the benefit of this approach on fistula healing has not been proven.

Supplemental Reading

Baker JP, Detsky AS, Wesson DE, et al. Nutritional assessment: a comparison of clinical judgment and objective measurements. N Engl J Med 1982;306:969–72.

Calam J, Crooks PE, Walker RJ. Elemental diets in the management of Crohn's perianal fistulae. JPEN 1980;4:4–8.

Christie PM, Hill GL. Effect of intravenous nutrition on nutrition and function in acute attacks of inflammatory bowel disease. Gastroenterology 1990;99:730–6.

Fukuci S, Seeburger J, Parquet P, et al. Nutrition support of patients with enterocutaneous fistulae. Nutr Clin Pract 1998;13:59–65.

Gonzalez-Huix F, Fernandez-Banares F, Esteve-Comas M, et al. Enteral versus parenteral nutrition as adjunct therapy in acute ulcerative colitis. Am J Gastroenterol 1993;88:227–32.

Jensen MB, Kissmeyer-Nielsen P, Laurberg S. Perioperative growth hormone treatment increases nitrogen and fluid balance and results in short-term and long-term conservation of lean tissue mass. Am J Clin Nutr 1998;68:840–6.

Klein S, Kinney J, Jeejeebhoy K, et al. Nutrition support in clinical practice: review of published data and recommendations for future research directions. JPEN 1997;21:133–56.

Lashner BA, Evans AA, Hanauer SB. Preoperative total parenteral nutrition for bowel resection in Crohn's disease. Dig Dis Sci 1989;34:741–6.

Rombeau JL, Rolandelli RH. Enteral and parenteral nutrition in patients with enteric fistulae and short bowel syndrome. Surg Clin North Am 1987;67A:551–71.

The Veterans Affairs Total Parenteral Nutrition Cooperative Study Group. Perioperative total parenteral nutrition in surgical patients. N Engl J Med 1991;325:525–32.

CHAPTER 96

LAPAROSCOPICALLY ASSISTED BOWEL RESECTION

MARK A. TALAMINI, MD

Laparoscopic surgery is changing the practice of abdominal and gastrointestinal surgery. This revolution began with laparoscopic cholecystectomy in 1989, which took the surgical world by storm. As a relatively easy operation to learn and perform, it was rapidly adopted by general surgeons. The advantages to patients were obvious, with dramatically shorter recovery times, far less pain, and a superior cosmetic result. With such spectacular success, general surgeons began to look for other arenas in which to apply this exciting new technology. Other frequently performed procedures that were obvious candidates were hernia repair, esophageal reflux surgery, and bowel resection.

The most common indications for bowel resection are tumor and inflammation. Laparoscopic resection for cancer is intriguing, but its development has been appropriately delayed while well-constructed randomized trials are being conducted. Laparoscopic resection for inflammation makes good sense, but has inherent technical challenges. The most common indications for bowel resection related to inflammation are diverticulitis and inflammatory bowel disease (IBD). Inflammation can make dissection difficult and potentially dangerous. The mesentery becomes foreshortened, thickened, and indurated. Important local structures can be drawn into the inflammation, moving them away from the normal anatomic course, rendering them difficult to recognize (the ureter being a prime example). Despite these challenges, innovative surgeons began to carefully apply laparoscopic technology to the resection of inflammatory diseases.

In considering a minimally invasive approach to bowel resection, two considerations are obvious. First, the tissue to be resected must be removed. Some creative approaches have emerged. One group removed sigmoid colon resections through the rectum using a colonoscope to grasp the tissue. Others have homogenized the tissue with a morcellizer. This may be problematic for the pathologist. Second, the bowel must be reanastomosed. This is the high-risk aspect of the procedure. A poorly constructed anastomosis places the patient at great risk. Whereas it is possible to anastomose the bowel using purely laparoscopic means, it is difficult and time consuming using current instrumentation.

The laparoscopically assisted procedure circumvents both of these problems. In this approach, the bowel is dissected free using laparoscopic tools. Then, a small incision is created and the bowel is eviscerated. The specimen is then resected on the abdominal wall, and the anastomosis performed using standard tools and techniques.

Surgeons have begun applying minimally invasive technology to colectomy for ulcerative colitis. In the most popular procedure, restorative proctocolectomy, at least some incision is needed to create the pouch. However, the incision can be small if the bulk of the colon dissection is performed laparoscopically. As this is already a long, technically challenging operation with little room for error, the minimally invasive approach has not yet been widely adopted.

Crohn's Disease

The indications for surgery in Crohn's disease are adequately discussed in other portions of this text. Briefly, acute indications include bleeding, obstruction, and, rarely, perforation. More chronic indications include fistulization, chronic obstruction, and perianal abscess. Perhaps the most frequent indication, and the most difficult to decide upon, is intractability. Should medical therapies be intensified, or should surgery be performed? Often such a decision is made in the setting of intermittent chronic obstruction, weight loss, and chronic pain. The decision requires balancing the risks of surgery against the potential advantages for each individual patient. It is this last indication (intractability) that may be modified by the introduction of minimally invasive surgery. If the pain, discomfort, disability, and disfigurement of surgery are significantly reduced by this approach, patients and their practitioners are more likely to opt for surgery.

Some common complicating factors in Crohn's disease can make the laparoscopic approach difficult. Fistulae into other intra-abdominal organs can be difficult or even dangerous to dissect and divide using laparoscopic instruments. Diseased bowel can be more difficult to assess laparoscopically, without the ability to feel structures or see them with three dimensional vision. Colonic disease, in particular, is difficult to assess and cannot be easily delivered out of the abdomen through a small incision for direct examination. Despite these potential problems, there are few situations in which a laparoscopic approach cannot be considered. As long as the surgeon is willing to convert to a conventional procedure if the dissection becomes difficult, all that can be lost is some operating room time. Those patients known to have badly adhesed abdomens from multiple previous procedures clearly would not benefit from such an approach, since intricate adhesiolysis would be required.

Technique

Preoperative Workup

Since laparoscopy limits direct examination of all abdominal bowel, preoperative evaluation is critical. With few exceptions, all patients undergo a computed tomography (CT), small bowel series, and colonoscopy (or barium enema). Patients need to be in good nutritional balance, and if they are not, interval home total parenteral nutrition (TPN) is used. Interval TPN often is used to allow inflamed tissues to settle down, increasing the likelihood of laparoscopic success. This approach increases the number of patients who can be considered for a laparoscopically assisted procedure.

Operating Room Specifics

The patient lies in a dorsal position if there is no sigmoid or perirectal disease, or with the legs in stirrups if there is. If possible, the arms should be tucked and protected, as the laparoscope often needs to be aimed from above down. Ports are placed according to the planned operation. The laparoscope is placed just above or below the umbilicus. Common convenient places for additional ports are just above the symphysis and midway between the umbilicus and the xiphoid, both in the midline. This arrangement allows for dissection of the terminal ileum and cecum or of the sigmoid colon.

The objective of the operation is to mobilize the target bowel enough for it to be delivered through a small incision onto the abdominal wall. The most common dissection necessary is of the terminal ileum, cecum, and ascending colon. This is accomplished by gently retracting the bowel toward the midline, revealing the attachments to the retroperitoneum. These attachments are then carefully divided with electrocautery or with the harmonic scalpel. Once the retroperitoneal space is opened near the pelvic brim, the ureter should be identified and avoided. The safest place to dissect during this phase is near the bowel itself, since it is to be removed. The bowel is ready to be eviscerated when the unaffected-appearing margins and the diseased segment all appear to reach the midline.

A small incision (1.5 to 2.0 inches) is then created in the midline on one side of the umbilicus. The midline is used because the mesentery is a midline structure, and

once mobilized, the bowel will stretch most easily from the midline. The diseased bowel and mesentery is then carefully delivered out of the wound onto the abdominal wall. This can be a difficult aspect of the procedure, because the mesentery often is thickened and indurated. Aggressive manipulation can initiate troublesome bleeding, so, if necessary, the incision can be enlarged to make room for evisceration of the mesentery as well as the bowel. Also, there may be additional attachments hindering evisceration. Often, they can be felt and divided through the incision, but if not, the incision must be extended.

At this stage, the resection and anastomosis is standard. More proximal or distal small bowel can be delivered segment by segment to evaluate directly most of the small bowel. If a strictureplasty is indicated, it too can be performed in this manner. The mesenteric defect is closed either out on the abdominal wall, using laparoscopy after the hole has been closed, or a combination of both. The abdomen is irrigated while the incision is still open. This takes on increased importance, as it is the only means of looking for bleeding. The irrigation fluid is carefully examined upon aspiration, and if it contains blood (particularly clots), then a search for unexpected bleeding may be necessary. The midline wound can be closed with interrupted sutures, all placed under direct vision. All of the wounds are infiltrated with bupivacaine for early postoperative pain control. The Foley and nasogastric tube are removed in the early postoperative period.

Future Directions

The future is bright for minimally invasive surgery in Crohn's disease. The current tools and means of visualization still are crude, but exciting enhancements are near. Robotic systems that eliminate tremor and use motion scaling for precise movements now are available. Sewing bowel with suture laparoscopically is quite difficult; many centers currently are exploring means of anastomosing bowel that are easier to accomplish. Thus, in the next decade, the ability to safely reconnect bowel will be markedly enhanced.

Single Institution Series

An initial series of 20 patients underwent ileocolonic resection by a laparoscopically assisted technique (1993 to 1995). Average age was 35 years, and 65 percent were female. Eighteen anastomoses were completed in 17 patients. The average incision length was 3.9 cm. There were two postoperative complications: one port site hematoma and one transient partial small bowel obstruction. When compared retrospectively to 36 patients with Crohn's disease resected by experienced IBD surgeons with a standard open technique, there was significantly less blood loss (14 mL vs 243 mL) with the laparoscopically assisted procedure, a more rapid return of bowel function (3.7 d vs 5.1 d), shorter length of hospitalization (5.9 d vs 8.1 d), less postoperative pain as measured by morphine equivalents, and a return to common activities of daily living 1 week sooner.

As of 1999, a total of 75 patients (average age, 38.5 yr) had undergone 77 attempted laparoscopic procedures. Indications for operation were obstruction (n = 58), fistula (n = 24), failure of medical management (n = 22), perineal sepsis (n = 4), and bleeding (n = 1). Fifty-one of the operations (66%) were completed laparoscopically; 30 were ileocecostomy, 15 were small bowel resections, strictureplasties in 5, fecal diversion in 6. Six included takedown of an enteric fistula. Thirty-four percent of the procedures had to be converted to an open procedure (incision over 2 inches in length). Of those who had to be converted to an open procedure, 52 percent had had a previous bowel resection compared with only 21 percent of patients in whom a laparoscopic technique was completed. This was because of adhesions in 23 of 26 patients. In five it was because of enteric fistula and in two it was because of the size of the inflammatory mass. Factors associated with the inability to perform the procedure laparoscopically included the fistulizing nature of the disease process, the presence of adhesions from previous procedures, continued need for steroids, and the presence of weight loss preoperatively. The mean operative time for the cases completed laparoscopically was 207 minutes, which is identical to the mean time indicated for 36 retrospective standard open procedures. Mean blood loss in this extended laparoscopic series was 133 cc. Postoperative complications included one pelvic abscess and one stroke. Time for passage of flatus and first bowel movement and time to discharge (5.7 d) were similar to times in the initial series.

Conclusion

Since societal costs can be significant in terms of insurance expenditure for an in-patient and time lost to business, a laparoscopically assisted approach may benefit some patients with Crohn's disease (and their health care provider). This approach is appropriate for virtually all patients with Crohn's disease. The only exceptions are those with known phlegmons, multiple strictures, or complex fistulae. However, the procedure is safe only if the surgeon is willing to convert to a standard surgical technique when difficulty is encountered or when the dissection becomes potentially dangerous. Obviously, no rules can be offered in this regard, since it depends upon the individual combination of the patient's diseased bowel state, the surgeon's skill level, and the sophistication of the surgeon's tools. In general, a laparoscopically assisted procedure is appropriate for nutritionally replete patients who have obstruction or intractable disease without complications.

Supplemental Reading

Bauer JJ, Harris MT, Grumbach NM, Gorfine SR. Laparoscopic-assisted intestinal resection for Crohn's disease. Which patients are good candidates? J Clin Gastroenterol 1996;23:44–6.

Canin-Endres J, Salky B, Gattorno F, Edye M. Laparoscopically assisted intestinal resection in 88 patients with Crohn's disease. Surg Endosc 1999;13:595–9.

Ogunbiyi OA, Fleshman JW. Place of laparoscopic surgery in Crohn's disease. Baillieres Clin Gastroenterol 1998; 12:157–65.

Reissman P, Salky BA, Edye M, Wexner SD. Laparoscopic surgery in Crohn's disease. Indications and results. Surg Endosc 1996;10:1201–3; discussion 1203–4.

Sardinha TC, Wexner SD. Laparoscopy for inflammatory bowel disease: pros and cons. World J Surg 1998;22:370–4.

Singh K, Prasad A, Saunders JH, Foley RJ. Laparoscopy in the diagnosis and management of Crohn's disease. Laparoendosc Adv Surg Tech 1998;8:39–46.

Thompson JS. The role of prophylactic cholecystectomy in the short-bowel syndrome. Arch Surg 1996;131:556–9; discussion 559–60.

CHAPTER 97

Surgery for Crohn's Disease: Strictureplasty

Scott A. Strong, MD

Crohn's disease is a chronic inflammatory condition of unknown etiology affecting the entire intestinal tract. No medical regimen has yet been developed that uniformly and reliably effects a cure, and operative therapy is by no means a panacea for this disease. Surgery usually is reserved for patients who have developed one or more disease complications or persons whose quality of life is significantly impaired despite appropriate medical therapy.

Rationale

The occurrence of skip lesions in the small intestine was identified soon after the earliest reports of regional ileitis appeared. In the past, a strictured segment of bowel separate yet near the principal area of involvement posed no significant technical challenge, as this was included in the resected or bypassed segment. Resection, either single or multiple, also was used for several short diseased segments located in the proximal small bowel. However, concerns about imminent short-bowel syndrome eventually were voiced when the recurrent nature of Crohn's disease was better appreciated. Thus, operations were avoided for patients with extensive jejunoileitis, and these individuals were arbitrarily treated with anti-inflammatory medications and hyperalimentation.

Patients afflicted by intestinal tuberculosis, similar to those with small bowel Crohn's disease, occasionally suffer from obstructive intestinal symptoms related to multiple strictures of the jejunum and ileum. In 1977, Katariya and colleagues reported using a novel operative technique described as "stricture-plasty" in patients with multiple tuberculosis strictures; the procedure effectively ameliorated obstructive symptoms while safely preserving the affected small bowel. Lee, of the John Radcliffe Hospital in Oxford, United Kingdom, successfully employed this nonresectional technique 2 years later in a 21-year-old woman with multiple small bowel strictures caused by Crohn's disease. Lee and Papaioannou subsequently reported their experience in nine patients in whom strictureplasty was performed for extensive Crohn's disease of the small bowel.

Timing

The surgeon caring for patients with Crohn's disease must understand the efficacy of appropriate medical therapy,

consider the patient's long-term prognosis, and conserve small bowel whenever possible, because repeated or massive resections can lead to short-bowel syndrome. Therefore, operative treatment is reserved for patients who develop a disease complication or fail their medical therapy. At the time of laparotomy, only those segments considered to be contributing to the patient's constellation of symptoms merit resection. However, if strictures are identified at operation, regardless of whether the surgeon believes them to be symptomatic, strictureplasty should supplement the primary procedure. This approach is justified because experience has proven that strictureplasty adds little to the morbidity of resection, and reoperation following strictureplasty is more likely to be necessary for new symptomatic strictures than for re-structuring of an old strictureplasty site.

Stricture Plasty Use

When it is realized that incision and suturing of diseased segments is the basis of the procedure, natural concerns arise regarding suture-line healing and the occurrence of intra-abdominal abscesses or fistulae. Aside from meticulous conduct of the procedure, prevention of such complications lies with patient selection. Indications and contraindications are listed in Table 97–1.

TABLE 97–1. Indications and Contraindications for Strictureplasty

Indications
    Stricture(s) in a patient who has undergone previous major resection(s) of small bowel (> 100 cm)
    Stricture in a patient with short-bowel syndrome
    Rapid recurrence of Crohn's disease manifested as obstruction
    Diffuse involvement of the small bowel with multiple strictures
    Nonphlegmonous, fibrotic stricture

Contraindications
    Colonic strictures
    Hypoalbuminemia (< 2.0 g/dL)
    Free or contained perforation of the small bowel
    Phlegmonous inflammation, internal fistula, or external fistula involving the affected site
    Multiple strictures within a short segment
    Stricture in close proximity to a site chosen for resection

TABLE 97–2. Reported Studies of Strictureplasty Experience

Study	Year	Center or City	Patients	Number of Operations	Strictureplasties
Pritchard et al	1990	Lahey Clinic	13	16	52
Spencer et al	1994	Mayo Clinic	35	36	71
Serra et al	1995	Toronto	43	57	154
Stebbing et al	1996	Oxford	52	76	241
Ozuner et al	1996	Cleveland Clinic	162	191	698
Hurst et al	1998	Chicago	57	60	109
Yamamoto et al	1999	Birmingham	111	111	285

Short-Term Outcome

Many centers have conducted comprehensive studies on 10 or more patients undergoing strictureplasty (Table 97–2). The typical patient treated by strictureplasty presents with symptoms related to small bowel obstruction unresponsive to medical therapy, even with 20 mg of prednisone daily. Nearly two-thirds of patients will undergo synchronous resection, most have three separate segments treated by strictureplasty, and more than 250 cm of small bowel remains after the procedure (Table 97–3).

The operation has proven to be safe, with a morbidity rate of about 15 percent and no mortality reported from the major series. The likelihood of septic complications, specifically, appears to be influenced by hypoalbuminemia and is nearly tripled when the preoperative serum albumin level is less than 2.5 g/dL (Ozuner et al, 1996). Therefore, a diverting stoma proximal to the sites of strictureplasty should be carefully considered in instances in which the patient's albumin value is less than 2.5 g/dL. Contrarily, steroid dosage, perforative or phlegmonous disease remote from the strictureplasty site, stricture length, number of strictureplasties, and need for synchronous resection do not significantly impact on the risk that the patient will experience a septic complication.

Although uncommon (~9%), hemorrhage can be particularly challenging to manage. Most instances of strictureplasty-site bleeding cease spontaneously without intervention. If hemorrhage persists, however, selective mesenteric angiography is performed and vasopressin is infused intra-arterially in a manner similar to that used for patients with diverticular hemorrhage. In the rare

event that bleeding is uncontrolled by the interventional radiologist or recurs, laparotomy typically is required to control the hemorrhage. Unfortunately, if reoperation is necessary, it is difficult to be certain of the specific bleeding site without opening the several strictureplasties.

Six months postoperatively, nearly all patients (98%) note relief of their obstructive symptoms and average 5 pounds of weight gain. Furthermore, most patients (~80%) have discontinued steroid therapy with the remainder averaging less than 10 mg of prednisone daily.

Long-Term Outcome

The Cleveland Clinic reported their experience with 162 persons undergoing 191 operations with 698 strictureplasties followed up for a mean of 42 months (Ozuner et al, 1996). The overall cumulative 5-year operative recurrence was 28 percent, and statistically similar between the strictureplasty alone (31%) and strictureplasty with resection (27%) groups. Moreover, of those requiring reoperation, 78 percent had new strictures or perforative disease at a location remote from the original strictureplasty site.

Yamamoto and colleagues (1999) reviewed 111 patients who underwent 285 primary strictureplasties. After a median follow-up of nearly 9 years, clinical recurrence occurred in 60 patients (54%), and 49 of these (44%) required reoperation.

At Oxford University, 241 strictureplasties were performed during 76 operations in 52 patients (Stebbing et al, 1996). After a median follow-up of 4 years, persons undergoing strictureplasty alone were no more likely to require reoperation than those who had undergone concomitant

TABLE 97–3. Strictureplasty Experience

Study	Year	Number of Operations	Strictureplasties	Strictureplasty Short:Long* (Number of Strictureplasties)	Alone:Resection† (Number of Operations)
Pritchard et al	1990	16	52	50:2	12:4
Spencer et al	1994	36	71	71:0	12:24
Serra et al	1995	43	136	127:9	11:32
Stebbing et al	1996	52	168	156:12	18:34
Ozuner et al	1996	191	698	617:81	52:110
Hurst et al	1998	60	109	90:19	—
Yamamoto et al	1999	111	285	236:49	65:46

*Short (<10 cm) versus long (>10 cm) strictureplasty; †strictureplasty alone versus strictureplasty with resection.

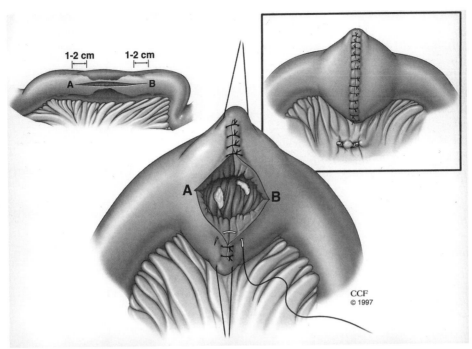

FIGURE 97–1. The type of strictureplasty is dependent upon the length of the stenotic segment. For strictures less than 10 cm in length, a Weinberg-Mikulicz (single layer) technique of strictureplasty is employed. A longitudinal enterotomy is made over the antimesenteric aspect of the stricture, and the defect is closed transversely.

resection at the first procedure; moreover, reoperation rates were similar after the first and second operations.

Technique

At the time of laparotomy, the stomach, duodenum, small intestine, and large bowel are examined. As the small bowel is traced from the duodenojejunal junction distally, suture tags are placed on segments affected by disease, with normal and diseased sites measured in relation to the ligament of Treitz.

In its classic form, Crohn's disease of the small bowel is easily recognizable. The involved segment is characteristically indurated, thick-walled, and constricted with omentum or adjacent bowel loops commonly adherent to the inflamed area. Skip lesions affecting short or long segments of small bowel occur in approximately 20 percent of cases. In ileal disease, frequently there is thickening of the mesenteric margin of the bowel, a fierce serositis or "corkscrew" appearance of the serosal vessels, and fat encroachment or wrapping on the sides of the intestinal wall. The scalloped appearance of the normal terminal ileal mesentery is lost, as the fat deposition between the terminal branches of the marginal vessels, vasa recta, is excessive. The proximal bowel above the strictured segment commonly is dilated and, with chronic obstruction, this bowel may be thickened because of muscular hypertrophy.

In some cases, these classic findings are absent. In these instances, the best guide to disease location is palpation along the mesenteric margin, as the margin of a diseased segment is invariably thickened in response to an overlying mesenteric ulcer. Even subtly strictured segments are easily recognized by this marginal thickening of the mesenteric angle. If doubt exists, or if the surgeon is inexperienced with strictureplasty, then calibration is a reasonable alternative for identifying strictured segments. Methods to quantify the caliber of a stricture through an open enterotomy include passage of a standard marble (16.5-mm diameter), 2-cm bougie, or Foley catheter with the balloon inflated to a 2-cm diameter. All of these techniques are time consuming and may contribute to intraoperative contamination.

For short strictures (≤ 10 cm), a linear antimesenteric incision is made, extending for about 2 cm beyond the stricture proximally and distally (Figure 97–1). The wound edges are carefully inspected and any bleeding meticulously controlled with electrocautery. The accompanying mesenteric ulcer is scrutinized and then biopsied to exclude an unrecognized malignancy. Stay sutures of 000 Vicryl or PDS are placed at the midpoint of the enterotomy site, along both edges, and lateral traction is applied to convert the longitudinal enterotomy into a transverse defect. The wound is closed transversely using an interrupted single layer of sutures. At the completion of the strictureplasty, a radiopaque titanium clip is applied to the mesenteric fat adjacent to the closure site. This marker allows for subsequent identification of strictureplasty sites during future contrast radiography of the small bowel.

The occurrence of long strictures may provide technical difficulties in performing a side-to-side (Finney) strictureplasty. Unless the bowel is supple enough to bend into a U-shape and still allow for a tension-free anastomosis, leakage and sepsis are likely to occur. The function of such segments remains unproven, and a remote risk of cancer, occurring later or coexisting, is present. In practice, the enthusiasm for preserving these long strictures by side-to-side strictureplasty is related indirectly to the length of remaining small bowel.

The Finney strictureplasty is commenced by incising along the antimesenteric margin in a manner similar to the Heineke-Mikulicz strictureplasty. However, instead of applying transverse tension on the enterotomy, the bowel is folded into a U-shaped configuration. The posterior portion of the strictureplasty is closed with a continuous 000 Vicryl or PDS, incorporating all layers of the bowel wall. Additional interrupted sutures are placed at about 1- to 1.5-cm intervals. The anterior layer is closed in a similar fashion while carefully inverting the mucosal layer, particularly at the apices of the enterotomy. Once again, a titanium clip is applied to the mesenteric fat to assist future operative or radiographic localization.

One of the concerns voiced regarding a Finney strictureplasty is that of bacterial overgrowth in the resultant large, diverticulum-like sac that extends from the intestine. Additionally, recurrent stricturing tends to occur within the afferent limb of bowel just proximal to the Finney-type diverticulum. Therefore, three alternative procedures have been proposed for the treatment of long strictures. Fazio and Tjandra (1993) described a method to treat multiple strictures in a segment measuring up to 25 cm in length. Another variation has been described by Sasaki et al (1996), in three patients with about 15-cm long disease segments, whereby a double Heineke-Mikulicz technique is employed. Perhaps the most helpful technique for strictures measuring more than 25 cm has been that devised by Michelassi (1996). He used a side-to-side, isoperistaltic, hand-sewn strictureplasty in three patients with severe Crohn's disease. However, resection of 15- to 20-cm lengths of bowel from the middle third of the diseased segment was required to facilitate performance of the side-to-side strictureplasty. This technique safely allows for a tension-free anastomosis and effectively eliminates the troublesome diverticulum associated with the Finney method.

Strictureplasty for fibrotic strictures at ileocolic or ileorectal anastomoses is just as safe and efficacious as resection with neo-anastomosis. And, although strictureplasty has been described for colonic narrowing, about 6 percent of colonic strictures are complicated by an underlying malignancy. Therefore, symptomatic colonic strictures should be resected rather than treated by strictureplasty. Strictureplasty for short duodenal strictures is described in the chapter on surgical management of Crohn's disease of the duodenum.

Summary

Strictureplasty remains relatively unchanged from its initial description almost two decades ago. Some variations have been suggested for relatively long strictures. Nearly all series attest to the short-term safety and efficacy of the technique, with long-term studies reporting competitive clinical and operative recurrence rates.

Editor's Note

Does medical therapy play any role after strictureplasty? Will any of our current anti-inflammatory or immuno-modulating agents influence scarring and fibrosis? Are some patients with jejunoileitis staying on azathioprine after strictureplasty? Does this influence results? What is the cause of the ulcer of the base of the mesentry at each strictured area? Is this pathologically different than the ulceration in Crohn's disease? As usual, I have more questions than answers. (TMB)

References

Fazio VW, Tjandra J. Strictureplasty for Crohn's disease with multiple long strictures. Dis Colon Rectum 1993;36:71–2.

Hurst RD, Michelassi F. Strictureplasty for Crohn's disease: techniques and long-term results. World J Surg 1998;22:359–63.

Katariya RN, Sood S, Rao PG, Rao PL. Stricture-plasty for tubercular strictures of the gastrointestinal tract. Br J Surg 1977;64:496–8.

Lee ECG, Papaioannou N. Minimal surgery for chronic obstruction in patients with extensive or universal Crohn's disease. Ann R Coll Surg Engl 1982;64:229–33.

Michelassi F. Side-to-side isoperistaltic strictureplasty for multiple Crohn's strictures. Dis Colon Rectum 1996;39:345–9.

Ozuner G, Fazio VW, Lavery IC, et al. How safe is strictureplasty in the management of Crohn's disease? Am J Surg 1996;171:57–60.

Ozuner G, Fazio VW, Lavery IC, et al. Reoperative rates for Crohn's disease following strictureplasty. Dis Colon Rectum 1996;39:1199–203.

Pritchard TJ, Schoetz DJ Jr, Caushaj FP, et al. Strictureplasty of the small bowel in patients with Crohn's disease. Arch Surg 1990;125:715–7.

Sasaki I, Funayama Y, Naito H, et al. Extended strictureplasty for multiple short skipped strictures of Crohn's disease. Dis Colon Rectum 1996;39:342–4.

Serra J, Cohen Z, McLeod RS. Natural history of strictureplasty in Crohn's disease: 9-year experience. Can J Surg 1995;38:481–5.

Spencer MP, Nelson H, Wolff BG, Dozois RR. Strictureplasty for obstructing Crohn's disease: the Mayo experience. Mayo Clin Proc 1994;69:33–6.

Stebbing J, Jewell D, Kettlewell M, Mortensen N. Long-term results of recurrence and reoperation after strictureplasty for obstructive Crohn's disease. Br J Surg 1996;82:1471–4.

Yamamoto T, Bain IM, Allan RN, Keighley MR. An audit of strictureplasty for small-bowel Crohn's disease. Dis Colon Rectum 1999;42:797–803.

CHAPTER 98

GASTRODUODENAL CROHN'S DISEASE: SURGICAL MANAGEMENT

PETER W. MARCELLO, MD, AND DAVID J. SCHOETZ JR, MD

Crohn's disease rarely involves the stomach or duodenum and usually is associated with more distal disease. There is also a chapter on medical management of gastroduodenal Crohn's disease. Gastroduodenal Crohn's disease affects between 0.5 percent and 4 percent of patients with idiopathic granulomatous enteritis and may predate the development of more distal disease in half of the patients (Nugent and Roy, 1989; Schoetz, 1992). Isolated duodenal Crohn's disease is uncommon. In a series of 89 patients with gastroduodenal Crohn's disease from the Lahey Clinic, 52 percent of patients had known distal Crohn's disease at the time the duodenal disease was identified. The diagnosis of duodenal and distal disease was made simultaneously in another 30 percent of patients. With a median follow-up time of 11.7 years (range, 6–14 yr), distal disease developed in 56 percent of patients with seemingly isolated duodenal Crohn's disease, and only 7.9 percent of patients remained without known ileal disease progression.

Symptoms and Evaluation

The symptoms of primary gastroduodenal Crohn's disease as described in the earlier cited chapter are initially nonspecific and often indistinguishable from peptic ulcer disease of the duodenum. Epigastric pain relieved by antacid, histamine$_2$ blocker, or ingestion of food is the most common complaint, with subsequent development of nausea, vomiting, and weight loss in two-thirds of patients when duodenal obstruction occurs.

Abnormal radiographic findings are identified in more than 90 percent of patients with gastroduodenal Crohn's disease. Thickened folds, nodular changes, and aphthous ulcerations occur initially (Miller et al, 1979) (Figure 98–1). As the disease progresses, cobblestoning, fissuring ulcers, and fibrotic changes may be observed, resulting in duodenal deformity and fixed luminal narrowing (Figure 98–2). Endoscopic and biopsy changes are described in the medical therapy chapter.

Surgical Indications

Medical therapy fails in one-third of patients with gastroduodenal Crohn's disease, and ultimately these patients require surgery. In a series of 22 patients undergoing surgery at the Lahey Clinic, refractory gastric outlet

obstruction was the primary indication in 77 percent of patients (Murray et al, 1984). Only 18 percent required intervention for persistent abdominal pain, and in only one patient was urgent surgery required for hemorrhage. Similar results were noted in a recent report from the Cleveland Clinic (Worsey et al, 1999). Of 34 patients requiring surgery, obstructive symptoms were noted in 94 percent, pain in 71 percent, bloating in 68 percent, and 65 percent of patients had significant (>20 lb) weight loss.

Another possible reason for operation is symptomatic gastroduodenal fistulas, which occurs less commonly than primary duodenal Crohn's disease. The majority of gastroduodenal fistulas arise from either recurrent ileocolic Crohn's disease or primary colonic disease and rarely from intrinsic duodenal disease. In a report of 14 cases of gastroduodenal fistulas from Crohn's disease, six arose from primary colonic disease, six from recurrent

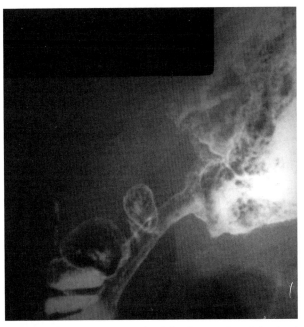

FIGURE 98–1. Barium study of distal stomach and duodenal sweep demonstrating gastroduodenal Crohn's disease, with conization of antrum and deformity of the duodenal bulb. There is luminal narrowing of the first portion of the duodenum, sparing of the second portion, and thickened folds and nodularity in the third portion of the duodenum.

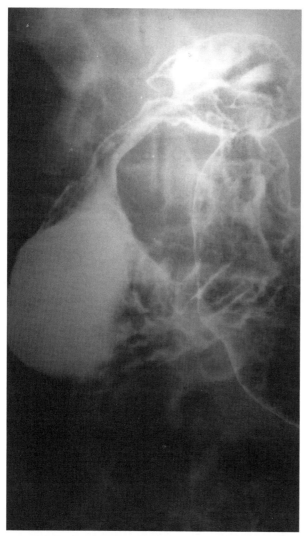

FIGURE 98–2. Fibrotic narrowing of the duodenum with pseudos-accularization. The saccular changes represent normal duodenal mucosa surrounded by circumferential and longitudinal Crohn's disease, resulting in luminal narrowing.

ileocolic disease, and only two cases developed from primary duodenal disease (Yamamoto et al, 1998).

Surgical Treatment

Intestinal bypass, with creation of a loop gastrojejunostomy to circumvent the obstructed duodenum, remains the procedure of choice in the majority of patients with gastroduodenal Crohn's disease. Preoperative differentiation between Crohn's disease and peptic ulcer disease is important because the performance of gastric resection in the setting of gastroduodenal Crohn's disease is associated with significantly higher morbidity. In the Lahey Clinic series (22 patients), a fourfold increase in serious complications was noted in patients who underwent resection compared with bypass alone.

Reoperation, both for complications of the gastrojejunostomy and recurrence of distal disease, is not uncommon when patients are observed for long periods of time. In a Cleveland Clinic series of 11 patients with gastroduodenal Crohn's disease followed up for 14 years, 7 of 10 surgically treated patients required further surgery directly related to duodenal disease, and 8 of the 11 patients required surgery for Crohn's disease of the distal bowel (Ross et al, 1983).

Role of Vagotomy

The role of vagotomy remains controversial in the surgical management of patients with gastroduodenal Crohn's disease. Of theoretic concern is the development of postvagotomy diarrhea in patients undergoing parasympathetic denervation by truncal vagotomy, particularly in patients who have had multiple small bowel resections or the loss of the ileocecal valve after ileocolic resection. However, results from various small series have not substantiated this anticipated complication.

The development of marginal ulceration following gastrojejunostomy may occur either with or without vagotomy. In the Cleveland Clinic series, in four of five patients (80%) undergoing bypass without vagotomy, marginal ulcers subsequently developed that required reoperation, resulting in the recommendation for routine vagotomy at the time of gastrojejunostomy. However, in the Lahey Clinic series, marginal ulceration occurred in three patients (33%) who underwent bypass with truncal vagotomy. Similar results were seen in patients undergoing bypass without vagotomy, with marginal ulcers developing in one of four patients (25%).

Based on these concerns for postvagotomy diarrhea and the observed incidence of marginal ulceration after bypass alone, gastrojejunostomy with highly selective vagotomy, which preserves autonomic innervation to the small bowel, is recommended for the initial surgical treatment of patients with primary gastroduodenal Crohn's disease.

Strictureplasty

Since the advent of strictureplasty for patients with small bowel Crohn's disease in the late 1970s, the indication for this technique has broadened to encompass isolated duodenal disease. Early small series noted favorable results (Table 98–1). However, two recent larger series have published opposing views of the role of strictureplasty for primary duodenal disease (Worsey et al, 1999; Yamamoto et al, 1999).

In a retrospective review, from Birmingham, England, of 13 patients undergoing duodenal strictureplasty (3 after a prior failed gastrojejunostomy), a high rate of complications and reoperation was reported (Yamamoto et al, 1999). Early complications, including anastomotic leakage and prolonged ileus, were seen in 6 patients (42%). Ultimately, 9 of 13 patients (69%) required a revisional procedure for either complications or recurrent

TABLE 98–1. Results of Strictureplasty for Duodenal Crohn's Disease

Author	Year	Number of Patients	Median Follow-up (mo)	Success (%)	Complications
Alexander-Williams and Haynes	1985	5	6	100	—
Poggioli et al	1997	3	—	67	1 (33%) Persistent obstruction
Eisenberger et al	1998	1	9	100	—
Yamamoto et al	1999	13	143	31	6 (46%) Anastomotic leak (n = 2) Persistent obstruction (n = 4)
Worsey et al	1999	13	42	100	2 (15%) Enterocutaneous fistula (n = 1) Persistent obstruction (n = 1)

stricture formation. The authors, therefore, concluded that the results of strictureplasty were not favorable.

In contrast are the results of strictureplasty recently published by the Cleveland Clinic (Worsey et al, 1999). In a retrospective review of 34 patients requiring surgery for duodenal Crohn's disease, the results of intestinal bypass performed in 21 patients were compared with primary strictureplasty in 13 patients. With a mean follow-up time of 8 years, operative complications developed in 2 of 21 patients undergoing bypass (16 with vagotomy), and only one patient required reoperation for recurrent disease. Although with a shorter follow-up time (mean, 3.6 yr), the results were similar for patients undergoing strictureplasty (5/13 with vagotomy), with two operative complications and one reoperation for recurrent stricture. The authors concluded that strictureplasty was safe and efficacious and should be considered an alternative to intestinal bypass in selected patients.

Strictureplasty should not be performed in the presence of active inflammatory disease; rather, it should be limited to those situations in which there is a fibrous stricture of limited length. Furthermore, great care must be taken to avoid injury to the common bile duct and ampulla of Vater.

Fistulas

The majority of gastroduodenal fistulas associated with Crohn's disease are a result of primary disease within the colon or recurrent distal ileal disease following a previous ileocolic resection. The duodenum becomes secondarily inflamed, and a fistula develops. In these patients in whom primary duodenal disease is not suspected, the duodenal fistula can be resected or débrided and the duodenum closed. If available, a tongue of omentum should be placed over the duodenal or gastric suture line to prevent re-formation. For a primary gastroduodenal fistula

from Crohn's disease, partial resection of the involved bowel is required. The site may be closed primarily if small, or alternatively, a duodenojejunostomy may be performed if the defect is large (Wilk et al, 1977). Omentum should be placed adjacent to the site of repair to prevent further fistula formation.

References

Eisenberger CF, Izbicki JR, Broering DC, et al. Strictureplasty with a pedunculated jejunal patch in Crohn's disease of the duodenum. Am J Gastroenterol 1998;93:267–9.

Miller EM, Moss AA, Kressel HY. Duodenal involvement with Crohn's disease: a spectrum of radiographic abnormality. Am J Gastroenterol 1979;71:107–16.

Murray JJ, Schoetz DJ Jr, Nugent FW, et al. Surgical management of Crohn's disease involving the duodenum. Am J Surg 1984;147:58–65.

Nugent FW, Roy MA. Duodenal Crohn's disease: an analysis of 89 cases. Am J Gastroenterol 1989;84:249–54.

Poggioli G, Stocchi L, Laureti S, et al. Duodenal involvement of Crohn's disease: three different clinicopathologic patterns. Dis Colon Rectum 1997;40:179–83.

Ross TM, Fazio VW, Farmer RG. Long-term results of surgical treatment for Crohn's disease of the duodenum. Ann Surg 1983;197:399–406.

Schoetz DJ Jr. Gastroduodenal Crohn's disease. Perspect Colon Rectal Surg 1992;2:145–54.

Wilk PJ, Fazio V, Turnbull RB Jr. The dilemma of Crohn's disease: ileoduodenal fistula complicating Crohn's disease. Dis Colon Rectum 1977;20:387–92.

Worsey MJ, Hull T, Ryland L, Fazio V. Strictureplasty is an effective option in the operative management of duodenal Crohn's disease. Dis Colon Rectum 1999;42:596–600.

Yamamoto T, Bain IM, Connolly AB, Keighley MR. Gastroduodenal fistulas in Crohn's disease: clinical features and management. Dis Colon Rectum 1998;41:1287–92.

Yamamoto T, Bain IM, Connolly AB, et al. Outcome of strictureplasty for duodenal Crohn's disease. Br J Surg 1999;86:259–62.

CHAPTER 99

MEASURES TO MINIMIZE POSTOPERATIVE RECURRENCES OF CROHN'S DISEASE

PAUL J. RUTGEERTS, MD, PhD, FRCP

There is no doubt that resection of diseased segments in patients with Crohn's disease induces long-lasting remission and greatly improves the quality of life. Although many of these patients feel that surgery has been postponed too long in their case, most clinicians think that surgery is advocated only in the presence of complications of the disease, including stenosis, abscess, and fistula. Intractable disease usually is not considered a surgical indication. Great differences exist among centers in policies concerning surgery for inflammatory bowel disease (IBD); some refer almost every patient for resection early in the disease course, whereas others delay surgery as long as possible.

The most important complication of bowel resection for Crohn's disease is recurrence of the disease. It has become clear that nearly all patients will suffer recurrence of Crohn's lesions leading to new symptoms after a variable length of time. Currently, these new lesions are detected early, but the question arises whether early detection improves long-term outcome. The focus in this chapter is on prevention of recurrence after "curative" resection (ie, after resection of all macroscopically diseased tissue). Local resections and bypass operations leaving macroscopic disease behind offer no chance of cure. It also has become clear in the early years of Crohn's disease treatment that radical surgery (large disease-free margins and removal of lymph nodes draining the region) does not protect against recurrence.

Prevention of recurrent Crohn's disease after resection of the diseased bowel is a completely different situation from maintaining clinical remission with the diseased bowel in place; therefore, combining studies on surgically induced and medically induced remission is not justified. The ultimate goal in the management of Crohn's disease should be to control the disease as early after diagnosis as possible to avoid surgery. Many clinicians believe that an early aggressive approach using immunomodulation and immunosuppression will make this goal achievable.

Natural History of Recurrent Crohn's Disease

Presymptomatic Phase

Systematic endoscopic study data are available only for the neoterminal ileum and ileocolonic anastomosis after ileal or ileocolonic resections. Recurrent lesions can be visualized as early as a few weeks to months after resection in the neoterminal ileum proximal to the anastomosis with a postanastomotic colon mostly free of macroscopic disease, although microscopic lesions can also be identified there. It is not clear what makes the ileal mucosa so vulnerable to recurrent lesions. Crohn's disease has been shown to be a disease that affects the entire intestine. In "normal" ileum, mucosal architectural changes, epithelial bridge formation, and goblet cell hyperplasia are present. Inflammatory lesions in the resection margins are not predictive of recurrence, but perineural inflammatory changes might be of importance. The combined presence of bacteria and bile acids, the break in the mucosa of the suture, reflux of colonic contents, and the organization of the mucosal immune cells may be contributing factors. Early recurrent lesions are described in 70 to 80 percent of the patients in the first year following surgery. In most cases, recurrence of tissue lesions precedes the appearance of recurrent clinical signs by several years, but eventually all patients with lesions develop recrudescence of Crohn's disease. This evolution over time was not previously appreciated largely because radiographic small bowel follow-through was too insensitive a method to detect early lesions.

Symptomatic Recurrence

The severity and extent of tissue recurrence predicts the time to clinical relapse. Patients without lesions or presenting only a few aphthous ulcers at ileocolonoscopy at 1 year are not at risk of early symptomatic relapse, but more than half of the patients presenting with diffuse aphthous or ulcerative ileitis will have symptomatic relapse within 1 to 3 years after operation. Patients with ulcers confined to the immediate preanastomotic region are presumably prone to develop fibrostenosis of the anastomosis.

There is convincing evidence that in patients with postoperative recurrence, the evolution of Crohn's disease mimics the natural evolution of Crohn's disease at its onset. The evolution goes from pre-ulcerative inflammation over lymphoid tissue to aphthoid ulcers to more extensive ulceration and nodularity, which result in complications, including stenosis and fissures that can be complicated by abscesses and fistulae. At some point, gastrointestinal (GI) symptoms recur, and it is conceivable that this symptom-free interval after surgery equals the presymptomatic phase at the onset of the disease.[*]

For assessment of recurrence rates, an actuarial analysis has to be used. This involves the calculation of the number of patients with recurrent disease divided by the number of patients at risk in each year of follow-up, allowing for recurrence in previous years.

Older follow-up studies report that symptoms recur after curative resection in about 10 percent of the patients per follow-up year. However, in the placebo groups of recent postoperative prevention drug studies, the symptomatic recurrence rates are higher, amounting to 23 to 26 percent at 1 year and about 40 percent at 2 years. The symptoms of recurrent disease are not always easily distinguishable from symptoms attributable to the postoperative state and to choleraic diarrhea. The baseline is the state at 3 months after resection. Most patients have recovered completely by that time. The Crohn's Disease Activity Index (CDAI) is an instrument that is not really valid in the postoperative setting.

The pattern of Crohn's disease remains unchanged after surgery in comparison with the preoperative situation. Patients who present with perforating disease (abscesses, fistulae) before surgery tend to develop the same complications after resection and will have early recurrent symptoms. When the disease is characterized by fibrostenosis prior to operation, the chances are that the disease will stay indolent after resection. The need for repeated surgery owing to complications of severe recurrence varies between 16 percent and 65 percent at 10 years overall.

A proportion of patients have chronic inflammation without complications that may or may not respond to anti-inflammatory therapy. It also is striking that the lengths of ileal involvement measured on small bowel radiographic examinations before and at the time of symptomatic recurrence are similar, whereas the extent of ileal lesions stays remarkably constant as long as the patient is not operated upon.

---

[*] Editor's Note: This presymptomatic phase is equivalent to the 1 or 2 years of diminished growth velocity before any symptoms are noted, which occurs in 40 percent of prepubescent adolescents. (TMB)

Risk Factors for Symptomatic Recurrence after Resection

The only independent factors generally reproduced in multivariate analysis are location of the disease prior to surgery, the pattern of the disease, and smoking status.

Location of Diseased Segment

The anatomic site of bowel resection is, without doubt, an important determinant of recurrence. The highest rates are found after resection for ileocolitis or ileitis involving an ileocolonic anastomosis. Lower rates are found after colonic resection with colocolic anastomosis. Surprisingly, Crohn's disease also recurs in the ileum after right colonic resection with ileocolonic anastomosis when the ileum was not diseased prior to surgery. The rate of symptomatic recurrence proximal to an ileostomy is lowest. It is not certain whether the rate is really lower or whether the evolution of recurrent lesions is slower. In all situations, a narrowed bowel seems to be associated with faster evolution.

Reoperation rates after resection with ileocolonic anastomosis range from 25 percent to 60 percent at 5 years and 42 percent to 91 percent at 15 years. After colocolic anastomosis, the rates range between 8.5 percent and 42 percent at 5 years and 22 percent and 40 percent at 15 years. The rate of reoperation for end ileostomies is still 25 percent at 5 years and 45 percent at 10 years. The rate of recurrence of Crohn's disease in the neoterminal ileum after ileorectal anastomosis seems comparable to that after more proximal ileocolonic anastomosis, but the disease more often spreads distally with anorectal complications as the main manifestation.

Behavior of Crohn's Disease

A good predictor of recurrence is the behavior of Crohn's disease, as described by studies of De Dombal and coauthors in Leeds and Greenstein et al (1988) in New York. In 1971, De Dombal and colleagues described a biphasic symptomatic recurrence graph with those with aggressive disease (fistulae, abscess) recurring early and those with a more indolent course recurring later. The Mount Sinai investigators distinguished perforating indications for resection from nonperforating indications. Perforating indications included acute free perforation, subacute perforation with abscess formation, and chronic perforation with intestinal fistula formation. Nonperforating indications comprised intestinal obstruction, medical intractability, hemorrhage, and toxic dilatation without perforation.

Operations for perforating indications in their retrospective analysis were followed by repeated resection twice as early as operations for nonperforating indications. Time to first reoperation was 4.7 years in the perforating group and 8.8 years in the nonperforating group.

TABLE 99–1. Results of Postoperative Recurrence Prevention Studies Using 5-Aminosalicylic Acid Formulations

Study	Year	Formulation	Dose (g)	Number of Patients	Duration (mo)	Mean Follow-up (mo)	Clinical Recurrence (%) Placebo	Clinical Recurrence (%) 5-ASA
Caprilli et al	1994	Asacol®	2.4	110	24	12	41	18
McLeod et al	1995	Salofalk®/Rowasa®	3.0	163	72	35(s)–29(p)	41	31
Brignola	1995	Pentasa®	3.0	77	12		26	18
Sutherland	1997	Pentasa®	3.0	66	12		23	10
Lochs	1997	Pentasa®	4.0	318	18		31	24

Asacol®, Procter & Gamble Pharmaceuticals, Phoenix, Arizona; Salofalk®, Axcan Pharma Inc., Minneapolis, Minnesota; Rowasa®, Solvay Pharmaceuticals Inc., Marietta, Georgia; Pentasa®, Ferring-Shire Pharmaceuticals Inc., Florence, Kentucky.

Time to second reoperation averaged 2.3 years for perforating versus 5.2 years for nonperforating indications. Second operations in the perforating indication group were undertaken for perforating indications again in 64 percent of the patients with ileitis and 77 percent of the patients with ileocolitis. A third resection in patients with perforating indications for second resection was carried out for perforating complications in 81 percent overall. Not all investigators have confirmed this dichotomy of Crohn's disease behavior. Fistulae and abscesses occurring secondary to strictures are sources of confusion.

Smoking Status

Generally, smoking has a deleterious effect on Crohn's disease. It is the major risk factor for clinical recurrence and reoperation. In an Italian series by Cottone, in 1994, the 6-year recurrence-free rate after surgery was 60 percent (95% confidence interval [CI] = 43–72) for nonsmokers, 41 percent (95% CI = 11–70) for ex-smokers, and 27 percent (95% CI = 17–37) for smokers.

The need for repeated surgery 5 years after surgery averages 20 percent in nonsmokers versus 36 percent in smokers as shown by Sutherland et al in 1990. At 10 years, these rates are 41 percent and 70 percent, respectively. The risk is particularly high in female smokers with small bowel disease (odds ratio [OR] = 9.2).

The risk of excisional surgery associated with smoking is increased only in patients not given immunosuppressive drugs, as shown by the French GETAID Group. Apparently, the effect of smoking can be antagonized by long-term immunosuppression, but patients should, of course, be convinced to quit smoking.

Prevention of Early Tissue Lesions

It is obvious that if the recurrence of new lesions in the remaining bowel can be prevented, symptomatic relapse also will be prevented; eventually this would lead to cure of the disease. To date, only one strategy has resulted in a long-term disease-free perianastomotic region. Diversion of intestinal contents through a proximal ileostomy protects the neoterminal ileum and ileocolonic anastomosis from recurrence, suggesting that luminal contents, probably the bacterial flora, trigger flares of Crohn's disease.

This is also strongly suggested by the finding that, in the same model, infusion of ileal contents through a normal diverted ileocolonic anastomosis after only 1 week would induce inflammation characterized by mixed inflammatory infiltrate and cytokine upregulation.

Therefore, prophylactic therapy after resection for Crohn's disease should aim primarily at keeping the remaining bowel completely free of Crohn's disease. A second endpoint could be the prevention of symptomatic recurrence. Researchers still are far from reaching the primary goal. Standard anti-inflammatory approaches with glucocorticosteroids (GCSs) or 5-aminosalicylic-acid (5-ASA) formulations are not able to prevent tissue recurrence. The new topically acting GCS budesonide did not prevent the development of new lesions at 1 year after resection. Therefore, standard GCSs or budesonide should be tapered and discontinued within 4 weeks after resection. Studies with 5-ASA formulations show that short term, the most severe endoscopic lesions can be prevented, but the evolution is only somewhat delayed. The problem with 5-ASA treatment may be the delivery of the highest concentrations at the site of the ileocolonic anastomosis.

Nitroimidazol antibiotics, including metronidazole (20 mg/kg/d) or ornidazole (1 g/d), are able to temporarily prevent endoscopic recurrence. They decrease the overall endoscopic recurrence rate and prevent severe lesions from developing as long as they are taken by the patient. There was some protective effect for 1 year after 3 months of therapy. Troublesome side effects prohibit long-term use of these antibiotics. Data are scarce but suggest that clinical relapse can also be prevented with these antibiotics.

Postoperative 6-mercaptopurine (6-MP) (50 mg/d) was more effective than placebo in preventing endoscopic and radiologic recurrence after 1 and 2 years. This modest dosage also was associated with clinical benefit.

Prevention Strategies

5-ASA Formulations

Prophylactic therapy with sulfasalazine has not (with one exception) been shown to be beneficial in preventing small bowel symptomatic recurrences. There are some

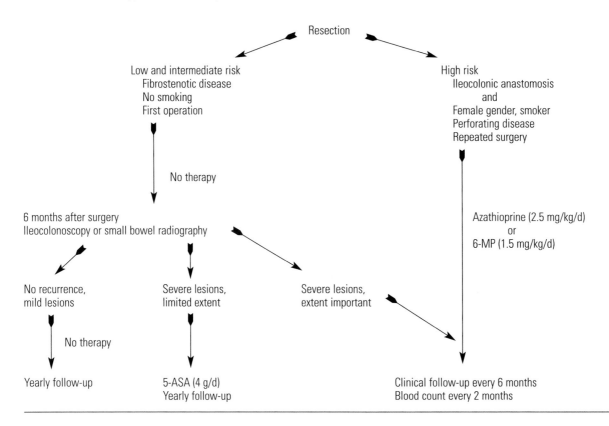

FIGURE 99–1. Algorithm for prophylaxis of Crohn's recurrence after resection. 5-ASA = 5-aminosalicylic acid; 6-MP = 6-mercaptopurine.

studies of postoperative clinical recurrence prevention with 5-ASA formulations (Table 99–1). They are heterogeneous with respect to the definition of recurrence, the location of the disease, and the duration of follow-up. A mild benefit for high doses of 5-ASA was observed. McLeod and co-workers (1995) noted a 37 percent risk reduction in the treatment group, which was of borderline significance. The study of Caprilli and colleagues, which reported the greatest benefit for 5-ASA, was not blinded and therefore may have been subject to bias.

A recent meta-analysis by Camma et al (1997), not including the data of Lochs, which are not yet fully published, shows a reduction of pooled clinical recurrence risk of 13 percent. This implies that eight patients would have to be treated with doses up to 3 to 4 g/d for a period of 2 to 3 years, at considerable cost, to prevent one clinical postoperative recurrence.

Small early trials have suggested that immunosuppresion with azathioprine (AZA) or 6-MP could efficaciously maintain surgically induced remission, especially in patients who had received AZA preoperatively. A large multicenter trial by Korelitz addressed this issue and compared 6-MP (50 mg/d) with Pentasa® (Ferring-Shire Pharmaceuticals Inc., Florence, Kentucky) (3 g/d) and placebo in a 2-year trial. Not only did 6-MP decrease the rate of endoscopic and radiologic recurrence but also the clinical recurrence rate at 2 years was significantly

decreased. However, the benefit was lower than expected. It is possible that too low a dose of 6-MP was used and that the drug may not have had its optimal activity immediately after surgery owing to the known slow onset of action of the drug. There is evidence of immune activation in the neoterminal ileum within weeks of anastomosis, which suggests starting therapy immediately postoperatively or even preoperatively.

A major drawback of prophylactic studies currently available is the lack of good patient selection at inclusion. Future studies should be designed in such way that only high-risk patients are included, so that the best prophylactic therapy can emerge. Not all patients should receive this type of treatment after bowel resection. Prophylactic immunosuppression therapy should be reserved for patients with severe extensive endoscopic or radiologic recurrence at 6 months or high-risk patients immediately postoperatively. For low-risk patients, colonoscopic or radiologic assessment at 6 months after resection is the determining factor in management (Figure 99–1).†

---

† Editor's Note: Figure 1 leaves some questions unanswered. If all ileocolonic anastomoses are high risk, presumably those operated for fibrotic disease are an exception. If a patient has undergone resection for active disease, I prescribe 5-ASA plus AZA for most. There is one study that suggests that budesonide may delay recurrences for a year in such patients. Those who needed AZA preoperatively will usually need it again. (TMB)

Management of Clinical Recurrence after Resection

It is imperative to treat patients with relapse due to disease recurrence in an aggressive manner. Therapy with 5-ASA alone is probably not adequate. Progression of the disease must be prevented since reoperation will lead to more diarrhea and deficiencies, which become more difficult to treat. Many symptoms that develop are not related to Crohn's disease itself. Initial treatment is a combination of budesonide 9 mg/d and azathioprine 2.5 mg/kg/d for 3 months and then steroids are discontinued and the patient continues on immunosuppression indefinitely. In as many as 60 percent of cases, the disease will remain controlled using AZA monotherapy; they may experience thorough tissue healing. If the disease flares despite AZA therapy, compliance should be verified, and dosage optimized, perhaps using 6-thioguanine nucleotide (6-TG) level before discontinuing Budesonide AZA should not be discontinued prematurely. Retreatment with budesonide is an option, but anti-tumor necrosis factor (TNF) antibodies (Remicade®, Centocor Inc., Malvern, Pennsylvania) may be helpful. The role of Remicade in postoperative management is yet to be determined.

Future Approaches

Immunosuppression and immunomodulation are attractive approaches to the prevention of recurrent Crohn's disease, and they have been suboptimally tested. Interleukin-10 (IL-10) is theoretically a good candidate for prevention of recurrence because of its immunoregulatory effects but one small study did not show efficacy for this cytokine in disease prevention. As mentioned, monoclonal antibodies to TNF (Remicade) should be effective for recurrence prevention, but data are lacking. Whether this therapy will be able to change the natural history of Crohn's disease remains uncertain. Combination therapies also are appealing. Ongoing studies include the combination of metronidazole and AZA for prevention of recurrent lesions in the tissue.[‡]

Conclusion

There are no clearly efficacious strategies to prevent symptomatic recurrence in all patients submitted to bowel resection for Crohn's disease. Glucocorticosteroids have no place, and the usefulness of prophylaxis with 5-ASA is borderline. Immunosuppression with Imuran® (Glaxo Wellcome, Research Triangle Park, North Carolina) or 6-MP is efficacious, but the protective effect may possibly be increased using induction therapy with metronidazole. It is likely that the use of anti-TNF strategies will change the picture in the future. There also is an important place for assessment of mucosal lesions with endoscopy or radiography in the planning of postoperative therapy.

References

Camma C, Giunta M, Roselli M, Cotone M. Mesalamine in the maintenance treatment of Crohn's disease: a meta-analysis adjusted for confounding variables. Gastroenterology 1997;113:1465–73.

Cottone M, Rosselli M, Orlando A, et al. Smoking habits and redurrence in Crohn's disease. Gastroenterology 1994; 106:543– .

Caprilli, Corrao G, Taodei G, et al. Prognostic factors for postoperative recurrence of Crohn's disease. Grappo Italiana per lo Studa del colone del Retto (GISC). Dis Colon Rectum 1996;39:335– .

de Dombel FT, Burton T, Goligher JC. Recurrence of Crohn's disease after primary excisional surgery. Gut 1971; 12:519–527.

Greenstein AJ, Lachman P, Sachar DB, et al. Perforating and non-perforating indications for repeated operations in Crohn's disease: evidence for two clinical forms. Gut 1988;29:588–92.

McLeod RS, Wolff BG, Steinhart AH, et al. Prophylactic mesalamine treatment decreases postoperative recurrence of Crohn's disease. Gastroenterology 1995;109:404–13.

Sutherland LR, Ramcharan S, Bryant H, Fick G. Effect of cigarette smoking on recurrence of Crohn's disease. Gastroenterology 1990;98:1123–8.

Supplemental Reading

Cameron JL, Hamilton SR, Coleman J, et al. Patterns of ileal recurrence in Crohn's disease: a prospective randomized study. Ann Surg 1992;215:546–52.

D'Haens G, Geboes K, Peeters M, et al. Early lesions of recurrent Crohn's disease caused by infusion of intestinal contents in excluded ileum. Gastroenterology 1998;114:262–7.

Griffiths AM, Wesson DE, Shandling B, et al. Factors influencing postoperative recurrence of Crohn's disease in childhood. Gut 1991;32:491–5.

Pallone F, Boirivant M, Stazi MA, et al. Analysis of clinical course of postoperative recurrence in Crohn's disease of distal ileum. Dig Dis Sci 1992;37:215–9.

Rutgeerts P, Geboes K, Peeters M, et al. Effect of fecal stream diversion on recurrence of Crohn's disease in the neoterminal ileum. Lancet 1991;338:771–4.

Rutgeerts P, Geboes K, Vantrappen G, et al. Predictability of the postoperative course of Crohn's disease. Gastroenterology 1990;99:956–63.

[‡] Editor's Note: This area is still evolving, with patient compliance still an important factor. I tend to use combination therapy because that is the approach I use for active disease. The groups that seem to be at highest risk are those operated early in their course for active disease and those operated for transmurally aggressive disease. (TMB)

CHAPTER 100

Diarrhea Following Small Bowel Resection

Lawrence R. Schiller, MD

The gastrointestinal (GI) tract is a long tube composed of segments with varied absorptive characteristics. The end result of this arrangement is the coordinated absorption of ingested food and drink and endogenous secretions that are added to the intestinal contents as part of the digestive process. In health, this mechanism is efficient. Of the 8 to 10 L of fluid passing the ligament of Treitz each day, 99 percent is absorbed, leaving a normal stool output of approximately 80 to 100 mL of water per day. Some excess capacity for absorption exists at each level of the intestine, and this allows some degree of compensation for abnormalities that occur at different levels.

In intestinal diseases, such as Crohn's disease and colitis, this normal orderly process is disrupted, and malabsorption of fluid and electrolytes may cause diarrhea. These intestinal diseases also may result in nutrient malabsorption and the consequences of malnutrition. Intestinal resection permanently removes one or more segments of the intestine. The extent of the absorptive defect depends upon which segment has been removed,

TABLE 100–1. Segmental Intestinal Function and Dysfunction with Resection

Functions	Dysfunctions with Resection
Jejunum	
High-capacity nutrient absorption	Markedly reduced nutrient absorption
High-capacity sodium and water transport	Flooding of lower bowel with fluid
Calcium and drug absorption	Reduced absorption
Ileum	
Nutrient salvage	Reduced nutrient absorption
Absorption of sodium against gradient	Reduced sodium and water transport
Vitamin B_{12} absorption	Reduced or absent vitamin B_{12} absorption
Bile acid reabsorption	Bile acid malabsorption: choleraic diarrhea, fat malabsorption
Ileal brake	Intestinal hurry
Colon	
Absorption of sodium against gradient	Reduced sodium and water transport
Short-chain fatty acid absorption	Osmotic diarrhea

TABLE 100–2. Mechanisms of Diarrhea after Intestinal Resection

Occurring Soon After Surgery	Occurring Some Time After Surgery
Loss of absorptive surface	Recurrent Crohn's disease
Bile acid malabsorption	Partial small bowel obstruction
Fatty acid malabsorption	Gastrocolic or enterocolic fistula
Loss of ileal brake	Small bowel bacterial overgrowth
Gastric acid hypersecretion	Medication-induced diarrhea
Fecal incontinence	Irritable bowel syndrome
Partial small bowel obstruction	Other causes of chronic diarrhea
Antibiotic-associated diarrhea	
Carbohydrate malabsorption	

how extensive the resection has been, and the ability of other segments to compensate for the missing functions of that segment (Table 100–1). For example, a small jejunal resection may be well tolerated, since more distal segments can compensate for the missing absorptive surface. On the other hand, distal ileal resection will reproducibly impair vitamin B_{12} and bile acid absorption, since no more distal segment of the intestine has the ability to compensate for these missing functions. There is a separate chapter on the short-bowel syndrome.

Differential Mechanisms of Postresection Diarrhea

Diarrhea can develop shortly after recovery from surgery and refeeding, or some time after recovery from surgery. The onset of diarrhea relative to the resection can be helpful in sorting through the mechanisms causing diarrhea and in developing appropriate management plans (Table 100–2).

Immediate Onset

Fluid and Electrolyte Malabsorption

When diarrhea develops in the immediate postoperative period as the patient is first being refed, several causes should be considered. First and foremost, the loss of the absorptive surface may critically reduce the capacity for intestinal transport. This is particularly true in the most common resection done for Crohn's disease, removal of the terminal ileum, ileocecal valve, and right colon. This part of the intestinal tract is specialized for absorbing sodium against a concentration gradient, whereas the residual jejunum and ileum can absorb fluid and sodium only when luminal sodium concentrations are over 80 to 100 mmol/L. In addition, loss of the ileocecal valve eliminates the major mechanism regulating colonic filling. This sort of resection may flood the lower part of the colon with salt and fluid beyond the absorptive capacity of the remaining colon, and diarrhea then results. Since surgeons are no longer resecting the entire ascending colon for ileocecal disease, the colonic aspect of this type of disease has been lessened.

BILE ACID MALABSORPTION

Another possible mechanism for development of diarrhea after ileal resection is bile acid malabsorption and bile acid–mediated inhibition of absorption by the colon. Ileal bile acid reabsorption usually is efficient: less than 5 percent of the bile acid entering the ileum enters the colon, because of the brisk absorption rate of bile acid by the healthy ileum. When this area is diseased or removed, more bile acid can enter the colon. If the luminal bile acid concentration exceeds 3 to 5 mmol/L, colonic sodium and water absorption is inhibited and net secretion may develop, producing diarrhea. This is a frequent mechanism of diarrhea when less than 50 cm of terminal ileum has been resected, because, in the absence of much water malabsorption, bile acid concentrations can become high enough to be cathartic in the colon. The bile acid synthesis rate increases to offset the losses and so steatorrhea does not develop.

STEATORRHEA

When longer segments of terminal ileum have been removed, water malabsorption in the small intestine dilutes bile acid concentration in the colon below the cathartic threshold. Bile acid malabsorption may be so profound that hepatic synthesis cannot compensate fully, and insufficient bile acid may be present in the duodenum to permit normal fat absorption. Delivery of fatty acids to the colon increases. Fatty-acid hydroxylation by colonic bacteria produces molecules that resemble ricinoleic acid, the active ingredient of castor oil, and diarrhea may result.

Additional mechanisms for diarrhea developing soon after resection include loss of the ileal brake, which ordinarily slows transit through the proximal intestine when excess nutrients enter the ileum; gastric acid hypersecretion, which complicates extensive small bowel resection; fecal incontinence; partial small bowel obstruction; and antibiotic-associated diarrhea, which may complicate the course of any patient after abdominal surgery. Carbohydrate malabsorption, such as that attributable to lactase deficiency, may be uncovered after intestinal resection.

Delayed Onset

When diarrhea develops weeks or months after resection, additional problems need to be considered. These include recurrent Crohn's disease, gastrocolic or enterocolic fistula, small bowel bacterial overgrowth, and medication-induced diarrhea.

RECURRENCE OF CROHN'S DISEASE

Recurrent disease must be the primary consideration for late-onset postresection diarrhea. Recurrence of Crohn's disease occurs in roughly 50 percent of patients after resective surgery over 10 years. Although the risk of recurrence is reduced by continuing mesalamine or some other form of therapy after resection, recurrent disease still may occur. Recurrences typically develop at the site of anastomosis. Diarrhea also can complicate recurrent disease, if the recurrence produces a gastrocolic or enterocolic fistula.

BACTERIAL OVERGROWTH

As a cause of diarrhea after resection, bacterial overgrowth is more likely to occur if the ileocecal valve has been removed or if there is an element of partial small bowel obstruction, blind loops, or diverticula that would encourage stasis and the growth of bacteria.

IRRITABLE BOWEL SYNDROME

A perplexing group of patients are those who develop a syndrome resembling irritable bowel syndrome (IBS), characterized by abdominal pain and loose stools on an intermittent basis. This situation actually may be irritable bowel syndrome, a common functional disorder, occurring in patients who have had surgery for inflammatory bowel disease (IBD). This is a difficult diagnosis to make in the presence of a history of IBD and surgery, but should be considered in this setting.[*] Likewise, any disease that produces chronic diarrhea might present after resection.

Evaluation of Diarrhea after Small Bowel Resection

The most important part of the evaluation of patients with diarrhea after resection is a careful history. As previously mentioned, the time of onset after surgery is an important clue to the possible cause of diarrhea. Recurrent Crohn's disease often produces the same group of symptoms that the patient originally had, particularly if the patient had systemic symptoms, such as weakness, arthralgia, or uveitis. Colonic disease may not have been recognized preoperatively. An accurate record of the frequency of evacuation and additional GI symptoms, such as bleeding, abdominal distention, nausea and vomiting, and weight loss, and a list of current medications provide key information. Physical examination should be directed

---

[*] Editor's Note: A simplistic view would be a large volume of fluid being introduced quickly into a spastic, but undiseased, left colon of a patient with an underlying irritable bowel syndrome plus Crohn's disease. Please see the chapters on the coexistence of IBS and IBD. (TMB)

TABLE 100–3. Treatments for Specific Conditions

Condition	Treatment
Loss of absorptive surface	Opiate antidiarrheals, fluid and electrolyte replacement
Bile acid malabsorption	Bile acid–binding agents (eg, cholestyramine)
Fatty-acid malabsorption	Bile acid replacement, low-fat diet
Loss of ileal brake	Opiate antidiarrheals
Gastric acid hypersecretion	Histamine₂-receptor antagonists
Fecal incontinence	Assess cause and treat abnormality if possible
Partial small bowel obstruction	Surgery
Antibiotic-associated diarrhea	Metronidazole, if due to *Clostridium difficile*
Carbohydrate malabsorption	Identify malabsorbed carbohydrate and omit from diet
Recurrent Crohn's disease	Anti-inflammatory or immunosuppressive drugs
Gastrocolic or enterocolic fistula	Surgery, infliximab
Bacterial overgrowth	Antibiotics: fluoroquinolone, metronidazole
Medication-induced diarrhea	Identify agent and discontinue
Irritable bowel syndrome	Low-dose tricyclic antidepressant, opiates, cellulose or psyllium in small amounts

at detection of complicating features, such as dehydration and evidence of activity of Crohn's disease. Routine laboratory testing, including a complete blood count, serum chemistries, thyroid-stimulating hormone (TSH), and stool microbiology tests to expose infectious causes of diarrhea, may be helpful.

Every patient with postresection diarrhea should have an evaluation for structural problems. Most important is small bowel radiography, which can show evidence of recurrent disease, fistula, and the length of the bowel remaining, and can give an approximate small bowel transit time. In some circumstances, particularly if an abdominal mass is present, computed tomography of the abdomen can be useful. Colonoscopic evaluation can show evidence of mucosal recurrence or anastomotic obstruction, but may not be as helpful as a well-done small bowel radiography series. As mentioned, colonic disease may have been present before ileal resection.

Analysis of stool collected as either a spot specimen or as part of a quantitative collection can be helpful for classifying the cause of diarrhea. Stool weight can give some idea of the absorptive capacity of the remaining gut and can help to distinguish conditions with low stool weight (eg, fecal incontinence, IBS) from those characterized by major water and electrolyte malabsorption. Electrolyte concentrations can be used to estimate fecal osmotic gap and allow one to categorize the diarrhea as being a secretory or osmotic process. One can also estimate electrolyte losses in the stool and more accurately replace these with intravenous fluid, if necessary. Assessment of fat excretion also is helpful. The presence of steatorrhea suggests the presence of bile acid deficiency in the duodenum, extensive proximal small bowel disease or resection, bacterial

overgrowth, or severe intestinal hurry. Carbohydrate malabsorption can be diagnosed if there is a large calculated fecal osmotic gap and if fecal pH is < 6. Additional tests on stool that may be useful include a fecal occult blood test, a stained smear for fecal leukocytes, and direct measurement of bile acid excretion.

Treatment

If a specific problem, such as bacterial overgrowth, is identified, specific treatment can be applied and may substantially improve the situation (Table 100–3). Often a specific treatable entity cannot be diagnosed and nonspecific treatment must be applied. Nonspecific treatment can provide significant improvement in symptoms and allow for use of the absorptive surface of the intestine in a more efficient fashion (Table 100–4).

Diet

If the patient has steatorrhea, a **reduction in fat intake** may help. However, fat is a useful source of energy calories, and replacement of fat by carbohydrate can actually generate a larger load of fluid entering the colon. In some cases, steatorrhea is attributable to insufficient duodenal bile acid concentration, and supplementation with exogenous bile acid (ie, **ox bile tablets**)* can improve fat absorption. When there is evidence of carbohydrate malabsorption, an effort should be made to identify the carbohydrate responsible. Often it will be lactose, and a

TABLE 100–4. Nonspecific Treatments for Postresection Diarrhea

Diet
  Steatorrhea: low-fat diet
  Carbohydrate malabsorption: reduce specific carbohydrate (eg, lactose)
  Frequent feedings
  Nutritional support: enteral or parenteral dietary supplements
  Lessen caffeine intake

Antidiarrheal medications
  Diphenoxylate with atropine tablets (up to 8/d in divided doses)
  Loperamide (up to 16 mg/d in divided doses)
  Codeine (up to 240 mg/d in divided doses)
  Deodorized tincture of opium (up to 80 drops [40 mg morphine] daily)
  Morphine (up to 40 mg/d in divided doses)

Stool modifying agents
  Psyllium, methylcellulose (up to 20 g/d in divided doses)
  Bile acid–binding agents (up to 20 g/d in divided doses)

Adjunctive medications
  Histamine₂-receptor antagonists (eg, cimetidine 300 mg qid)
  Anticholinergic drugs (eg, propantheline 15 mg qid)

Replacement therapy
  Fluid and electrolytes (oral rehydration solution, intravenous solution)
  Magnesium, calcium
  Parenteral vitamin B₁₂, fat-soluble vitamins

---

* Editor's Note: Drs Little, Schiller and Fordtran have used Oxbile tablets experimentally. I do not have information on a commercial source. (TMB)

lactose-free diet is needed. Frequent feedings use the absorptive surface of the intestine on a more continuous basis and may result in better fractional absorption of fluid, electrolytes, and nutrients. In some cases, malabsorption may be so severe as to require nutritional support with enteral or parenteral supplements. These are not routinely needed but ought to be considered in patients with postresection diarrhea who are substantially malnourished.

Antidiarrheal Medications

Opiate antidiarrheal medications can be extremely helpful in patients who have postresection diarrhea owing to a loss of mucosal surface area. Slowing the progress of luminal fluid through the intestine allows more time for each of the remaining segments to reabsorb water and electrolytes; thus, the total amount absorbed can increase. Less potent antidiarrheals, such as diphenoxylate or loperamide, may not be sufficiently active for some patients. Deodorized tincture of opium, codeine, or morphine may be required. However, even potent opiates cannot substitute for specialized absorption defects, such as inability to absorb vitamin B_{12} or bile salt.

Stool Modifying Agents

Fiber supplements can improve stool consistency but may increase total stool weight and water losses. Bile acid–binding agents (eg, cholestyramine) are of use in patients with proven or suspected bile acid malabsorption and may also help some individuals with fatty acid–induced diarrhea. If used for an empiric trial, a large dose (20 g/d in divided doses) should be tried and reduced to the lowest possible dose, if effective.[†] Bile acid–binding resins may bind other drugs and should be given at least 2 hours before or after other agents.

Adjunctive Medications

Several additional medicines can be of help in patients with postresection diarrhea. Histamine2-receptor antagonists can be used to reduce acid secretion and the amount of fluid and electrolytes entering the upper intestine. This class of drugs is particularly useful in patients with gastric acid hypersecretion, but may help other patients by reducing fluid loads. Proton pump inhibitors may not work as well in patients with postresection diarrhea, because all oral proton pump inhibitors are marketed in time-release capsules to bypass gastric acidity, and there may not be sufficient time for the medication to be absorbed. In contrast, histamine2-receptor antagonists are administered in a rapidly absorbable form and can inhibit acid secretion substantially. Anticholinergic

medications can be used as antitransit and antisecretory medications and can improve the efficiency of other antidiarrheal drugs.

Replacement Therapy

Another important aspect of therapy is to replace malabsorbed substances. These include water and electrolytes, when diarrhea leads to dehydration, sodium chloride and magnesium, if diarrheal losses have been too extreme, and vitamin B_{12}. Oral rehydration solutions may be used to replete sodium chloride but may cause stool output to increase. Repletion of magnesium is problematic, since it is a poorly absorbed ion, and efforts to replace it by giving it orally often result in worse diarrhea. Intermittent parenteral administration of magnesium may be needed in some individuals. Patients with postresection diarrhea also should be considered for parenteral vitamin B_{12} administration and replenishment of fat-soluble vitamins. Since both vitamin B_{12} and fat-soluble vitamins may be stored within the body, it may take some time for overt deficiencies to develop and prophylactic supplementation should be considered early in individuals who have had substantial resections. The chapter on short-bowel syndrome (#102) includes further details on replacement therapy.

Supplemental Reading

Arrambide KA, Santa Ana CA, Schiller LR, et al. Loss of absorptive capacity for sodium chloride as a cause of diarrhea following partial ileal and right colon resection. Dig Dis Sci 1989;34:193–201.

Fine KD. Diarrhea. In: Feldman M, Scharschmidt BF, Sleisenger MH, eds. Sleisenger and Fordtran's gastrointestinal and hepatic diseases. Pathophysiology, diagnosis, management. 6th Ed. Philadelphia: WB Saunders, 1998:128–52.

Fine KD, Schiller LR. AGA technical review on the evaluation and management of chronic diarrhea. Gastroenterology 1999;116:1464–86.

Gruy-Kapral C, Little KH, Fordtran JS, et al. Conjugated bile acid replacement therapy for short-bowel syndrome. Gastroenterology 1999;116:15–21.

Hammer HF, Fine KD, Santa Ana CA, et al. Carbohydrate malabsorption. Its measurement and its contribution to diarrhea. J Clin Invest 1990;86:1936–44.

Little KH, Schiller LR, Bilhartz LE, Fordtran JS. Treatment of severe steatorrhea with ox bile in an ileectomy patient with residual colon. Dig Dis Sci 1992;37:929–33.

Schiller LR. Review article: anti-diarrhoeal pharmacology and therapeutics. Aliment Pharmacol Ther 1995;9:87–106.

Schiller LR, Bilhartz LE, Santa Ana CA, Fordtran JS. Comparison of endogenous and radiolabeled bile acid excretion in patients with idiopathic chronic diarrhea. Gastroenterology 1990;98:1036–43.

[†] Editor's Note: Some physicians start with 4 g in the morning plus loperamide before meals and in the evening. This is adequate in some patients. (TMB)

CHAPTER 101

HYPEROXALURIA AND NEPHROLITHIASIS

WILLIAM A. ROWE, MD, CNSP

Hyperoxaluria associated with inflammatory bowel disease (IBD) is referred to as enteric hyperoxaluria in the urologic literature. Enteric hyperoxaluria occurs not only with IBD, but also with short-bowel syndrome, jejunoileal bypass, and other malabsorption states. Enteric hyperoxaluria is distinct from other forms of hyperoxaluria, including the rare primary hyperoxaluria, which is a hepatic enzyme disorder, and the more common metabolic hyperoxaluria, an increase in red blood cell oxalate exchange.

The finding of renal stones in association with IBD occurs with a frequency ranging from 1 percent to 5 percent. Most studies noting coincidental findings of nephrolithiasis were on the low end of the spectrum; however, higher figures are noted in studies specifically designed to look for nephrolithiasis as a complication of IBD (Deren et al, 1962). Not all kidney stones found in patients with IBD are oxalate stones. Chemical analysis of a passed stone or of the urine must be made before enteric hyperoxaluria can be assumed to be the cause of the nephrolithiasis.

Pathophysiology

Selection of treatment for hyperoxaluria and oxalate nephrolithiasis is aided by an understanding of the mechanisms of oxalate stone formation. Hyperoxaluria is defined as urinary oxalate excretion of greater than 45 mg/d. If more than 80 mg/d is present, primary or enteric hyperoxaluria is likely. Mild-to-moderate elevations may occur from dietary intake of oxalate-rich foods.

The basic mechanism of calcium-oxalate stone formation is that increases in the concentrations of urinary calcium and oxalate render the urine supersaturated with respect to stone-forming salts, with subsequent precipitation. This precipitation may or may not be symptomatic, but even when the kidney stones are asymptomatic, renal damage from the nephrolithiasis may occur.

Perhaps the major contributor to the formation of a calcium-oxalate precipitation in patients with IBD is dehydration. Low urine volume occurs from inadequate fluid intake or from dehydration secondary to diarrhea This concentrated urine contributes to stone formation by rendering the urine supersaturated with respect to stone-forming salts.

There are multiple defects that account for the increased intestinal absorption of oxalate in enteric hyperoxaluria. Fat malabsorption leads to calcium- and magnesium-soap formation, which limits the amount of divalent cations available to complex oxalate within the intestinal lumen. This, in turn, raises the intraluminal pool of free oxalate available for absorption. Oxalate absorption can be increased further directly by the action of bile salts and fatty acids on the intestinal mucosa since bile salts and fatty acids increase the permeability of intestinal mucosa to oxalate. The colon appears to be a major site of oxalate absorption. Oxalate excretion is the result of excess oxalate absorption. Small incremental increases in oxalate excretion markedly raise the activity product of the ions in the urine, making urinary oxalate more important than calcium in determining calcium-oxalate supersaturation.

Urinary oxalate comes from two sources: 80 to 90 percent of urinary oxalate is synthesized in the liver; the remainder comes from dietary oxalate. Of the hepatically synthesized oxalate, approximately 40 percent is derived from the metabolism of ascorbate (vitamin C), and the remainder is derived directly or indirectly as a metabolic end product of glycine or glyoxylate metabolism. Normal amounts of dietary ascorbate do not cause an increase in urinary excretion of oxalate, but in some individuals increases in urinary oxalate occur following the ingestion of 1 to 2 g of ascorbate (two to four 500-mg vitamin C tablets). Pyridoxine (vitamin B_6) is a cofactor necessary for enzymatic shunting of metabolic products away from oxalate production, so that deficiency of pyridoxine leads to increased formation and excretion of oxalate. Although vitamin B_6 supplementation may help a patient deficient in this cofactor, there is no evidence that "megadosing" with vitamin B_6 is of any therapeutic value. Thus, hyperoxaluria can occur from a defect in oxalate synthesis, dietary overindulgence in high-oxalate foods, or excess vitamin C intake. The dietary causes alone account for only a small percentage of increased urinary oxalate.

The concentration of urinary electrolytes other than calcium and oxalate also plays a role in oxalate nephrolithiasis. Urinary citrate tends to be low, especially in patients who are hypokalemic or have intracellular acidosis. Urinary magnesium is low from formation of magnesium-oxalate complexes and magnesium–fatty acid soaps.

Clinical Presentation and Evaluation

Renal stones often are asymptomatic; when this is the case, such as when nephrolithiasis is found incidentally, medical attempts at dissolution are appropriate. However, when the stone becomes symptomatic, more aggressive intervention is warranted. Nephrolithiasis classically presents as renal colic. Unfortunately, in patients with IBD a high index of suspicion is necessary, because the pain associated with the kidney stone may easily (and erroneously) be attributed to the underlying IBD. Microscopic hematuria is suggestive of the diagnosis.

Patients with enteric hyperoxaluric nephrolithiasis are considered at high risk for developing recurrent stones, and thus a thorough urologic evaluation is generally indicated. Urologic consultation is warranted for the evaluation and to assist in designing an optimal prevention strategy. An evaluation for enteric hyperoxaluria or nephrolithiasis typically includes serum evaluations of calcium, phosphate, and parathyroid hormone, as well as urinary calcium (both fasting and after calcium load), urinary uric acid, citrate, oxalate, magnesium, and pH.

Treatment of Nephrolithiasis

The treatment for acute, symptomatic nephrolithiasis is initially narcotic analgesia with copious hydration in an attempt to help the patient pass the stone spontaneously. If this is unsuccessful, a urologist is consulted, and the stone can be removed transureterally, surgically, or by using extracorporeal shock wave lithotripsy (ESWL). Performed under general anesthesia, the goal of ESWL treatment is to fragment the stone into a size that can easily be passed by the patient; ESWL should not present any greater risk for a patient with IBD than any alternative procedure. Once alleviation of the acute nephrolithiasis event is accomplished, it then becomes necessary to prevent stone recurrence.

Medical Management of Hyperoxaluria

The medical management of enteric hyperoxaluria is undertaken in patients with asymptomatic hyperoxaluric nephrolithiasis as well as in those in whom stones have been removed, to prevent recurrence. The treatment options available often depend upon the activity of the IBD, other treatments being administered or considered, and the nutritional status of the patient. The basic treatment options call for **increasing hydration status, treating malabsorption, lowering saturation levels** of calcium and oxalate, and possibly **preventing dietary indiscretion** (Table 101–1).

TABLE 101–1. Summary of Treatment Options for Enteric Hyperoxaluria

Category	Treatment Options
Hydration	Goal: 2 L urine output per day
Treat malabsorption	Treat underlying IBD
Electrolyte management options	Potassium citrate 30–60 meq/d* Urocit-K® (Mission Pharmacol Urologicals, San Antonio, TX) 2 to 4 tabs tid (5 meq/tab) Calcium citrate 0.25–1.0 g/qd* Citracal® (Mission Pharmacol Urologicals, San Antonio, TX) 1 tab/qd (OTC) Magnesium oxide 400 mg/qd or bid* Beelith® (Beach Pharmaceuticals, Tampa, FL) 1 tab/qd (with food)†
Dietary	Avoid vitamin C supplements Supplement vitamin B6 (many multivitamins) Avoid rhubarb, spinach, beets, peanuts, chocolate, parsley, celery, tea, coffee

*There may be contraindications; † Beelith® also contains vitamin B6.

Hydration

The most profound influence on the risk of formation of renal stones is hydration status. Concentrated urine will always be at higher risk of allowing crystal growth and aggregation than will dilute urine. The patient should be encouraged to increase fluid intake to maintain urine output greater than 2 L/d. It may be advantageous to actually have the patient measure urine output, especially in patients who have undergone ileostomy, in whom increased hydration also increases ileostomy output. For those patients without diarrhea, a urinary output of 2 L/d generally can be obtained by drinking 10 large (10 oz) glasses of water per day. In those patients with IBD on hyperalimentation, free water in the total parenteral nutrition solution can easily be increased.

The use of oral rehydration solution to increase hydration in patients with hyperoxaluria (and nephrolithiasis) must be done with caution. The increased sodium and bicarbonate intake may adversely affect the solubility product of calcium and oxalate and increase the likelihood of stone formation. However, it is likely that this risk would be more than offset if the urinary output increased substantially. This is a situation in which urine output and periodic monitoring of urinary calcium and oxalate concentrations would be warranted.

Correct Malabsorption

The next most effective intervention is the treatment of underlying malabsorption. Since enteric hyperoxaluria can arise in a number of conditions other than IBD, the treatment of the malabsorption depends upon the underlying disease and interventions that have been performed. Immune suppression in patients with IBD often is beneficial in the treatment of hyperoxaluria; it must be borne in mind that corticosteroids increase urinary calcium excretion, which would increase the risk of calcium-oxalate stone formation. Enteric hyperoxaluria in a patient with IBD is clearly one situation in which long-term use of immunomodifiers, such as azathioprine (AZA) or 6-mer-captopurine (6-MP), would be preferable to multiple short courses of corticosteroids. In some patients, especially if a portion of the terminal ileum has been resected, cholestyramine may be beneficial. Pancreatic enzymes also may be beneficial in isolated instances. A decrease in dietary fat intake may be necessary.

Since much dietary oxalate appears to be absorbed in the colon, colectomy for underlying IBD occasionally may be curative of enteric hyperoxaluric nephrolithiasis as well. However, there are multiple reports of nephrolithiasis in patients with ileostomies, although the types of stones frequently are not chemically identified or are identified as uric acid stones. The majority of excreted oxalate is not from direct oxalate absorption; therefore, colectomy primarily for the treatment of hyperoxaluric nephrolithiasis cannot be recommended.

Selective Electrolyte Management

Magnesium and citrate play an inhibitory role in calcium nephrolithiasis. Citrate lowers the urinary saturation of calcium oxalate by forming a more soluble calcium-citrate complex. In addition, citrate may directly inhibit calcium oxalate and phosphate crystallization.

Magnesium increases the solubility product of calcium oxalate and calcium phosphate. In addition, oral magnesium supplementation can be used to complex oxalate in the lumen and to correct hypomagnesuria, but may exacerbate diarrhea. This latter problem may significantly limit the use of oral magnesium for the treatment of hyperoxaluria. Of note, the urinary chemical profile is improved most (from an oxalate stone prevention standpoint) when magnesium oxide is taken with food.

Oral administration of moderate amounts of calcium (0.25 to 1.0 g/d) can bind calcium in the intestinal lumen, but may increase urinary calcium in some patients. Calcium citrate is theoretically advantageous; calcium binds oxalate in the intestinal lumen, and citrate helps correct metabolic acidosis and hypocitruria. Use of calcium citrate also has the benefit of helping to prevent bone dimineralization.

Combinations of electrolytes are also available. Potassium citrate 30 to 60 meq/d (in patients with normal renal function) can correct hypokalemia and metabolic acidosis as well as increase urinary citrate levels. A recent clinical trial demonstrated that a combination potassium-magnesium citrate is an effective prophylaxis against recurrent calcium oxalate nephrolithiasis, reducing the risk of recurrence by 85 percent (Ettinger et al, 1997). This latter agent is not yet commercially available.

Allopurinol, commonly used to treat uric acid stones, is not thought to have any effect, either beneficial or adverse, on calcium oxalate stones. Thiazide diuretics, used to decrease urinary calcium concentration in a variety of renal stones, increases urinary oxalate and should not be used in patients with oxalate stones. Phosphate-containing compounds, which tend to increase both urinary calcium and oxalate, are generally avoided in hyperoxaluria as well.

Dietary Intervention

For a patient with calcium oxalate stones, it is wise to avoid dietary excess of oxalate. The main direct dietary sources of oxalate are rhubarb, spinach, beets, peanuts, chocolate, parsley, celery, tea, and coffee.[*]

Of greater importance is the indirect dietary source of oxalate, which is protein (Table 101–2). As a rule of thumb, most patients do well with a protein intake of 1.0 to 1.2 g of protein per kilogram of body weight per day. This assumes well-controlled, quiescent IBD. However, because IBD causes a protein-losing enteropathy, this author is reluctant to restrict protein intake for any patient with any significant degree of IBD activity.

TABLE 101–2. Diet and Stone Risk

Dietary Item	Effect on Stone Risk
Protein	↑ ↑ ↑
Salt	↑ ↑
Oxalate	↑
Calcium	↑ or ↓
Phosphate	↑ or ↓
Magnesium	↓
Citrate	↓ ↓
Fluids	↓ ↓ ↓

References

Deren JJ, Porush JG, Levitt MF, Khilnani MT. Nephrolithiasis as a complication of ulcerative colitis and regional enteritis. Ann Intern Med 1962;56:843–53.

Ettinger B, Pak CYC, Citron JT, et al. Potassium-magnesium citrate is an effective prophylaxis against recurrent calcium oxalate nephrolithiasis. J Urol 1997;158:2069–73.

Supplemental Reading

Dobbins JW, Binder HJ. Importance of the colon in enteric hyperoxaluria. N Engl J Med 1977;296:298–301.

Goldfarb S. Diet and nephrolithiasis. Annu Rev Med 1994; 45:235–43.

---

* Editor's Note: Although Dr. Rowe, the author, correctly puts dietary oxalate intake into perspective (in Table 101–2) as a minor factor in hyperoxaluria, some patients with unusual diet habits want detailed information on the oxalate content of foods. Therefore, we have taken the liberty of including Table 101–3, which lists the oxalate content of a variety of foods. This is not intended to decrease the emphasis on the other therapeutic factors that are stressed in the chapter. (TMB)

Larsson L, Tiselius HG. Hyperoxaluria. Miner Electrolyte Metab 1987;13:242–50.

Meyer JL, Smith LH. Growth and calcium oxalate crystals. II. Inhibition by natural urinary crystal growth inhibitors. Invest Urol (Berl) 1975;13:36.

Pak CY, Holt K. Nucleation and growth of brushite and calcium oxalate in urine of stone-formers. Metabolism 1976;25:665–73.

Parivar F, Low RK, Stoller ML. The influence of diet on urinary stone disease. J Urol 1996;155:432–40.

Tiselius H, Almgard LE. The diurnal excretion of oxalate and the effect of pyridoxine and ascorbate on oxalate excretion. Eur Urol 1977;3:41–6.

TABLE 101–3. Oxalate Content of Various Foods*

Food Group	Moderate Oxalate Content (2–10 mg/serving)	High Oxalate Content (>10 mg/serving)
Beverages	Coffee, any kind (8 oz) Cranberry juice (4 oz) Grape juice (4 oz) Orange juice (4 oz) Tomato juice (4 oz) Nescafe powder	Cocoa Draft beer, stout Juices containing berries Ovaltine and other beverage mixes Tea
Protein	Sardines	Baked beans canned in tomato sauce Peanut butter Soybean curd (tofu)
Vegetables and fruits	Asparagus Broccoli Carrots Corn Cucumber, peeled Green peas, canned Lettuce, iceberg Lima beans Parsnips Tomato, 1 small Turnips	Beans: green, wax, dried Beets: tops, root, green Celery Chives Collards Dandelion greens Eggplant Escarole Kale Leeks Mustard greens Okra Swiss chard
	Apples Apricots Black currants Cherries, red sour Orange Peaches, Alberta Pears Pineapples Plums, Damson Prunes, Italian	Blackberries Blueberries Concord grapes Dewberries Fruit cocktail Gooseberries Lemon peel Lime peel Raspberries Red currants Rhubarb Strawberries Tangerines
Breads and other starches	Cornbread Spaghetti, canned in tomato sauce Sponge cake	Fruit cake Grits, white corn Soybean Wheat germ
Miscellaneous	Chicken noodle soup, dehydrated	Chocolate, cocoa Nuts Peanuts Pecans Pepper (in excess of 1 tsp/d) Tomato soup Vegetable soup

Modified from Ney DM. The low diet book for the prevention of oxalate stones. San Diego, California: University of California, 1981, and UCLA manual of clinical dietetics. Los Angeles: University of California, 1986.

*Editor's Note: This list of oxalate content was added to this chapter for physician and patient information but the minor role of dietary intake of oxalates and the major importance of other factors should not be obscured by the presence of this list. (TMB)

CHAPTER 102

Clinical Management of Short-Bowel Syndrome

Alan L. Buchman, MD, MSPH, and Joseph Sellin, MD

The absorptive capacity of the small intestine has significant reserve capacity, and small resections are of little or no clinical consequence. However, patients with Crohn's disease who undergo multiple intestinal resections may develop what is known as short-bowel syndrome. The definition of short-bowel syndrome may vary, but generally implies either malabsorption or the necessity for specific nutrient therapies. Depending upon the length and health of the remaining intestine, as well as the presence or absence of the ileocecal valve or colon, such patients may require various oral supplements, intravenous fluids, or even total parenteral nutrition (TPN). Bowel length may be difficult to determine because most commonly used methods such as barium contrast studies and intraoperative measurement are imprecise. In addition, there is significant individual variation in the adaptive response to differing lengths of residual intestine. Younger individuals, especially neonates, have a much greater capacity to adapt than adults.

Several factors are important for ensuring optimal adaptation. Following a massive resection, the bowel hypertrophies; it grows slightly in length, but more importantly, villus number and size and crypt depth all increase; intestinal absorptive surface area increases significantly. In addition, colonic hypertrophy occurs, which leads to increased colonic fluid and electrolyte absorption. These may be hormone-mediated responses, possibly mediated by enteroglucagon, glucagon-like peptide II, secretin, cholecystokinin, and various growth factors. The adaptation process may continue for up to 2 years in humans. The health of the remaining bowel also is significant. Unfortunately, Crohn's disease can recur regardless of how little bowel remains.

Generally, virtually all digestion and nutrient absorption are completed within the first 100 to 150 cm of jejunum in a normal individual. The minimum length of residual small bowel necessary to avoid parenteral nutrition is approximately 100 cm of healthy bowel in the absence of an intact colon and 60 cm with an intact colon. Patients who have less than 100 cm of residual jejunum often exhibit significant fluid loss with food. However, there is a large interpatient variability. Equivalent proximal resections are much better tolerated than massive distal resections, because remaining ileum can take over much of the function of jejunum. In contrast, residual jejunum is incapable of either vitamin B_{12} or bile salt absorption. In addition, studies in the dog have shown that the hypermotility associated with massive bowel resections returns to normal faster with more proximal resections.

Medical Treatment Strategies

Treatment of Excessive Fluid Losses

Massive fluid and electrolyte losses often occur frequently during the first week or two following a massive small bowel resection, but may improve over the ensuing months. During this postoperative period, patients usually require parenteral fluids and nutrition. It also is important to institute enteral nutrition as soon as possible to hasten the intestinal adaptive response. Transient gastric hypersecretion perhaps related to hypergastrinemia also occurs for the first 6 to 12 months following a massive intestinal resection. Histamine$_2$ (H$_2$) antagonists and proton pump inhibitors are useful for decreasing jejunal fluid and potassium losses during the first 6 to 12 months. These medications all are absorbed in the proximal jejunum. If transit time is significantly decreased, medication absorption is correspondingly decreased, and larger doses may be necessary. Medications such as loperamide, diphenoxylate, codeine, or tincture of opium (listed in order of increasing need) may be important to slow motility and increase nutrient contact time. Loperamide hydrochloride or diphenoxylate in doses up to 16 mg may be required to control fluid losses. If not adequate, codeine sulfate (30 to 60 mg tid) or tincture of opium (10 drops bid tid) may be necessary. High dose of calcium (2.4 to 3.6 g/d of elemental Ca) also may be useful for decreasing diarrhea, probably because of increased binding of fatty acids. Octreotide is rarely necessary except for some patients with high output jejunostomies. Its use should be avoided if possible because of an association with pancreatic insufficiency, malabsorption, decreased intestinal adaptation, and cholelithiasis.

Because of the predilection of Crohn's disease for ileocecal segments of intestine, resection is common. Should the ileocecal valve be resected, intestinal transit time also will be decreased. It has been hypothesized that either the distal ileum or the colon acts as a "brake" and exhibits a negative effect on duodenal motility, perhaps mediated via peptide YY. Malabsorption is increased because of the decreased contact time for nutrients with the luminal surface epithelium. In addition, bacterial colonization of the small intestine may occur, increasing diarrhea. This results because of the competition from bacteria for the available nutrients, such as vitamin B_{12}. D-lactic acidosis is a rare complication of bacterial overgrowth, but may result in serious sequelae, including ataxia, dysarthria, ophthalmoplegia, nystagmus, stupor, and coma. It may develop when simple carbohydrates, such as glucose and lactose, are malabsorbed and are fermented by anaerobic flora. Bacteria deconjugate bile salts, leading to decreased reabsorption and increased fecal losses, which leads to increased bile salt loss. Therefore, fewer bile salts are available for micelle formation and normal fat digestion in the proximal intestine. Diarrhea may worsen in patients who have had > 100 cm of ileum resected and in whom part or all of the colon remains, in part because bile salts stimulate cyclic adenosine monophosphate (cAMP) and calcium-mediated chloride secretion. Unabsorbed long-chain fatty acids also may stimulate colonic electrogenic anion secretion.

Treatment of bacterial overgrowth or D-lactic acidosis may be undertaken with either metronidazole or tetracycline. Unfortunately, the use of broad-spectrum antibiotics also may contribute to the worsening of diarrhea, because of either *Clostridium difficile* or non–*C. difficile*-associated diarrhea. Antibiotic use also may be associated with vitamin K deficiency, because normal gastrointestinal flora synthesize at least half of the body's daily requirement.

Enhancement of Absorption

One of the most important factors for the promotion of intestinal hypertrophy and optimal adaptation of the remaining segment is the provision of **enteral feeding** as soon as possible postoperatively. The presence of growth factors, such as epidermal growth factor, in the salivary glands and esophagus makes oral feeding preferable. However, except for certain patient groups, there is no need for either special diets or dietary restrictions. What is important is that the patient consume as much energy and nitrogen as possible. This may mean upward of 4,000 to 6,000 kcal and 150 g of nitrogen daily. Depending on the absorptive capacity of the remaining intestine (and colon), much of this may not be assimilated. Bolus feedings should always be avoided, and the patient should be instructed to "graze" throughout the day. Although initial nonblinded studies of glutamine and growth hormone use suggested improved adaptation and absorption, two more recent double-blinded, placebo-controlled studies cast doubt on whether either has any potential influence on bowel adaptation in humans. Studies with glucagon-

like peptide II (GLP-II) are underway, and the results are eagerly anticipated.

Diets and Specific Nutrient Requirements

All diets should be lactose-free, as the intestine will have lost a significant portion of its surface area and, therefore, its capacity to synthesize disaccharidase following a massive resection. In addition, patients should avoid consumption of caffeine-containing products and osmotically active medications or sweeteners (sorbitol for example) that increase fluid secretion, stimulate motility and lead to a further decrease in intestinal transit.

Oral Rehydration Solution

Water should be avoided since additional fluid and electrolyte losses may result. Isotonic fluids such as oral rehydration solution (ORS) should be used instead. Oral rehydration solutions are useful for the maintenance of normal hydrational status in short-bowel syndrome as well as acute diarrhea. Such solutions are based on the mechanism of the sodium-glucose cotransporter, whereby both solutes are actively absorbed together by the enterocyte. Water is pulled in with both sodium and glucose (solvent drag). Oral rehydration solution does not decrease fluid losses but does enhance fluid absorption. Recent data actually suggest that hypotonic ORS (but not water) may be preferential because of the ability of these solutions to enhance intestinal water absorption (without sodium absorption). Sodas and juices are hypertonic and should be avoided. An attempt should be made to have the patient consume dry solids first, followed by isotonic liquids an hour later. However, this may be difficult in practice.

Fats

Human studies have shown no beneficial effect from high-fat or high-carbohydrate (in the absence of a colon) diets, or so-called elemental diets (small peptide or free amino acid-based enteral formulas) on stool weight or energy, nitrogen, electrolyte, or mineral absorption. Dietary fat restriction decreases steatorrhea but does not increase fat absorption. Medium-chain triglycerides (MCT) are absorbed independently of bile salts and may provide a useful energy loss in patients with significant steatorrhea. However, they are expensive, are often unpalatable (despite modern recipes), cannot be used with cooking oil because of a low smoke temperature, may worsen diarrhea in excessive doses (> 40 g/d), and may have an adverse effect on intestinal adaptation. There have been a few case reports that suggest replacement of bile salts with ox bile may lead to improvement in long-chain triglyceride absorption. Dietary fat should not be replaced with MCT as essential fat (linoleic acid) is not supplied. To prevent essential fatty-acid deficiency, linoleic acid must constitute at least 2 to 4 percent of the total

absorbed calories. It is presently unclear whether lino-
lenic fatty acid is essential as well.

Oxalates

Residual colon becomes an important instrument for
nutrient digestion and absorption. Therefore, dietary recommendations may vary depending on whether colon is
present. Unlike the patient with a jejunostomy, dietary fat
intake should be restricted in the patient with remaining
colon, although not to the extent as to render the diet
unpalatable. Patients also should be provided with a diet
low in oxalate content. See the preceding chapter on
hyperoxaluria and nephrolithiasis. A table on oxalate
content in foods has been added to that chapter.

Foods such as chocolate, tea, cola, spinach, celery, and
carrots should be avoided, as should dehydration.
Although some of the vitamin C in the TPN solutions
may be converted to oxalate with a resultant hyperoxaluria, otherwise, patients without a colon are theoretically not at increased risk for oxalate nephrolithiasis.

Short-Chain Fatty Acids

In the normal individual, aside from fluid and limited
calcium absorption, the colon has little importance nutritionally. However, in short-bowel syndrome with significant carbohydrate malabsorption, the colon plays a much
greater role nutritionally. Soluble fibers (eg, pectin, but
less so soy, oats or wheat bran, and not lignin) and starch
are metabolized by normal colonic flora to the short-
chain fatty acids (SCFAs): acetate, butyrate, and propionate. These SCFAs (most notably butyrate) are the
preferred fuel for the colonocyte, stimulate sodium and
water absorption (although bicarbonate secretion may
increase), and may account for upward of 1,000 kcal daily
in energy absorption. Therefore, the residual colon and a
diet containing substantial amounts of soluble fiber,
complex carbohydrate, and some insoluble nonstarch
polysaccharides provide an opportunity for colonic
energy salvage. Patients with a colonic mucus fistula
should be reanastomosed as soon as possible.

Fat-Soluble Vitamins

For the patient who can be maintained without parenteral nutrition, regardless of the presence or absence of
a colon, various vitamin and mineral supplements often
are necessary (Table 102–1). Fat-soluble vitamins (A, D,
E, and K) should be routinely monitored in non-TPN-
dependent patients, or in those who are only partially
TPN dependent. Vitamin A (10,000 to 50,000 U/d), vitamin D (1,600 U DHT/d), or vitamin E (30 U/d) supplements may be necessary. In the presence of significant
steatorrhea, the water-soluble forms of vitamin A and E,
as well as the 25-OH$_2$ D$_3$ form, may be preferable.
Patients with significant renal insufficiency may require
supplementation with 1,25-OH$_2$D$_3$. Since vitamin D

TABLE 102–1. Vitamin and Mineral Supplements for Patients with Short-Bowel Syndrome

Supplement	Requirement
Vitamin A	10,000–50,000 units daily
Vitamin B$_{12}$	300 μg subcutaneously monthly for those with terminal ileal resections or disease
Vitamin C	200–500 mg daily (except with oxaluria)
Vitamin D	1,600 units DHT daily; may require 25-OH or 1,25 (OH$_2$)-D$_3$
Vitamin E	30 IU daily
Vitamin K	10 mg weekly
Calcium	See text
Magnesium	See text
Iron	As needed
Selenium	60–100 μg daily
Zinc	220–440 mg daily (sulfate form)
Bicarbonate	As needed

*The table lists rough guidelines only. Vitamin and mineral supplementation must be routinely monitored and tailored to the individual patient because relative absorption and requirements may vary.

enhances intestinal calcium absorption, simultaneous
calcium supplementation also should be provided.
Adequate sun exposure also may be an inexpensive alternative to vitamin D supplementation.

The serum calcium should be monitored as well as vitamin A and D concentrations because toxicity can result
from excessive intake of any of these. Vitamin E is
thought to be essentially nontoxic, although the clotting
activity may be further suppressed in patients taking war-
farin simultaneously. Adequacy of supplementation
should be routinely monitored by measurement of serum
vitamin A, vitamin D (25-OH), and vitamin E concentrations. Vitamin E concentration may vary in relation to the
serum total lipid concentration. Therefore, total serum
lipids should be measured simultaneously, and the ratio
of vitamin E to total serum lipids actually should be used
as the index of vitamin E status. Because enteric bacteria
synthesize much of the daily vitamin K requirement
(approximately 1 mg/d), in addition to that contained in
the diet, supplementation is not usually necessary,
although the prothrombin time should be monitored.

Calcium

Adequate calcium intake is important, especially because
of the adverse effects on bone of cytokines, vitamin D
malabsorption, and the medications often used to treat
Crohn's disease (corticosteroids, cyclosporine, Tacrolimus, methotrexate). In the absence of jejunal Crohn's
disease or jejunal resections, most non-Jewish, white
patients with Crohn's disease will *not* be lactose intolerant. Unfortunately, many patients are convinced they are
and their dairy product intake is limited. This in turn may
severely limit calcium intake. For the patient who is truly
lactose intolerant, perhaps unrelated to Crohn's disease or

their resection, calcium supplements are recommended. This may take the form of certain antacids, yogurt (where the lactose is already hydrolyzed), lactaid-containing milk or ice cream, or hard cheeses (lactose is concentrated in the whey portion of cheese). Calcium supplementation of 1,000 mg daily should be routinely provided. Bone mineral density should be routinely followed in these patients, with consideration for biphosphonate (Fosamax®, Merck, West Point, New Jersey; Actonel®, Procter & Gamble Pharmaceuticals, Cincinnati, Ohio) therapy for those with increased fracture risk.

Water-Soluble Vitamins

Deficiencies of water-soluble vitamins are rare, even in patients with short-bowel syndrome. However, they may occur, and therefore it is important that patients ingest one or two B-complex vitamin supplements and 200 to 500 mg of vitamin C daily. Vitamin B_{12} should be administered at a dose of 1,000 μg intramuscularly every 3 months in patients who have had significant gastric or ileal resections, or in those who have active Crohn's disease in their remaining terminal ileum. The adequacy of vitamin B_{12} supplementation is best measured by following the serum methylmalonic acid concentration. In the absence of sufficient vitamin B_{12}, the methylmalonic acid concentration remains elevated, because it will not be metabolized to succinyl coenzyme A. Similarly, folate is required for the metabolism of homocysteine to methionine. The Schilling test is not a test to determine vitamin B_{12} status, but to determine why a particular patient is vitamin B_{12} deficient. Once either neuropathy or megaloblastic anemia is present, deficiency probably has been present for some time. Although the B vitamins essentially are nontoxic, excessive vitamin C ingestion has been associated with calcium oxalate nephrolithiasis.

Iron

Iron deficiency in Crohn's disease more commonly reflects ongoing blood loss rather than iron malabsorption even in short-bowel syndrome. Therefore, supplementation is not routinely necessary in the absence of active Crohn's disease or gastrointestinal hemorrhage or significant duodenal resection. Serum ferritin should be monitored, although it will be elevated as an acute-phase reactant in active Crohn's disease.

Zinc

Zinc supplements are routinely necessary because of the significant fecal losses (17 mg/L). To put these losses in perspective, standard TPN solutions typically provide 2 mg of zinc daily. Usually one or two 220-mg zinc sulfate tablets are sufficient. Although there is considerable debate on the appropriate test for measurement of zinc status, the serum concentration should be followed. Zinc is bound to albumin; therefore, the serum zinc concentration may be depressed in the presence of a low serum albumin, although physiologic zinc status may be normal. Unfortunately, no conversion factor is available. Zinc deficiency also has been associated with increased diarrhea, which may be ameliorated with zinc supplementation.

Other Replacements

Patients with excessive fecal volume losses also are losing significant amounts of bicarbonate, magnesium, and selenium. Replacement of bicarbonate can be accomplished with BiCitra® (Alza Corp., Palo Alto, California) or sodium bicarbonate tablets. This may be necessary to maintain normal acid:base status and to help prevent development of osteoporosis. Magnesium replacement may be difficult because of the cathartic effect of all currently available oral supplements and the poor bioavailability of the enteric-coated tablets. Replacement via injection is painful; periodic intravenous replacement may be required. Because the vast majority of magnesium is found intracellularly, measurement of serum concentration may not accurately reflect magnesium status. Therefore, 24-hour urine magnesium should be routinely followed. Values above 70 mg daily suggest adequate magnesium stores.

Selenium status can be followed by measurement of the plasma selenium concentration by a laboratory experienced in the measurement of this trace metal. It can be supplemented (60 to 120 μg/d) if necessary. Deficiency has been associated with cardiomyopathy, macrocytosis, myositis, and pseudoalbinism. Copper deficiency is rare, as most excretion is biliary in origin. Deficiency has been associated with anemia, cardiomyopathy, neutropenia, neuropathy, osteoporosis, retinal degeneration, and testicular atrophy.

Complications of Short-Bowel Syndrome

Complications of short-bowel syndrome include dehydration (which may result in uric acid nephrolithiasis), generalized malnutrition, electrolyte disturbances, specific nutrient deficiencies, calcium-oxalate nephrolithiasis, and cholelithiasis. Those patients with significant malabsorption requiring long-term TPN are at additional risk for hepatic steatosis and cholestasis with potential progression to cirrhosis, either acalculous or calculous cholecystitis, metabolic bone disease, nephropathy, and central venous catheter-related problems, including infection and occlusion (thrombotic and nonthrombotic).

Total Parenteral Nutrition

Patients are most likely to require parenteral nutrition and fluids initially following massive bowel resection. This continues for at least 7 to 10 days, perhaps as long as 1 to

2 years during the adaptation process, and permanently if bowel surface area and adaptation is insufficient. Patients should be provided with 30 to 33 kcal/kg/d (or use indirect calorimetry with an added activity factor) and 1.0 to 1.5 g/kg/d of amino acids. Energy is provided as dextrose (3.4 kcal/mL) and lipid emulsion (1.1 kcal/mL for the 10% and 2.0 kcal/mL for the 20% form). Requirements for young children and neonates are substantially greater. Electrolytes, minerals, vitamins, and trace metals also are needed.

Baseline fluid requirements approximate 1 mL/kcal. Additional fluid to replace gastrointestinal losses usually is required. Initially this replacement fluid (0.5% normal saline) should be provided intravenously. When oral intake is possible, ORS and antimotility agents should be used, although some intravenous replacement fluid may be required. Histamine$_2$ blockers can be added directly to the TPN solution. Fluid status, weight, sodium, potassium, magnesium, and bicarbonate status should be monitored carefully. Once patients have met their prescribed goal for nutritional support, their nutritional status may be monitored by following the total lymphocyte count, visceral protein status (prealbumin; note that the half-life of albumin is approximately 20 days so short-term changes in visceral protein status would be difficult to detect), and nitrogen balance. Acid:base status can be adjusted by controlling the ratio of chloride to acetate and by controlling stool losses (and therefore bicarbonate losses) to some extent.

Central Catheter

A single-lumen, tunneled catheter should be placed with the catheter tip in either the superior or inferior vena cava in preparation for home TPN once it has been determined that the patient will be unlikely to absorb sufficient energy or fluid for at least 6 weeks. In general, both single-lumen and tunneled catheters have substantially lower risk of infection compared to their nontunneled counterparts, although a properly cared for percutaneously inserted central catheter (PICC) may be an exception. Preferably, the catheter should be used only for TPN and fluids. Blood draws should be obtained peripherally, and each time the catheter is used, connected or disconnected, it must be cleaned appropriately. Alcohol alone is not bactericidal. Patients should be instructed on proper catheter care and dressing changes and the prompt recognition of a catheter-related infection (eg, fever, perhaps only during the TPN infusion or chills during catheter flushing for catheter sepsis; erythema; purulence or tenderness at the exit site, indicating a cuff infection; or erythema over the site of the subcutaneous tunnel tract, indicating a tunnel infection). The selected reading section contains information on catheter care and complications. There is a specific chapter on TPN.

Patients should be prepared for home TPN by cycling their TPN and fluids so that they are received overnight. This allows maximal rehabilitation potential during the day and later enables the patient potentially to return to work. Because it may take some time for the pancreas to fully adapt to the increased insulin requirements from the infused dextrose, compression of the total volume of TPN from a 24-hour infusion to a 10- to 12-hour overnight infusion should take place slowly, typically by 2-hour nightly increments. Some patients may require the addition of regular insulin to their TPN (starting with 0.5 to 1.0 µg dextrose) or an increase in the percentage of lipid calories (with a decrease in the dextrose calories), at least initially. When the TPN infusion for a given 24-hour period has been completed, it should be tapered off over a 30-minute period. Because the half-life of insulin is longer than that of dextrose, patients with substantial amounts of insulin in their TPN may require a 1-hour taper. Once the patient is stable at home, laboratory monitoring should be less frequent (as infrequently as three to four times yearly for long-term patients), and the TPN volume adjusted downward as the patient's bowel adapts and normal fluid and nutritional status is maintained.

Surgical Management and Intestinal Transplantation

There have been numerous reports of various bowel lengthening procedures and other methods aimed at prolonging bowel transit time and nutrient–epithelium contact time. These have included the use of aperistaltic segments; attempts to increase surface area by "butterflying" the bowel, for lack of a better description; colonic interpostion; reversed intestinal segments; and recirculating small bowel loops. Although there are a few case reports of at least temporary success, none of these procedures has been considered routinely successful. All have been associated with the potential for significant morbidity.

Small intestine transplantation has been proposed by some as a potential "cure" for patients with short-bowel syndrome who require home TPN. It is not a cure for inflammatory bowel disease, although simultaneous bone marrow transplantation may have therapeutic potential. Unfortunately, the published 1-, 2-, 3-, and 4-year survival rates are 62 to 83 percent, 48 percent, 47 percent, and 37 percent, respectively. Although about 78 percent of survivors are able to successfully discontinue TPN, the overall survival rates compare poorly with that of home TPN. The 3-year survival rate for home TPN patients with Crohn's disease is approximately 90 percent. Therefore, small bowel transplantation should be reserved exclusively for patients with coexistent hepatic failure in whom combined small bowel-liver transplantation is necessary. The next chapter is on small bowel transplantation.

Supplemental Reading

Buchman AL. The clinical management of short bowel syndrome: steps to avoid parenteral nutrition. Nutrition 1997;13:907–13.

Buchman AL. Handbook of nutritional support. Philadelphia: Mosby, 1997.

Grant D. Current results of intestinal transplantation. The International Intestinal Transplant Registry. Lancet 1996; 347:1801–3.

Ladefoged K, Christensen KC, Hegnhoj J, Jarnum S. Effect of a long-acting somatostatin analogue SMS 201-995 on jejunostomy effluents in patients with severe short bowel syndrome. Gut 1989;30:943–9.

MacMahon RA. The use of the World Health Organization's oral rehydration solution in patients on home parenteral nutrition. J Parenter Enteral Nutr 1984;8:720–1.

McIntyre PB, Fitchew M, Lennard-Jones JE. Patients with a high jejunostomy do not need a special diet. Gastro-enterology 1986;91:25–33.

Messing B, Pigot F, Rongier M, et al. Intestinal absorption of free oral hyperalimentation in the very short bowel syndrome. Gastroenterology 1991;100:1502–8.

Nightingale JMD, Walker ER, Farthing MJG, Lennard-Jones JE. Effect of omeprazole on intestinal output in the short bowel syndrome. Aliment Pharmacol Ther 1991;5:405–12.

Nordgaard I, Hansen BS, Mortensen PB. Importance of colonic support for energy absorption as small-bowel failure proceeds. Am J Clin Nutr 1996;64:222–31.

Scolapio JS, Camilleri M, Fleming CR, et al. Effect of growth hormone, glutamine, and diet on adaptation in short-bowel syndrome: a randomized, controlled trial. Gastroenterology 1998;113:1074–81.

Intestinal Transplantation

Kenneth K.W. Lee, MD, FACS, and Kareem Abu-Elmagd, MD, PhD, FACS

Surgical conservatism is a guiding principle in the management of Crohn's disease, but complications of the disease may necessitate multiple intestinal resections. When the cumulative resections are extensive (short-bowel syndrome) or combined with dysfunction of the remaining intestine, intestinal failure may result. Parenteral nutrition provides life-sustaining treatment of irreversible intestinal failure and remains primary therapy for this condition, but in some patients complications may ensue that prevent its indefinite use. In these instances, intestinal transplantation is the only effective alternative.

Overview of Intestinal Transplantation

Human intestinal transplantation was first attempted nearly 40 years ago, but limited success was first possible when cyclosporine-based immunosuppressive therapy became available. Following its introduction in 1989, experimental studies demonstrated the efficacy of Tacrolimus and supported its subsequent use in clinical intestinal transplantation. This has resulted in significant improvements in graft and recipient survival and elevated intestinal transplantation from an experimental to a proven, albeit challenging, therapy for end-stage intestinal failure.

Survival

At the Sixth International Symposium on Small-Bowel Transplantation, in October 1999, the Intestinal Transplant Registry reported on 443 patients who underwent 471 intestinal transplants between 1985 and May 1999. For transplants performed after February 1995, 1-year patient and graft survival have been approximately 62 percent and 56 percent, respectively; 3-year survival has been approximately 49 percent and 43 percent. Full graft function with nutritional autonomy has been achieved in 78 percent of all survivors and in 80 percent of patients surviving more than 6 months after transplantation. Although overall survival for patients on home parenteral nutrition has been estimated to be 85 percent at 3 years, the use of intestinal transplantation as a salvage therapy for patients failing on parenteral nutrition prevents a meaningful comparison of these results.

Costs

Cost-effectiveness and quality-of-life analysis support intestinal transplantation as an alternative to chronic parenteral nutrition. The average costs in our institution of isolated intestinal and combined liver and intestinal transplantation currently are $132,285 and $214,716, respectively. In comparison, based on Medicare data for 1992, the average yearly cost of home parenteral nutrition exclusive of the cost of related hospitalizations, medical equipment, and nursing care was $150,000. Therefore, intestinal transplantation becomes cost effective 2 years after transplantation.

Despite these improvements in graft and recipient survival and quality-of-life and cost benefits, the morbidity and mortality associated with intestinal transplantation remain substantial. As such, parenteral nutrition remains the primary treatment for irreversible intestinal failure, and intestinal transplantation should be considered only for patients whose nutritional and metabolic condition cannot be maintained by this means.

Isolated versus Composite Grafts

Experimentally as well as clinically, the cumulative risk of graft loss due to rejection is higher for isolated intestinal grafts than for combined liver-intestinal grafts. In a series of 104 consecutive transplants from our institution, the incidence of rejection was 92 percent for isolated intestinal grafts compared with 66 percent for composite grafts during the first 30 days after transplantation. Although the cumulative rejection rate of the intestine in a composite graft approached that of isolated intestine, the rate of graft loss from rejection was less than half of that for isolated intestine. However, despite these apparent benefits of composite liver-intestinal grafts, isolated intestinal transplantation is preferred in the absence of irreversible liver failure, because, in the event of failure, the graft can be removed and the patient returned to parenteral nutrition. Isolated intestinal transplantation may be considered in patients who (1) have fluid and electrolyte abnormalities that cannot be adequately controlled on parenteral nutrition, (2) lack adequate venous access for continued long-term parenteral nutrition, (3) have frequent episodes of parenteral nutrition-related sepsis, or (4) develop moderately severe, but potentially reversible, liver dysfunction from chronic parenteral nutrition. When irreversible liver failure develops, combined liver-intestinal transplantation is necessary.

With these guidelines, the number of potential intestinal transplant recipients is relatively small, and there is no shortage of available donors for isolated intestinal transplantation. The availability of an appropriate liver donor is limiting when combined liver-intestine transplantation is necessary, because current organ allocation schemes pool liver and liver-intestine recipients together. ABO blood group matching is necessary, but, to date, the importance of human leukocyte antigen matching has not been firmly established for intestinal transplantation. Among the initial 104 intestinal transplants, the incidence of intestinal rejection was similar for both positive and negative lymphocytotoxic crossmatch grafts, although the mean number of rejection episodes was higher in positive crossmatch grafts. Living-related intestinal transplantation has been reported, but until tissue matching is clearly demonstrated to be beneficial for intestinal transplantation, it remains unclear that the risk to the donor is justified, except in the case of identical twins with a nonheritable cause of intestinal failure. Transplantation from a cytomegalovirus (CMV)-positive donor to a CMV-negative recipient has been associated with less favorable outcomes, and accordingly such donor-recipient mismatches are avoided.

When possible, venous outflow from isolated intestinal grafts is directed into the native portal circulation, as this reestablishes a normal intestine-liver axis. Experimentally, portal venous drainage also confers immunologic benefits upon the small intestine. However, under the intensive immunosuppressive regimens used in clinical intestinal transplantation, this probably minor effect is not evident, and systemic venous drainage has not been observed to increase the risk of graft rejection or graft loss.

Immunosuppression

Currently, immunosuppression for intestinal transplantation is based upon **Tacrolimus** and **prednisone**. Adjunctive **cyclophosphamide**, **mycophenolate mofetil**, or **azathioprine** has also been used. Maintenance immunosuppression has been individualized according to the patient's clinical course and reduced whenever possible. Recently, perioperative administration of **daclizumab**, an **anti-interleukin-2 (IL-2) alpha receptor antibody**, has decreased the incidence of rejection episodes. When such episodes occur, they are treated by adjustments of Tacrolimus dosage or supplemental prednisone and, if necessary, OKT3. Results of investigation of the possible tolerogenic effect of concurrent infusion of donor bone marrow indicate that these infusions are safe and not associated with a heightened incidence of graft-versus-host (GHV) disease, as had been feared. Nevertheless, no differences in the overall incidence, frequency, or median time of onset of the first rejection episode have been noted.

Small-Bowel Rejection

Fever, abdominal pain, distention, diarrhea or increased stoma output, leukocytosis, or acidosis may signal acute small-bowel rejection. Malabsorption and electrolyte abnormalities also may occur as a consequence of mucosal injury. Although absorption tests have been validated for the diagnosis of acute rejection in experimental models, in clinical intestinal transplantation they have not yet provided additional useful information in comparison to histologic analysis alone. In most centers, endoscopy with mucosal biopsies is performed for routine graft surveillance and as clinically indicated. Endoscopic findings during acute rejection may be variable, in part resulting from the often patchy character of acute rejection. Ulcers are associated with more severe rejection; other endoscopic findings include granularity, friability, erythema, and edema. Histologic criteria of acute rejection consist of crypt injury; mucosal infiltration, primarily by mononuclear cells; and increased crypt apoptosis. Using these criteria, acute rejection can be identified reliably and distinguished from other pathologic processes affecting the transplanted intestine.

Chronic rejection also may occur and is usually marked clinically by evidence of graft dysfunction. As in other allografts, a progressive obliterative arteriopathy occurs but may be absent in superficial mucosal biopsies. Mural fibrosis, mild apoptosis, perivascular inflammation, and a range of mucosal alterations that may include reparative changes or persistent ulceration also are seen. Accurate diagnosis of chronic rejection often requires full-thickness graft biopsies and consequently the incidence of chronic rejection typically is underestimated.

Graft-versus-Host Disease

Transfer of large amounts of donor lymphoid tissue in the intestinal allograft also creates the potential for development of GVH disease. However, immunosuppressive regimens necessary to prevent graft rejection usually also suffice to prevent clinical GVH disease. When suspicious lesions arise in the skin, gastrointestinal tract, or other target organs, such as the lungs, liver, or bone marrow, biopsies studied by routine histopathology or immunohistologic staining for human leukocyte antigen (HLA) may help to establish a diagnosis of GVH disease.

Lymphoproliferative Disease

As with other solid organ transplants, lymphoproliferative disease may occur following intestinal transplantation. The incidence has been lower for isolated intestinal transplantation than for combined liver-intestine or multivisceral transplantation. The Intestinal Transplant Registry has reported 8 percent and 14 percent incidences of lymphoproliferative disease after isolated intestine or combined liver-intestine transplantation, respectively, with median follow-up of 3 and 2.5 years. **Lymphoma** has been the cause of death in 14 percent of patients identified by the registry. In our initial series of 104 transplants, lymphoma was the cause of death in 6 of 36 patients.

The University of Pittsburgh Experience

At the University of Pittsburgh Medical Center, 135 intestinal transplants have been performed in 128 patients through October 1999, comprising 29 percent of the worldwide experience. As found by the Intestinal Transplant Registry, survival has been better in more recent experience (Figure 103–1). Several factors have contributed to this improved survival, including better immunosuppression management, better recipient selection, exclusion of the colon from the transplanted graft, avoidance of CMV mismatched isolated grafts, and careful Epstein-Barr virus monitoring.

Survival

Detailed analysis of the first 104 intestinal transplants performed in 98 patients from 1990 through 1997 (37 isolated intestine, 50 combined liver-intestine, and 17 multivisceral transplants) showed that overall cumulative patient survival was 72 percent at 1 year and 48 percent at 5 years. With mean follow-up of 40 ± 29 months (range, 1 to 94 mo), 31 patients were alive beyond the third postoperative year and 18 beyond the fifth postoperative year. Cumulative 5-year survival was best in patients between 2 and 17 years of age (68%). Technical failures resulted in increased mortality in children less than 2 years old. Graft survival rates at 1 year and 5 years were 64 percent and 40 percent, with no differences observed between isolated and composite grafts. Of current survivors, 93 percent were at home, fully active, and completely off parenteral nutrition. Parenteral nutrition was necessary in the remaining patients because of chronic graft dysmotility or recent episodes of moderate to severe graft rejection.

Graft Removal

Graft removal may be necessary for treatment of refractory acute or chronic rejection. Less commonly, it is performed for treatment of immunosuppression-related lymphoma, infection, or primary graft failure. Isolated grafts can be removed and the patient returned to parenteral nutrition, but there is a substantial mortality associated with the graft enterectomy; inasmuch as intestinal transplant recipients usually are failing parenteral nutrition, there also is substantial morbidity and mortality associated with resuming parenteral nutrition. In the authors' series of intestinal transplants, 13 isolated grafts were removed from 12 patients; graft removal was prompted by rejection in 8 patients (6 acute, 2 chronic).

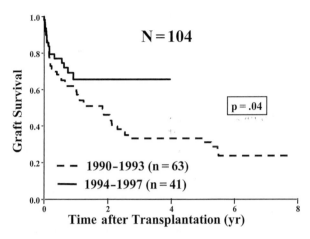

FIGURE 103–1. Patient survival according to time, showing significant improvement in survival during the later period.

Retransplantation was performed in three of these patients, but two of these patients died within 5 months of retransplantation; one patient is well after a repeat isolated intestinal transplant. Among the other nine patients, two died of sepsis following graft removal and another five died of total parenteral nutrition (TPN)-related complications without having undergone retransplantation. Four recipients of composite liver-intestine grafts have undergone retransplantation (two liver-intestine, one multivisceral, one isolated liver) with only one survivor after 3 months.

In the series of 98 patients undergoing 104 intestinal transplants, 36 additional deaths occurred with intestinal grafts remaining in place. The causes of death were infection (n = 15), technical or management errors (n = 8), B-cell lymphoma (n = 6), rejection (n = 5), and other (n = 2). At the time of death, however, 18 of these patients had achieved and maintained full nutritional autonomy, and 6 had partially functioning intestinal grafts.

Intestinal Transplantation for Crohn's Disease

Approximately two-thirds of intestinal transplants to date have been performed in children, but in children intestinal failure rarely results from Crohn's disease. Among adults undergoing intestinal transplantation, Crohn's disease has been the cause of intestinal failure in about 20 percent of patients. Among adults identified in the 1999 report of the Intestinal Transplant Registry, Crohn's disease was the cause of intestinal failure in 16 percent of patients, second only to ischemia (19%). Crohn's disease also has been the second most frequent cause of intestinal failure leading to intestinal transplantation in the Thomas E. Starzl Transplantation Institute, affecting 11 of 48 (23%) adults transplanted between May 1990 and December 1998. Nine patients received isolated intestinal transplants, because of frequent line sepsis (n = 8), persistent fluid and electrolyte disturbances (n = 5), lack of central venous access (n = 4), and progressive liver dysfunction (n = 2); two patients received composite liver-intestinal grafts because of coexisting liver failure. This represents the largest single center experience with intestinal transplantation for Crohn's disease.

With mean follow-up of 30 months, 5 (45%) of these 11 patients are alive: 4 with fully functioning grafts (3 isolated, 1 composite liver-intestine) and 1 on parenteral nutrition following a graft enterectomy performed for chronic rejection and CMV enteritis. One patient died from pancreatitis and liver failure after undergoing a graft enterectomy for severe acute rejection. The remaining five deaths of patients with fully or partially functioning grafts in place were attributable to pulmonary embolus (n = 1), acute respiratory disease or pneumonia (n = 1), technical complication (n = 1), narcotic overdose (n = 1), and unknown causes (n = 1). Acute rejection occurred in 10 of the 11 intestinal grafts; the mean number of rejection episodes per graft was 4.5 (0 to 17).

The possibility that immunologic dysregulation may contribute to the pathogenesis of Crohn's disease has prompted concern that intestinal transplantation for Crohn's disease would be more prone to graft rejection. Experience with transplantation for Crohn's disease fails to substantiate this concern. Results with transplantation for Crohn's disease are poorer than the results in the overall series; however, this comparison is skewed by the better results achieved in children. When graft survival rates are stratified according to the cause of intestinal failure among adults, the best results have been achieved in Crohn's disease (Figure 103–2).

Crohn's disease does pose certain technical challenges for intestinal transplantation. Typically, recipients have undergone numerous prior abdominal operations for treatment of their Crohn's disease; in the authors' series, a median of 10 (2 to 19) prior operations had occurred. Loss of domain within the abdominal cavity and extensive abdominal wall defects that require plastic reconstruction are also common.

Crohn's Disease in Transplanted Intestine

In this series of transplants performed for Crohn's disease, active Crohn's disease arising in either the transplanted intestine or the native gastrointestinal tract has not been observed. One case of apparent occurrence of Crohn's disease in the transplanted intestine has been reported. In this patient, graft biopsies obtained 7 months after transplantation showed noncaseating mucosal epithelioid granulomas in addition to acute rejection. A segmental intestinal resection performed 14 months after transplantation because of small-bowel obstruction also showed histologic lesions compatible with Crohn's disease. In addition to noncaseating granulomas, other findings in the allograft biopsies consistent with, although not

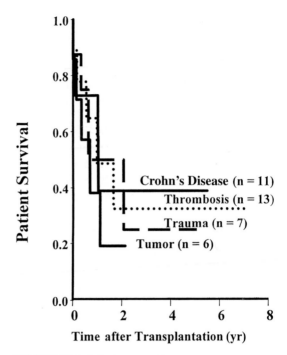

FIGURE 103–2. Patient survival according to the cause of intestinal failure, showing best survival in patients with Crohn's disease.

diagnostic of, Crohn's disease included transmural inflammation, goblet cell hyperplasia, and aphthous ulceration. Other causes for the development of granulomas, such as tuberculosis, sarcoidosis, fungal infection, and foreign body reactions, could not be identified, suggesting that this was a bona fide occurrence of Crohn's disease in the transplanted intestine.

This case indicates that the recipient milieu may foster development of Crohn's disease in the transplanted intestine. The occurrence of Crohn's disease despite the intensive immunosuppression given in conjunction with the intestinal transplant suggests that **nonimmunologic factors**, such as infection or enteric microflora, may be important in the development of Crohn's disease. As the etiology of Crohn's disease becomes more fully elucidated, the risk of recurrent Crohn's disease in the transplanted intestine or remaining native gastrointestinal tract will become better defined. Presently, however, the risk is not such as to preclude transplantation for these patients.

Conclusion

Nutritional support by means of parenteral nutrition remains the first line of treatment for patients suffering from intestinal failure attributable to Crohn's disease. However, in patients who cannot be maintained on long-term parenteral nutrition, intestinal transplantation should be considered. The morbidity and mortality of intestinal transplantation, though still significant, continue to decline, and long-term survival with nutritional autonomy presently can be achieved in nearly one-half of adult patients undergoing intestinal transplantation for Crohn's disease. Future advances in the prevention and treatment of acute and chronic rejection as well as post-transplantation infections will further reduce the risks of intestinal transplantation, leading to earlier isolated intestinal transplantation before irreversible liver failure has occurred and increasing the overall usefulness of intestinal transplantation.

Supplemental Reading

Abu-Elmagd K, Reyes J, Fung JJ, et al. Evolution of clinical intestinal transplantation: improved outcome and cost effectiveness. Transplant Proc 1999;31:582–84.

Abu-Elmagd K, Reyes J, Todo S, et al. Clinical intestinal transplantation: new perspectives and immunological considerations. J Am Coll Surg 1998;186:512–27.

Intestinal Transplant Registry data. Presented at the 6th International Symposium on Small-Bowel Transplantation, Omaha, Nebraska, October 1999.

Kaufman SS, Wisecarver JL, Ruby EI, et al. Correlation of mucosal disaccharidase activities with histology in evaluation of rejection following intestinal transplantation. Pediatr Transplant 1998;2:134–8.

Lee KK, Stangl MJ, Todo S, et al. Successful orthotopic small bowel transplantation with short term FK 506 immunosuppressive therapy. Transplant Proc 1990;22:78–9.

Lee RG, Nakamura K, Tsamandas AS, et al. Pathology of human intestinal transplantation. Gastroenterology 1996;110:1820–34.

Sustento-Reodica N, Ruiz P, Rogers A, et al. Recurrent Crohn's disease in transplanted bowel. Lancet 1997;349:688–91.

Tzakis AG, Thompson JF. Current status of diagnosis of small bowel rejection [editorial]. Pediatr Transplant 1998;2:87–8.

CHAPTER 104

Management of Postoperative Fistulae

Walter A. Koltun, MD

Fistulae formation after operation for Crohn's disease (CD) can be classified as those occurring soon after operation, usually on the same hospital admission, or those occurring later, usually after at least several weeks. An early fistula is almost invariably attributable to technical factors related to the surgical procedure itself, whereas a late fistula most commonly represents recrudescence of the underlying Crohn's disease. Therefore, treatment depends on the fundamental understanding of the cause of the fistula. In addition to the more conventional anastomotic enterocutaneous fistula, there are certain special types of fistulous complications specifically associated with CD and surgery, including the peristomal fistula, persistent perineal sinus (or nonhealing perineal wound), and the ileal pouch fistula in patients with previously unrecognized Crohn's disease.

Early Postoperative Fistulization

The occurrence of anastomotic complications after intestinal resection for CD is relatively low, with many studies showing only a 0 to 4 percent incidence of early postoperative fistulization. Principles of anastomotic creation are no different than in the patient who does not have inflammatory bowel disease (IBD): a tension-free anastomosis with a good vascular supply and the avoidance of anastomosis in the septic, malnourished patient. Typically, the anastomosis is done in healthy bowel after resection of gross disease, but even in the case of strictureplasty, where diseased fibrotic bowel is sutured, the incidence of fistulization or leak is surprisingly low (5 to 10%). Therefore, management of such early fistulae is similar to that in the patient without IBD. If the patient appears septic, with metabolic deterioration and poor control of the leaking succus, prompt reoperation with stoma creation at the site of leak or more proximally is necessary. If the patient is stable, then appropriate wound management, bowel rest, intravenous hyperalimentation, and broad-spectrum antibiotics (for no more than 7 to 10 d) are instituted. Antifungal prophylaxis is appropriate and longer-term metronidazole is desirable owing to its demonstrated benefit in the treatment of spontaneous CD fistulae. Radiographic study of the fistula may be performed, especially if an associated intra-abdominal collection or abscess is suspected. In this circumstance, computer tomography (CT)

with percutaneous drainage may help convert a poorly controlled fistula into one for which surgery can be avoided. A retrograde water-soluble contrast study is worthwhile, to rule out downstream obstruction that could have caused the anastomotic leak in the first place and then be inhibiting its subsequent healing.

The issue of steroid and other immunosuppressive management is critical. Since the patient's Crohn's disease should have been addressed at the original surgery, the goal should be the discontinuance of all immunosuppressive medication that could further complicate sepsis. In the case of suspected steroid-dependent patients, a 5- to 7-day taper using dexamethasone is instituted, during which time an adrenocorticotropic hormone (ACTH) (Cortrosyn) stimulation test is done. If adequate adrenal function is documented, steroids are discontinued, recognizing the possible need for future occasional steroid supplementation at times of stress. Other adjuvant therapies can include nasogastric decompression, histamine$_2$ (H$_2$) blockade, and the institution of somatostatin, to further decrease fistula drainage volume. Once sepsis is controlled, the fistula should heal within 30 days; persistence beyond this time frame reflects a poor chance for spontaneous closure. Factors adversely affecting the success rate of such nonoperative care include foreign body within the fistula tract, radiation, a short fistula tract or its epithelialization, the presence of malignancy, proximal location of the fistula, and a large associated tissue defect. Even if the fistula does not completely heal, delayed operation, using these techniques, can facilitate interval re-exploration, minimizing subsequent bowel resection and possibly avoiding stoma creation.

Late Fistula Formation

Late fistula formation after surgery most often is attributable to recurrent Crohn's disease and commonly occurs in patients with a history of previous fistula formation. Management focuses on controlling the underlying CD and the administration of medications shown to benefit fistula healing, specifically metronidazole, 6-mercaptopurine (6-MP), or azathioprine (AZA), and more recently, a tumor necrosis factor (TNF) antagonist (infliximab). These medications frequently provide control and improvement in the symptoms associated with the fistula (whether enteric, enterocutaneous, or perianal) but rarely "cure" the fistula in the long term, especially when medications are discontinued. Eventual definitive surgery is frequently required, but can hopefully be done under optimized circumstances, using these medications to decrease inflammation, edema, and secondary tissue injury associated with the fistula. Further discussion of such CD-associated fistula management is provided elsewhere in this text.

Peristomal Fistula Management

The creation of a temporary or permanent stoma is a common surgical therapy in CD. Studies show that patients with Crohn's colitis have an approximately 15 to 40 percent chance of stoma creation. This figure is even higher in those with significant perianal disease. Rate of stoma complications and, specifically, fistula formation are higher in patients with CD, compared to ulcerative colitis or cancer, and in those with a colostomy, as opposed to an ileostomy. The incidence of ileostomy fistulization in the patient with CD has been reported to be about 7 or 8 percent and can be related to perioperative technique, in which case, the fistula occurs soon after stoma creation. With recurrence of CD, the fistula occurs months to years after surgery.

Immediate postoperative fistulization often is believed to be attributable to the injudicious placement of serosal-to-skin stabilizing stitches, placed to elevate or prolapse the stoma for the purpose of facilitating appliance adhesion. Avoiding such suturing, or tethering the serosa to the subcutaneous fat as opposed to the skin, is recommended by some. Conservative management of such an early postoperative fistula with accommodating pouching techniques may lead to spontaneous healing, but more frequently, an interval surgical revision, at 8 to 12 weeks, is necessary. This can be accomplished usually by a local peristomal incision as a day surgical procedure, provided the intestine is healthy, well perfused, and without signs of CD.

Late fistula formation is attributable to recurrent Crohn's disease and mandates workup of the entire intestinal tract for synchronous disease. Conservative therapy with metronidazole, 6-MP, or TNF antagonists can be used to temporize, but eventually surgery is required. Usually, the distal segment of intestine involved with the stoma is diseased, and therefore, surgical resection requires major laparotomy and intestinal resection. Not infrequently, patients present with acute peristomal inflammation, tenderness, and purulent drainage. Hospital admission, CT to document site of abscess and rule out herniation or intra-abdominal extension should be done. Intravenous antibiotic therapy, including metronidazole, is instituted and a local drainage procedure is then done in the operating room, recognizing the potential for injury to adjacent bowel. The incision is performed either immediately adjacent to the mucocutaneous junction of the stoma or several centimeters away, to facilitate pouching and control of both stoma and fistula. Once the acute sepsis has been controlled and subsides, further intestinal workup can be performed in anticipation of definitive surgery. If the stoma site has concurrent herniation or there is extensive local sepsis and fistula tracking, transposition of the stoma to another abdominal quadrant is necessary.

Persistent Perineal Sinus

Although not strictly speaking a fistula, the persistent perineal sinus, or nonhealing perineal wound, in the CD patient after proctectomy behaves similarly in many ways. Acute dehiscence is frequently attributable to perioperative technical issues, whereas prolonged lack of healing reflects persistent "systemic" CD activity. Its reported incidence varies, owing to differences in investigator definition, but approximates 30 percent in patients with CD undergoing proctectomy. Factors associated with a greater chance of nonhealing are perianal sepsis, rectal involvement with CD, extrasphincteric or wider operative dissection, steroid use, and fecal contamination at operation. Avoidance of the problem is the best advice for treatment. Therefore, preparation of the patient with CD for proctectomy involves the advance drainage of any sites of perianal abscess and control of fistulae with indwelling setons, prolonged preoperative use of oral metronidazole or ciprofloxacin, and control of systemic CD activity, preferably with nonsteroidal medications. At the time of operation, antibiotic irrigation of the rectum and wound, attempt at intersphincteric dissection, placement of omental or gracilis pedicle flaps to fill the dead space, and definitive wound closure with the placement of transabdominal drains are recommended.

Postoperatively, in the patient with CD with a nonhealed perineal wound who has failed conservative wound packing care, treatment should focus on control of systemic CD and consideration of operative débridement and placement of gracilis flaps from the legs. Abdominal rectus flaps should be avoided, because of the possibility of compromising future stoma management. In a woman, a search should first be made to rule out a vaginal communication. The author has had experience with three patients who spontaneously healed their persistent perineal wounds after a transvaginal repair of previously unrecognized vaginal fistulae.

Ileal Pouch Fistula

Presently, the ileal pouch-anal anastomosis (IPAA) is not prospectively recommended for patients with Crohn's colitis, owing to relatively high rates of complication and pouch failure. However, after-the-fact diagnosis of CD in patients having had the IPAA for either presumed ulcerative colitis or indeterminate colitis is sometimes

attributable to and associated with specific fistulous complications. Such fistulae usually present late, at least 6 months after pouch use and as such are infrequently the result of surgical error. Management of such a fistula involves a critical review of the original pathology, the institution of local care (skin emollients and antifungal therapy), and, usually, an examination under anesthesia to clearly identify the fistula course and treat any associated sepsis with drainage or seton placement. Flexible endoscopic evaluation with pouch and small-bowel biopsies to detect histopathologic signs of CD should be performed. Similarly, small-bowel radiologic studies may make the definitive diagnosis of Crohn's disease. Without pathognomic findings of CD, fistula management involves the use of oral metronidazole and conventional surgical care. This sometimes requires fecal diversion and flap repair of the fistula or the interposition of tissue (omental or leg gracilis flap). If CD is documented or strongly suspected, then early institution of 6-MP and infliximab can be successful. The author's personal experience is with three patients, all of whom have responded well to 6-MP therapy after having had recrudescence of fistulous disease after initial surgical management including fecal diversion. In two of three, 6-MP was started when another diverting stoma was in place. After healing of the fistulae, the stomas were closed and both patients are asymptomatic approximately 2 and 4 years later, without recurrence of fistulae. The third patient had institution of 6-MP without a second diverting stoma. Presently, he is asymptomatic but has a persistent, albeit small, external fistulous opening. Overall, the reported pouch failure rate (resulting in a permanent stoma) in patients with such postoperative fistulous complications associated with the diagnosis of indeterminate colitis or CD approximates 30 percent.

Editor's Note

This chapter illustrates the patient care opportunities for surgical, medical, nutritional, nursing, and plastic surgery cooperation. (TMB)

Supplemental Reading

Grobler SP, Hosie KB, Affie E, et al. Outcome of restorative proctocolectomy when the diagnosis is suggestive of Crohn's disease. Gut 1993;34:1384–8.

Hashemi M, Novell JR, Lewis AA. Side-to-side stapled anastomosis may delay recurrence in Crohn's disease. Dis Colon Rectum 1998;41:1293–6.

Ozuner G, Fazio VW, Lavery IC, et al. How safe is strictureplasty in the management of Crohn's disease? Am J Surg 1996;171:57–60.

Ozuner G, Hull T, Lee P, Fazio VW. What happens to a pelvic pouch when a fistula develops? Dis Colon Rectum 1997;40:543–7.

Post S, Herfarth C, Schumacher H, et al. Experience with ileostomy and colostomy in Crohn's disease. Br J Surg 1995;82:1629–33.

Ricart E, Panaccione R, Loftus EV, et al. Successful management of Crohn's disease of the ileoanal pouch with infliximab. Gastroenterology 1999;117:429–32.

Yamamoto T, Bain IM, Allan RN, Keighley MR. Persistent perineal sinus after proctocolectomy for Crohn's disease. Dis Colon Rectum 1999;42:96–101.

CHAPTER 105

Surgery for Crohn's Colitis

ROGER D. HURST, MD, MARCOVALERIO MELIS, MD, AND FABRIZIO MICHELASSI, MD

The surgical treatment of Crohn's disease (CD) affecting the colon and rectum is a particularly challenging endeavor. Crohn's disease of the colon and rectum manifests with a wide variety of anatomic distributions, diverse complications, and clinical patterns, for which the optimal surgical management must be individualized for each patient's specific situation. Further confounding the complexities regarding the surgical management of colorectal CD is the lack of large, prospective studies to help guide the surgeon in formulating the optimal surgical strategies for the differing clinical presentations. Most studies regarding the surgical treatment of colorectal CD involve small numbers of patients reported in a retrospective fashion. On many issues, the literature is conflicting. Prospective studies are rare and randomized control trials are virtually unheard of. However, from the cumulative clinical experience, it is clear that recurrence after segmental resection of colorectal CD is frequent and occasionally rapid. Additionally, patients with colorectal CD are at risk for requiring a permanent stoma. Hence, the risk for substantial life-long morbidity in these patients is high.

Indications for Operation

Colorectal CD is a chronic debilitating and potentially life-threatening disease. The mainstay of therapy is based upon medical management; surgical treatment is required when medical treatment fails and in the presence of septic complications, obstruction, cancer, hemorrhage, and toxic megacolon.

Failure of Medical Management

Failure of medical management to adequately control disease activity and its symptoms is the most common indication for surgical management of Crohn's colitis. Failure of medical treatment of colorectal CD occurs when the response to therapy is inadequate, when the disease progresses during maximal and optimal regimens, when medical treatment results in unacceptable complications, or when the patient cannot be weaned from corticosteroids within a reasonable time frame.

Fistulae and Abscesses

The frequency of fistulae and abscesses requiring surgical management for colorectal CD varies, but it has been reported to be the indication for operation in up to 25 percent of patients undergoing surgery for Crohn's colitis. Fistulae are diagnosed preoperatively at the time of radiographic contrast studies. Asymptomatic coloenteric fistulae do not require surgical treatment. However, fistulae may be a marker of severe colorectal CD where other indications exist for surgical treatment. Fistulae become the indication for surgery if they cause discomfort or embarrassment to the patient, such as colocutaneous or rectovaginal fistulae, or if their presence is associated with significant complications, such as colovesical fistulae.

Intra-abdominal abscesses related to colorectal CD are an infrequent complication and, in the authors' experience, have been the indication for operation in only 10 percent of patients with disease limited to the colon and rectum. The diagnosis of intra-abdominal abscess occasionally is suggested by the classic symptoms of chills and fever with leukocytosis and a palpable mass; yet most commonly, patients just fail to improve on medical treatment. The diagnosis is confirmed with abdominal and pelvic computed tomography (CT). The presence of an abscess is an absolute indication for surgery with resection of the diseased segment. Small abscess cavities that can be completely drained and débrided do not preclude a primary anastomosis if the anastomosis can be located away from the abscess site. In some cases, however, the location and size of the abscess may hinder attempts at primary anastomosis. To minimize the need for a stoma, attempts at preoperative percutaneous drainage of larger abscesses often are worthwhile. Surgical resection of the diseased intestinal segment still is warranted even after successful percutaneous drainage because the abscess is likely to recur or to result in an enterocutaneous fistula.

Perforation

Free perforation of the colon with diffuse peritoneal contamination is an infrequent complication of CD. Perforation of the colon has been reported to occur in 1.3 percent of cases of Crohn's colitis or ileocolitis. Free perforation is an indication for urgent surgical intervention and is associated with high morbidity and mortality. The clinical situation in which perforation typically occurs is in patients with severe or fulminant disease. Often these patients are receiving intensive medical therapy, including

496 / Advanced Therapy of Inflammatory Bowel Disease

high-dose corticosteroids, which can mask the typical symptoms and physical findings of peritonitis. A high index of suspicion for this uncommon complication is necessary in the clinical setting of fulminant disease.

Obstruction

Chronic or severe Crohn's colitis can result in some degree of stricture formation with luminal compromise. Whereas symptomatic strictures often are an indication for surgery in managing small bowel Crohn's disease, symptomatic colonic obstruction is relatively uncommon and represents the indication for surgical intervention in only about 10 percent of cases of colorectal CD. High-grade or extensive Crohn's strictures can be difficult to distinguish from malignancy. Thus, even when asymptomatic, Crohn's strictures of the colon should be investigated to rule out the possibility of malignancy, and any lesion that carries a suspicion for cancer should be resected.

Cancer or Cancer Risk

Patients with CD are estimated to have a risk of colorectal cancer that is 6 to 20 times that of the normal population. When present, colorectal cancer is an obvious indication for surgical resection. In addition, patients with Crohn's colitis may be found to harbor mucosal dysplasia on colonoscopic biopsies. The finding of dysplasia indicates that the patient is at substantial risk for the presence or the subsequent development of colorectal adenocarcinomas. Thus, as in ulcerative colitis (UC), colonic mucosal dysplasia in patients with CD is seen as an indication for surgical resection. Unfortunately, few data exist regarding the natural history of dysplasia in patients with CD, and the appropriate extent of resection in these cases is not entirely clear. During surgery for colonic dysplasia, the segment of colon and rectum affected by active CD should be removed. However, extensive resection of normal colon under these circumstances probably is not required.

Hemorrhage

Massive lower gastrointestinal (GI) hemorrhage is an uncommon complication of colorectal CD, but when present, it often mandates surgical intervention. Robert et al (1991) reported severe GI hemorrhage in 17 of 929 cases of Crohn's colitis. Although medical control of severe hemorrhage can be accomplished in up to half of the cases, massive rebleeding is common. On the other hand, rebleeding after successful surgical resection occurs in only 10 percent of cases and may be associated with a high risk for morbidity and even mortality. Surgical treatment, therefore, is indicated even if conservative measures are effective at initially controlling the bleeding.

Toxic Megacolon

Crohn's colitis occasionally can result in the development of toxic megacolon, although it is much less frequent than with UC. Toxic megacolon as an indication for surgical treatment has been reported to be as high as 19 percent among patients undergoing surgery for Crohn's colitis. However, with improvement in medical treatment and with optimal collaboration and communication between medical and surgical specialists, the authors have not seen a case of toxic megacolon in the last 500 consecutive patients undergoing surgery for treatment of CD at the University of Chicago. When present, toxic megacolon requires urgent colectomy.

Preoperative Evaluation and Preparation

When planning surgical therapy, the surgeon should confer with the patient and the family so that they understand the nature of the proposed operation, the necessity for surgery, the treatment options, operative hazards, and possible complications as well as the anticipated benefits. Prior to operation, a complete assessment of the GI tract is necessary to determine the extent of involvement with CD. The small intestine should be evaluated with either a small bowel follow-through or preferably an enteroclysis. If the patient has a palpable abdominal mass or is suspected of having an abdominal or pelvic abscess, preoperative CT of the abdomen and pelvis is recommended. The colon should be fully evaluated with colonoscopy. It is particularly important to make note of the distal limit of disease and to note the condition of the rectum. A healthy rectum and sphincter mechanism almost always enable the patient to avoid a permanent ostomy. On the other hand, rectal involvement with CD places the patient at high risk for a permanent stoma.

When performing surgery on the colon, it is important to obtain a meticulous mechanical preparation of the bowel. Cleansing the colon of fecal material lessens the likelihood for infectious complications and maximizes the primary healing of colonic anastomoses. In most instances, adequate colonic preparation can be achieved with standard polyethylene glycol or Fleet phosphosoda enema.*

The optimal regimen for prophylactic antibiotics in the setting of elective colon surgery is controversial; however, most surgeons agree that broad-spectrum intravenous antibiotics affording coverage for aerobes and anaerobes should be given prior to making the skin incision. In clean to contaminated cases, antibiotics should be continued for 24 hours after surgery. For contaminated cases, antibiotics should be continued until the sepsis has cleared, and the white blood cell count and the temperature curve have returned to normal. For patients who have been on steroid therapy, stress doses of intravenous hydrocortisone should be administered in the perioperative period.

---

* Editor's Note: Oral phosphate solutions can cause aphthous ulcers. (TMB)

For patients who require an intestinal stoma, the optimal location of the ostomy should be determined prior to operation. Preoperative consultation with an enterostomal therapist should be obtained to assist in the placement of the proposed stoma. (Refer to a separate chapter by an ostomy nurse.) Ideally, the ostomy should be placed over the left or right rectus muscle on a flat area away from deep skin folds and bony prominences. The surface of the abdomen should be evaluated in both the sitting and standing positions; this often demonstrates skin folds and creases not evident in the supine position. The patient's belt line also should be identified, and the stoma should be placed below it. Once the optimal position for the proposed stoma has been identified, it should be marked with an indelible marker.

Extent of Resection

One of the most controversial issues regarding the surgical management of colorectal CD is the optimal extent of resection. Although it has been established that radical excision of grossly normal small intestine has no advantage with respect to the risk of recurrent disease, it appears that under particular circumstances, radical resection of grossly normal colon in patients with colorectal CD may result in a lowered risk for recurrence compared to less extensive resections. Recurrence of disease within grossly normal residual colon is common but recurrence in the small bowel after a proctocolectomy for colorectal CD is substantially less frequent. The entire residual colon and rectum may be at high risk for a postsurgical recurrence, and it has been suggested that this risk is greatest in the portion of colon proximal to the area of resected disease. For this reason, resection of normal proximal colon with ileocolonic anastomosis has been advocated as a means of lessening the likelihood of recurrence and hence the need for further surgery. This is the case, for instance, when the transverse colon and splenic flexure are diseased and the right colon and hepatic flexure are grossly normal. Yet, the aim of lessening recurrence rates needs to be balanced with the functional side effects of larger resections. When the disease is limited to a short segment of the left colon or rectum, an abdominal colectomy or a proctocolectomy may lead to excessive loss of absorptive surface area such that unacceptable diarrhea may result. Under such circumstances, a segmental resection with colocolonic anastomosis or an abdominoperineal resection with a left-sided colostomy may be preferable, even if the risk for recurrence is higher.

Surgical Strategies

The choice of operation for colorectal CD is dependent on multiple variables, including the distribution of disease, the extent of involvement, previous resections, rectal compliance, and adequacy of fecal continence.

Management of Common Anatomic Patterns of Colorectal Crohn's Disease

CECAL DISEASE

Crohn's disease involving the cecum almost always is associated with a disease pattern that predominates in the ileum with some limited involvement of the proximal colon. Terminal ileal disease with limited involvement of the cecum tends to behave much like disease limited to the terminal ileum. Under such circumstances, surgical resection should encompass the margins of gross disease with anastomosis between the neoterminal ileum and the proximal ascending colon.

DISEASE OF THE RIGHT COLON

Disease involving the entire right colon can occur along with ileal disease or it may occur in isolation. Extensive involvement of the right colon as a form of ileocolic disease is less common than the ileocecal pattern. Isolated involvement of the right colon without involvement of the ileum is an unusual pattern of disease. Surgical treatment involves standard right hemicolectomy encompassing the gross limits of the disease in the colon and ileum, with anastomosis between the ileum and the proximal transverse colon.

Following a right hemicolectomy, the anastomosis often rests in close proximity to the duodenal loop, and recurrent disease may result in a dense phlegmon adherent to the duodenum with or without a fistulous communication. Secondary involvement of the duodenum with CD recurring at the anastomosis or at the pre-anastomotic ileum can place a patient at substantial risk for significant morbidity should the need for surgical treatment of the recurrent disease arise. Therefore, it is worthwhile to make an effort to protect the duodenum by interposing omentum between the duodenum and the anastomosis. If the patient has no substantial omentum, an attempt should be made to allow the anastomosis to rest in a position away from the duodenum.

DISEASE INVOLVING THE RIGHT AND TRANSVERSE COLON

Crohn's disease involving both the right and transverse colon is best treated with an extended hemicolectomy encompassing the limits of gross disease. Occasionally, the anastomosis between the proximal descending colon and the ileum can result in an awkward alignment of the bowel loops such that kinks or twisting of the intestine may occur. Under such circumstances, a more extensive colectomy with an ileosigmoid anastomosis may be necessary.

EXTENSIVE COLITIS WITH RECTAL SPARING

Extensive colitis or pancolitis with sparing of the rectum is a common pattern of colorectal CD and occurs in approximately 20 percent of the population with Crohn's colitis. If the rectum is free of involvement, according to gross endoscopic inspection, if the anal sphincters are adequate, according to history, and if perianal disease is absent or controlled according to physical examination, total abdominal colectomy with ileorectal anastomosis can be performed. This procedure can result in good long-term function and enables many patients to avoid an ileostomy and maintain acceptable bowel function. However, some patients may experience frequent and loose stools to the point that incontinence may develop after ileorectal anastomosis. Additionally, any degree of recurrence in the rectum may result in significant deterioration of bowel function requiring further medical or even surgical intervention. To make this operation worthwhile, 10 to 14 cm of rectum should be free of disease. For elderly patients with questionable sphincter function, total proctocolectomy with permanent ileostomy often is a wiser option.

CROHN'S PROCTOCOLITIS

Extensive involvement of the colon and rectum requires total proctocolectomy with permanent ileostomy. In most cases, this can be performed in a single step. However, for patients who also display significant and active perianal disease, a two-stage procedure may be required. At the first operation, the intra-abdominal colon and a majority of the rectum are removed, leaving a short rectal stump. At the same time, perineal abscesses are drained and fistulae are laid open. This approach removes the diseased colon and rectum without creating a perineal wound that may be difficult to heal in the presence of active perianal sepsis. After the perineal sepsis has cleared and the perineum has healed by secondary intention, the short Hartmann's pouch is removed through a perineal approach. At this second stage, primary closure usually can be accomplished, avoiding any persistent perineal wounds.

As most surgeons consider CD to be a contraindication to restorative surgery, ileal pouch-anal anastomosis (IPAA) procedures have been performed unwittingly in patients whose diagnosis of CD was made only after the restorative proctocolectomy. Various reports indicate that recurrence of CD within the pouch is common, and removal of the pouch often is necessary. Patients who do not suffer from uncontrollable recurrence of disease do well and typically experience good pouch function. Even so, many surgeons argue that the length of small bowel that is lost in case of pouch excision does not warrant the risk of intentionally performing IPAA in patients with CD. In addition, CD of the pouch can result in pouch-vaginal or pouch-perineal fistulae, notoriously difficult complications to heal even with pouch excision. Postsurgical scarring combined with Crohn's-related pelvic inflammation and sepsis can make pouch excision difficult, with a risk for heavy bleeding and even pelvic autonomic nerve injury. For all of these reasons, IPAA

should not be performed in patients with an established diagnosis of CD. However, Panis et al (1996) identified a subset of patients with CD who, in their experience, are at low risk for recurrence after IPAA. They reported that patients with CD limited to the colon and rectum without any small bowel or perineal manifestations are at low risk for pouch failure after IPAA. After 5 years of follow-up, only 2 of their 31 patients required pouch excision. Four additional patients experienced recurrent CD, but their pouches were salvaged. It remains difficult to recommend IPAA to a patient with known CD; however, with further experience and data, a restorative procedure may become an option in carefully selected younger patients without small bowel disease or perianal manifestations.

CROHN'S PROCTITIS

Crohn's disease limited to the rectum is an unusual pattern of disease. In general, surgical management of Crohn's proctitis mandates proctectomy. However, the extent of the proximal resection is controversial. Performing an abdominal perineal resection with an end-sigmoid colostomy has been associated in some reports with a high risk for stomal complications compared to total proctocolectomy with the Brooke ileostomy. Additionally, experience suggests that the residual colon may be at high risk for recurrent disease. For these reasons, total proctocolectomy with ileostomy is at times recommended for CD limited to the rectum and distal colon. This is particularly true for patients who have no history of small bowel CD. Patients who have undergone prior small bowel resection or older patients may be at high risk for a high output ileostomy and, therefore, may benefit from attempts to preserve the colonic absorptive capacity. These patients may be better treated with proctectomy and end-colostomy.

Removal of the anorectum is best carried out along the plane between the internal and external sphincters. This intersphincteric dissection allows for a perineal closure that is associated with fewer complications and better healing than wider dissections that encompass the entire sphincter mechanism. Frequently, fistulae from perineal CD traverse the intersphincteric plane, and a wider dissection is required to encompass the diseased tissue. Occasionally, perineal scarring is so severe that very wide dissection with extensive loss of perianal skin and subcutaneous tissues is required. Resultant wounds often are too large for primary closure and require advanced tissue transfer techniques, such as gluteal flaps, gracilis flaps, or myocutaneous rectus abdominis pedicle flaps.

Sexual dysfunction is a much-feared complication from surgical proctectomy. However, with meticulous attention to maintaining the dissection close to the rectal wall, sexual complications after proctectomy for CD are relatively uncommon. Impotence occurs in approximately 1 to 2 percent of male patients. Retrograde ejaculation is more common and occurs in up to 5 percent of males. Sexual dysfunction in the female mostly is limited to dyspareunia and is seen in 30 percent of cases. Typically, however, dyspareunia is temporary and minor. Female fertility is not appreciably diminished after total proctocolectomy, and the procedure does not preclude full-term pregnancy with normal vaginal delivery. Complications related to the abdominal stoma unfortunately are common and include stomal necrosis, peristomal hernias, prolapse, and stricture. Lifetime risk for patients to require surgical revision of their stoma to deal with one or more of these complications approaches 25 percent.

SEGMENTAL CROHN'S COLITIS

When CD involves limited and isolated segments of the colon, surgical management is controversial. There is little argument that segmental involvement of the right colon should be managed by right colectomy with ileotransverse anastomosis. For segmental disease involving the transverse colon, an extended right hemicolectomy probably is an easier procedure to perform than a segmental transverse colectomy, and it responds to the concerns of lessening the recurrence rate by avoiding a colocolonic anastomosis. For disease in the descending or sigmoid colon, the appropriate surgery is more controversial. Whereas some studies have indicated that segmental colonic resection with colocolonic anastomosis can be performed with overall good results, others have shown a risk for early recurrence of disease. Even if the risk for recurrence is higher with segmental resection, for some patients the benefits of preserving the absorptive surface may outweigh the higher risk of recurrence. When the disease is limited to a short segment of the left colon, a segmental colectomy with colocolonic anastomosis may be preferable, even if the risk for recurrence may be somewhat higher. This is particularly true for older patients or patients who have undergone significant previous small bowel resection. It has been argued that younger patients with no previous small bowel resections may be better treated with resection of the diseased segment of colon and the normal proximal colon with creation of an ileosigmoid or ileorectal anastomosis.[†]

Emergency Surgery

Severe fulminant colitis, toxic megacolon, severe hemorrhage, colonic perforation, and sepsis require emergent surgical intervention. Under such circumstances, inadequate bowel preparation, peritoneal contamina-

tion, or the patient's overall poor condition may preclude safe anastomosis. Additionally, in the presence of peritoneal contamination or severe medical debilitation, the extensive pelvic dissection of a proctectomy should not be performed. Often, in emergency situations, the operation needs to be designed in a staged fashion, with the initial goal of stabilizing the patient and thereby allowing completion of the surgical therapy once the patient's medical condition has improved. In the urgent setting, resection with temporary ileostomy formation often is required. If the rectum is free of disease, the GI continuity can almost always be reestablished at a later date. For disease involving both the colon and the rectum, abdominal colectomy with end-ileostomy should be performed in the urgent setting. The diseased rectum is left behind as either a Hartmann's pouch or a mucous fistula. This approach allows the patient to recover from the acute illness, and the rectum can then be removed at a later date when the patient's condition has improved and the proctectomy can be performed under safer conditions.[‡]

Once a diverted rectal stump has been created, it can be removed on an elective basis; however, a diverted rectal stump should not be left in place for an extended period, because disease activity in the excluded rectum typically progresses and may result in complex abscess and fistula formation such that subsequent excision of the rectum may be exceedingly difficult and associated with a high risk for complications. An excluded rectal stump carries a high risk for development of adenocarcinoma over the long term and for this reason alone elective excision of excluded rectal stumps is indicated in patients with CD.

After diversion of the fecal stream, the activity of disease within the rectum may appear to subside. This may entice the surgeon to attempt a takedown of the stoma with an ileorectal anastomosis. However, clinical experience has shown that disease activity within the rectum often rapidly recurs after the reestablishment of intestinal continuity. Attempts at salvage of the rectum under these circumstances are not worthwhile.

Long-term Results

At the University of Chicago, 161 colectomies for CD limited to the colon were performed between 1986 and 1998. After a mean of 48 months follow-up, the postsurgical recurrence rate has been 10 percent. Breakdown of the data by procedure demonstrates some common observations regarding the natural history of Crohn's colitis (Table 105–1). The experience from these patients supports the contention that the residual colon is at risk for recurrent disease. This is particularly true when colon

---

[†] Editor's Note: There are few data on the role of "prophylactic" medical therapy after colonic resection. Mesalamine in large doses (3 g or more) seems to be best for ileal or ileo-right colon disease. I have started or continued azathioprine in a number of patients with colonic resection for active disease, but there are few data on this approach. Whether Remicade® (Centocor Inc., Malvern, Pennsylvania) will be useful postoperatively in selected patients is not known. (TMB)

[‡] Editor's Note: Some "conservative" surgeons "protect" colonic anastomoses in areas of diseased colon with a diverting ostomy even in elective operations. This conservative approach could be helpful for surgeons who are not as experienced in IBD surgery as these authors. (TMB)

TABLE 105–1. Postsurgical Recurrence of Crohn's Disease

Procedure	Number	Recurrences (%)	Recurrence Location	Mean Time to Recurrence (mo)
Right colectomy	42	2 (5)	2 colon	54.0
Segmental colectomy	19	7 (37)	6 colon; 1 small bowel	24.4
Abdominal colectomy	22	1 (5)	1 small bowel	30.6
Proctectomy with colostomy	11	3 (27)	3 colon	25.2
Proctocolectomy with ileostomy	68	3 (4)	3 small bowel	55.2

proximal to the resected segment is preserved. The most frequent and the quickest recurrences happen after segmental resection with colocolonic anastomosis or proctectomy with end-colostomy (37% and 27% surgical recurrence, 24 and 25 months, respectively). Eleven of the 13 recurrences occurred in the remaining colon. Complete extirpation of the colon and rectum resulted in the lowest rate of recurrence in these patients.

References

Panis Y, Poupard B, Nemeth J, et al. Ileal pouch-anal anastomosis for Crohn's disease. Lancet 1996;347:854–7.

Robert JR, Sachar DB, Greenstein AJ. Severe gastrointestinal hemorrhage in Crohn's disease. Ann Surg 1991;213:207–11.

Supplemental Reading

Bauer JJ, Gelernt IM, Salky B. Sexual dysfunction following proctocolectomy for benign disease of the colon and rectum. Ann Surg 1983;197:363–7.

Berry AR, de Campos RDE, Lee ECG. Perineal and pelvic morbidity following perimuscular excision of the rectum for inflammatory bowel disease. Br J Surg 1986;73:675–7.

Block GE, Michelassi F, Tanaka M, et al. Crohn's disease. Curr Probl Surg 1993;2:173–265.

Greenstein J, Mann D, Heimann T, et al. Spontaneous free perforation and perforated abscess in 30 patients with Crohn's disease. Ann Surg 1987;205:72–5.

Jirsch DW, Gardiner GW. Crohn's disease in an isolated rectal stump. Dis Colon Rectum 1980;23:426–9.

Metcalf AM, Dozois RR, Kelly KA. Sexual function in women after proctocolectomy. Ann Surg 1986;204:624–7.

Michelassi F, Testa G, Pomidor W, et al. Adenocarcinoma complicating Crohn's disease. Dis Colon Rectum 1993;36:654–61.

Sagar PM, Dozois RR, Wolff BG. Long-term results of ileal pouch-anal anastomosis in patients with Crohn's disease. Dis Colon Rectum 1996;39:893–8.

Sanfey H, Bayless TM, Cameron JL. Crohn's disease of the colon. Is there a role for limited resection? Ann Surg 1984;147:38–42.

Stern HS, Goldberg SM, Rothenberger DA, et al. Segmental versus total colectomy for large bowel Crohn's disease. World J Surg 1984;8:118–22.

Tjandra JJ, Fazio VW. Surgery for Crohn's colitis. Int Surg 1992;77:9-14.

Trnka YM, Glotzer DJ, Kasdon EJ, et al. The long-term outcome of restorative operation in Crohn's disease: influence of location, prognostic factors, and surgical guidelines. Ann Surg 1982;196:345–55.

CHAPTER 106

PERIANAL DISEASE

ALON J. PIKARSKY, MD, AND STEVEN D. WEXNER, MD

The reported incidence of perianal involvement in patients with Crohn's disease ranges from 18 to 94 percent. This variation is a consequence of case selection and differences in criteria used to define anal lesions. The incidence increases with more distal Crohn's disease, involving over 80 percent of patients with Crohn's proctitis. Anorectal lesions occur as the only manifestation of Crohn's disease in 5 to 10 percent of patients.

Assessment

Anorectal lesions in the setting of inflammatory bowel disease (IBD) may be the only way to differentiate between Crohn's disease and ulcerative colitis. In general, any atypical lesion should be regarded as resulting from Crohn's disease and not ulcerative colitis. Multiple lesions, painless lesions, eccentric lesions, and wounds that fail to heal after surgical intervention all are features that raise the possibility of Crohn's disease. It is particularly critical to distinguish between mucosal ulcerative colitis and Crohn's disease if the patient is being considered for a colectomy for colonic IBD. In this instance, a history of suppurative anorectal disease as opposed to fissures is particularly relevant. Whereas the latter condition can occur with chronic diarrhea, the former greatly raises the index of suspicion for Crohn's disease in the absence of any other features to help distinguish between the two idiopathic IBDs. A total abdominal colectomy with ileostomy may be the preferred mode of management, allowing the pathologist the opportunity to review the entire specimen to help make a differentiation. In addition the patient can be monitored for the progression of any anal manifestations prior to further surgical intervention.

The **history** should include bowel habits, type and duration of perianal disease, and any pharmacologic intervention, with the duration and dose of such therapy. The patient should be queried regarding evacuatory difficulties, which may be secondary to anal stenosis or stricture, and conversely regarding any symptoms of incontinence, which may be attributable to prior fistula surgery. The use of an incontinence score is helpful to objectify any complaints of fecal incontinence.

Inspection should include assessment of perianal skin for excoriation, evaluation of any skin tags and fissures, and, if possible, digital examination and anoscopy. In the presence of a stenosis, acute separation, or tenderness caused by any other etiology, the examination may be best performed under general anesthesia. Suspicious ulcers may be biopsied, suppuration drained, and stenoses gently digitally dilated.

Clinical Evaluation

If office evaluation is possible, proctosigmoidoscopy should be performed to evaluate any rectal or rectosigmoid inflammation. In selected instances, other adjunct studies, such as anal manometry, rectal compliance and capacity measurement, anal electromyography, pudendal nerve terminal motor latency assessment, and anal ultrasonography may be of value. The latter technique is particularly useful to assess any underlying sphincteric injuries attributable to prior fistula surgery or vaginal delivery. Delineation of fistula tracts and elucidation of occult internal openings may be facilitated by injection of hydrogen peroxide during anal ultrasonography. Furthermore, if any sphincter division or restorative resections are contemplated, anal manometry and the adjunct assessments of rectal compliance and capacity measurement are valuable preoperative procedures. In addition to manometry, ultrasonography, and these other investigations, the extent of proximal disease needs to be delineated. Upper gastrointestinal radiographic evaluation with small-bowel series and colonoscopy with biopsy form the cornerstones of this assessment. On occasion, computer tomography and other specialized investigations may be of value.

The approach to the anorectal manifestations of Crohn's disease is based on aggressive medical therapy combined with conservative surgical therapy. Traditionally, surgeons advised against aggressive intervention in these patients. John Alexander-Williams noted, "The major reason for fecal incontinence in patients with Crohn's disease is more often the aggressiveness of the surgeon rather than the aggressiveness of the disease."

Therapeutic Alternatives

The surgical strategy for treating perianal Crohn's disease depends on the chronicity of the problem, the presence of suppuration, the condition of the rectum, and the status of any small-bowel disease (Figure 106–1). Certain

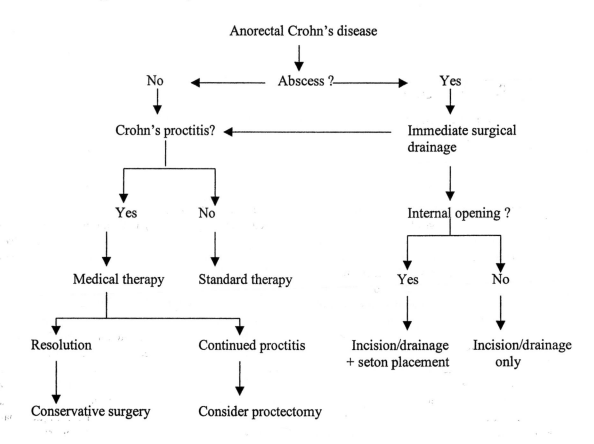

FIGURE 106–1. Algorithm for surgical treatment of perianal Crohn's disease.

conservative interventions can be employed without fear of disease exacerbation, regardless of the specific manifestation of perianal Crohn's disease. As examples, stool softeners, psyllium bulking agents, topical steroids, antidiarrheal agents, steroid and 5-aminosalicylic acid (5-ASA) suppositories, with or without enemas, and warm sitz baths are all useful adjuncts. It is critical to remember that the aim of the management of perianal Crohn's disease may not necessarily be to eradicate the condition but rather to preserve the anus with an acceptable level of function. Thus, repeated gentle anal dilations, even including home self-administered daily anal dilations, may be preferable to fecal diversion with or without proctectomy. The use of a chronic indwelling seton, although potentially inconvenient to the patient, may be far more acceptable than a fistulotomy, which can produce an unhealed wound, fecal incontinence, or both.

Even though the loop ileostomy may be constructed as a "temporary" stoma, it should always be undertaken with a technique that will allow it to be permanently situated. If the patient has experienced a poorly constructed temporary stoma, he or she may be loathe to undergo a permanent one even if such a creation would offer significant benefit. Conversely, having experienced a well-constructed, easy-to-manage stoma, the patient may be more accepting of this potentially inevitable consequence of Crohn's disease.

The authors do not routinely employ diverting stomas but strongly consider them under certain circumstances. Specifically, a patient in whom a high transsphincteric or rectovaginal fistula has failed to respond to advancement flap therapy may be best served by construction of a laparoscopic loop ileostomy prior to repeating the flap procedure or to interposing a gracilis muscle. The patient with high-grade stenosis but an otherwise normal rectum may be well served by a temporary stoma. Patients with progressive anal suppuration and sepsis, despite appropriate ongoing evaluation and management but who refuse proctectomy with permanent stoma, may again be advised to undergo at least temporary fecal diversion for symptomatic relief. Regardless of the indication for a stoma, patients should be counseled preoperatively by an enterostomal therapist to help facilitate and expedite the recovery process. In addition, the enterostomal therapist can select the optimal position for the stoma.

Control of Intestinal Disease: Local versus Proximal Therapy

Controversy exists over the influence of proximal intestinal disease on the course and outcome after surgical intervention for perianal Crohn's disease. Attempts to heal perianal manifestations by proximal diversion of the fecal stream have had variable rates of success. Although transient induration of rectal and perianal disease may be achieved, long-term failure is noted in most cases. However, several authors do advocate control of proximal disease prior to any attempt to operate upon the perianal manifestations. The present authors advocate preliminary control of the intestinal disease before primary local therapy of complex perianal lesions. Such treatment may be either medical or surgical, including proximal intestinal resections and fecal diversion. In these cases, the success attributed to the proximal resection of disease results mainly from control of diarrhea. Therefore, every attempt is made to achieve quiescence of proximal disease by means of medical therapy, including immunomodulation and control of diarrhea.

Proctectomy in Crohn's Disease

In the presence of severe Crohn's proctitis that has not responded to medical management, concomitant severe perianal disease is an indication for initial proctectomy. Other indications in the absence of Crohn's proctitis are less agreed upon, as most patients can be managed with relative success for long periods of time. Fecal incontinence may be another indication; all other indications are relative. Refractory, severe, and intractable disease should be considered individually in each patient. Patients with a young age of disease onset, with fistula as the first manifestation of perianal disease, or with more than three perianal lesions during follow-up, as well as those with individual rectal involvement by Crohn's disease, have been identified at high risk for proctectomy.

The overall cumulative probability of proctectomy in patients with perianal Crohn's disease has been estimated to be 10 percent at 10 years, increasing thereafter by 1 percent each year. In those patients who need a proctectomy, there is no advantage in preserving the rest of the colon. Isolated severe proctitis with an unaffected colon is a rare occurrence, and the preferred procedure is a total proctocolectomy with an end ileostomy.*

Technique and Problems

Sexual Dysfunction

Autonomic nerve injury, especially in young male patients, is always a feared consequence of proctectomy. Accordingly, in patients with Crohn's disease an intersphincteric dissection is performed along the intersphincteric groove, leaving the external anal sphincter intact. This technique, combined with perimuscular excision of the rectum, leaves an intact pelvic muscular support for the remaining pelvic structures. The resultant perineal incision has a better cosmetic appearance, and the likelihood of sexual dysfunction is markedly decreased.

---

* Editor's Note: Some patients with rectal CD seemingly do quite well with a left-sided solostomy and continued medical therapy. (TMB)

Perineal Wound Nonhealing

Following proctectomy for Crohn's disease, nonhealing of the perineal wound occurs more commonly than following proctectomy for cancer. The intersphincteric proctectomy is one of the means to prevent this complication. It results in a smaller wound and less pelvic dead space than does an oncologic proctectomy. Some authors advocate leaving the pelvic floor open for drainage in these cases, to allow healing by secondary intention. The authors routinely close the pelvic floor in a layered fashion, leaving a large irrigating sump drain in the pelvis through the abdominal wound. The drain is removed once the irrigated fluid returns clear in decreased amounts, in most cases after 48 hours.

In the majority (85%) of patients, the wound heals by primary intention. In the remaining patients, slow healing by secondary intention occurs. Only a small proportion of the patients develop a persistent perineal sinus. A variety of topical therapies can be attempted, such as gauze packing, curettage, and Silastic foam dressings. Metronidazole therapy usually is not successful in inducing healing of these sinuses. A few patients may respond favorably to curettage followed by fibrin glue instillation. Others may require complex procedures, including skin grafts, gracilis muscle or other myocutaneous flap interposition grafts, or resection of the sacrococcygeal bone. In any event, with the appearance of a persistent perineal sinus, an ultrasound, small-bowel series, and computed tomography should be performed prior to any surgical intervention. These studies will define the problem and help differentiate between a pelvic sinus and any enteric communication.

Treatment of Specific Conditions

Fissures

Anal fissures in Crohn's disease usually are not associated with increased sphincter resting pressure, and the overshoot phenomenon is not demonstrated during manometry. For painless acute fissures, medical therapy is employed. There is no justification for surgical intervention unless the fissure is painful or persists, and both events are rare.

Persistent or painful fissures pose an underlying problem. These patients should undergo examination under anesthesia to exclude an associated abscess or ulcer as the cause for pain. When an abscess is found, it should be adequately drained. The base of the fissure or ulcer found should be débrided and biopsied if indicated. Anal dilation is not recommended with the technique; it is painful and can contribute to subsequent incontinence.

The vast majority of fissures can be treated successfully in a conservative manner. Methods employed include a combination of local measures and stool modulating agents. The former include sitz baths, topical steroids, 5-ASA suppositories, and occasionally, 0.25 percent Xylocaine (Astra USA Inc., Westborough, Maryland)

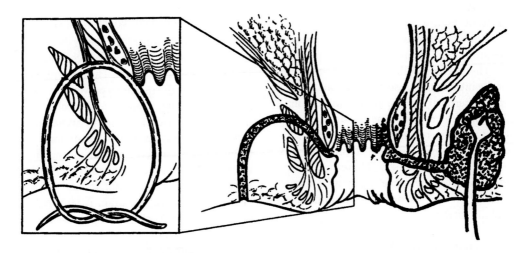

FIGURE 106–2. Abscess with associated fistula treated by placement of a seton and mushroom catheter.

ointment. The sitz baths should consist of warm water without any additives. They should be taken upon awakening, after each bowel movement, upon returning home at the end of the day, and prior to retirement for the evening. The stool modulating regimen should include stool softeners and psyllium bulking agents. If diarrhea is a significant component, antimotility agents, such as loperimide or diphenoxylate, should be employed. The goal is to achieve soft, effortless stool with the frequency ranging from one bowel movement every 3 days to three bowel movements per day.

More recently, other conservative measures have been suggested, although none have been reported to date in patients with Crohn's disease. Specifically, topical application of nitric oxide (isosorbide dinitrate) had variable success for the treatment of ischemic anal fissure. Similarly, botulinum toxin injection also has had some role in patients without Crohn's disease. In select circumstances, these agents may be tried. Ultimately, sphincterotomy may be considered if persistent posterior midline anal fissures are unresponsive to medical therapy. However, the patient must be cognizant of the potential risk of incontinence. As potential safeguards to hopefully limit the chance of incontinence, patients may be advised to undergo preoperative anal manometry and ultrasound evaluation. Differentiation in this treatment regimen is between the anal fissure and anal ulcer. Sphincterotomy should be assiduously avoided in cases of anal ulcer.

Abscesses

Abscesses are common in Crohn's disease, and complete surgical drainage is always indicated. Establishing free drainage is important even if the amount of purulence is limited. Simple de novo rectal abscesses can be treated by incision and drainage, and in the majority of patients, this can be performed under local anesthesia as an outpatient procedure. However, complete drainage should

never be compromised to limit the extent of the procedure. Following drainage of a painful abscess in patients with Crohn's disease, a painless, well-tolerated fistula will appear. If the associated fistula is obvious, a drawing seton or even multiple setons are placed to establish long-term drainage. Blind sinuses and abscess cavities are maintained open by placement of a mushroom catheter in the abscess cavity (Figure 106–2). Fistulotomy during abscess drainage is not recommended.

No attempts are made to forcefully probe fistula tracts or to reveal "occult" internal openings. Certain techniques can help facilitate identification of the internal opening. Specifically, prior to drainage of the abscess, an anoscope can be placed in the anal canal. Gentle pressure applied upon the fistula may allow purulence to exude at the internal opening at the dentate line. Knowledge of Goodsall's rule in this respect is helpful. Once the cavity is drained, gentle injection of hydrogen peroxide, curettage of the cavity while "following" the granulation tissue by digital palpation, and gentle probing are all useful adjuncts. However, care must be taken not to create false passages or new internal openings. In inflamed edematous tissue, it is easy to convert an intersphincteric or low transsphincteric fistula into a high transsphincteric or extrasphincteric one. The consequences of such misadventure are obviously significant. Abscesses left undrained may lead to extensive tissue destruction, and therefore, antibiotics should be regarded only as an adjunct to definitive therapy. Intraoperative endorectal ultrasonography may be used during surgery to define exact locations and extent of clinically unsuspected collections. When in doubt, an examination under anesthesia with needle localization of any abscess cavities should be undertaken.

Fistulae

Although some perianal fistulae in Crohn's disease may be complex, the majority are simple. Overall, approximately

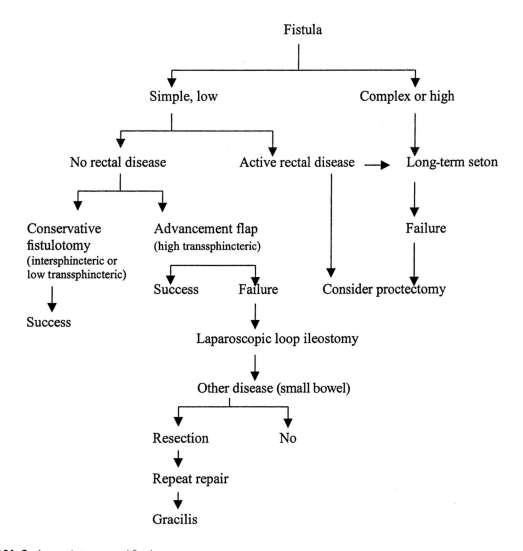

FIGURE 106–3. Approach to anorectal fistula.

85 percent of patients with Crohn's proctitis have fistulae; in some patients, the fistula is asymptomatic, and in others, the fistula manifests with only minimal tenderness and pain. Two dramatically opposed views have been espoused regarding the surgical treatment of fistulae in Crohn's disease.

The conservative approach (Alexander-Williams) states that these fistulae often spontaneously heal and that surgical intervention frequently does not result in healing and may instead result in incontinence. The opposite approach regards surgery as safe and effective provided the fistula is intersphincteric or transsphincteric and there is no coexisting rectal disease. The treatment of fistulae should be individualized; only symptomatic fistulae require operative treatment (Figure 106–3).

Standard surgical therapy of simple low fistulae in Crohn's disease by means of fistulotomy results in satisfactory healing rates; incontinence is rare and the proctectomy rate is low. In cases of complex fistulae involving large portions of the sphincter muscle, standard techniques may result in high rates of incontinence. In these patients, it is preferable to place a seton or multiple setons without dividing any sphincter muscle. This technique is particularly suitable for high anorectal fistulae with coexisting sepsis.

These setons can be made of any minimally reactive material, including suture material, pediatric feeding tubes, rubber vessel loops, and other materials. Since these setons will remain in place for long periods as drains rather than being used as "cutting" setons, they should be nonreactive material. It is not uncommon for patients with extensive perianal Crohn's disease to prefer an existence with multiple chronically drained setons in well-formed, well-drained tracts than to undergo a proctectomy with permanent stoma.

Rectovaginal Fistulae

Rectovaginal fistulae are uncommon in Crohn's disease, occurring in 5 to 10 percent of women with Crohn's proctitis. Unlike other etiologies, in many patients with

Crohn's disease these fistulae do not commonly result in severe incontinence, although the majority of patients complain of intermittent vaginal discharge and gas passage through the vagina. Fistulae that occur as a result of severe rectal disease usually present in the midportion of the rectovaginal septum as suprasphincteric. Some fistulae are the result of infected anal glands, and in these cases, the tract can be superficial, transsphincteric, or suprasphincteric. Fistulae resulting from an infected bartholinian abscess are low anovulval. These fistulae carry a poor prognosis even after fecal diversion and often result in proctectomy. A more unusual etiology is an intestinal loop communicating with the posterior fornix in the pouch of Douglas. This type of fistula can result from a diseased loop of sigmoid or a leaking intestinal anastomosis.

Medical management, consisting of antibiotics and immunosuppression, does not result in healing of rectovaginal fistulae. The authors do not use it as sole treatment, but it is important to induce remission of intestinal and rectal disease prior to attempted repair. Although some authors have advocated staged seton fistulotomy of transsphincteric fistulae, the risk of incontinence is great, and it is not recommended.

Those high fistulae arising from diseased intestine in the pouch of Douglas are treated by resection of the diseased segment, often by a laparoscopic approach. In cases of a sphincter defect, as detected by endoanal ultrasound, an overlapping sphincter repair may yield better closure rates. Routine diversion of the fecal stream is not recommended, unless the operation is a repeat one. Even then, initial failed repair is not necessarily indicative of a permanent stoma. Repeat repairs have been successful, with preliminary temporary diversion. In cases where there is loss of healthy tissue in the perineal body, a repeat repair consists of an anal advancement flap with interposition of a gracilis muscle between the rectum and the vagina. This later approach is used also for rectourethral fistulae complicating Crohn's disease and for recurrent pouch vaginal fistulae. There is a separate chapter on rectovaginal fistulae.

Incontinence

In Crohn's disease, incontinence usually is the result of previous surgical intervention rather than disease progression. Active disease with loose stools as well as severe proctitis with loss of rectal compliance can contribute to incontinence. Control of intestinal disease and frequently treating proctitis can help improve continence even with concomitant sphincter muscle dysfunction. At times, incontinence is the result of unrelated causes, such as obstetric injuries, and in these circumstances, as long as rectal and intestinal disease are controlled, sphincter repair can result in a good outcome.

Once again, anal sphincter repair need not be accompanied by temporary fecal diversion. However, repeat sphincter repairs would generally be an indication for diversion. These operations should be undertaken only by surgeons well versed in the treatment of incontinence and after detailed counseling of the patient about the potential adverse sequalae, such as permanent stoma in case of failure. As a prerequisite to sphincter repair, these patients should undergo thorough anorectal physiologic testing to ensure adequacy of both pudendal nerves; absence of multifocal injury, as noted by both anal ultrasound and anal electromyography; and the potential for improvement in manometric pressures. Moreover, rectal capacity and compliance should be acceptable, because successful muscular repair distal to a noncompliant small-volume rectum may offer no symptomatic relief. Patients with incontinence and severe proctitis are probably better treated by fecal diversion, perhaps as a total proctocolectomy.

Anorectal Strictures

Anorectal strictures can result from chronic abscess, fistulae, ulcerations, and multiple surgical interventions. They occur in 5 percent of patients with perianal Crohn's disease. The symptoms related to strictures are those of urgency, tenesmus, incontinence, and difficult evacuation. Obstruction is a rare occurrence, because the patients usually experience loose bowel movements. Short, annular strictures (less than 2 cm) can resolve after one or two sessions of digital or proctoscopic dilation. Longer, tubular strictures are the result of defunction atrophy. These strictures are less responsive to dilation, are progressive, and eventually require fecal diversion or proctectomy.

Strictures that do not respond to conservative nonoperative therapy may necessitate fecal diversion, possibly as permanent proctectomy. The results of anoplasty for the treatment of anal stenosis in patients with Crohn's disease has not been overwhelmingly positive. In general, the use of stool softeners, some psyllium bulking agents, fluid, and anal dilations is adequate.[†]

Hemorrhoids

Hemorrhoids are uncommon in Crohn's disease, whereas edematous perianal skin tags are common and are often confused with external hemorrhoids. On a rare occasion, hemorrhoids may become symptomatic, so that some form of therapy is indicated, but symptoms fluctuate and a very conservative approach is recommended. Hemorrhoidectomy in Crohn's disease is associated with a high rate of complications from sepsis, stenosis, fistulae, and unhealed wounds, often resulting in proctectomy. Therefore, it is best to avoid surgery for hemorrhoids in these patients. The most important aspect of the treatment of "hemorrhoids" in patients

---

[†] Editor's Note: Anecdotally, four of my patients with ulcerations of the side of the rectal stricture have required less dilatations on Remicade® infusions. The concept of post-dilatation immune suppression is discussed in the next chapter. (TMB)

with Crohn's disease is the differentiation of hemorrhoids from anal skin tags. Because of the high incidence of unhealed wounds and ultimate stenosis in these patients, it is best to maintain a long-term conservative therapeutic approach rather than surgery.

There are three other chapters on perianal Crohn's disease in this text including Rectovaginal Fistula in Crohn's Disease,* Perianal Crohn's Disease: Medical Therapy,* and Fistulizing Crohn's Disease.

Fecal Diversion

Temporary fecal diversion may improve patient comfort and allow better healing of complex repairs. In these cases, the preferred mode of diversion is a loop ileostomy, with an everted proximal and flush distal limb; this technique offers virtually complete fecal diversion. It is easy for the patient to maintain and for the surgeon to subsequently reverse. A laparoscopic approach is preferable, even if a concomitant band resection is indicated. Sheets of carboxymethylcellulose-sodium hyaluronate bioresorbable membrane (Seprafilm™, Genzyme Corp., Cambridge, Massachusetts) are placed around the ileostomy site to facilitate future takedown. Diversion using a colostomy should be discouraged, because Crohn's disease may involve the stoma and thus complicate its management.‡

Supplemental Reading

Alexander-Williams J, Buchmann P. Perianal Crohn's disease. World J Surg 1980;4:203–8.

Beck DE, Wexner SD, eds. Fundamentals of anorectal surgery, 2nd Ed. London: WB Saunders, 1998.

Cohen JL, Stricker JW, Schoetz DJ, Coller JA. Rectovaginal fistula in Crohn's disease. Dis Colon Rectum 1989;32:825–8.

Hughes LE. Clinical classification of perianal Crohn's disease. Dis Colon Rectum 1992;35:928–32.

Hull TL, Fazio VW. Surgical approaches to low anovaginal fistula in Crohn's disease. Am J Surg 1997;173:95–8.

Makowiec F, Jehle EC, Becker HD, Starlinger M. Perianal abscess in Crohn's disease. Dis Colon Rectum 1997;40:443–50.

Regimbeau JM, Panis Y, Marteau P, et al. Surgical treatment of anoperineal Crohn's disease: Can abdominoperineal resection be predicted? J Am Coll Surg 1999;189:171–5.

Sangwan YP, Schoetz DJ, Murray JJ, et al. Perianal Crohn's disease: results of local surgical treatment. Dis Colon Rectum 1996;39:529–35.

Sardinha TC, Wexner SD. Laparoscopy for inflammatory bowel disease: pros and cons. World J Surg 1998;22:370–4.

Scott A, Hawley PR, Phillips RKS. Results of external sphincter repair in Crohn's disease. Br J Surg 1989;76:959–60.

‡ Editor's Note: Whether long-term immunodilator use with a left-colon colostomy will be an acceptable alternative remains to be determined. (TMB)

CHAPTER 107

ENDOSCOPIC MANAGEMENT OF SMALL BOWEL, ANASTOMOTIC, AND COLONIC STRICTURES IN CROHN'S DISEASE

RICHARD A. KOZAREK, MD

Historically, refractory disease and obstruction are the most common indications for surgery in Crohn's disease, and obstruction refractory to medical management is the most common indication for reoperation. Whereas strictureplasty has been extensively used in the surgical realm in an attempt to preserve bowel length, series studying balloon dilation in an attempt to avoid an operation altogether are limited. In whom should dilation be attempted? What are the data regarding concomitant corticosteroid injections into the stricture? Should concomitant oral corticosteroids or immunosuppressive agents be used?

Presentation

Strictures in inflammatory bowel disease (IBD) can be symptomatic (obstipation, pain, and distention in small bowel; colonic or anastomotic stenoses; nausea, vomiting, and postprandial pain with gastroduodenal strictures). Alternatively, they may simply be radiographic or endoscopic areas of narrowing that preclude subsequent tissue sampling by virtue of their small diameter. However, in the case of a significant stenosis, the onus is on the clinician to ensure that this stricture is benign; proof of benignity, in turn, may be based upon radiographic, endoscopic or histologic, or clinical parameters (Table 107–1). Significant stenoses may include long stenoses, those with mass effect, and presence at an anastomosis. Endoscopic proof requires adequate tissue sampling, which, in turn, may require use of a pediatric colonoscope or small-caliber upper endoscope or dilation to bypass the stenosis. Clinical concerns regarding stricture malignancy have primarily reviewed

TABLE 107–1. Diagnostic Approach to Obstructing Strictures in Crohn's Disease

Rule out malignancy and extrinsic compression by abscess
  Barium contrast studies
  Abdominal computer tomography

Endoscopic or histologic assessment
  Pediatric colonoscope
  Upper endoscope
  Balloon dilation to allow full scope inspection or tissue sampling

Clinical parameters

TABLE 107–2. Therapeutic Approach to Obstructing Strictures in Crohn's Disease

Therapeutic Approach	Medication or Procedure
Medications	Corticosteroids
	Immunosuppressive agents
	Infliximab ± antibiotics
Balloon dilation	With or without corticosteroid injection
One-time or sequential	Radial incision
	Possible expandable stent insertion
	Pharmacologic control of Crohn's disease
	(eg, steroids, immunosuppressives, 5-ASA)
Surgery	Resection
	Strictureplasty

colorectal strictures in ulcerative colitis (UC) as opposed to Crohn's disease. For instance, Gumaste and colleagues (1992) found 70 separate colonic strictures in 59 of 1156 (5%) patients with UC. Seventeen of these 70 strictures (24%) proved malignant. Three clinical features suggested malignancy: (1) appearance late in the disease course (61% malignancy after 20 yr of disease vs 0% before 10 yr); (2) location proximal to the splenic flexure (86% malignancy proximal to the splenic flexure, 47% sigmoid, and 10% rectum); and (3) symptomatic large bowel obstruction (100% malignancy vs 14% of those without). These results cannot be generalized to patients with Crohn's stenoses, not only because of the relatively lower risk of malignancy in this setting but also because of the higher incidence of obstruction as part of the disease process. Even an associated mass may simply be bowel-wall and mesenteric thickening. A diagnosis of small-bowel cancer is more often an incidental finding at surgery than a consequence of fastidious endoscopic biopsy.

Management

The management of Crohn's disease strictures is not done in endoscopic isolation (Table 107–2). The majority of patients are already taking 5-aminosalicylic acid (5-ASA) or broad-spectrum antibiotics, such as metronidazole or ciprofloxacin, and a subset is taking immunosuppressives

TABLE 107–3. Factors That Determine Candidacy for Stricture Dilation

Ideal Candidate	Poor Candidate
Short stricture (< 4 cm)	Acutely and completely obstructed patient
Anastomotic stenosis	Long stricture (≥ 5 cm)
Absence of mass: PE/CT	Multiple strictures
Moderate stenosis (5–10 mm)	Associated extraluminal or intraluminal fistula or deep ulceration
Prolonged interval from surgical intervention	Associated malignancy
	Tight stenosis (< 1–2 mm)
	Ileal strictures, nonoperated patient
	Acutely angulated stenosis
	Recently created anastamosis

or corticosteroids. Patients who develop symptomatic low-grade obstructive symptoms may or may not undergo limited barium contrast or computed tomographic (CT) studies, but instead are often offered a trial of or an increased dosage of corticosteroids. Those already taking a significant steroid dose or who have proven refractory to steroids or immunosuppressives should be considered as potential candidates for infliximab infusion. Patients who are steroid intolerant or nonresponders and individuals who have ongoing or rapidly recurring obstructive symptoms despite infliximab infusion should undergo radiographic and endoscopic evaluation with consideration of endoscopic or surgical treatment. Table 107–3 outlines ideal and suboptimal candidates for balloon dilation. The patient who becomes totally obstructed acutely is usually better handled medically or surgically as is the individual with multiple long stenoses. Likewise, patients with an internal or external fistula originating within the stricture (as determined by CT or radiography) probably should not undergo dilatation therapy for fear of disrupting an established fistulous tract. Finally, dilatation of a malignant Crohn's stricture in a candidate who is a good surgical risk is not recommended unless the aim is simple luminal enlargement to allow adequate bowel preparation for resective surgery.

Dilation Technique

As much information as possible about the stricture should be obtained prior to dilation. This may require traversing the stenosis with a diagnostic endoscope or, in ileal and some ileocolonic stenoses, injecting contrast through an endoscopic retrograde cholangiopancreatography (ERCP) catheter to outline stricture length, angulation, and luminal size. Fluoroscopic visualization adds an important measure of safety to attempted dilation. Not only does it allow fluoroscopic visualization of contrast injection, it also ensures effective dilation by documentation of balloon waist effacement. Finally, in acutely angulated stenoses, in which a guidewire may initially be passed as a luminal finding or straightening maneuver, fluoroscopic visualization ensures that the balloon shaft parallels the wire.

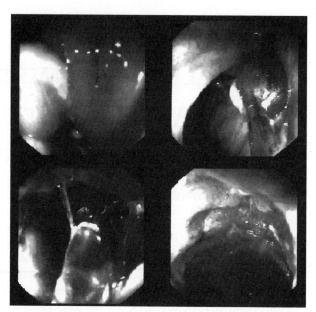

FIGURE 107–1. Balloon dilation of short anastomotic stricture. Lower right, terminal ileum.

Although recent technologic advances have led to the introduction of dilating balloons that have a variable diameter contingent upon inflation pressure and that can be inserted over a guidewire, no known report exists of them having been used for Crohn's strictures. Instead, the vast majority of stenoses have been dilated with through-the-scope (TTS) hydrostatic balloons. The use of a TTS dilator requires endoscopic approximation of the stricture size and selection of a balloon that is several millimeters larger. Both balloon and dilator shaft should be coated with silicone, and negative pressure should be applied to the balloon, using a 10- to 20-mL syringe. These measures, as well as using a therapeutic endoscope and avoiding excessive angulation of the endoscopic tip, allow dilator passage until all or part of the balloon is visualized. The balloon is centered in the stenotic anastomosis or stenosis using a combination of endoscopic and fluoroscopic control (Figures 107–1, 107–2, and 107–3). As noted, the latter also helps prevent damage of more proximal bowel wall related to excessive pressure of the balloon tip or extreme balloon angulation.

Although air can be used for inflation, a 10 to 25 percent contrast solution allows better visualization fluoroscopically and more uniform balloon dilation (see Figure 107–3). Technical efficacy in dilation requires obliteration of the balloon waist. The lb/per square inch (atmospheres [atm]) vary for 15-mm and 10-mm balloons (see manufacturer's instructions). The author uses between 30 and 40 lbs/sq inch (2–3 atm) for 15 and 10 mm balloons, respectively. Low-profile balloons with bursting pressures between 4 atm and 8 atm also have been marketed. Although theoretically these may be more efficacious, data concerning their use have been sparse. There are no data that demonstrate that 2 minutes of continued

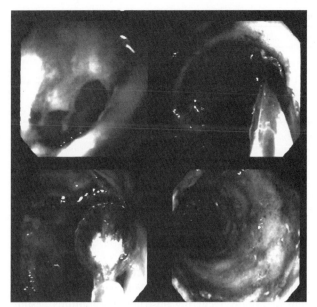

FIGURE 107–2. Tight ileocolonic stricture treated with balloon dilation. Lower right, severe ileitis.

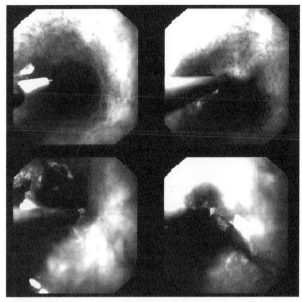

FIGURE 107–4. Circumferential triamcinolone injection in a patient with Crohn's disease with refractory sigmoid stenosis.

inflation are advantageous over 15 seconds once a balloon waist has been effaced. This author generally uses 30 to 60 seconds of dilation and subsequently redilates a second or third time, after repositioning the balloon. Once dilation has been effected, complete evacuation of the balloon and straightening of the scope tip are required to allow retrieval. Additional larger dilating balloons can subsequently be used, but the degree of luminal enlargement in a single session remains a matter of common sense and is contingent on the size of the initial

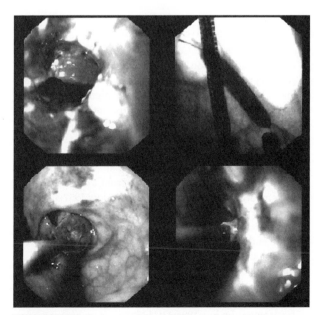

FIGURE 107–3. Impacted Asacol® (Procter & Gamble Pharmaceuticals, Cincinnati, Ohio) tablet in ileocolonic stricture in patient with acute small-bowel obstruction. Treatment consisted of disimpaction and balloon dilation.

stenosis, presence and degree of active ulceration, and patient discomfort with initial dilation. As such, the ultimate goal is to dilate with a 15- to 18-mm balloon followed by complete endoscopic inspection of more proximal bowel. This goal sometimes requires two or three dilating sessions separated by a several-day interval, if the obstruction is acute, or a several-week interval, if it is chronic.

In addition to balloon dilation, three additional endoscopic methods of treating Crohn's stenoses have been described. The first, described by Rolny (1993), includes multiple radial cuts in short strictures, using either a contact-tip laser or electrocautery, a technique previously applied to "defiant" lower esophageal rings. Caution should be used regarding application of this technique, because, in contrast to Schatzki rings, most Crohn's strictures are associated with active and transmural inflammation.

The second method includes circumferential (four-quadrant) corticosteroid injections, using a sclerotherapy needle (Figure 107–4). Applied to refractory keloids or esophageal reflux stenoses, this procedure usually entails injection of 40 to 180 mg of triamcinolone either concomitantly or in lieu of dilation (Ramboer et al). This method is used in patients who develop recurrent obstructive symptoms rapidly or in those individuals who are intolerant of or refuse oral corticosteroids.

The final approach, reported by Matsuhashi and colleagues (1997), includes placement of a self-expandable metallic stent following dilation. This has been used infrequently; its use is discouraged unless the patient is a prohibitive operative risk or placement is done under an investigational protocol.

TABLE 107–4 Summary of Reports of Balloon Dilation for Anastomotic and Ileocolonic or Gastroduodenal Stenoses

Author	Year	Number of Patients	Successful Dilation	Successful Treatment	Complications (%)	Follow-up (mo)
Couckayt et al	1995	55	70/78	34/55 (62%)	11	12
Ramboer et al*	1995	13	11	11/13 (85%)	0	7
Rolny	1993	27	27	18/27 (66%)	15	7–38
Linares et al	1988	33	33	17/33 (51%)	NS	NS
Matsuhashi et al †	1997	2	2	2/2 (100%)	0	1–5

*Includes radial cautery incisions; †includes expandable stent placement; NS = not specified.

Results

Tables 107–4 summarizes some of the experience to date using balloon dilation for anastomotic and ileocolonic or gastroduodenal stenoses, respectively. One thing is clear upon literature review: studies have been sparse and there have been multiple publications from the same groups using an expanding database. For example, the Leuven group (Couckayt et al, 1995) described dilation of 27 patients with anastomotic ileocolic strictures. They later updated their experience to 55 patients with 59 anastomotic stenoses, with technically successful dilation in 70 percent of the 55 patients, although 6 patients sustained contained (n = 4) or free (n = 2) perforations, the latter 2 requiring surgery. Of the 55 patients, 34 (62%) were free of obstructive symptoms after one (n = 20), two (n = 13), or three (n = 1) dilations. Rolney (1993) reported treatment of 27 patients with Crohn's disease with anastomotic strictures, of whom two developed bleeding and two developed acute perforations related to concomitant radial electrocautery incisions.*

In contrast, Linares and colleagues (1988) reported their experience of dilating 33 anorectal strictures in patients with Crohn's disease using a variety of techniques. Approximately one-half of these patients experienced short- or long-term relief. Comparable results have been shown using balloon dilation of gastroduodenal stenoses in Crohn's disease, although series have been small and the need for repeated dilation over time variable.

What to do after the balloon has been inflated has been a contentious issue. As one is dealing with a local inflammatory and fibrotic process in the setting of immune and cytokine activation, it would appear logical to treat this process much as one would treat acid peptic stenoses, with histamine[2] (H_2) blockers or proton pump inhibitors in conjunction with medications to eradicate *Helicobacter pylori*, if applicable, following dilation of an obstructed pylorus. As such, use of topical 5-ASA products, systemic corticosteroids, or immunosuppressives all appear reasonable. To date, a single study has addressed this issue (Raedler et al, 1997). In that series, 30 patients with high-grade stenoses of less than 4 cm (rectosigmoid, n = 8, ileocecal, n = 22) were randomized to receive a combination of budesonide 9 mg/d plus azathioprine 100 mg/d or

placebo after dilation and prospectively followed for 1 year. At that time, 53 percent of the placebo group and only 20 percent of the patients treated with combination therapy (p = .021) developed stenosis recurrence.

Conclusion

Balloon dilation of Crohn's strictures, particularly anastomotic ones, appears reasonable in patients with persistent or rapidly recurring obstructive symptoms despite good medical therapy. The approach should be used prior to additional surgical intervention in most patients unless there is an acute obstruction with potentially compromised bowel, uncertainty about concomitant malignancy, or an associated fistula within the stenosis. Although yet to be proven, concomitant injection of a long-acting corticosteroid should be considered in patients intolerant of or unwilling to take oral corticosteroids, those who develop an anastomotic stricture within 6 months of surgical resection, or those patients who rapidly restenose following a technically successful balloon dilation. Finally, radial electrocautery is contraindicated in these patients, and use of expandable prostheses clearly is investigational.

References

Couckayt H, Gevers AM, Coremans G, et al. Efficacy and safety of hydrostatic balloon dilation of ileocolonic Crohn's strictures: a prospective long-term analysis. Gut 1995;36:577–80.

Gumaste V, Sachar DB, Greenstein AJ. Benign and malignant colorectal strictures in ulcerative colitis. Gut 1992;33:938–41.

Linares L, Moreira LF, Andrews H, et al. Natural history and treatment of anorectal strictures complicating Crohn's disease. Br J Surg 1988;75:653–5.

Matsuhashi N, Nakajima A, Suzuki A, et al. Nonsurgical strictureplasty for intestinal strictures in Crohn's disease: preliminary report of two cases. Gastrointest Endosc 1997;45:176–8.

Raedler A, Peters I, Schreiber S. Treatment with azathioprine and budesonide prevents recurrence of ileocolonic stenosis after endoscopic dilatation in Crohn's disease. Gastroenterology 1997;112:A1067.

Ramboer C, Verhamme M, Dhondt E, et al. Endoscopic treatment of stenosis in recurrent Crohn's disease with balloon dilation combined with local corticosteroid injection. Gastrointest Endosc 1995;42:252–5.

Rolny P. Anastomotic strictures in Crohn's disease: a new field for therapeutic endoscopy. Gastrointest Endosc 1993;39:862–4.

* Editor's Note: Success rate is greatest for anastomatic strictures dilated over 7 years after surgery. (TMB)

Supplemental Reading

Matsui T, Hatakeyama S, Ikeda K, et al. Long-term outcome of endoscopic balloon dilation in obstructive gastroduodenal Crohn's disease. Endoscopy 1997;29:640–5.

Ouzner G, Fazio VW, Lavery IC, et al. How safe is strictureplasty in the management of Crohn's disease? Am J Surg 1996; 171:57–60.

Schreiber S, Nikolaus S, Raedler A, Taber B. Stricture formation in Crohn's disease. Res Clin Forum 1998;20:87–100.

American Society for Gastrointestinal Endoscopy. The role of colonoscopy in the management of patients with inflammatory bowel disease. Gastrointest Endosc 1998;48:689–90.

CHAPTER 108

RECTOVAGINAL FISTULAE

TRACY L. HULL, MD, FACS

Women with Crohn's disease have about a 3 to 5 percent incidence of developing a rectovaginal fistula. This problem can be devestating for some women, and it is difficult to eradicate. Most are true anovaginal fistulae, as they arise from the anal canal and fistulize into the vagina, perineal body, or labia. However, some are true rectovaginal fistulae from proximal disease, such as ileal disease, penetrating the upper vagina. This chapter discusses only true anovaginal fistulae, referring to them as rectovaginal fistulae (RVF), since this is the conventional misnomer.

When a woman presents with complaints consistent with RVF, a thorough history should be done. Precise symptoms need to be clarified; they can range from infrequent gas per vagina to stool running down her leg. Additionally, bowel symptomatology, comorbid conditions, associated Crohn's disease, obstetric history (delivery method, use of forceps, episiotomy, or tearing), and problems with fecal incontinence need to be defined. For instance, some women do not find their fistula symptoms distressing and they do not wish to undergo aggressive treatment, whereas other women "cannot live with the problem."

The location of the fistula is determined by physical examination. A high fistula is more difficult to treat than a low fistula. Associated anal disease, palpable induration, rectal disease, and sphincter integrity are specifically noted. If the examination is too painful for the patient to endure, examination under anesthesia may be necessary to determine the extent of disease. Painful examination may signal sepsis in the region, and drainage with a seton or mushroom catheter may be needed. (See Chapter 106)

If a patient has classic RVF symptoms, but the internal opening cannot be found, a tampon can be placed in the vagina and the patient given methelene blue per rectum. If a fistula is present, the tampon will be stained in less than 15 minutes.

If the patient has not had a full bowel evaluation in recent months, a small-bowel series and barium enema or colonoscopy can be used to define additional disease that may affect treatment approaches. If preoperative incontinence is found by history, or an anterior anal muscle weakness is noted on physical examination, manometry is strongly recommended. Incontinence that is attributable to destroyed sphincter muscles secondary to Crohn's disease may prompt different treatment goals than incontinence and a fistula from an obstetric type injury.

After all of the information has been gathered, realistic goals of surgery must be discussed. For instance, it would be unrealistic to discuss a curative surgical repair in a woman with severe colorectal disease, but a seton may palliate symptoms and delay an ileostomy for a long period. In treatment planning, the physician weighs the patient's symptoms and treatment goals against her general condition and results of the physical examination.

Medical Treatment and Drainage

All patients found to have rectovaginal fistulae need to have any sepsis drained as the first line of any treatment option. This can be done with a loosely tied flexible seton or a mushroom catheter. For patients with mild-to-moderate symptoms, medical treatment can be considered. These are usually patients with a small fistula. Antibiotics such as ciprofloxacin (500 mg bid) and metronidazole (250–500 mg tid) work well, particularly for women with suppuration or pain despite seton drainage. In some cases, antibiotic therapy decreases symptoms from associated Crohn's disease elsewhere and makes further treatment of the RVF unneeded. At times, extended courses of antibiotic therapy (several months) are given.

Steroids do not usually help this problem. If there are symptoms from associated disease elsewhere in the gastrointestinal tract, steroids may reduce those symptoms and make the fistula symptoms seem less severe, thus delaying further treatment.

Imuran® (Glaxo Wellcome, Research Triangle Park, North Carolina) has been reported to cause closure of some fistulae and should be considered, especially for women who have few other options. However, for many patients who have experienced difficulty while taking Imuran, with no relief of symptoms, earlier surgical intervention may have been beneficial. It has been this author's experience that the postsurgical rate of infection was seemingly higher in patients concurrently taking Imuran. Therefore, it is preferable that Imuran therapy be

---

* Editor's Note: Imuran is prescribed postsurgically for some patients by physicians who believe that it may provide a degree of prophylaxis. (TMB)

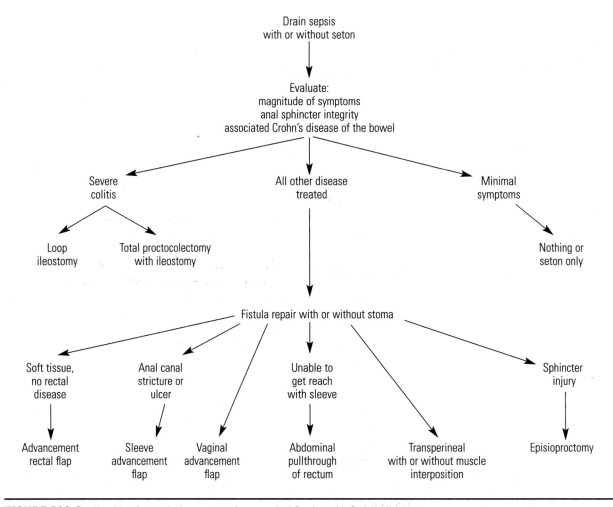

FIGURE 108–1. Algorithm for surgical treatment of rectovaginal fistulae with Crohn's disease.

discontinued at least 4 weeks prior to planned surgery for fistula closure.*

Perhaps, infliximab will be the optimal medical therapy for some of these women, but the only published report did not include any women with rectovaginal fistulae. When infliximab is prescribed at the Cleveland Clinic, the patient is given the first dose of medication, and then the seton is removed prior to the second dose. It remains to be seen if this has long-term healing benefit. Perhaps other biologic treatments will be more effective and make surgical intervention obsolete.†

Surgical Management

Fecal Diversion

Fecal diversion is considered in women who have persistent sepsis despite seton drainage. A loop ileostomy usually is done, particularly if there is any colonic involvement. Ileostomy alone does not allow the fistula to

"heal." The symptoms may decrease, but when the stoma is closed, the fistula recurs. Therefore, the stoma must be combined with other treatment if fistula healing is the goal. Additionally, ileostomy can be combined with bowel resection (ie, terminal ileal resection) and fistula repair, if needed. When doing a fistula repair, the author prefers to use a stoma for repeat surgery, when the repair did not go well technically, for complicated repairs, or for a sleeve or transabdominal repair. In some women who need proctocolectomy, a laparoscopic loop ileostomy prior to colon removal gives them the opportunity to experience a stoma without the emotional finality of it. It also allows inflammation to decrease in the perineum, which may decrease the chance of an unhealed perineal wound.

Proctectomy

At RVF presentation, some women have severe proctocolitis along with anal disease. They have few options; proctocolectomy may be the only choice. Perineal wound healing may be delayed in this group of patients. It may be necessary to consider a staged operation that removes the rectum after a period of fecal diversion, either

---

† Editor's Note: The role of immunomodulators and infliximab is evolving with time and experience. (TMB)

TABLE 108–1. Comparisons of Treatments for Rectovaginal Fistulae with Crohn's Disease

Procedure	Advantages and Indications	Disadvantages and Contraindications
Medical treatment with or without drainage	Aggressive surgery not needed Drainage will decrease pain	Probably does not cure fistula
Fecal diversion	Allows resection of diseased bowel at the same time; allows patient to adjust to stoma	Does not cure fistula
Proctectomy	Done with severe colonic and anorectal disease	Permanent stoma May have problems with perineal wound healing
Advancement rectal flap	Can be done with mild-to-moderate rectal disease Stoma not mandatory Does not burn bridges	Do not do with severe anorectal disease, anal stricture, anal sepsis
Transvaginal advancement flap	Can do with anal stricture Allows nondiseased tissue to be used Does not burn bridges or stretch sphincter muscles	Do not do with sepsis
Rectal sleeve advancement flap (transanal or transabdominal)	Can be done with anal canal ulceration and anal canal stricture Must have near-normal rectum	Major procedure Increases sphincter stretch If reach is not sufficient with the transanal approach, transabdominal approach is used Do not do with perianal sepsis Avoid with fecal incontinence
Episioproctomy	Anterior sphincter weakness with the fistula or fecal incontinence as a result of a sphincter problem Stoma not mandatory	Do not do with severe anorectal disease, high fistula, sepsis Divides the anal sphincters, which could increase problems with incontinence if healing does not occur
Fibrin glue	Does not burn bridges Minor procedure Fistula tract must be greater than 1 cm long	Long-term success is unknown Must drain all sepsis before using

through an initial loop ileostomy or a subtotal colectomy with ileostomy and mucous fistula.

Surgical Fistula Closure

Women who qualify for surgical closure of fistulae must have all sepsis drained, and anorectal disease must be relatively quiescent. There is debate over the extent to which colonic and small-bowel disease interfere with fistula closure. Intuitively, it seems appropriate to resect severe small-bowel disease and have all other Crohn's disease under good medical control before embarking on surgical RVF closure. Figure 108–1 shows an algorithm for treating RVF. Table 108–1 provides a comparison of treatment procedures.

FLAP REPAIR

Flap repair is the most common type of repair and, of these, the *advancement rectal flap* is the most popular. Approaching the problem from the anorectum seems logical, as it represents a shunt between the high-pressure anorectum (25 to 85 cm H_2O) and the low-pressure vagina (atmospheric). It requires that there be minimal or no rectal disease (some mild granularity is acceptable, but ulceration is a contraindication), no anal stricture, and a pliable anal canal and rectum. The patient should undergo a full bowel cleansing and receive intravenous antibiotics preoperatively and postoperatively. After

adequate regional or general anesthesia, the patient is placed in the prone position. A semicircular incision is made that encompasses the anal side of the fistula, and a flap is raised. The flap consists of the mucosa, submucosa, and a few fibers of the internal anal sphincter. The flap is mobilized for at least 4 cm proximal to the fistula. The fistula is cored out and closed in layers, leaving the vaginal side open for drainage. The distal flap is trimmed and then advanced down and sewn in place. An advantage of this procedure is that it divides no sphincter muscle. Experience has been that 60 percent of women were healed intially after this repair.

Transvaginal advancement flaps are preferred by some. Proponents believe that this procedure avoids manipulation of diseased rectal tissue. Most incorporate raising the flap in a manner similar to the above-described technique for the transanal approach. The anal opening is closed and the levator muscles are approximated. The flap is trimmed and closed in a manner similar to the transanal approach. Some surgeons who do this type of repair believe that the interposing of the levator muslces between the rectal wall and the vaginal mucosa is the key to success with this procedure.

The *rectal sleeve advancement* is probably the most complicated of the flap repairs. This repair is indicated for certain women with anal canal ulceration or associated fistula in ano, but without rectal disease. Again, after a full bowel preparation and intravenous antibiotics, the patient receives adequate general anesthesia and is placed in the prone position. The mucosa is stripped from the anal canal. Next, the full thickness of rectum is mobilized from the transanal approach cephalad to allow the rectal cuff to reach the dentate line with minimal tension. If the cuff of rectum will not reach, a transabdominal approach is needed. The fistula is handled as described for the advancement rectal flap. The cuff of rectum is sewn to the dentate line after the distal edge has been trimmed. Usually, this type of repair is done in conjunction with a stoma. Typically, it also is done in cases of failed previous repair of RVF. Healing has been achieved in 66 percent of cases with this approach.

TRANSPERINEAL REPAIR

When the sphincter muscles have a defect, with or without fecal incontinence, a transperineal repair should be considered. This repair is termed an episioproctomy and is similar to a fourth degree obstetric injury. The anal canal must be soft and pliable for success with this repair. A probe is passed through the fistula, and all tissue above the probe is divided. Then the sphincter ends are dissected free and suture overlapped to repair the sphincter defect and at the same time close the fistula. The rectal mucosa, perineal skin, and vaginal mucosa are closed. This repair apparently produces excellent results.

Some practitioners prefer a different transperineal repair that is approached by dividing the perineal body transversely and dissecting out both internal openings and closing them. Then muscle, usually levator (but can be gracilis if the levators are not acceptable), is mobilized and interposed between the anorectal wall and the vaginal wall. Authors who prefer this approach feel it eliminates dissecting in the diseased anorectum; however, the internal opening must still be addressed in the anus, which may have significant disease.

TRANSABDOMINAL REPAIR

In select cases, the rectum cannot be mobilized transanally. Sometimes, this can be anticipated from the preoperative examination of the anal area, and at other times the rectal sleeve advancement flap simply will not reach during that operation. (Therefore, all patients undergoing a sleeve are told of the possibility of needing a transabdominal approach.) In these situations, an abdominal incision is made, and the rectum is mobilized from the abdominal approach and advanced down and out the anus. It can be trimmed and sewn to the dentate line immediately or pulled through the anus for about 10 cm and left extending from the anus for about a week. After 5 to 7 days, the rectal end is amputated and sewn to the dentate line. Sometimes, the delayed closure technique is preferable, because it gives the bowel a chance to adhere to the fistula and seal over the repair before sutures are placed.

Fibrin Glue

Fibrin glue has been used successfully to close some fistulae in patients with Crohn's disease. For optimal results when using fibrin glue, the fistula should have a tract longer than 1 cm; therefore, RVF may be a poor candidate. This treatment in a few women with a long fistula tract that exited from the labia or perineal body achieved about a 45 percent closure rate. It can be considered, because it does not require major surgery and does not rule out any procedure that might be necessary for future repairs.

Supplemental Reading

Cintron JR, Park JJ, Orsay CP, et al. Repair of fistulas-in-ano using autologous fibrin tissue adhesive. Dis Colon Rectum 1999;42:607–13.

Hull TL, Fazio VW. Rectovaginal fistula in Crohn's disease. In: Phillips RKS, Lunniss PJ, eds. Anal fistula. London: Chapman and Hall, 1996:143–62.

Hull TL, Fazio VW. Surgical approaches to low anovaginal fistula in Crohn's disease. Am J Surg 1997;173:95–8.

Present DH, Rutgeerts P, Targan S, et al. Infliximab for treatment of fistulas in patients with Crohn's disease. N Engl J Med 1999;340:1398–405.

Sher ME, Bauer JJ, Gelerent I. Surgical repair of rectovaginal fistulas in patients with Crohn's disease: transvaginal approach. Dis Colon Rectum 1991;34:641–8.

CHAPTER 109

Fate of Excluded Bowel

BRET A. LASHNER, MD

Bypass surgery for Crohn's disease is a traditional and time-honored method of treatment. The jejunum, ileum, or colon can be excluded, either temporarily or permanently, depending on the indication. In general, the activity of the Crohn's disease decreases in the excluded bowel. The fate of the loop excluded from the digestive stream is different for each of these segments of bowel. Prominent complications are as follows: from a bypassed duodenum, marginal ulceration and strictured anastomose; from a bypassed jejunum or ileum, possible small bowel malignancy; and from a bypassed colon, diversion colitis.

Duodenum

Duodenal Crohn's disease is rare, occurring in less than 2 percent of patients with Crohn's disease. Most of those can be adequately treated medically with anti-inflammatory agents and proton pump inhibitors. Rarely, though, a patient needs surgery for obstructive symptoms characterized by early satiety, upper abdominal pain, vomiting, and weight loss. For strictures in the first and second portion of the duodenum, a gastrojejunostomy with vagotomy is therapeutic, and for strictures in the third and fourth portions of the duodenum, a duodenojejunostomy without vagotomy provides adequate drainage. Bypass surgery for duodenal Crohn's disease is becoming less necessary as surgeons are acquiring better experience with strictureplasties of the duodenum. Strictureplasties in the bowel, including the duodenum, are named after the corresponding pyloroplasty: Heineke-Mikulicz procedure for short strictures, Finney procedure for long strictures, and Jaboulay procedure for short strictures in the proximal duodenum. The Jaboulay procedure creates a "double pylorus" and a bypassed, nonexcluded loop.

The most common complications of creating a gastroenterostomy are ulceration and stricture at the gastrojejunostomy site, usually at or distal to the anastomosis. This marginal ulceration could be attributable to a hypersecretory state. Patients who have a concomitant small-bowel resection usually develop hypergastrinemia and are prone to peptic ulcer disease. A vagotomy and the use of proton pump inhibitors minimize that risk. A highly selective vagotomy rather than a truncal vagotomy could minimize the risk of both marginal ulceration and postoperative diarrhea. Reoperation following gastro-

jejunostomy for Crohn's disease is common. Approximately 25 percent of patients need reoperation by 5 years, and a majority need a second surgery by 15 years.

Jejunum and Ileum

When an inflammatory mass is so situated as to make it impossible to remove safely, a bypass of the mass is sometimes the best and most expeditious surgical approach. Otherwise, resection is the preferred surgery for an inflammatory mass. However, resection was not always the preferred strategy. Bypass surgeries were commonly done for both inflammatory and stricturing Crohn's disease since it was the simplest procedure to relieve symptoms. However, publication of an article in 1978 describing seven cases of small-bowel cancer in the excluded loop of patients with Crohn's disease had a major impact even though the cancer risk is probably the same in nonexcluded strictures. Currently, bypass surgery is only rarely done, and only in patients with a high risk of mortality from surgery. Small-bowel cancer in an excluded loop rarely has been reported, with only 22 cases reported as of 1989. The pathogenesis of cancer in Crohn's disease has not been elucidated fully, but it has been theorized that the presence of chronically active disease fosters genetic changes responsible for the malignancy.

Not all excluded ileal loops present problems to the patient. The most famous patient with an excluded loop because of Crohn's disease was President Dwight D. Eisenhower, whose medical history has been published in great detail. President Eisenhower was diagnosed with Crohn's disease of the terminal ileum in May 1956, by small bowel radiography, at the age of 66 years, near the end of his first term as president. Approximately 1 month later, he presented with abdominal pain and vomiting and was found to have complete small-bowel obstruction. On June 9, 1956, at 2:20 am, President Eisenhower was taken to surgery; dense adhesions were noted from an appendectomy 33 years earlier, but the obstruction was attributed to "chronic, dry type of regional enteritis." There was mesenteric thickening, lymph node enlargement, and proximal small bowel dilatation. An ileotransverse colostomy was fashioned, about 12 to 15 cm proximal to the region of Crohn's disease. He had an uneventful recovery, won a second term in office, and had small-bowel radiography in 1958, 1960, 1961, 1963, and 1965, all of which showed barium passing through the bypass and the excluded loop with no visible abnormal pathology. In 1966, he underwent cholecystectomy, but the bypassed loop could not be inspected visually because of dense adhesions. In 1967, he began to have repeated attacks of intestinal obstruction, which resolved with conservative management. In February 1969, another bout of small-bowel obstruction occurred, which did not resolve with a Cantor tube. At surgery, a loop of small bowel 18 inches proximal to the bypass was adherent to the abdominal wall, causing the obstruction. The excluded loop showed "burned out ileitis." Approximately 1 month later, on March 29, 1969, President Eisenhower died of cardiac complications following surgery. At postmortem examination, the excluded loop showed changes of quiescent Crohn's disease with "thick-walled, fibrotic, burned-out, dry type of chronic ileitis which had remained essentially unchanged since the creation of the ileotransverse colostomy 13 years previously." There was no cancer seen. Such was the fate of President Eisenhower's excluded loop. The disease had beome inactive in the excluded loop.

It is well known that exclusion from the fecal stream of a diseased segment of bowel with bypass surgery, or the less effective method of bowel rest with parenteral nutrition, is likely to induce remission in Crohn's disease. Still, there are patients who do not respond to bypass surgery and suffer typical complications of Crohn's disease, such as perforation and sepsis. Unfortunately, excluded segments only rarely can be brought back into the fecal stream. Recurrence following reanastomosis (with the need for additional surgery) is exceedingly high. Recurrence also is high following refeeding after an extended period of parenteral nutrition. Because of the complications of the bypassed loop, such as perforation, sepsis, and cancer, and the high risk of recurrence following reanastomosis, resection is preferred to bypass for Crohn's disease.

The jejunoileal bypass procedure for morbid obesity may theoretically serve as a model for understanding some complications of bypass surgery for Crohn's disease. In the jejunoileal bypass, 40 cm of jejunum from the ligament of Treitz is anastomosed to the sigmoid colon to create fat malabsorption from a short-bowel syndrome. The bypassed loop can develop intussusception, volvulus, fascial hernias, or bacterial overgrowth with dilatation, in the excluded-loop syndrome. A more curious and severe complication is hepatic failure from nonalcoholic steatohepatitis, the so-called NASH syndrome. Fatty infiltration of the liver, a lymphocytic infiltration, bridging necrosis, and fibrosis with cirrhosis are characteristic findings of the natural history of NASH. A poor prognosis is related to ballooning degeneration, Mallory hyaline, and perisinusoidal fibrosis. This sequence is not common in patients with Crohn's disease, perhaps because bypasses rarely are done.

The fecal stream is trophic for small-bowel mucosa. Therefore, segments excluded from the fecal stream will become atrophic and prone to develop perforation and bleeding. If short-bowel syndrome is induced with the creation of the excluded loop, hormones that facilitate the adaptive process in the in-stream bowel, such as glucagon, epidermal growth factor, prostaglandins, and growth hormone, could delay the atrophic process in the excluded bowel. There have been interesting reports of patients with short-bowel syndrome whose adaptation process was enhanced with the combination of growth hormone, glutamine (a preferred enterocyte fuel source), a high-carbohydrate diet, and fiber for 3 to 4 weeks. Although these results could not be repeated in a separate randomized clinical trial, it might be reasonable to try such therapy, at least growth hormone and glutamine, for bypassed Crohn's disease patients, to prevent atrophy when a temporary bypass procedure is being done.[*]

Colon

Diverted colonic segments in Crohn's disease usually occur following subtotal colectomy, in preparation for ileorectal anastomosis, or following diversion to allow perianal disease to heal. The fecal stream delivers important nutrients to colonocytes, and the absence of these nutrients can lead to diversion colitis in a minority of these patients. In vitro, colonocytes preferentially metabolize short-chain fatty acids over glucose or ketone bodies. Short-chain fatty acids (ie, butyrate, propronate, and acetate) are produced by the metabolism of undigested carbohydrates by colonic bacteria. The symptoms and signs of diversion colitis are similar to those of ulcerative colitis: hematochezia, urgency, and continuous superficial ulcerations with friability, and possibly an exudate throughout the diverted segment. Replacement of short-chain fatty acids via an enema preparation has been therapeutic for patients with diversion colitis. The odoriferous enema, which can be made by most compounding pharmacies, consists of a 100 mM solution of butyrate or a 100-mM combination of butyrate, propionate, and acetate that is made isosmolar with a neutral pH by the addition of sodium hydroxide and sodium chloride. Typically, one 60-mL enema is instilled twice daily. Once the colonic segment is returned to the fecal stream, the short-chain fatty acid enemas no longer are necessary.

When a subtotal colectomy is done in preparation for an ileorectal anastomosis, surgeons wait approximately 3 to 6 months for the acute inflammatory process to subside. Endoscopic examination of the excluded rectal

---

[*] Editor's Note: This assumes that the effect of glutamine is systemic rather than luminally directed, as with short-chain fatty acids in the colon. Growth hormone and a high-protein diet reportedly led to improvement in active CD as compared to controls (N Engl J Med 2000). (TMB)

pouch is done to remove scybala or a mucus plug for the patient's comfort and for evaluating for diversion colitis, Crohn's colitis, or carcinoma. For diversions to treat perianal fistulae, the interval to reanastomosis may be longer than 6 to 12 months to allow immunosuppressive therapy to reach maximal therapeutic efficacy, in an effort to minimize the chance of recurrence. Whether Remicade® (Centocor Inc., Malvern, Pennsylvania) (anti-tumor necrosis factor) infusions increase the chance of successful reanastomosis remains to be determined. Currently, successful reconnection is the exception.

Rarely, a blowhole colostomy is done for patients with toxic megacolon who are too ill to have a subtotal colectomy.[*] In such a procedure, an ileostomy is placed and the colostomy is made (often in the transverse colon or cecum) to decompress a dilatated colon. In patients with ulcerative colitis who have a blowhole colostomy, the fate of the excluded colon is tenuous; the colostomy should not be closed. Such patients would be at high risk for recurrence of megacolon and require total proctocolectomy (possibly with an ileal pouch-anal anastomosis) when their medical condition permits. Interestingly, the colon may be salvaged in patients with toxic megacolon due to antibiotic-associated colitis if vancomycin is instilled through the blowhole colostomy.

Supplemental Reading

Cook SI, Sellin JH. Short-chain fatty acids in health and disease. Aliment Pharmacol Ther 1998;12:499–507.

Greenstein AJ, Sachar D, Pucillo A, et al. Cancer in Crohn's disease after diversionary surgery: a report of seven carcinomas occurring in occluded bowel. Am J Surg 1978;135:86–90.

Haas BA, Fox TA, Szilagy EJ. Endoscopic examination of the colon and rectum distal to a colostomy. Am J Gastroenterol 1990;85:850–4.

Harig JM, Soergel KH, Komorowski RA, Wood CM. Treatment of diversion colitis with short-chain fatty acid irrigation. N Engl J Med 1989;320:23–8.

Hughes CW, Baugh JH, Mologne LA, Heaton LD. A review of the late General Eisenhower's operations: epilog to a footnote to history. Ann Surg 1971;173:793–9.

Scolapio JS, Camilleri M, Fleming CR, et al. Effect of growth hormone, glutamine, and diet on adaptation in short-bowel syndrome: a randomized, controlled study. Gastroenterology 1997;113:1074–81.

Senay E, Sachar DB, Keohane M, Greenstein AJ. Small bowel carcinoma in Crohn's disease: distinguishing features and risk factors. Cancer 1989;63:360–3.

Vanderhoof JA, Langnas AN. Short-bowel syndrome in children and adults. Gastroenterology 1997;113:1767–78.

Wolff BG, Nyam CNK. Bypass procedures. In: Michelassi F, Milsom JW, eds. Operative strategies in inflammatory bowel disease. New York: Springer, 1999:268–78.

Worsey MJ, Hull T, Ryland L, Fazio V. Strictureplasty is an effective option in the operative management of duodenal Crohn's disease. Dis Colon Rectum 1999;42:596–600.

---

[*] Editor's Note: Blowhole colostomies were described by Dr Turnbull at The Cleveland Clinic but, currently, are not commonly employed. (TMB)

CHAPTER 110

INFLAMMATORY BOWEL DISEASE GENETICS

STEVEN R. BRANT, MD, AND JUDY H. CHO, MD

Is Inflammatory Bowel Disease Genetic?

One of the difficulties for patients accepting their diagnosis of inflammatory bowel disease (IBD) is that there is no specific etiology. Both genetic and environmental factors have been implicated. Within the environment of Western industrial countries, the greatest risk for developing IBD is genetic.

Several studies have compared the risk of developing IBD in relatives of patients with IBD compared to relatives of controls. Overall, 15 to 20 percent of patients have a family history of IBD. Inflammatory bowel disease is found 5 to 12 times more frequently in relatives of people who have Crohn's disease (CD) or ulcerative colitis (UC) than in relatives of normal controls. Family IBD history for patients with CD most often has been CD, and for patients with UC most often has been UC. However, the cross disease association may be considerable. For example, in the Johns Hopkins series of 554 consecutive patients with CD, a family history of UC was present in 5 percent and a family history of CD in 17 percent. A Danish study found that first-degree relatives of people with UC have an 8 times greater risk than that of the general population of developing UC and 1.72 times greater risk of developing CD. Comparative figures for CD–CD and CD–UC in the Danish population were 10.00 and 3.85, respectively.

That familial aggregation is primarily genetic rather than from a shared environmental etiology, such as an infectious agent, is suggested by a lack of increased risk to spouses, and the observed aggregation of IBD occurring among relatives raised separately. The most rigorous epidemiologic evidence for a genetic etiology of IBD, especially CD, comes from carefully controlled studies of twins. In the Swedish twin registry, proband pairwise concordance was 58.3 percent for CD in identical (monozygotic) twins and 3.9 percent in fraternal (dizygotic) twins. Dizygotic twin concordance is not much different from that in nontwin siblings. This suggests that genetic factors predominate over a more similar environment shared among fraternal twins than among nontwin siblings. The proband pairwise concordance for UC in monozygotic twins was 6 percent as compared to 0 percent for dizygotic twins, indicating a more significant genetic component for CD compared to UC and correlating with more extensive IBD family history observed for CD than for UC probands in most studies. However, the twin data also show that IBD cannot be completely explained by genetics. The lack of complete concordance in monozygotic twins may be attributable to the unaffected twin not being exposed to an environmental trigger or risk factor or, alternatively, the presence of a protective environmental effect. It is not known whether sporadic, nonfamilial cases of IBD are genetic. However, especially for CD, the twin data suggest that the majority of cases result from some genetic influence. It is extremely rare to encounter monozygotic twins in whom one has CD and the other UC, suggesting that the net genetic susceptibility factors causing CD and UC are different.

Additional evidence that IBD is genetic is that there is consistently elevated risk in Ashkenazi Jews (2 to 9 times) in comparison with their non-Jewish neighbors, irrespective of diet and religious observance. Inflammatory bowel disease is more common in some diseases that are solely of genetic etiology, notably Turner's syndrome, pachydermoperiostosis, Hermansky-Pudlak syndrome, and glycogen storage disease IB (Table 110–1). One of these genetic syndromes noted in a patient with gastrointestinal symptoms should raise suspicion for IBD. Inflammatory bowel disease also is more common in patients with ankylosing spondylitis, psoriasis, and multiple sclerosis, multifactorial diseases for which, as for IBD, there is strong evidence for genetic susceptibility. Inflammatory bowel disease, primarily UC, coexisting with primary sclerosing cholangitis (PSC) is so common (50 to 70%) that patients with PSC should always be evaluated for IBD. The colitis may be asymptomatic, and significant dysplasia and colon cancers have been found in asymptomatic patients with PSC.

Finally, as noted, IBD cannot be completely explained by genetics. There is an over 10-fold less frequent occurrence of IBD in non-Western industrialized nations. The potential tremendous effect of environment in Western industrial nations is demonstrated by the observation that the rate of UC in West Indians living in England is similar to that of the ancestral Caucasian population and is believed to be far greater than that in the Caribbean. Similarly, the prevalence of IBD in Ashkenazi Jews has been much greater in the United States and Western

TABLE 110–1. Diseases Associated with Inflammatory Bowel Disease

Disease	Association with IBD	Recent Genetic Progress
Genetic diseases		
Turner's syndrome	Significant association with CD and UC, especially with abnormal rather than absent X chromosome	Suggestive genetic linkage in IBD on X chromosome reported
Pachydermoperiostosis	Familial association with CD	Possible variant of psoriatic distal interphalangeal arthritis
Hermansky-Pudlak syndrome (HPS)	Atypical granulomatous colitis	HPS gene an organelle transmembrane protein
Glycogen storage disease, IB	Neutrophil-monocyte dysfunction associated with CD phenotype	Genetic linkage on chromosome 11q23
Autoimmune-associated diseases*		
Ankylosing spondylitis (AS)	Axial spondyloarthropathy, male predominance; higher prevalence in IBD	IBD associated AS associated with HLA-B*27 and DRB1*0101
Psoriasis	Population prevalence 2%; higher psoriasis prevalence in CD (10%)	Genetic linkage in MHC region; psoriasis locus found in same region of chromosome 16 as CD locus *IBD1*
Multiple sclerosis (MS)	IBD prevalence 4% among patients with MS. Common clustering of genetic linkage reported between MS and IBD.	TNF and TNFR implicated in animal models of MS and IBD; associations with HLA DR15, DR4, and DQ6 reported

*For primary sclerosing cholangitis, the most common autoimmune disease associated with IBD, see the relevant chapter.
HLA = human leukocyte antigen; TNF = tumor necrosis factor; MHC = ?

Europe than in Israel. As nations increase their westernization, a steady increase first in UC incidence and then in CD incidence is observed. Inflammatory bowel disease was increasing in the United States until the past two decades. The exact environmental inciting effect is unknown, but an attractive theory is that parasitic diseases, common in less industrial nations and more common in the United States prior to the 1970s, may somehow be protective against IBD development. Preliminary evidence suggests that CD may be ameliorated by introduction of parasites. However, some studies have suggested that measles and other infections may trigger IBD; these data will need to be reconciled. Within the environment of Western industrial nations, the only consistently measurable risk factor for CD has been smoking, which appears to be protective for UC. Several other environmental risk factors have been postulated but remain unproven, notably nonsteroidal anti-inflammatory drugs (NSAIDs), birth control pills, and measles.

Defining the Risk in Offspring

Inflammatory bowel disease is a complex genetic disorder with no defined mode of inheritance (ie, dominant versus recessive). The presence of two or more susceptibility genes likely is required for there to be an inherited risk of IBD. The empirical risk of IBD developing in the offspring of a parent with IBD ranges from 0 to 2.5 percent. The difficulty with using the empirical risk is that the risk of developing IBD is cumulative, reaching the median age sometime in the third decade. Most offspring in study populations likely are juveniles. Optimum estimates can be developed only after long-term follow-up of offspring from a large population cohort. Data from two studies that have estimated the lifetime risk to offspring and siblings (assuming a life expectancy of 70 yr) corrected by

age-specific incidence data are summarized in Table 110–2. Note that these studies represent only two specific population sets, and the risk to offspring and siblings found for any study likely is affected by the overall relative geographic incidence.

Genetic Counseling

In practice, patients are counseled with the following information. There are no established guidelines for IBD risk to offspring of affected parents. The lifetime risk to children of a parent with IBD ranges between 5 percent and 10 percent, and half of the risk will be reached during the third decade of life. The risk tends to be higher if the parent has a family history of IBD, developed IBD at an early age, or is of Ashkenazi Jewish ancestry. The risk of IBD to a child of parents who both have IBD, whether or not it is CD or UC, may be as high as 50 percent. The only known study (from New York City) involved 19 couples in which both partners had IBD. Among the 23 children who were 20 years of age or older, 12 (52%) developed IBD, usually CD. There are insufficient data to estimate risks for counseling of patients with IBD not of European (Caucasian) ancestry. The reduced familial disease aggregation in these groups would suggest that the data generated from Caucasians would represent the upper limits of risk unless a non-Caucasian patient already has a family history of IBD.

Sibling Risk

Risks to siblings are similar. When siblings are concerned about developing IBD, they should be counseled accordingly, taking into account their age and subtracting the past years of risk. Guidance also should be given to avoid potential risk factors. Risk to parents because their child developed IBD and risk to second-degree relatives of a

TABLE 110–2. Estimated Lifetime and Empirical IBD Risk to Offspring and Siblings of Patients with IBD

Study	Probands	Percentage of Relatives at Risk (Empirical Risk)		
		Offspring	Siblings	All First Degree
Los Angeles, USA				
Jewish probands with CD	134	7.4 (1.8)	16.8 (8.0)	7.8 (4.5)
Jewish probands with UC	157	7.4 (1.9)	4.6 (2.4)	4.5 (2.6)
Non-Jewish probands with CD	124	0.0 (0.0)	3.0 (7.0)	5.2 (2.7)
Non-Jewish probands with UC	112	11.0 (2.3)	0.9 (0.4)	1.6 (0.9)
Belgium[*]				
Belgian probands with CD	640	10.4 (2.3)	4.9 (3.0)	4.8 (2.8)

[*]Risk to siblings is for CD; all other risks are for all IBD (CD and UC).

proband with IBD are less than the sibling and offspring risk. Currently, there are no genetic markers or tests (such as small bowel permeability, antineutrophil cytoplasmic antibodies [ANCA] or anti-*Saccharomyces cerevisiae* antibodies [ASCA]) for potential identification of relatives at greater risk for developing IBD that are beyond the investigative stages. The implications of a positive ANCA or ASCA test in an asymptomatic relative of a proband with IBD are unknown. It is likely that in the population of asymptomatic relatives, the positive predictive value of these tests is very low; therefore, use of these tests is not indicated in asymptomatic individuals. Thorough evaluation of relatives of patients with IBD is recommended, with greater suspicion if they should develop symptoms that overlap with IBD.

Genetic Implications on Management

In a 1996 study, the mean age at diagnosis in 432 patients with CD without a family history of IBD was 26.7 years, and in 120 patients with CD with a family history of IBD, the mean age at diagnosis was 22.5 years. Patients with CD with a family history of IBD are more likely to have small bowel than colonic disease; complications of perforation, abscess, and fibrostenotic disease; and, perhaps, more extra-intestinal manifestations.

These findings suggest that CD in families is more likely to be severe, to involve complications, and to occur at a younger age than that found in patients without a family history of IBD. The presentation and course of CD in relatives are important considerations. Inflammation may occur at a variety of sites, usually categorized as duodenojejunoileitis; distal ileum; ileum and right colon (ileocolitis); and colon only. Furthermore, there are apparently three distinct types of transmural aggressiveness of the inflammation: inflammatory, fistulizing-perforating, and fibrostenotic-stricturing. After 8 years following diagnosis, the patterns of site and type tend to remain stable for the course of the disease. It should be noted that (1) the occurrence of fistulae in perianal disease is not considered "fistulizing" disease; (2) a fistula upstream of a stricture is believed to result secondarily from the stricture, and, thus, the disease type is classified

as stricturing and not fistulizing; and (3) surgical or medical intervention may prevent fistulae from occurring.

In a series of 60 consecutive families, concordance was noted within two members for site in 86 percent and inflammatory type in 82 percent of families; these variables in one relative with CD tended to predict the disease course in another affected family member. Especially impressive was the finding that a relative of a proband with fistulizing disease had over 100 times the likelihood of also developing fistulizing rather than inflammatory or stricturing disease. Concordance for site as well as for age at onset was greatest among siblings. The concept of concordance for site of disease within two affected relatives also has been confirmed in French and Canadian populations. These predictions have important clinical implications, because more than 50 percent of patients with fistulizing and fibrostenotic disease require surgical intervention by 8 years following diagnosis, whereas less than 20 percent of patients with inflammatory disease require surgical intervention during the same time frame. Most useful is to guard against and anticipate the possibility of perforation in a patient who has a relative with that complication.

There also are important nongenetic associations with disease type: younger age of onset is associated with stricturing disease and small bowel disease, and it is inversely associated with inflammatory disease. Jewish ethnicity, smoking, and NSAID use are important risk factors for fistulizing disease, again including perforating disease.

Potential Gene Markers

At present, no gene abnormality has been unequivocally demonstrated as partly responsible for development of CD or UC. However, recent evidence from several linkage studies and a large collaborative study proves the existence of a CD gene or genes at genetic locus *IBD1* in the pericentromeric region of human chromosome 16. This molecular genetic evidence establishes that a significant proportion of familial CD has an underlying genetic cause. Interestingly, loci for psoriasis, lupus, and the autosomal dominant granulomatous autoimmune disorder, Blau syndrome, also map to pericentromeric chromosome 16. However, *IBD1* can explain only a minor portion of the overall familial CD risk, perhaps more in families with disease occurring before adulthood. Strong but not yet established linkage evidence exists for loci about chromosomes 12 (*IBD2*), 1p, and the major histocompatability locus on chromosome 6p (*IBD3*). Recent data suggest that the *IBD2* locus may be more important for UC genetic risks.

Multiple candidate genes have been studies. Most extensive is the major histocompatibility complex (MHC) class II alleles. Human leukocyte antigen (HLA) DRB1*1502 (DR2) is associated with risk of UC in Japanese and Ashkenazi Jews, but the allele is rare in non-Jewish Europeans with UC. A Crohn's disease–HLA association is less tentative, with strongest evidence coming from HLA DRB3*0301. Several studies have suggested that HLA alleles may explain variations in phenotypic expression of UC. For example, DR2 is more pronounced in Japanese with extensive colitis and DR103 (DRB1*103), with extra-intestinal manifestations. One difficulty with HLA associations is that there are multiple immune-associated genes in the region that are in linkage disequilibrium. Therefore, allelic HLA association may only be a surrogate marker for the actual disease-causing allele on a nearby gene. Within the MHC region are the tumor necrosis factor (TNF) genes TNF-α and TNF-β. Anti-TNF-α antibodies have been effective in treating CD, particularly CD fistulae. Early reports suggest that specific TNF alleles can predict response to the medication, but larger studies are needed, and a recent Japanese study shows strong evidence of an association with TNF-α promoter polymorphisms and CD.

There are provocative but not yet well-replicated associations of several other candidate genes and IBD, notably interleukin (IL)-10, natural resistance-associated macrophage protein (NRAMP)1, IL-1 receptor antagonist, transporter associated with antigen processing (TAP)2, T-cell receptor B, and intracellular adhesion molecule-1 (ICAM-1). Currently, the only clinically established genetic markers are HLA-B27, helpful in establishing coexisting ankylosing spondylitis, and HLA-B8 and DR3 associated with 60 to 80 percent of primary sclerosing cholangitis.

Supplemental Reading

Bayless TM, Tokayer AZ, Polito JM II, et al. Crohn's disease: concordance for site and clinical type in affected family members: potential hereditary influences. Gastroenterology 1996;111:573–9.

Bennett RA, Rubin PH, Present DH. Frequency of inflammatory bowel disease in offspring of couples both presenting with inflammatory bowel disease: differences between Jews and non-Jews. Gastroenterology 1991;100:1638–43.

Cho JH, Brant SR. Genetics and genetic markers in IBD. In: Podolsky D, ed. Current opinion in gastroenterology. Vol. 14. Philadelphia: Lippincott, Raven, 1998:283–8.

Orholm M, Munkholm P, Langholz E, et al. Familial occurrence of inflammatory bowel disease. N Engl J Med 1991; 324:84–8.

Peeters M, Nevens H, Baert F, et al. Familial aggregation in Crohn's disease: increased age-adjusted risk and concordance in clinical characteristics. Gastroenterology 1996;111:597–603.

Polito JM II, Childs B, Mellits ED, et al. Crohn's disease: influence of age at diagnosis on site and clinical type of disease. Gastroenterology 1996;111:580–6.

Tysk C, Lindberg E, Janerot G, Floderus-Myrhed B. Ulcerative colitis and Crohn's disease in an unselected population of monozygotic and dizygotic twins: a study of heritability and the influence of smoking. Gut 1988;29:990–6.

Yang H, McElree C, Roth M-P, et al. Familial empiric risks for inflammatory bowel disease: differences between Jews and non-Jews. Gut 1993;34:517–24.

CHAPTER 111

MANAGING PATIENTS' CONCERNS

GABRIELE MOSER, MD, AND DOUGLAS A. DROSSMAN, MD

The inflammatory bowel diseases (IBDs), because of their unpredictable effects, can burden a patient's life-style, especially for those with more severe or chronic disease activity who are living "from bathroom to bathroom." The issues that some patients with IBD must face include (1) experiencing difficult social problems regarding diarrhea, fear of fecal incontinence, and flatulence; (2) managing abdominal pain; (3) physical or psychological effects on sexual functioning; and (4) addressing the financial, psychological and physical (role, functioning) effects of frequent hospitalizations and painful procedures. Even usually commonplace experiences, such as having an endoscopy, may be fraught with concerns: "Will they find cancer?" "Will it hurt?" Patients do not always volunteer even very important concerns: fear of disability, financial hardship, self-appearance, and even the unpredictable course of the illness. Clinical observations indicate that these kinds of worries and concerns related to IBD and its consequences may affect health status. Thus, to manage the concerns of patients with IBD, it is necessary to understand the impact of these chronic disorders on the emotional and psychosocial status of patients.

Disease-Related Concerns and Information About IBD

To assess IBD-specific worries and concerns, Drossman et al (1991) developed a questionnaire containing 25 items of concern related to IBD, the Rating Form of IBD Patient Concerns (RFIPC). All patients were asked questions in the following format: "Because of your condition, how concerned are you with...?" Each item was rated by the patient from 0 to 100 (0 = not at all, 100 = a great deal) on a visual analogue scale. To find cross-cultural variations in the impact of this chronic condition, the RFIPC was administered to 2002 patients with IBD in eight countries. Having surgery, having an ostomy, the uncertain nature of the disease, and medication side effects each were rated among the first five in importance in six of eight countries. A relation was found between disease-related concerns of patients with IBD and their information level about IBD. Lower information level was associated with greater concerns (Moser, 1995). In this context, it is important to know that more than 60 percent

of patients with IBD consider themselves insufficiently informed about the disease. In addition, the burden of uncertainty about possible complications or necessary interventions is greater when the patient feels uninformed. Patients are able to adjust to their disease much more readily when they are informed about its nature and effects. Therefore, the provision of adequate information that can address the concerns of patients may lead to better adjustment to the illness and possibly to improved outcome.

Subjective Experience of Living with Inflammatory Bowel Disease

About 90 percent of patients with IBD are able to lead an almost normal life and to remain within the workforce and engage in gainful employment. However, more than 50 percent of patients with Crohn's disease feel that exacerbations of their disease strain their professional and personal life, and, probably as a result, up to 30 percent of patients actively conceal their illness from employers. Thus, disease activity does not fully explain the patient's illness experience, and the illness experience needs to be actively elicited by health care professionals. There are several chapters on support systems, including a chapter on an IBD nurse advocate.

Adaptation to Illness and Use of Unconventional Therapies

Factors that help patients adapt to their illness include (1) accurate information about IBD, (2) having a sense of control over the illness, and (3) strong social support. It also is important to understand that patients are seeking benefit from alternative medicine and treatments. Certain concerns, including having surgery, being treated as different, and feeling out of control, seem to influence the decision to use unconventional therapies (Moser, 1996). Actively eliciting the concerns and expectations of patients in clinical practice may help them to choose more effective treatment strategies and possibly avoid the use of unproven and expensive alternative therapies. Asking patients in a nonjudgmental fashion about the reasons for their use of complementary medicine can be helpful. Most show dissatisfaction or skepticism toward conventional medicine because they do not experience adequate control of their health care, and they seek, and may receive, a higher degree of participation in care giver–patient relationship with the practitioners of alternative medicine. However, the powerful effect of an effective physician–patient relationship also can be implemented by the traditionally trained physician. There is a separate chapter on alternative therapies.

Experience with Stress and Exacerbation of Inflammatory Bowel Disease Symptoms

When asked about possible causes for the onset of their disease, the majority of patients with IBD believe that psychosocial stress is an important reason for the exacerbation of their disease. Yet only a few prospective studies address the influence of major life events on biologic disease activity, and these have yielded contradictory results (Drossman, 1999). Some patients need to be relieved of feelings of self-blame. There also may be attitudes communicated through simplistic psychoanalytic theories when somatic symptoms have been interpreted as symbolic of unresolved conflicts. It is helpful to ask patients for their "illness model," the possible causes for the onset or exacerbation of their disease. In doing so, a great deal can be learned about relevant concerns and psychosocial factors affecting the patient's life. If patients believe that some life events may have contributed to the exacerbation of their disease, one can take the opportunity to discuss this further and indicate that reducing stress or solving problems can be beneficial to some patients. The question as to whether or not stress precipitates a clinical relapse remains open, but it is important to recognize that the exacerbation of symptoms need not be an inflammatory response. Symptoms typical for irritable bowel syndrome may explain some of the clinical presentations in IBD (Bayless, 1990). For patients with Crohn's disease, clinical indices have been found to be only weakly linked with endoscopic and biologic factors. Perceived stress might relate to perceived symptoms virtually independent of the severity of the inflammatory process. This makes it important to ask, "What makes you feel better or worse?"

Psychological Disturbances

Children and adolescents with IBD comprise a population at high risk for developing a comorbid psychiatric condition. Lack of self-reliance and a tendency to rely on others when ill is an understandable concomitant of the disease, especially when illness begins in adolescence and hampers the normal process of maturation and separation of family to achieve personal autonomy. The degree of psychological difficulties seems to correlate with the disease severity. Admixtures of anger, depression, denial, and anxiety all are common and normal reactions to

living with IBD. The subgroup of patients who do not develop effective coping styles may show varying combinations of maladaptive symptoms, such as depression, chronic anxiety, and denial of illness, and some show social withdrawal or have difficulties with moving away from the "sick" role (Kaplan, 1996). It is important to identify those patients with severe psychological difficulties who require psychological counseling. The need for psychotherapy and psychopharmacologic treatment are generally the same for patients with IBD as for anyone else. Psychotherapy for the IBD patient is not recommended for the purpose of preventing a relapse or for maintenance of remission. Patients and psychotherapists should have realistic goals for the treatment. Psychotherapy is indicated if there is psychological suffering and motivation on the part of the patient. The few prospective studies on psychotherapy for patients with IBD have found no influence on the biologic course of IBD in the long run, but have shown it to be effective in reducing anxiety and depression and improving quality of life and ability to cope with stress (Jantschek et al, 1999).

Clinical Management of Patients with Inflammatory Bowel Disease and the Role of the Physician in Adjustment to Inflammatory Bowel Disease

The assessment of psychosocial factors in IBD is an essential part of treatment, because poor quality of life and the burden of the disease experienced are important predictors of health care use by patients with IBD. Crucial variables in determining psychosocial well-being are:

- the severity of the underlying illness
- current life stress and daily hassles
- personality characteristics
- problems unrelated to IBD (eg, job demands, insufficient health care system)
- quality of social supports
- coping with the disease

If the psychological concomitants of the illness are not addressed, patients may feel misunderstood by their physicians.

Recommendations for Clinical Practice

Ask about disease-related worries and concerns. Encourage patients to talk about difficult-to-share concerns and problems, their frustrations with treatments, and their use of unconventional medicine. Use nondirective, open-ended questions to which the patient does not answer with "yes," or "no" but instead describes his or her attitude and concerns. If they exist, acknowledge your own challenges and frustrations in treating IBD, so the responsibility to resolve difficult situations is shared.

Be aware of the patients' fear of endoscopic or other procedures. Recommend appropriate sedation or analgesics for endoscopies or painful procedures. Involve the patient and (if they want) family members or partner in treatment decisions. Provide the best level of information to ensure that the patient is a well-informed partner in discussions of treatment plan.

Assess the patient's quality of life and adaptation to the illness. Ask what the patient does or does not do (related to the illness) every day and become aware of disability and maladaptive coping strategies, such as denial of illness. Patients who deny or minimize the illness may not seek medical care at the time of an acute exacerbation or during a difficult phase of the disease. This can increase the risk of complications or need for surgery. Look at the role of the family and physician relationships. Ask who is providing social support and who the patient talks to about difficulties (toilet seeking, problems in sexual life), and recognize feelings of isolation, maladaptive coping, or excessive dependence on others.

Address patient's emotions by communicating your understanding.

- Empathize. ("That seems sad for you." "I can imagine that must have been quite upsetting." etc.)
- Show positive regard. ("You've really dealt remarkably well with this.")
- Support a partnership. ("Together, I think we can get on top of this.")

Provide psychological support whenever the patient needs it. Generally, psychological support is best given by persons closely connected to the patient and by the treating physician. Support groups (national foundations) may be helpful to the majority of patients to reduce the feeling of isolation with these socially difficult symptoms. They help to promote common concerns, and this improves quality of life.

Recognize the indications for psychotherapy and psychopharmacologic treatment. Do not overlook psychiatric comorbidity. Ask about depressive symptoms such as sadness (tendency to cry), feeling hopelessness or guilty, lack of motivation, and maladaptive perceptions ("Being a burden on others"). Fatigue and lack of energy both may be a result of anemia and signs of depression. Some patients have difficulty expressing their feelings and fantasies (alexithymia). Do not force the patient to speak about his or her emotional situation; modify your communication style to match that of the patient. Try to create a trusting clinical environment so the patient will feel able to disclose thoughts and feelings.

Cooperate with psychiatrists or psychotherapists. Whenever psychological treatment is necessary, consult specialists who are experienced with patients with IBD.

In general, the patient with IBD needs a physician who is aware of and can address some of the psychosocial aspects of the illness. A patient-centered interviewing style with nondirective, open-ended questions is the best approach to capture the personal aspects of the patient's story.

References

Bayless TM, Harris ML. Inflammatory bowel disease and irritable bowel syndrome. Med Clin North Am 1990;74:21–9.

Drossman DA. Psychosocial factors in ulcerative colitis and Crohn's disease. In: Kirsner JB, Shorter RG, eds. Inflammatory bowel disease. 5th Ed. Baltimore: Williams & Wilkins, 1999.

Drossman DA, Leserman J, Li Z, et al. The Rating Form of IBD Patient Concerns: a new measure of health status. Psychosom Med 1991;53:701–12.

Jantschek G, Zeitz M, Pritsch M, et al. Effect of psychotherapy on the course of Crohn's disease. Scand J Gastroenterol 1999;33:1289–96.

Kaplan M. The psychiatric treatment of patients with Crohn's disease. In: Prantera C, Korelitz BI, eds. Crohn's disease. New York: Marcel Dekker, 1996:455–65.

Moser G, Tillinger W, Sachs G, et al. Disease-related concerns: a study on outpatients with inflammatory bowel disease (IBD). Eur J Gastroenterol Hepatol 1995;7:853–8.

Moser G, Tillinger W, Sachs G, et al. Relationship between the use of unconventional therapies and disease-related concerns: a study of patients with inflammatory bowel disease. J Psychosom Res 1996;40:503–9.

Supplemental Reading

De Boer AGEM, Sprangers MAG, Bartelsman JFW, de Haes HCJM. Predictors of health care utilization in patients with inflammatory bowel disease: a longitudinal study. Eur J Gastroenterol Hepatol 1998;10:783–9.

Smith RC, Hoppe RB. The patient's story: integrating the patient- and physician-centered approaches to interviewing. Ann Intern Med 1991;115:470–7.

Steiner-Grossman P. The approach to the inflammatory bowel disease family. In: Kirsner JB, Shorter RG, eds. Inflammatory bowel disease. 4th Ed. Baltimore: Williams & Wilkins, 1995:985–94.

CHAPTER 112

Life-Style Issues and Inflammatory Bowel Disease

Richard P. Rood, MD, FACP

Inflammatory bowel diseases (IBDs), ulcerative colitis, and Crohn's disease are chronic diseases that can afflict patients at various times of their lives. As a practicing gastroenterologist specializing in IBD, and as an IBD patient myself for almost 30 years, I have lived with the ramifications of the disease and had the opportunity to counsel patients who also are living with either ulcerative colitis or Crohn's disease. In this chapter, I hope to give the benefit of my experience so other practitioners will be able to gain insight into living and functioning with IBD, and how we, as treating physicians, can become more effective practitioners for this unique group of patients. One does not necessarily have to walk the walk in order to talk the talk, but insights, from trained observers who have had these experiences, can be the basis for invaluable lessons.

Certainly, living with IBD redefines a normal lifetime routine. The patient never knows when their "time is up," (ie, when a period of remission is about to run out). Patients can have adverse effects from the simplest ailments. For example, a gastrointestinal viral illness may attack an entire family and spontaneously resolve in 24 to 48 hours in most normal family members. However, the patient with IBD may be incapable of compensating for the diarrhea and emesis-induced fluid and electrolyte losses and require a hospital admission for significant rehydration.

Life-Style Changes

Patients with IBD must identify the location of the nearest restroom when they enter a building. The unpredictability of the disease often dictates that plans have to be modified. A patient with IBD might feel uncomfortable going camping with his or her children, not knowing what type of facilities are available and where they are located. Certainly, not all buildings or venues have adequate numbers of restroom facilities. A patient with IBD may have done his due diligence in locating the closest restroom facility only to find that there is a single toilet stall and a long line around the corner. There is actually a guidebook *Where To Go, A Guide to Manhattan's Toilets,* by Vicki Rovere, with over 450 listings and maps.

Living with IBD is like a never-ending roller coaster ride in the dark. You may be coasting along just fine, but you never know when a sharp turn, peak, or valley is right in front of you. Once you take a plunge, you do not know how long it will take to get back to that comfortable coasting position again. When you are at a peak, you are feeling great, in command of your body and your life, but those sharp turns and sudden plunges can shake you to your core. How long will it take to get back on your feet, to feel better, get back to work, or get back to school? Too many and too frequent wild rides can really challenge your confidence and your attitude, and leave those around you shaken as well.

As with any chronic illness, treating only the symptoms and complications of these diseases may not meet all of the needs of the individual patient. The treating physician must take into account that the individual patient does not live in a vacuum; rather, he or she generally functions as part of a larger group, specifically their family, work, or school environment. The impacts of the patient on his family and the family on the patient are important influences on the success of treatment. In addition to just being themselves, they are also spouses, parents, and children. All of these relationships define who they are. In the past, it was possible to isolate the patient in the hospital for evaluation and treatment, often admitting the patient for "a complete evaluation." A concentrated effort could be made toward assisting the patient's adjustment and coordinate the family interaction. However, times have changed. Lengths of hospital stay are shorter and more is evaluated in the ambulatory setting, often taking longer, and instead of the nurse playing the role as early supporter to the newly diagnosed patient, or the patient requiring major medical intervention, the family plays a more pivotal role in the delivery of care.

The success or failure of a particular treatment plan also is predicated on the ability of the family, or support system, to understand the situation and become the surrogate nurse for these patients. So often this unique aspect of care is taken for granted. Physicians forget that these family members are just that, caring family members. It is important to bring them into the process early to affect the best therapeutic outcome. When I make the initial diagnosis of IBD or make significant changes in the course of treatment, I request to meet and discuss this information with the supporting family, parent, spouse, or child. An informed, educated support structure has the best chance of affecting a successful outcome.

The life-style issues that need to be addressed in the individual patient are dependent upon the stage of that patient in life. The issues that need to be dealt with in childhood are different from the problems of early adulthood. Physicians must acknowledge these differences to customize therapy for the individual patient.

Children and Adolescents

Children and adolescents are faced with the normal growth and development milestones to achieve. However, the added ramifications of a chronic disease can be nearly insurmountable. Children with IBD have to deal with issues in school, with teachers and peers. I recently had to write a letter on behalf of one of my young patients to educate the classroom teacher about his disease, asking that when the patient needed to use the restroom that it be done in such a way that the child did not stand out and an issue not be made of the event. Apparently, the teacher thought that this child, suffering from active Crohn's disease, was just like all of her other students and could wait for the next break in the schedule to use the restroom. It was important that the child be supported so he maintained as normal a classroom experience as possible. Teachers make adjustments for students who are hearing, visually, speech, or developmentally impaired, so with proper education, they need to adjust for the student with chronic diarrhea. A Crohn's and Colitis Foundation of America (CCFA) brochure for teachers can be helpful.

Adolescence adds its unique problems. Adolescents are greatly influenced by their peers. Conforming to and fitting into the social arena are important. For these reasons, special care needs to be taken with this group of patients. A child with chronic diarrhea, abdominal pain, growth and sexual retardation, and acne and moon face from steroid therapy will feel different from his or her peer group. How this is handled by the family and school and supported by the physician is important in the overall development of these young patients. It would be best to anticipate some of these situations and possibly role-play with the child, rather than having the child face the situation alone. How does the 13-year-old adolescent with Crohn's disease and an ileostomy deal with gym, showers, and toilets with open stalls? I fervently believe that the method of handling these situations is education and support. The parent and physician can educate the teacher and school and form the basis for support. Additional assistance can come from mutual support groups within the CCFA and, when appropriate, the United Ostomy Association (UOA). Both of these groups have age-appropriate brochures and books that can serve as excellent resources for the patient, family, and school. Through the CCFA and the UOA, children and parents

can interact and brainstorm answers to these challenging circumstances.

Young Adulthood

Although dating starts in adolescence, it hits high gear in young adulthood. This is the time when one looks toward building long-term relationships. Once again, education is important. Following a CCFA education meeting, I was approached by a young woman who lamented that she had ulcerative colitis and had been treated surgically with a proctocolectomy and ileoanal anastamosis. She had attempted several relationships with gentlemen and when she told them of her illness, these relationships rapidly chilled. One could say that the problem was related to the ignorance of the gentlemen she was dating. I was told by another young woman who underwent emergency proctocolectomy and end ileostomy for toxic megacolon that her own gastroenterologist, who had cared for her for several years, told the impressionable, postoperative young woman in her twenties, that maybe someday someone would marry her. Here is an example of a seemingly educated professional who had no idea how to handle the situation. As it turned out, this individual survived the experience in spite of her physician.

Adulthood

As one matures further into adulthood, additional issues arise. Beyond the family and educational environment, the individual patient with IBD must deal with issues of financially supporting his or her family and interacting within the workplace. As with any person with a chronic illness, the patient with IBD often can have problems with endurance, absenteeism, and, therefore, job performance during times of active disease. As I considered the type of medical practice I would enter into as a gastroenterologist who has IBD, I needed to consider what safeguards would be available for my patients should I suddenly become ill. What would I do with a schedule full of patients already prepared for their colonoscopies? I had to build in a coverage situation, so that I would have partners who could assist in the rare event that I might become suddenly dehydrated and unable to adequately function.

Partners and employers, in general, are willing and capable of temporarily adjusting workloads and responsibilities to assist the patient with IBD. When employers and co-workers are ignorant regarding the problems associated with IBD, or are unwilling to adjust the work environment, problems can occur. One of my patients with Crohn's disease worked for a medial equipment manufacturer on an assembly line. She had frequent spells of diarrhea while at work. Her employer decided that the method of handling this was to follow my patient into the restroom to make sure that her symptoms were legitimate. Unfortunately, this occurred prior to the Americans with Disabilities Act, and my patient was given no option but to resign and attempt, in vain, to obtain disability compensation.

Admittedly, most of the time patients with IBD do not have these problems, especially when the patients are in remission. What happens when the patient becomes ill, requires extended hospitalization, or requires extended recovery from surgical procedures? First of all, can he or she get or afford adequate health insurance coverage? The patient or his or her family may be locked into larger corporate employment to obtain and maintain insurance benefits. There is a useful chapter on insurance and disability. Even if insurance plans are available, they may be prohibitively expensive or offer only limited coverage. I took care of a certified public accountant who suffered from Crohn's disease. He owned his own small accounting firm but could not obtain health insurance. He was forced to close his firm and apply for Medicaid to afford proper medical treatment. The employed individual not living with a chronic illness generally has some safeguards against financial ruin in the event of illness. In addition to health insurance, they often have benefit packages that can include access to disability and life insurances. I have cared for a young, employed patient with Crohn's disease whose employer did not offer health insurance and who had been turned down for coverage by multiple insurance underwriters. This patient would be a candidate for immunomodulator therapy, yet resources are not available to properly manage his disease. This situation demonstrates the influence of financial security upon successful medical therapy. Unfortunately, as patients recover from surgery or experience periods of active disease, they will have to deal with all these financial issues. How do we handle these problems? Funds are available in communities for the uninsured or underinsured patient. Clinical trials can be found that might be available for these patients, and pharmaceutical firms do have compassionate-need programs for patients unable to afford medications.

Elderly Patients

Elderly patients experience IBD similarly to other adult patients with similar problems in the workplace, established family, and spousal relationships. The problem arises when the elderly patient with IBD begins to lose his independence and requires assistance and even supervision. Once again, the familial support structure becomes essential to the success of medical therapy. Often, medication regimens are complicated, and the patient may get confused about instructions or be unable to read instructions placed on medication bottles. Dosages and adverse events of medical therapy may vary, depending on other comorbid conditions and medications. Practitioners need to remain vigilant about the living environment of the patient. Functional status also has an impact on determining which medications can be used in the individual

patient. A widowed, arthritic patient with distal proctitis will likely be incapable of administering enema-instilled medications, such as mesalamine or hydrocortisone, unless help is available. It is helpful to try to anticipate some of the needs of the patient in advance by educating the family as well as other support agencies. Networking with other elderly patients within the CCFA can lead to invaluable support for the individual patient and family. Why not take advantage of the experience of someone else and learn from it? The treating physician needs to be aware of the resources that are available for the mature patient with IBD in his community. The chapter on IBD in the elderly provides information on management issues unique to this population.

Concluding Remarks

It would be absurd to think that practicing gastroenterologists can solve all of these problems; certainly, we cannot. Most of these societal issues are outside our control. However, we need to acknowledge the prejudices against patients with chronic diseases, such as ulcerative colitis and Crohn's disease, occurring in society as a whole. These prejudices have a significant impact on the health of our patients. I do not believe that the practicing physician must know the answers to all of society's shortcomings. However, I would hope that the compassionate physician would know where to direct his or her patient when situations such as these arise. I challenge the physician to be the patient's advocate; it is likely that we are the last patient advocates remaining. Once again, support from organizations such as the CCFA can be invaluable. I hope that my experience, as both a patient with IBD and a practicing gastroenterologist, has given other physicians the insight necessary to assist patients with IBD to avoid some of the bumps on the roller coaster of life with IBD. There are several chapters on support services and on behavioral therapy. Chapter 113, "Inflammatory Bowel Disease Nurse Advocate," also may be informative.

Supplemental Reading

Rovere V. Where to go. A guide to Manhattan's toilets. New York: Vicki Rovere, 1991.

Stein SH, Rood RP, eds. Inflammatory bowel disease: a guide for patients and their families. 2nd Ed. Philadelphia: Lippincott-Raven Publishers, 1999.

Other Sources

Crohn's and Colitis Foundation of America, National Headquarters, 386 Park Avenue South, 17th Floor, New York, New York 10016-8804. Phone: 800 932-2432. Website: *www.ccfa.org*

United Ostomy Association, Inc., 36 Executive Park, Suite 120, Irvine, California 92714-6744. Phone: 800 826-0826. Website: *www.uoa.org*

Inflammatory Bowel Disease Nurse Advocate

Sharon A. Hunt, BSN, RN

Many patients with Crohn's disease or ulcerative colitis report frequent encounters with health care providers who know little about inflammatory bowel disease (IBD) and how to manage it. One such patient, Blaine Franklin Newman, vowed to help others avoid that distress. The resultant endowment gift gave rise to and continues support of the Inflammatory Bowel Disease Nurse Advocate position at The Johns Hopkins Hospital.

The primary goal of this position is to responsibly address the multidisciplinary needs of this unique patient population. Patients ranked effective communication of health-related information second to clinical skill as the most crucial element of outpatient care. Responding to patient perception, the "advocate" model prioritizes the essentials of improved communication, patient education, and accessibility to the health care system. Using a collaborative approach, the IBD Nurse Advocate functions as a "physician extender." This approach to practice promotes productivity and effective use of personnel, and positively impacts on patient outcomes.

Essential and Complementary Skills

The skills and qualities essential to assess, plan, implement, evaluate, and modify mutually derived treatment plans include but are not limited to the following:

1. Oral and written communication skills.
2. Self-confidence as evidenced by a strong theory foundation and the ability to participate in decision-making.
3. Organizational skills that incorporate flexibility to coordinate multidisciplinary involvement.
4. Professional maturity that recognizes the legal responsibilities of Practice Acts, safety, documentation, and scope of care.

Desired complementary skills, knowledge, and experience include:

- Ostomy knowledge and care
- Experience with long-term care of chronic illness
- Endoscopy knowledge
- Outpatient and office experience
- Patient education experience
- Research experience
- Nutritional counseling experience

Primary Responsibilities

Participation in scheduled IBD outpatient clinics is the highest priority of this position because of its measurable impact on both patients and physicians. Using a customized IBD patient intake form (Figure 113–1), the Nurse Advocate performs assessment interviews on designated new patients and all returning patients. The returning-patient interview averages 15 minutes. Details focus on interim medical and psychosocial status, compliance with previously prescribed treatment plans, and diagnostic study updates. Much of the time is spent discussing symptoms, a modified disease activity index, actual medications used, adverse events, and the need for prescriptions and testing. The Crohn's Disease Activity Index (CDAI) of the Harvey-Bradshaw score can be incorporated in the interview form. After presenting the assessment, the Nurse Advocate assists the physician with the patient physical examination. Treatment plans are mutually established and documented. Patient privacy and confidentiality are maintained throughout the visit. The Nurse Advocate promotes patient compliance with the prescribed treatment plan through patient education and written instructions. Additional responsibilities include the coordination of surgical, nutritional, and ostomy service appointments when indicated. The inflammatory bowel disease Nurse Advocate has been involved in an average of 1,200 outpatient visits per year.

The second most crucial function of the IBD nurse advocate is to serve as a patient resource and physician liaison via telephone communication. Accessibility to the health care team promotes optimum patient outcomes, compliance, and satisfaction. Verbal correspondence is documented to ensure continuity of care and legal awareness. It should be noted that any modification of treatment plan must be physician-approved prior to implementation.

One of the essential ingredients for advocacy is knowledge. A strong emphasis is placed on educating patients, staff, and others within and outside the immediate practice. The IBD Nurse Advocate is expected to be a spokesperson for the IBD center at inservices and at local and national conferences and symposia. This role requires a current command of the various aspects of IBD, including, but not limited to, current resources, insurance issues

Patient Name:_____ History #: _____

Clinic Physician: _____ Date: _____

DX: Crohns   UC   collagenous colitis   IBD   IBS   celiac   other _____

Significant Dates:
Date of Dx _____
Last visit_____   Surgery 1) _____
UGI / Sm Bowel _____   2) _____
Colonoscopy _____   3) _____
    findings: _____

Vital Signs: T _____   BP _____ / _____   HR _____   Weight: _____ (> <) Prev. wt _____ [_____]

WELL in between ILL / PAR Energy: _____ (scale of 1–10)
Appetite:_____ lactose intolerance   fat intolerance   high/low fiber   carbonated beverages   gum / caffeine / gassy foods
Do you smoke?____Yes_____No_____
Upper GI sx : indigestion / heartburn / reflux   Intervention_____effective: Yes No

Bowel characteristics: Frequency: _____ formed / loose / liquid / urgency / incontinence / nocturnal / constipation / ribbon / float / marble / pellet / blood / mucous

SX: pain / cramping / gas / distention / noise / other_____

Extra-intestinal sx: joint pain / mouth ulcers / abscess / fistula / other: _____

Medications:

Prednisone: dose: _____ Start date:_____ Stop date:_____-
Budesonide (dose) _____ Start date_____

Azulfidine / sulfasalazine 500 mg _____ _____ Folic acid 1 mg _____
Asacol 400 mg _____Pentasa 250 mg_____

Imuran (azathioprine) 50 mg _____ start date:_____ Purinethol / 6-MP (6-mercaptopurine)_____
Methotrexate 25 mg/15 mg Start date: _____ Week # _____
CSA (100 mg) _____ Start date:_____
Remicade candidate: Yes   No   comment:_____

Cipro 500 mg _____ Flagyl / Metronidazole 250 / 500 mg _____ Tetracycline _____
Bently / dicyclomine 10 mg _____ Levsin 0.125 mg _____

Prilosec 20 mg _____ Propulsid 10 mg _____ Zantac 150 mg _____ Pepcid _____

Fiber Con _____ Metamucil _____ Citracil _____
Questran / Colestid (cholestyramine) 4 g _____other: _____
Loperamide 2 mg (immodium) _____ Lomotil _____ DTO _____

Topicals: Rowasa (4 g enema / 500 mg suppository)
          Cortenema
          Cortifoam / Proctofoam / Proctocort / Anusol-Hc

Misc. meds: _____
NSAIDS : Yes / No

Prescription refills? _____

Family Hx: _____

FIGURE 113–1. A customized intake form for patients with inflammatory bowel disease.

CHAPTER 113

and their implications, and the latest treatment modalities. The emergence of biologic therapies demands additional attention, extending the role of the Nurse Advocate. The administration and monitoring of these therapies require program design, coordination of services, instruction, and supervision. Participation implies the responsibility to share experiences, and the Nurse Advocate is involved in continuing education and in the drafting of formal publications.

Research is a natural extension of the role of the IBD Nurse Advocate. The IBD Nurse Advocate participates in the coordination of duties and responsibilities in research trials as directed by the primary investigator and may be responsible for the design and implementation of research projects.

Measuring Role Impact

Investigators have demonstrated that collaborative practice can increase compliance, increase patient satisfaction, and improve efficiency while decreasing costs, missed appointments, and hospitalizations. The author's team practice was able to increase annual revenue through an increased number of new and returning-patient visits. This growth pattern has been sustained over time, exceeding original projections. Additionally, there were increased numbers of endoscopic procedures and surgical referrals as a result of coordination of care, which in turn generated additional revenues for the medical institution.

Increased patient satisfaction was validated using a team-designed survey tool. The survey consisted of 24 questions, which reviewed patient perception of the efficacy of the IBD Nurse Advocate. The format was multiple choice, for ease of completion, with space provided to add a narrative comment if desired. Completed surveys strongly supported the role of the IBD Nurse Advocate.

Telecommunication

Patient use of the IBD Nurse Advocate via telecommunication further demonstrates acceptance of the position as well as perceived benefit for patients. Over 3,000 calls were logged during the first 2 years of availability. The time required of the Nurse Advocate in this function is proportionate to the potential time saved by the physician. This telephone forum has been a valuable source of information, contributing suggestions for practice modifications to meet patient needs. In the future, e-mail presumably will occupy a larger role in communication.

Community Outreach

Professional growth results when shared commitment and mutual respect meet the needs of patients. It fosters a sense of purpose and a compassion that searches for expression. An ideal channel for this energy is through the Crohn's & Colitis Foundation of America (CCFA). A partnership of professionals and laypersons, the CCFA is dedicated to optimizing therapy and finding a cure for IBD. The organization sponsors educational programs, research, publications, and support groups. Complementing the professional role of the IBD Nurse Advocate with active volunteer service creates a synergy with immeasurable returns.

Summary

The success of the IBD Nurse Advocate role has exceeded expectations. The impact on the author's practice was immediately visible and attracted the attention of other health professionals who have modeled the position to accommodate their needs. Establishing industry standards for patient advocacy is a progressive responsibility. True collaboration is essential to the success of any expanded role. Written job descriptions are of paramount importance to identify strengths and limitations and to establish responsibilities and boundaries of authority. The downside to this experience was in underestimating the growth potential of the position. Patient use has exceeded capacity. Patient and practice needs have to be identified, prioritized, and scheduled to be realistically achieved.

Acknowledgment

The author and the IBD group at Johns Hopkins are grateful to Ms. Zoralyn Stahl, the Blaine Franklin Newman family and their medical advisor, Dr. Charles Warfield, and to the Johns Hopkins Hospital for their encouragement and support of this important position.

Supplemental Reading

Baldwin D. Some historical notes on interdisciplinary and interprofessional education and practice in healthcare in the USA. J Interprof Care 1996;10:173–87.

Henneman E, Lee J, Cohen J. Collaboration: a concept analysis. J Adv Nurs 1995;21:103–9.

Laine C, Davidoff F, Lewis C, et al. Important elements of outpatient care: a comparison of patients' and physicians' opinions. Ann Intern Med 1996;125:640–5.

CHAPTER 114

CROHN'S & COLITIS FOUNDATION OF AMERICA: INFORMATION AND SUPPORT SERVICES

MARJORIE MERRICK, DIRECTOR OF RESEARCH AND EDUCATION

The Crohn's & Colitis Foundation of America (CCFA) is an organization of laypersons, medical professionals, and professional staff who are dedicated to conquering Crohn's disease and ulcerative colitis. This dynamic partnership is the cornerstone of the foundation and has been responsible for its rapid growth over the years. The National Headquarters of the CCFA is located in New York City, and the foundation has over 50 chapters across the country.

When the foundation was established in 1967, our single goal was to find the cure for Crohn's disease and ulcerative colitis, collectively known as inflammatory bowel disease (IBD), by raising money for medical research. It was quickly apparent, however, that to realize our primary goal, CCFA needed to combat the pervasive ignorance and misinformation about IBD among both laypersons and medical professionals by creating educational programs that would provide accurate, up-to-date information about IBD.

In addition, the majority of our members either suffered from IBD or had family members afflicted with these diseases. Whereas their support was essential to our medical research program, they, in turn, needed supportive services to help them cope with the profound impact of IBD on their lives.

Following are some of the ways CCFA can help people with IBD and the professionals who care for them.

Publications

Over the years, CCFA has developed a wealth of patient education materials. To ensure that the most accurate, up-to-date information is disseminated, all materials must be reviewed and approved by the medical experts who participate on our National Scientific Advisory Committee (NSAC). Many of our materials are free for the asking, some are available for purchase, and others are provided as a benefit of membership.

Each year, more than a million brochures are distributed free of charge to patients, physicians, and hospitals. These easy-to-read brochures provide general information about the diseases, diet and nutrition, complications,

surgeries, emotional factors, and guides for parents, teachers, and children and teenagers. In addition, for persons looking for more detailed information on the diseases in general, coping techniques, or pediatric IBD, CCFA has three books covering these topics available for purchase. There is a complete list of these publications at the end of this chapter.

All CCFA lay and professional members receive *Foundation Focus*, the foundation's national magazine. Published three times a year, *Foundation Focus* contains articles and special features on research, medical therapy, and surgery, as well as updates on national and chapter programs. Many CCFA chapters also publish newsletters for their local membership.

The IBD community is intensely interested in what is happening in research. In addition to research updates in *Foundation Focus* and on our Website, CCFA circulates *Under the Microscope*, a six-page newsletter that is published once a year and highlights the most productive research areas as well as CCFA-supported research endeavors. Last, our *Annual Research Report*, which is an integral part of our *Annual Report*, features an overview of what is happening in research, explains our different grant programs, and includes descriptions of each of the types of research grants and training awards currently funded by the CCFA as well as articles about the investigators.

Both health care professionals and lay members may subscribe to the professional journal of the CCFA, *Inflammatory Bowel Diseases*. This quarterly peer-reviewed publication offers original articles on the "cutting edge" of basic and clinical research in IBD. Readers also find review articles, selected summaries, and the popular "Controversies in IBD," in which experts debate the pros and cons of selected topics. *Inflammatory Bowel Diseases* has been accepted by *Index Medicus*, enabling scientists to electronically access the contents from all issues of the journal.

Website

In 1996 CCFA joined the electronic revolution by creating an extensive, award-winning Website (http://www.ccfa.org). Thousands of people from around the world now visit the Website every month. The very latest news appears in the "Weekly Feature" and "News Update," both of which are changed each week.

The divisions within the Website offer a plethora of information. Comprehensive, up-to-the-minute information about IBD may be found in four areas:

- The "Library" contains a host of articles on every aspect of IBD, including diagnosis and treatment, complications, coping day-to-day, insurance issues, etc.
- In the "Research" section, visitors learn about the latest developments in basic and clinical research. There are articles on every major field of investigation, plus a complete list of current CCFA-funded grants.
- "Ask the Specialist" is a bulletin board where visitors may post questions about IBD, which are answered by volunteer physicians.
- The "Find-a-Doctor" directory contains all of the doctors and health care professionals affiliated with CCFA. Although this is not a form of accreditation, it is an invaluable resource to persons who are moving or traveling to other parts of the United States and who need to identify a gastroenterologist with a special interest in treating IBD.

Other areas on the site include:

- "Physician's Resource Room": This site is designed especially for the needs of physicians and other health professionals involved with people with IBD. Visitors to this site can find articles about IBD therapies, including treatment guidelines, and diagnostic techniques; a calendar of IBD-related medical meetings; summaries of medical meetings; information concerning current CCFA research awards and the guidelines and application forms for our grant programs; tables of contents for every issue of our journal, *Inflammatory Bowel Diseases*; links to other professional sites; a list of our current medical leadership; the full text of our popular "Q&A about Crohn's Disease" and "Q&A about Ulcerative Colitis"; a glossary; an online order form; and information about becoming a professional member of CCFA.
- "Links" to related organizations or Websites: These include medical organizations and agencies; medical journals; physician sites; sites for people with IBD, by people with IBD; message boards and IBD chats; international organizations and information in other languages; clinical trial information; miscellaneous references.
- "Legislative Affairs": Visitors to this site can read about advocacy programs of the CCFA; review the basics of legislation, such as how a bill gets passed into law; access key government documents; and learn how they can become involved.
- "CCFA Programs": This section contains basic information about the foundation and what we have to offer.
- "Chapters & Events": Find a complete listing of our

chapters around the country and a calendar of their education and fund-raising events.
- "Membership and Donations": Become a member or make donations online by using this secured section.
- "CCFA Bookstore": Our books may be purchased online through this secured section.
- "Contact CCFA": Got a question? Send it directly to us.
- "Overseas Foundations": This listing of Crohn's and colitis foundations in other countries is especially valuable for people traveling abroad and for those seeking information in other languages.

Education Programs

Chapters of the CCFA regularly hold patient education meetings that are developed in cooperation with the Chapter Medical Advisory Committee (CMAC). These meetings cover a variety of topics, such as a general overview of IBD, medical and surgical therapies, extraintestinal manifestations, nutrition, and coping techniques. Many programs are only an hour or so in duration, although some chapters offer "IBD Days." Chapters also may offer programs or weekend camps for children and adolescents with IBD.

The CCFA also provides educational opportunities for medical professionals by hosting symposia focused on the most current developments in diagnosis and treatment of IBD, which will, in turn, improve patient care. Most local chapters host at least one professional education symposium per year. Chapters also have the opportunity to host one or both of the two accredited professional education workshop series that have been developed by members of the Professional Education Committee of the NSAC. The long-running "Pathologic and Endoscopic Diagnosis in Inflammatory Bowel Disease" workshop is open to pathologists, clinicians, and endoscopists. This full-day workshop focuses on clinical, endoscopic, and pathologic correlation in the diagnosis of IBD, with special attention given to dysplasia in IBD, and emphasizes the importance of teamwork between endoscopist and pathologist in gathering and interpreting endoscopic and biopsy data. The second series, "Inflammatory Bowel Disease Update and Management: New Perspectives in Diagnosis and Treatment," is a full-day workshop geared for nurses. This course explores the definition and differentiation of Crohn's disease and ulcerative colitis, discusses laboratory tests and procedures used to diagnose IBD, gives an overview of medical and surgical treatment and management of ostomy patients, and explores the psychosocial issues of living with IBD.

A complete listing of chapter programs may be found in the "Chapters and Events" section of CCFA Website.

Support Groups

As with any chronic disease, people with IBD face psychological and social adjustments. They will tell their doctors about bowel symptoms but may not feel comfortable discussing their concerns about how the disease affects their day-to-day life and often feel as though no one really understands what they are going through. Chronic pain, weakness, diarrhea, and bleeding are not easy topics to discuss, even with family and close friends, much less at social gatherings. To exacerbate the situation, IBD sufferers also must deal with concerns about self-image and sexual function, possible surgery, unpleasant side effects from medications, swings in emotions and frequent absences from work or school. Family members, friends, physicians, the clergy, and peer organizations, such as CCFA, are essential sources of support for those afflicted with IBD.

Many people with IBD find solace and practical information by joining a self-help or mutual support group. It is not unusual that participation in a support group may be the first time they have ever met and talked with another person with Crohn's disease or ulcerative colitis. Sharing anxieties and problems in coping with IBD with others who also have personal experience with the diseases can be extremely beneficial. Whatever problem someone is facing, there is usually someone in the group who has "been there, done that" and is able to give practical hints in how to successfully deal with the situation.

Chapters of the CCFA host over 300 support groups throughout the United States. Most of these groups meet monthly, and a few meet on an 8-week basis. Some are true "rap sessions" where everyone shares their experiences with the group, whereas others have a more structured format that addresses a specific topic each week. Every group has a facilitator who acts as a gatekeeper to ensure that discussions remain on track and everyone has an opportunity to speak. The CCFA recently implemented a national training program for facilitators to ensure adherence to basic guidelines, such as confidentially, no one may give medical advice, and personal physicians are not mentioned by name.

The support group setting gives members a wonderful opportunity to share coping techniques, to explore practical solutions to the unique problems faced by IBD sufferers, and to learn how to better communicate with their physicians. Group members may discuss how IBD affects family members and friends, and thereby gain a better realization that they truly are not alone in dealing with their disease. There is a chapter on support groups for ileostomy and ileoanal pouch patients.

Other Supportive Services

The national office of the CCFA provides staff to answer the questions of patients that come in by telephone, mail, and e-mail. Some chapters also provide telephone support by trained volunteers who offer emotional support and information about IBD. There is a chapter outlining the most commonly asked questions that come to the CCFA "hot line."

Hospital visitation is another supportive service offered by some CCFA chapters. A patient may request a visit from a trained patient volunteer. The trained visitor follows the same basic policies and procedures as a support group facilitator. Contact your local CCFA chapter office to see if this service is offered in your area.

Research

Education and supportive programs for the layperson and health professional are two vital components of the mission of the CCFAs, and both go far toward improving the quality of life for those with IBD. However, our ultimate goal is to cure and prevent Crohn's disease and ulcerative colitis, and only basic and clinical research can achieve that goal.

The commitment of the CCFA to IBD research has surpassed $50 million and is steadily growing. A rigorous peer review is used to evaluate applicants for our grants, and we fund the work of both established investigators and promising young researchers. Over 35 individual grants and first awards, 10 fellowships, and 10 career development awards are funded each year.

In 1990, CCFA invited 40 of the world's scientific experts to evaluate the state of the art in IBD research and to outline the needs and future directions in disciplines such as immunology, microbiology, genetics, and animal models. The result was the landmark document, "Challenges in IBD Research," which became the map for CCFA research programs. The document has been updated twice and has shown an interesting trend. In 1990, each area of research was segregated. By 1997, the boundaries have blurred considerably and collaboration between disciplines is now commonplace.

The CCFA was instrumental in discovering that a strain of mice at The Jackson Laboratories spontaneously developed a type of ulcerative colitis that closely resembled human disease. The Foundation's support of this mouse colony helped lead to the genetic knockout models that are so crucial to current investigations.

One of the biggest challenges facing clinical researchers is that of acquiring sufficient numbers of patients to make their study or drug trial statistically significant. To meet this need and expedite the process, CCFA established the Clinical Research Alliance, a consortium of major IBD research centers that are linked to a central data management center. Like the spokes of a wheel, hospitals and private practitioners may affiliate with the member institutions and participate in the studies undertaken by the Alliance.

The whole area of genetic research is advancing at a rapid pace. The CCFA not only has supported a series of workshops focused on the genetics of IBD but also is developing a genotype-phenotype cell-line bank as a resource for researchers.

Every 12 to 18 months, the CCFA hosts a scientific meeting focused on specific areas of interest such as immune–nonimmune cell interaction in IBD, microbiology and genetics, animal models, cancer and surveillance, and signal transduction. Outstanding senior and junior investigators are invited to participate in these 2- to 3-day meetings.

Fund-Raising Efforts

How does the CCFA do all of the above? Through contributions from individuals, foundations, and corporations. For fiscal year 1998, total contributions and revenue exceeded $19 million. More than 82 cents of every dollar the foundation spends goes directly into research and education programs. The CCFA consistently meets the standards set by such organizations as the National Charities Information Bureau and the Better Business Bureau.

You can help. Become a professional member. Encourage your patients and their families to join and become actively involved with chapter activities. Every dollar contributed, every hour volunteered, brings us closer to making IBD a disease of the past.

Conclusion

The rise of managed care makes the mission of the CCFA more critical than ever. Physicians have less and less time to spend educating their patients and have come to rely on the CCFA to help fill this gap with unbiased, scientifically sound information. Patients, their families, and their friends turn to the CCFA for answers to the myriad questions that always seem to arise *after* they have left the doctor's office, or that they were simply too embarrassed to ask. The Foundation's research programs are instrumental in forging rapidly toward the cure.

But, perhaps most important of all, the CCFA offers everyone, lay person and professional alike, a chance to take an active part in the fight against IBD. Together, we can hasten the day when no one has to suffer with these devastating diseases.

Supplemental Reading

Benkov KJ, Winter HS. Managing your child's Crohn's disease or ulcerative colitis. Master Media, 1996.

Hanauer S. Inflammatory bowel disease: a guide for patients and their families. Philadelphia: Lippincott Raven, 1998.

Steiner-Grossman P. The new people . . . not patients: a source book for living with inflammatory bowel disease. New York: Crohn's & Colitis Foundation of America Inc., 1997.

Other Resources

Crohn's & Colitis Foundation of America, Inc.
  Toll-free hotline: 800 343-3637
  Website: *http://www.ccfa.org*

National Headquarters:
  Crohn's & Colitis Foundation of America, Inc.
  386 Park Avenue South, 17th floor
  New York, NY 10016-8804
  Phone: 800 932-2423 or 212 685-3440
  Fax: 212 779-4098

Brochures available free of charge:
  A Guide for Children and Teenagers
  A Parent's Guide
  A Teacher's Guide
  Living with IBD (booklet for teenagers)
  Questions and Answers about Complications
  Questions and Answers about Crohn's Disease
  Questions and Answers about Diet and Nutrition
  Questions and Answers about Medications
  Questions and Answers about Pregnancy
  Questions and Answers about Surgery
  Questions and Answers about Ulcerative Colitis

CHAPTER 115

Pediatric Patient and Family Support

Maria I. Clavell, MD, Robert D. Baker, MD, PhD, and Susan S. Baker, MD, PhD

Management of inflammatory bowel disease (IBD) in the pediatric population is a twofold challenge for the clinician. The first challenge is to recognize that the impact of the disease extends beyond the individual patient and embraces the family unit. The second challenge is to deal with the profound effect IBD has on the process of growth and development at the physical and psychological levels occurring in children and adolescents. The clinician plays a vital role providing (1) education about medical aspects of the disease process; (2) therapy, combining drugs, nutrition, or surgery; (3) coordination of various medical specialists; and (4) guidance that promotes the development of effective coping skills to handle the disease.

Advances in the biomedical field involving medications, nutrition, and surveillance allow for early interventions that enhance the quality of life of patients with IBD. At the same time, there are multiple resources available that offer information, a sense of connection, and hope for individual children, adolescents, and their families. The combined effort of families, health care providers from several disciplines, and outside support networks will lead to the successful integration of children and adolescents into day-to-day activities, as well as their appropriate physical and psychological growth and adjustment.

Pediatric Inflammatory Bowel Disease

Crohn's disease and ulcerative colitis manifest themselves in the pediatric population with signs and symptoms similar to those in older individuals. Despite the increasing prevalence of these disorders in the pediatric population, multiple questions remain to be elucidated regarding their origin, course, and management. An important distinction is that children and adolescents have not completed their physical or cognitive maturity; therefore, any chronic disease can have a profound impact on the patients at both levels.

Diagnosis

The diagnosis of IBD produces in the patients and their families a multitude of powerful emotions. It is a relapsing chronic illness even in the presence of good compliance with medical therapy. There is no cure for Crohn's disease, and the surgical treatment to cure ulcerative colitis is radical.

There is a varied range of emotions, including shock, fear, anxiety, guilt, relief, ignorance, denial, anger, and disbelief. As with any chronic and severe diagnosis, it is not infrequent for families to go through several stages of grief. The unpredictability of the clinical course is difficult for families to accept or understand. Additional concerns include the possibility of additional family members developing IBD in the future. Since 30 percent of pediatric patients have a positive family history of IBD, genetic aspects are important issues. Questions that patients and families ask about genetics are discussed in a separate chapter. The increased risk of colonic malignancy in those patients diagnosed with IBD is another important issue. The misinformation in the general population regarding these disorders may result in a sense of alienation of the patients and their families.

From the time of the initial diagnosis, it is essential to establish a comprehensive plan for patient care; in other words, a background must be provided for the individuals to learn to live full, productive lives with their diagnosis. Achieving a better understanding of this condition will enhance therapeutic compliance and at the same time decrease levels of anxiety that are known to affect disease exacerbations.

Education

The physician plays an important role as the most reliable source of information for the patient and family regarding the disease. The information should be complete and at the same time concise and appropriate for the level of education of the individuals. Adequate reinforcement is needed throughout subsequent encounters. Education is an essential step that helps the individuals understand and live with their disease, but also assists in educating patient's contacts at home, at school, and in the community about these conditions. Currently, a variety of sources of information are available through the Internet, ranging from medical research and therapeutic trials and the Crohn's & Colitis Foundation of America to alternative medicine to bulletin boards for patients and families. The depth and topics vary from those suited for health care providers to those appropriate for lay people.

Care Givers

A caring sympathetic doctor has a positive influence and creates a sense of confidence at a time when many families are undergoing significant stress and strain. Patients and their families need to be taken care of and viewed as whole individuals. Inflammatory bowel disease has an effect that goes beyond the gastrointestinal tract and beyond the individual patient, especially in pediatric patients in whom nutrition, growth, and development can become significantly affected by these diseases. Secondarily, self-image and self-confidence concepts become important issues in the management of pediatric patients. Body image in childhood and adolescence is discussed in a separate chapter.

In the case of children with IBD, particular attention must be given to maintain the sense of dignity and privacy of patients; this is vital in younger children as well as adolescents. Discussion of some topics, such as elimination, can be particularly embarrassing, but at the same time is extremely important to provide the adequate care they need. They should be approached in a direct and objective fashion. There are many questions and concerns about areas of day-to-day living that are equally of concern to them. Sometimes, it is necessary to understand clues about areas and topics patients are afraid to bring up. That is one of the important functions of support systems. Children and families can develop a sense of isolation when faced with the diagnosis of IBD. In addition, it may be simply embarrassing for them to discuss this with friends, extended families, and school contacts.

It is important to understand that the impact of IBD on the everyday life of patients goes beyond the complaints of abdominal pain and diarrhea. The interest and concern of the care giver foster a positive relationship that enhances the compliance of the patient with the recommended therapy. Compliance is essential for the long-term management of IBD. Patients need to be motivated to follow their medical regimes when they begin to feel well to decrease the likelihood of a relapse, and patients need to remain motivated to comply with recommendations even if there is partial response to therapy or in spite of side effects of medications.

Comprehensive Care

A team approach is the most successful way to intervene with patients diagnosed with IBD. Input from nutritionists, nursing specialists, psychologists, and social services is essential to complete the care and management of these children and their families.

Support Groups

The role of support groups is tremendous for patients and families with IBD; these may include other people with IBD, who are able to share similar experiences, or individuals close to the families. In general, the size and or composition of the group depends on the level of comfort of the families. Support groups also become a forum for the education of newly diagnosed patients. They have the opportunity to relate to other individuals sharing a similar experience who can understand the problems they currently are facing. These peers become models for their adaptation to life with a chronic disease. Support groups can range from chat rooms and message boards on the Internet to a group of a few individuals in an informal setting to more formally structured groups. There is a separate chapter on support groups.

A comprehensive approach that integrates support systems along with medical interventions is important to ensure the adjustment that is essential for the patient's compliance with therapeutic regimes to control IBD activity.

Children

There are several issues to take into consideration, including age of onset, severity of symptoms, developmental state, and degree of disruption of day-to-day activities when dealing with children with IBD. Understanding the cognitive and psychological development of children assists in communicating with the patients to help them in the coping process, and this cognitive stage will determine the best approach regarding education about IBD.

Feelings of guilt, helplessness, and fear are natural and vary according to chronologic age. Younger children of age 7 years or less interpret the disease and all related procedures as a punishment for wrongdoing. Children are exposed to a variety of new interactions, including doctors' visits, tests of several varieties, and even more invasive procedures, including hospitalizations and surgery. In addition, their privacy is constantly invaded. Every effort should be made to carefully protect the privacy of every patient. All of these cause significant anxiety, which increases with the outpatient care, as children do not understand the concept of chronic illnesses. Young children do not have a clear concept of death, and this may become an underlying fear that they have difficulty verbalizing. Children between 7 and 10 years view disease as a result of germs and become increasingly concerned about these. They focus more on their appearance and ability to perform activities. Impairments on any of these will profoundly affect their self-esteem.

Separation from family and peers is another important issue for younger children. All of these issues can lead to regressive behavior as a coping mechanism. Children should receive information appropriate for their intellectual capacity. They should be encouraged to talk about their disease, and professional help through nursing specialists, counselors, or psychologists is useful in the process of education and coping.

Children should be encouraged to participate in age-appropriate activities, including school attendance and sports participation. Physicians will make specific recommendations if limitation of activities is needed for limited time periods. It is beneficial for children to maintain age-appropriate contacts and to maintain a sense of normal life as much as possible. Unhealthy adaptive patterns may become manifested as externalizing or internalizing behaviors.

Adolescent Experience

Multiple issues affect the adolescent patient with IBD. Issues related to achievement of independence, identity, sexuality, and becoming indistinguishable from peers are threatened by the constant reminders of a chronic disease. These facts markedly affect their compliance with therapy and their ability to achieve age-appropriate goals. A goal for adolescent patients with IBD is a progressive transfer of more responsibility concerning their care. The process should advance under adequate but not overzealous or lax supervision. On the other hand, adolescents have a more complete cognitive understanding of their disease, as they progress in their understanding of abstract concepts. Sexuality and body image issues are discussed in another chapter.

Parent

The adjustments of the child and of the family unit are closely intermingled. Having a child diagnosed with a chronic medical disease causes turmoil in a family unit. Multiple anxieties and fears develop and cause strains in parents and siblings. Effective communication patterns and family involvement are positive factors in the mutual adjustment process. Enmeshment, rejection, and over-protectiveness are counterproductive for both families and patients; however, they are commonly seen patterns. A multidisciplinary intervention is an effective means to achieve healthy adaptive patterns for the family.

It is common for parents to develop a sense of isolation that is greatly relieved once they communicate with other families affected by IBD. Unfounded feelings of guilt and helplessness should be dispersed with adequate education about the disease. Other particular concerns from the parental standpoint are the financial effects of the disease in the short and long term, especially if there is need for a parent to stay at home, costs of medications and tests, etc. In addition, the effect of a chronic disease on long-term insurance coverage procurement is a current concern of many families. Education is a process that continues throughout all of the physicians' interactions with patients and their families. It is essential for families to be well informed, interested, and motivated to know about IBD.

Support Systems

It is essential for patients and families to establish connections beyond the health care providers to assist in the adjustment and coping process. Each family should decide the type of support group best suited for their circumstances. These may include other families with IBD. Support groups composed by IBD patients and families provide a setting in which newly diagnosed families can talk to peers. These groups become sources of information on day-to-day living activities that families may not feel comfortable discussing with doctors. These groups provide models for coping with IBD in eveyday life.

Formal meetings, telephone conversations, or even computer interactions have allowed the integration of individuals in a variety of support groups, with the goal of helping them live with IBD. There are support networks intended specifically for pediatric patients and their families. In addition, there are materials intended for children that are particularly beneficial. Since the coping skills of patients and their families are dynamic and change with time and circumstances, they must be continually reviewed to identify maladaptive patterns.

Conclusion

The diagnosis of a chronic IBD can be devastating for patients and families. They are faced with an overwhelming challenge that initially may threaten the foundations of their stability as individuals and families. Physicians play a key role in educating patients, families, and communities. Through compassion, kindness, and the use of a supporting and caring network system integrating families, health care providers, and community resources, patients can manage not only to get by but to live normal, fulfilling lives. The ultimate goal for children with IBD is to learn to live with IBD. Education, multidisciplinary interventions, and the developments in the medical field allow for a positive outlook on the quality of life of children with IBD and their families.

Supplemental Reading

Bayless TM. Current management of inflammatory bowel disease. 3rd Ed. Toronto: B.C. Decker Inc., 1989:305–23.

Benkov KJ, Winter HC. Managing your child's Crohn's disease or ulcerative colitis. Master Media, 1996.

Eiser C. The psychology of childhood illness. New York: Springer Verlag, 1985:60–80.

Hanauer S. Inflammatory bowel disease: a guide for patients and their families. Philadelphia: Lippincott Raven, 1998.

Hugel K. Young people and chronic illness. Free Spirit, 1998.

Lansdown R. Children in hospital: a guide for families and carers. Oxford: Oxford University Press, 1996:48–9.

Mullen BD, McGinn KA. The ostomy book: living comfortably with colostomies, ileostomies, and urostomies. Bull Publishing, 1992.

Northam EA. Psychosocial impact of chronic illness in children. J Paediatr Child Health 1997;33:369–72.

Polito JM II, Childs B, Mellits ED, et al. Crohn's disease: influence of age at diagnosis on site and clinical type of disease. Gastroenterology 1996;111:580–6.

Pope A, McHale S, Craighead WE. Self-esteem enhancement with children and adolescents. New York: Pergamon, 1988.

Steiner-Grossman P. The new people...not patients: a source book for living with inflammatory bowel disease. Revised Ed. New York: Crohn's and Colitis Foundation of America, Inc., 1997.

Thompson JR, Gustafson KE. Adaptation to chronic childhood illness. Washington, DC: American Psychological Association, 1996.

Vernon D, et al. Psychological responses of children to hospitalization and illness. Springfield, IL: Charles C. Thomas, 8–58.

Other Sources

Crohn's & Colitis Foundation of America, Inc.
386 Park Avenue South, 17th Floor
New York, NY 10016-8804
Tel: 800 932-2423 or 212 685-3440
e-mail: info@ccfa.org.
<www.ccfa.org>

National Digestive Diseases Information Clearinghouse
2 Information Way
Bethesda, MD 20892-3570
E-mail: nddic@info.niddk.nih.gov

Pediatric Crohn's and Colitis Association, Inc.
P.O. Box 188 Newton, MA 02168
Tel: 617 244-6678

Reach Out for Youth with Ileitis and Colitis, Inc.
15 Chemung Place
Jericho, NY 11753
Tel: 516 822-8010

United Ostomy Association, Inc.
36 Executive Park Suite 120
Irvine, CA 92714
Tel: 800 826-0826 or 714 660-8624

CHAPTER 116

Nutritional Consultation and Guidance

Allen L. Ginsberg, MD

The etiology and pathogenesis of ulcerative colitis and Crohn's disease are poorly understood. The reason that people who develop these disorders develop symptoms when they do is not understood. Therefore, it is only natural that patients and physicians alike would attempt to control and even cure inflammatory bowel disease (IBD) through dietary measures. This chapter focuses on issues that commonly arise during patient visits. There are other chapters on nutrition and IBD as well as a chapter on alternative health approaches.

A brief computer Web search for colitis diets reveals advertisements for such books as the "Colitis Cookbook" and the "Culinary Couples Creative Cookbook." Well-meaning warnings can be found to avoid "foods that kill," such as aspartame, sugar, fats, refined foods, processed foods, fried foods, smoked foods, meat, and cheese. There are proponents of low-carbohydrate diets, high-carbohydrate diets, Atkins diets, protein power diets, anabolic diets, high-fiber diets, and low-fiber diets. There is even a detailed diet cure for ulcerative colitis that begins with a "juice fast" limiting oral intake to dilute papaya juice or raw cabbage and carrot juice, with strict admonition to avoid citrus. Gradually, an unconventional diet with numerous restrictions is added.

Ulcerative Colitis

Unfortunately, there is no good evidence to suggest that ulcerative colitis is caused by diet. Bowel rest alone, with total parenteral nutrition, elemental diet, or even diverting ostomy, will decrease the number of bowel movements but does not result in bowel healing or disease remission. Thus, diet manipulation does not play a primary role in the management of patients with ulcerative colitis.

Athough there is no such thing as a "colitis diet," many patients do have individual dietary idiosyncrasies. Any food that repeatedly produces unpleasant gastrointestinal symptoms or aggravates the symptoms of IBD should be avoided. It makes no sense, however, to tell Mrs. Jones what Mr. Smith cannot eat. Just because Mr. Smith cannot tolerate spicy foods, tomatoes, or alcohol does not mean that these items will produce symptoms in Mrs. Jones. It is bad enough to have to live with a chronic premalignant disease of unknown cause without also having physicians imposing restrictive diets that have no proven benefit or scientific basis. There is a separate chapter on dietary considerations in ulcerative colitis including a discussion of short-chain fatty acids.

Crohn's Disease

In contrast to ulcerative colitis, dietary and luminal factors may play a role in initiating and perpetuating Crohn's disease activity. Both total parenteral nutrition and enteral nutrition with an elemental diet have been shown to control disease activity in up to 75 percent of patients with active, uncomplicated Crohn's disease (Greenberg et al, 1988). In some studies, these approaches have been found to be as efficacious as corticosteroids in inducing remission. There are other chapters on nutrition and Crohn's disease in both adults and children.

Although induction of disease remission using parenteral nutrition or elemental diets can be readily accomplished, the identification of specific dietary triggering factors that must be avoided poses a daunting challenge. Patients with partial bowel obstruction will have symptoms of pain triggered by eating almost any solid food. When disease is clinically active, almost any food passing through inflamed bowel may produce cramping pain or diarrhea. In contrast, when the disease is in complete remission and the bowel is healed, if a dietary factor is responsible for inflammation, repeated exposure may be necessary to produce enough inflammation to produce symptoms.

Exclusion Diets

It is possible that in a small subset of patients with Crohn's disease, elimination of specific dietary antigens may allow control of disease activity. In a 1989 report (Ginsberg and Albert), a patient with severe steroid-dependent Crohn's disease was described in whom total remission was induced with a nonelemental formula diet of known composition (Ensure Plus®, Ross Division, Abbott Laboratories, Abbott Park, Illinois). Corticosteroids were withdrawn and laboratory studies, including sedimentation rate, returned to normal. Food challenges revealed that milk precipitated disease activity and a strict milk-free diet maintained clinical and laboratory remission without any medications for over 5 years. Jones et al (1985), in uncontrolled studies, claimed that exclusion diets allowed 51 of 77 patients to maintain remission for up to 51 months.

Specific Dietary Measures

In a 1999 study (Riordan et al), there was a lower rate of relapse in patients on an elimination diet (62%) than in those tapered off prednisone (79%). However, in another study (Pearson et al, 1993), rechallenges with offending foods could be confirmed in only 25 percent of patients. It is not warranted to put all patients on elimination diets.

Although dietary manipulation with exclusion or other diets cannot cure or prevent relapses in ulcerative colitis and are useful for only a small minority of patients with Crohn's disease, some specific dietary measures are useful for individual patients with both disorders. Anything that can aggravate symptoms, such as lactose intolerance, should be addressed.

Lactose

It can be revealing to have patients avoid milk, cheese, and ice cream for 10 days and then challenge themselves with a cheese pizza and a milk shake to determine if lactose intolerance is contributing to symptoms.

Fiber

Some patients with colitis limited to the rectosigmoid colon find that the addition of fiber in the form of psyllium or bran is helpful. This is especially true of patients who tend toward constipation or who have irritable bowel syndrome in addition to IBD. Other patients, especially those with chronic left-sided disease and some patients with Crohn's disease, find that fiber, including fresh fruit and vegetables, aggravates their symptoms, perhaps because more fecal material must pass through the inflamed or narrowed intestine. Although no data are available, patients with Crohn's disease with strictures ought to avoid corn, popcorn, raw broccoli, cauliflower, water chestnuts, and spaghetti squash, which potentially can block the narrowed lumen. The role of fiber supplements or the need for a low-fiber diet can best be evaluated in the individual patient by trial and error.

Specific Nutrients

Nutritionally complete well-balanced diets are appropriate. Specific vitamins and minerals deserve mention.

Potassium

Patients treated with corticosteroids often require potassium supplements because of loss of potassium in stool and urine. Bananas, raisins, and orange and tomato juice offer rich sources of potassium.

Calcium and Vitamin D

There is an increased incidence of osteoporosis in patients with Crohn's disease. Corticosteroids and avoidance of milk products further contribute to osteoporosis seen in IBD. Oral calcium supplements are appropriate. In addition, calcium should be combined with vitamin D and biophosphonate (Actonel®, Procter & Gamble Pharmaceuticals, Cincinnati, Ohio, or Fosamax®, Merck, West Point, New Jersey) therapy in patients treated for prolonged periods with corticosteroids. There is a separate chapter on osteopenia and osteoporosis.

Iron

Iron deficiency anemia is common in IBD, and iron supplementation may be required. However, oral iron can be poorly tolerated and can result in severe cramping in patients with active Crohn's disease. Some patients inappropriately have been given corticosteroid therapy for cramps caused by oral iron preparations. The chapters on hematologic complications or extra-intestinal manifestion discuss the therapy of iron deficiency anemia, including use of erythropoietin.

Caloric Supplementation

Patients with IBD may be underweight and malnourished. Laboratory testing may reveal low serum albumin and cholesterol. Enteral dietary supplementation with high-calorie formula products, such as Ensure, may be useful.

Fish Oil

A role for fish oil as an enteric supplement in IBD has been suggested. N-3 fatty acids in fish oil may exert an anti-inflammatory effect by decreasing production of leukotriene B_4 and thromboxane A_2. Two controlled trials in patients with ulcerative colitis have shown a reduction in rectal leukotriene B_4 and a modest steroid-sparing effect (Stenson et al, 1992; Hawthorne et al, 1992). In selected Italian patients with Crohn's disease in clinical remission, a novel enteric-coated fish oil preparation reduced the relapse rate by more than 50 percent compared to placebo (Belluzzi et al, 1996).

References

Belluzzi A, Brignola C, Campieri M, et al. Effect of an enteric-coated fish-oil preparation on relapses in Crohn's disease. N Engl J Med 1996;334:1557–60.

Ginsberg AL, Albert M. Treatment of patient with severe steroid-dependent Crohn's disease with nonelemental formula diet: identification of possible etiologic dietary factor. Dig Dis Sci 1989;34:1624–8.

Editor's Note: There are more details on nutritional aspects of IBD in other chapters in this text. There is also a chapter on alternative medicines and approaches. Growth hormone injections and a high-protein diet were seemingly helpful in a small controlled trial in CD (N Engl J Med 2000). (TMB)

Greenberg GR, Fleming CR, Jeejeebhoy KN, et al. Controlled trial of bowel rest and nutritional support in the management of Crohn's disease. Gut 1988;29:1309–15.

Hawthorne AB, Daneshmend TK, Hawkey CJ, et al. Treatment of ulcerative colitis with fish oil supplementation: a prospective 12 month randomised controlled trial. Gut 1992;33:922–8.

Jones VA, Dickinson RJ, Workman E, et al. Crohn's disease: maintenance of remission by diet. Lancet 1985;2:177–80.

Pearson M, Teahon K, Levi AJ, Bjarnason I. Food intolerance and Crohn's disease. Gut 1993;34:783–7.

Riordan AM, Hunter JO, Cowan RE, et al. Treatment of active Crohn's disease by exclusion diet: East Anglian multicentre controlled trial. Lancet 1993;342:1131–4.

Stenson WF, Cort D, Rodgers J, et al. Dietary supplementation with fish oil in ulcerative colitis. Ann Intern Med 1992; 116:609–14

Supplemental Reading

Griffiths AM, Ohlsson A, Sherman PM, Sutherland LR. Meta-analysis of enteral nutrition as a primary treatment of active Crohn's disease. Gastroenterology 1995;108:1056–6.

Kelly DG, Fleming CR. Nutritional considerations in inflammatory bowel diseases. Gastroenterol Clin North Am 1995;24:597–611.

Lewis JD, Fisher RL. Nutrition support in inflammatory bowel disease. Med Clin North Am 1994;78:1443–56.

CHAPTER 117

QUESTIONS FREQUENTLY ASKED OF A SUPPORT SERVICE

ALETHEA TRINKAUS, MPH

Today, more than ever, people are becoming educated about inflammatory bowel disease (IBD) and questioning their medical treatment. Whether they are the patient, the partner, or parent of a patient, ultimately, they are seeking to better understand the disease and what they can do to help fight it.

In this age of the Internet, patients are searching for the most recent and reliable information available. However, not all IBD-related Websites offer information grounded in scientific fact, and patients can come across potentially harmful misinformation. The Crohn's & Colitis Foundation of America, Inc. (CCFA) is the only foundation dedicated to providing patients, their families, and their friends with the most accurate and up-to-date information on Crohn's disease and ulcerative colitis. Since the launch of the CCFA Website (*http://www.ccfa.org*), just 3 years ago, the number of patient phone calls and e-mails has skyrocketed, providing a clear picture of what patients want to know and the confusion that still exists regarding these diseases.

In recent years, patient questions have become increasingly focused and detailed, often questioning their physician's choice of treatment. All of the foundation's literature is reviewed by its medical advisors, but it is important to know that there are no physicians on staff and the foundation is unable to provide medical advice or opinions. Questions relating to dosages, medical opinions, and so on always are referred back to the treating physician.

Following are some of the questions that CCFA receives daily from patients all over the world and the responses given to these questions.

How Did I Get This Disease?

This is the most frequently asked question and one of the toughest to answer. Currently, the origin of Crohn's disease and ulcerative colitis is unknown. Research has made great strides in understanding the factors believed to contribute to the cause of IBD. A complex interaction of genetic susceptibility, an overactive immune response system, and environmental factors have come to the forefront of research. Researchers now believe that the cause is probably not just one factor but a combination of factors.

What we *are* certain of is that IBD is *not* caused by stress or nerves. Even today, many believe that Crohn's disease and ulcerative colitis are "nervous diseases." This may be attributable, in large part, to the confusion of the differences between irritable bowel syndrome (IBS), which for years has been referred to as "colitis" ("spastic colitis" or "mucous colitis") and IBD. The use of the word colitis at diagnosis often causes confusion for a patient who finds out that the word is used to describe different diseases. Actually, IBS is not a *true* colitis; it is a functional disorder, stemming from a hyperreactive muscular component of the bowel. In contrast, IBD is a chronic disorder, causing structural damage to the bowel wall. Much of the confusion may be avoided by a simple change in the terminology. The foundation receives calls each day from patients who do not know what "type of colitis" they have or assume that IBS and IBD are the same condition. The CCFA refers IBS patients to the International Foundation for Functional Gastrointestinal Disorders, located in Milwaukee, Wisconsin (Tel: 888 964-2001).

What Is the Difference Between Crohn's Disease and Ulcerative Colitis?

Many patients call wanting to know the differences between Crohn's disease and ulcerative colitis. Aside from mailing literature and providing the Website address, we also try to explain some of the basic differences.

Crohn's disease is an inflammation of the lining of the intestine that can occur anywhere from the mouth to the rectum, but most often occurs in the lower part of the small intestine (ileum) and large intestine (colon). With Crohn's disease, all layers of the intestine are involved, and there often are patches of healthy bowel between patches of diseased bowel. There is no known cure for Crohn's disease.

Ulcerative colitis also is an inflammation of the lining of the intestine, but is limited to the large intestine (colon) and affects only the innermost lining (mucosa) of the intestinal wall in a continuous manner. The "cure" for ulcerative colitis is a proctocolectomy (removal of the colon and rectum). Unlike Crohn's disease, which can recur after surgery, ulcerative colitis does not recur once the colon is removed.

Is There a Specific Diet I Should Follow?

Patients often are frustrated when their physician does not provide them with a specific diet. Many are confused when their physician tells them to eat "whatever they want." We try to explain that each person's disease is individual; what one can tolerate another cannot, and they must learn their tolerance to foods on a trial-and-error basis. Along with literature, we provide patients with some general nutritional rules they may find helpful.

Many patients with IBD, to some degree, are lactose intolerant and will need to monitor their consumption of foods containing lactose. Patients should avoid popcorn and any type of nut, as these may cause obstruction. We also explain that they may find it difficult to digest foods high in fiber, such as raw fruits and vegetables, and that a low-fiber diet *may* help decrease symptoms and pain. Although patients would prefer to be given a cookbook with recipes, they are usually receptive to these general guidelines and are grateful to know that there are several articles on nutrition under "Diet, Nutrition, and Fitness," in the Library on the CCFA Website.

How Does Stress Affect My Disease?

Although stress is not known to be the cause of IBD, it will tend to exacerbate it and may possibly cause a flare. Many patients say that when their stress increases, they tend to flare, and if they are able to keep their emotions under control, their symptoms seem to lessen. Of course, stress cannot be completely avoided, but understanding the relation between the two is important. Often, patients just need to hear that they did not do anything to cause their disease.

Everyone chooses different ways to decrease their stress levels. Often, becoming involved in a local chapter of the CCFA or a support group, or entering an on-line IBD chat group, such as those found under "Links" on the CCFA Website, allows patients to share their experiences, find support, and know that they are not alone.

Is There a Genetic Component to This Disease and Will My Children Get It?

The world of genetics research in IBD is moving so quickly that it is often difficult to keep up. The genetic aspect of IBD is more complicated than most genetic disorders, and researchers are racing to discover the genes that determine whether one is likely to develop IBD. Although a large percentage of patients do not have any relatives with IBD, research has shown IBD to have a genetic component. The differences in the frequency of disease among ethnic groups and studies performed on families in which IBD is prevalent are two of the ways this is shown. American Jews of European descent are four to five times more likely to develop IBD than the general population. Several studies have found that the average *actual* risk to a first-degree relative of a patient with IBD is approximately 2 to 6 percent. This increases significantly if both parents suffer from Crohn's disease or ulcerative colitis. There is a chapter on genetics and IBD in this text.

The CCFA has participated in a series of International IBD Genetics Workshops held since 1997. One of the foundation's initiatives in IBD genetics research is the development of the DNA and Cell Line Bank, which will collect and store a large number of DNA samples from a number of well-characterized patients. This bank will act as a resource for researchers across the country.

Are There Alternative Therapies That I Can Try?

Not surprisingly, this is quickly becoming one of the most frequently asked questions. Patients are concerned not only about the immediate side effects of their medications but also about the long-term effects. Most patients need to understand that, with a few exceptions, most of the medications used to treat IBD have been around for a while and have a proven track record. The long-term effects of new medications, such as Remicade® (Centocor Inc., Malvern, Pennsylvania), are not yet known, but the CCFA explains that, with the help of their gastroenterologist, patients can make an informed decision about their treatment.

However, patients are becoming more and more willing to explore alternative therapies, and there are many to choose from. The CCFA refers to them as adjunct therapies, because whatever a patient would like to try must be checked by their gastroenterologist and must be used in conjunction with their traditional therapy. Many believe that herbal, holistic, or natural therapies cannot be harmful. Usually out of frustration, patients consider abandoning their traditional therapy completely and trying a herb someone has recommended. They do this without realizing that they may be doing more harm than good. The CCFA explains that the decision is theirs to make and general literature is on the Website, but they should always consult with their physician before making any changes. The chapter on alternative medications and approaches provides more information on this subject.

Will I Develop Colon Cancer?

Some patients seem to be less concerned that they have Crohn's disease or ulcerative colitis and more concerned with their chances of developing cancer. It is important for them to understand that the majority of patients with IBD never develop colorectal cancer. Depending on the extent of their disease and the length of time they have had it, there is a small risk, which increases over time. Fewer than 5 percent of patients with ulcerative colitis develop colon cancer and even fewer patients with Crohn's disease do so. The CCFA tells patients that, after having the disease for 8 to 10 years, it is critical that, they stay in contact with their gastroenterologist and be periodically screened (usually every 1 to 2 yr). Studies are ongoing as to when patients should be screened, how often, and the type of screening procedure that should be performed. We stress that this is one of the most preventable types of cancer and is one of the most curable when detected early. The CCFA has good information on cancer in IBD in the Library section of the Website. There are four chapters on dysplasia and colon cancer in ulcerative colitis and in Crohn's disease in this edition.

I Am Having Problems With Insurance, What Can I Do?

There are several situations a patient with IBD may encounter when it comes to insurance problems, and none of them are easy. It is important for a patient to be as well educated as possible about his or her situation and rights. The CCFA Website has informative articles in the Library, under "Medical Central." Insurance laws differ from state to state; patients should contact their State Insurance Commissioner's Office for additional information and assistance. The Website of the National Association of Insurance Commissioners is *http://www.naic.org*. The chapter on insurance and patient advocacy issues provide specific information (Chapter 118).

Editor's Note

Our purpose for including this important chapter is to highlight for the physicians and nurses, as well as support groups, the unanswered questions your patients may have when they leave your office. Those issues should be addressed either directly or by personally pointing out the answers in a brochure or by referring patients to a Website. (TMB)

Supplemental Reading

Stein SH, Rood, RP. Inflammatory bowel disease: a guide for patients and their families. New York: CCFA/Lippincott, Williams & Wilkins, 1999.

Steiner-Grossman P, Banks PA, Present DH. The new people . . . not patients: a source book for living with inflammatory bowel disease. Iowa: CCFA/Kendall Hunt Publishing, 1992.

Other Sources

Crohn's & Colitis Foundation of America, Inc. Website: *http://www.ccfa.org*.

Brochures available free of charge:
Questions and Answers about Ulcerative Colitis
Questions and Answers about Crohn's Disease
Questions and Answers about Diet and Nutrition
Questions and Answers about Emotional Factors

International Foundation for Functional Gastrointestinal Disorders (IFFGD)
P.O. Box 17864
Milwaukee, WI 53217
414 964-1799
888 964-2001
Fax: 414 964-7176
http://www.iffgd.org

National Association for Insurance Commissioners Regional and State Offices
http://www.naic.org/

National Digestive Disease Information Clearinghouse (NDDIC)
2 Information Way
Bethesda, MD 20892-3570
301 654-3810
Fax: 301 907-8906
http://www.niddk.nih.gov

United Ostomy Association, Inc. (UOA)
19772 MacArthur Blvd., Suite 200
Irvine, CA 92612-2405
800 826-0826
Fax: 949 660-9262
http://www.uoa.org

CHAPTER 118

INSURANCE AND DISABILITY ADVOCACY ISSUES IN INFLAMMATORY BOWEL DISEASE

DOUGLAS C. WOLF, MD

There are approximately 1 million patients with inflammatory bowel disease (IBD) in the United States. Whereas good data do not exist on the number of individuals with IBD who are uninsured, the numbers are significant. It is estimated that there are 44.3 million uninsured Americans in a population of approximately 225 million. This provides an approximation of 16.3 percent of the population of the United States being uninsured. Some patients with IBD are insured but, because of preexisting condition exclusions, do not have insurance that covers the IBD. It is estimated that there are 25 million insured individuals with preexisting medical conditions. Others, who have insurance, may have high deductibles such that the insurance is basically "catastrophic coverage" and are underinsured as a result. Although full disability in the IBD population is unusual, certain levels of partial disability are more common. There is little agreement on what constitutes disability in IBD, in part because it often appears to be a hidden disability, but objective criteria do exist. The following is a summary on the subject of insurance and disability issues in the IBD population with emphasis on how physicians can be better advocates for their patients with IBD. The key to being a good advocate is to be knowledgeable about the issues and to be able to offer facts and guidance to patients with their many insurance and disability-related issues.

Vulnerable Age Peak

The peak age of onset of Crohn's disease and ulcerative colitis coincides with the peak distribution of the uninsured population. Of the uninsured population, 15.4 percent are under 18 years of age. Over 50 percent of the uninsured population are between the ages of 18 and 34 years. Individuals between the ages of 18 and 23 may continue on their parent's health insurance if they are true dependents (ie, living in their home) or if they maintain full-time student (college) status. This can vary depending on the wording of the particular plan. Parents should understand the coverage options of their particular policy prior to their child's eighteenth birthday. Many individuals leave home at this age, and their jobs may not offer insurance or other related benefits. It is easily understandable how one's health coverage can lapse. Once it lapses, it can be difficult reestablishing health care cover-

age. There may be a 12-month delay for coverage of preexisting conditions. If one is taking an individual health insurance policy, there is no guarantee of acceptance, and no limit established on the policy premium.

New Health Insurance Policies

When a patient with IBD requests coverage with a new individual health insurance policy, it is likely that they will be turned down. Key to this determination is the status of the patient's disease. A patient with no hospitalizations over the past 3 years may qualify but likely would pay a higher rate. A patient with multiple hospitalizations within the last year or so likely would be denied coverage. When coverage is obtained, the risk-adjusted premium may amount to several multiples of a standard policy rate. The insurance company wants to avoid any situation in which it is likely to lose money. An insurance agent or broker can help a patient find the best rate. Although insurance consultants are available to make recommendations, these individuals may charge an hourly rate or other fee, and this should be understood.

Changing Employment

When a patient has an active or chronic medical condition, it is usually best to be employed by a company that provides major benefits. The most valuable major benefit is group health insurance. If one works for a company with more than 20 employees, then group coverage generally applies. It would seem acceptable to work for a lower wage, if otherwise unavailable benefits became available as part of the compensation package. Self-employed individuals should contact trade groups, associations, the local Chamber of Commerce, or other groups that may offer group health programs.

Increasingly, in this day and age, employees change jobs and do not stay with the same employer "for life." As a result, transitional insurance programs are needed. Short-term health policies and conversion options exist, and they can be engaged for 6 months, possibly with one renewal option. Preexisting conditions may be excluded. If one is leaving employment and there is a lapse prior to reemployment, a group medical plan can be converted to an individual plan, for which the full premium is paid.

The Consolidated Omnibus Budget Reconciliation Act (COBRA) of 1985 represented the first national employer mandate to address the portability problems associated with the loss of employment-related health insurance. Often, a COBRA option can be exercised, whereby the group coverage is maintained for the period between jobs, and the premium is 102 percent of the basic coverage cost. Under COBRA, continuation of coverage for a period of 18 months can be exercised if coverage is lost because of a "qualifying event," such as voluntary or involuntary employment termination. If the qualifying event is family related, such as the divorce, legal separation, or death of an insured worker, then coverage is offered for 36 months. The option to continue coverage must be exercised within 60 days of the qualifying event. Certain conditions must be met before an employer is required to offer COBRA coverage. Any company with a group insurance plan and 20 or more full-time or part-time employees during 50 percent of the business days in the preceding year must offer continuous coverage following a qualifying event.

In August 1996, the Kassenbaum-Kennedy Health Insurance Reform Bill was passed and became known as the Health Insurance Portability and Accountability Act (HIPAA). The impact of HIPAA is broad in scope, but its primary function is to provide continuity in health care coverage when one changes jobs. Its major provision is to prevent gaps in coverage that could expose individuals to preexisting condition exclusions. Although HIPAA applies to those in both group and individual health care plans, the requirements for those desiring individual coverage are more stringent than for those wanting to enter the group market. It has no impact on the uninsured, the unemployed, or on health insurance cost. Nonetheless, it allows portability of a health care plan when one changes, leaves, or loses his or her job, and this is an important benefit for anyone with a chronic illness, such as a patient with IBD.

Under HIPAA, if one loses or leaves a job but has been continuously insured for the previous 12 months, one can purchase an individual insurance policy. Every insurer must offer two policy options, and exclusions for preexisting conditions have been severely curtailed. Key HIPAA provisions include no ineligibility for health-related status, same rates for those with and without medical problems, and continuity for preexisting conditions.

Whereas the details of HIPAA may seem complicated, the general message is clear. Patients changing jobs should obtain details about how HIPAA may apply to them and their families. A certificate of coverage needs to be obtained from the previous employer. This hopefully will lessen the occurrence of "job lock," where one is afraid to change jobs because of fear of losing health care coverage.

Managed Care

The majority of health plans currently offered are managed care plans. These plans, offered by most major insurers, attempt to manage cost of care. Plans may limit access to care, particularly subspecialty access, by limiting covered services or may limit other services, such as certain prescription drug coverage. Choice of physician is often restricted, as is choice of hospital. The restrictions can have a significant impact on the patient with IBD. Whereas prescription drug coverage often is provided, a particular brand may not be on the managed care formulary. A telephone call or letter to the medical director may be needed to obtain approval for the use of nonformulary medication.

Benefits Programs

Medicare

Patients who are 65 years of age or older, or those who have received Social Security Disability Insurance benefits for 2 years, are eligible for Medicare. Medicare is made up of Part A, which covers inpatient care or other facility care, and Part B, which covers physician care and several other services and some supplies that Part A does not cover.

In a standard Medicare policy, medications are not covered services on an outpatient basis, with the exception of some infusion medications, which require nursing administration. The only current example is infliximab.

Medicare Managed Care (Health Management Organization [HMO]) policies currently are available, and although some of these have offered prescription drug coverage (a benefit valuable to all recipients, but especially IBD patients), prescription drug coverage is being offered less often, because of the added expense. Physician choice and other features also are restricted in Medicare Managed Care.

Medicaid

Medicaid is a state-run program for patients with low income and limited resources. Medicaid programs often service the pediatric population with chronic illnesses such as IBD. For information about Medicaid eligibility in your state, contact the welfare office, which may have a specific name, such as Department of Family and Children Services. Many states also are funding insurance coverage for children through the Children Health Insurance Program Services (CHIPS) legislation. This insurance provides coverage for children of low-income parents who do not qualify for Medicaid.

High-Risk Insurance Pools

High-risk insurance pools provide coverage to people who are unable to obtain private health insurance because of a preexisting condition, such as Crohn's disease or ulcerative colitis. People who do not have insurance available through their place of employment typically use this. Not all states offer high-risk insurance pools. Every state has its own criteria for eligibility and these vary from state to state. The following are usual requirements:

- proof of ineligibility for Medicare or Medicaid
- proof that you were rejected by a private insurer
- proof of your inability to obtain coverage comparable to that offered by the state plan

To determine if this is available in your state, one should call the State Department of Insurance or the National Association for Insurance Commissioners at 816 842-3600.

Family and Medical Leave

Patients and family members of patients with IBD should be aware of the Family and Medical Leave Act (FMLA). Employers covered by the FMLA must, pursuant to a written company policy, give an eligible employee the right to take unpaid leave for up to 12 work weeks in a year if his own medical condition or that of a family member makes him unable to perform his job. To be eligible, the employee must:

- have worked for this employer for at least 12 months
- have completed at least 1,250 hours of service during the previous year
- work at a site within a 75-mile radius of 50 employees of the company

The following are qualifying criteria for a chronic condition such as IBD:

- Requires periodic hospital visits for treatment
- Continues over an extended period of time
- May cause episodic rather than continuous incapacity

The law protects any employee from being disciplined or discharged for requesting or using FMLA leave. A patient who is experiencing a flare-up or a family member who is providing support or comfort to a patient may take leave. If the leave is foreseeable, 30 days notice must be given. If the leave is unforeseeable, then 2 working days notice is needed. The employee may be responsible for paying 100 percent of his or her medical insurance premiums while on leave, depending on an employer's written FMLA policy. Although FMLA protects most employees, "key employees," who are exempt from overtime laws and are among the highest paid, may be subject to certain qualifications at the time of their job restoration.

Disability Programs

Social Security Disability Benefits

If a patient's IBD has progressed so that it seems unlikely that the patient will be able to continue to work or function for a sustained period, then an application to the Social Security Administration is appropriate. Patients can get applications for Social Security Disability from

TABLE 118–1. Listing of Impairments: Chronic Ulcerative or Granulomatous Colitis (5.06)

A. Recurrent bloody stools documented on repeated examinations and anemia manifested by hematocrit of 30% or less on repeated examinations; or

B. Persistent or recurrent systemic manifestations, such as arthritis, iritis, fever, or liver dysfunction, not attributable to other causes; or

C. Intermittent obstruction due to intractable abscess, fistula formation, or stenosis; or

D. Recurrences of findings of A, B, or C above after total colectomy; or

E. Weight loss as described under 5.08 of the Social Security Disability Criteria

the local Social Security Office. Brochures are available and assistance is provided. Social Security offers a toll-free number (800 772-1213) for information, including the location of the nearest Social Security Office. The Website is *http://www.ssa.gov*. The treating physician must submit a report to Social Security, documenting the nature and features of the disability. Reapplication is part of the process, and the greatest frequency of approval occurs upon repeated reapplication, when the case is presented at a hearing before a Social Security Administrative law judge. Although an initial application may be initiated by the patient or family, reapplications are most successful if the assistance of a disability attorney or related professional is sought.

There are two ways in which the application of a patient with IBD may be approved. The first way is when criteria are met or exceeded in the "Listing of Impairments." Table 118–1 lists the necessary impairments in chronic ulcerative or granulomatous colitis and Table 118–2 lists the necessary impairments in Crohn's ileitis or regional enteritis. Criteria for disability based on weight and laboratory values are more lengthy and necessitate review of the "Listing of Impairments," which may be obtained from the Social Security Office.

The second way disability can be justified is by demonstrating that the symptoms, such as diarrhea, pain, or fatigue, preclude full-time employment. There are no specific criteria for this, and a thorough description of the nature of the symptoms and their ramifications is needed. Proper documentation in the medical record is important since the entire medical record will be

TABLE 118–2. Listing of Impairments: Regional Enteritis (5:07)

A. Persistent or recurrent intestinal obstruction evidenced by abdominal pain, distention, nausea, and vomiting and accompanied by stenotic areas of small bowel with proximal intestinal dilation; or

B. Persistent or recurrent systemic manifestations, such as arthritis, iritis, fever, or liver dysfunction, not attributable to other causes; or

C. Intermittent obstruction due to intractable abscess or fistula formation; or

D. Weight loss as described under 5.08 of the Social Security Disability Criteria

reviewed multiple times. A thorough summary letter is necessary as part of the disability application. It should reflect the level of symptoms and disability contained in the medical record.

Returning to Work after Social Security Disability

Patients who recover from their disability can try to return to work or train for a new career. Increasingly, individual clinical responses to immunotherapy (eg, azathioprine or 6-mercaptopurine), biologic therapy (eg, anti-tumor necrosis factor or infliximab), or surgery are restoring the health of patients with IBD. The Social Security Administration offers work incentives that allow the patient to continue to receive monthly benefits for a set period of time while returning to work or while entering a vocational training program. These programs allow a patient to attempt work reentry and to determine whether they are able to work on a regular basis, without risking or reapplying for benefits. Work incentives differ with Social Security Insurance (SSI) and Social Security Disability Insurance (SSDI). Detailed information is available from the Social Security Administration.

The American Disabilities Act

The American Disabilities Act (ADA) was enacted in 1991 and revised with major amendments in 1995. This federal legislation has implications during the hiring process and throughout employment. Employers may not base their decisions to hire an individual based on their disabilities. Once an employer has knowledge that an employee is disabled, the employer is required under the ADA to provide reasonable accommodations to the affected employee. For an individual with IBD, the accommodations may be relatively simple: more time for necessary visits to the restroom and flexible time schedules for diet or rest. Extra time off may be needed for exacerbations or hospitalizations. Each case depends on a set of variables, and the employee's needs must be balanced by the ability of the employer to provide the requested accommodations.

Education for the Disabled Patient with Inflammatory Bowel Disease

The All Handicapped Children's Act of 1975 guarantees a free public education for all children with disabilities. If a child is unable to attend school because of a disabling chronic illness, home schooling or in-hospital instruction must be provided. This usually is needed for limited periods of time. It is best if students and parents work together with teachers and the school system to help provide this benefit. The Crohn's & Colitis Foundation of America (CCFA) brochure, "A Teacher's Guide to Crohn's Disease and Ulcerative Colitis," is helpful in this dialogue.

The 1973 Rehabilitation Act, Section 504, addresses discrimination in higher education. This ruling covers any program or activity that receives financial assistance from the United States Department of Education, and this includes public school districts, institutions of higher education, and other state and local education agencies. Medical information can be requested only after the student has been accepted to a school and, once obtained, cannot be used to exclude a student from school activities. Additional information can be obtained from the Office for Civil Rights, Department of Health and Human Services, Washington, DC 20201.

Disability Insurance

Individual disability insurance is **difficult to obtain** once a diagnosis of IBD has been made. If insurance is available, a significant surcharge may apply. Group disability insurance is often part of the benefits package of large companies. If one has disability insurance, it is best to maintain it, and this may be possible even when one changes jobs. However, HIPAA and other related legislation applies to health insurance and not to disability or other insurance.

Summary

It is important for the treating physician to be knowledgeable about health care and disability issues to provide the best guidance for all patients with IBD. Some tips for these patients include:

1. If you have health insurance, do not let it lapse.
2. If you do not have health insurance, look into the options available to obtain it.
3. Have regular visits with the doctor, as insurers look favorably on patients who have regular visits, and this will also help you to stay well.
4. Take medication as prescribed, because your condition likely will not improve on its own, even if the use of medication temporarily disallows eligibility to an insurance plan.
5. If possible, choose a job with group insurance and portable benefits.
6. For parents of children with IBD, anticipate their need for modified coverage prior to their eighteenth birthday. Determine with your insurance agent or benefits representative what the best options are for the teenager prior to turning 18 so that no lapse in coverage occurs.

Editor's Note

This is a useful chapter and we are indebted to Dr Wolf for assembling this information. Since staying out of the hospital for 3 years can be one criterion for a patient with IBD to obtain health insurance, albeit at an increased premium, this is another incentive for both physician and patient compliance with long-term remission maintenance programs. This includes adjustments in medications and doses at the onset of relatively minor symptomatic recurrences, before an incapacitating relapse is addressed by hospitalization. (TMB)

Supplemental Reading

Niecko TE, Schafermeyer KW, Martin BC. The Health Insurance Portability and Accountability Act of 1996: the issue of portable health care coverage. J Manage Care Pharma 1999;5:1–8.

Toner R. Why Washington rediscovered the health care crisis. The New York Times, October 10, 1999.

Other Sources

Crohn's & Colitis Foundation of America, Inc. Website. *http://www.ccfa.org/medcentral/library/legal/.* Accessed 10/20/99.

Crohn's & Colitis Foundation of America, Inc.: A teacher's guide to Crohn's disease and ulcerative colitis. [pamphlet]

Social Security Administration, Disability evaluation under Social Security "listing of impairments." Publication #64-039;1998.

United States Department of Education, Office of Civil Rights. Rehabilitation Act of 1973 (Section 504).

CHAPTER 119

SEXUAL ADJUSTMENTS AND BODY IMAGE

Paula Erwin-Toth, MSN, RN, ET, CWOCN, CNS

The effect of inflammatory bowel disease (IBD) on body image, sexuality, and sexual functioning ranges from minor to profound. Physical and psychosexual adjustments depend on the extent and progress of the disease, side effects of medications, and individual variables. No one responds to a chronic illness in exactly the same way; however, there are some interventions the physicians and health care professionals caring for these patients can implement to assist patients facing difficulties with body image and sexual adjustments. Detailed interventions and therapies relating to sexual counseling are beyond the scope of this chapter. Persons with persistent or severe sexual adjustment difficulties or a history of sexual trauma should be referred to a licensed sex therapist specializing in sexuality and chronic illness.

Discussion Opportunities

The most important intervention is to give the patient permission and encouragement to discuss matters related to body image and sexuality in a supportive, unhurried manner. In a busy clinical practice, this is often easier said than done. The benefits to patients in their overall adjustment to IBD as well as adherence to the medical regime can be enhanced by attention to this important topic. A brief statement relating to coping, body image, and sexuality as it relates to IBD can open the door to discussion. The age, gender, and sexual orientation of the patient are important considerations. Whether they are or have been sexually active, married or single, divorced or widowed can provide helpful baseline information. Some authors suggest that this type of data can be gathered from a brief questionnaire, but others claim that this type of personal disclosure is best obtained on a one-to-one basis.

Body Image

Body image is defined as the way in which we view ourselves within the context of our physical being. Body image is a component of self-concept, but the sense of self has an even more all-encompassing presence in an individual. For example, children born with birth defects have no inborn knowledge that they are different from other children; despite profound problems, many can be raised with a good self-concept that enables them to cope with the fact of their physical challenges and to feel positive

about themselves and their bodies. Conversely, the literature is filled with evidence of body-image and self-concept disorders in persons with no outward physical challenges, indeed, many with what others consider highly attractive physical characteristics. It is important for the clinician to ascertain the patient's pre-illness and present body image and self-concept patterns. This information can provide clues as to the duration and extent of the problem.

Coping Mechanisms

Gaining insight into successful and unsuccessful coping mechanisms the patient has developed can assist in developing a plan of care. **Locus of control**, a concept frequently applied in studies of patients with diabetes mellitus, has applicability to persons living with IBD. Determining an individual's locus of control in life and management of disease can provide valuable information as well. Does the person view himself or herself as helpless over fate? These individuals demonstrate a sense of little to no control and no desire or perceived ability to exert control over their lives, disease, or therapies. They are said to have an external locus of control and may need specific advice and exercises to address their issues regarding body image and sexual adjustment.

Individuals with an internal locus of control demonstrate a sense of mastery over self and events. When IBD does not respond the way they want it to, such patients may need to undertake some general coping and relaxation strategies to enhance adjustment to the unpredictable nature of the disease. Events beyond their direct control can pose coping difficulties for these patients in all aspects of their lives.

Sexual Adjustment Problems

Sexual adjustment problems and IBD can be related to three key areas: the **disease process** itself, **side effects of medications**, and **psychosexual or psychosocial influences**. The duration and extent of the disease has a direct impact on sexual adjustment. Frequent stools, abdominal pain, fatigue, and perianal skin problems ranging from irritation to fistulae are some of the most common problems related to body image and sexual adjustment. Problems with extra-intestinal manifestations of IBD, pelvic floor dysfunction, dyspareunia, and tenesmus can interfere with normal sexual functioning. Patients who require abdominal stomas or who experience enterocutaneous fistulae or other skin problems benefit from the interventions of an enterostomal therapy nurse for physical and psychological rehabilitation. There is a separate chapter on enterostomal therapy.

The myriad of medications used to treat the condition can alleviate or control many of the symptoms of IBD. Unfortunately, the side effects of these same medications can create a whole new set of difficulties for the patient. Mood swings, loss of libido, impotence, vaginal dryness, and weight gain are only a few of the complications patients may experience as a result of medications used to treat IBD. Concerns regarding sexual activity and reproduction are common in relation to both the disease and the treatments. Use of budesonide, a rapidly metabolized steroid with less side effects, is discussed in two separate chapters.

Stages of Life

Individual psychosexual and psychosocial characteristics determine how a patient is able to adjust to the progress of the disease and therapies. Erikson's Theory of Psychosocial Development can provide some insight into developmental crises and tasks people face at various stages of their lives. Since IBD can occur at almost any time across the life span, it is important for the clinician to consider the potential effects of IBD in patients of all ages. Even those with longstanding disease will face new challenges as they age and the progress of their disease changes. These challenges will in turn have an impact on body image and sexual adjustment.

Infancy and Childhood

A sense of trust versus mistrust is being established in infancy. Although diagnosis of IBD in this age group is relatively rare, parents have reported that children diagnosed with IBD demonstrated gastrointestinal difficulties in infancy. Separations and discomfort caused by physical symptoms and medical tests may interfere with an infant's ability to trust and potentially threaten parent–child bonding.

Toddlers are said to be developing a sense of autonomy versus shame. At this stage, IBD presents particular challenges, as the child attempts to gain mastery over himself and his environment, especially toilet training. A sense of self and burgeoning body image can be at odds with the symptoms and management of IBD.

Preschoolers are developing initiative versus guilt. A diagnosis of IBD at this stage could lead a child to believe his efforts at increased independence and inventiveness are being thwarted or punished. As children enter the school-age years, the developmental crisis experienced is industry versus inferiority.

These years are instrumental, as a child develops a sense of pride and accomplishment, an emphasis on peer relationships, and a heightened self-concept and body image. During these years, IBD can disrupt education and recreational activities critical to normal development. The chapter on the pediatric patient and family support addresses some of these issues.

Adolescence

During the teen years, IBD is particularly challenging for the young person establishing a sense of identity versus identity diffusion. Efforts to establish greater independence from parents and strong peer relationships and a strong emphasis on body image, sexual attractiveness, and potential sexual activity can be thwarted by the disease and associated therapies. Young adults face further issues relating to establishing a sense of intimacy versus isolation. The presence of IBD could potentially interfere with their ability to establish a meaningful relationship with another, establish a career, and further their independence from their parents. A protracted illness may leave a young adult with conflicting emotions and desires.

Middle Years

During the middle years, IBD occurs at a time when adults are establishing generativity versus stagnation. This is generally a time of maximum earning potential, launching of offspring to adulthood, and caring for aging parents, combined with the onset of menopause and perceived loss of youth and vitality. At this stage of life, IBD can present with particular difficulties, as patients are coping with multiple challenges. Concerns over sexual attractiveness and sexual function can be of special significance during mid-life.

Older Adults

Older adults said to be undergoing ego integrity versus despair can be especially vulnerable to the physical, sexual, and financial aspects of living with IBD. The need to maintain social contacts, including intimate relationships, can be adversely affected by IBD. Potential loss of self-esteem and social isolation can be devastating to seniors coping with IBD.

Risk Factors for Adjustment Difficulties

High-risk indicators for sexual adjustment difficulties in patients with IBD include lack of social support, family or relationship dysfunction, history of alcohol or drug abuse or eating disorders, and history of coping difficulties. On an intrapersonal level, persons with low self-esteem or other self-concept disturbances, including expressions of powerlessness or hopelessness, high or mild anxiety, anger or depression, are at high risk. The socioecomomic impact of IBD cannot be overlooked. Financial worries related to employment and insurance difficulties can combine to erode self-esteem and have a negative impact on intimate relationships.

Communication Patterns

Establishing and maintaining effective communication patterns is essential to overall coping with IBD and enable the patient to make successful sexual adjustments as they live with the disease. Active listening is the cornerstone of successful two-way communication. The permission, limited information, specific suggestions, intensive therapy (PLISSIT) model can be a useful guide to the clinician providing sexual counseling and rehabilitation.

The first step, **permission**, opens the door to frank discussion of the patient's sexual concerns. In the second step, **limited information**, the clinician provides factual information related to the patient's current condition. The third phase, **specific suggestions**, focuses on interventions tailored for the patient's specific needs and concerns. Finally, if the clinician determines deep-seated or complex sexual problems, the fourth phase, **intensive therapy**, should be considered. Intensive therapy will require the interventions of a licensed sex therapist, psychologist, psychiatrist, or, in the case of some conditions such as a rectovaginal fistula, a surgical consultation.

Sexual adjustments to IBD are as varied as the symptoms and patients themselves. It is the responsibility of the clinician to address patient concerns regarding body image and sexual adjustments in an open, individualized manner. Changes in the patient's physical, developmental, intrapersonal, or socioeconomic status will signal the need for the clinician to modify the plan of care to optimize the patient's body image and sexual functioning.

Editor's Note

The concept of an IBD nurse advocate is discussed in a separate chapter. The issues in this chapter on sexuality and body image could be addressed by nursing personnel as well as, if not better than, by the physicians. (TMB)

Supplemental Reading

Annon JS. The PLISSIT model: a proposed conceptual scheme for the behaviorial treatment of sexual problems, Sex Educ Ther 1972;2:1.

Benirschke R. Alive and kicking. San Diego: Firefly Press, 1996.

Engstrom I. Family interaction and locus of control in children and adolescents with inflammatory bowel disease. J Am Acad Child Adolesc Psychiatry 1991;30:913–20.

Erikson E. Childhood and society. 2nd Ed. New York: WW Norton, 1993.

Erwin-Toth P. Enterostomal therapy. In: Corman M, ed. Colon and rectal surgery. 4th Ed. Philadelphia: Lippincott-Raven, 1998.

Erwin-Toth P. The effect of childhood ostomy surgery between the ages of 6 and 12 years on psyshosocial development during childhood, adolescence, and young adulthood. J Wound Ostomy Continence Nurs 1999;26:77–85.

Kane S. Women's issues in inflammatory bowel disease. Foundation Focus. Magazine of the Crohn's & Colitis Foundation of America, 1999; Summer:16–18.

Konen JC, Summerson JH, Dignan MB. Family function, stress, and locus of control. Relationships to glycemia in adults with diabetes mellitus. Arch Fam Med 1993;2:393–402.

CHAPTER 120

ROLE OF CLERGY AND THE PATIENT WITH CHRONIC DISEASE

RABBI MURRAY SALTZMAN, DDS, DHL, DD

He had been a remarkably good physician. His appearance revealed obvious discomfort. Breathing with effort, he coughed, sometimes violently. As a diagnostician, he knew better than anyone else that death was not far off. I sensed that he was somewhat astonished by his own need to talk to me, his rabbi, as the end drew near.[*]

Spiritual Presence

He emphasized his rationalistic perspective. How ironic, this situation. He could not count the times he had offered comfort to patients as they dealt with the reality of a debilitating disease ravaging their bodies. The echo of his own voice lending supportive hope and courage was clearly heard. But now he needed to hear and feel a caring spiritual presence doing this for him. He could not do it for himself. I think he was a little embarrassed. He was glad I was there.

What is the spiritual presence this competent physician and bright and good man sought? How do you define spiritual presence in another human being, be it clergy, physician, or friend?

Integrity

I think a spiritual presence is projected by an image of integrity. Occasionally, there is confusion between "telling the truth" and integrity. Not everyone who tells the truth conveys integrity. Truth can destroy life when it is insensitively delivered. A physician who tells the truth about a terminal illness and also crushes the human spirit with hopelessness and despair does not inspire the patient's ability to cope with reality. To help a patient cope with the reality of illness is a function of the clergy or the physician. Integrity compels the speaker of truth to couch it in a manner and with phrases that may help to evoke courage, resiliency, and hope. Even when confronting a terminal illness, there may still be hope of infusing the remaining life with quality. Such hope is often a saving ray of light in an otherwise dark, despairing tunnel.

The healing team of physician and clergy manifests integrity by approaching the patient as a whole person. The patient is more than a malfunctioning body. Family, vocation, interests, fears, hobbies, and idiosyncrasies make up the composite of a whole person. Each may be explored as a component in a rapport-building communication. This sharing process promotes mutual understanding, trust, and confidence—the elements of integrity.

It is vital to understand where the patient is coming from emotionally and spiritually. In my experience, the personality does not undergo fundamental alteration when one is under stress. We tend only to intensify the traits we already possess. Someone who has never handled life realistically or maturely will be less able to do so when exposed to the stress of dangerous illness.

The opposite is also true. One who normally has been realistic will become even painstakingly so at times of crisis. The patient will quickly conclude how he or she is being perceived. We all want to be perceived during illness as we were perceived when healthy. Integrity grants the patient the right to be the person he or she has been throughout his or her life.

Compassion

A spiritual presence also projects an image of compassion. Just as integrity does not simply translate into truth, so compassion does not simply suggest pity. Pity brings the patient no benefit, because it is emotionally crippling and spiritually immobilizing.

Despite the presence of serious illness, life can continue to include dynamic emotional and spiritual growth. Growth is possible when the patient copes with illness by maintaining autonomy. When serious illness strikes, we all may want to surrender to despair. Initially, we may not relish continued autonomy. In despair, however, we lose the ability to exercise critical decision-making capacities. We retard life's dynamic potential. To reverse the flight into despair, we must offer compassion, not pity. Whereas pity may serve to diminish identity, compassion helps to confirm it.

Our compassion should not become indulgent appropriation of the patient's responsibilities, tasks, or decisions. Neither the clergy nor the family should inhibit the patient's efforts to maintain a familiar life style. Latent spiritual and emotional resources are unleashed when compassion is supportive of autonomy. "You can do it" is far better than "Let me do it for you."

---

[*] This chapter appeared in the first edition of this book in 1989.

Certainly, in the time closely following the discovery of serious, life-threatening illness, the initial response may often be one of anger, shock, unwillingness to accept the news, tears, dejection, or hopelessness. Compassion from physician and clergy encourages the individual undergoing trauma to be in touch with those feelings and to ventilate them. Once he or she is beyond the initial impact, the patient can begin to manage reality and its inevitable consequences. The helping person must recognize that both the patient and his or her family experience this initial trauma. Both require compassion.

How else is compassion demonstrated? Perhaps it is merely physical contact, such as holding the hand of the patient even without speaking. Compassion requires the clergy or physician to move from behind the desk and sit or stand in close proximity. Perhaps even the simple gesture of an arm over the shoulder can communicate caring. Most significantly, compassion gives credence and appropriateness to the expression of fear-laden emotion.

More often than not, death is not the source of fear. It is pain. Reassurance about minimizing pain, when possible, is helpful. The articulation of one's fear avoids wastefully expending energy in a cover-up. The release of untapped resources, in the face of illness, is the result of the forthright expression of emotions. The patient is enabled to move beyond immobilizing fear once having verbalized it.

Faith

This is the point at which the physician or clergy, as spiritual persons themselves, can influence a patient's response to a diagnosis of serious illness. Linked to the expression of integrity and compassion is faith. Faith is the third dimension a spiritual presence offers a patient to help cope with disease.

Faith can empower the seriously ill individual with energy for creative living. Creative living musters inner resources perhaps never before experienced. Illness does not deprive us of our spiritual and emotional potential. Illness does not negate the mediation of laughter, love, joy, beauty, companionship, curiosity, or, indeed, hope itself. Even during the course of illness, we may attain new heights of emotional and spiritual growth.

Faith, for some, is an expectation that we can miraculously transform or overcome the forces of nature. Prayer, faith's vehicle, is then viewed as a magic wand to generate healing that contradicts or, at best, astonishes the rational processes of nature. There are those who believe that faith can accomplish anything and everything.

My interest is not to engage here in theological argument about faith and prayer. This is not a treatise on theology but an exposition of the personal convictions of one rabbi about how to unleash human resources to realistically cope with serious illness. Unrealistic efforts for miraculous and supernatural interventions ultimately can do more harm than good, or so I believe.

Faith demonstrated by the helping person should prompt growth and hope, courage and resiliency in the patient. This mitigating faith is defined in a thoughtful mediation:

Prayer invites God to let His presence suffuse our spirits, to let His will prevail in our lives. Prayer cannot bring water to parched fields, nor mend a broken bridge, nor rebuild a ruined city; but prayer can water an arid soul, mend a broken heart, and rebuild a weakened will.

Faith, as I view it, is not planted in the soil of theological absolutes. Faith suggests that life has meaning and that beyond life there is also an infinite reality in which we can place our trust and confidence. Faith permits us to entertain life's paradoxes and ambiguities. Faith entitles us to grieve at life's inevitable conclusion without placing ourselves in an emotional dead end.

The physician or cleric does not have to feel that he or she must provide all of the answers. Some eternal questions have no answers. Life beyond death is one such issue. In any case, the patient should appeal to his or her own faith orientation, without having to contend with a contrary view from the physician or clergy. Tolerance of the patient's beliefs is the most helpful posture.

To the angry and hostile inquiry, "Why me?," we need not respond by rationalizing that God, by bestowing extraordinary suffering, has some mysterious design for us. We can allow the patient the right to question the benevolence of life as suffering imposes unremitting pain. The faith of the healing person allows the admission that sometimes seemingly unreasonable accidents intrude upon the more usual experience of life's orderliness. We simply may never understand why irrational incidents occur in the lives of some and not others.

In short, faith does not insulate life from the sudden and irrational onslaught of disease and illness. Faith does not shield us from perturbing questions. It can, however, liberate the spirit and intelligence to grow and flourish even in times of utmost trial.

A wholesome, mature faith thus arouses confidence in our value as human beings. No one escapes the inner realization of weakness and fragility. To overcome the erosion of self-worth, we require the healing balm of faith. Whether or not we are ill, physician, clergy, and patient alike can share in a positive faith that uncompromisingly honors life.

The human spirit is of infinite value, incandescent and eternal because it loves and cares. Faith tells us we are precious because we were fashioned in the image of God with intelligence to discern between good and evil. Faith emboldens us to believe we are worthy of healing and life. But, if God so wills it, faith helps us to acknowledge that we are also worthy of returning from whence we came, to eternal peace.

While the language and imagery of faith are not easily verbalized by the average physician, the clergy can impart them. The physician should encourage the patient to consult with the cleric. On occasion, a conference with the family's cleric can help the physician to know how to be most helpful. Similarly, the cleric's behavior can be guided by contact with the physician.

A caveat to this exposition of faith is necessary. Superstition responds to a deep-seated human conviction that we are not in total control of our destinies. How true this is! Faith can thereby be reduced at times to superstitious dependency. When an individual is under great stress, with peace of mind at risk, it is not the time to suggest that his or her prayer or actions are inappropriate. Accept the person where he or she is. Then go forward with gentleness to transmit confidence and self-esteem. This helps to liberate mind and spirit from superstition's imprisoning grip.

Confidence and Self-Esteem

Confidence and self-esteem result when the physician and cleric, as spiritual persons trusted and valued by the patient, express friendship by cultivating a genuine relationship. Warmth and interested listening convey to the anxious, frightened person that a respected and admired physician or cleric also respects and admires him or her.

The spiritual presence of clergy and physician is crucially supplemented by the family. The family's supportive presence cannot be underestimated. The three dimensions of a spiritual presence—integrity, compassion, and faith—reinforce the strength of physician, clergy, and family when dealing with a medical crisis. Then the period of severe illness is not irretrievably submerged under despair and anguish. It can be a moment when our humanity nobly unfolds at the same time that we are confronted by our impending mortality. The irony of life inexorably bound to death is forever with us.

CHAPTER 121

APPRECIATION OF PSYCHOSOCIAL FACTORS

RAY E. CLOUSE, MD

Psychosocial factors are important in any chronic medical disorder, and inflammatory bowel disease (IBD) is no exception. The emotional reaction to illness can become more dominant than the inciting gastrointestinal problems, taking on a life of its own. Acknowledging the potential emotional toll of IBD is routine by clinicians, and further raising of such awareness is not the intent of this chapter. Psychological impairment, whether the result of chronic illness or an independent event, has great potential for influencing the presentation and course of the patient with IBD. Appreciation of these effects is often less robust, yet an exploration of their relevance to the individual patient may lead to additional, helpful interventions. The emotional contribution to the symptomatic state often, sadly, is passively accepted, leaving an important therapeutic area undermanaged.

Optimal treatment of the patient with IBD often, not occasionally, requires a comprehensive approach that includes attention to active psychological issues. In the author's opinion, failure on the part of the clinician to address these factors and intervene when appropriate is one of the key reasons why patients with IBD require escalating treatment and referral to tertiary centers. Appreciation of their importance can be gained by considering the prevalence of emotional disturbances in patients with IBD, ways in which emotional disorders can influence the presentation and course of the gastrointestinal disorder, and the potential impact of psychiatric treatment on outcome of the medical illness.

Prevalence of Psychiatric Disorder in Inflammatory Bowel Disease

Although anecdotal observations once fueled a debate over the psychosomatic origin of ulcerative colitis, the contemporary scientific literature has put this issue to rest. From the standpoint of psychiatric diagnosis, patients with ulcerative colitis are as resilient as the general population in resisting the presentation of anxiety and affective disorders, even in the face of chronic medical illness. Many stressful aspects of this disease, including its long duration, potential for severe symptoms, need for corticosteroids, and even need for colectomy, do not appear to induce major depressive episodes any more frequently than the usual stressors of daily life in the general population. Fewer than 20 percent of the population with ulcerative colitis report persistent symptoms required to make the psychiatric diagnosis of depression. Nevertheless, subclinical depression is undoubtedly prevalent, and major depression, when it does occur, must be taken seriously.

Crohn's disease may enhance susceptibility to psychiatric disorder, particularly depression. Major depressive episodes are reported by as many as 36 percent of patients with Crohn's disease, a rate significantly exceeding that found in ulcerative colitis or in medically well subjects. Neither IBD diagnosis appears particularly predisposing to other psychiatric illnesses, and the rates should be expected to parallel those seen in the general population or in groups with chronic medical disease. Prevalence data do not establish directional causality. Higher rates of depression in Crohn's disease could be related to negative effects of the bowel disorder on emotional functioning or, as an alternative explanation, depression could induce changes in the presentation and course of Crohn's disease, thereby increasing representation of depressed patients with Crohn's disease in the clinic populations under investigation. A third plausible explanation is that other external factors (eg, genetic susceptibility) favor the expression of both depression and Crohn's disease in the same patient.

Knowing the precise explanation for the co-occurrence of a psychiatric disorder with IBD is unessential. It simply behooves the clinician to remain aware of the reasonable likelihood of co-occurrences, especially in patients with Crohn's disease. Depression tends to be a relapsing disorder, whether associated with medical illness or not. Precipitants of emotional change, including severe stress or corticosteroids, may induce episodes of significant depression with greater likelihood in patients with histories of prior episodes. Prophylaxis against relapse is not uniformly necessary or recommended, but maintaining an open channel of communication regarding both gut and emotional symptoms is important.

TABLE 121–1. Interactions of Depression with Inflammatory Bowel Disease

Interaction Mechanism	Example
Cognitive or behavioral	Excessive focusing on abdominal pain or discomfort, medication noncompliance
Overlapping symptoms	Fatigue, altered appetite, weight loss
Precipitation of functional gastrointestinal symptoms	Bloating, urgency, pain, other symptoms of irritable bowel syndrome
Effect on quality of life	Impaired vitality, decreased social functioning

Effects of Psychological Dysfunction of Inflammatory Bowel Disease

Psychosocial factors can influence IBD in many ways. Better understood interactions include the potential effects of depression on the presentation and course of gastrointestinal illness (Table 121–1). Anxiety and depression, not always to the level of definable psychiatric diagnosis, surface intermittently. The accompanying cognitive alterations can be sufficient to influence the behavior of the patient regarding the somatic disease. Anxiety can lead to a misinterpretation of symptom significance. The anxious patient with IBD may insist on additional testing to exclude cancer or other concerning diagnoses. Acquiescence to additional testing is the easiest tack for the clinician, but reassurance is often inadequate for the persistently anxious patient. Open discussions when psychological factors are the driving forces precipitate resolution or intervention with psychotropic medications or formal psychotherapy when required. Similarly, cognitive abnormalities from depression result in unnecessary focusing on unpleasant thoughts and sensations. As for anxiety, reassurance following unrevealing tests typically fails to manage the dysphoric mood, especially if many or severe symptoms of depression are present.

Besides influencing the perception of medical illness, emotional factors alter the clinical presentation of IBD in more direct ways. The patient with comorbid IBD and psychiatric disorder often cannot determine the relative contribution of either to the global symptomatic state: he or she presents to the doctor, explains current symptoms, and expects the physician to determine an appropriate intervention. Because many patients with IBD seek help from clinicians whose primary interests are in somatic (or, more specifically, gastrointestinal) illnesses, psychological contributions to the presentation may be overlooked. A disorder of emotional dysfunction can confound the interpretation of IBD activity through at least three mechanisms: (1) by producing overlapping symptoms with IBD, (2) by inducing or exacerbating symptoms of functional gastrointestinal disorder, and (3) by simultaneously interfering with quality of life. Although possible through stress-related effects on inflammatory cell function, a significant effect of emotional factors (eg, depression or stressful life events) toward exacerbating disease activity in IBD has not been established.

Each of these mechanisms is best exemplified by considering the potential effects of depression on the presentation of a patient with Crohn's disease. Depression is expressed by somatic manifestations that accompany the defining cognitive abnormalities (eg, dysphoric mood, anhedonia, pessimism, and guilt). Fatigue, reduced appetite, nausea, and weight loss are common; accentuation of abdominal pain and other abdominal discomforts also occurs. These manifestations of depression sufficiently overlap with measures of inflammatory activity that both the patient and physician are easily confused. In fact, symptoms of depression are sufficient alone to elevate the Crohn's Disease Activity Index from normal well into the active range. The confound introduced by overlapping symptoms of depression with IBD is potentially of great significance.

Emotional factors also are important in precipitating symptoms of functional gastrointestinal disorders. Longitudinal surveys of subjects without IBD demonstrate the close relation of functional gastrointestinal symptoms with anxiety and affective disorders; these symptoms also co-segregate with anxiety and affective disorders in families. Expectedly, anxiety and affective disorders are more prevalent in patients seeking care for functional gastrointestinal disorders than in suitable comparison groups. Although the mechanisms underlying this association remain unclear, accentuation of functional gastrointestinal symptoms through emotional effects is accepted. Patients with IBD are not protected from these effects, although establishing the prevalence of irritable bowel syndrome (IBS), for example, in patients with IBD is difficult—a problem largely related to semantics. A rate at least equal to that in the general population (15 to 20%) would be expected. Because anxiety and depression appear to be important contributors to symptom production in IBS, then an overrepresentation of IBS might be expected in IBD, at least in the Crohn's disease subset. This appears to be the case in this author's practice. To substantiate presumptions that functional gastrointestinal symptoms are important, it may be necessary to establish their temporal relation to stress, to determine their relation to anxiety and depression episodes, or simply to seek the entire cluster of typical symptoms that define a functional disorder. This mechanism further exemplifies the importance of discussing psychosocial factors in optimal management of the IBD patient. There are two chapters in this text on the coexistence of IBS and IBD.

A third direct mechanism by which psychological factors contribute to the IBD presentation is through their independent effects on quality of life. An important indicator of a patient's successful struggle with IBD is found in the response to questions like "How are you doing overall?" "Are you getting along okay?" "Is [your IBD] interfering very much with your life?" Together, the patient and I know that such broader measures of quality of life will influence the extent of evaluation, need for medication change, the efforts taken to close a fistula, and whether surgery, for example, should be considered. Quality of life is an established determinant of health care use in the patient with IBD but cannot be predicted by disease activity alone. A physician's care would be inadequate if he or she ignored the influences of psychosocial factors on patient evaluation of quality of life. Clinical depression influences all aspects of daily functioning and often is used as a comparison standard for impaired quality of life. The effects of this psychiatric illness and other emotional disturbances on global health perception and quality of life in the patient with IBD are easily perceived and cannot be overemphasized.

Potential for Intervention

The provided examples outline at least superficially the potential importance of psychosocial factors in the patient with IBD. In many cases, the described interactions lead to specific intervention. Psychosocial issues should be discussed from the outset. Few patients resist such a discussion, especially if the focus is on understanding the patient's global health in the context of appreciating both psychological and physical contributors. The patient can be asked outright how he or she is handling the illness. The physician then works backward from a broader functional assessment to determine the significance of emotional factors. Whenever a patient is doing poorly, it is important to establish whether physical or emotional illness is the greatest contributor. Keep in mind the confounding nature of symptoms, but an abbreviated, directed psychiatric interview usually will uncover additional cognitive symptoms of anxiety or affective disorder, for example, if they are present. Because most primary care physicians and subspecialists in internal medicine have become familiar with managing anxiety and affective disorder using contemporary psychotropic agents, referral to a mental health professional as discussed in a separate chapter is not commonly required. Simply initiating a discussion of psychosocial factors in the interview setting is helpful, a maneuver of proven efficacy in reducing health care use by patients with functional gastrointestinal disorders. Patients with IBD who desire additional counseling often have increased needs for empathic support.

Several specific scenarios may help demonstrate techniques used by the author in practice. A patient with Crohn's disease seeks another opinion for persistent right lower quadrant pain. Repeated evaluations have not shown any significant finding other than modest ileitis without obstruction, abscess, or other significant complication. The symptom did not improve with a tapering course of corticosteroids and even may have worsened. On evaluation, the patient is found to be very impaired from this problem. He has stopped working and is considering applying for disability benefits. Further questioning reveals unequivocal evidence of active depression. In cases such as this, the degree of disability and functional impairment exceeds what one might expect from the gastrointestinal findings. The importance is explained of managing depression using contemporary antidepressants to induce global improvement. Although many contemporary antidepressants, particularly the selective serotonin reuptake inhibitors, can exacerbate gastrointestinal symptoms initially, side effects typically abate within several weeks of treatment. Walker and colleagues (1995, 1996) have shown that depressed patients with Crohn's disease are significantly impaired by general measures of vitality and functioning compared with nondepressed patients with similar Crohn's disease activity. Following only 4 weeks of antidepressant therapy, the previously depressed patients begin to approach the scale scores of the nondepressed subset. There is no excuse for accepting depression as an expected outcome of chronic medical illness and leaving it untreated. This is an antiquated concept.

A more typical scenario is the patient with IBD who appears also to have functional gastrointestinal symptoms. This possibility remains overlooked or is deemed impossible by many physicians. Inflammation in the gut may be an important initiating factor in IBS and other functional gastrointestinal disorders. This is stressed in one of the chapters on IBS and IBD. However, Gwee and colleagues (1996) showed that psychosocial factors remain the most important determinants toward producing the manifestations of IBS following acute infectious diarrhea, suggesting that an **interaction** of inflammation and psychological factors is most relevant in producing the symptomatic state. Anxiety, depression, and somatization tendencies were the significant psychological factors in that study, the same psychological characteristics that appear operational in promoting symptom production in other studies of the functional gastrointestinal disorders. Consequently, an interaction may underlie the inflammation of IBD and emotional factors to induce manifestations of functional gastrointestinal symptoms in IBD patients. When symptoms persist after adequate anti-inflammatory intervention, appear in the face of anxiety or depression, follow severely stressful events, or reappear spontaneously in a patient with typical functional symptoms that antedated the diagnosis of IBD, a therapeutic trial directed at functional symptoms is in order. Tricyclic antidepressants are the recommended principal approach in such cases (eg, amitriptyline, nortriptyline, imipramine, desipramine). The tricyclic antidepressants are the most effective medications available today for treating IBS, functional dyspepsia, and functional chest pain. The medications are particularly useful for pain management, but other symptoms (eg, urgency, bloating, incomplete evacuation) also respond. If significant anxiety or depression is not in the picture, a low-dose regimen may suffice. Targeting a daily dose to 30 to 75 mg is a reasonable goal. The use of low-dose antidepressant therapy for this purpose requires a considerable amount of cautious dose manipulation and drug change, as side effects interfere with use in more than a third of patients. Detailed methods for successful use of psychotropic medications for managing functional gastrointestinal disorders can be found in the supplemental readings.

Summary

Psychosocial factors undoubtedly are important in every patient with IBD. Their appreciation by the clinician may be most relevant to patients in whom emotional functioning is influencing the presentation and course of gastrointestinal symptoms or significantly contributing to impaired quality of life. The mechanisms by which psychological dysfunction can influence manifestations of IBD are multiple. Fortunately, most patients are amenable to disclosing their emotions and freely discussing the activity of emotional symptoms. Unfortunately, the patient alone cannot determine fully the impact that emotional factors may be having on the gastrointestinal illness. A careful clinical evaluation can help in this regard, and interventions directed both at correcting emotional disturbances and reducing the inflammation of IBD often provide an optimal approach to patient management.

References

Gwee KA, Graham JC, McKendrick MW, et al. Psychometric scores and persistence of irritable bowel after infectious diarrhoea. Lancet 1996;347:150–3.

Walker EA, Gelfand AN, Gelfand MD, Katon WJ. Psychiatric diagnoses, sexual and physical victimization, and disability in patients with irritable bowel syndrome or inflammatory bowel disease. Psychol Med 1995;25:1259–67.

Walker EA, Gelfand MD, Gelfand AN, et al. The relationship of current psychiatric disorder to functional disability and distress in patients with inflammatory bowel disease. Gen Hosp Psychiatry 1996;18:215–9.

Supplemental Reading

Clouse RE. Psychotropic medications for the treatment of functional gastrointestinal disorders. Clin Perspect Gastroenterol 1999;2:348–56.

Irvine EJ. Quality of life in inflammatory bowel disease and other chronic diseases. Scand J Gastroenterol 1996; 221(Suppl):26–8.

North CS, Alpers DH. A review of studies of psychiatric factors in Crohn's disease: etiologic implications. Ann Clin Psychiatry 1994;6:117–24.

North CS, Alpers DH, Helzer JE, et al. Do life events or depression exacerbate inflammatory bowel disease? A prospective study. Ann Intern Med 1991;114:381–6.

North CS, Clouse RE, Spitznagel EL, Alpers DH. The relation of ulcerative colitis to psychiatric factors: a review of findings and methods. Am J Psychiatry 1990;147:974–81.

Ramchandani D, Schindler B, Katz J. Evolving concepts of psychopathology in inflammatory bowel disease. Implications for treatment. Med Clin North Am 1994;78:1321–30.

Talal AH, Drossman DA. Psychosocial factors in inflammatory bowel disease. Gastroenterol Clin North Am 1995; 24:699–716.

Turnbull GK, Vallis TM. Quality of life in inflammatory bowel disease: the interaction of disease activity with psychosocial function. Am J Gastroenterol 1995;90:1450–4.

CHAPTER 122

Psychiatric Complications of Inflammatory Bowel Disease

Mark L. Teitelbaum, MD

Psychiatric disorders often complicate the course of inflammatory bowel disease (IBD). About one-half of patients with active Crohn's disease suffer from a diagnosable psychiatric disorder, a proportion that is significantly increased compared with that among patients suffering from other chronic medical illnesses. About one-quarter of patients suffering from ulcerative colitis likewise suffer from a diagnosable psychiatric disorder. However, this proportion is not significantly greater than the proportion of patients with psychiatric disorder suffering from other chronic medical illnesses. For many years, some psychiatrists and some gastroenterologists thought that there was a casual relation between psychiatric disorder and IBD. There is no solid evidence to support this notion. Nevertheless, since psychiatric disorder is an important source of suffering in its own right, it needs to be recognized and treated. The common psychiatric disorders found in association with IBD include delirium, depression, anxiety, and personality disorders. Each is discussed with emphasis on current concepts in management. The role of the psychiatrist in IBD is to assist the gastroenterologist in the recognition, diagnosis, and treatment of these conditions.

Delirium

Delirium is a psychiatric syndrome characterized by an alteration in the patient's state of consciousness and cognitive impairment. It is most commonly found in hospitalized patients who are very ill and carries with it a high mortality rate. Drugs, infections, and metabolic disturbances, such as fluid and electrolyte imbalance, are all common contributors. A decrease in the patient's ability to concentrate often is the first sign of delirium. As delirium worsens, the patient becomes drowsy, confused, disoriented, inattentive, and distractible. Complicating features, such as agitation, depressed or anxious mood, hallucinations and delusions, and even suicidal behavior may appear. Diffuse slowing of the electroencephalogram (EEG) helps confirm the diagnosis. The treatment of delirium involves aggressive treatment of the underlying medical condition, psychological management, and pharmacologic intervention.

Treatment of the Underlying Medical Condition

Vigorous search for occult causes of delirium is often required. Discontinuance of possibly offending medications should always be considered after a careful review. Patients getting more than 40 mg of prednisone a day are at increased risk for becoming delirious. This can occur even in patients with no history of psychiatric illness.

Psychological Management of the Delirious Patient

Frequent attempts by the physician and staff to talk with the patient are helpful. At these times, he or she can be oriented, as well as reassured. This should be direct and straightforward, pointing out to the patient where he or she is, why he or she is in the hospital, and what is happening to him or her. A clock in the room and a calendar on the wall also can be of help. Visits by family should be encouraged. Placing familiar objects from home in the patient's room also can be recommended. Keeping a light on in the room at night can help reduce perceptual ambiguity. In an intensive care unit (ICU) with glass partitions around the beds, talking about a patient within his or her view should be avoided to reduce the patient's tendency toward misinterpretation.

Pharmacologic Treatment of Delirium

Severe agitation, hallucinations, and delusional thinking are indications for pharmacologic intervention. For most patients, 1 to 2 mg of haloperidol (Haldol) given by mouth two or three times a day will usually suffice. In the elderly, small doses (0.5 mg) of haloperidol given twice a day often are effective. For the patient who is having most difficulty at night, the bulk of the daily haloperidol dose can be given at bedtime. In an emergency, parenteral haloperidol can be administered intramuscularly or intravenously in similar doses at intervals of 20 or 30 minutes until the patient is calm. Once the delirium has resolved, haloperidol should be maintained until it is believed that the underlying medical problem has been treated adequately; then it can be tapered over several days.

Depression

Mild lowering of mood, simple discouragement, or demoralization are common reactions to medical illness and its accompanying losses. These reactions often are self-limited and only rarely interfere with medical treatment. Serious mood disorder also may complicate IBD. Depressive illness is a psychiatric syndrome characterized by persistent disturbances in mood, self-attitude, vital sense, and motivated behaviors. The mood of the patient may be described as "sad," "blue," "down-in-the-dumps," "dejected," or even "empty." Self-attitude change may be experienced as a lowering of self-esteem, a loss of confidence, or even frank feelings of worthlessness or guilt. Vital sense alterations usually are reported as the subjective experience of lowered energy, fatigue, and inefficient or slow thinking. Disturbances in motivated behaviors take the form of sleep disturbance, especially early morning awakening, loss of appetite with weight loss, and loss of sexual interest. History of episodes of depression as well as a family history suggestive of depressive illness help support the diagnosis. Inquiries about suicidal thoughts and intent should be made during the initial interview of any patient who is thought to be depressed. The treatment of depression involves consideration of setting, psychological management, and drug treatment.

Inpatient versus Outpatient Treatment of the Depressed Patient

The majority of depressed patients seen by the physician in everyday practice can be treated as outpatients. Indications for inpatient treatment include depression with psychotic features, high suicide risk, lack of family or other social support network, malnutrition or dehydration requiring parenteral support, or other complicating medical conditions that require inpatient treatment. Psychiatric consultation should be considered in such circumstances.

Psychological Management of the Depressed Patient

Psychological management of the depressed patient involves support and education aimed at combating lowered self-esteem, pessimism, and guilt. The offering of regular follow-up appointments and of time to listen mobilizes powerful forces against failing self-esteem and hopelessness. By simply offering his or her time and empathy to a depressed patient, the physician is communicating the belief not only that the patient is worth the time and effort but also that there is a future for the patient. Straightforward explanations that depression is treatable and invariably gets better also are helpful in combating hopelessness.

Pharmacologic Treatment of Depression

Most patients suffering from depressive illness require pharmacologic treatment with an antidepressant along with psychological support. Paroxetine (Paxil), one of the newer selective serotonin reuptake inhibitors (SSRI), is an excellent drug with which to begin treatment. For most adult patients, treatment can be initiated with a dose of 20 mg each morning. The majority of patients respond to this dose. Elderly patients, as well as those with compromised renal or hepatic function, should be started on 10 mg a day. After 3 or 4 weeks at the initial dose, some improvement is generally noted. If not, the dose can be increased to 40 mg a day for most adults or to 20 mg a day for older patients. The patient should know that full improvement may take 6 to 8 weeks. Psychiatric consultation should be considered when there is lack of adequate response to such an intervention.

Once depressive symptoms have resolved, it is the author's practice to maintain a therapeutic dose of paroxetine for about 1 year before entertaining the possibility of gradually discontinuing the drug. Patients often want to stop treatment earlier, but this should be discouraged, because the risk of relapse is high in the first year. Some patients can be successfully taken off antidepressant medication after this period of time. However, others tend to relapse and may require long-term maintenance treatment.

Common side effects of paroxetine are insomnia, weight gain, nausea, and sexual dysfunction. Insomnia, which may be a symptom of the patient's depression, can be induced or worsened by most SSRIs. Drugs such as trazodone (Desyrel) 50 to 100 mg or diphenhydramine (Benadryl) 25 to 50 mg, given at bedtime, can alleviate this problem. Weight gain, the mechanism of which is unknown, is a common reason for noncompliance with this drug. In some instances, it is a helpful side effect. For most patients, careful attention to diet and regular exercise are needed to moderate this effect. Nausea is generally transient but sometimes requires a reduction in dosage. Sexual dysfunction also is a common reason for noncompliance. In men, retarded ejaculation is the most common form of this disturbance. Where premature ejaculation had been a problem prior to treatment, this side effect is a "blessing in disguise." In women, inhibition of orgasm is the problem encountered most frequently. Many remedies have been suggested—none truly satisfactory. For some patients, skipping their dose on a day intercourse is expected can be of help.

Anxiety

Mild anxiety and fear are common accompaniments of serious medical illness. For the patient, exposure to a strange environment, separation from family and home, the specter of pain, surgery, and even death are threats that can understandably provoke both of these unpleasant mood states.

Serious anxiety disorder may complicate IBD as well. Typical findings of tension, apprehension, worry, and fear often associated with poor concentration, insomnia, and fatigue suggest the diagnosis of an anxiety disorder. Some patients may give a history of acute attacks of panic during which they fear that something terrible is going to happen, that they are going to die, lose control of themselves, or go crazy. Such episodes often are accompanied by signs of sympathetic arousal with rapid heart rate, sweaty palms, elevation of blood pressure, and complaints of weakness, dyspnea, and lightheadedness. Many patients with panic attacks may develop secondary fears about being alone, driving a car, leaving their homes, or going to places where help is not readily available should they become panicky. This can sometimes result in a patient becoming housebound. The treatment of patients with anxiety disorders usually involves both psychologic and pharmacologic measures.

Psychological Management of the Anxious Patient

Most mild anxiety responds readily to a supportive doctor–patient relationship in which the physician can educate, reassure, and enhance the patient's sense of security. Patients with more severe anxiety or panic attacks need to understand that they have an illness that requires treatment with medication. They also need to understand that they will not go crazy or die during a panic attack, and that even untreated, most episodes of panic abate within several minutes. Once panic attacks have been sufficiently blocked pharmacologically, psychological support is still required, as patients generally need to be encouraged to begin activities that were previously avoided out of fear.

Pharmacologic Treatment of Anxiety

Diazepam (Valium) is an excellent drug for treatment of moderate to severe anxiety and can be started in doses of 2 to 5 mg given two to four times a day. If needed, the dose can be gradually raised until the desired effect is achieved. The long half-life of this drug makes it possible to give the bulk of or even the entire dose at bedtime. This is particularly helpful when anxiety is contributing significantly to insomnia or a once-a-day dose is more convenient. Once anxiety symptoms have improved, an attempt should be made to gradually reduce the dose and discontinue the drug over several weeks to 2 or 3 months. Diazepam is not able to block panic attacks, however. Fortunately, antidepressants can.

Paroxetine (Paxil) is an effective antipanic agent. Some patients suffering from panic attacks are exquisitely sensitive to antidepressants and may experience an increase in jitteriness when treatment is initiated. This may lead to noncompliance. It is recommended, therefore, to start at a lower dose than when treating depression. The patient can be started on 5 mg of paroxetine each morning, by cutting a 10-mg tablet in half, and the dose increased by 5-mg increments every few days until a total dose of 20 mg a day is reached (10 mg for the elderly or debilitated). Most patients have effective blocking of their panic attacks at this dose. As with treatment for depres-

sion, it may take several weeks for the full antipanic activity of paroxetine to be apparent. Once panic attacks have abated, a therapeutic dose of paroxetine should be maintained for at least a year. Psychiatric consultation should be considered if a patient does not respond to such an intervention.

Personality Disorder

Personality disorder can make patient management more difficult, because the patient's characteristic and habitual ways of reacting to life circumstances and dealing with people produce difficulties and suffering for both himself or herself and others. Adjusting to chronic illness, disability and pain, compliance with a complicated treatment regimen, dealing with an ileostomy, and coping with the many other challenges of being a patient all may be problematic. Often, it is the ability of the physician to relate to and therefore influence the patient that makes the difference between success or failure of treatment. Psychiatric consultation should be considered if the patient's problems adjusting to illness are thought to be attributable to aspects of his or her personality, are interfering with treatment, and have exhausted the resources of the gastroenterologist.

Management of the Histrionic Patient

The histrionic patient tends to be self-dramatizing, emotionally labile, seductive, dependent, and vain. To maintain a relationship with such a patient requires that the physician provide sufficient time and attention to ensure that the patient feels cared about. A kindly, paternal attitude generally is experienced as supportive. The patient's tendency to complain about nonspecific physical symptoms sometimes complicates management. It is important to recognize that hysterical complaints may commingle with symptoms of physical disease. Complaints about nonspecific physical symptoms often are best understood as meaningful communication by the patient that his or her needs for attention, care, and appreciation are not being met. Regularly scheduled visits rather than "as-needed" visits may be sufficient to reduce this behavior. Setting limits on unneeded diagnostic procedures, dangerous therapeutic interventions and "doctor shopping" often is necessary. Over time, the patient can be encouraged to talk about his life circumstances in an attempt to clarify emotional difficulties that might be dealt with directly.

Some histrionic patients develop chronic pain that has no adequate somatic explanation. Addiction to opiates or benzodiazepines may complicate matters. The management of such a patient usually begins with detoxification. A specialized pain treatment unit is an excellent place for this undertaking. Once detoxified, management of the patient with chronic pain can focus on alternative coping strategies and "getting on with life." There are two chapters on chronic pain management.

Adjusting to an ileostomy can be difficult for the histrionic patient, because of the patient's vanity. Fears that loss of beauty will invariably lead to loss of love or even abandonment can be aroused. The sensitivity of the gastroenterologist to this issue can be crucial for the histrionic patient's acceptance of the ileostomy and successful coping with it. Sometimes helping the patient's spouse or significant other to understand the patient's fears is useful as well. The chapter on body image and sexuality, written by a stomal therapist, also is helpful.

Management of the Obsessive Patient

The obsessive patient tends to be perfectionistic, overly intellectual, stubborn, and doubting. The patient's need for perfection and control can be a problem, because illness is not always predictable and medical treatment often is less than perfect. Such patients respond to these events with anxiety, worry, hypochondriacal brooding, and a tendency to become increasingly preoccupied with details. The physician will do best with such a patient by attempting to forge a relationship in which the patient is an equal partner or collaborator. Appealing to the patient's intellect and reason with frequent logical explanations often is required to help the obsessive patient cope. Sometimes, gentle confrontation and encouragement to "get to the point" during history taking and other discussions is required to help the patient stop endlessly focusing on details and start dealing directly with the situation at hand. A collaborative doctor–patient relationship of equal partners also tends to prevent the endless power struggles that obsessive patients tend to get into with people.

The obsessive patient may have trouble accepting an ileostomy at first, as these patients have great difficulty with change of any kind. Emphasizing the fact that the patient's control over his bowel function will be greatly improved by the ileostomy is generally a strong motivator for the obsessive patient to go ahead.

Management of the Antisocial Patient

The antisocial patient tends to be impulsive and exploitative, seems to have a lack of concern for others, has difficulty abiding by rules and regulations, and often is in conflict with authority. Such patients often are the most difficult for the physician to deal with. Managing his or her own anger and critical judgment of the patient's behavior are important if a relationship is going to be established. Firm limit-setting on destructive behaviors is needed from time to time. If the physician suspects that alcohol or drug abuse is complicating treatment of the patient's IBD, confrontation is needed, and firm insistence upon obtaining appropriate treatment should follow. Because the antisocial patient is very slow to develop trust in others, complete openness and honesty in all matters is crucial to the development of a workable doctor–patient relationship.

An ileostomy can be a challenge for the antisocial patient, because complying with any regimen often is a problem. Confrontation by the physician that involves warning of negative consequences rarely influences the patient; however, rewards often are motivators. Sometimes, the reward of continued care by the physician has to be made contingent upon the patient's compliance.

Editor's Note

If you do not recognize some of your patients here, you either do not see many patients or you do not talk with them. (TMB)

Supplemental Reading

Depaulo JR. Depression. In: Stobo JD, Hellmann DB, Ladenson PW, et al, eds. The principles and practice of medicine. 23rd Ed. Stamford, CT: Appleton and Lange, 1996:922–6.

Helzer JE, Chammas S, Norland CC, et al. A study of the association between Crohn's disease and psychiatric illness. Gastroenterology 1984;86:324–30.

Helzer JE, Stillings WA, Chammas S, et al. A controlled study of the association between ulcerative colitis and psychiatric diagnosis. Dig Dis Sci 1982;27:513–8.

Hoehn-Saric R, McCleod DR. Clinical management of generalized anxiety disorder. In: Coryell W, Winokur W, eds. The clinical management of anxiety disorders. New York: Oxford, 1991:79–100.

Teitelbaum ML. Psychological responses to illness. In: Stobo JD, Hellman DB, Ladenson PW, et al, eds. The principles and practice of medicine. 23rd Ed. Stamford, CT: Appleton and Lange, 1996:946–8.

Tune L, Folstein MF. Post-operative delirium. Adv Psychosom Med 1986;15:51–68.

CHAPTER 123

Psychological Perspectives on the Care of Patients with Inflammatory Bowel Disease

David H. Edwin, PhD

It is much more important to know what sort of a patient has a disease than what sort of disease a patient has.
                                   Attributed to Sir William Osler

This comment was made in an era when diagnosis was less firmly rooted in anatomy, physiology, and molecular biology than it currently is, and much less directed to tiers of rational and empirical treatment. Nonetheless, it is true now, as it was then, that the patient is more than simply a host to the disease, and that empathic, behavioral, and social factors play a major role in the individual's response to illness and treatment. To understand "the patient with the disease" requires at least four distinct perspectives, each of which reveals and obscures different aspects of our patients' lives, and all of which are essential for effective care of the ill as well as the troubled (Table 123–1). The *disease* method focuses attention on the "broken" organ or system and on the disruptions of life that attend the illness and its treatment. The *trait* method draws attention to normal and extreme differences in universal human attributes, such as intellect and personality, and how they emerge as strengths and vulnerabilities in life circumstances such as illnesses. The *behavior* method deals with the purposeful actions that individuals choose or "fall into" and their consequences in health and illness. The *life story* method draws attention to the ongoing process in which people make sense of their lives as they unfold and shape these—for better and sometimes for worse—into autobiographies that stretch into the future. This chapter explores the perspectives of the psychologist in understanding and caring for "the patient with the disease."

The Disease Perspective

The burdens and challenges of inflammatory bowel disease (IBD) do not need elaboration here. The myth still persists in some quarters, despite an utter absence of empirical support, that ulcerative colitis (UC) and Crohn's disease (CD) are specific expressions of certain pathologic personality types. In fact, even the more plausible hypothesis relating emotional stress to illness exacerbations remains at best equivocal; it is supported by retrospective surveys and (weakly) by a few prospective studies, but more frequently reinforced by anecdotal experience and the commonsense assumption that stress *must* take its toll. Epidemiologic studies have not demonstrated a higher incidence or prevalence of major psychiatric illness in patients with IBD than in patients with other chronic illnesses. There is, however, considerable evidence that depressed or otherwise psychiatrically ill patients with IBD (and other chronic illnesses) fare more poorly in terms of clinical course and social-vocational adaptation than those without psychiatric illness. Finally,

TABLE 123–1. Psychological and Psychiatric Perspectives

Perspective	Focus	Strategies
Disease What the patient *has*	UC and CD symptoms and treatment side effects Other medical illnesses, symptoms, and treatment effects Primary psychiatric illnesses, symptoms, and treatment effects	Identification of symptoms and syndromes Treatment or specialty referral
Dimension Who the patient *is*	The patient's personal status with respect to basic human attributes	Guidance for adaptation to stressful aspects of life
Behavior What the patient *does*	Poor personal skills and resources Poor choices with unintended consequences	Increasing adaptive skills Decreasing or stopping negative behaviors
Life story What it all *means*	Changes and disruptions in the meanings underlying personal lives	Reformulation of the life story "script"

TABLE 123–2. Some Implications of the Five Factors for Patient Care Strategies

Personality Factor	High	Low	Strategic Implications
Neuroticism (N)	Tend to be unhappy Tend to be pessimistic Tend to be disappointed, angry	Tend to be stable, consistent Tend to be optimistic Tend to be accepting, content	High N: often resist reassurance, overemphasize side effects, are less satisfied with treatment outcomes than low N; focus on objective outcomes and indices, rather than self-report and satisfaction.
Extroversion (E)	Social, engaging Emotionally reactive Present oriented Quick to react, dramatic Quick to recover	Quiet Emotionally reserved Future oriented Slow to react, moderate Slow to recover	Low E: may be difficult to draw out High E: provide emotional rather than factual accounts 'How do I feel now?' vs 'How will I feel in the future?' Hi E: may respond impulsively, then simmer down; treatment response may be quick but transient Low E: may not react for some time
Openness (O)	Open to new formulations, ideas Willing to try new treatments Psychologically minded	Suspicious of new ideas Reluctant to try new treatments Apsychological	Low O: may be skeptical and resistant to new approaches or to psychological referral Hi O: may be accepting and eager, but if low C (below) may not follow directions and may "doctor-shop"
Agreeableness (A)	Friendly, easy to relate to Acquiescent	Skeptical, questioning May provoke staff	High A: may make excellent first impression, regardless of C (below) Low A: may alienate care givers
Conscientiousness (C)	Adherent to treatment Organized	Nonadherent Disorganized	High C: may be better motivated, organized, and compliant but may take reversals more to heart

the immunosuppressive medications used to treat IBD, most notoriously corticosteroids, are not psychiatrically benign. Emotional ability as well as depression, hypomania, and frank delirium, is reported among patients taking these agents, and the first three may persist after the drug is tapered.

The role of the psychologist from this perspective starts with the identification of psychiatric illness by history and mental state examination. Frank affective illness, whether or not it appears in the context of illness exacerbation, usually responds to any of the numerous antidepressant medications, which can be administered by a variety of routes. Although medication is often necessary for these patients, it is rarely sufficient. These patients may be quick to blame themselves for the depth of their emotional distress and may require considerable help and support in coming to understand the nature of the affective illness and its implications for themselves and, possibly, their families. On the other hand, patients with demoralization (the understandable emotional reaction to serious adversity) are generally not helped by these medications, although they are, of course, vulnerable to all of the side effects. Their difficulties respond more readily to the methods and interventions described below.

The Dimensional Perspective

Even (perhaps *especially*) in the absence of psychiatric illness, individuals differ from one another in important ways. Patients with modest intellect may have difficulty understanding what physicians try to teach them about their illnesses and their treatment. They may have difficulty with emergent situations and even with the routine variability of symptoms. Their medications may be difficult for them to track and take at proper times; at other times, they may take two and three times their prescribed

doses. Careful teaching may require an appreciation of cognitive deficiencies, which may also reveal the need to rally the support of family and community resources. Physicians and nurses often develop considerable sensitivity and expertise in this area.

Patients also vary widely in their persisting patterns of behavior and emotional reactivity and in their vulnerabilities to specific environmental challenges. Most often, it is in this area that psychologists provide unique perspectives and interventions. A few general observations about personality may be helpful, followed by a discussion of some specific problems and how they may be ameliorated (Table 123–2). Contemporary personality research suggests five major dimensions of personality, along which all people are arrayed; each of these factors has some impact on illness behavior in general.

Neuroticism-stability describes the general tendency to be more often unhappy (sad, angry, embarrassed, hopeless, self-doubting, as opposed to stable or satisfied) than others under the same circumstances. Patients higher in neuroticism tend to be more severely affected by their symptoms, more vexed by their treatments, and less satisfied with their outcomes.

Extroversion-introversion describes a range of general emotional, behavioral, and social reactivity; it reflects a sort of "psychological Brownian movement." More extroverted patients react quickly and intensely to their circumstances, good or bad. Their emotions tend to pervade and dominate their experiences in life, but are often remarkably inconsistent: events affect them intensely, but often transiently. More introverted individuals are less prone to react quickly and dramatically, but more likely to nurture worries and discontents for long periods.

Openness reflects interest in new ideas and experiences of all kinds. Patients high in openness are more willing than others to consider a variety of approaches to their problems, including "host-centered" rather than "symptom-centered" options. Thus, they are more willing to consider psychological, behavioral, and "alternative" treatment strategies than their less open counterparts, who regard discussions of stress and support as attributions of personal weakness.

Agreeableness reflects the degree to which the patient is friendly, trusting, and confiding, as opposed to questioning, critical, and even belligerent. It goes without saying that agreeable patients at least start out easier and are more gratifying to care for, but if they are high in neuroticism or low in conscientiousness, they may soon exhaust their doctors with their neediness or their inability to follow through on their care plans.

Conscientiousness describes the degree to which patients are motivated, organized, consistent, and self-disciplined. Conscientious individuals process information carefully with the intent to "get it right"; they persevere despite distraction or adversity. Less conscientious individuals may have good intentions but fail to plan and organize their lives to accommodate the requirements of their treatment, and may soon be distracted or discouraged, becoming essentially "noncompliant." On the other hand, there is some evidence that highly conscientious patients may take treatment reversals personally, as though they had somehow failed in their responsibilities.

Obviously, patients high in neuroticism are among those most frequently referred for psychological care or consultation. Those who are also highly extroverted tend to be dramatic in their complaints and behaviors, and in their overwhelming experience of their negative emotions, may be the most prone to contemplate self-harm. Similarly, they may respond with injudicious enthusiasm to small improvements, whereas they may be utterly crushed by inevitable reversals. They need to be reassured, assisted with "reality testing," and redirected toward the long-run view, which does not come easily to them when they are distressed. On the other hand, those who are more introverted may worry their physicians with their quiet pessimism and reluctance to acknowledge small gains, as though to look at these would be to risk evaporating them. They may be refractory to reassurance but respond to an approach that emphasizes a succession of treatment options and contingency plans.

Patients low in conscientiousness also are frequently referred to psychologists, as they can be vexing to manage despite the initial impressions they may make. They may forget appointments or arrive late, and yet expect to be seen promptly. They tend to neglect scheduled bloodwork or other procedures, and have difficulty following medication regimens. When they are high in openness and agreeableness, they may respond warmly and enthusiastically to each new treatment plan, but quickly become disillusioned when results are not immediately

forthcoming. They may do well if support and structure can be developed, from their families or others, in a nonjudgmental manner that acknowledges their motivation but deals forthrightly with their casual disorganization and apparent passivity.

Patients with difficult personality traits may be especially vulnerable to chronic illness in at least two ways. They may develop disabling anxiety and demoralization that exacerbate the impact of their symptoms, and they may allow their life plans to be disrupted by their illnesses more than needs to be the case. The first category of difficulty is discussed from the behavioral perspective, and the second is discussed from the perspective of the life story.

The Behavioral Perspective

Human behavior can be understood as a product of motivation and intention: people act to maintain or bring about a desirable state of affairs or to avoid or terminate an undesirable one. In some cases, owing to personality vulnerabilities or deficient learning opportunities, patients lack essential skills of one kind or another and make choices that frustrate these intentions rather than serve them. This is most clearly evident in patients who become derailed in managing their anxiety or demoralization, and in those who have trouble successfully managing their drives and impulses.

Management

Anxiety and demoralization are inevitable in life, and particularly in the lives of individuals with these illnesses that affect some of the most intimate human functions in the most awkward, painful, and utterly unpredictable ways. As discussed elsewhere in this volume, psychotropic medication may be the appropriate response to syndromic major depression or panic disorder. There are also a variety of psychological techniques for managing anxiety, depression, and pain; like medications, they really represent "trade-marked" variations on a smaller number of basic themes (Table 123–3). The first category of these is addressed at the intensely unpleasant state of muscular and visceral arousal that accompanies subjective apprehensiveness, either chronic or acute. **Progressive muscle relaxation** engages the patient in tensing and then relaxing successive muscle groups, starting with the hands or feet and moving through to the scalp and facial muscles. The patient learns to recognize and control the physical concomitants of anxiety and to manage episodes of pain and, in the process, gains a sense of competence and mastery. Other methods of accomplishing the same end include *hypnosis, self-hypnosis,* and *autogenic training,* with affirmations of well-being ("Every day in every way I'm getting better and better"); commercially produced self-help courses and tapes are available, but optimal practice would allow the psychologist to help the patient choose and learn a method along with the rationale for its

TABLE 123–3. Basic Cognitive and Behavioral Treatment Strategies

Technique	Target Problems
Relaxation methods and related treatment*	Anxiety, fearfulness
Systematic desensitization	Pain management
Flooding	Learned or condition avoidance
Thought stopping	
Anxiety management	
Stress Inoculation	**Preparation for Inevitable Reversals**
Cognitive restructuring	Social withdrawal
Cognitive and cognitive behavior therapy	Interpersonal problems
Rational emotive therapy	Depression and demoralization
Social skills training	Social skills deficits
Group therapies	Stigmatization
Support groups	Resource and coping deficits
	Isolation and alienation
	Need for confrontation
Counseling	Life-meaning issues
Insight and relationship-oriented psychotherapy	Life-stage task interruption
	Relationship problems
	Failure of other psychological therapies

*Progressive relaxation, guided imagery, meditation, hypnosis, biofeedback, etc.

use. *Biofeedback* management of surface temperature, electrodermal conductivity, and muscle tension in specific regions (eg, frontalis muscles) may be used to induce generalized relaxation as well; biofeedback may have the disadvantage of inducing a dependency on assistive devices, but may have the added benefit in some cases of allowing the training of specific muscle groups that might otherwise be difficult to address (eg, sphincter function).

It is important to remember that relaxation techniques themselves are not enduring in their effects, so that a comprehensive program for the patient's use of these techniques is the crucial factor. In practice, relaxation exercises often are coupled with either imagined or, preferably, in vivo confrontation of provocative stimuli, often social events or medical procedures. Patients thus learn that they can relax and prevail in challenging circumstances, generalize the techniques to other challenges, and increase their general sense of competency.

Another major category of techniques (eg, cognitive therapy, cognitive behavior therapy, rational emotive therapy) is directed at the set of perceptions, cognitions, and beliefs that may constrain the ability of patients to cope with the challenges and opportunities they encounter. The central assumption of these methods is that individuals often are more handicapped by their systematically distorted perceptions and erroneous beliefs about circumstances than by the objective circumstances themselves. In these forms of treatment, the therapist carefully elicits erroneous perceptions or beliefs, as for example:

They can all tell right away that I am sick.
I could tell right away he wouldn't be interested.
I'm damaged goods—no one would ever want me.

If I can't graduate on time with my class, my life is ruined.
I'll never have children—or be able to care for them.

Other errors of thinking include selective perception of negative information, overgeneralization, and "catastrophizing." The therapist helps the patient to make these often unacknowledged cognitions explicit and then to reassess them and their emotional implications:

Many potential mates may want a "perfect" partner, and that may make my search harder. But I only need to find one, and that is not impossible.
If I don't date much, I may be disappointed. But there will be things I can do to cope. For example . . .
There are many ways to have children . . .

Often, the best advice, inspiration, and motivation may derive from contacts with other patients in hospital visitations, support groups, and other forums. Patients may be able to challenge one another more forthrightly than their care takers can and offer them more concrete guidance:

Come on, you can believe that if you want but it wasn't true for me and it doesn't have to be true for you.
When John and I were dating, I used to bring along two magazines in case I had an attack—one for me and one for him.

The Life Story Perspective

People understand their lives as evolving stories, *biographies* that make sense and move along in meaningful ways. Each person's story has both general and unique aspects. The general aspects reflect, for example, the theme in contemporary culture that illnesses should be transient and ultimately overcome. Those of us who spend our days with patients forget this: illness can be experienced as a failing, a blemish, and evidence of weakness or culpability. It produces a spoiled identity and has little place in the normative life stories that most younger individuals expect to live out. The very fact of a chronic illness makes people uneasy, and patients afflicted with chronic illness early in life often feel like a disappointment to their families, unworthy of a professional career, marriage, or parenthood.

Each patient is deeply invested in his or her own evolving autobiography, which reflects a particular reading of the details and meanings of his or her history, leading with novelistic force to a projected future. These subjective autobiographies may be reasonable and based in reality or not, and they may provide an effective basis for making choices or not. In any case, disruptions of the patient's life story are experienced as psychological crises, and they may require considerable effort to resolve. Some patients accommodate these resolutions with a minimum of disorganization in their behavior and relationships, whereas others become more disorganized and unhappy.

Some behave in ways that are destructive to themselves and their families. The reconstruction of a more realistic and effective autobiography from the remainder of one that has become untenable is the fundamental task of traditional psychotherapy.

Summary

Inflammatory bowel disease by its nature is chronic but unpredictable and may strike at times when patients are organizing their lives in crucial areas of identity, career, and family. Using a methodologic approach, medical and psychiatric illnesses and their consequences can be identified and treated. Patients can be guided in developing their strengths and avoiding their vulnerabilities to make the most of the opportunities that are open to them. Behaviors can be shaped—reduced or eliminated, enhanced or expanded—to improve adaptation to less-than-perfect circumstances. Life stories can be rewritten to engender futures that accommodate realistic limitations and understandable aspirations. It is the role of the psychologist to assist patients in achieving satisfying and rewarding personal, vocational, and family lives despite the formidable challenges of illness.

Reference

McHugh PR, Slavney PR. The perspectives of psychiatry. 2nd Ed. Baltimore: Johns Hopkins University Press, 1998.

CHAPTER 124

STRESS MANAGEMENT

H. RICHARD WARANCH, PHD

Living a stress-free life is unrealistic. Stress is a normal part of life. When stress is mild to moderate, it may motivate a person to try harder and perform better. It is when stress is severe and prolonged that problems develop. Since stress cannot be completely eliminated, a more practical goal is to learn to deal with stress actively and effectively. Stress management is not a specific treatment technique applied to an illness called "stress." Rather, stress management refers to a general treatment approach that may combine many techniques to help to improve a broad category of health and behavioral problems.

Five steps are followed in designing an appropriate stress management program for an individual:

1. Assess the individual's problem(s)
2. Educate
3. Increase healthy behaviors
4. Increase healthy thinking
5. Teach relaxation techniques

Assessment

Each person with symptoms or behaviors that appear to be stress related (eg, headaches, insomnia, anxiety) presents with a different history and set of circumstances that must be assessed before treatment can begin. For example, Joe is a 40-year-old, married man, who was referred by his neurologist for biofeedback and relaxation training. His presenting symptoms were chronic left-sided facial pain and low back pain. Medical records from the neurologist and the patient's internist summarized his medical history in scrupulous detail and his lack of response to multiple medications as well as acupuncture, chiropractic treatment, and treatment by a dentist specializing in temporomandibular joint dysfunction (TMJD). Magnetic resonance imaging (MRI), blood work, and physical examinations were all essentially normal. Notably absent from the medical reports was information about Joe's lifestyle. An interview revealed that Joe worked in a family construction business. He typically worked 7 days a week and 14 to 16 hours per day. He rarely took a day off, and he had taken only one 4-day vacation in 11 years of marriage. He believed that he personally had to supervise every job and each of his employees or something would go wrong. Joe had always been a

hard worker and somewhat of a perfectionist about work, but he became even worse after his father died a year earlier. His father was the founder of his company and after his father's death Joe felt even more responsibility for all aspects of the business. Also, he now assumed responsibility for taking care of his elderly mother. Joe was about 25 pounds overweight, did not exercise, and often ate fast food on the run. Given his history and life style, it was not surprising to me that Joe's symptoms did not improve with conventional medical treatment. My recommendation to Joe was that he needed to make some life-style changes rather than pursue biofeedback treatment.

Education

Most people who present with stress-related symptoms are given a brief overview of the basic stress mechanism as described in the early 1900s by Walter B. Cannon. Cannon introduced the theory that humans react to stressful events (stressors) with physical preparation to fight or flee. He proposed that our prehistoric ancestors developed a nervous system that responded to life-threatening events by preparing the body to do battle or to run away. He called this mechanism the "fight-flight" response. So, faced with perceived danger, heart rate and blood pressure skyrocket, the liver pours out glucose to be converted into energy, breathing becomes deeper and more rapid, and blood is diverted from nonessential functions to the brain and muscles. This is precisely what our prehistoric ancestors needed to survive when faced with acute, relatively short-term, physical threats.

Civilization, by contrast, presents a host of everyday events that may be perceived as stressors. For example, traffic jams, commuting, household and car repairs, unexpected bills, and long work hours may elicit the same response in us as the sight of a saber-toothed tiger did in our prehistoric ancestors. Human beings are equipped to deal with such stressors, if they do not happen too often. However, our bodies were not meant to deal with prolonged chronic stress. When stressful events happen repeatedly over a lifetime, the effects multiply and compound.

Unfortunately, the implied promise that technology would somehow increase leisure time and make people more relaxed has certainly not materialized. If anything,

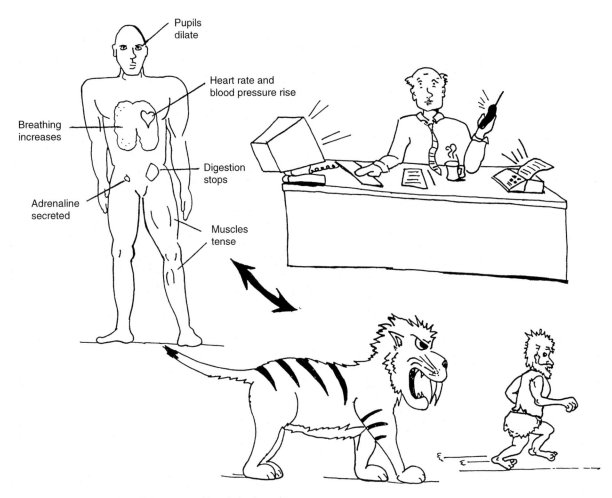

FIGURE 124–1. Cannon's fight-flight response (description in text).

technology has added to stress level and eaten away at leisure activities. My patient, Joe, complained that whenever he misses a day at work he returns to dozens of e-mails, faxes, and voice mails waiting for his immediate response.

Figure 124–1 illustrates Cannon's fight-flight mechanism comparing prehistoric with modern man. I keep a copy of this picture in my office and I actually show it to patients in explaining how stress can play a significant role in contributing to their specific problem.

Increasing Healthy Behaviors

It is well known that it is unhealthy to abuse alcohol, drugs, and nicotine; to have an unhealthy diet; to be overweight; to constantly work long hours; and to rush and to lose one's temper. At the same time, everyone knows that it is healthy to exercise, to get an adequate amount of sleep, and to schedule time for relaxation and recreation. Once the physician determines that a problem exists for a particular patient, practical and realistic recommendations must be presented. Merely telling a patient to "quit smoking" or "lose weight" will unlikely result in behavioral

changes. Rather, if appropriate, the patient should be referred to a specific program (eg, Weight Watchers or a stop-smoking program) and some articles or books to read may be suggested. Follow-up with phone calls and scheduled appointments is important. Changing behavior is not easy and must be done gradually and in small steps.

Increasing Healthy Thinking

When I first saw Joe he was about 10 minutes late for his appointment, which was fairly typical for him. In leaving his office, he left with barely enough time to make our appointment as long as there was no traffic. However, there was traffic and he admitted to getting very tense and frustrated and to driving somewhat recklessly in an attempt to get to the appointment on time. He also admitted to such thoughts as "I should have left earlier," "I shouldn't be taking time away from my office anyway," "I know something will go wrong while I'm gone," and "I know this will be a waste of time anyway." Joe's self-talk is meant to illustrate that how we think or talk to ourselves can determine how we feel and what actions we decide to take. Some explanations we give ourselves are positive and empowering. Others arouse anger, feed our frustration, or lead to feelings of depression or anxiety. Shakespeare's Hamlet put it succinctly in saying, "There is nothing either good or bad but thinking makes it so." Our internal dialogue has been called "self-talk" by rational emotive theorist Albert Ellis and "automatic thoughts" by cognitive theorist Aaron Beck. Most people talk to themselves quite differently than they talk to others. In talking to others, we are usually rational and objective and able to describe events as cause and effect relations. However, in talking to ourselves, we can be subjective and irrational. We usually are unaware of the continuing chatter in our heads, so we do not connect our negative feelings with our negative thoughts. Learning to change self-talk is the focus of cognitive therapy, and self-help books, such as *Feeling Good* and *The Feeling Good Handbook*, by David Burns, can help a person learn to increase healthy thinking.

Learning to Relax the Body

Relaxation responses can counteract the fight-or-flight response. Relaxation can be achieved through a number of different approaches. For patients with more severe problems, there are psychologists and social workers who work with individuals, using a variety of relaxation techniques. For patients with mild to moderate problems, there are formal classes in meditation and yoga. For patients with mild problems, there are self-help books and CDs. Merely making a referral to a psychologist or a recommendation to enroll in a yoga course is not likely to be effective without a follow-up plan from the physician. Patients can be taught the following relaxation exercise. The physician should actually demonstrate the technique to a patient and then give him or her a handout describing the technique as follows.

Diaphragmatic Breathing

Diaphragmatic breathing involves learning to use the diaphragm, rather than the shoulders and chest muscles, to draw air into the lungs. This allows more efficient breathing with less muscular work. It allows you to relax the neck and shoulder muscles while breathing.

Training Procedures for Diaphragmatic Breathing

Use a recliner. A recliner or high-backed chair with arms is ideal initially because the entire body is supported and musculature tension is reduced. Once learned, diaphragmatic breathing can then be used in a variety of settings and with different postures to help you relax.

Hand placement. Place your right hand on your stomach, between the bottom of your rib cage and your naval. Place your left hand on your chest, just below your collar bone.

Loosen restrictive clothing. Unbutton your pants and loosen your belt. Research has demonstrated that people take in less oxygen when they are wearing restrictive clothing around their abdomen.

Baseline breathing. First, just breathe regularly and simply pay attention in a passive manner to your breathing. Notice the air passing through your nostrils and, at the same time, notice the rise and fall of your hands as you inhale and exhale. **Remember, do not try to control your breath, but simply sustain your awareness through the entire inhalation and exhalation cycle.** For now, all other thoughts apart from the sensations of breathing are distractions. Whenever your mind wanders—whether to thoughts, sounds, or other sensations—bring your mind back to paying attention to your breathing.

Diaphragmatic breathing practice. As you inhale, imagine your stomach to be a balloon that inflates, lifting your right hand. As you exhale, the balloon deflates and your right hand falls. Your left hand remains still as your right hand rises and falls.

Feedback. Do not try to force it. Just attend to the motion of your hands and the feelings in your chest. Allow your right hand to rise and fall while your left hand remains still.

Slow breathing. Next, slow your breathing by pausing very briefly at the top and bottom of each breath. Just a second or so. Do not hold your breath or pause so you are uncomfortable. Aim for one breath about every 6 or 7 seconds.

Tension release. Each time you exhale, let your whole body become limp all over and allow it to sink deep in your chair.

Repeat the word "calm." Some people find it helpful to anchor their mind on the breath by silently repeating a word with each exhalation. I like the word "calm," but any word that is personally meaningful (e.g., "peace," "one," or "uhm") could be used. If you use a word along with the breath, try to keep the actual sensation of breathing in the foreground of your awareness, and the word itself in the background, a quiet whisper in the mind.

Placement of hands at sides. After one or two sessions with the hands on your chest and abdomen, the hands can usually be placed on the arms of the chair or in your lap.

Some difficulties. For most people, diaphragmatic breathing is awkward and uncomfortable initially. As in learning any new skill, with consistent practice, most people can become proficient and comfortable with this new style of breathing.

Practice. To become comfortable with the technique, you should try to practice at least 5 to 10 minutes once or twice a day. Most people find that one convenient time to practice is in bed just prior to going to sleep. However, relaxed breathing aims for a state of relaxed alertness and if you are too drowsy you might fall asleep. So, practicing at the end of the work day or before dinner might be better. Once you have mastered the technique and can do it rather quickly, you can begin using it when feeling stressed. However, without regular practice in nonstressful situations first, diaphragmatic breathing is not likely to be very helpful when you feel stressed.

When feeling stressed. Diaphragmatic breathing will be most useful if you can catch symptoms early. Once in the midst of a full-blown anxiety attack or a severe migraine, diaphragmatic breathing is not likely to be very helpful. However, taking 5 to 10 minutes to practice breathing at the onset of such symptoms may serve to actually abort the symptoms or delay their occurrence.

Supplemental Reading

Burns D. Feeling good: the new mood therapy. New York: William Morrow, 1980.

Burns D. The feeling good handbook. New York: Penguin, 1989.

Other Sources

Stress management tapes and books:

ISHK Book Service, Department T-52, P.O. Box 176, Los Altos, CA 94022

New Harbinger Publications, 2200 Adeline, Suite 305, Oakland, CA 94607. Tel: 415 465-1435

Whole Person Associates, 210 West Michigan, Duluth, MN 55802-1908. Tel: 1 800 247-6789

Behavioral Pain Management

Harry S. Shabsin, PhD

Ulcerative colitis and Crohn's disease are the major idiopathic inflammatory diseases of the bowel. In addition to symptoms of diarrhea, rectal bleeding, and weight loss, abdominal pain is described by more than 75 percent of patients with inflammatory bowel disease.[*]

Inflammatory bowel disease was initially considered a psychosomatic disorder related to obsessive-compulsive, passive-dependent, and alexithymic (difficulty expressing emotion or feelings) personality characteristics because of the high incidence of these traits in patients with this disorder. However, the theory that psychological traits contribute to the development of inflammatory bowel disease remains to be proved, and the mechanism by which personality traits might affect gastrointestinal physiology resulting in inflammatory bowel disease has not been shown. Consequently, emphasis has shifted to an organic explanation in which inappropriate immune system responses, bacterial contagions, and or diet are hypothesized to account for the development of the disease.

Although psychological characteristics have not been shown to cause inflammatory bowel disease, patients having this disorder have been found to be more hypochondriacal, depressed, anxious, obsessive-compulsive, and nonassertive than normal control populations in many studies, even though there are some exceptions. In addition, patients with inflammatory bowel disease have been reported by some investigators as being similar to patients diagnosed with psychosomatic disorders such as spastic colitis on measures of anxiety, neurotic tendencies, or affective disorders. These findings have led to the conclusion that the interaction between emotional stress and psychological characteristics can affect the onset or exacerbation of symptoms associated with inflammatory bowel disease. As a consequence, behaviorally based treatments useful in the management of chronic pain arising from other disorders can be applied in the treatment of pain associated with inflammatory bowel disease.

Recognizing Patients with a Chronic Pain Syndrome

Chronic pain is usually defined as pain lasting for 6 months or longer or pain failing to respond to medical

or surgical management, excluding symptoms associated with a terminal illness such as cancer. Patients who continually complain of pain or who habitually fail to respond to medical treatments may be suffering from a chronic pain syndrome in which environmental stresses and behavioral components contribute to complaints of pain. However, identifying this type of patient is not always straightforward, especially since psychological profiles, which might be helpful in this regard, are typically unavailable. There are, however, certain physical or behavioral signs, listed below, that are useful in identifying patients whose chronic pain complaints may be related to personality characteristics.

Physical and Behavioral Signs

1. Pain complaints continue in the absence of physical findings or are out of proportion to the amount of tissue pathology.
2. The description of pain is given in a vague or inconsistent fashion.
3. Symptoms are described in an emotional or dramatic fashion.
4. Discrepancies are found between observed behavior and reported pain.
5. Overreaction occurs during physical examination.
6. There is inappropriate patient use of antianxiety or narcotic-analgesic medication.
7. Symptoms result in decreased work, social, or family responsibilities.
8. The patient shows evidence of a poor ability to express feelings or emotion.
9. The patient shows evidence of depression or poor self-esteem.
10. The patient experiences an anxious mood or chronic stress.
11. There is heightened worry, focus, or concern about symptoms.
12. Legal action related to symptoms has occurred.

Although none of these signs guarantee that psychological components contribute to chronic pain, they are all indications that nonmedical conditions are influencing symptom complaints. When such signs are recognized in patients with inflammatory bowel disease, there are a

---

[*] This chapter appeared in the first edition of this book in 1989.

number of helpful strategies the physician can employ to help the patient.

Physician-Patient Relationship

For the patient with inflammatory bowel disease, the development of a supportive relationship with the physician is often helpful in decreasing chronic abdominal pain. The overall aim of such a relationship is to assist the patient in developing a sense of independence and control over his or her symptoms. Several suggestions are offered below that are useful in achieving this goal.

Acceptance of the Patient

Acceptance of the patient's symptoms, personality traits, and style of interacting with those around him or her is helpful in establishing a positive therapeutic relationship. This increases patient confidence in the care being received and improves compliance with medical or behavioral advice. An important aspect in developing such a relationship is to allow enough time for the patient to talk about worries or concerns involving his or her illness or to discuss personal issues that may be causing anxiety or emotional distress. Patients with chronic abdominal pain, including those with inflammatory bowel disease, often report feeling better after being allowed to talk to their physician in a supportive atmosphere. For the patient with inflammatory bowel disease, establishing a therapeutic relationship may be particularly important because the loss of personal relationships has been hypothesized to be highly stressful for this type of patient and has often been retrospectively reported to be related to the onset or exacerbation of symptoms.

Providing Information and Encouragement

Many patients with a chronic medical condition have misconceptions or irrational beliefs about their symptoms and the pain they experience. This may lead to exaggerated fears about being unable to cope with their illness or a belief that their symptoms are becoming worse, even when they are faced with evidence to the contrary. Such feeling can lead to increased anxiety or despair, which, in turn, can cause increased complaints of pain and more frequent requests for medical attention. In addition, the experience of chronic pain often leads to decreased social, family, or work-related activities. In such situations, patients can begin to feel they are no longer productive or are becoming a burden on others. The patient who begins to think this way often also begins to experience increased feelings of isolation, helplessness, or depression.

Providing encouragement helps to decrease behavioral disabilities related to the stress a patient can experience when faced with chronic pain. Patients should be advised to keep busy. Whenever feasible, they should be directed to return to work. They should also be encouraged to be physically and socially active and to engage in regular exercise programs, if possible. Being active helps the patient to feel better about himself or herself and acts as a distraction from medical problems.

It is also important to find out the meaning a particular patient's symptoms have for him or her. Once this is accomplished, misconceptions and unrealistic worries can be dispelled by providing information about the nature of inflammatory bowel disease and the symptoms that result from this disorder, going over realistic expectations a patient should have about his or her illness and discussing unrealistic concerns a patient may have. Providing this type of information helps the patient to overcome unnecessary fears or disability related to inflammatory bowel disease. In many instances, it is the misconceptions a patient has about the disease or a fear of making his or her condition worse, rather than the level of pain or actual symptoms, that cause restrictions in social and professional activities. Although it may require persistence and patience, reassurance and proper guidance by an authoritative and supportive figure are very helpful in decreasing pain and behavioral disabilities associated with a chronic illness.

Behavioral Pain Management for Inflammatory Bowel Disease

Unfortunately, not all patients with chronic pain or behavioral disabilities respond to helpful suggestions. When a patient continues to display a decreased level of functioning that seems out of proportion to physical findings or seems to be related to personality traits more than organic pathology, that person may be thought of as displaying "illness behavior." In such cases, referral for behavioral pain management to help the patient decrease the symptoms and disability associated with chronic illness is appropriate. Because sensitivity to pain is a multidimensional process, behavioral pain management programs utilize a variety of treatment methods, some of which are described below, to address psychological states, personality characteristics, and social situations that are known to affect pain perception.

Stress Management

Patients with chronic abdominal pain often report that their symptoms increase with the onset of emotional stress. Stress management is an umbrella term for an assortment of strategies designed to increase a patient's ability to cope with stressful situations without undue emotional arousal. Depending on the particular patient, this type of therapy may take the form of problem solving (ie, teaching the patient productive ways of analyzing problems), and teaching patients to be more assertive in expressing their needs and feelings, improving communication skills, or helping the patient attain important goals through the use of improved interpersonal skills. Helping patients develop a sense of mastery over their personal lives many times generalizes to increased feelings of control over their symptoms and results in a decrease in physical complaints. The chapter on stress management reviews some of these changes.

Somatic Anxiety

Heightened anxiety levels are related to increased pain perception under a variety of situations, including chronic illness. As such, an important component of any pain management program should be the reduction of anxiety related to chronic pain or illness. Patients sometimes become so focused on their condition that their symptoms become a major source of concern and they become unresponsive to simple encouragement. In such instances, a behavioral treatment based on a psychotherapeutic technique termed "cognitive restructuring" is an effective means of decreasing inappropriate anxiety arising from a medical disorder such as inflammatory bowel disease. Cognitive restructuring provides patients with alternative ways of conceptualizing the meaning of their symptoms and is particularly useful for treating patients with chronic pain. In brief, patients are asked to record cognitions about their illness with emphasis on emotional or illness-related thought concerning pain or other symptoms. They are then instructed to replace negative health perceptions with positive conceptualizations about their illness. Over time, patients who originally conceived of their symptoms as horrible or unbearable events find themselves accepting their illness with a greater sense of control and much lower levels of anxiety or emotional trauma. This reduction in anxiety and the accompanying improvement in mood it brings about are effective ways of reducing or eliminating chronic complaints of pain associated with illnesses such as inflammatory bowel disease.

Biofeedback

Biofeedback is the process of providing information about biologic activity to an individual. Typically, electrodes or electronic transducers are attached to the body, and signals of interest are sent to appropriate equipment for amplification and processing. This equipment then produces auditory or visual information (biofeedback) about the occurrence of specific physiologic events. Commonly used forms of biofeedback provide patients with information on heart rate, blood pressure, hand temperature, striated muscle tension, galvanic skin response, or electroencephalographic activity. The most useful of these modalities for treating chronic abdominal pain are hand temperature and musculoskeletal activity. The goal of biofeedback in the treatment of chronic abdominal pain is to teach patients to reduce the physiologic arousal that often accompanies the onset of pain. In learning to decrease levels of arousal, patients are often able to decrease the intensity and duration of chronic pain symptoms and, at times, to eliminate pain altogether.

Relaxation Training

Relaxation training consists of systematic physical or mental exercises designed to promote an increased awareness of levels of autonomic arousal or striated muscle tension. This treatment is aimed at enabling an individual to develop the ability to decrease physiologic arousal voluntarily in a concise and orderly fashion. Relaxation exercises are similar to biofeedback in intent except that they do not require electronic equipment to monitor biologic activity. Instead, they rely on the spontaneous effect their use produces to promote increased levels of relaxation. Two commonly used relaxation procedures are Jacobson's progressive muscle relaxation exercises, which involve tensing and relaxing various muscle groups of the body, and autogenic training, which uses phrases to promote feelings of heaviness or warmth that are normally found during periods of relaxation. Research has shown relaxation procedures to be an effective treatment for reducing abdominal pain in patients with inflammatory bowel disease. A recent controlled study of 40 patients with ulcerative colitis randomly assigned to treatment and no-treatment groups found that patients given progressive relaxation training reported significantly less intense and less frequent pain as well as less distress from their symptoms when compared with patients not receiving relaxation training. The accompanying chapter, "Stress Management," provides more details on this methodology.

Behavior Therapy

Behavior therapy uses an assortment of strategies for altering a person's behavior and has been successfully employed in treating a variety of disabilities ranging from phobias to conduct disorders. The usefulness of behavior therapy in the treatment of chronic pain lies in its ability to reduce or eliminate illness behavior and time spent by the patient in the helpless or "sick" role. Behavior modification is also helpful in decreasing pain behaviors such as complaints about symptoms, displays of pain affect, the use of ineffective remedies (eg, holding a pillow or heating pad over the abdomen), or asking others for assistance in tasks the patient can perform but does not because of illness.

One beneficial behavioral therapy for treating pain and illness behavior is termed "desensitization." Desensitization involves having a person engage in some anxiety-producing behavior at a level that does not cause any appreciable amount of concern. The individual next attempts to accomplish the targeted behavior or activity, stopping each time anxiety becomes too great, until the goal of therapy is achieved. This procedure may take anywhere from a few days to several months to complete, depending on the activity and the amount of anxiety it produces. Eventually, individuals can achieve goals that were initially too anxiety provoking for them to even consider. For patients with inflammatory bowel disease, desensitization is particularly useful in helping individuals return to work, increasing physical activities such as housework or athletic pursuits, or decreasing social isolation resulting from fears of embarrassment related to alterations in bowel habits. As patients increase activities, they begin to experience a decrease in somatic sensations as they focus their attention on socializing or work instead of their symptoms. This combination of increased activity with decreased attention to symptoms is very effective in diminishing or eliminating pain arising from chronic medical conditions such as inflammatory bowel disease.

Family Therapy

Family members and close friends can also play an important role in decreasing chronic pain if they are included as part of a behavior modification program. It is normal and appropriate to treat persons with acute illnesses with a special deference and to provide them with dependent care typically given to the sick. However, this type of care can serve to promote pain and illness behavior in the patient with a chronic condition by providing secondary gain for having symptoms. For the patient with chronic pain, secondary gain typically occurs when he or she receives special attention because of symptoms, experiences decreases in work or care-taking responsibilities because of illness, or is provided with gifts or favors to help him or her feel better.

Behavior modification should involve family members or friends by asking them to stop thinking of the patient as a "sick" person. Those who interact with the person who complains of chronic pain are asked to encourage the patient to be more active by not doing things for him or her because he or she is in pain. They are also asked to ignore pain behaviors such as grimacing, rubbing, or sighing. Instead, attention is given to the patient for being active, taking care of himself or herself, or interacting with others without pain behaviors. In addition, solicitous inquiries to the patient about his or her health are to be avoided, as they serve as reminders of chronic pain and tend to shift or maintain the patient's attention on somatic symptoms. Verbal complaints of pain are also ignored, and conversations with the patient should not include discussions of pain or other symptoms. Besides aiding the patient directly, this type of behavior therapy also benefits family members and friends by providing them with guidance on how they can help the patient with chronic pain to feel better.

Use of Narcotic-Analgesic Medications

The management of chronic pain requires careful scrutiny of the use of narcotic-analgesic pain medication for controlling symptoms. Narcotic analgesics not only decrease pain but also exert psychotropic effects related to the reduction of anxiety and the elevation of mood. These psychotropic effects provide the potential for strong secondary gain. If patients find the use of narcotic analgesics helpful to them in coping with their illness or in decreasing emotional stress related to difficult situations, their pain complaints may be reinforced rather than relieved by the use of narcotics. Under such conditions, pain complaints become more associated with the rationale for obtaining narcotic analgesics than with the physiologic transmission of pain signals by the body. In cases of abdominal pain, the situation is complicated even more by the fact that narcotics alter bowel motility in such a fashion as to produce many of the same pain complaints they may have originally been prescribed to eliminate. Because of both the psychological and physiologic ramifications of using narcotic-analgesic medications to treat chronic pain, their use in the treatment of symptoms arising from inflammatory bowel diseases or any other chronic gastrointestinal illness should be carefully assessed from both a behavioral and a medical standpoint. Withdrawal from narcotic analgesics alone has been reported to be an effective treatment for relieving chronic abdominal pain in some situations.

Case Report

The following case report highlights some of the behavioral strategies discussed above and illustrates the successful treatment of chronic pain in a patient with inflammatory bowel disease.

The patient was an intense and intelligent young graduate school student awaiting the results of the certification examination he had recently completed. He had a diagnosis of Crohn's disease and had undergone several hospitalizations and one abdominal surgery in the past 2 years. Each of his Crohn's disease flare-ups had been preceded by increased abdominal pain. At the time of his referral, he was using prednisone for control of his Crohn's disease and was taking 50 to 60 analgesic tablets per week for his abdominal pain. The patient was anxious about his abdominal pain, since he feared it meant an exacerbation of his illness and a return to the hospital. He discussed his symptoms frequently with his wife of 2 years but not with others, except for his physicians. His wife was overprotective and asked him often throughout the day how he was feeling. She was also very worried about his symptoms and advised him frequently about his diet and self-care. Although the patient appreciated his wife's concern, he appeared to resent her interference with his care of himself. He also overutilized his analgesic medication in dealing with daily stresses. For instance, he doubled his analgesic medication whenever he became worried about the results of his examination, and in one instance he tripled the prescribed dosage during a 5-day period when he was suffering from a cold. He often reported that his abdominal pain symptoms intensified during periods of increased anxiety or interpersonal conflicts.

The treatment program for this patient consisted of stress management to help him deal more productively with anxiety about his illness and with conflicts he experienced in his interactions with others. Behavior modification was also employed by having his wife let her husband take care of himself without interference on her part. She was also instructed to stop asking her husband how he felt and to cease engaging in discussions with him about his illness or symptoms. Finally, the patient was weaned from his analgesic medication over a 3-month period while being provided with biofeedback and relaxation exercises as an alternative pain management procedure. At the end of 4 months of treatment, the patient's pain complaints had decreased markedly, to the point that he no longer needed analgesic medication of any kind and, with his gastroenterologist's consent, he was decreasing his use of prednisone.

In considering this case, several factors should be noted. First, both the patient and his wife were well motivated and were able to understand and carry out the behavioral program with only a minor amount of difficulty. Unfortunately, this is not always the case, especially when the use of narcotic-analgesic medication or other behavioral situations resulting in secondary gain are involved. In such situations, it may require a psychotherapist familiar with chronic pain syndromes to successfully carry out a behavioral pain management program. Second, the close relationship between this patient's pain complaints and increased levels of anxiety makes it likely that some of his abdominal pain complaints were related to alterations in colonic motility in response to stress rather than to his Crohn's disease. This type of gastrointestinal response is typical of patients with irritable bowel syndrome and, as was noted by this patient's gastroenterologist, he probably had abdominal pain arising from both irritable bowel syndrome and inflammatory bowel disease. Regardless of other organic problems that might

exist, the contribution of stress to symptom complaints should always be evaluated in patients with chronic abdominal pain. Not to do so may decrease the effectiveness of medical management in helping the patient with chronic illness and pain function to the fullest potential.

Supplemental Reading[**]

Block A, Kremer E, Gaylor M. Behavioral treatment of chronic pain: the spouse as a discriminative cue for pain behavior. Pain 1980;9:243–52.

Chapman S, Brena S. Pain and society. Ann Behav Med 1985;7:21–4.

Degossely M, Koninckx N, Lenfant H. Ulcerative rectocolitis: autogenous training. On several serious cases. Acta Gastroenterol Belg 1975;38:454–63.

Fava G, Pavan L. Large bowel disorders 1. Illness configurations and life events. Psychother Psychosom 1976-77;27:93–9.

Karush A, Daniels G, O'Connor J, Stern L. The response to psychotherapy in chronic ulcerative colitis. 1. Pretreatment factors. Psychosom Med 1968;30:256–76.

Liedtke R, Freyberger H, Zepf S. Personality features of patients with ulcerative colitis. Psychother Psychosom 1977; 28:187–92.

McMahan A, Schmitt P, Patterson JP, Rothman E. Personality differences between inflammatory bowel disease patients and their healthy siblings. Psychosom Med 1973;35:91–103.

Sandgren J, McPhee M, Greenberger N. Narcotic bowel syndrome treated with clonidine. Ann Intern Med 1984; 101:331–4.

Shabsin, HS and Whitehead, W. Psychophysiological disorders of the gastrointestinal tract. In Linden W. ed. Biological barriers in behaviorial medicine. New York: Plenon Press.

Shaw L, Ehrlich A. Relaxation training as treatment for chronic pain caused by ulcerative colitis. Pain 1987;29:287–94.

Sheffield BF, Carney WP. Crohn's disease: a psychosomatic illness. BMJ 1976;128:446–50.

Turk D, Meichenbaum D, Genest M. Pain and behavioral medicine: a cognitive-behavioral approach. New York: The Guilford Press, 1983.

Whitehead W, Schuster M. Gastrointestinal disorders: behavioral and physiological basis for treatment. New York: Academic Press, 1985.

[**]Editor's Note: This list was compiled for the first edition in 1989. (TMB)

Pain Management

Julio A. Gonzalez, MD, and Peter S. Staats, MD

Although pain frequently is considered only a symptom of disease, it can be extremely debilitating, and is a major reason patients seek physicians' services. Pain is the major cause of disability in the United States and costs the American people more than cancer and heart disease combined. Yet until recently, attention has been concentrated only on curing the disease, and little attention has been given to symptom control. Training of physicians in pain management has been sparse, with only 2 hours allocated in most medical schools to pain management instruction.

To provide comprehensive pain management, it is important to understand the disease process, the biologic basis of pain, and the emotional state of the patient. This involves a comprehensive evaluation of the patient, assessing the source of nociception, spinal processing that may be occurring, the emotional state of the individual, and abnormal or destructive behaviors associated with pain.

The first goal in pain management is to establish an accurate diagnosis; then, an attempt is made to cure the disease, and thus eliminate sources of nociception whenever possible; finally, strategies to minimize the suffering associated with pain are developed and implemented. When it is not possible to cure the disease, the management of pain becomes paramount. A thorough understanding of pain, its neural substrate, and the options available for its treatment currently are considered part of good medical practice.

Definitions and Taxonomy of Pain

The International Association for the Study of Pain (IASP) defines pain as "an unpleasant sensory and emotional experience associated with actual or potential tissue damage, or described in terms of such damage." The definition recognizes that pain is not only a sensory experience but an emotional response as well, and it can be altered with affective and cognitive responses. This definition of pain also indicates that it is subjective and dependent on patient reports of pain. There are no laboratory reports, imaging studies, or any other objective measure that accurately correlates with the patient's pain. Physicians are entirely dependent on patient reports when assessing the severity of pain. Nociception refers to the physiologic process of activation of specialized neural pathways, specifically by tissue-damaging or potentially tissue-damaging stimuli.

Pain, in contrast to nociception, is a conscious experience, and although the stimulus-induced activation of afferent neural pathways may play an important role, other factors may influence the overall perception of pain. The experience of pain, particularly chronic pain, often results in suffering. Suffering results from a multitude of factors, including loss of physical function, social isolation, family distress, and a sense of inadequacy or spiritual loss.

This chapter focuses on chronic abdominal, visceral pain that (1) persists beyond either the course of an acute disease or a reasonable time for an injury to heal, (2) is associated with a chronic pathologic process that causes continuous pain, or (3) recurs at intervals of months or years. Some investigators use the arbitrary duration of 6 months or more to designate pain as being chronic, but this is not appropriate, because there are many acute diseases or injuries that heal in 2, 3, or 4 weeks, or, at most, 6 weeks. In such conditions, if pain is still present after a cure should have been achieved, it must be considered chronic pain.

The abdomen is one of the most frequent sites of regional chronic pain, and the differential diagnosis can be challenging. Abdominal pain can arise from both visceral and somatic etiologies and also can be confused with referred pain from the thoracic cavity. One of the most difficult diagnostic dilemmas for the practicing physician in treating pain is to distinguish between chronic visceral and chronic somatic pain. Even though many patients with chronic pain have pain from visceral structures, current knowledge about visceral pain arises largely from the studies of the cutaneous and peripheral nervous system. Unfortunately, there is an underlying misconception that occurs when visceral pain is simply considered as a variant of somatic pain. Visceral pain is probably generated by different biologic or neurologic substrate and abides by different principles.

Visceral pain is difficult to locate and usually radiates away from the affected organ. It frequently is associated with hyperalgesia or spasm of the overlying somatic tissue. These features can probably be explained by the fact that there is a small number of nerve afferents subserving a wide anatomic area. Also, the visceral afferent and the somatic structures input converge in the spinal cord at the same level ("viscerosomatic convergence").

Visceral pain can be induced by distention and contraction of the hollow visceral wall, stretching of the capsule, formation or accumulation of algogenic substances, ischemia, direct action of chemical stimuli on compromised mucosa, and traction or compression of ligaments, vessels, or mesentery. Visceral afferents may undergo a change in function similar to somatic nociceptors, that is, they can be sensitized, and hyperalgesia may ensue.

Pain Pathways

Nociceptive impulses from the jejunum and ileum are transmitted by sympathetic afferent nerves through the least and lesser splanchnic nerves, and from there through the superior mesenteric and part of the celiac plexi to enter the spinal cord at the T8 to T12 levels. Impulses from the cecum, ascending colon, and right half of the transverse colon are transmitted by sympathetic afferent nerves that pass through the least and lesser splanchnic nerves, and from these to the inferior mesenteric and superior mesenteric plexi to enter the spinal cord at the T10 to L2 levels.

Nociceptive impulses from the left half of the transverse colon and from the descending colon and rectum arrive at the spinal cord by two different pathways. Some of them are carried by afferent fibers that accompany sympathetic fibers to the lower thoracic and lumbar sympathetic trunks, and others course with the parasympathetic nerves through the pelvic plexus and pelvic nerves (nervi erigentes) and then enter the spinal cord at the S2 and S4 levels.

In a few people, afferent sensation can also be carried by the vagus nerve, because midbowel visceral pain can be felt after spinal cord transection above T1 as well as after bilateral splanchnic nerve resection (Figure 125B–1).

Characteristics of the Pain Produced by Inflammatory Bowel Disease

The two major diseases included in the inflammatory bowel disease (IBD) terminology are Crohn's disease (CD) and ulcerative colitis (UC). Crohn's disease is a frequent cause of both acute and chronic abdominal pain, particularly in young people. Either the small or large intestine or both are involved. Ulcerative colitis does not involve the small intestine and does not skip over areas of normal colonic mucosa, as CD does. The pathogenesis of IBD remains unknown, but multiple pathogenic mechanisms have been postulated, including immune, infectious, and psychological factors.

In CD, pain is produced by either intestinal inflammation or intestinal obstruction. Inflammatory pain can be referred anywhere in the abdomen, depending on the

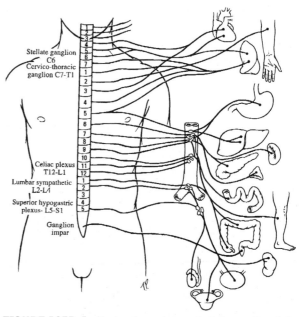

FIGURE 125B–1. Nociceptive and sympathetic innervation of visceral structures. Anatomic location of the visceral plexi is listed on the far left.

location of the area of inflammation. Nevertheless, pain mostly is referred to the right lower quadrant, because the terminal ileum and cecum are the segments most frequently involved. Most of the time, the pain is described as constant and achy, sometimes radiating to the anterior aspect of the right thigh. It is not necessarily related to bowel movements, but eating can make it worse. When the pain is caused by obstruction, patients describe it as cramping and located in the periumbilical region. It can be superimposed on the continuous achy pain produced by inflammation and is often relieved by bowel movements. Patients with CD in whom pain is caused by transmural inflammation note a worsening of left lower quadrant pain with bowel movements. Associated symptoms could include nausea and vomiting; diarrhea, which can be bloody; fever; and weight loss. Anal and rectal symptoms are common. Perianal pain due to fistula, fissure, or perianal abscess is found in about 40 percent of the patients at some time during their illness.

In UC, signs and symptoms are similar to those seen in patients with CD. Nevertheless, in most cases pain is referred to the left lower quadrant of the abdomen and usually described as cramping. Diarrhea and urge to defecate are common issues; bowel movements often relieve the pain. In UC, perianal pain is not as common as it is in CD. Extra-intestinal complications, including arthritis, skin and liver involvement, conjunctivitis, uveitis, and oral ulcerations, also can be seen in patients with CD or UC. Patients with UC and with CD have an increased risk for the development of colon carcinoma, and those patients with change in the character of their diarrhea or abdominal pain should be investigated for this complication.

Establishing the etiology of pain can be difficult, and when patients do not respond to conventional treatment, the diagnosis should be reassessed. Because of the viscerosomatic convergence and the development of hyperalgesia, patients with true visceral etiologies can develop secondary myofascial pain, which can be more painful than the original visceral pain. It is important to carefully assess the abdominal musculature, looking for trigger points and painful muscles. When these are found, injection therapy and physical therapy can be useful.

Some pain may have a primary somatic or neuropathic etiology. Neuropathic pain easily can be confused with visceral pain. Diabetic neuropathy, intercostal neuralgia, and spinal cord injury all can present with dull, achy complaints as seen with visceral pain.

Slipping Rib Syndrome

One of the most commonly missed diagnoses is slipping rib syndrome. This disease involves a disarticulation of the T8 to T11 rib. It is diagnosed in patients who have had some sort of trauma to the abdomen (which could include surgery), who experience pain with palpation, and in whom lifting the anterior margin of the rib reproduces pain. The diagnosis is confirmed with diagnostic blocking (temporarily anesthetizing) of the affected ribs. If the pain is relieved after the block, a somatic source is presumed.

Pain Management

Effective pain management in patients with gastroenterologic diseases requires an understanding of the variety of approaches that are effective in chronic pain. A diagnosis is established and a pharmacologic or surgical intervention designed to improve the disease state is attempted. However, if these fail or do not adequately relieve pain, a wide variety of effective pain management approaches are available. These include pharmacologic manipulation, psychological approaches, and alternative interventional approaches that can be effected to treat chronic pain. Most of the pharmacologic interventions can be performed by primary care specialists.

It is important to remember that pain is not only a biologic event but also a psychological event that follows the principles of emotional responding. The realms necessary to understand patients with chronic pain include the biologic underpinning, learning, behavior, cognition, emotion, personality, and social environment. A comprehensive treatment of patients with chronic visceral pain should be multidisciplinary, including therapies directed at affecting the psychological modifiers of pain (guided imagery, biofeedback, semantic therapy, rehabilitation, etc.). There are two separate chapters on behavioral management of pain and others on psychiatric and on psychological approaches.

After other possible causes of abdominal pain have been ruled out, treatment must involve a multidiscipli-

nary approach, including gastroenterologists, surgeons, psychologists, and nutritionists. Ideally, appropriate management of the underlying disease effectively controls pain.

Medical Therapies

Opioids

Opioids should be used judiciously in the management of IBD. The decreased intestinal motility associated with these agents can precipitate toxic megacolon in patients undergoing severe attacks of CD or UC. On the other hand, opioids (eg, codeine, loperamide, diphenoxylate with atropine) are helpful in managing chronic diarrhea and cramping. Other anticholinergic agents, such as dicyclomine, can relieve intestinal cramping in some patients.

Appropriate medical or surgical therapy is important to help minimize opioid use. Patients with disease limited to the rectum and descending colon often benefit from topical administration of mesalamine or hydrocortisone enemas or suppositories. Surgery is indicated in cases of significant intestinal obstruction, unhealed fistulae, drainage of abscesses, repair of intestinal perforation, massive hemorrhage, or toxic dilatation of the colon unresponsive to medical therapy.

Specialists in pain medicine are consulted in cases of severe pain that have not responded to basic pharmacologic therapy. For the patient who is undergoing acute exacerbation of IBD, the two major pain treatment options are parenteral opioid therapy and central nerve blocks, particularly, epidural administration of local anesthetics or opioids. As mentioned, opioid therapy must be judiciously evaluated and probably avoided in patients with high risk of developing toxic megacolon. Continuous epidural analgesia may be an option in patients who do not have concomitant coagulation disorders, sepsis, or hemodynamic instability.

The recommendations for chronic pain treatment usually follow the World Health Organization (WHO) guidelines for pain therapy in which adjuvant agents and nonopioid analgesics are used first. This often is followed with the addition of weak opioids and then potent opioids. If these medications fail, invasive therapies, including intrathecal therapy and autonomic nerve blocks, may be of benefit.

RISKS OF OPIOD THERAPY

In spite of being one of the oldest medical treatments, opioids remain one of the safest approaches to managing pain. Physicians frequently are concerned with (1) creating addiction, (2) respiratory depression and other side effects, and (3) the legality of opioid use. These fears are attributable to an inadequate knowledge of the topic. Addiction frequently is confused with physical dependence.

Traditional definitions of addiction often have included criteria that reflect expected physiologic responses to opioids, such as physical dependence and tolerance, as well as behavioral responses that might be expected in patients with pain who are appropriately using opioids for pain relief.

Physical dependence is a physiologic state in which abrupt cessation or marked decrease of the opioid or administration of an opioid antagonist results in a withdrawal syndrome. Physical dependence is an expected occurrence in all individuals in the presence of continuous use of opioids, and it does not, in and of itself, imply addiction.

Tolerance is a form of neuroadaptation to the effects of chronically administered opioids and is manifested by the need for increasing or more frequent doses of the medication to achieve the initial effects of the drug. It does not, in and of itself, imply addiction.

Addiction is characterized by a persistent pattern of dysfunctional opioid use that may involve adverse consequences associated with the use of opioids, including loss of control over their use or preoccupation with obtaining opioids despite the presence of adequate analgesia. These phenomena may be accompanied by distortions in thought, chiefly denial, and a tendency to relapse once in recovery.*

Pseudoaddiction is a phenomenon that needs to be distinguished from true addiction. Pseudoaddiction occurs in individuals who have severe, unrelieved pain and who become intensely focused on finding relief for their pain. Sometimes such patients may appear to observers to be preoccupied with obtaining opioids, but their preoccupation is with finding pain relief, rather than using opioids per se. When effective analgesia is obtained, the previous behavior resolves.

A previous history of addiction or medication abuse increases the risk of addiction. It is not known what, if any, level of risk exists of inducing addiction in individuals with no family or personal history of addiction when using opioids for pain treatment. Available data suggest that such occurrence is extremely low.

Nonsteroidal Anti-inflammatory Drugs

Nonsteroidal anti-inflammatory drugs (NSAIDs) have been used to provide analgesia for a wide range of acute and chronic pain processes. These agents that involve both peripheral and central sites of action for analgesia interfere with prostaglandin production and are valuable in the control of inflammatory responses. This may result in

---

* Editor's Note: Chronic opioid use complicates the evaluation of recurrent abdominal pain. Sigmoid spasm, increased incomplete fecal evacuation, distention, and increased pain is a vicious cycle, especially in individuals with a history of IBS. Suicide attempts have been reported in a few of these patients. (TMB)

decreased sensitization. However, their use has been related to an increased risk for developing erosions and ulcerations at the level of the intestinal mucosa. Their use in patients with IBD remains controversial. In theory, the new cyclo-oxygenase 2 (COX-2) inhibitors, Celebrex® (Searle Pfizer, Skokie, Illinois) and Vioxx® (Merck Research Laboratories, Whitehouse Station, New Jersey) could be safer for patients with IBD, but limited data are available.

Tricyclic Antidepressants

Tricyclic antidepressants (TCAs) have been used for many years to provide analgesia for many chronic pain syndromes. These agents block presynaptic reuptake of the neurotransmitters norepinephrine and serotonin at the level of the dorsal horn of the spinal cord. Descending inhibitory systems for pain transmission are then facilitated. This beneficial effect is independent of mood effects. Sedation often is a useful side effect for patients with poor sleep patterns. Recommendations for use of TCAs include titration to desired effect, as well as prompt serum level determination when evidence of toxicity is present.

Anticonvulsants

Anticonvulsive agents have been used to provide analgesia for typical neuropathic pain states. Mechanisms of action include alteration of sodium and potassium conductance to create a stabilizing effect on neuronal membranes and increase γ-aminobutyric acid (GABA) activity. Although these agents have not been identified in the literature as ideal agents for visceral pain, pain physicians at the Johns Hopkins Pain Center have begun applying them for the treatment of chronic pelvic pain. The rationale is based upon evidence of sensitization of visceral organs, and results to date have been promising.

Intraspinal Opioids

Opioids are effective for visceral pain, and the risk for developing toxic megacolon is probably extremely low in a chronic pain setting. To date, they are an important component of the treatment of chronic, nonmalignant visceral pain. Intrathecal opioid therapy has proved to be effective, with lower systemic levels and, therefore, less inhibition of intestinal motility. Analgesia can be achieved with extremely low doses by delivering the opioid directly to the spinal cord. The dorsal horn of the spinal cord (substantia gelatinosa) has opiate receptors that are known to modulate nociceptive transmission. Patients with chronic pain can receive opiates continuously via an implanted infusion pump, placed in the abdomen, that is connected to a catheter implanted into the spinal fluid. This approach should be reserved for patients who have inadequate relief or intolerable side effects with systemic analgesics.

Neurolytic Blocks

The visceral afferents can be temporarily anesthetized with local anesthetics or semipermanently destroyed using a variety of toxic approaches. Local anesthetic nerve blocks involve placing bupivacaine (Marcaine®, AstraZeneca, Wayne, Pennsylvania) directly onto the visceral plexi, which are known to contain nociceptive afferents. Bupivacaine temporarily interrupts neural transmission by binding to sodium channels.

Neurolytic blocks of the visceral afferent pathways are well described in the literature for both cancer and non-cancer pain. Excellent success rates have been reported with neurolytic blocks for celiac and superior hypogastric plexi neurolysis. Although well accepted for cancer pain, the use of neurolysis for chronic visceral pain is controversial in regard to risks and outcome. Because of the procedure-associated risks, and unclear outcomes in patients with long life expectancies, this approach should be reserved for patients who have failed the more conservative, reversible approaches.

Conclusion

Pain remains one of the most debilitating and disabling symptoms associated with IBD. The physician must have a thorough understanding of nociceptive and visceral afferents to optimally treat patients with pain. The treatment of pain is part of good medical practice and can improve outcome and patient satisfaction. The risks of treating patients with pain are minimal.

Supplemental Reading

Bonica JJ. The Management of Pain. 2:1146–1213.
Panchal SJ, Staats PS. Visceral pain: from physiology to clinical practice. J Back Musculoskeletal Rehabil 1997; 9:233–45.

CHAPTER 126

FITNESS PROGRAMS

PETER NIELSEN

In life, there is always opportunity. Sometimes, we see it; sometimes, we are too afraid to see it. Usually, fear comes with knowing that opportunity means facing up to change. At the time, I did not realize it, but I look back now and see that I was blessed with the opportunity to be a vehicle to touch the lives of many people. These are people of every sort, from persons with physical handicaps or serious challenges to meet, to top-ranking athletes who have attained the pinnacle of performance in their fields. It always has been my desire to help people learn from the experience of others—and from the mistakes made by other people, including me. One lesson I learned painfully was that opportunity is adversity turned inside out. I discovered that when you are in a situation that cannot be avoided but must be dealt with, it is the attitude we take that permits us, as William Faulkner said, not only to endure but also to prevail.

Challenges

Those challenges, those bad moments in life, are our opportunities to make something more and better of ourselves. For me, my response to adversity took the form of building for myself a healthier life style. Much of what I discovered on that journey was learned from others. But as much as I have wanted to share these insights and concepts with others, I realized long ago that I was unable to do it alone. I wanted to light in others that same spark that had been kindled in me, the spark that saved my life.

Surgery

I lost 2.5 feet of my intestine and went from 145 pounds to 86. I believed that I had been dealt a "bad deck of cards." I did not feel normal. In 1977, I spent Christmas in Long Island College Hospital for what was supposed to be a weekend of tests. Lying there, I got my wake-up call: they said they were doing exploratory surgery, and I woke up with a pouch on my side, and tubes coming out of me. I realized that there is no perfect person. I had to appreciate every gift that God had given me; I needed to stop the self-pity and start developing a purpose: fitness.

The treatments I underwent before my surgery had a powerful effect on my body. There were many days when I could barely move. I worked consistently on my diet and adhered to a steady fitness plan, which included cardio-vascular activity and weight lifting. Keeping my plan constant helped me tremendously to get through flare-ups, relieve pain, and increase self-love.

Opportunities

After going through all of these negatives, I turned these adversities into opportunities. I feel like a fitness dynamo. I work out every day and have never felt healthier. I have a stronger commitment and love for physical activity because the illness had limited the most basic movement and activity. I appreciate how important it is to take care of our precious bodies.

I realize there are days when I will feel like a dynamo, and days when I feel lethargic. Sometimes, I will have a fissure, or blood in my stool. I know that thin line, and I need to respect it. Know your limitations! When I do feel good, I need to take advantage and get moving. Do not get defeated if you have to miss a workout. It is part of the program.

Fitness Training

In the beginning, my medications nauseated me and I could not work out. I spoke with my doctors and realized I could work out early in the morning and take my medications at night. As far as how fitness training affects my illness, exercise is wonderful, because it builds up the immune system. Catabolic steroids tear down muscle and bone density, and when you get moving, with your doctor's approval, you can build it back up. It has made me strong enough to endure my bouts. Fitness is a great thing. It gives me the self-confidence that I need to fight Crohn's disease. Crohn's disease affects men and women like me, in their twenties, when self-esteem and confidence are very important. I tell my family that if I am not working out, I am not feeling well. If I am feeling well, I will be found exercising. Encouragement from family and friends is the mainstay of fighting inflammatory bowel disease (IBD), but fitness and well-being are personal. Only you can change your life style.

Nutrition Awareness

When you look at a well-prepared dish of food, what you see is something delicious, perhaps shrimp scampi or linguini with clam sauce. Another way of looking at it

600 / Advanced Therapy of Inflammatory Bowel Disease

would be to see complex carbohydrates and cholesterol. The difference between those two visions is huge. I do not want you to lose the pleasure that comes with the first vision, and there's no reason you should, but if you want to be nutritionally fit, you will have to start seeing the world of food through both lenses. Looking through the analytic lens, I know exactly what goes into my body every day. I know by the gram, and in some cases by the milligram, what nutrients are stoking my fire. I do not know how far you plan to go down the road toward personal nutrition awareness. Even if you are serious, you will not have to count grams of protein quite as closely as I do. You will not have to be as stopwatch precise as I am with my meals. You will not have to pass up quite as many "reward" treats as I do.

Nevertheless, whether you are into a serious athletic regimen or barely exercising, you should have at least a working knowledge of basic nutrients. You should know what they do *for* you and *to* you. You should know how to structure a healthy dietary regimen to fit your tastes and your life style.

Water

Water is the "forgotten" nutrient. Many people are dehydrated and do not even know it. Not everyone who is tired, moody, and fatigued is dehydrated, of course, but those are symptoms. In one sense, water is not a nutrient at all. Nutrients, the raw materials for fueling our bodies and building new cells, are found in food. But water is crucial to virtually every basic function of the body, from temperature regulation to blood circulation, metabolism, immune system function, and waste elimination. The fact that something so basic can be so misunderstood, or ignored, shows just how far out of touch the average person is with his or her own body and its maintenance.

Take, for example, the matter of weight control, which always seems to be the one area where the average American picks up at least a passing interest in nutrition. If you are overweight, or if you have fluid retention problems, you should be drinking more water. If you keep your body adequately supplied with water, it will actually speed up your metabolism. When the body is not being given enough water, it sees that as a threat to survival and, like a camel, begins to hold on to every drop. Drink more water, and the body will release the excess. Water also suppresses appetite, and naturally helps the body metabolize stored fat; overweight people with a larger metabolic load need more water than thin people.

Every body, thin or fat, needs plenty of water every day. The average person loses about 2 cups daily through perspiration (temperature control), even without unusual physical exertion. Another 2 cups disappear in the respiration process. The intestines and kidneys together use about 6 cups a day. That is about 10 cups

total, not counting water loss through perspiration during any heavy exercise. Some of the water loss is replaced through the food we eat, liquid or solid. The bottom line, however, is that the average person should be drinking at least 6 to 8 cups of water each day. To be more specific, divide your body weight by two. That gives you the number of ounces of water you should be drinking. Divide that by eight to get the number of cups.

Be grateful to your kidneys, nature's filtering department. If you could somehow survive without them, you would need to drink 2,500 gallons of water every day just to flush out the system. The fact is millions of Americans do not come close to drinking their daily quota of water. Their rationale is that the oceans of pop, coffee, beer, and liquor-soda combinations they knock down every day will do the trick. Well, there are some serious problems with that idea. Alcohol and caffeine, besides depleting the body of vitamins and minerals, are natural diuretics, meaning they actually lead to fluid elimination and dehydration.

There are many degrees of dehydration, of course. We are not talking about someone dying in the desert as his body runs dry. Lesser levels of dehydration occur when you do not take in enough water to replace all that is lost through breathing, urination, and exercise. You did not have to be perspiring profusely or urinating frequently to be losing water. If you work in a stuffy house or office building, you lose large amounts of fluid invisibly. You can lose 2 pounds of water in the rapidly circulating cabin air of a 3- to 4-hour airplane flight. Stress, as well as alcohol and caffeine, acts as a diuretic. In other words, you can be dehydrating yourself on a normal day.

Speaking athletically, or in terms of any kind of physical performance, 75 percent of muscle tissue is water. Dehydrate a muscle by 3 percent and you lose 10 percent of contractual strength and 8 percent of speed. Dehydration increases blood viscosity. Thicker, more concentrated blood stresses the heart. Your arteries become less able to provide muscles with nutrients and oxygen and to eliminate accumulated wastes. So you do not need to be a scientist, rocket or otherwise, to figure out that dehydration is a common cause of poor athletic performance.

On the more cerebral side, dehydration can produce a minuscule but crucial shrinkage of the brain. Deprive yourself of enough water and your concentration and coordination will be affected. In other words, you need those 6 to 8 cups a day whether you are pumping iron in a gym or crunching numbers at a desk. People often say, "No problem; I drink tons of water with my meals." Well, that is exactly the wrong way to consume your quota of water. It dilutes your food and makes for less efficient absorption of nutrients. Milk is an acceptable drink with meals, because milk becomes a semisolid in the stomach. But you should avoid drinking water beginning 15 minutes before a meal and for 30 to 60 minutes after a meal, to give your stomach time to begin the digestive process. Thirst, by the way, is a poor barometer of whether or not you need water. It is best to make drinking water a habit. (You'll find that 90 percent of the battle with a dietary regimen is nothing but habit, so give it a chance.) Best of all, water is almost habit forming. It is not all that excessive to carry a squirt bottle with you and to drink water throughout the day. This is now very socially acceptable.

Fitness

Fitness is the best gift; it has given me a better quality of life, self-love, and understanding, especially about the preciousness of health. It is an incredible vehicle, especially for someone with Crohn's disease. But a person with IBD needs a specific program and special attention in many areas. It is best to go to a place that does personal training with an exercise physiologist. He or she will understand, for example, what exercises are appropriate for the person who has either a vertical or a horizontal surgical scar.

If you say you can't, you probably are right. If you say you can work through the pain, the depression, and the disease, then you will. I am living proof that you can have tremendous quality of life and reach whatever goal you want if you say you can.

Editor's Note

Peter Nielsen was a competing bodybuilder and weight lifter who now operates a series of fitness centers in the Detroit area. He is a former Mr. America and Mr. Universe. He has inflammatory bowel disease. We thank him for this essay, which you may wish to share with patients. (TMB)

CHAPTER 127

ALTERNATIVE PATIENT CARE METHODS

ROBERT J. HILSDEN, MD, MSC, FRCPC

Gastroenterologists frequently encounter patients who are using or want to use an alternative therapy to treat their inflammatory bowel disease (IBD). The patient may have learned of the therapy through friends or family, books, the media, or the Internet or may have seen a complementary practitioner. Managing these situations can be difficult for gastroenterologists as they may not be knowledgeable about the therapy and are likely to be hesitant to support a therapy without strong scientific evidence of its efficacy and safety. This chapter reviews what is currently known about the use of alternative and complementary therapies by patients with IBD and provides practical guidelines for informing and counseling patients about them. Finally, some useful sources of information on complementary therapies are listed.

Complementary Therapies

The term complementary therapies (CT) is used herein to refer to the diverse collection of health systems and diagnostic and therapeutic modalities that are not part of the conventional Western medical system. Examples of CT include alternative medical systems (homeopathy, traditional Chinese medicine, Ayurveda), products derived from nature (phytotherapy), orthomolecular medicine (high-dose vitamin C, coenzyme Q10), pharmacologic interventions (antineoplastons), manipulative and physical therapies (chiropractic, massage), and various procedures and devices (colonic lavage, bioresonance).

Practitioners of complementary therapies often have a quite different view of disease and its treatment than conventional physicians. They usually place a strong emphasis on holism, vital forces, and naturalism. A holistic approach is characterized by an emphasis on diagnosing and treating illness through an understanding of the whole person (body, mind, and spirit) and how the individual interacts with the world around them. The concept of a vital energy or life force plays an important role in many alternative medical systems. Disease may be seen as the result of a blockage or disruption of the vital energy or an imbalance between two opposing forces (eg, ying and yang). Treatments are directed at restoring a healthy balance and flow in these forces and stimulating the self-healing potential of the body. Naturalism emphasizes man's intimate relationship with the natural world and

relies on detoxification (often through fasting) and natural remedies (herbs, vitamins) to improve and maintain health. These philosophies often lead to highly individualized treatments.

In many alternative medical systems, the patient plays a more active role in his or her treatment. The patient may be seen as the primary agent of healing, helped by the guidance of the practitioner. The patient-centered focus of CT along with the common emphasis on health and well-being, rather than on disease, may be particularly appealing to patients.

Use of Complementary Therapies by IBD Patients

Patients with IBD commonly use CT. Recent studies have reported that approximately 40 to 50 percent of patients with IBD have used or are using some form of CT. In a study conducted in Calgary, Alberta, Canada, commonly used therapies included herbs (aloe vera, cat's claw, ginseng), chiropractic manipulation, diets (gluten-free diet, carbohydrate-specific diet), and biologics-probiotics (*Lactobacillus acidophilus*). Investigators in other parts of the world have shown that different therapies are more common, including homeopathy, prayer, and exercise. Therefore, the patients' cultural background and what is available locally are likely to be important determinants of the therapy chosen by a patient. A complementary practitioner may provide these therapies, but more commonly, patients self-treat with any of the therapies that are readily obtainable at health food stores or drug stores, by mail order, or over the Internet.

Patients with IBD use CT for their IBD and also for concomitant medical conditions or general health promotion. Important factors leading patients to use CT for their IBD are dissatisfaction with their conventional medical treatments, especially a lack of effect or side effects; of medical treatments; and a desire to avoid surgery. However, other factors also are important, including a patient's health beliefs, culture, and knowledge and their previous experiences with CT. Some patients' health beliefs may be more compatible with CT, and therefore, they may use them early during the course of their disease. Others may be comfortable with conventional medicine and only seek out CT when they believe they have seen the limitations of conventional medicine.

Combination Therapy

In general, patients do not abandon conventional medicine in favor of complementary therapies. Instead, they tend to use both, often hoping for a synergistic effect or that the complementary therapy will ameliorate or prevent side effects from the conventional medicine. Many patients report using conventional medicine when their disease is very active and use complementary therapies to try to maintain remission or when they have chronically but moderately active disease that is not responding to usual treatments.

Perceived Benefits

Patients report obtaining a number of benefits through the use of CT. One of the most common benefits is a greater sense of being in control of their disease. They also frequently feel that by using CT they have taken a more active role in the management of their disease. Often these benefits over-shadow any improvement in their symptoms resulting from their use of CT. Therefore, a patient may not appreciate any improvement in their disease but may still be satisfied with their use of CT because of their increased sense of control. It is important for the gastroenterologist to understand this because it helps explain why rational patients demonstrate, what is from the gastroenterologist's perspective an irrational health behavior, the use of an unproven therapy. Understanding patients' use of CT requires looking beyond symptoms to the impact the disease and its treatment has on every aspect of patients' lives.

Health Beliefs

The degree of satisfaction with a CT is partly associated with the patient's health beliefs. Patients whose health beliefs are more congruent with complementary medicine are more likely to report a high degree of satisfaction with the CT they used than patients whose health beliefs are more congruent with conventional medicine.

Patients frequently exclude their gastroenterologist when deciding to use a CT and then often do not inform the physician about using it. Patients often indicate that they withhold this information because they are afraid of their physician rejecting their use of CT or because they do not see their physician as being knowledgeable about these therapies.

In summary, patients with IBD commonly use CT as part of the treatment of their disease in combination with their conventional medicines; they often do so because of problems they have had with their conventional treatments, and they frequently do not include their physician in the decision-making process.

Efficacy and Safety of Alternative Treatments

One of the main problems facing both patients and physicians is the lack of information on the safety and efficacy of CT. In fact, patients rated CT as one of their most important information needs. In general, there are no major safety concerns with the common forms of therapy (herbs and nutritional supplements) used by patients with IBD. Potential risks include allergic reactions; contamination or mislabeling of herbal products; nutritional deficiencies, resulting from restrictive diets; and neck and spine injury resulting from spinal manipulation. However, physicians and patients should be aware that some therapies are associated with the risk of serious side effects attributable to the therapy's chemical constituents (eg, hepatic veno-occlusive disease from herbs, such as comfrey, that contain pyrrolizidine alkaloids), contamination with heavy metals (reported with some medicines prepared in Asia), and the potential risk for toxicity to a fetus.

Medication Interactions

The potential for interactions between complementary and conventional medicine exists but is poorly documented for most therapies. **Many herbs can affect the absorption or metabolism of conventional medicines. Patients on immunosuppressants or other medications with a narrow therapeutic window should be especially careful.**

There is even less information available on the efficacy of common forms of CT used by patients with IBD. Many CTs based on traditional healing practices have a rich folk history supporting their use; however, there is little, if any, direct scientific evidence supporting the benefits of most forms of CT. Much of the evidence to which patients and physicians have access is anecdotal. Some controlled trials of specific therapies have been conducted, but these often are reported in journals unfamiliar to practicing physicians, are flawed, and examine treatments not widely used or available. There is a body of ethnopharmacology and basic science research on some herbal products that supports a possible role in the treatment of IBD. For example, aloe vera gel has been shown to attenuate inflammation in the trinitrobenzene sulfonic acid (TNBS) colitis model, and cat's claw has been shown to suppress nuclear factor κB (NF-κ-B) expression. However, anti-inflammatory effects in humans have not yet been demonstrated.[*]

Approach to the Patient Using or Wishing to Use a Complementary Therapy

Counseling patients about CT use is important and can help the patient make a more informed choice. To be effective, it must be done in a sensitive and nonjudgmental fashion. As with any attempt to modify health behavior, gastroenterologists should avoid an authoritative

---

[*] Editor's Note: Bromelain, a proteolytic enzyme extracted from the pineapple stem, was reportedly helpful in two patients with UC (Kane and Goldberg, 2000). (TMB)

"advice-giving" or direct persuasion approach, because this can push the patient into a more resistant and defensive position. This is not to say that physicians must agree with their patients' use of CT. Patients often recognize that they are obtaining only one side of the story from those promoting a complementary therapy. However, they want more than just a "No, don't use it" from their gastroenterologist. They value their gastroenterologist as an information source and want an open discussion of the potential value or risks associated with a therapy, even if ultimately the gastroenterologist disagrees with their use of it.

Dr. David Eisenberg has written a valuable article on advising patients who seek alternative medical therapies. It is directed toward the patient who is seeking care from a complementary practitioner. Even though most patients with IBD self-treat with complementary therapies rather than see a complementary practitioner, Eisenberg's guidelines are still appropriate. Below are the steps recommended for use when counseling a patient.

Patient Counseling

Documenting Use of Complementary Therapies
Determining current and past use of CT should be part of the routine medical history for all patients. There are several reasons for doing so. First, use of a CT may be an indication that the patient is dissatisfied with current treatment either because the desired benefits are not being achieved or because he or she is suffering side effects. Second, the use of potentially dangerous therapies can be discovered. Third, potential drug–CT interactions can be anticipated. Finally, the effects of the CT, either good or bad, will not be misconstrued as resulting from a conventional treatment.

Patients are reluctant to reveal their use of CT, especially if they view their gastroenterologist as being intolerant or uninformed. This is not the correct time to use terms such as quackery, fraudulent, or unconventional therapies. I routinely ask the patient whether they (1) use herbal or natural therapies, (2) have made any dietary changes, and (3) use any other therapies for their IBD. There is no evidence that inquiring about CT use will lead a nonuser to begin using one of these therapies.

Determine Reasons for Seeking Complementary Therapy
A patient who is using or considering using a complementary therapy should be asked about their reasons for doing so. This is important because determining specific areas of dissatisfaction with their conventional treatment could allow modifications to be made. Again, careful questioning is required, as the patient may be reticent to reveal issues that they feel may be perceived as criticism by their gastroenterologist. Open-ended questions such as "What do you see as the potential benefits of using this therapy?"

and "Do you have any concerns about your current treatment for your IBD that is leading you to consider this new therapy?" allow the patient to openly discuss their perspective on their treatment. It also is valuable to obtain some sense of the patient's health beliefs. Patients who are firm believers in the principles of complementary medicine are unlikely to be convinced not to use one. On the other hand, patients who are more comfortable with conventional medicine may seek alternatives because they are experiencing problems, and they may be willing first to try a modification in their conventional medical treatment.

Explore the Patient's Knowledge and Source of Information about the Complementary Therapy
Many sources of information available to the patient, for example, books and Internet sites, provide an overly optimistic and one-sided account of the effectiveness of a therapy and often are based only on testimonials. Often information about safety is not provided. The patient's understanding of how the therapy works and its potential benefits and harms should be determined. Some patients have very realistic expectations. They may understand that their chance of obtaining some benefit is low but they are willing to try it on the off chance that they do benefit. However, many patients have unrealistic expectations and expect a quick cure. In the short time available for counseling a patient, it is impossible and impractical to teach them the principles of scientific medicine and the randomized controlled trial. However, the patient should be encouraged to define realistic treatment goals and to reevaluate their use of a therapy after a set period.

Many patients often believe that CTs are without risk, often because they are "natural" therapies. This belief often is promoted by advertisements for the therapy. Therefore, the patient may not have considered the possibility of side effects. Physicians should ask patients whether they know the possible side effects of a therapy and should warn patients about the possibility of interactions with alcohol or other drugs. The patient and the physician may have difficulty finding any specific information about the risks of these with a given product. Patients should be encouraged to think of any therapy in terms of a trade-off between potential benefits and potential risks. Often patients think more about the potential benefits and neglect to consider whether they are willing to incur the risks of a CT, including its cost.

Determine How the Patient will Obtain and Use the Therapy
If the patient is seeing or will be seeing an alternative practitioner, the gastroenterologist can provide the patient with questions he or she should ask the practitioner. These would include (1) Is the practitioner licensed and what was his or her training? (2) How experienced is he or she in treating patients with IBD? (3) When can the patient expect from the treatment in

terms of benefits and side effects? (4) What is the basis for these expectations? and (5) What will be the cost of the treatment?

Patients should not start a number of different therapies, especially a combination of conventional and complementary therapies, at the same time. If this is done, it will be impossible to determine which therapy resulted in any benefits or side effects.

Finally some method for monitoring for side effects should be agreed upon. This will depend upon the potential risks associated with a therapy.

Information Sources About Complementary Therapies

There are a variety of valuable information sources available for physicians, although none of them are specifically focused on IBD. Patients should not rely too heavily on the advice or recommendations provided by employees of health food stores or other stores selling herbal and nutritional supplements. Often only the owner or the manager of the store has much experience and knowledge about the therapies. Other employees may have relatively little training and may not be able to distinguish between treatments safe and appropriate for IBD and those more commonly used for other gastrointestinal complaints. Many general intestinal remedies sold at health food stores contain laxatives.

Following are several sources of information on CT that I find useful. I have chosen these because they critically review therapies and provide supporting evidence for any claims made. All of them are relatively inexpensive (at least compared to medical textbooks).

The Honest Herbal (by V.E. Taylor, PhD. Pharmaceutical Products Press). This comprehensive book provides a wealth of critical and referenced information on many herbs. The author describes the putative active ingredients, recommended uses, and supporting evidence of efficacy for each herb and also debunks unwarranted claims.

The Complete Book of Symptoms and Treatments (E. Ernst, Editor. Element Books Limited). This book is divided into three sections: (1) symptoms and disorders, (2) therapies used in complementary medicine, and (3) diagnostic techniques used in complementary medicine. Within the symptoms and disorders section, therapies used for a variety of medical conditions are discussed. There is a section on gastrointestinal conditions, although neither ulcerative colitis nor Crohn's disease is specifically included. Each therapy is given a rating as to the likelihood of achieving a therapeutic benefit, and potential risks are listed. The level of evidence supporting

any benefits (ie, case reports, clinical trials) is given, but unfortunately no references are provided.

Professional Handbook of Complementary and Alternative Medicines (by C.W. Feltrow and J.R. Avila. Springhouse Publishers). This book describes the chemical components, actions, reported uses, and suggested doses of many herbs and alternative medicines. The authors also list potential adverse events and drug interactions. The book is less critical of claims made about the efficacy of the treatments than the two books previously mentioned.

Herb Contraindications and Drug Interactions (by F. Brinker. Eclectic Medical Publications). This book describes known and speculated side effects, contraindications, and drug interactions of herbs. The book is well referenced and indexed.

Websites: Quackwatch (*www.quackwatch.com).* Described as "Your guide to health fraud, quackery, and intelligent decisions."

Supplemental Reading

Carty E, Ballinger A, Azooz O, et al. Does topical aloe vera reduce the severity of trinitrobenzene sulphonic acid (TNBS) colitis in rats? Gastroenterology 1998;114:A948.

Crone CC, Wise TN. Use of herbal medicines among consultation-liason populations. Psychosomatics 1998;39:3–13.

Eisenberg DM. Advising patients who seek alternative medical therapies. Ann Intern Med 1997;127:61–9.

Hilsden RJ, Scott CM, Verhoef MJ. Complementary medicine use by patients with inflammatory bowel disease. Am J Gastroenterol 1998;93:697–701.

Hilsden RJ, Meddings JB, Verhoef MJ. Complementary and alternative medicine use by patients with inflammatory bowel disease: an Internet survey. Can J Gastroenterol 1999; 13:327–32.

Hilsden RJ, Verhoef MJ. Complementary and alternative medicine: evaluating its effectiveness in inflammatory bowel disease. Inflamm Bowel Dis 1998;4:318–23.

Kane S, Goldberg MJ. Use of bromelain for mild ulcerative colitis. An Intern Med 2000;132:680.

Moser G, Tillinger W, Sachs G, et al. Relationship between the use of unconventional therapies and disease-related concerns: a study of patients with inflammatory bowel disease. J Psychosom Res 1996;40:503–9.

Rawsthorne P, Shanahan F, Cronin NC, et al. An international survey of the use and attitudes regarding alternative medicine by patients with inflammatory bowel disease. Am J Gastroenterol 1999;94:1298–303.

Sandoval-Chacon M, Thompson JH, Zhang X-J, et al. Anti-inflammatory actions of cat's claw: the role of NF-κB. Aliment Pharmacol Ther 1998;12:1279–89.

CHAPTER 128

Fertility and Pregnancy in Inflammatory Bowel Disease

Douglas G. Moss, MD

The peak incidence of the development of inflammatory bowel disease (IBD) occurs during the reproductive years and, therefore, is a common concern for the practicing obstetrician. Often, the first issue discussed when consulting a new patient with Crohn's disease or ulcerative colitis is their reproductive future. Couples frequently introduce concerns about how their condition will impact the probability of conception. They wonder if their illness will negatively impact a future pregnancy and if pregnancy will negatively impact their disease. The ultimate concern is whether the outcome of a pregnancy will be successful and whether they can give birth to a healthy baby. This chapter focuses on gynecologic and obstetric issues in these challenging patients.

Fertility and Inflammatory Bowel Disease

Early reports have suggested that patients with both Crohn's disease and ulcerative colitis have reduced fertility. Later reports have suggested that only patients with Crohn's disease are subfertile. When controlling for patients who voluntarily decided not to become pregnant, Hudson and colleagues (1997) demonstrated that patients with IBD had similar fertility rates to their age-matched controls. In that retrospective study of over 400 IBD patients, significantly higher infertility rates were noted only in women who had undergone surgery for their IBD. In many cases, this was secondary to fallopian tube dysfunction.

At the Mount Sinai Medical Center, which is a major referral center for Crohn's disease and ulcerative colitis, fertility prospects are presented in a positive way to young patients with IBD. Women who are referred with a history of either Crohn's disease or ulcerative colitis whose gastroenterologist gives them the go-ahead to become pregnant are reassured and do not undergo an infertility workup unless the diagnosis of either primary or secondary infertility is made (no conception after 1 year of unprotected sex). In women with a history of surgery for their IBD, particularly surgery involving the ileum and colon, a workup is initiated sooner with particular attention to tubal-factor infertility. A hysterosalpingogram is an extremely helpful study in this regard and can be accomplished safely in these patients if antibiotic prophylaxis is used. If the diagnosis of tubal disease is made, many of these patients can become pregnant using various assisted reproductive technologies, such as in vitro fertilization.

Male-factor infertility in IBD has been reported secondary to sulfasalazine therapy, which may affect sperm count motility and morphology. This easily can be treated by discontinuation of this therapy.

Pregnancy and Inflammatory Bowel Disease

Patients with IBD who desire pregnancy can be encouraged provided their disease is in remission either spontaneously or through drug therapy. Many studies demonstrate that patients with Crohn's disease or ulcerative colitis in remission are equally as likely to experience recurrence of disease during pregnancy as they are if not pregnant, over the same time period. Approximately one-third of patients with ulcerative colitis experience recurrence during their pregnancy if they were in remission at conception, whereas, if conception occurs during active disease, two-thirds either stay active or get worse. The course of Crohn's disease during pregnancy is similar to ulcerative colitis in that patients with active disease at conception tend to remain active or get worse and those who are in remission do well. As with many medical diseases, women with IBD have the highest recurrence risk in the first trimester and during the puerperium. Patients with IBD who have ileostomies should be reassured that the distending abdomen in pregnancy rarely leads to related complications.

The gastroenterologist should order the necessary diagnostic tests. Endoscopic procedures and radiographic studies can be accomplished safely in pregnancy. Minimizing radiation exposure is important; however, animal studies do not demonstrate adverse fetal effects when the embryo has been exposed to less than 25 rads. In those patients who become pregnant with active IBD or whose disease becomes active during pregnancy, a favorable outcome can be achieved by working closely with a gastroenterologist, using aggressive medical therapy. Marion and colleagues (1996) reported successful treatment of five pregnant patients with severe IBD using intravenous cyclosporine. None of the five women required surgery during the pregnancies and four of five delivered healthy babies. Surgical treatment should be reserved for acute situations, because it is associated with a high risk of both maternal and neonatal morbidity and mortality. Hill and co-workers (1997) described six cases of acute exacerbation of Crohn's disease that required surgical intervention. In that series, all of the patients recovered and five of six (83%) had healthy babies.

First Trimester Considerations

Women with IBD should pay particular attention to their nutritional requirements at and around conception. Patients should be screened for anemia, as they may be iron, B_{12}, and folate deficient. Of particular concern may be folic acid absorption. Folate deficiency may be associated with neural tube defects in the developing fetus. Patients with IBD may have increased requirements secondary to poor absorption or to sulfasalazine therapy.

Embryogenesis occurs during the first trimester of pregnancy (week 1 to week 12). Many patients with Crohn's disease or ulcerative colitis express great concern over producing newborns with congenital defects. Many studies in the literature have shown that patients with IBD produce offspring with congenital defects at the same rate as the general population (0 to 3%.)

The developing embryo is most sensitive to potential teratogens during the first trimester. During weeks 2 to 4, harmful exposures tend to be embryolethal. It is called an "all or none" phenomenon, because exposure either destroys the developing embryo or has no effect. Weeks 4 to 11 are most critical with regard to organ development; exposure at this time can be most damaging. Many patients with IBD are kept in remission by the diligent use of drug therapy under the watchful care of their gastroenterologists. In addition, many of these patients have a history of first trimester exposure to ionizing radiation.

Ionizing Radiation

Many patients, either accidentally or because deemed necessary for diagnostic and management purposes, have been exposed to radiation in their first trimester. As previously stated, exposure during weeks 2 to 4 is less concerning as it either destroys the developing embryo or has no effect on it. During the critical weeks 4 to 11, exposure to very high doses of radiation has been shown to cause multiple organ damage. In animal studies, this risk of damage has not been demonstrated with exposure of less than 5 rads.

5-Aminosalicylic Drugs

Sulfasalazine is effective through its 5-aminosalicylic acid (5-ASA) component. It is linked to a sulfapyridine moiety to facilitate transport to the colon where its diazo-linkage can be metabolized by bacterial flora. Although first trimester exposure probably is safe, some reports in the literature warn of possible teratogenic effects. Furthermore, sulfasalazine may interfere with folic acid absorption and may lead to various maternal toxicities. All of this probably is secondary to its sulfapyridine component. In pregnancy, therefore, it is probably better to use the 5-ASA drugs, such as mesalamine (Asacol®, Procter & Gamble Pharmaceuticals, Cincinnati, Ohio), olsalazine (Dipentum), and mesalamine (Pentasa®, Ferring-Shire Pharmaceuticals, Florence, Kentucky). Diav-Citrin and colleagues (1998) prospectively studied 146 women who had first trimester exposure to mesalamine. There was no increase in the number of major malformations compared to their control group.

Antibiotics

Metronidazole often is the antibiotic of choice for treatment of perirectal abscess and fistulae from Crohn's disease. Although not yet recommended in the United States for use during the first trimester in pregnancy, it is widely used in Europe for many conditions in pregnancy. Many studies demonstrate its safety during the first trimester of pregnancy. Other commonly prescribed antibiotics can be used with safety during the first trimester of pregnancy; these include the penicillins and the cephalosporins. Some authors believe that ciprofloxacin, commonly used in IBD, should not be used in pregnancy; others believe that it is acceptable, if needed. As with most medications, few data are available.

Corticosteroids

Obstetricians have much experience with steroids in pregnancy. Many diseases require their liberal use throughout the first trimester and embryogenesis. Animal studies have reported evidence of increased risk of spontaneous abortion and cleft palate. However, many human studies show no evidence of congenital defects associated with first trimester exposure. Patients who require steroid treatment during the first trimester of pregnancy are reassured that their pregnancy is unlikely to be adversely affected by its use.

Immunosuppressive Agents

Azathioprine, cyclosporine, and 6-mercaptopurine (6-MP) all have been used to treat IBD. Immunosuppressive agents often can be used to treat and maintain patients with Crohn's disease or ulcerative colitis who have failed traditional therapy. Although animal models have implicated their teratogenicity, all three drugs have been used in pregnancy with success. Francella and collegues (1996) studied 450 patients with IBD who had received 6-MP; among them, 155 had conceived at least one pregnancy after developing IBD. In this study, there was no difference in the number of spontaneous abortions or congenital anomalies in patients who stopped 6-MP prior to conception, stopped it during pregnancy, or continued throughout pregnancy compared to those never on the drug. It is their conclusion that 6-MP is safe in the first trimester of pregnancy. There are differences of opinion among physicians on this topic.

Methotrexate

Although effective in some patients with Crohn's disease, methotrexate is contraindicated in the first trimester of pregnancy secondary to its high incidence of teratogenicity.

Other Medications

Medications such as antidiarrheal agents, antispasmodics, and histamine2 blockers often are necessary to treat mild exacerbations of the patient with IBD. These agents should be used if necessary; no detrimental effects have been described in association with their use in pregnancy.

Second Trimester Considerations

The first trimester of pregnancy often is the most taxing, as women tend to have nausea, decreased appetite, and extreme fatigue. As the twelfth week is completed, the second trimester brings with it some relief as many of these symptoms disappear.

Patients with Crohn's disease or ulcerative colitis generally do well in the second trimester of pregnancy. The risk of recurrence at this time is unlikely if the patient's disease is in remission. Particular attention is paid to general nutrition at this stage and approximately an 11-pound weight gain is expected during these 12 weeks. Patients with IBD who are not gaining weight appropriately should have nutritional supplements added to their diet. For patients who require surgical intervention, the second trimester tends to be the safest time to operate for both the mother and the developing fetus. Acute episodes of IBD, such as perforation or obstruction, may require surgery irrespective of fetal age.

Genetic screening usually is offered during the second trimester, and many patients express a desire to do additional screening because of their condition. Although it is well known that there is a familial pattern of inheritance with IBD, to date there has been no specific gene defect isolated. Family history seems to be the most important risk factor. Yang and colleagues (1992) observed a 5.2 percent and 7.8 percent lifetime risk of Crohn's disease and a 1.6 percent and 4.5 percent lifetime risk of ulcerative colitis in offspring of one parent affected with IBD in gentile and Jewish populations, respectively. When both parents are affected, this risk seems to be greatly increased. Patients are greatly reassured when told of the relatively low risk of transmission. As far as other genetic defects, patients with IBD are no different then the general population and are counseled the same way. There is a chapter on genetic aspects of IBD.

Although congenital abnormalities do not seem to be increased in patients with IBD, patients maintained on drug therapy or exposed to ionizing radiation all undergo fetal surveillance through directed ultrasound by a board-certified perinatologist in the mid-second trimester. Patients who received corticosteroids in the first trimester, for example, can be reassured, since sonography can easily detect midline defects, such as cleft palate.

Finally, it is important to encourage patients maintained on medications for IBD to continue as advised by their gastroenterologist throughout the second trimester. Medical therapy should be maximized as needed at this time, because fetal effects are less a consideration after embryogenesis. Exposure to ionizing radiation during weeks 12 to 16 targets the central nervous system as critical development occurs. High-dose exposure could lead to microcephaly and mental retardation. Low-dose exposure is of little concern, because risk is minimal.

Third Trimester Considerations

Patients with IBD tend to do well in the final trimester of their pregnancy (week 24 to delivery) if they have been in remission throughout. Again, particular attention is directed to the nutritional status of these patients, and an additional 11-pound weight gain is expected during this time. In pregnancy, the recommended daily allowance requires the addition of 300 kcal to the normal daily diet. Some patients with IBD may have additional requirements secondary to deficiencies in absorption. Requirements will vary, and patients should be assessed individually.

All patients are screened for anemia in the beginning of the third trimester. In normal pregnancies, the maternal plasma volume increases steadily from 10 weeks to about 30 to 34 weeks by about 50 percent, whereas the red blood cell mass increases only around 25 percent by term. Therefore, a physiologic anemia normally occurs. Many patients with IBD are anemic to begin with and find that by the third trimester, their mild-to-moderate anemia has become severe. Porter and Stirrat (1986) retrospectively analyzed 82 pregnant women with IBD and found lower hemoglobin levels in these women than in their matched control groups. In women with hematocrits below 30 percent, a formal anemia workup is indicated. The vast majority of anemia in pregnancy (approximately 75%) is related to iron deficiency. Once diagnosed, ferrous sulfate 325 mg three times daily is given. Folate deficiency is the most common cause of megaloblastic anemia in pregnancy and is rarely seen before the third trimester. Vitamin B_{12} deficiency is extremely rare in pregnancy but should be considered in those patients with IBD who might have impaired absorption. If anemia is diagnosed and specific therapy is only mildly helpful, the fetus should be monitored for growth retardation by serial sonographic measurements.

Once a pregnancy reaches 24 weeks, viability is assigned to the fetus. In other words, the unborn child becomes a patient. Many studies in the literature show an increase in the number of preterm births in women with Crohn's disease or ulcerative colitis. Baird and associates (1990) found around a two- to threefold elevated risk for preterm delivery in both diseases. Although neonatal outcome was not addressed in their study, other investigators have found similar results, implying a significant increase in neonatal morbidity and mortality. In the author's practice, pregnant patients with IBD undergo frequent cervical examinations throughout the third trimester. Evidence of preterm labor can hopefully be detected early and managed aggressively. In addition, all babies are delivered in a hospital with a level-three nursery, thus ensuring optimum care for the preterm infant. Most patients with IBD who are in remission should be reassured, as they are likely to deliver a healthy neonate at term. Reports show that the rate of normal healthy offspring born to women with IBD equals that of the general population.

Patients maintained on drug therapy should be encouraged to continue throughout the third trimester. If a patient is on sulfasalazine in the third trimester, her pediatrician should be informed, as there may be a small risk of kernicterus. Although animal studies have associated corticosteroids with intrauterine growth retardation, human studies have failed to demonstrate this association. This may be because cortisol is rapidly metabolized into the much less active cortisone by the human placenta and both prednisone and prednisolone barely cross the placenta at all. Nonetheless, as stated previously, all patients on corticosteroids should be serially monitored by ultrasound.

Delivery

With good prenatal care, most patients with IBD can expect to have normal labor and delivery. Many patients with IBD have strong associations between impending hospitalization and the very worst experiences with their disease. In these patients, the thought of going to the hospital to labor triggers painful memories of their illness. It is important to emphasize to these patients that the pain they will feel in labor is not a signal of any illness. Although this seems implicit, discussing these fears well before labor may reduce anxiety and, therefore, improve the entire birthing experience.

Patients with ulcerative colitis can expect normal labor and delivery. Cesarean section should be done for obstetric indications only. Currently, many young patients with chronic ulcerative colitis treated surgically undergo ileoanal anastomosis (IAA) as an alternative to the traditional proctocolectomy and ileostomy. Initially, patients who had undergone IAA routinely had elective cesarean

sections to preserve the anastomotic integrity. Currently, patients are offered the opportunity to deliver vaginally if they are so motivated. Scott and colleagues (1996) reported a series with no pouch-related complications in women who had undergone IAA who were allowed to deliver vaginally. Most patients delivered vaginally, and cesarean sections were performed for obstetric indications only. They concluded that vaginal delivery is safe in this population of patients.

The mode of delivery in patients with Crohn's disease is controversial among practicing obstetricians. In patients with active perineal disease, it is wise to completely avoid that area during childbirth, and since the actual delivery process itself is often associated with episiotomy or other perineal trauma, this certainly could exacerbate the condition. In these patients, a planned cesarean section should be performed. In patients in whom vaginal delivery is unavoidable, such as in a precipitous delivery, episiotomy should be avoided if possible. If unavoidable, mediolateral episiotomy is preferable, to reduce the risk of rectal involvement. If either episiotomy is done or there is a laceration, diligent perineal care should follow, to reduce complications. In women without active disease but with a history of perineal involvement, controversy exists with respect to mode of delivery. Brandt and associates (1995) surveyed patients with Crohn's disease who had undergone vaginal deliveries and discovered that 17.9 percent of women developed perineal disease after delivery without a preexisting history. The number of patients in the survey with a preexisting history of perineal disease was too small to evaluate (n = 5); however, none had recurrence after delivery. Many of the patients who developed perineal disease had episiotomies. When evaluating a patient for vaginal delivery, two factors are considered: (1) patient motivation after risks and benefits are described and (2) evaluation of the risk of perineal trauma during birth. A motivated patient who is expected to deliver easily may be allowed a vaginal trial. Her history of previous labors, if applicable, her pelvic size, and the estimated fetal weight should be taken into consideration. During delivery, episiotomy or other perineal trauma should be avoided by carefully guiding the expulsion of the presenting fetal part. An effective epidural anesthetic often is helpful in this regard.

Puerperium

As previously stated, patients who have done well throughout their pregnancy generally do well in the postpartum period. Again, vigorous attention should be focused on care of the perineum in all patients with Crohn's disease. Irrigating the perineum with warm water at least three times daily and after voids and bowel movements is important. The risk and benefits of breast-feeding should be discussed with women who are maintained on medications for their IBD. Patients maintained on immunosuppressive drugs should be discouraged from nursing, because their effects are unknown. Patients who require corticosteroids can feel free to nurse, because only small amounts are secreted in the breast milk. The 5-ASA component of sulfasalazine or one of the other 5-ASA drugs concentrates in the colon, and systemic absorption is rare. Although data are limited, patients on these medications can be encouraged to nurse if motivated, since no untoward effects have been described.

Conclusion

Women who have suffered with Crohn's disease and ulcerative colitis usually are able to live normal productive lives. In many cases, this is attributable to advances both medically and surgically. Integrating these advances into the care of the patient with IBD has enabled many who have been unable to get pregnant, either by choice or professional recommendation, to conceive, have healthy pregnancies, and deliver healthy babies. Obstetricians and gastroenterologists need to recognize this and relay it to patients in an encouraging manner. There is another chapter on pregnancy and IBD, written from a gastroenterology viewpoint. There are additional references with that chapter.

References

Baird DD, Narendranathan M, Sandler R. Increased risk of preterm birth for women with inflammatory bowel disease. Gastroenterology 1990;99:987–94.

Brandt LJ, Estabrook SG, Reinus JF. Results of a survey to evaluate whether vaginal delivery and episiotomy lead to perineal involvement in women with Crohn's disease. Am J Gastroenterol 1995;90:1918–22.

Diav-Citrin O, Park Y, Veerasuntharam G, et al. The safety of mesalamine in human pregnancy: a prospective controlled cohort study. Gastroenterology 1998;114:23–8.

Francella A, Dayan A, Rubin P, et al. 6-mercaptopurine (6-MP) is safe therapy for child-bearing parents with inflammatory bowel disease (IBD): a case controlled study. Gastroenterology 1996;110:909.

Hill J, Clark A, Scott NA. Surgical treatment of acute manifestations of Crohn's disease during pregnancy. J R Soc Med 1997;90:64–6.

Hudson M, Flett G, Sinclair TS, et al. Fertility and pregnancy in inflammatory bowel disease. Int J Gynecol Obstet 1997; 58:229–37.

Marion JF, Rubin PH, Lichtiger S, et al. Cyclosporin is safe for severe colitis complicating pregnancy [abstract]. Am J Gastroenterol 1996;91:1975.

Porter RJ, Stirrat GM. The effects of inflammatory bowel disease on pregnancy: a case-controlled retrospective analysis. Br J Obstet Gynecol 1986;93:1124–31.

Scott HJ, McLead RS, Blair J, et al. Ileal pouch-anal anastomosis: pregnancy, delivery, and pouch function. Int J Colorectal Dis 1996;11:84–7.

Yang H, McElrece C, Roth MP, et al. Familial imperic risks for inflammatory bowel disease: differences between Jews and non-Jews [abstract]. Gastroenterology 1992;102:31.

Supplemental Reading

Brent RL. Environmental factors: radiation. In: Brent RL, Harris MI, eds. Fogarty International Series on preventive medicine. Vol. 3. DHEW Publ. No. 76-853. Bethesda, MD: National Institutes of Health, 1976:179.

Dekaban AS. Abnormalities in children exposed to x-radiation during various stages of gestation: tentative timetable of radiation injury to the human fetus. Part I. J Nucl Med 1968;9:471–7.

Korlitz B. Inflammatory bowel disease and pregnancy. Gastroenterol Clin North Am 1998;27:213–24.

Rosa EW, Baum C, Shaw M. Pregnancy outcomes after first trimester vaginitis drug therapy. Obstet Gynecol 1987; 69:751–5.

CHAPTER 129

PREGNANCY AND INFLAMMATORY BOWEL DISEASE

DANIEL H. PRESENT, MD

Inheritance

One large multicenter study reported that, in a first-degree relative of a non-Jewish proband, the lifetime risk of developing Crohn's disease was 5.2 percent, with the risk to siblings being 7 percent and to parents, 4.8 percent. With Jewish probands, the lifetime risk was higher, 7.8 percent overall, with the risks to siblings of 16.8 percent; to parents, 3.8 percent; and to offspring, 7.4 percent. We estimate the overall risk in Crohn's disease of having a child with inflammatory bowel disease (IBD) was between 5 and 10 percent. With ulcerative colitis, the risks were lower; however, if both parents had IBD, the risk of a child developing IBD was 36 percent. For children who had reached 20 years of age, the risk was 50 percent. If both parents had Crohn's disease or if one parent had Crohn's disease and the other had ulcerative colitis, Crohn's disease was the more likely occurrence in the child. There are no data on the risk if one spouse had IBD and a first-degree relative of the other spouse also had IBD. There is a separate chapter on IBD genetics and the questions frequently asked by patients.

Fertility

There is a separate chapter, by an obstetrician, on fertility in patients with IBD. In ulcerative colitis, approximately 90 percent of patients are able to conceive. In case-controlled studies, there has been an increase in voluntary childlessness, greater than seen among controls.

In a large case-controlled study of 275 patients with Crohn's disease (matched for age), there was a significant reduction in fertility and pregnancy in women between the ages of 18 and 45 years. The authors pointed out that medical advice against conception may have played a role, but it appeared that patients with Crohn's disease practiced less birth control than control patients, and still there was a 42 percent rate of inability to conceive as compared to 28 percent in controls. This subfertility may be related to multiple factors, including active bowel disease with debility of the patient, lack of sexual desire because of disease activity, the presence of perianal fistulae associated with patients' fears about delivery, fallopian tube occlusion, and, finally, medical advice from physicians.

Smoking also may have an effect on fertility. It has been shown that fetal growth may be reduced by smoking alone, and several studies suggest that smoking may activate Crohn's disease. However, stopping smoking may activate ulcerative colitis. Most women prefer to stop smoking before they become pregnant, and they often are surprised to find that their ulcerative colitis will exacerbate. I strongly advise women to maximize their preventive medical therapy (whether it be 5-aminosalicylic acid [5-ASA] or 6-mercaptopurine [6-MP]) before stopping smoking. Hopefully, they can discontinue cigarettes and try to conceive while still remaining in remission.*

There have been few studies of infertility in relation to IBD in males. Sulfasalazine decreases sperm count and alters motility, resulting in a number of abnormal sperm forms. There is a single study that shows a decrease in family size among patients with Crohn's disease whether or not the male took sulfasalazine or steroids. More recent studies have not confirmed any diminished capacity to reproduce in males with IBD.

Influence of Ulcerative Colitis and Crohn's Disease on Pregnancy

Two large retrospective reviews encompassing several thousand patients show normal births in 83 percent of patients, which is directly comparable to the normal population. The rate of congenital abnormalities and spontaneous abortions and stillbirths appears to be similar to that seen in healthy patients.

Results of case-control studies show only minor differences, such as birth weight being statistically less in children born to women who have been affected by Crohn's disease. Prematurity also has been shown to be somewhat increased in women with Crohn's disease. The mode of delivery was similar in both groups. Patients who are in clinical remission at the time of conception can be advised that, if they remain in remission, IBD will have little effect on the pregnancy and should not influence obstetric management.

---

* Editor's Note: Excellent advice. The combination of stopping smoking and increasing physical exercise, with a resultant use of nonsteroidal anti-inflammatory drugs (NSAIDs), was associated with a severe recrudescence of disease in one of my patients. (TMB)

Obstetricians believe that pregnancies in patients with IBD are potentially high risk and that close monitoring including early ultrasound examination is indicated for both the mother and the fetus. There is an increased risk of premature delivery in patients with IBD who have active disease or who have developed colitis during pregnancy; therefore, more frequent examinations are indicated. At weeks 32 and 34, the fetus is carefully monitored for hypoxia related to placental insufficiency. Variability of fetal heart rate diminishes with hypoxia, and in this situation the obstetrician may have to consider early delivery.

It is advisable that an obstetrician, not a midwife, be in charge of the case, and if the patient has active IBD, monitoring in a tertiary care setting is appropriate. If there are any complications, a perinatologist should be available for consultation.

The mode of delivery (vaginal or caesarean section) should be considered. In a recent population-based study of 572 births in patients with IBD, it has been shown that statistically there are more elective cesarean sections among patients with ulcerative colitis and Crohn's disease as compared to the general population. This may be related to the fear of perineal rupture, with subsequent weakening of the anal sphincter, in patients who already have increased frequency of bowel movements. Studies in women not affected by IBD who suffer a rupture show that anal incontinence is high (over one-third) 5 years after a repair of the rupture.

In a survey done by the Crohn's & Colitis Foundation of America, it was shown that almost 18 percent of patients without a prior problem developed perineal disease postpartum. This usually was associated with an episiotomy. Crohn's patients should be advised to have a cesarean section if the child is large and the obstetrician believes that an episiotomy will be required, or if there is significant perianal disease. In those patients who have undergone ileoanal anastomosis with a proximal pouch, cesarean section is advisable in that significantly altered bowel function has been observed after a vaginal delivery in such cases. A pouch vaginal fistula can be a major problem for this type of patient. Another view is expressed by an obstetrician in the preceding chapter.

Activity of Disease and the Influence on Pregnancy

The management of the IBD depends on whether the disease is in remission or is active at the time of conception. In Miller's review (1986) of over 500 pregnancies in eight large series, if the women had inactive ulcerative colitis at the time of conception, approximately one-third relapsed during gestation and puerperium. This relapse rate was similar to that seen in nonpregnant patients. The majority of relapses occurred in the first trimester. This may be related to the fact that women prefer to discontinue all medication when they are planning to become pregnant. If they discontinued sulfasalazine, they lost the maintenance effect of this agent when they became pregnant. If fulminant disease occurs, it must be treated aggressively.

Miller also reported a series comprised of 227 women who conceived while their ulcerative colitis was active. The activity persisted in 24 percent of patients and worsened in 45 percent, indicating that almost 70 percent of patients will have a poor course, and this certainly reduces the chances of a normal delivery, since disease activity often leads to prematurity and low birth weight. The major priority would be to establish a remission before the patient conceives rather than having to deal with managing active disease during pregnancy.

The data are much the same with respect to Crohn's disease. In Miller's review, among 186 pregnancies in which the Crohn's disease was inactive at the time of conception, relapse occurred in 27 percent. This rate is similar to that in nonpregnant patients. As in ulcerative colitis, relapse appeared to be most common in the first trimester and postpartum. Again, this may have been related to whether medications were continued or discontinued. Several small series, comprising 93 pregnancies in women with active Crohn's disease, showed that the activity continued in one-third and worsened in one-third. Therefore, the overall risk of having a poor pregnancy is about 65 percent when the patient with Crohn's disease becomes pregnant with active disease. The question arises: Is there a minimum time period during which a patient should be in remission before becoming pregnant? No specific answer can be offered; nevertheless, the longer the remission, the more likely it is that the patient will do well after becoming pregnant. In ulcerative colitis, remission can be clearly evaluated with blood studies and a colonoscopy, whereas in Crohn's disease, it is more difficult to define remission, because endoscopy often shows activity even though the patient clinically is well. It would be ideal in Crohn's disease if the acute-phase reactants, such as C-reactive protein (CRP) and erythrocyte sedimentation rate (ESR), were normal at the time of conception.

In summary, it is absolutely essential that the physician communicate clearly to the patient that she should be in remission before attempting to conceive, and that medications that are keeping her in remission should not be discontinued either prior to conception or during the first trimester.

One cannot predict whether the course of the IBD will be the same in subsequent pregnancies, and therefore, it is not necessary to discourage subsequent pregnancies when the first has been complicated by activity. Fulminant disease, although rarely occurring during pregnancy, is associated with increased fetal and maternal mortality. Several anecdotal reports indicate that when the onset of IBD occurs during pregnancy, the disease is more severe.

Assessment of Disease Activity in Pregnant Patients with Inflammatory Bowel Disease

Standard laboratory studies, such as ESR, hemoglobin, and albumin, become abnormal during pregnancy, and therefore they have limited value. On the other hand, if the patient is in the first trimester and the ESR has gone up over 100 mm/hr and the albumin has sunk below 3.0 g, there is an obvious suggestion of disease activity. Diagnostic ultrasound appears to be safe, and recent studies with magnetic resonance imaging (MRI) also suggest that this may be a way to assess disease activity. There is a separate chapter on use of abdominal ultrasound to assess IBD status. There always is the concern about radiation dosage, and although it is advisable to avoid the use of radiography, if there is an acute or semi-acute complication, then the risk to the fetus of abdominal radiography is minimal (0 to 3 cases in 10,000 women exposed to abdominal radiography during the first 4 mo of pregnancy). Limited radiation does not induce labor or result in congenital abnormalities.

Flexible sigmoidoscopy is a simple and safe way to evaluate the patient with ulcerative colitis. Colonoscopy should be considered only in cases of life-threatening lower gastrointestinal bleeding or when the only alternative therapy is surgery. However, some believe that a full colonoscopy can be performed safely in almost all pregnant patients.

Indications for surgical intervention during pregnancy include obstruction that cannot be relieved medically, perforation, and massive bleeding. If an abscess develops, it must be drained. Fetal mortality is reportedly as high as 50 percent with colectomy.

Patients with ileostomies are capable of pregnancy, but stomal prolapse is a possibility. Pregnancy can be achieved in a patient who has undergone ileal pouch-anal anastomosis; however, this can be associated with increased bowel movements and leakage, especially in the third trimester. Fortunately, there is usually a return to normal postpartum function several months after delivery. In this group of patients, cesarean section is advisable, with a colorectal surgeon standing by at the time of the procedure.

Effects of Inflammatory Bowel Disease Medications on Pregnancy

The use of medications in pregnancy is a major concern of physicians of patients with IBD who plan to conceive. Most drugs do cross the placenta, and women usually want to avoid "all" drugs during pregnancy. There have been few studies of drugs in semen, but many drugs are known to be excreted into the semen, and there is potential risk of a male-mediated teratogenetic effect. Pharmaceutical companies rarely test products in pregnant women. The advice found in the *Physician's Desk Reference* (PDR) is basically a medicolegal disclaimer, and the Food and Drug Administration (FDA) classification can be ambiguous and difficult to interpret because of the lack of data. Animal studies, some with high dose, often are used to try to establish the risk to humans. If malformations occur rarely, it may take a prolonged period of observation for epidemiologic studies to demonstrate that a drug is toxic to the fetus. Koren and colleagues (1998) pointed out that 35 years after the recognition of the serious congenital anomalies that thalidomide caused in fetuses, fewer than 30 drugs have been shown to be teratogenic in humans, and even fewer currently are being used clinically. The issue of the use of drugs in pregnancy is lacking evidence-based proof for either safety or lack of safety. If stopping a medicaton because of lack of data leads to a relapse in the mother during pregnancy, this is a serious problem. To quote Dr. David Sachar, "The greatest risk to pregnancy is active disease—not active medicine." Medications that are used in the therapy of IBD are classified according to their safety for use during pregnancy in Table 129–1 and during breast-feeding in Table 129–2.

Nonspecific Symptomatic Agents

Acetaminophen has not been reported as being associated with fetal abnormalities and appears to be safe during pregnancy and breast-feeding. On the other hand, reports on aspirin ingestion have shown conflicting data on teratogenesis, and high doses appear to be associated with prolonged labor. Low doses may be of some value in coagulation disorders, such as deep vein thrombosis; however, there is also a risk of intracranial bleeding. Approximately 20 percent of the maternal dose of salicylate passes into

TABLE 129–1. Safety during Pregnancy of Medications Prescribed for Inflammatory Bowel Disease

Safe to Use When Indicated	Probably Safe*	Probably Not Safe*	Contraindicated
Oral mesalamine	Corticosteroids	Tetracycline	Methotrexate
Topical mesalamine	Olsalazine	Sulfonamides	
Sulfasalazine	Azathioprine		
Certain antibiotics	6-Mercaptopurine		
(ampicillin, cephalosporins)	Cyclosporine		
	Metronidazole		
	Ciprofloxacin		

*Limited data available.

TABLE 129–2. Safety during Breast-Feeding of Medications Prescribed for Inflammatory Bowel Disease

Safe to Use When Indicated	Probably Safe*	No Data Available	Contraindicated
Oral mesalamine	Topical mesalamine	Azathioprine	Methotrexate
Sulfasalazine		6-Mercaptopurine	Cyclosporine
Corticosteroids		Metronidazole	
		Ciprofloxacin	

*Limited data available.

the breast-milk. There is no contraindication to either acetaminophen or salicylates in breast-feeding.

Prostaglandins do play a significant role in the development of the fetus, and the nonsteroidal anti-inflammatory drugs (NSAIDs) are contraindicated, especially during the third trimester. Steroids may affect fetal blood vessels and produce pulmonary hypertension and bleeding. Their use in nursing is questionable and, therefore, they should not be taken by the mother at that time.

Among antidiarrheals, codeine has not been associated with fetal abnormalities and appears to be safe in breast-feeding. Questions have been raised about drug withdrawal in the newborn; however, this rarely is seen. No known reliable data exist on the use of loperamide (Imodium®) in pregnancy; however, diphenoxylate hydrochloride with atropine sulfate (Lomotil®) has resulted in increased malformations in a small number of infants. There also is a question of inhibition of lactation. In summary, acetaminophen appears to be the best drug available for pain control and, if required, codeine is probably the best medication for diarrhea.

Sulfasalazine

Sulfasalazine has been available for over 60 years, and there have been no studies demonstrating any harmful effects in pregnancy. It can affect male fertility by reducing sperm density and motility, as well as causing morphologic abnormalities. This occurs in perhaps 50 percent of males taking the drug and is rapidly reversed (within 6 to 8 wk) when sulfasalazine is discontinued and the patient switched to mesalamine in comparable dosages.

There have been no reports of increased fetal malformations related to sulfasalazine, and although it readily crosses the placenta, minimal amounts are secreted in breast-milk. A theoretic risk of kernicterus with displacement of bilirubin from plasma protein has been postulated; however, this has not been observed clinically. Sulfasalazine interferes with folic acid metabolism; therefore, because folates are important for neural tube development, 1 mg of folic acid twice a day is prescribed for both males and females who are taking sulfasalazine and are considering conception.

Mesalamine

Animal studies have demonstrated that mesalamine poses no risk to the fetus. In two recently published studies (123 and 165 pregnancies, respectively), 242 of the 288

subjects were taking mesalamine during the first trimester (mean doses, ~ 2 g/d). In one study, 20 percent were taking ≥3.2 g/d. Neither study demonstrated an increase in malformations compared to the teratogenic risk among the general population.* Currently available data indicate that mesalamine is not a teratogenic risk and is safe for use in pregnancy. Only one child has been reported to have had renal insufficiency, with biopsy showing interstitial fibrosis and tubular atrophy. This child improved over 6 months. There are rare allergic diarrheal reactions in infants who have received 5-ASA transferred through breast-milk. No teratogenicity has been seen in animal studies using topical 5-ASA, whether given as suppositories or enemas; there is poor absorption, ranging from 10 to 24 percent. These agents have been available for many years without fetal abnormalities being observed.

Antibiotics

Antibiotics frequently are needed during pregnancy for intercurrent infection, and although there have been few rigorous controlled trials, ampicillin, the cephalosporins, and erythromycin generally are considered to be safe in pregnancy. Trimethoprim is teratogenic; sulfonamides also may produce teratogenicity and kernicterus; and tetracycline has been associated with cataracts, liver necrosis, and dental discoloration.

In animals, no teratogenicity has been observed with ciprofloxacin, although arthropathy has been seen in immature animals, with an effect on growing cartilage. In a small study of 38 pregnancies, no fetal abnormalities were observed, although increased cesarean sections were performed. A larger study of 307 pregnancies in which 55 patients took ciprofloxacin during the first trimester showed no congenital abnormalities.

Metronidazole rapidly crosses the placental barrier, and it is a carcinogen in rodents, causing pulmonary, hepatic, and mammary tumors. There are no well-controlled trials in pregnancy; however, there have been several reports in which metronidazole has been used to treat vaginal trichomoniasis during the first trimester. One study of over 1,000 patients showed no increased risk of birth defects with a single course of metronidazole. No data exist regarding patients with Crohn's disease

---

* Dr. Present reminds us that congenital anomalies are observed in up to 3% of healthy patients. (TMB)

on prolonged high dosages; however, most obstetricians believe that it is safe to prescribe metronidazole in the second and third trimesters. Reports to date indicate that metronidazole during the first trimester is not associated with birth defects.

In summary, ampicillin and the cephalosporins are safe, especially for fistulizing complications in Crohn's disease, and ciprofloxacin and metronidazole probably are safe. The risk in breast-feeding is uncertain with the latter two agents and, therefore, it is not advisable.

Steroids

Patients, in general, have not been as concerned about taking corticosteroids during pregnancy as they have about taking immunomodulators. However, corticosteroids have been associated with an increased incidence of spontaneous abortions, cleft palate, and stillbirths in mice, yet teratogenicity is unusual in humans. High doses of steroids also have been associated with retardation of fetal growth. Prednisone and prednisolone poorly cross into the fetal circulation, and it is rare to observe adrenocortical insufficiency. Adrenocorticotropic hormone (ACTH) has been used successfully in several small series with no negative effects on pregnancy or the fetus. Steroids have been shown to be safe in other disorders, such as rheumatoid arthritis, lupus, and asthma. In a large survey of 531 pregnant patients, the complication rate has been shown to be increased with the use of steroids; however, this occurred in patients with severe, active IBD and was mostly thought to be disease-related rather than medication-related. Once again, in very sick patients the risk to the fetus of the active disease is greater than that of corticosteroids, and steroids should be used as needed in pregnant patients with IBD, if they are moderately to severely ill, in the same way as they are used in nonpregnant patients with active IBD. The amount of steroids received by the nursing infant is minimal, and when used in low dosages appears to be safe.

Immunomodulatory Drugs

There has been great reluctance to use 6-MP or azathioprine (AZA) in patients with IBD who are pregnant. The use of immunosuppressives in women with transplants is not contraindicated during pregnancy, and animal and human studies show that immunosuppressants are not carcinogenic. There is an increase in lymphoproliferative disorders in transplant patients; however, this may be related more to the transplant than to the drugs used for immunomodulation. There also is concern for growth retardation and prematurity in transplant patients. This occurs predominantly in female infants, and is possibly related to the health of the mother. Chromosomal abnormalities have occasionally been observed in adults and their children, but in long-term follow-up in patients who received AZA, the abnormalities have disappeared.

Azathioprine is rapidly converted to 6-MP and is transmitted through breast-milk.

The data on 6-MP and AZA in patients with IBD are limited to a small retrospective study of 16 pregnancies in 14 women. The results demonstrated no perinatal problems, no congenital abnormalities, and no increase in neonatal or childhood infections. Among 155 patients with IBD who conceived at least one pregnancy, the results were similar. Group A had taken 6-MP or AZA prior to pregnancy, improved, discontinued the drug, and then conceived. Group B1 were those patients who conceived while on these drugs, and then stopped taking them when they found out they were pregnant. Group B2 patients conceived while on the drug and continued taking the drug throughout pregnancy. These were compared to Group C patients who had IBD and who conceived but did not receive 6-MP or AZA until after their children were born. This study of 325 pregnancies showed that 6-MP used before conception, at conception, or during pregnancy was not directly associated with any statistically significant increase in prematurity, spontaneous abortion, congenital abnormalities, neonatal or childhood infections, or neoplasia. Several other small studies have found chromosomal abnormalities on amniocentesis, and therapeutic abortion was therefore advised. Other reports suggest that the children of men with IBD who have been recently taking 6-MP have an associated increased in congenital abnormalities.

Patients probably are safe when conceiving on 6-MP. If they have had a long and protracted course of severe disease before the 6-MP was instituted, they should continue the drug throughout the pregnancy. The risk of relapse is a greater risk to the fetus than the risk of 6-MP toxicity. On the other hand, if the patient has been in a prolonged remission for many years and is strongly against taking this drug during pregnancy, she should be allowed to stop the 6-MP. No data are available regarding 6-MP or AZA in nursing, although anecdotal experience with fewer than six patients has shown it to be safe.

Methotrexate and Cyclosporine

Methotrexate produces oligospermia during therapy and is contraindicated during pregnancy. The drug causes chromosome damage and is teratogenic. It is also contraindicated in breast-feeding women.

Among infants of male transplant recipients who had taken cyclosporine, there was a low birth weight in 4 percent and prematurity in 10 percent. No specific congenital abnormalities were observed. Among infants of 233 female transplant recipients, low birth-weight was seen in almost 40 percent and prematurity in almost 60 percent; however, the survival rate in these children still was greater than 90%. No congenital abnormalities were seen in the infants of female transplant recipients. Breast-feeding should be avoided.

There are only six cases reported in the literature of patients who have received intravenous (IV) cyclosporine for severe exacerbation of their IBD during pregnancy. Five of the six patients had a live birth. No colectomies were acutely required; however, several patients ultimately required an elective colectomy. No congenital abnormalities were observed. However, these numbers are small. The risks associated with cyclosporine must be weighed against the high rate of fetal mortality associated with colectomy.

Infliximab

As of the time of writing of this chapter, Centocor Inc., Malvern, Pennsylvania, had been notified of seven pregnancies in patients who have recently taken infliximab. There has been one spontaneous abortion, one therapeutic abortion, and one normal child born. Four pregnancies are still in utero.

The half-life of infliximab is approximately 9 days, and the drug disappears from the bloodstream in 10 to 12 weeks. If there is concern about timing of conception, it should probably be attempted at 3 months after an infusion, which should avoid exposure to the circulating antibody.

Editor's Note

This chapter, despite editing, is longer than most. Dr. Present has a lot to say on this topic, and we are interested in his opinion. Some of his references are listed in the previous chapter, which also deals with fertility and pregnancy in IBD. (TMB)

References

Koren G, Pastuszak A, Ito S. Drugs in pregnancy. N Engl J Med 1998;338:1128–37.

Miller JP. Inflammatory bowel disease in pregnancy: a review. J Royal Soc Medicine 1986;79:221–5.

Supplemental Reading

Albengres E, Le Louet H, Tillement JP. Immunosuppressive drugs and pregnancy: experimental and clinical data. Transplant Proc 1997;29:2461–6.

Alstead EM, Ritchie JK, Lennard-Jones JE, et al. Safety of azathioprine in pregnancy in inflammatory bowel disease. Gastroenterology 1990;99:443–6.

Connell WR. Safety of drug therapy for inflammatory bowel disease in pregnant and nursing women. Inflamm Bowel Dis 1996;2:33–47.

Diav-Citrin O, Park YH, Veerasuntharam G, et al. The safety of mesalamine in human pregnancy: a prospective controlled cohort study. Gastroenterology 1998;114:23–8.

Francella A, Dayan A, Rubin P, et al. 6-Mercaptopurine (6-MP) is safe therapy for child-bearing patients with inflammatory bowel diseae (IBD): a case-controlled study. Gastroenterology 1996;110A:909.

Jarnerot G, Into-Malmberg MD. Review. Fertility, sterility, and pregnancy in chronic inflammatory bowel disease. Scand J Gastroenterol 1982;17:1–4.

Marteau P, Tennenbaum R, Elefant E, et al. Foetal outcome in women with inflammatory bowel disease treated during pregnancy with oral mesalazine microgranules. Aliment Pharmacol Ther 1998;12:1101–8.

Mogadam M, Dobbins WO, Korelitz BI, et al. Pregnancy in inflammatory bowel disease: effects of sulfasalazine and corticosteroids on fetal outcome. Gastroenterology 1981;80:72–6.

Sachart D. Exposure to mesalazine during pregnancy increased preterm deliveries and decreased birthweight [commentary]. 617 Gut 1998;43:316.

Yang H, McElree C, Roth MP, et al. Familial empirical risks for inflammatory bowel disease: differences between Jews and non-Jews. Gut 1993;34:517–24.

CHAPTER 130

COLITIS IN THE ELDERLY

JAMES J. FARRELL, MB, AND LAWRENCE S. FRIEDMAN, MD

The spectrum of pathophysiologic conditions associated with diarrhea in the elderly is broad and includes inflammatory diseases of the colon (Table 130–1). Colitis in the elderly, defined arbitrarily as an age greater than 65 years, merits particular attention because the diagnostic possibilities and the course and prognosis of colitis in the elderly differ from those in younger patients. Determining the cause of colitis is particularly challenging because the number of diagnostic considerations increases with advancing age.

Diarrhea in the elderly may lead to serious morbidity and even death. In the United States, the majority of all diarrheal deaths occur in the elderly, particularly the "old elderly" (above age 85 yr). The relatively high case-fatality rate is attributable in part to the high frequency of comorbid illnesses in elderly patients and the intolerance of elderly persons to the cardiovascular and metabolic complications of diarrhea. Use of oral rehydration solutions, which have been so successful in treating dehydration and preventing diarrheal deaths in children, has been useful in the elderly (Bennett and Greenough).

Clinical Presentation

The clinical presentation of colitis in elderly patients is similar regardless of the cause. Typical symptoms include crampy lower abdominal pain and frequent bowel movements, which are characteristically small in volume. Tenesmus (rectal urgency), blood in the stool (microscopic or visible), and fever also suggest colonic inflammation. The detection of polymorphonuclear neutrophils in large numbers on microscopic examination of stool ("fecal leukocytes") suggests direct tissue invasion or mucosal disruption and provides confirmatory evidence of colonic inflammation. Because the spectrum of symptoms associated with colitis is limited, data from the history and physical examination must be interpreted in the context of microbiologic analysis of stool specimens (stool culture and examinations for *Clostridium difficile* toxin and ova and parasites), the appearance of the colonic mucosa (radiographic or endoscopic), and, often, the histopathology of the colorectal mucosa.

Differentiating among infectious, ischemic, and ulcerative or Crohn's colitis may be particularly difficult in an older patient. Often symptoms of colitis in the elderly do

TABLE 130–1. Causes of Colitis in the Elderly

Infectious pathogens
  Salmonella species
  Shigella species
  Campylobacter jejuni
  Escherichia coli O157:H7
  Clostridium difficile
  Entamoeba histolytica

Ischemic colitis
Inflammatory bowel disease (ulcerative colitis, Crohn's colitis)
Microscopic (collagenous and lymphocytic) colitis
Segmental colitis associated with diverticulosis
Radiation therapy

Drugs
  Ischemic colitis:
    Digitalis
    Vasopressin
    Psychotropic drugs
    Estrogens
    Danazol

  Idiosyncratic colitis
    Nonsteroidal anti-inflammatory drugs
    Phosphate soda oral preparations
    Gold compounds
    Methyldopa
    Flucytosine
    Isotretinoin
    Allopurinol

not immediately suggest an inflammatory disorder, let alone inflammatory bowel disease (IBD), for several reasons, including a blunted response to pain; poor communication owing to impaired cognition, hearing, or vision; fear of the medical system; a focus on cancer as the most likely cause of altered bowel function or gastrointestinal bleeding; and the misconception that IBD rarely has its onset in old age. Physical signs in the elderly may be atypical as a result of altered sensory perception, related in part to the use of a variety of medications or the presence of coexisting systemic disease. A delay in diagnosis is common in older patients with IBD and may result in complications or inappropriate treatment. The diagnostic evaluation of colitis is generally unaffected by age. Although many clinicians are reluctant to perform invasive testing in older patients, age alone (in the absence of concurrent illnesses) does not appear to confer additional risk to endoscopic or radiologic evaluation. In fact, appropriate, expeditious diagnostic testing is particularly important in older patients presenting with atypical symptoms.

Infectious Colitis

Infectious colitis is common in the elderly and should be the initial diagnostic consideration in an elderly patient with colitis, especially of recent onset. The risk of infection is increased in the elderly, because of waning immunity, institutional living, and, perhaps, decreased gastric acid production caused by longstanding *Helicobacter pylori* gastritis. *Salmonella* species have been responsible for the largest numbers of nursing-home outbreaks of colitis and cause greater morbidity and mortality in the elderly than in the young. Similarly, the frequency and severity of hemorrhagic colitis caused by *Escherichia coli* O157:H7 and pseudomembranous colitis is increased in older people, especially those in nursing homes.

In general, infectious colitis rarely persists longer than 4 weeks, although infections caused by *Yersinia*, *Campylobacter*, *Mycobacterium tuberculosis*, *Entamoeba histolytica*, and *Schistosoma* species may persist for several months in some cases. Multiple cultures of stool and blood and repeated fecal microscopic examination for ova and parasites should be obtained routinely. Special cultivation techniques may be required to identify *E. coli* serotype O157:H7, *Campylobacter*, *Yersinia*, and *Vibrio* species. In one prospective study of patients with diarrheal illness of short duration in whom the presumed diagnosis was idiopathic IBD, extensive laboratory investigations ultimately revealed an infectious etiology in 38 percent of cases.

Verocytotoxin-producing *E. coli* serotype O157:H7 is an important cause of infectious colitis in the elderly. The spectrum of clinical manifestations includes asymptomatic infection, nonbloody diarrhea, hemorrhagic colitis, hemolytic-uremic syndrome (HUS), thrombotic thrombocytopenic purpura (TTP), and, occasionally, death. Epidemics in the general population and outbreaks in nursing homes result from undercooked infected ground beef and direct person-to-person transmission. *Escherichia coli* O157:H7 strains are not invasive but produce high levels of cytotoxins, which have been implicated in the pathogenesis of HUS and TTP as well as hemorrhagic colitis. Older age is a risk factor for *E. coli* O157:H7 colitis and increases the risk of HUS, TTP, and death, with mortality rates of 18 to 35 percent in the elderly; in 10 reported major outbreaks, all fatalities occurred in the elderly.

The most frequent symptoms of *E. coli* O157:H7 colitis are severe crampy abdominal pain and tenderness, occasionally with vomiting, in the absence of a high fever. The stools may be grossly bloody. Fecal leukocytes often are absent, and stool cultures fail to reveal a pathogenic organism unless specific cultivation techniques are requested. On sigmoidoscopy or colonoscopy, the rectum and sigmoid may appear normal, but erythema and edema become increasingly pronounced in more proximal portions of the colon. On barium enema, thumbprinting, resulting from submucosal edema rather than hemorrhage, is common. The clinical features of *E. coli* O157:H7 colitis often are mistaken for noninfectious colitis, especially ischemic colitis. In the past, emergency colectomy has been done in some elderly patients mistakenly thought to have fulminant ulcerative colitis. The optimal treatment of *E. coli* O157:H7 infection is unknown. Despite susceptibility of the organism to most antimicrobial agents in vitro, the duration of illness, typically 8 to 10 days, is not reduced significantly by antimicrobial therapy. Antidiarrheal drugs may prolong the disease and should be avoided.

Clostridium difficile colitis affects the elderly more frequently and more severely than younger patients. This gram-positive spore-forming bacillus frequently is isolated from the stool of hospitalized patients and the hands of health care personnel. The organism is transmitted readily among residents of long-term care facilities and has become endemic in some facilities. Antibiotic use may result in antibiotic-induced diarrhea, colitis, or pseudomembranous colitis. The frequency of isolating *C. difficile* cytotoxin in stool specimens from patients with antibiotic-associated diarrhea increases with age. Factors that predispose to infection and to pseudomembranous colitis in the elderly include decreased colonic motility; an age-related reduction in the renal excretion of antibiotics, resulting in elevated biliary and enteric antibiotic levels; and a diminished or absent antibody response to toxigenic *C. difficile*.

Pseudomembranous colitis should be suspected when diarrhea develops abruptly in a hospitalized patient or soon after antibiotic use. The onset of colitis may be delayed up to 6 weeks following completion of a course of antibiotics. Pseudomembranous colitis has been reported in the absence of antibiotic exposure; fecal stasis and hypochlorhydria may play a role in these cases. Clinical features include fever; leukocytosis, which is sometimes marked; and crampy abdominal pain. Occasionally, elderly patients may present with malnutrition owing to protein-losing enteropathy in the absence of overt diarrhea.

The diagnosis of pseudomembranous colitis usually is confirmed by a positive assay for the cytotoxin of *C. difficile* in stool or by endoscopic visualization of pseudomembranes (raised yellow plaques on an inflamed mucosa). Pseudomembranes may be absent on sigmoidoscopy but evident in the more proximal colon on colonoscopy in about 20 percent of cases.

Treatment with oral metronidazole (250 mg four times a day) or vancomycin (125 mg four times a day) for 10 to 14 days is effective in most cases, but relapses may occur in up to 20 percent of cases. Prolonged therapy and tapering regimens may be curative in these instances. For cases refractory to standard medical care, the use of rifampin, cholestyramine, intravenous immunoglobulin, or capsules containing the yeast *Saccharomyces boulardii* may be considered. There is a separate chapter on infectious agents complicating IBD.

Ischemic Colitis

Ischemic colitis is predominantly a disease of the elderly and results from diminished or absent inferior mesenteric arterial blood flow. A specific precipitating event often is not identifiable. The presence of congestive heart failure, cardiac arrhythmias, systemic emboli to other organs, vasculitis, or diabetes should suggest the possibility that acute or subacute colitis is ischemic in nature

The sudden onset of mild, crampy left lower quadrant pain followed by bloody diarrhea within 24 hours is typical of ischemic colitis. There may be associated nausea, vomiting, and tenesmus. Localized abdominal tenderness may occur over the involved colonic segment; fever, leukocytosis, and signs of peritoneal irritation suggest colonic infarction or impending perforation. Toxic dilatation occurs rarely. A colonoscopy or barium enema usually can confirm the diagnosis of ischemic colitis but must be performed with caution so as not to worsen the ischemic damage. Computed tomography (CT) can be helpful. Endoscopic visualization of infarction or gangrene is diagnostic of ischemic colitis. Ulceration, friability, erythema, edema, and focal hemorrhage are nonspecific findings. The histologic appearance of ischemic colitis is most specific early in the course of the illness when coagulative necrosis, submucosal edema, and hemorrhage are noted. As ischemia becomes chronic, histologic differentiation from IBD may be difficult, because superficial ulceration is a prominent finding in both entities. The rectum typically is spared in ischemic colitis, in contrast to ulcerative colitis (UC) and infectious colitis. The involved bowel is sharply demarcated from uninvolved bowel and does not contain skip lesions. The "watershed" areas of the splenic flexure and sigmoid colon traditionally are believed to be the most vulnerable to ischemia, owing to their potentially poor collateral circulation; however, any portion of the colon may be affected. Thumb-printing due to submucosal hemorrhage and edema may be noted on a plain abdominal radiograph or barium enema 2 to 3 days after the onset of symptoms; however, submucosal hemorrhage also can be seen with infectious diarrhea. Resolution of these findings within several days after the initial insult is strongly supportive of a diagnosis of ischemic colitis. Angiography seldom reveals acute arterial obstruction and rarely is helpful.

Most episodes of ischemic colitis are confined to the colonic mucosa and are mild and self-limited; recovery usually is complete, and recurrences are notably rare. In general, the treatment of ischemic colitis consists of supportive care and fluid replacement. In a minority of cases, ischemia is severe, leading to infarction with full-thickness necrosis of the colonic wall. Pneumatosis may be seen on flat plate or CT scan. Even with prompt surgical intervention, the mortality rate in such cases exceeds 50 percent. In some patients, the course of ischemic colitis lasts weeks or months and may result in the formation of a colonic stricture. Strictures that produce no symptoms should be observed, as some of these will resolve over the next 12 to 24 months without specific therapy. Strictures that cause obstructive symptoms will require either endoscopic dilatation or surgical resection.

Diverticulitis

The incidence of diverticular disease and its complications increases with age. Colonic diverticula are present in 35 to 60 percent of people over age 60. Whereas the majority of patients with diverticular disease remain asymptomatic, some may present with chronic constipation or bowel irregularity, acute left lower quadrant pain and tenderness with a mass on examination (diverticulitis), or gross rectal bleeding.

Because diverticulosis is so common and the presentation of Crohn's disease (CD) may mimic that of diverticulitis, CD is frequently misdiagnosed as diverticulitis in the elderly. Moreover, over 50 percent of patients with late-onset IBD have concomitant diverticulosis, and diverticulitis may actually be precipitated by extension of IBD, especially colonic CD, into a diverticulum. Similarities in the clinical manifestations of diverticulitis and CD make the two disorders difficult to distinguish and frequently cause diagnostic confusion and a delay in diagnosis. Clinical features favoring CD include the insidious onset of symptoms, perianal disease, previous history of colonic resections, and fistula formation in atypical locations (including perineal, low rectovaginal, flank, and thigh fistulae). Bleeding associated with diverticular disease generally is brisk and self-limited and occurs in the absence of diverticulitis, whereas distal CD is more typically associated with the frequent passage of small amounts of blood, often with diarrhea. Extraintestinal complications, such as arthritis or pyoderma gangrenosum, favor a diagnosis of CD but may rarely occur in patients with diverticulitis. Endoscopic findings suggestive of CD include mucosal inflammation with friability, granularity, and ulceration, whereas endoscopically normal mucosa is typical of diverticulitis.

The preoperative recognition of underlying CD in patients with both conditions appears to reduce surgical operative mortality. Conversely, failure to recognize that presumed diverticulitis may in fact be CD or a combination of both diseases often leads to a poor surgical outcome, especially in the elderly. The diagnosis of CD may not become evident until after an operation for presumed diverticulitis. In these patients, surgery for presumed diverticulitis may be followed by persistent symptoms, delayed wound healing, disruption of the anastomosis, fistula formation, sepsis, and a high frequency of recurrent disease in the remaining rectum and colon.

A syndrome of "segmental colitis" in association with sigmoid diverticulosis has been described predominantly in elderly patients. This syndrome is characterized by rectal bleeding, diarrhea, and abdominal pain. Colonoscopy reveals patchy mucosal erythema and hemorrhage involving a segment of the colon, usually the sigmoid, containing diverticula. Biopsy of the involved mucosa shows chronic active colitis without granulomas, whereas grossly uninvolved areas are histologically normal. The inflammation does not extend into the diverticula and is limited to the sigmoid colon, sparing the rectum and proximal colon. This syndrome appears to be distinct from diverticulitis, CD, or UC and usually resolves spontaneously or responds to therapy used to treat IBD, such as sulfasalazine or corticosteroids. However, in a few cases, features typical of UC may eventually develop. The cause of segmental colitis is unknown. Mucosal redundancy with prolapse and use of nonsteroidal anti-inflammatory drugs (NSAIDs) have been proposed as possible contributing factors. Pathologists now use the term "diverticular colitis" to describe the condition of some of these patients.

Collagenous and Lymphocytic Colitis

Collagenous and lymphocytic colitis, referred to collectively as microscopic colitis, are rare disorders characterized by chronic watery diarrhea and a normal endoscopic appearance to the colonic mucosa despite histologic evidence of mucosal inflammation. There is a separate chapter on collagenous and microscopic colitis. Up to 80 perent of the reported cases of collagenous colitis have been in women with a mean age of 60 years. Both men and women are affected equally in lymphocytic colitis. In both disorders, the diarrhea is generally secretory in nature, up to 4 liters or more daily, and is made worse by eating. Patchy colonic involvement is common, and multiple biopsy specimens from different segments of the colon may be required to confirm the diagnosis. In collagenous colitis, colonic mucosal biopsies reveal a distinctive thickened collagen layer (7 to 100 μm thick [normal < 3 μm]) beneath the surface epithelium and an inflammatory infiltrate, primarily of lymphocytes and plasma cells, in the lamina propria. A prominent lymphocytic infiltration of the epithelium and lamina propria without an underlying collagen band is characteristic of lymphocytic colitis.

Treatment is empirical. Bismuth subsalicylate (two tablets four times daily for 8 weeks) has been reported to lead to clinical and histologic resolution in a high percentage of cases. Cholestyramine also may have some efficacy. Otherwise, sulfasalazine and other 5-aminosalicylates have been

the mainstays of therapy. Corticosteroids (including budesonide) may be tried for refractory disease. Symptomatic treatment involving bulkage and antidiarrheal agents may be helpful in patients with mild symptoms. Spontaneous remission often occurs within 3 years of onset, but some patients have persistent, disabling symptoms. Therapy is discussed in Chapter 132.

Inflammatory Bowel Disease in the Elderly

Although often regarded as a disease of young adults, IBD occurs with greater frequency in the elderly than is generally appreciated. The age distribution of IBD is bimodal; after an initial peak in incidence in the third decade, there is a second increase in the incidence of both UC and CD between the sixth and eighth decades of life. Late-onset disease accounts for about 12 percent of cases of UC and 16 percent of cases of CD. The prevalence of IBD in the elderly is not explained by misdiagnosis of other conditions, such as ischemic colitis. The clinical features of IBD in the elderly differ little from those in younger patients. However, there is a tendency for both CD and UC to involve the distal colon in older patients. As a consequence, the disease often is milder and less complicated than in younger patients. However, in the elderly, presenting symptoms of IBD often are presumed to be attributable to another cause, and, initially, the correct diagnosis is sometimes overlooked.

Ulcerative Colitis

For many elderly patients, UC is a relatively mild illness, because the colonic inflammation often is limited to the rectum or sigmoid colon (ulcerative proctitis and proctosigmoiditis). This distribution of disease is generally associated with fewer systemic manifestations, better response to medical therapy, and less need for surgery than more extensive UC. Involvement of the entire colon (pancolitis) is less common in elderly than in younger patients. In one large, multinational survey, about 12 percent of patients over 60 years of age had pancolitis compared to 27 percent of those under age 60.

Older patients appear to be more likely than younger patients to present with a severe initial attack, associated with a relatively high fatality rate. In one large community-based study, 14 percent of patients over 70 years of age had a severe initial attack of UC, compared to 3 percent of adults aged 30 to 69 years. Severe first attacks contributed to a mortality rate of 19 percent in the elderly, compared to only 3 percent for the entire study population. Although advanced age clearly is an important risk factor for mortality during initial attacks of UC, overall mortality rates have, in fact, declined significantly with improved medical and surgical therapy, and for the vast majority of elderly patients who survive a severe first attack of UC or who undergo early surgery, the prognosis appears to be better than that for younger patients.

Most elderly patients with UC respond favorably to medical management, perhaps even better than their younger counterparts. Once in remission, relapse appears to be less frequent in the elderly, regardless of the severity of the initial attack. In one study, only 40 percent of patients over 70 years of age at the time of a first attack of UC experienced a relapse within 5 years of presentation, compared to 80 percent of those under age 30.

The extent and duration of colitis are risk factors for the development of colorectal neoplasia in patients with UC. Because pancolitis is relatively uncommon in the elderly and the duration of disease is relatively short, older patients with UC may be at risk for colonic cancer on the basis of their age per se, rather than UC. In fact, the relative risk of colonic cancer may be lower in older patients with UC than in younger patients. Sporadic adenomas may be difficult to distinguish from more ominous colitis-related dysplastic masses in elderly patients with UC. In general, colonoscopic polypectomy is appropriate for isolated adenomas, but colectomy should be considered when mucosal biopsies adjacent to the adenoma also show dysplasia. This issue is discussed in the chapter on colonoscopic surveillance for dysplasia.

Crohn's Disease

Crohn's disease presenting in the older person (especially older women) has a propensity for limited involvement of an isolated left colonic segment or the rectum. Whereas CD is limited to the colon in about 25 percent of all patients with CD, in older patients, this proportion approaches 60 percent. In contrast, disease affecting the terminal ileum and ascending colon is the most common pattern of CD in younger adults. Older patients with late-onset CD rarely have a positive family history of IBD, and the pathogenesis may be more environmental than genetic.

Complications such as intestinal obstruction, perforation, and fistula formation are less common with colonic involvement than with small bowel CD. Consequently, surgery is necessary less often in older patients than in younger patients. Furthermore, colonic disease, especially segmental or distal colitis, appears to be more responsive to drug therapy. Elderly patients with ileal or ileocolonic CD occasionally require intestinal resection but generally tolerate surgery well and appear to have low rates of postoperative recurrence. Thus, the consequences of CD in older patients may be less severe than in the young.

Treatment of Inflammatory Bowel Disease

The principles of medical and surgical management of IBD are the same regardless of the age of the patient. Nonetheless, there are several important considerations when treating elderly patients with IBD. Because severe initial attacks of UC can be associated with high mortality

rates in the elderly, early colectomy, before malnutrition and deconditioning develop, may be preferable to prolonged medical treatment; attempts to avoid the risks of surgery with protracted medical management may actually lead to an increased mortality rate. A conventional ileostomy is generally favored following colectomy in older patients, because the anal sphincter-saving surgical procedures, such as an ileal pouch-anal anastamosis, often have poor functional results in older patients.

The most commonly used medications in the treatment of IBD include sulfasalazine, mesalamine (5-aminosalicylic acid), and corticosteroids, which generally are well tolerated in older patients. However, corticosteroids also have a higher risk of complications in the elderly, particularly accelerated bone loss and fractures, hypertension, and diabetes. Distal colitis tends to be more refractory to topical therapy in older than in young patients, and affected elderly patients are more likely to require systemic therapy. The immunosuppressive agents azathioprine and 6-mercaptopurine generally are well tolerated in the elderly, although some authorities have argued against their use in older patients on the theoretic grounds that they may further impair the immune dysfunction associated with aging and result in an increased risk of infection or possibly malignancy. Metronidazole can be effective in CD, but its use may be limited by the occurrence of peripheral neuropathy. Clinical studies of infliximab have not included sufficient numbers of older patients with CD to determine whether this drug has a role in the elderly. There is a separate chapter on anti-tumor necrosis factor medications.

Others Causes of Colitis in the Elderly

Other conditions may mimic IBD clinically, radiographically, and endoscopically in older patients. The acute and chronic effects of radiation injury, especially if limited to the rectum, may result in abdominal cramps, bleeding, and tenesmus. The diagnosis is seldom difficult if a history of prior radiation therapy is known. The diagnosis is confirmed by colonoscopy with biopsy; mucosal telangiectases are characteristic. Treatment is symptomatic and may include laser therapy or topical application of formalin to reduce bleeding. There is a chapter on radiation enterocolitis.

Ileocecal carcinoma, lymphoma, and carcinoid tumors may, on occasion, resemble CD. Involvement of the colon by systemic diseases, such as vasculitis or amyloidosis, rarely may suggest a diagnosis of IBD. Drugs associated with ischemic colitis include digitalis, vasopressin, psychotropic drugs, estrogens, and danazol. Drugs associated with idiosyncratic colitis include NSAIDs, gold compounds, methyldopa, flucytosine, isotretinoin, and allopurinol.

Use of NSAIDs is particularly prevalent in older persons. With long-term exposure to these compounds, ulceration and fibrotic strictures of the small intestine or colon may develop. A variety of lesions have been described, including solitary ulcers (occasionally leading to colonic perforation), diffuse colitis, and diaphragm-like colonic strictures. Associated clinical features include diarrhea, profound weight loss, and hypoalbuminemia. Occasionally, an incorrect diagnosis of CD may be made. Typically, NSAID-induced colitis resolves promptly on withdrawal of the offending drug and recurs with rechallenge. In addition to causing colitis de novo, NSAIDs have been reported to provoke relapses of previously quiescent IBD. The next chapter in this text is devoted to NSAID-induced enterocolitis.

Approach to the Elderly Patient with Colitis

After initial stabilization and adequate rehydration, a history and physical examination should focus on elucidating the cause of the colitis. Information about previous episodes, recent travel, exposure to possible infectious agents, major medical illnesses, including vascular disease, previous radiation therapy, and current medications should be obtained. Findings of cardiac disease on physical examination suggest that the new onset of colitis may be ischemic in origin. Extra-intestinal features, such as erythema nodosum, pyoderma gangrenosum, arthritis, or iritis, favor a diagnosis of IBD.

Before specific therapy is instituted, stool samples should be obtained for culture and microscopic analysis, including a *C. difficile* toxin assay and, if indicated, examination for ova and parasites. The rectal and sigmoid mucosa should be examined by sigmoidoscopy with mucosal biopsies. The mucosal abnormalities seen on sigmoidoscopy (or colonoscopy, if indicated) usually are nonspecific and consist of erythema, edema, focal hemorrhage, loss of normal vascular pattern, granularity, ulceration, and friability. However, infarction or gangrene are specific for ischemic colitis, and pseudomembranes are characteristic of *C. difficile* infection. Biopsies should be obtained from both diseased and normal-appearing mucosa.

It may be safe to institute corticosteroid therapy when an infectious etiology has been ruled out and IBD is suspected. However, histologic confirmation is generally necessary to distinguish ischemic colitis from IBD. Surgical intervention may be indicated for cases refractory to medical therapy and for complications of severe colitis, including perforation and obstruction.

Supplemental Reading

Akerkar GA, Peppercorn MA. Inflammatory bowel disease in the elderly. Practical treatment guidelines. Drugs Aging 1997;10:199–208.

Bennett RG, Greenough, WB III. Diarrhea in the elderly, in *Principles of Geriatric Medicine and Gerontology*. Huzzard, WR, et al., eds. McGraw-Hill, New York 1999:1507–1517.

Greenwald DA, Brandt LJ. Colonic ischemia. J Clin Gastroenterol 1998;27:122–8.

Grimm IS, Friedman LS. Inflammatory bowel disease in the elderly. Gastroenterol Clin North Am 1990;19:361–89.

Peppercorn MA. Drug-responsive chronic segmental colitis associated with diverticula: a clinical syndrome in the elderly. Am J Gastroenterol 1992;87:609–12.

Polito JM II, Childs B, Mellits ED, et al. Crohn's disease: influence of age at diagnosis on site and clinical type of disease. Gastroenterology 1996;111:580–6.

Slutsker L, Ries AA, Greene KD, et al. *Escherichia coli* O157:H7 diarrhea in the United States: clinical and epidemiologic features. Ann Intern Med 1997;126:505–13.

CHAPTER 131

Nonsteroidal Anti-inflammatory Drugs, Enterocolonic Ulceration, and Inflammatory Bowel Disease

Simon Smale, BMBS, MRCP, and Ingvar Bjarnason, MD, MSc, FRCPath, DSc

Nonsteroidal anti-inflammatory drugs (NSAIDs) cause damage throughout the gastrointestinal tract. Whereas there is much awareness of the fact that these drugs cause gastric and duodenal ulcers, with potential for catastrophic bleeding and perforation, it is becoming increasingly recognized that NSAIDs cause small bowel inflammation (NSAID enteropathy), which may require treatment. Rarely, NSAIDs cause colitis, but their use is associated with an enhanced risk of appendicitis in the elderly and diverticular complications (fistulae and abscesses). The use of NSAIDs in patients with inflammatory bowel disease (IBD) is challenging because they may cause relapse of disease. This chapter outlines an approach to treatment of the damage of NSAIDs to the small bowel and management of patients with IBD who require NSAIDs.

Nonsteroidal Anti-inflammatory Drug Enteropathy

Sixty percent of patients on long-term conventional NSAIDs develop NSAID enteropathy. The diagnosis is based on the clinical history and measurement of inflammatory markers in feces ([111]indium-labelled white cells, fecal calprotectin or lactoferrin concentrations) or by direct visualization (erosions and ulcers) at enteroscopy. Most patients are asymptomatic from the enteropathy because the inflammation is low grade. However, patients bleed from the site of inflammation in the small bowel, and this contributes (along with many other factors) to iron deficiency anemia. There also is protein loss that may lead to hypoalbuminemia, and somewhat less frequently the inflammation progresses toward stricturing (diaphragm strictures).

Only a selected subgroup of patients taking NSAIDs with the most severe complications are likely to find their way to a gastroenterology specialist. These fall into three broad clinical categories where the main problem is iron deficiency, hypoalbuminemia, or strictures. Irrespective of the particular clinical category, the first-line management for these problems is similar. The initial aim is to

discontinue the NSAID that the patient is taking or change over to a non-NSAID analgesic (paracetamol, acetaminophen) and to encourage the rheumatologist who is treating the patient to consider introducing or increasing a second-line agent that might reduce NSAID requirement, as well as physiotherapy. Although these measures are commendable, they are not particularly practical, because these patients often have severe arthritis that demands adequate anti-inflammatory and pain relief. The patient who cannot do without NSAID therapy usually can be switched from a conventional acidic-NSAID to the nonacidic pro-NSAID nabumetone (Relafen®, SmithKline Beecham, Philadelphia, Pennsylvania) (1 g twice a day) or given a large dose of aspirin with a proton pump inhibitor for maximal gastric protection. The rationale for these measures is that nabumetone, being a nonacidic pro-NSAID, does not cause small bowel problems in man, presumably because it has no "topical" effect (detergent action, NSAID-phospholipid interaction, or uncoupling of mitochondrial oxidative phosphorylation) during drug absorption, and its active metabolite is not excreted in bile. Similarly, aspirin mostly is absorbed before it reaches the small bowel, and it is not excreted in bile; therefore, it does not affect the small intestine in man, given at normal doses.

With the recent introduction and availability of preferential (selective, highly selective) cyclo-oxygenase-2 (COX-2) inhibitors, the choice of NSAID for these patients certainly is changing. Some of the COX-2 preferential agents (nimesulide; Celebrex®, Searle and Pfizer Inc., Skokie, Illinois; Vioxx®, Merck Research Laboratories, Whitehouse Station, New Jersey) not only are nonacidic (and therefore do not have the damaging topical action), but they only decrease gastric and intestinal mucosal prostaglandins by 10 to 30 percent, at most, at full therapeutic doses (COX-1 dependent function). They do not affect platelet function (COX-1 dependent) and are remarkably safe in experimental animals. Available data suggest that the same holds true for man with regard to both the gastroduodenal mucosa and the small bowel. Therefore, a case can be made for initiating treatment in a rheumatoid patient, at the time of diagnosis, with these COX-2 preferential agents, because of their substantially improved gastrointestinal tolerability. A patient who is experiencing difficulties while on NSAID therapy should be switched to one of the new agents. It remains to be seen whether NSAID enteropathy, once established (which may be COX-2 driven, as is the case with many other inflammatory conditions), is perpetuated by these drugs; available data suggest that they do not by themselves cause small bowel damage.

Iron Deficiency Anemia

Iron deficiency anemia (hemoglobin less than 10 g/dL) is a common problem in the patient on NSAIDS with rheumatoid arthritis or osteoarthritis. Initially, a malignancy needs to be ruled out. Following endoscopy and colonoscopy, neither of which usually show pathology sufficiently severe to explain the iron deficiency, the question of NSAID enteropathy with bleeding is raised, and possible management is considered. In addition to the general measures, changing to a non-NSAID analgesic, a less toxic NSAID regime, or addition of a second-line agent, the preference of the authors in these cases is simply to document the severity of the inflammation using fecal calprotectin, without further investigation. Fecal occult blood testing is unhelpful, and chromium 51 tagging of red blood cells is too time consuming to undertake for routine purposes in such patients. Iron deficiency is corrected by oral or parenteral iron (preferably not parenteral in patients with rheumatoid arthritis as intravenous iron may cause a flare-up of their joint disease) or, in selected cases, by blood transfusion. If the inflammation is significant (fecal calprotectin of more than 30 mg/L; normal upper limit, 11 mg/L), then treatment of the intestinal inflammation with *metronidazole* 400 mg three times a day for 2 weeks is commenced. This is followed by metronidazole 400 mg twice a day for a further 4 to 24 weeks. The length of treatment depends to some extent on fecal calprotectin responses (although it is not essential to monitor these for patient management) and to some extent on the severity and persistence of the iron deficiency anemia. A beneficial response, namely, a 50 percent reduction in fecal calprotectin, is usually seen within 2 weeks. If there are contraindications to metronidazole, there are other options, such as a broad-spectrum antibiotic against anaerobic bacteria (one of the cephalosporins), misoprostol 200 µg four times a day for 4 to 6 weeks, or sulfasalazine 1 g two to three times a day for 6 months or more, which have been shown to decrease inflammation and the associated blood loss in NSAID enteropathy. The threshold for giving sulfasalazine is somewhat low in patients with rheumatoid arthritis because this treatment has a disease-modifying effect on the joints and may, thereby, indirectly reduce the

need for NSAIDs. If the patient is on methotrexate, it is worth considering the use of another disease-modifying agent. Although not well studied in man, it is clear that methotrexate causes villus blunting at moderate doses in experimental animals. It is possible that similar damage occurs in man, in which case iron absorption may be decreased, which would contribute further to the anemia.

More rarely (in the authors' practice, one to two cases a year), patients are admitted with a clinically obvious, acute, and severe small bowel bleed as evidenced by a sudden drop in hemoglobin, passage of semifresh blood, or melena and normal gastroscopy and colonoscopy. Apart from immediate resuscitation measures, these patients need careful and considered investigation. A high-quality small bowel barium enema (enteroclysis) in some cases (about 50%) shows a significant abnormality (nonspecific and sometimes resembling that of IBD), if not a well-defined ulcer crater or craters. Push enteroscopy may show ulcers in the proximal jejunum, whereas a sonde enteroscopy may detect more distal ulcers. When discrete ulcers are documented in these bleeders and, for that matter, in patients in whom no morphologic change is found but in whom there is overwhelming clinical suspicion for a small bowel bleed, surgery is recommended as antibiotic treatment; when tried, it has not been successful. The small intestinal resection specimens have shown multiple (numbering 3 to 12) small bowel ulcers with a nonspecific histology. Postoperative recovery has in all cases been excellent, and the simple modification of the NSAID treatment, detailed above, has been successful, in that none of these patients has had a recurrence of bleeding. Postoperatively, these patients receive a COX-2 selective agent.

Hypoalbuminemia

About 10 percent of patients with severe rheumatoid arthritis who are admitted to hospital have hypoalbuminemia. When serum albumin drops below 20 g/L (normal, 35 to 45 g/L), most patients have peripheral edema, which is most distressing. In the past, hypoalbuminemia in patients with rheumatoid arthritis was ascribed to decreased synthesis by the liver or renal side effects of second-line agents, gold in particular. (NSAIDs are rarely associated with significant glomerular damage). Nevertheless, most patients on NSAIDs with hypoalbuminemia have no evidence of liver disease, and usually there is no significant proteinuria. Traditional symptomatic treatment with diuretics and fluid restriction often leaves these patients dehydrated and tired and is in fact without much effect on the peripheral edema.

In the past, intestinal protein loss was documented by the chromium 51-labeled albumin technique, but this no longer is practical because it prolongs the duration of hospitalization. Currently, intestinal inflammatory activity is quantitated by the fecal calprotectin method, and provided that there is significant inflammation (intestinal protein loss parallels the inflammatory activity), metronidazole is administered by the same protocol as for the patients with iron deficiency anemia related to NSAID enteropathy. This protocol, along with stopping NSAID intake, results in marked improvement in the hypoalbuminemia (approaching 30 g/L) within 2 to 3 weeks of treatment, and resolution of associated symptoms occurs at the same time.

There are no particular risk factors for this complication of NSAID enteropathy, and most patients subsequently do well on aspirin or nabumetone (Relafen), without recurrence of hypoalbuminemia. Preferential COX-2 inhibitors can be prescribed following healing of the intestinal inflammation. Most patients on NSAIDs with hypoalbuminemia have had rheumatoid arthritis. The osteoarthritic patients on NSAIDs with hypoalbuminemia have had coexisting anemia and often have a history of diarrhea. In general, this symptom complex is more suggestive of NSAID-induced small intestinal strictures.

Strictures

Patients on conventional NSAIDs get characteristic if not pathognomic small bowel strictures termed diaphragm disease. These usually are multiple, thin, and remarkably concentric septate-like projections that may narrow the lumen to a millimeter or less. The strictures usually are located in the mid-small intestine, although cecal strictures have been described in patients on sustained-release NSAIDs. These occur equally in rheumatoid and osteoarthritic patients.

The symptoms of strictures are twofold. First, patients present with systemic symptoms, such as weight loss, some diarrhea (may be severe), anemia, and hypoalbuminemia. When investigated, they often have severe intestinal inflammation, and diaphragm strictures can be documented on enteroscopy. Second, patients present with intermittent, subacute small intestinal obstructive symptoms. Inflammatory activity is only moderate as assessed by fecal markers, and it is suspected that this represents a fibrotic end-stage of the inflammatory lesion. In either case, the diaphragms can be difficult to document. Radiology may suggest changes resembling classic Crohn's disease, but more often, the films are reported as normal, the problem being that the diaphragms are only 2 to 4 mm thick and do not distort the bowel wall appreciably. Enteroscopy provides the best chance of obtaining a preoperative diagnosis. Nevertheless, many of the patients have been referred for surgery simply on the basis of symptoms (in the pre-enteroscopy era). Stricureplasty is a better option than straightforward resection, because the strictures may occur throughout the small intestine. Postoperatively, conventional NSAID

treatment should be avoided. Where this has not been possible, most patients have done well without recurrence of symptoms. Nevertheless, two patients who were lost to follow-up after surgery resumed their normal NSAID intake only to be re-admitted 10 years later with similar symptoms and strictures requiring re-operation.

Nonsteroidal Anti-inflammatory Drug-Induced Colonic Damage

Rarely, NSAIDs affect the "normal" colonic mucosa. There are fewer than 30 case reports of NSAID-induced colitis, and most of these were attributable to mefenamic acid (Ponstel®, Parke-Davis), which is notorious for causing diarrhea. These cases usually have occurred in the setting of longstanding ingestion of fenamates, which was otherwise not associated with any apparent problems. Diarrhea then became a problem, but because the patients did not associate the diarrhea with the drug, they continued with the treatment only to develop urgency and frank bloody diarrhea. Results of rectal biopsies in these cases often have been assessed as ulcerative colitis, although the term nonspecific colitis is more characteristic. Symptoms resolve within days of cessation of the fenamates, and the patients tolerate other NSAIDs well. This suggests that factors other than simple inhibition of prostaglandin production may be the mechanism. The suggestion that NSAIDs are a significant risk factor for the development of collagenous colitis appears no longer to be tenable. Rectally administered NSAIDs are notorious for causing rectal urgency and bleeding. The pathology has not been studied in detail, but most patients make an uneventful recovery when they stop the treatment or when the route of administration is altered. Rectal strictures requiring surgical resection after NSAID rectal suppositories and indeed after non-NSAID drugs, such as paracetamol (acetaminophen), containing suppositories, have been described.

Nonsteroidal Anti-inflammatory Drugs in Inflammatory Bowel Disease

There is no firm evidence that NSAIDs cause classic IBD, nor is there support for the suggestion that NSAIDs are a significant risk factor for the development of IBD. Nevertheless, these issues are controversial, because in some gastroenterology centers it has been suggested that as many as 20 to 50 percent of patients with newly diagnosed proctitis or colitis may be on NSAIDs. Simple withdrawal of the NSAID may or may not relieve symptoms in these patients. It is better established that NSAID treatment in patients with IBD can cause a relapse of disease, and those who work closely with rheumatologists will encounter patients that have IBD and rheumatoid arthritis requiring NSAID treatment. These patients often have a symptomatic chronically active form of IBD that is difficult to control by conventional treatment, and, indeed, many of these patients become corticosteroid-dependent or are subjected to colectomy if they have ulcerative colitis. Ingestion of NSAIDs in patients with IBD certainly is a practical problem, but how frequently are IBD patients taking NSAIDs?

Many IBD patients may require NSAIDs because of arthritis or fractures secondary to osteoporosis. See the chapters on arthritis and on osteoporosis. Before detailing their management, there is an interesting side issue. It is now widely acknowledged that about 60 percent of patients with classic human leukocyte antigen (HLA)-B27-positive ankylosing spondylitis have histologic ileitis. It has been suggested that the ileitis may represent subclinical Crohn's disease, but this is a highly controversial issue. Radiology of the terminal ileum invariably is normal; if not, then the diagnosis is Crohn's disease associated with ankylosing spondylitis. These patients do not usually have gastrointestinal symptoms, even when taking NSAIDs (other than dyspepsia), and the presence and type of ileal inflammation seen on biopsies obtained during ileocolonoscopy seem to give prognostic information about the course of the spondylitis. Five to eight percent of these patients, almost all of whom require NSAIDs, go on to develop classic IBD, as demonstrated by abnormal radiology of ileum or histologic abnormalities on colonic biopsies. Although the ileitis of classic ankylosing spondylitis differs fundamentally from the inflammation of NSAID enteropathy, it is possible that NSAIDs have some deleterious effect on this inflammation, but, as yet, no study has addressed this issue satisfactorily.

In the case of a patient with IBD and severe peripheral pauciarticular arthritis, it is clear that the arthritic activity parallels the intestinal inflammatory activity. It is relatively easy to treat the intestinal disease aggressively (with corticosteroids, elemental diets, etc.) and, thereby, bring the joint inflammation and pain under control. In a matter of 1 or 2 weeks, symptoms of intestinal disease and the arthritis resolve. Non-NSAID analgesics can be prescribed to control joint pain. Even if the analgesic effect is suboptimal, patients often are reassured that adequate pain relief will occur within a short time. However, this strategy is not successful in the other two types of arthropathy (peripheral nonsymmetric polyarthritis and spondylitis) or in patients with IBD with rheumatoid arthritis because the course of the arthritis is independent of the activity of the intestinal disease. In the case of spondylitis or ankylosing spondylitis-associated back pain in patients with IBD, it is important to have close collaboration with the rheumatologists. Many patients can altogether avoid NSAIDs provided that an integrated and aggressive combination treatment regimen can be implemented involving exercise, physio- and hydrotherapy, and sulfasalazine (2 to 3 g/d). It is important for these patients

to be on sulfasalazine rather than 5-aminosalicylic acid preparations. The reason for this is that while both drugs reduce or modify the intestinal inflammation, the sulfapyridine moiety of sulfasalazine has a disease-modifying effect on the spondylitis and perhaps more so on the peripheral arthropathy itself, thereby somewhat decreasing the need for pain control or anti-inflammatory action.

There remains a small group of patients with spondylitis who still require NSAIDs and also the somewhat larger group of patients with rheumatoid arthritis and IBD. The therapeutic options here are limited indeed. The COX-2 preferential agents have minimal, if any, advantage over conventional NSAIDs in these patients, because the mechanism of relapse almost certainly relates to the COX-2 action of both classes of drugs rather than the topical action. Other new preparations, such as esterified NSAIDs with a nitric oxide-releasing moiety, theoretically will be equally problematic in these patients, but this is an educated guess rather than a fact. However, one possibility is to try the R-enantiomers of flurbiprofen rather than the racemate of S-flurbiprofen (Ansaid®, Pharmacia and Upjohn, Peapack, New Jersey). The rationale here is that the R-enantioner, which is not significantly converted over to the S-enantiomer in man, has no significant effect on the COX enzymes, but is still purported to have a powerful analgesic action. This form of treatment remains speculative and untested in man.

The management of these patients is difficult and indeed unsatisfactory. The use of gold, especially oral gold, in patients with rheumatoid arthritis and IBD is discouraged as this drug has major gastrointestinal side effects as well as being a recognized cause of colitis. Sulfasalazine (1 g three times a day) may be beneficial for both the arthritis and the IBD. Similarly, if methotrexate has not been tried as a disease-modifying agent in patients with rheumatoid arthritis and Crohn's disease, weekly muscular injections should be considered. The relatively rapid onset of action will minimize the need for NSAIDs. Those who still require NSAIDs can be given a conventional NSAID of their choice. The reason for not placing these patients on a well-tolerated NSAID is that all NSAIDs are equally damaging to patients with IBD, and they can receive the one that is most efficacious for the arthritic symptoms. The only exception to this practice is that delayed- or sustained-release formulations of NSAIDs should not be prescribed for patients with colonic disease, and there is a slight preference to give patients with small bowel Crohn's disease nabumetone (Relafen) (2 g/d), because it does not have topical action. Since the NSAIDs often lead to deterioration of the gastrointestinal symptoms, these patients may require additional and aggressive treatment for symptomatic IBD. Most patients are placed on azathioprine (Imuran®, Glaxo Wellcome Inc., Research Triangle Park, North Carolina) (2 mg/kg initially) although the benefits are not seen for a few months. Corticosteroids are effective to counteract NSAID-induced aggravation of IBD, but most patients with severe joint disease become steroid dependent (requiring 10 to 20 mg prednisolone/d) in the long term. When the long-term steroid treatment complications start setting in, consideration of the difficult choice between continuing this treatment and performing a colectomy in patients with ulcerative colitis is necessary.

At present, there is no perfect answer for the small number of patients who require NSAIDs and have significant IBD activity despite all of these measures. A sympathetic ear is sometimes the only thing offered. It is astonishing how brave, uncomplaining, and resolute many of these rheumatoid or spondylitic patients are, despite IBD activity scores that would otherwise demand hospitalization.

Patients with a few isolated aphthous ulcers are sometimes mistakenly labeled as having Crohn's disease. Some have taken NSAIDs.*

Supplemental Reading

Bjarnason I, Hayllar J, Macpherson AJ, Russell AS. Side effects of nonsteroidal anti-inflammatory drugs on the small and large intestine. Gastroenterology 1993;104:1832–47.

Bjarnason I, Hayllar J, Smethurst P, et al. Metronidazole reduces inflammation and blood loss in NSAID enteropathy. Gut 1992;33:1204–8.

Hayllar J, Price AB, Smith T, et al. Nonsteroidal anti-inflammatory drug-induced small intestinal inflammation and blood loss. Effects of sulfasalazine and other disease-modifying antirheumatic drugs. Arthritis Rheum 1994;37:1146–50.

Sigthorsson G, Tibble J, Hayllar J, et al. Intestinal permeability and inflammation in patients on NSAIDs. Gut 1998;43:506–11.

Tibble J, Sigthorsson G, Foster R, et al. NSAID enteropathy: a new simple diagnostic test. Gut 1999;45:362–6.

Wallace JL. Nonsteroidal anti-inflammatory drugs and gastroenteropathy: the second hundred years. Gastroenterology 1997;112:1000–16.

---

* Editor's Note: There are anecdotal reports of patients with irritable bowel syndrome (IBS) who are taking a modest number of NSAIDs daily and whose condition is erroneously labeled as Crohn's disease because of a few scattered aphthous ulcers in the ileum. In retrospect, some may have taken oral phosphate soda preparations prior to colonoscopy. These oral preparations are known to be associated with colonic aphthous ulcers. In others, NSAIDs may be responsible for the ulceration. Most patients are given oral 5-ASA preparations. Follow-up colonoscopies are negative and the diagnosis is "nonspecific inflammation." (TMB)

CHAPTER 132

Collagenous and Lymphocytic Colitis

Marcia Cruz-Correa, MD, and Francis M. Giardiello, MD

Microscopic colitis is a term encompassing collagenous and lymphocytic colitis. It denotes the absence of endoscopic (macroscopic) abnormalities in the presence of microscopic histopathology.

Collagenous and lymphocytic colitis are clinicopathologic syndromes that represent distinct, possibly autoimmune, forms of idiopathic inflammatory colonic bowel disease. Both disorders present as chronic, watery, noninfectious diarrhea in middle-aged patients with negative radiographic and endoscopic studies. Collagenous colitis predominantly occurs in women; lymphocytic colitis is found equally in both genders. Often there is intermittent, crampy, diffuse abdominal pain, and, not surprisingly, some patients have a previous diagnosis of the irritable bowel syndrome (IBS). Routine blood studies generally show normal results, but abnormalities in Westergren sedimentation rate and eosinophil count are not uncommon. Abnormalities in complement levels, serum immunoglobulins, and perinuclear antineutrophil cytoplasmic antibodies (pANCA) may be found. Although stool studies are negative for pathogens and blood, **up to 55 percent of patients have white blood cells in stool samples.** Some patients also have thyroid disease, inflammatory arthropathies, pernicious anemia, urethral fibrosis, vitiligo, and small bowel villus atrophy.

Colorectal Biopsy

Although macroscopically, the colonic mucosa may appear normal, the diagnosis of these disorders is based on microscopic examination of colorectal biopsies. Diffuse colitis is present with lymphocytic infiltration of the surface epithelium and lamina propria. Also, surface epithelial damage is found, with stratification and occasional detachment of the surface epithelium. The distinctive histopathologic finding in collagenous colitis is a characteristic band of collagen beneath the surface epithelium in colonic mucosa. The banding is most consistently noted in the right and transverse colon. Rectal biopsies may show little or no collagen banding, in contrast to samples taken in the more proximal colon.

In lymphocytic colitis, the histopathology is similar to that in collagenous colitis, except that collagenous thickening does not occur. Because of the clinical and histopathologic similarity in these disorders, currently, they are considered to be a single category of inflammatory bowel diseases (IBD), "collagenous-lymphocytic colitis," for purposes of treatment. A "Cracking" of the colonic mucosa has been seen during colonoscopy in a few patients.

Diarrheal Mechanism

The pathogenesis of chronic diarrhea in collagenous-lymphocytic colitis is multifactorial. Primarily, diarrhea appears to result from net colonic fluid secretion. This occurs from decreased luminal absorption secondary to damaged surface epithelium and collagen deposition, combined with a continued normal rate of secretion from intact crypts. In some patients, small bowel dysfunction has been noted, including bile salt wasting, fatty acid malabsorption, small-bowel net secretion, and, rarely, villous atrophy. These additional abnormalities may exacerbate the diarrhea. Underlying IBS and thyroid disease must also be considered as possible elements in the diarrheal diathesis.

Management Concepts

Limited experience exists in the treatment of collagenous-lymphocytic colitis. There are single case reports and several small series, but no randomized controlled studies from which to draw firm conclusions. The concepts one can use to guide therapy can be extracted from the literature and the personal experience of others. Table 132–1 outlines the management approach used by the authors.

Symptomatic Therapy

In patients with symptomatic collagenous-lymphocytic colitis, several factors should be considered. Since colonic absorption is decreased in all patients and small bowel secretion has been noted in some patients, dietary secretagogues, such as caffeine- or lactose-containing foods, should be eliminated from the diet. Because of possible association between collagenous colitis and nonsteroidal anti-inflammatory drugs (NSAIDs), these agents should be discontinued. If steatorrhea is documented, a low-fat diet may be helpful. In the presence of bile salt malabsorption, binding resins, such as cholestyramine, have been useful. Some patients are helped by bulking agents

TABLE 132–1. Management Approach

Eliminate secretagogues (lactose, caffeine, fat) and stop NSAIDs. Rule out thyroid dysfunction. Use antimotility agents and binding agents (psyllium or cholesypane).

Trial of bismuth subsalicylate (262 mg, 3 tablets in am, 2 tablets at noon, 3 tablets in pm, each day for 8 weeks)

If no resolution,

Add 5-ASA drugs with or without antimotility agents for 1 to 2 months (Asacol, 1,200 to 1,600 mg three times/d or Azulfidine, 1 g four times/d)

If no resolution,

Add adrenal corticoid (prednisone, 20 to 40 mg/d; budesonide 3 mg three times/d or 9 mg in am)

If no resolution,

Rule out small bowel disease, steatorrhea

If no resolution,

Immunosuppressive therapy (methotrexate or azathioprine)

If no resolution,

Surgery (diverting ileostomy or colectomy)

and by antidiarrheal medications, such as loperamide hydrochloride (Imodium®, McNeil, Fort Washington, Pennsylvania), diphenoxylate hydrochloride, and atropine (Lomotil®, Searle, Chicago, Illinois), deodorized tincture of opium, or codeine.

Antibacterial Agents

Patients with collagenous colitis have been treated with antibacterial agents with positive results. Fine and Lee reported an open-label trial of bismuth subsalicylate (Pepto Bismol [Procter & Gamble Pharmaceuticals, Phoenix, Arizona], eight chewable 262-mg tablets/d for 8 wks) in 12 patients with collagenous or lymphocytic colitis. Eleven patients had resolution of diarrhea and histopathologic changes without recurrence 7 to 28 months after treatment. No side effects were reported. However, there are two case reports of bismuth nitrate (used for treatment of gastritis) causing dementia, both of which resolved after discontinuation of the drug. Response rates of 60 percent have been seen with metronidazole (250 mg three or four times a day) and with erythromycin.

Sulfasalazine and Other 5-Aminosalicylates

Sulfasalazine has been used as the initial anti-inflammatory agent at a dose of 2 to 4 g/d in divided doses with meals and at bedtime. The full dosage should be achieved slowly, starting with one tablet (0.5 g) daily and adding one tablet per day until the desired dosage is achieved. This may help avoid nausea and, perhaps, headaches. Abatement of diarrhea in 1 to 2 weeks with sulfasalazine as a single agent has been noted in 50 percent of patients. The maintenance therapy dosage usually is the same as that used to achieve remission.

In persons who are unresponsive or have a history of sulfa allergy or sulfasalazine intolerance, large doses of other 5-aminosalicylic acid (5-ASA) compounds may be used. The higher doses of Asacol® (Procter & Gamble Pharmaceuticals, Cincinnati, Ohio) are 1,200 to 1,600 mg three times a day, and Pentasa® (Ferring-Shire Pharmaceuticals Inc., Florence, Kentucky) 1,000 mg twice to four times a day. Patients who respond usually improve within 2 to 3 weeks. The maintenance dose usually is similar to that required to achieve remission. Since collagenous-lymphocytic colitis usually involves the proximal colon, 5-ASA enemas and suppositories can only be considered adjunctive to oral therapy.

As a guide to therapy, repeat colonic biopsies usually are taken after 2 to 3 months of treatment to assess resolution of collagen banding and the inflammatory infiltrate in the surface epithelium and lamina propria. If clinical and histologic benefit is evident, 6 to 12 months of empirical treatment has been given in an attempt to maximize histologic improvement. Subsequently, it may be possible to taper the sulfasalazine or 5-ASA with continued attention to dietary factors and the use of antidiarrheal agents in some but not all patients. Diarrhea may recur after the cessation of sulfasalazine or 5-ASA.

Adrenocorticoids

If no clinical improvement is noted after 2 to 4 weeks of bismuth subsalicylate or 5-ASA therapy, adrenocorticoid medication, usually prednisone, is added. Dramatic resolution of diarrhea has been noted within 5 days of the start of treatment in 80 to 90 percent of individuals. Histologic improvement has been seen in some patients. Disappearance of the collagen banding and repair of the surface epithelial damage also has been documented in some patients with collagenous colitis.

Most individuals have been treated as outpatients with prednisone in a morning dosage of 20 to 40 mg. Occasionally, a patient with more than 2 L of stool a day has been hospitalized and treated with intravenous prednisolone (60 mg/d) or hydrocortisone. Once control of diarrhea has been achieved, patients have been maintained on 20 to 30 mg of prednisone for 2 to 3 months, and repeat colonic biopsies have been obtained. After 2 to 3 months, a change to an alternate-day dose or discontinuation of prednisone may be attempted. However, diarrhea recurs in most patients. In these cases, small doses (10 to 15 mg) of prednisone daily or alternate-day steroids have been administered with success. The antibacterial and other anti-inflammatory products are continued to minimize prednisone dosage and the adverse side effects.

Recently, budesonide, a topical corticoid released in the small intestine and in the ascending colon has been incorporated in the treatment of collagenous colitis, which can be most obvious in the right colon. Budesonide has a topical effect and a low bioability of about 10 percent. This drug is therapeutically similar to prednisone, but with many less side effects. In an open-label pilot trial, budesonide (3 mg tid) was given to seven patients with collagenous colitis. Clinical improvement was achieved within 10 days of initiation of budesonide in all patients and maintained after dose reduction. In three patients, no diarrhea recurred within 7, 12, or 15 months after treatment when budesonide was terminated. In these patients, colonic biopsies showed marked histologic improvement. Further studies and long-term follow-up are warranted. The chapter on topically active steroids in patients with IBD provides further details about the use of budesonide in right-sided colitis.

The therapeutic approach described has produced symptomatic improvement in most patients and histologic improvement in some. However, in only a few patients has there been total histologic reversal, even in those who are asymptomatic for many months. Therefore, questions still remain as to the duration of therapy and the usefulness of histologic appearances as a guide to treatment.*

Other Agents

Several case reports have suggested improvement with octreotide therapy. Also, methotrexate has been used with dramatic reduction of symptoms in a patient refractory to antidiarrheal, 5-ASA, and corticosteroid agents. Case reports documenting improvement of collagenous colitis have been noted with azathioprine, chlorpheniramine (histamine, antagonist), quinacrine, mepacrine, ketotifen (mast cell stabilizer), and with small bowel diversion via an ileostomy.

Surgery

Colectomy, performed in a few patients, has eliminated diarrheal symptoms and, in one case, extra-intestinal manifestations of collagenous colitis. Diverting ileostomy has led to a presumably temporary regression of the clinicopathologic findings in eight women with collagenous colitis unresponsive to medical therapy (sulfasalazine, mepacrine, corticosteroids, mesalamines, Flagyl® [Searle, Skokie, Illinois]). A sigmoidostomy was performed in one patient. Postoperative diarrhea ceased in all patients, with histologic resolution of the collagen layer. The ileostomy was reversed in three patients after a diversion period of 4 to 15 months, and clinical symptoms and the abnormal collagen layer recurred in all three individuals.

---

* Editor's Note: In my experience with perhaps 20 patients, those who require anti-inflammatory drug therapy usually have to stay on higher doses of mesalamine, bismuth, and perhaps budesonide plus the various symptomatic antidiarrheal measures outlined in this chapter. Because of the prominent role of the lymphocytic infiltration, one assumes an alteration of the immune–inflammatory cascade is involved and, as stated, may be the future focus of therapy in unresponsive patients. (TMB)

Other Considerations

Villous atrophy of the small bowel has been documented in some patients with lymphocytic or collagenous colitis. This probably represents another disease entity rather than concomitant celiac disease. Several patients with collagenous colitis have been given gluten-free diets without improvement. In any event, attention to the role of the small bowel as a source of fluid seems appropriate in an unresponsive patient with collagenous-lymphocytic colitis. A few patients have responded to oral beclomethasone, a topically active steroid with rapid hepatic metabolism. Collagenous-lymphocytic colitis should be considered in a patient with refractory celiac disease and diarrhea. Because thyroid disease has been noted in association with this syndrome, hypo- or hyperthyroidism should be corrected.

Long-Term Outlook

Long-term experience is limited, but retrospective examination of patients with collagenous-lymphocytic colitis reveals a benign and chronic course. Although the authors have noted one patient with granulomatous colitis (Crohn's disease), there appears to be no association with Crohn's disease or ulcerative colitis.

There are a few reports of rectal or colonic cancer in elderly patients with coexistent collagenous colitis, but these must be considered coincidental. In a recent study by Chan and colleagues, 117 cases diagnosed as collagenous colitis were reviewed. No cases of colorectal cancer were found during a mean follow-up period of 7.0 years after the diagnosis of colitis, and the relative risk of colon cancer in collagenous colitis patients was similar to the general population.

We have been serving as an unofficial registry for patients with collagenous-lymphocytic colitis in the hope that uniform collection of histologic and clinical records will speed the accumulation of meaningful data. If additional research provides further clues to the nature of collagenous-lymphocytic colitis, such as an autoimmune etiology, therapeutic guidelines may become clearer.

References

Fine KD, Lee EL. Efficacy of open-label bismuth subsalicylate for treatment of microscopic colitis. Gastroenterology 1998;114:29–36.

Chan JL, Tersinette AC, Offerhaus GJA, et al. Cancer risk in collagenous colitis. Inflamm Bowel Dis 1999;5:40–3.

Supplemental Reading

Bohr J, Tysk C, Eriksson S, et al. Collagenous colitis: a retrospective study of clinical presentation and treatment in 163 patients. Gut 1996;39:846–51.

Fernandez-Bañares F, Salas A, Forne M, et al. Incidence of collagenous colitis: a 5-year population-based study. Am J Gastroenterol 1999;94:418–23.

CHAPTER 133

RADIATION ENTEROCOLITIS

CHOON JIN OOI, MD, CHRISTOPHER G. WILLETT, MD, AND DANIEL K. PODOLSKY, MD

Management of radiation injury to the small and large intestine continues to present challenges to gastroenterologists, radiation oncologists, and surgeons alike. With many oncology protocols now employing radiation therapy either as adjuvant or curative therapy, the collateral effects of radiation on rapidly proliferating tissues are increasingly important issues. The normal intestinal mucosa and, to a lesser extent, intestinal vascular and interstitial connective tissue compartments are sensitive to ionizing radiation. Consequently, this may be especially problematic in tissues already affected by inflammatory bowel disease (IBD), because of the varying amount of coincident injury and inflammation as well as the hyperproliferative state of the epithelium. In addition, whole-body irradiation is part of the preparative phase of allogeneic bone marrow or stem cell transplantation, which has been used in a few patients with Crohn's disease and leukemia. The effects of that type of radiation are discussed in the chapter on stem cell transplantation.

Intestinal Intolerance

Intestinal intolerance frequently is the major limiting factor in the radiation treatment of tumors in both the abdomen and pelvis. Currently, it is well known that small and large intestinal complications are dependent on radiation therapy techniques and better use of the modality should enable further reductions in adverse events. In general, acute complications are correlated with the amount of irradiated bowel and the fraction size. The risk of long-term complications is correlated with the severity of acute events, although the absence of an acute event per se does not preclude the development of chronic radiation syndrome. In addition, chronic events also are dependent on the total surface area of bowel irradiated, fraction size, and the total amount of radiation. Prior abdominal surgeries, cholecystectomy, pelvic inflammatory disease, hypertension, and diabetes mellitus have been documented as risk factors increasing the likelihood of the development of chronic events.

Risk with Coexistent Inflammatory Bowel Disease

Although it often has been said that patients with IBD (Crohn's disease and ulcerative colitis) may have an increased frequency of intestinal complications of radiotherapy, there is a paucity of primary data from which conclusions can be drawn. Prior studies have been limited to case reports describing the outcome of one to five patients subjected to external-beam radiation therapy. These reports have documented toxicities from radiation in a small number of patients and, on that basis, have advised avoidance of this modality, when possible. However, none of these studies provides reliable assessment of incidence or prevalence in either absolute or relative terms for patients with IBD compared to those without IBD.

A confounding factor limiting the ability to draw firm conclusions is the heterogeneous nature of IBD patients, both with respect to underlying disease and the radiation treatment protocols used. Thus, available data do not permit any assessment of differential sensitivity between patients with Crohn's disease compared with those with ulcerative colitis. Nonetheless, a recent study of 28 patients cared for at the Massachusetts General Hospital lends further credibility to the assumption that a significant number of patients with IBD suffer from increased morbidity as a result of conventional radiotherapy. On the other hand, proper treatment planning to titrate the dose, limit the radiation field by individualized custom-blocking techniques, and avoid intestinal irradiation, appears to decrease adverse events (Table 133–1).

Pathogenesis of Radiation Enterocolitis

The pathogenesis of radiation enterocolitis remains to be fully elucidated. Energy dissipated from ionizing radiation therapy can release toxic radicals, including reactive oxidative metabolites, which can destroy cell integrity and inhibit proliferative renewal. Histopathology reveals transient loss of mucosal cells and infiltration of the lamina propria with neutrophils and plasma cells. In the small intestine, mucosal atrophy can result in malabsorption of various substances, including fat, carbohydrate, protein, bile salts, lactose, and vitamin B_{12}. In the large intestine, watery diarrhea results from poor fluid absorption. However, histologic changes correlate poorly with symptoms and functional changes.

Pathologic specimens of intestinal tissue affected by chronic radiation injuries show obliterative endarteritis

TABLE 133–1. Severe Toxicity by Type of Inflammatory Bowel Disease and Treatment Parameters

	Number of Patients	Severe Acute Toxicity	Severe Late Toxicity	Total Severe Toxicity
Total patients	n = 28	n = 6 (22%)	n = 8 (29%)	n = 13 (46%)*
IBD type				
Crohn's disease	10	3 (30)	1 (10)	4 (40)
Ulcerative colitis	18	3 (17)	7 (39)	9 (50)*
		p = NS	p = NS	p = NS
Prior IBD surgery				
Yes	19	4 (21)	4 (21)	8 (42)
No	9	2 (22)	4 (44)	5 (56)*
		p = NS	p = NS	p = NS
IBD status at EBRT				
Quiescent	16	3 (19)	6 (38)	9 (56)
Active	12	3 (26)	2 (17)	4 (33)*
		p = NS	p = NS	p = NS
EBRT technique				
Specialized	16	4 (25)	2 (13)	6 (38)
Conventional	12	2 (17)	6 (50)	7 (58)*
		p = NS	p = .02	p = NS

* One patient developed both severe acute and late toxicity. EBRT = external-beam radiation therapy; NS = not significant. Adapted from Willet CG et al.

in the small vessels of the intestinal wall, submucosal fibrosis, and lymphatic dilatation. It is thought that these initial subclinical events may eventually lead to progressive ischemia of the intestinal wall, which subsequently results in necrosis, ulcerations, bleeding, perforation, fistula, or stricture formation.

Prevalence

Acute Complications

Nearly all patients subjected to abdominal or pelvic irradiation experience transient acute bowel symptoms. Diarrhea occurs in almost all patients. The symptoms appear to be a function of the dose rate and fraction size rather than the total dose. Up to 20 percent of patients may suffer from acute symptoms severe enough to warrant discontinuation of the treatment modality. In 28 patients with IBD (10 with Crohn's disease and 18 with ulcerative colitis), 22 percent experienced severe acute toxicities requiring discontinuation of planned therapy. Although the rate of severe acute toxicities was higher in patients with Crohn's disease (30%) compared to those with ulcerative colitis (17%), this did not reach statistical significance. Furthermore, the activity status of IBD at the time of radiation therapy did not affect or predict severe acute complications. In addition, the rates of severe acute toxicities were compared between patients treated with specialized protocols to alleviate bowel irradiation by adjusting daily dose fractions, limiting field size, and avoiding irradiation of normal gut. There was no difference in the incidence of severe acute events in patients with IBD when subjected to either specialized or conventional radiation protocols.

Chronic Complications

From data involving patients with noninflammatory bowel disease with long-term severe small bowel complications, it would appear that the frequency of such events ranges from 4 to 29 percent. The increased incidence of such events seems to correlate with a higher dose fraction, bigger total dose, and larger radiation fields. Data on patients with ulcerative colitis support these impressions. Notably, 39 percent of the patients with ulcerative colitis developed late toxicities following external-beam radiation therapy, which required laparotomy because of small or large bowel complications (eg, obstruction or fistulae). Only one patient with Crohn's disease developed severe late toxicities. This may be due to a greater number of patients with ulcerative colitis undergoing conventional radiation techniques that did not attempt to minimize the size of radiation fields or employ special surgical techniques to avoid small and large bowel irradiation. Similar to the observations with severe acute complications, IBD activity status did not correlate with or predict the development of subsequent severe chronic syndromes.

Diagnosis

Acute radiation enterocolitis usually is a clinical diagnosis. The symptoms include diarrhea, nausea, abdominal cramps, and tenesmus of varying severity. These conditions usually are transient and resolve within a few weeks of completion of radiation treatment. In the setting of IBD, it may be difficult to distinguish between a concomitant disease flare and primary radiation injury. The endoscopic findings may be similar, including inflamed, edematous, and friable mucosa. However, the two entities may sometimes be distinguished by histopathologic features, such as classic findings of focal inflammation and granulomas in Crohn's disease and architectural distortion in association with acute and chronic inflammation more frequently observed in ulcerative colitis. Thus, the assessment of an experienced gastrointestinal pathologist sometimes can help resolve this diagnostic dilemma.

The diagnosis of long-term complications may be more difficult, particularly since the latent period between radiation therapy and subsequent development of complications may range from months to years. Potential symptoms include those of obstruction, perforation, bleeding, malabsorption, diarrhea, and fistulae. In addition, symptoms can be progressive, and patients who manifest one complication have an increased risk of developing further chronic events with time.

Treatment

Acute Radiation Enterocolitis

Symptoms usually are mild and self-limited, and they largely respond to antispasmodics, anticholinergics, or opiates. Anecdotal reports also have documented successful use of cholestyramine, a bile sequestering agent, in alleviating diarrhea. In addition, buffered acetylsalicylate acid was shown to improve bowel symptoms in patients undergoing curative radiotherapy for gynecologic malignancies in a double-blind placebo controlled study by Mennie and colleagues (1975). The use of elemental diet and parenteral nutrition have been shown to be superior to normal diets in the management of acute intestinal events during radiotherapy. However, severe symptoms would mandate a discontinuation of radiation treatment.

Management may be problematic when a concomitant flare of IBD is suspected. If diagnostic biopsies are obtained, management is dependent on the predominant lesion. Usual therapies for Crohn's disease and ulcerative colitis include oral and topical mesalamine or steroids, with immunomodulators reserved as second-line drugs. It may be wise, if possible, to defer completion of the course of radiotherapy until the acute IBD activity is well controlled.[*]

Chronic Radiation Enterocolitis

The management of chronic complications is difficult and frequently unsatisfactory. Close consultation with a surgeon often is appropriate. Chronic radiation damage occurs most commonly following radiotherapy for malignant prostatic or gynecologic lesions. The rectum and rectosigmoid colon most commonly are involved, owing to their proximity to pelvic organs and their relative immobility. In such lesions, treatments include low-residue diets

---

[*] Editor's Note: If my memory is correct, radiation was once proposed as therapy for IBD. (TMB)

and steroid suppositories. Damage to large intestine often is associated with significant injuries to the distal part of the small intestine. A hysterectomy allows a loop of small intestine to enter the pelvis and thus be at risk in the radiation field. When the small bowel is involved, antispasmodics, anticholinergics, broad-spectrum antibiotics, cholestyramine, and salazopyrine have been used, but only anecdotal reports of the benefits of these agents have been available. The use of a low-fat, low-residue, lactose-free, or elemental diet has been reported to be useful in selected patients. In a randomized study comparing total parenteral nutrition (with or without methylprednisone) to enteral nutrition for severe chronic small bowel enteritis, it was found that parenteral nutrition enhanced by the use of methylprednisone was superior in eliciting improvement in nutritional, radiologic, and clinical parameters. Previous cholecystectomy seemingly increases the risk of chronic diarrhea.

In patients with fistulization or small bowel obstruction not responding to conservative medical management, treatment is surgical, with a morbidity and mortality ranging from 10 to 80 percent. Gastrointestinal bypass without extensive resection of the involved bowel has less mortality.

Novel techniques, including the use of argon lasers for mucosal telangiectatic vessels, have been used with some success. Its superficial penetration without aggravating further mucosal ischemic injury has been superior to Nd:YAG laser therapy, which potentially can cause transmural necrosis.

Prevention

In the treatment of most pelvic malignancies, the therapeutic index of radiation therapy is narrow. The majority of neoplasms in the pelvis are relatively insensitive to radiotherapy, requiring high-dose radiation. This increases the potential for injury to surrounding normal tissue. In the setting of concomitant IBD, conclusions from the authors' study suggest that these patients tend to have frequent severe acute and chronic complications from irradiation. In view of this, radiotherapy in this setting should be applied judiciously. Sites of bowel involvement in Crohn's disease or ulcerative colitis should preferably be delineated, either by imaging or endoscopy, before the initiation of radiation treatment. Inflamed areas should not be included in the treatment field, if possible. As mentioned, a previous hysterectomy places more small bowel at risk.

For patients with IBD undergoing surgery for colorectal malignancies and judged to require postoperative irradiation as part of adjuvant therapy, placement of clips to delineate the tumor or tumor bed and surgical maneuvers to mobilize small and large bowel away from the proposed radiation field are useful. These surgical efforts could include omentoplasty or the use of Dexon or Vicryl mesh. Additional strategies include limiting the radiation field, total dose reduction and scheduled breaks during therapy. In some instances, patient positioning in prone or decubitus position may be helpful.

In some colorectal cancer patients, 5-fluorouracil-based chemotherapy is added as an adjuvant to irradiation. 5-Fluorouracil itself can result in gastrointestinal adverse events, and it is thought that 5-fluorouracil could exacerbate diarrhea in patients with IBD, resulting in severe or life-threatening symptoms. Although few data exist, a study from Memorial Sloan-Kettering Cancer Center by Tiersten and Saltz (1996) did not find a statistical difference in the development of severe diarrhea between patients with active IBD and those with inactive disease when treated with 5-fluorouracil. Furthermore, the incidence of diarrhea did not seem to correlate with concurrent radiation, though more studies are required.

When caring for patients with prostatic cancers and concomitant adjacent Crohn's disease or ulcerative colitis, the use of brachytherapy or neoadjuvant hormonal therapy may permit a reduction in the total external-beam radiation dose.

References

Mennie AJ, Dalley VM, Dineen LC, et al. Treatment of radiation-induced gastrointestinal distress with acetylsalicylate. Lancet 1975;2:942–3.

Tiersten A, Saltz L. Influence of inflammatory bowel disease on the ability of patients to tolerate systemic fluorouracil-based chemotherapy. J Clin Oncol 1996;14:2043–6.

Supplemental Reading

Buchi K. Radiation proctitis: therapy and prognosis. JAMA 1991;265:1180.

Willett CG. Radiation enteritis. In: Morris P, Wood W, eds. Oxford textbook of surgery. 1st Ed. Oxford: Oxford University Press, 1994:997–8.

Willett CG, Ooi CJ, Zeitman A, et al. Acute and late toxicities of patients with inflammatory bowel disease undergoing irradiation for abdominal and pelvic neoplasms. Int J Radiat Oncol Biol Phys 2000;46:995–8.

Yeoh EK, Horowitz M. Radiation enteritis. Surg Gynecol Obstet 1987;165:373–9.

CHAPTER 134

COLITIS AND ENTERITIS IN IMMUNOCOMPROMISED INDIVIDUALS

GARY I. KLEINER, MD, PhD, AND LLOYD MAYER, MD

To maintain homeostasis, a unique gut-associated lymphoid tissue tightly regulates immune responses in the gastrointestinal (GI) tract. Not only is the gut the largest lymphoid organ in the body but also the demands upon it far exceed those of other lymphoid organs. Unlike the spleen and lymph nodes, numerous antigens constantly bombard the immunologically active cells in the loose connective tissue stroma (lamina propria). This underscores the need for some mechanism of immunologic control in the mucosa-associated lymphoid tissues (MALT). It is easy to envision how defects in the regulation of this system could result in an active inflammatory disease. Hence, it is not surprising that patients with immunodeficiency, resulting from immunoregulatory defects, can present with GI abnormalities.

Immune responses may be subdivided into either cellular or humoral responses. The failure to produce antibodies has obvious implications for host defense mechanisms. In the GI tract, the major immunoglobulins (Ig) are the secretory Igs (IgA and IgM). These antibodies impede the binding of luminal antigens to the intestinal epithelium by forming immune complexes, targeting the epithelial cell attachment site on bacteria and viruses. Antibody deficiency, particularly of secretory Igs, might disrupt the mucosal barrier function in the GI tract and facilitate the uptake and penetration of antigens. Studies have shown that there is increased macromolecule uptake from the GI tract into the circulation in the setting of immunoglobulin deficiencies. Increased concentrations of dietary antigens have been detected in the circulation of patients with hypogammaglobulinemia.

Primary Immunodeficiency

In patients with primary immunodeficiency, there may be defects in either the humoral (B-cell) or the cellular (T-cell) arm. Although there are many forms of congenital antibody deficiency, including *IgA deficiency* (the most common form with an incidence of between 1/200 and 1/700), *the hyper-IgM syndrome, Bruton's agammaglobulinemia*, and *severe combined immunodeficiency*, the most common form of this disorder associated with clinical disease is *"acquired" agammaglobulinemia*, also termed *common variable immunodeficiency (CVI)*. The term "acquired" reflects the late onset (after 3 years of

TABLE 134–1. Defects Implicated in Common Variable Immunodeficiency

Defect	Implication
B-cell defects	Maturation arrest of B cells at an immature non-antibody secreting stage Failure to secrete synthesized antibody Failure of isotype switch
T-cell defects	Excessive suppressor cell activity Ineffective T-cell help Cytokine deficiency
Monocyte defects	Defective T cell–monocyte interaction Processing defect

Alone or in combination, any of these defects can result in ineffective antibody production

age) of disease rather than knowledge of the actual insult leading to the absence of circulating immunoglobulin. Common variable immunodeficiency is a *heterogeneous disorder* that can result from abnormalities in *B-cell activation, B-cell maturation, T-cell help, T-cell suppression, or accessory cell dysfunction* (Table 134–1). It occurs most frequently in the second or third decade of life. In the majority of cases, the exact pathogenetic mechanism remains unclear.

Common Variable Immunodeficiency

Patients with CVI most often present with recurrent infections of the upper and lower respiratory tracts, including sinusitis, bronchitis, and otitis media, although there is a greater incidence of autoimmunity and malignancy, reflecting an immunologically dysregulated state. Infection occurs most commonly with encapsulated organisms including *Haemophilus influenzae* and *Streptococcus pneumoniae*, reflecting the B-cell defect in this patient population. Antibody is essential in host defense against encapsulated organisms, and, as a consequence, B-cell defects are associated with recurrent infections with these organisms. Defects in T cells also can be found in CVI, and T cell-associated infections, including infection with *Pneumocystis* can be seen together with infections with encapsulated organisms. Many of the recurrent infectious disorders, including bronchiectasis, may be prevented with early use of intravenous gamma globulin. The differential diagnosis includes other conditions, such as allergies, anatomic abnormalities (deviated septum), adenoid hyperplasia, cystic fibrosis, and immotile cilia syndrome. These also can result in recurrent infections, and must be ruled out by the appropriate diagnostic tests. Human immunodeficiency virus (HIV) also should be considered in the differential diagnosis, since recurrent infections with encapsulated organisms can be an early feature.

Laboratory Evaluation

Laboratory evaluation for CVI entails measurement of *quantitative immunoglobulins* (IgG, IgA, IgM) and IgG subclasses. The World Health Organization (WHO) definition of CVI requires a significant reduction in two or more isotypes, most often IgG and IgA. IgG subclass deficiency can be as significant as reduction of total IgG if the subclass affected is a major contributor to humoral immune responses (eg, IgG1 and IgG2). The deficiency of IgG subclasses including IgG2 and IgG4 either alone or in combination with IgA deficiency is associated predominantly with recurrent upper respiratory infections but not with gastrointestinal disease. Lymphocyte numbers usually are within the normal range, although there are patients with reduced or nearly absent total B cells. Such patients may reflect a select subgroup of CVI, acting more like patients with Bruton's agammaglobulinemia (X-linked agammaglobulinemia, failure of pre-B cells to differentiate).

In addition to the absolute immunoglobulin levels, *functional antibody measurements* also are required. The inability to synthesize antibodies in response to an antigenic challenge is the best marker to evaluate overall B-cell function and represents the major indication for *intravenous gammaglobulin replacement therapy*. In some patients, an inability to respond to specific antigens is seen even though there are normal levels of circulating antibodies, and this is termed *antibody deficiency syndrome*. Both *protein* and *polysaccharide* vaccines are chosen for immunization because they represent two broad categories of antigens that have different requirements for antibody production. *Protein antigens* are T cell dependent and require T-cell help and processing by accessory cells, such as monocytes and dendritic cells, to drive B cells to differentiate into antibody-producing plasma cells, whereas *polysaccharides* with multiple repeating epitopes are T cell independent and require less T-cell help.

Immunization to assess B-cell function in the evaluation of suspected antibody deficiency is performed using *pneumococcal vaccine*, which contains 12 of the most common polysaccharides from the capsule of the pneumococcus, and *H. influenza B* capsule vaccine. *Pre- and post-immunization titers* are obtained, the postimmunization titer after a 3- to 6-week interval. A *fourfold rise* in antibody to seven of the pneumococcal polysaccharides and *H. influenzae* is considered a normal response.

TABLE 134–2. Gastrointestinal Complications of Common Variable Immunodeficiency

Infectious	Inflammatory	Neoplasia
Giardia *Cryptosporidium*	Nodular lymphoid hyperplasia Sprue-like disorder Pernicious anemia Aphthous stomatitis Inflammatory bowel disease Malacoplakia of the colon Ménétrier's disease	Adenocarcinoma Intestinal lymphoma

Protein antigens commonly used include tetanus toxoid, influenza A and B, and diphtheria toxoid. At least a fourfold increase in antibody titer 2 to 4 weeks after immunization is expected.

Common variable immunodeficiency is a heterogeneous disorder that likely reflects a large mix of pathogenetic processes. Intrinsic defects in T cells, in B cells, or in both can give rise to the same clinical phenotype (hypogammaglobulinemia and recurrent infections); however, the nature of the specific defect in any given patient may render that patient more or less susceptible to associated disorders (malignancy, autoimmunity, chronic inflammatory disease).

Gut Manifestations

The global nature of the immune defects in CVI also affects the mucosal immune system. Gastrointestinal problems are common in CVI and can be divided into three groups: infectious, inflammatory, and neoplastic (Table 134–2). The major reported GI manifestations in CVI include nodular lymphoid hyperplasia, giardiasis, and sprue-like disorders. Almost all of the alimentary tract may be affected in CVI.

Nodular Lymphoid Hyperplasia

A characteristic hallmark of CVI is *nodular lymphoid hyperplasia*, defined as discrete micronodules consisting of lymphoid aggregates confined to the lamina propria and superficial submucosa. Although these nodules occur predominantly in the small intestine, they may also occur in colon. Multiple, small, discrete lymphoid nodules involving variable segments predominantly in the small intestine and rarely in the large intestine are seen radiologically. The hyperplasia may be associated with mucosal flattening and occasionally may cause obstruction.

Four distinct clinical groups of lymphoid hyperplasia are recognized: focal lymphoid hyperplasia of the stomach, focal lymphoid hyperplasia of the rectum, focal lymphoid hyperplasia of the small intestine, and nodular hyperplasia of the GI tract. Focal lesions are single and variably circumscribed. In contrast, nodular lymphoid hyperplasia of the GI tract associated with CVI is more diffuse and is characterized by discrete mucosal nodules that affect variable segments of the intestine. Nodular lymphoid hyperplasia is not specific for CVI and may be a normal finding in young children.

Nodular lymphoid hyperplasia (NLH), in which prominent germinal centers develop in lymphoid tissue, presumably a compensatory B-cell proliferative response to increase the precursor pool of antibody-producing cells, may be part of a greater syndrome of Peyer's patch enlargement, adenopathy, and splenomegaly. Diagnosis is made by endoscopy, small bowel enteroscopy, or double-contrast barium studies. Nodular lymphoid hyperplasia occurs mainly in CVI and to a lesser extent in selective IgA deficiency. *Giardia lamblia*, which can cause diarrhea and malabsorption in CVI, once was thought to be the etiologic agent of NLH; however, antibiotic therapy does not result in resolution of the nodules, which may persist for years.

Giardia lamblia

Giardia lamblia used to be one of the most common causes of diarrhea and malabsorption in CVI. The parasite is transmitted in the form of cysts from person to person or in water. Ingested cysts excyst, giving rise to trophozoites that colonize the duodenum and jejunum. Symptoms consist of watery diarrhea and abdominal bloating, along with excessive flatus and foul smelling stool, beginning 1 to 3 weeks after ingestion of the cysts. Abdominal cramping and bloating are common complaints. The natural course of infection leads to resolution of the diarrhea in 1 to 4 weeks. Although diagnosis sometimes is determined by positive enzyme-linked immunosorbent assay (ELISA) or the presence of cysts and trophozoites in the stool, a duodenal or jejunal aspirate may be necessary to demonstrate the parasite.

The pathophysiology of *Giardia*-related diarrhea and malabsorption is not well understood. The trophozoite can invade the mucosa, directly disrupting the absorption of fats and carbohydrates. Direct epithelial cell damage mediated by *Giardia*, including disaccharidase deficiency, altered levels of enteropeptidases, and decreased vitamin B_{12} absorption is common. Either mechanical irritation of the epithelium, with increased epithelial turnover, or epithelial damage secondary to a T-cell response to the parasite may account for the mucosal damage. The extent of epithelial damage mediated by *Giardia* is related to duration of infection. Although antibodies to *Giardia* are produced in normal individuals infected with this parasite, the T cell is required for eradication of the organism. Patients with CVI have a much more prolonged course of infection with *Giardia*, which may last months to years (possibly related to T-cell defects). Eradication generally results in reversal of the symptoms, although residual lactose intolerance and intestinal irritability may persist. Metronidazole (250 mg orally three times a day for 1 week) is frequently successful in treating this infection. Given the difficulty of confirming diagnosis, empirical treatment with metronidazole often is begun following complaints of the onset of a diarrheal illness, as a therapeutic test for *Giardia* infection.

Idiopathic diarrhea and malabsorption not associated with *Giardia* have been reported in CVI as well. Bacterial overgrowth with anaerobic coliform organisms can occur. However, eradication of the bacterial organisms does not always improve the diarrhea or malabsorption. Other approaches include cholestyramine, which has been reported to reduce diarrhea in selected patients with CVI with malabsorption. Interestingly, *Shigella* and *Salmonella* infections, the most common causes of bacterial diarrhea in normal hosts, are not seen frequently in patients with CVI. Other pathogens, including *Cryptosporidium* and *Coccidioides,* have been implicated as causes of diarrhea in some antibody-deficient patients.

Far more frequently seen is malabsorption not related to *Giardia* infection or overgrowth. Small bowel biopsy reveals flattened villi with lymphocytic infiltration in a pattern resembling that of celiac sprue. In contrast to classic celiac disease, plasma cells are absent in the cellular infiltrate in CVI, suggesting a T-cell–mediated mechanism. In this respect, the intestinal lesion associated with CVI is similar to that seen in pernicious anemia. Immunoglobulin A deficiency more frequently is associated with a form of celiac disease that is responsive to a gluten-free diet. However, despite the histologic similarity to celiac disease, gluten-free diets in CVI have not had much success. Patients with intractable sprue-like illness have required more aggressive forms of therapy (after failure of dietary intervention). These approaches include the use of immunomodulators, such as azathioprine (AZA) and 6-mercaptopurine (6-MP), at low doses (50 to 100 mg/d) or in severe cases, agents such as steroids. In many of these patients, alternate-day steroids can be used with success. Concerns over the use of immunomodulating agents, such as steroids and AZA, are alleviated in part by the concomitant use of intravenous gammaglobulin (although steroid use may be more problematic). Although anecdotal at this time, the incidence of infectious complications in patients treated in this manner does not appear to be any greater than their nontreated counterparts.[*]

Recurrent aphthous stomatitis and oral thrush are associated with CVI in patients with T-cell deficiencies. The mechanism for the aphthous ulcer is unknown, although overproduction of macrophage-derived cytokines has been implicated. These patients respond well to sucralfate suspension two to three times a day in a swish and swallow regimen. Viral esophagitis, although common in T-cell deficiencies such as HIV, is rare in CVI.

---

[*] Editor's Note: Beclomethasone, a poorly absorbed and rapidly metabolized corticosteroid, is reportedly helpful in graft-versus-host disease (see the chapter on stem cell transplants) and might be helpful in this situation. (TMB)

The most common autoimmune intestinal disease in patients with CVI is pernicious anemia. In non-immunodeficient patients, the average age at onset of pernicious anemia is 60 years, whereas in CVI, the average age is between 20 and 40 years. Gastric atrophy is present both in patients with CVI and in those without CVI, with lymphocytic infiltration of the lamina propria.

However, although plasma cells are present in non-immunodeficient patients, they are absent in patients with CVI. Ninety percent of patients with pernicious anemia have an anti–parietal-cell antibody, and 60 percent have an anti–intrinsic-factor antibody. In contrast, in CVI-associated pernicious anemia, anti–parietal-cell antibodies are not seen, suggesting a T-cell–mediated mechanism. Pernicious anemia is more common in IgA deficiency than in CVI, although the reasons for this finding are unclear. These patients are treated no differently than patients with pernicious anemia without associated immunodeficiency.

Inflammatory Bowel Disease in Patients with Common Variable Immunodeficiency

For some time, immunologists have reported an association of inflammatory bowel disease (IBD) (ulcerative colitis [UC] and Crohn's disease [CD]) with patients with primary immunodeficiency, specifically, CVI. The incidence of IBD in patients with CVI at the Mount Sinai Medical Center, New York, has been reported to be 5.4 percent. In patients with CVI, chronic GI problems are more likely to occur in those with other autoimmune phenomena, such as autoimmune hemolytic anemia, thrombocytopenia with antiplatelet antibodies, neutropenia, thyroid dysfunction, or pernicious anemia.

ROLE OF T CELLS IN INFLAMMATION

It has become clear that absent or functionally defective T cells are responsible for intestinal inflammation, as demonstrated by cytokine knockout mice. In these models, generally those cytokines involved in suppression (interleukin-10 [IL-10], transforming growth factor-beta [TGF-β]) or in early T-cell regulation (IL-2) are more likely, in their absence, to cause disease. These findings suggest that regulatory T cells are important in maintaining intestinal homeostasis. In the absence of such a T cell, inflammation ensues. Based on these observations, it appears that T cells are the key participants in the development of bowel inflammation. A number of other recently described models involving transfer of specific T-cell subpopulations (CD45RB^h into SCID mice) have supported the concept that dysregulation of T cells results in an IBD-like presentation.

PATHOGENESIS OF INFLAMMATORY BOWEL DISEASE

While these animal models have been informative, they have been developed at a time when the understanding of human IBD is increasing. Inflammation in IBD appears to be a three-tiered event: triggering, activation, and inflammation and injury. There is evidence that bacterial and viral antigens aid in the initial triggering of the disease. A common clinical scenario is the development of IBD after an intestinal insult, such as turista, amebic colitis, or viral gastroenteritis. The second event appears to be the excessive activation of the intestinal immune system, with potentially aberrant activation of CD4+ T cells in the lamina propria. There is a fair amount of evidence that these CD4+ T cells are central to the process as they not only exist in the colon or small intestine but also are found in the peripheral circulation. These activated T cells secrete cytokines that promote the third phase of this process, nonspecific inflammation and tissue injury (epithelial cell destruction, fluid secretion, fibrosis, smooth muscle proliferation). Cytokine secretion appears to be critical to the inflammation seen in IBD. Treatment of fulminant UC with the cytokine inhibitor cyclosporine shuts down the inflammatory process. Similar results have been reported in CD. The profile of cytokines present in the lamina propria appears to be different in UC compared to CD. There is an increase in interferon-gamma (IFN-γ) and IL-2 by both protein and mRNA in CD tissues.

Colitis in Common Variable Immunodeficiency

The colitis seen in patients with CVI has variably been characterized as resembling graft-versus-host (GVH) disease, lymphocytic colitis, and UC. Common features are increased lymphocytes in the surface epithelium, similar to lymphocytic colitis; acute inflammatory cells in crypt epithelium and lamina propria; and, in severe cases, loss of crypts, similar to UC and GVH disease.

There is recent evidence from two laboratories that patients with CVI with more profound defects in T-cell function may have distinct clinical phenotypes. Mechanic and colleagues (1997) and Hermaszewski and Webster (1993) described a diffuse granulomatous disease in patients with CVI who had severe T-cell dysfunction. This disorder was manifest by cutaneous granulomas, sarcoid-like lung lesions, and granulomatous hepatitis. No infectious etiology was identified in these patients, and there was clear-cut evidence of macrophage activation (eg, high angiotensin converting enzyme [ACE] levels). Although granulomas are the hallmark of CD, none of these patients had intestinal inflammation.

For patients with CVI who have concomitant IBD, anti-inflammatory treatment is identical to that for conventional IBD, including 5-aminosalicyclic acid (5-ASA), AZA, or 6-MP, and steroid (or 5-ASA) enemas. More novel therapies have not been attempted, because most patients respond to one or more of these approaches. Antibiotics rarely help, and the majority of patients have mild disease. Owing to the underlying T-cell immunodeficiency, oral steroids for such patients should be avoided if at all possible. Beclomethasone is discussed in the chapter on stem-cell transplantation.

Common variable immunodeficiency also is associated with an increase in malignancy, particularly lymphoma and adenocarcinoma. There is a 47-fold increase in the incidence of GI malignancies in comparison with the general population. Cunningham-Rundles and Bodian (1989) noted an incidence of lymphoma of 11 percent; some cases involved the bowel, but there were no primary GI malignancies.

Rarer GI associations include malacoplakia, a chronic granulomatous disease that affects the urinary tract but can cause colonic stricture. Pneumatosis intestinalis and Ménétrier's disease also have been reported in CVI.

Gastrointestinal Tract Disease in Other Immunodeficiency Disorders

In addition to CVI, other immunodeficiency states have been associated with GI complications. Bruton's agammaglobulinemia and X-linked immunodeficiency, with arrest at the pre–B-cell stage of B-cell differentiation, occasionally have been associated with recurrent *Salmonella* infections, chronic diarrhea, and malabsorption. Nevertheless, patients with X-linked agammaglobulinemia rarely present with GI complaints. Intractable diarrhea and oral moniliasis characterize severe combined immunodeficiency, a combined T- and B-cell disorder. Massive diarrhea and failure to thrive are common. The small intestine is devoid of lymphocytes and displays flattened villi. There may be crypt abscesses and pigment-containing macrophages, similar to those seen in Whipple's disease. Infection with HIV-1, aside from multiple opportunistic infections, also is associated with chronic diarrhea of unclear etiology (possibly tumor necrosis factor alpha [TNF-α]).

Certain intestinal disorders themselves have been associated with immunodeficiency. Intestinal lymphangiectasia results in the rupture of dilatated lymphatics into the intestinal lumen, resulting in loss of lymphocytes, fat, and protein. The patients present with severe fat malabsorption and hypoproteinemia. The immunodeficiency here is secondary, rather than related to lymphocyte maturation defects, as seen in the previously described disorders. Malabsorption syndromes and CVI have an associated zinc deficiency that has been reported to decrease cell-mediated immunity.

Therapy

Therapy to prevent infections in patients with hypogammaglobulinemia requires intravenous gamma globulin replacement. Doses of 300 to 500 mg/kg of body weight at intervals of 3 to 4 weeks are necessary to restore circulating levels. However, because intravenous Ig preparations contain IgG but not IgA (the principal secretory antibody in the gut and lung), gamma globulin therapy only partially restores the antibody deficiency and, generally, has no effect on the intestinal disorders associated with CVI. Oral gamma globulin has been tried in an attempt to deliver more immunoglobulin to the gut. However, gastric acid, luminal proteases (pepsin or papain), and bacterial enzymes destroy much of it. As a result, this therapy has been relatively ineffective. Patients in whom specific intestinal disorders arise should be treated in a similar fashion to those individuals who have the disease but are not immunodeficient. This may include the use of immunomodulator therapy, but in the presence of restoring humoral immunity with intravenous gamma globulin, such therapies are generally well tolerated.

Conclusion

When patients present with GI disorders that are resistant to conventional therapies (eg, gluten withdrawal in celiac sprue) or autoimmune GI disease, which occurs at a young age, immunoglobulin levels should be measured to rule out immunodeficiency as a cause. Because there is a high prevalence of recurrent giardiasis, sprue-like disorder, NLH, and IBD in immunodeficient patients, patients with these GI diseases should be screened for hypogammaglobulinemia. Early diagnosis and treatment may reduce the morbidity and mortality associated with immunodeficiency.

For immunodeficient patients who present with diarrhea or malabsorption, efforts should be made to seek the cause of these problems, because common causes, such as giardiasis and celiac disease, are treatable. There need not be concerns about treating these patients with potentially immunosuppressive agents (steroids or AZA), because the immunodeficiency is generally controlled with intravenous Ig. Owing to the increased risk of malignancy in immunodeficient patients, periodic GI evaluation in patients with primary immunodeficiency has been advocated, with a view to early detection and treatment of these malignancies.

Editor's Note

A list of 42 references can be requested from the author. E-mail: *gkleiner@smtplink.mssm.edu.*

References

Cunningham-Rundles C, Bodian C. Clinical and immunologic analyses of 103 patients with common variable immunodeficiency. J Clin Immunol 1989;9:22–33.

Hermaszewski R, Webster A. Primary hypogammaglobulinemia: a survey of clinical manifestations and complications. Q J Med 1993;86:31–42.

Mechanic L, Dikman S, Cunningham-Rundles C. Granulomatous disease in common variable immunodeficiency. Ann Intern Med 1997;127:613–7.

Supplemental Reading

Ammann A, Ashman R, Buckley R, et al. Use of intravenous gamma-globulin in antibody immunodeficiency: results of a multicenter controlled trial. Clin Immunol Immunopathol 1982;22:60–7.

Cunningham-Rundles C, Siegal F, Smithwick E, et al. Efficacy of intravenous immunoglobulin in primary humoral immunodeficiency disease. Ann Intern Med 1984;101:435–9.

Cunningham-Rundles C, Bodian C. Common variable immunodeficiency: clinical and immunological features of 248 patients. Clin Immunol 1999;92:34–48.

Reinhold D, Ansorge S, Grungreiff K. Immunobiology of zinc and zinc therapy. Immunol Today 1999;20:102–3.

Sperber K, Mayer L. Gastrointestinal manifestations of common variable immunodeficiency. Immunol Allergy Clin North Am 1988;8:423–34.

Spickett G, Webster A, Farrant J. Cellular abnormalities in common variable immunodeficiency. Immunodefic Rev 1990; 2:199–219.

Washington K, Stenzel T, Buckley R, Gottfried M. Gastrointestinal pathology in patients with common variable immunodeficiency and X-linked agammaglobulinemia. Am J Surg Pathol 1996;20:1240–52.

CHAPTER 135

Lymphoma in Inflammatory Bowel Disease

Sharon Masel, MD, and Stephen B. Hanauer, MD

Lymphoma may either mimic or complicate ulcerative colitis (UC) and Crohn's disease (CD), and the understanding of this relationship is of importance to physicians. There is significant overlap between the symptoms, signs, and the radiologic and endoscopic appearance of intestinal lymphoma and inflammatory bowel disease (IBD). Small intestinal lymphoma may mimic CD and colonic lymphoma may mimic both colitis and colonic adnocarcinoma. Intestinal lymphoma also may complicate IBD; therefore, awareness of its association, clues to its presence, and knowledge of appropriate diagnostic investigations (and their shortcomings) are critical to patient management.

Primary Intestinal Lymphoma

Lymphoma may involve the gastrointestinal tract either primarily or as a manifestation of disseminated systemic disease. Primary gastrointestinal lymphoma is defined as a tumor involving the gastrointestinal tract without evidence of peripheral lymphadenopathy, splenomegaly, abnormal chest radiographs, or abnormal peripheral white blood cell count and differential. Although accounting for only 1 to 4 percent of gastrointestinal malignancies, the gastrointestinal tract is the most frequent site of extranodal lymphoma. The stomach is the most commonly involved site in Western countries, followed by the small bowel and then the colon.

Malt Lymphoma

A significant proportion of gastric lymphomas are associated with the presence of *Helicobacter pylori* and are, most commonly, a low-grade mucosa-associated lymphoid tissue or "MALT" lymphoma. The stomach normally does not contain lymphoid tissue but, in the presence of *H. pylori*, lymphoid tissue is acquired in the gastric mucosa. When of low grade, these MALT tumors may regress with eradication of the *H. pylori* organism but may transform into high-grade lymphomas, at which time their growth is autonomous and no longer responsive to *H. pylori* eradication. Low-grade gastric MALT lymphomas have a favorable prognosis.

Mediterranean Lymphoma

In the Middle East and Mediterranean regions, the small bowel is the most common site of gastrointestinal lymphoma. The incidence of small bowel lymphomas increases, as one progresses distally in the small bowel toward the ileum, corresponding to the amount of lymphoid tissue in the bowel wall. In Westernized countries, small bowel lymphomas are discrete tumors, whereas in "developing" countries, they tend to diffusely involve the bowel wall. The diffuse variant appears to be a distinct entity and also is referred to as **Mediterranean lymphoma, alpha chain disease, or diffuse primary small intestinal lymphoma.** Proliferating Immunoglobulin (Ig) A-secreting B lymphocytes intensely infiltrate the small bowel lamina propria and sometimes regional lymph nodes. The association of this lymphoma with geographic regions of poor hygiene and endemic parasitic infection suggests infection as a possible predisposing factor. Although no causative organism has been isolated, **tetracycline** has been shown to cause regression of the lymphoid infiltrate if administered at a pre-lymphomatous stage and can result in complete remission.

Incidence

The incidence of primary intestinal lymphoma has dramatically increased in Westernized countries over recent years, doubling from 1985 to 1990 in the United States. This has been attributed to the increased number of immunocompromised patients (with HIV infection and post-transplantation) as well as immigration from the Middle East and Mediterranean regions. It has increasingly become recognized that CD and celiac disease are associated with an increased risk for the development of small bowel lymphomas, and colonic lymphomas have been reported to be increased in both ulcerative and Crohn's colitis. More recently, an increased incidence of extra-intestinal lymphomas has been reported to complicate both CD and UC.

Association of Inflammatory Bowel Disease and Lymphoma

Both Hodgkin's disease (HD) and non-Hodgkin's lymphoma (NHL) have been reported in CD and UC.

Although earlier studies suggested that lymphoma associated with IBD tended to occur at sites of chronic intestinal inflammation, more recently, a predominance of extra-intestinal lymphomas has been identified in studies of large IBD cohorts. A study from Mount Sinai Hospital, New York, reported nine lymphomas in an IBD population of 2,636, all of which were extra-intestinal. This risk of approximately 341/100,000 is greatly in excess of the United States population incidence of lymphoma of approximately 18/100,000. Similarly, a series from the Cleveland Clinic found an increased incidence of lymphoma in their UC population, although with a p value of .06, this did not reach statistical significance. In contrast to the reports from these tertiary IBD centers, three population-based studies have reported no evidence of an increased risk of lymphoma associated with IBD. In our own series from the University of Chicago, the estimated risk of lymphoma among nearly 5,000 IBD patients extrapolates to approximately 104/100,000, with all cases being extra-intestinal NHLs.

The association between UC and colonic lymphoma first was reported in 1928 by Bargen. Subsequently, more than 30 cases of lymphoma, predominantly NHL, have been reported in UC. The potential risk factors for colonic lymphoma in UC are similar to those for colonic adenocarcinoma and include extensive and longstanding colitis. However, the development of extra-intestinal lymphoma appears to be independent of these features and has occurred subsequent to curative proctocolectomy and ileoanal anastomosis. Hodgkin's disease accounts for less than 20 percent of lymphomas reported in UC. Two-thirds of the cases of lymphoma in UC have been multicentric and four cases have been associated with concomitant colonic adenocarcinoma.

Hughes described an ileal reticulum cell sarcoma occurring in the setting of CD in 1955 and first reported the association between lymphomas and CD. Several subsequent isolated reports of ileal lymphomas followed including the reported potential association of CD with Hodgkin's disease. Confirming a true association, however, has proved difficult due to the relative infrequency of the two diseases, their similar clinical and radiologic characteristics, and occasional lack of histologic confirmation of the diagnosis. Case reports remain small in number and include a preponderance of NHL (both intestinal and extra-intestinal) compared to HD.

Celiac Disease and Lymphoma

Patients with celiac disease also are at greater risk than the general population for the development of malignancies, particularly lymphoma. These usually are T-cell lymphomas. The relative risk remains uncertain due to imprecision of the diagnosis of celiac disease in the literature, lack of histologic confirmation, and inconsistent accounts of clinical response to gluten withdrawal.

Diagnosis of lymphoma complicating celiac disease is difficult, although abdominal pain, bleeding, and fever are uncommon in celiac disease and should raise the suspicion of complicating lymphoma. Similarly, suspicion should be raised in patients with changes in the pattern of their disease or in those who are unresponsive to a gluten-free diet. Small bowel barium studies and CT may be useful if ulcerations or mesenteric or retroperitoneal adenopathy is identified, but usually are not diagnostic. Even endoscopy and biopsy may fail to confirm the suspicion of intestinal lymphoma that may require a laparotomy and a full-thickness sampling. Tissue diagnosis is essential as both symptoms and physical findings are nonspecific and intra-abdominal lymphadenopathy has been documented in uncomplicated celiac disease. Extra-intestinal lymphomas also have been reported in association with celiac disease, as have adenocarcinomas of the small bowel, oropharynx, esophagus, and breast. The pathogenic process underlying the development of lymphoma in celiac disease remains uncertain, although it has been proposed that the passage of environmental carcinogens across the damaged and more permeable intestinal mucosa may be involved in disease initiation.

Pathogenesis of Lymphoma in Inflammatory Bowel Disease

There have been a number of hypotheses proposed to explain the apparent relationship between IBD and lymphoma. Non-Hodgkin's lymphoma clearly is related to immune suppression as shown by the increased associations with organ transplantation, AIDS, and congenital immunodeficiency. Other autoimmune and chronic inflammatory diseases such as rheumatoid arthritis have increased risk of lymphomas that are independent of immunosuppressive drug therapy and thought to be directly related to the underlying disease state. Similar to rheumatoid arthritis in IBD, it may be the underlying immunologic defect or the chronic inflammatory state itself that may predispose to lymphoma. The increased incidence of lymphomas complicating UC, CD, and celiac disease suggests the possibility of common etiopathogenic events despite the different patterns of mucosal immune responses in the different disease states. In contrast to the association between NHL and immune suppression, HD accounts for 34 percent of lymphomas in the general population but only 3 percent of lymphomas in the transplant population, and does not appear to be associated with immune-suppressed states.

Potential Role of Immune-Suppressant Medication on Lymphoma Development in Inflammatory Bowel Disease

The role of immune-suppressant medication in the development of lymphoma in IBD remains controversial. An increased incidence of lymphoma has been observed in patients with autoimmune and chronic inflammatory diseases, including IBD, on immune-suppressant medication. Kinlen (1985) was the first to describe an increased risk of lymphoma in a large prospective study of 1,349 patients with "autoimmune" disease, including 280 patients with IBD. This increase in NHL was supported by a subsequent study of 1,600 nontransplant patients on immune-suppressant medication that identified six cases of NHL compared to an expected 0.55.

Large series of IBD patients, however, have failed to identify an increased risk attributable to the most commonly used immune-modifying agents: azathioprine and 6-mercaptopurine. In a series of 755 patients treated with azathioprine at St. Mark's Hospital, London, over a 30-year period, no cases of lymphoma were identified. However, in a series of patients treated with 6-mercaptopurine in New York, 1 of 396 patients developed a cerebral NHL—the cerebrum being a site most often associated with immune compromise. A case report of a reversible Epstein-Barr virus-related lymphoma in a patient with CD on azathioprine raises concern of a similar pathogenesis of lymphoma in IBD as in the transplant population. Reassuringly, in the series from Mount Sinai Hospital, New York, none of the nine patients with lymphomas had received azathioprine or 6-mercaptopurine. Similarly, in our own series of six lymphomas diagnosed in patients with IBD, no patient had been treated with immune suppressant medication.

Cyclosporine, Tacrolimus, and mycophenolate all have been associated with lymphoma development in transplant patients. However, there have not yet been reports of lymphoma development in IBD patients treated with these more potent immune suppressants. Cyclosporine in UC has been recommended only for short-duration therapy, and this may be a reason for the lack of association of its use in IBD and lymphoma development.

With the recent advent of therapy directed at tumor necrosis factor-α (TNF-α) there has been concern regarding the potential development of lymphomas in both IBD and rheumatoid arthritis patients. Of the first 394 patients with rheumatoid arthritis and CD treated with infliximab (chimeric monoclonal anti-TNF-α antibody) followed for 6 months to 3 years, 1 case of NHL was seen in a patient with CD and 4 in those patients with rheumatoid arthritis. All 5 patients had long-standing chronic disease and prior therapy with steroids, azathioprine, or methotrexate. There are not yet sufficient data to determine the risk imparted by the specific antibody therapy directed at TNF.

Diagnosis of Lymphoma in Inflammatory Bowel Disease

Crohn's disease and lymphoma of the small bowel may produce indistinguishable symptoms and findings on physical examination. Similarly, colonic lymphoma may mimic both colitis and colonic adenocarcinoma. Radiologic investigations, therefore, are relied upon but often are inconclusive due to nonspecific findings and the absence of pathognomonic features of either IBD or lymphoma. In most cases where suspicion arises, a histopathologic diagnosis is required. As with celiac disease, when a patient with IBD develops a change in the pattern of disease or fails to respond to medical therapy, alternative diagnoses or complications including lymphoma should be considered.

Symptoms of small bowel lymphoma include nonspecific abdominal pain in 70 to 80 percent and weight loss in 30 percent. A change in bowel habit, nausea, vomiting, lethargy, and fever may also occur. Malabsorption is uncommon but is seen in lymphoma secondary to celiac disease. An abdominal mass is palpable in 40 to 60 percent of patients; lymphadenopathy and hepato- or splenomegaly usually are absent. Up to 25 percent of patients with small bowel lymphomas present with intestinal perforation. Obstruction is seen more commonly with small than with large bowel lymphomas.

As there are no truly distinguishing clinical or radiologic features between CD and small bowel lymphoma, the diagnosis of a superimposed lymphoma often is delayed considerably. Crohn's disease also is associated with an increased incidence of small bowel adenocarcinoma, and these, too, rarely are diagnosed preoperatively. Most are identified during surgery performed to investigate refractory symptoms.

Upper gastrointestinal series with small bowel follow-through are abnormal in 90 percent of patients with small bowel lymphoma but rarely are diagnostic. Radiologic features include aneurysmal dilatation of the bowel wall with diffuse thickening and displacement of adjacent loops. Similar to the appearance of CD, lymphomas may be associated with aphthous and linear ulceration, fistulous tract formation, stricturing, or the demonstration of a distinct mass in the intestinal wall. Enteroclysis may improve the diagnostic yield of small bowel lesions. Terminal ileal tumors also may be detected at colonoscopy, and duodenal tumors at gastroscopy; small bowel enteroscopy is becoming increasingly available to provide both visualization and a tissue biopsy of more proximal small bowel lesions. Computed tomography remains more useful in the staging workup of intestinal lymphoma than in the demonstration of the primary lesion.

Colonic lymphomas also present insidiously and diagnosis usually is late. Obstruction, perforation, and bleeding are less common as compared with small bowel lymphomas. Increased or refractory symptoms of diarrhea or bleeding may herald malignant transformation, though differentiation between lymphoma and adenocarcinoma is difficult. Systemic symptoms of fever and weight loss may be present. Most often, symptoms are ascribed to a flare in colitis and not uncommonly the lymphoma is diagnosed incidentally on biopsy at colonoscopy. Barium enema is abnormal in up to 80 percent of colorectal lymphomas but rarely is diagnostic, particularly in the setting of preexisting UC. Endoscopic biopsy with immunohistochemical staining for tumor markers is the definitive diagnostic test.

Conclusion

Intestinal lymphomas are uncommon but both intestinal and extra-intestinal lymphomas appear to be of increased incidence in chronic inflammatory bowel disease states, including IBD. The relationship between immune-modifying therapy used in IBD and the development of lymphoma remains controversial. The differential diagnosis between IBD and lymphoma, either complicating IBD or occurring independently, is difficult. Most intestinal lymphomas diagnosed in the setting of IBD have been unanticipated and were found incidentally at the time of surgery performed for IBD indications or only subsequently in the histopathology of the resected specimen.

Supplemental Reading

Connell WR, et al. Long-term neoplasia risk after azathioprine treatment in inflammatory bowel disease. Lancet 1994; 343:1249–52.

Ekbom A, et al. Extracolonic malignancies in inflammatory bowel disease. Cancer 1991;67:2015–9.

Greenstein AJ, et al. Lymphoma in inflammatory bowel disease. Cancer 1992;69:1119–23.

Kinlen LJ. Incidence of cancer in rheumatoid arthritis and other disorders after immunosuppressive treatment. Am J Med 1985;78:44–9.

Larvol L, Soule JC, Le Tourneau A. Reversible lymphoma in the setting of azathioprine therapy for Crohn's disease [letter]. N Engl J Med 1994;331:883–4.

Mir-Madjlessi SH, et al. Colorectal and extracolonic malignancy in ulcerative colitis. Cancer 1986;58:1569–74.

Persson PG, et al. Crohn's disease and cancer: a population-based cohort study. Gastroenterology 1994;107:1675–9.

Present DH, et al. 6-Mercaptopurine in the management of inflammatory bowel disease: short- and long-term toxicity. Ann Intern Med 1989;111:641–9.

Sandborn WJ, Hanauer SB. Antitumor necrosis factor therapy for inflammatory bowel disease: a review of agents, pharmacology, clinical results, and safety. Inflamm Bowel Dis 1999;5:119–33.

Trier JS. Celiac sprue. N Engl J Med 1991;325:1709–19.

GASTROINTESTINAL COMPLICATIONS IN STEM CELL TRANSPLANTATION

LINDA A. LEE, MD, AND GEORGIA VOGELSANG, MD

Stem cell transplantation (SCT) is the standard of care for the treatment of many hematologic malignancies, pediatric solid tumors, inherited disorders, and aplastic anemia. It also is being used to treat many autoimmune disorders in experimental situations. Several patients with Crohn's disease and leukemia have remitted or remained in remission after allogeneic bone marrow transplantation. Complications related to SCT are becoming more widely recognized. Gastrointestinal complications of SCT result from preparative regimen toxicity, infection, and acute and chronic graft-versus-host (GVH) disease, which may be difficult to diagnostically separate and are therefore addressed in this chapter.

Overview of Stem Cell Transplantation

The aim of SCT is to eradicate malignancy, a defective immune system, or disordered hematopoiesis by replacing stem cells with the patient's own (autologous) stored stem cells or those from a selectively matched human leukocyte antigen (HLA)-identical (allogeneic) donor. Although GVH disease and immunodeficiency occur more commonly after allogeneic transplantation, toxicity from the preparative regimen arises in both allogeneic and autologous transplants. Before transplantation, a preparative regimen is administered to rid the host of malignant or defective cells as well as to decrease the likelihood of donor stem cell rejection in allogeneic SCT. Protocols for SCT vary, depending upon the disease, but often include total-body irradiation and chemotherapy. The day of stem cell infusion into the host is designated as day 0, whereas the days prior to infusion, during which the preparative regimen is administered, are designated day 4, day 3, and so on.

Toxic Injury

Most transplant centers vary the preparative regimen based on the disease. Thus, the expected toxicity of the preparative regimen depends on the combination of agents administered and the overall condition of the patient. Patients who have been heavily treated or have comorbid medical conditions have more toxicity from the preparative regimen. Protocols often include cyclophosphamide and total-body irradiation (TBI) (1,100 cGy to 1,400 cGy),

which, in combination, injure the intestinal mucosa. Total-body irradiation at high doses (> 1,200 cGy) induces damage to DNA, particularly in rapidly dividing cells that are found in the crypts. The impaired regenerative capacity of the crypt epithelium leads to villous blunting and loss of brush-border enzyme activity; the patient may become lactose intolerant. If the regenerative capacity is severely impaired, ulceration may develop and lead to fluid and electrolyte losses. High doses of TBI have been associated with an increased likelihood of developing intestinal GVH disease in animal models. Cyclophosphamide may itself induce mucositis, diarrhea, and, rarely, hemorrhagic colitis.

Diarrhea related to toxicity induced by the preparative regimen may last until day 15 after SCT. To eliminate superimposed bacterial infection in the evaluation of diarrhea, stool cultures should be obtained. Once infectious etiologies are ruled out, antidiarrheal agents, such as loperamide, may be initiated. Nausea, vomiting, and anorexia occur commonly during the preparative regimen. Prophylactic antiemetics routinely are given, and the 5-hydroxytryptamine-3 serotonin receptor antagonists, such as granisetron, appear to offer significant protection from radiation-induced vomiting. If the mucositis, nausea, and vomiting are severe, total parenteral nutrition frequently must be instituted. Studies are underway to determine whether addition of glutamine to enteral or parenteral feedings alters morbidity from SCT.

Infection

Evaluation of post-transplant diarrhea, which affects 43 percent of patients after day 20, must prompt a consideration of infectious etiologies. Although GVH disease remains the most common cause of diarrhea after day 20 in allogeneic SCT, viral and bacterial pathogens must be sought in all patients. The most likely bacterial pathogen is *Clostridium difficile*, and despite the variables that contribute to the infection, namely, use of broad-spectrum antibiotics and an immunocompromised state, the infection usually responds to standard therapy with metronidazole or vancomycin. Parasites rarely are found in SCT patients, although rare case reports of amebiasis and giardiasis exist.

Viral infection, particularly that caused by cytomegalovirus (CMV), significantly affects mortality in this patient population. Although some transplant groups use prophylactic ganciclovir, the side effect of marrow toxicity has made this a difficult practice. Many groups now employ serologic detection of CMV early antigen as an indication to initiate ganciclovir therapy, even before overt CMV disease develops in CMV-seropositive patients. In the absence of prophylaxis, CMV may occur 30 to 100 days after SCT in 70 percent of seropositive recipients and up to 40 percent of seronegative recipients, but is rare in seronegative patients maintained on seronegative blood products. Cytomegalovirus may infect epithelial and endothelial cells anywhere in the gastrointestinal (GI) tract and give rise to diarrhea, abdominal pain, or GI bleeding. Ulceration may occur, probably as a result of local ischemia induced by CMV infection of endothelial cells and vasoconstriction. The most sensitive methods for the diagnosis of CMV involvement of the gut are centrifugation culture, polymerase chain reaction, and in situ hybridization using biopsy specimens. Routine histology may be insensitive and routine viral culture may take 2 weeks to provide a result.

Other viruses, such as adenovirus, rotavirus, and astrovirus, have been identified as pathogens in SCT patients. Adenoviral infection, with its poor prognosis, manifests as a multisystemic disease, with pneumonitis, cystitis, and enteritis occurring concurrently. No adequate treatment is presently available. Rotavirus infection may be diagnosed by enzyme-linked immunoabsorbent assay (ELISA) of the stool or by electron microscopy. Frequently, it is a self-limited infection, but administration of intravenous immunoglobulin in children with refractory infection has led to reports of therapeutic response. The significance of astrovirus as a pathogen remains unclear but was the virus identified most frequently in SCT patients in one study. Finally, visceral varicella zoster infection may cause abdominal pain, diarrhea, nausea, vomiting, abnormal liver function tests, and fever. It is unclear from the case reports that dot the literature if the symptoms always arise from true viral infection of tissues of the gut or if the symptoms really stem from compromise of GI motility secondary to disseminated viral infection. However, electron microscopy positively identified the presence of varicella zoster viral particles in the gastric biopsy in one report. The abdominal pain may be the presenting symptom of disseminated varicella zoster infection and can be so severe that it has sometimes resulted in exploratory laparotomy. Abdominal pain may precede the vesicular skin eruption by up to 2 weeks, which contributes to the difficulty in making the diagnosis. The symptoms of visceral varicella zoster infection respond to acyclovir.

Neutropenic enterocolits, or **typhilitis**, may occur in recipients of SCT. Although the pathogenesis remains ambiguous, typhilitis is thought to arise from cytotoxic injury to the mucosa of the terminal ileum, cecum, or right colon, followed by superimposed bacterial or fungal infection. Infection may lead to perforation and an acute abdomen. Symptoms and physical signs may be nonspecific, but the diagnosis should be entertained in any patient with fever, neutropenia, and abdominal pain. Abdominal radiography and computed tomography demonstrate thickening of the right side of the colon and possibly pneumatosis intestinalis. Typhilitis may be managed conservatively with broad-spectrum antibiotics. Development of peritoneal signs warrants surgical consultation and intervention.

Gastrointestinal Bleeding

Significant GI bleeding may occur post-transplant and contributes to higher mortality associated with SCT. Most significant GI bleeding arises from the upper GI tract. More specifically, the site of bleeding is the antrum where there is generalized hemorrhage from the mucosa, but rarely is ulceration seen. Biopsies have demonstrated a chemical gastropathy characterized by foveolar hyperplasia, reactive epithelial changes, edema, and vascular congestion. Bipolar electrocoagulation is of limited efficacy, and significant quantities of blood products are required to support the patient. Gastric vascular ectasia (watermelon stomach) frequently has been reported in these patients and may be amenable to laser therapy. Occasionally, bleeding occurs as a consequence of GVH disease or peptic ulcer disease.

Graft-versus-Host Disease

At its simplest level, GVH disease arises from the recipient's immune recognition of minor antigenic differences between donor and recipient. In those who obtain severely lymphocytic depleted grafts, GVH disease is rare. Increased numbers of infused lymphocytes, increased disparity between donor and host (as in unrelated donor transplants), and inflammatory cytokine production (as in sepsis) raise the risk of GVH disease. Acute GVH disease presents after the patient engrafts and arises from activation of donor T cells in response to host. Both tissue damage from the preparative regimen and T-cell activation contribute to the release of inflammatory cytokines, such as interleukin-2 and tumor necrosis factor-alpha (TNF-α) and gamma (TNF-γ). Cytokines, in turn, trigger a cascade of more intense inflammatory events. In the presence of these cytokines, natural killer and cytotoxic T cells mediate injury to three organ systems: skin, gut, and liver. Skin is the organ most commonly involved in GVH disease. Gut or liver involvement usually is seen with skin disease, but it is possible to have isolated organ involvement.

Clinical Manifestations

Patients with gut GVH disease present with abdominal pain, nausea, and vomiting or diarrhea. The physical

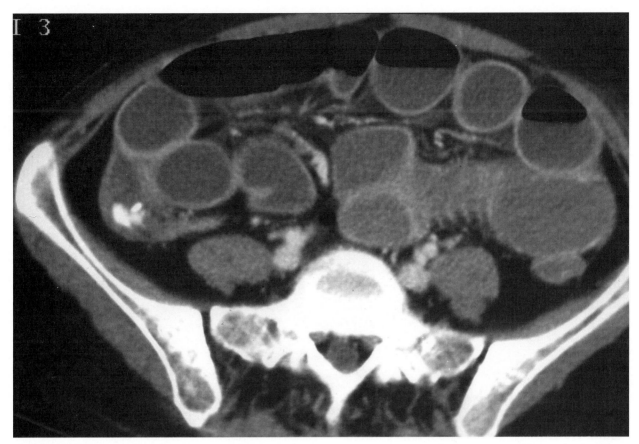

FIGURE 136–1. Radiologic appearance of advanced acute graft-versus-host disease in the gut. Computed tomographic scan showing dilatated loops of small bowel with thickened walls and air-fluid levels.

examination or history may reveal rash or serum elevations in the alkaline phosphatase and direct bilirubin that are consistent with GVH disease involvement of the skin and liver. Initially, the rash involves the hands, feet, and ears. It initially may resemble a drug-related eruption, but as the GVH disease progresses, it becomes confluent and, in severe cases, leads to blisters. The abdominal pain seen in gut GVH disease usually is severe. It often is associated with cramping, requiring narcotics for control of the pain. Nausea and vomiting may indicate gastric involvement, whereas diarrhea suggests small bowel or colonic involvement. A secretory diarrhea, at times in excess of 3 L/d, represents defects in salt and water resorption in the distal small bowel and colon. Careful attention to fluid and electrolyte replacement is required, especially in small children. When mucosal sloughing is present in the most severe form of gut GVH disease, the diarrhea may be described as "stringy" and composed of protein exudates. Acute GVH disease is graded by several clinical criteria, one of which is the volume of diarrhea. Volumes less than 500 cc/d usually are associated with grade 1, whereas those in excess of 1500 cc are characteristic of grade 3 GVH disease. Significant GI blood loss may result from mucosal ulceration associated with GVH disease and, as mentioned, is associated with a poor prognosis. Abdominal

bloating, gastroparesis, and gastroileitis may occur and are indicative of severe injury. Abdominal radiography may show dilatation of the small bowel with air-fluid levels. A characteristic "ribbon sign" observed on computed tomography of the abdomen reflects widespread mucosal edema, small bowel dilatation, and loss of normal gut topography (Figures 136–1 and 136–2). Because of the gut denudation, these patients are at extreme risk for disseminated bacterial infection. Most groups treat such patients with empirical antibiotic coverage for gram-negative and anaerobic organisms.

Histologic Diagnosis

The diagnosis of GVH disease must be made by histology. Thrombocytopenia may dissuade the endoscopist from obtaining biopsies of the mucosa, but biopsies probably can be safely obtained if platelet counts are over 50,000/mm^2. The endoscopic appearance of the gastric or intestinal mucosa may be normal or demonstrate nonspecific erythema or edema. In more advanced cases, ulceration that progresses to frank mucosal sloughing can be seen. Histology of the gastric mucosa demonstrates apoptotic cells, or in the intestinal mucosa, apoptotic cells within the crypt epithelium, vanishing crypts, and sometimes crypt abcesses (Figure 136–3). A lymphocytic infiltration of the lamina propria usually is present. Antral

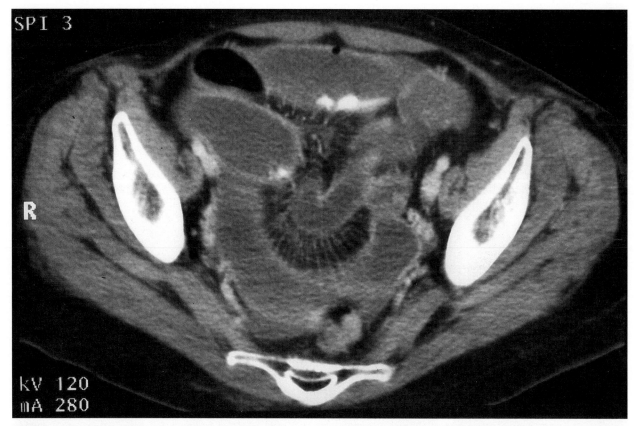

FIGURE 136–2. Computed tomographic scan showing thickened bowel wall, fluid accumulation, and mesenteric changes.

biopsies correlate well with the severity of GVH disease in the duodenum and the colon, even if the presenting symptom is diarrhea. However, since CMV and other infections may coexist with acute GVH disease, evaluation of the colon is extremely important in patients with diarrhea.

Management

Treatment of acute GVH disease consists of increasing immunosuppressive therapy. All patients, except for recipients of markedly lymphocyte-depleted grafts, are started on prophylactic cyclosporine or Tacrolimus at the time of the SCT. If GVH disease occurs, patients usually receive solumedrol 2 mg/kg/d intravenously, initially for 3 to 7 days, and then are placed on a steroid taper. Oral *beclomethasone*, a topically active steroid, when used in conjunction with oral prednisone or intravenous prednisolone has been reported to improve anorexia, nausea, vomiting, and diarrhea in patients with intestinal GVH disease. If there is no improvement on steroids, repeat endoscopy and biopsy should be considered before second-line treatment is initiated, because the risk of opportunistic infection is high. Also, in patients with severe gut damage from GVH disease, extensive mucosal injury certainly will require weeks to heal, during which time diarrhea may persist. Unfortunately, most immunosuppressive agents are associated with an increased risk of opportunistic infection, and GVH disease itself is

immunosuppressive. Investigational drugs directed at controlling cytokine-induced effects, include pentostatin, anti-IL2, and anti-TNF-α. Salvage therapy in GVH disease has been disappointing.

Diarrhea Management

The control of symptomatic diarrhea can be difficult in these patients. Antidiarrheal agents initiated at high doses often are ineffective in reducing the volume of diarrhea. In a nonrandomized pilot study, octreotide at 500 µg intravenously every 8 hours for 7 days has been reported to induce complete resolution of diarrhea in 71 percent of patients with grade 3 or 4 GVH disease. Patients were treated with an intense immunosuppressive regimen simultaneously. The high rate of response was attributed in part to the early initiation of therapy. Octreotide is thought to act by stimulating water and electrolyte absorption, a process that can take place only if the gut epithelium has not sloughed. A possible complication of octreotide used long term is gallbladder stasis and predisposition to gallstone formation.

Chronic Graft-Versus-Host Disease

Chronic GVH disease affects 40 percent of patients surviving to day 100 post-transplant. Chronic GVH disease affects skin, liver, eyes, mouth, and gut, and the clinical manifestations differ from those seen in acute GVH

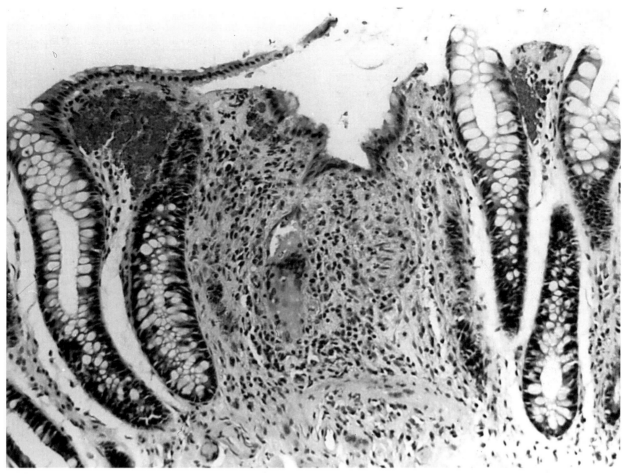

FIGURE 136–3. Histologic appearance of graft-versus-host disease in the sigmoid colon. Apoptotic cells and vanishing crypts are characteristic features.

disease. Chronic GVH disease arises from a dysregulation in autoimmunity, similar to that seen in collagen-vascular disease, which it clinically resembles. Damage to the thymus may predispose to development of autoreactive cells.

Chronic GVH disease of the gut most commonly presents with anorexia, cachexia, nausea, and vomiting. Oral involvement with chronic GVH disease is one of the most common manifestations. Patients may have extensive leukoplakia, ulceration, and dysphagia. Secondary viral and fungal infections are common and often present with an increase in pain without a clinically significant change in appearance of the mouth. Besides treatments of oral infection, treatment of isolated oral GVH disease should start with local therapy. In many cases, decadron swishes will contain the process. Liquid cyclosporine swishes, intraoral psoralen plus ultraviolet A (PUVA), and intralesional injection with steroids also have been used alone or in conjunction with systemic therapy for patients with multisystem disease.

Late post-transplant diarrhea often is ascribed to chronic GVH disease. In the current era of lymphocyte depletion and immunosuppression, actual active gut involvement is rare. However, infection and drug-induced inflammation, particularly that attributable to mefetil, occur frequently and should be sought aggressively. Malabsorption from pancreatic enzyme deficiency also may present following transplantation, because TBI has been noted to induce chronic pancreatitis. As in the case of diarrhea immediately following transplantation, ascertaining an etiology of malabsorption is the first step in treatment.

Oral chronic GVH disease may contribute to the anorexia and weight loss because it may cause ageusia, difficulty swallowing, and an inability to open the mouth. Anorexia and weight loss also may be mediated in part by high levels of circulating TNF-α, but it is important to exclude structural and functional abnormalities of the gut. Patients may have scleroderma-like gut involvement and present with esophageal, gastric, and small bowel dysmotility secondary to submucosal fibrosis, esophageal reflux, and proximal esophageal web formation. Small bowel strictures may lead to delayed small bowel transit, bacterial overgrowth, and steatorrhea. Biopsies may show changes suggestive of inactive inflammatory disease and usually do not possess the pronounced inflammatory infiltrate seen in acute GVH disease. Focal fibrosis in the submucosa and in the serosa may occur. Biopsy of gut mucosa is not as informative in acute GVH disease, and, therefore, barium studies may prove more useful.

Esophageal webs and strictures respond to endoscopic dilatation. Systemic treatment thus far has been aimed primarily at the skin manifestations, which commonly include joint contractures, hypo- and hyperpigmentation, and sclerodermatous changes. Administration of anti-TNF-α antibody, as is used in rheumatoid arthritis and Crohn's disease, may one day prove effective in treating some of the GI symptoms related to chronic GVH disease. Increasing immunosuppression to address the skin and oral changes may likewise improve the GI disease.

Supplemental Reading

Abbott B, Ippoliti C, Bruton J, et al. Antiemetic efficacy of granisetron plus dexamethasone in bone marrow transplant patients receiving chemotherapy and total body irradiation. Bone Marrow Transplant 1999;23:265–9.

Bilgrami S, Feingold J, Dorsky D, et al. Incidence and outcome of *Clostridium difficile* infection following autologous peripheral blood stem cell transplant. Bone Marrow Transplant 1999;23:1039–42.

Cox GJ, Matsui SM, Lo RS, et al. Etiology and outcome of diarrhea after marrow transplantation: a prospective study. Gastroenterology 1994;107:1398–407.

David DS, Tegtmeier BR, O'Donnell MR, et al. Visceral varicella-zoster after bone marrow transplantation: report of a case series and review of the literature. Am J Gastroenterol 1998;93:810–3.

Ippoliti C, Champlin R, Bugazia N, et al. Use of octreotide in the symptomatic management of diarrhea induced by graft-versus-host disease in patients with hematologic malignancies. J Clin Oncol 1997;15:3350–4.

McDonald GB, Bouvier M, Hockenberry DM, et al. Oral beclomethasone dipropionate for treatment of intestinal graft-versus-host disease: a randomized, controlled trial. Gastroenterology 1998;115:28–35.

Nevo S, Enger C, Swan V, et al. Acute bleeding after allogeneic bone marrow transplantation: association with graft-versus-host disease and effect on survival. Transplantation 1999;67:681–9.

Ponec R, Hackman R, McDonald G. Endoscopic and histologic diagnosis of intestinal graft-versus-host disease after marrow transplantation. Gastrointest Endosc 1999;49:612–21.

Snover D. Graft-versus-host disease of the gastrointestinal tract. Am J Surg Pathol 1990;14:101–8.

Song H, Kreisel D, Canter R, et al. Changing presentation and management of neutropenic enterocolitis. Arch Surg 1998;133:979–82.

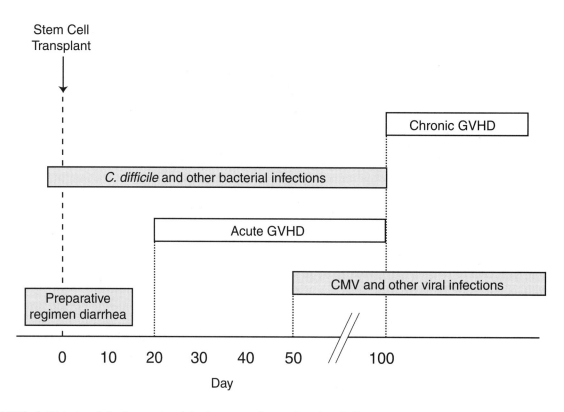

FIGURE 136–4 Etiologies of diarrhea on days following stem-cell transplantation. CMV most commonly occurs around day 50, but may present as early as day 30. Day 100 separates acute GvHD from chronic GvHD, although they are in fact distinct pathologic entities.

CHAPTER 137

BEHÇET'S DISEASE

DAVID B. HELLMANN, MD

In 1937, Dr. Hulusi Behçet, a Turkish dermatologist, described the syndrome that bears his name as a triad of recurrent mouth ulcers, genital ulcers, and eye inflammation. Although these features are among the most salient, Behçet's disease is now known to be an inflammatory disorder of unknown cause that can affect multiple organ systems, including the gastrointestinal (GI) tract. The disease most commonly affects people living along the ancient Silk Route, which includes Japan, Korea, Iran, Saudi Arabia, Turkey, and Greece. The disease is 100 times less common in the United States of America, where only 1 of 500,000 people is affected. Most patients develop the disease in their twenties and thirties, but some present during childhood. Whether the disease predominates in men or women varies from country to country. In the author's experience, chiefly with American patients, women more commonly are affected than men.

Pathogenesis

Although the cause of Behçet's disease is not known, genetic and environmental factors appear to influence the expression of the disease. In Asia, up to 80 percent of patients with Behçet's disease have the human leukocyte antigen (HLA)-B51 allele. The prevalence of this allele is much reduced in Americans with Behçet's disease. The observation that Behçet's disease rarely develops in Japanese who have immigrated to Hawaii suggests that environmental factors are involved in pathogenesis. The frequent finding of vasculitis in lesions of Behçet's disease and the demonstration of overactive neutrophils in patients with this disorder indicate why Behçet's disease often is considered to be an autoimmune disorder.

Diagnosis and Clinical Features

Since no single symptom, finding, or laboratory test is pathognomonic, the diagnosis of Behçet's disease depends on the patient meeting a set of established clinical criteria (Table 137–1). The pathergy phenomenon, development of sterile pustules 24 to 48 hours following a skin prick with a sterile needle, is a much less helpful criterion in Americans who, in contrast to Turkish patients, rarely demonstrate this reaction. The criteria for the diagnosis of Behçet's disease are not an exhaustive list of the clinical features seen in the disorder.

Additional features seen in some patients include gastrointestinal disease, peripheral arthritis (usually nondeforming, oligoarticular, large joint, and asymmetric), sacroiliitis, epididymitis, thrombophlebitis (may be migratory), or large vessel vasculitis (occasionally with bruit, stenosis, or rupture). Although oral lesions are the most frequent presenting symptoms, disability most often results from, in descending order of frequency, uveitis (causing blindness), central nervous system (CNS) disease (causing stroke and dementia), and GI disease.

Gastrointestinal Disease

Approximately 10 to 25 percent of patients with Behçet's disease develop GI involvement. Gastrointestinal Behçet's disease is important because patients who have it often are acutely ill, have a worse prognosis than patients without

TABLE 137–1. Criteria for the Diagnosis of Behçet's Disease*

Finding	Description
Recurrent oral ulceration	Minor aphthous, major aphthous, or herpetiform ulcers observed by the physician or patient that have recurred at least three times over one 12-month period
Recurrent genital ulceration	Aphthous ulceration or scarring observed by physician or patient
Eye lesions	Anterior uveitis, posterior uveitis, or cells in the vitreous on slit-lamp examination; or retinal vasculitis detected by an ophthalmologist
Skin lesions	Erythema nodosum observed by the physician or patient, pseudofolliculitis, or papulopustular lesions; or acneiform nodules observed by the physician in a postadolescent patient who is not receiving corticosteroids
Positive pathergy	Test interpreted as positive by the physician at 24 to 48 hours (see text)

*For the diagnosis to be made, a patient must have recurrent oral ulceration plus at least two of the other findings in the absence of other clinical explanations. (Reproduced with modification from Sakane T, Tekeno M, Suzuki N, Inaba G. Behçet's disease. N Engl J Med 1999;341:1284–91.

TABLE 137–2. Distinguishing between Behçet's Disease and Inflammatory Bowel Disease

Features	Comment
Recurrent oral ulcers, genital ulcers (more common in Behçet's), peripheral arthritis, spondylitis, thrombophlebitis, anterior uveitis, erythema nodosum	Common to both
Posterior uveitis	Favors Behçet's disease
Meningoencephalitis and pathergy phenomenon	Unique to Behçet's disease (pathergy rare in Western Caucasians)
HLA-B51	Favors Behçet's disease
Ileocecal predominance of ulcers	Favors Behçet's disease
Few but large ulcers of the colon	Favors Behçet's disease
Granulomatous inflammation of gut	Unique to Crohn's disease

HLA = human leukocyte antigen

GI involvement, and usually require chronic therapy. With regard to the timing, GI involvement may be evident when Behçet's disease is first diagnosed or, more typically, may emerge a year or more later. Gastrointestinal Behçet's disease even has been seen to develop as many as 10 years after the initial oral and genital ulcers. Most patients with GI Behçet's disease also have active disease in other organ systems. Some patients with previous multisystem Behçet's disease present with isolated GI disease.

Behçet's disease can affect any portion of the GI tract, from the mouth to the anus, and therefore, can present in a wide variety of ways. Gastrointestinal Behçet's disease most commonly presents as aphthous ulcers that preferentially involve the ileum and cecum. At least 75 percent of patients with GI Behçet's disease have lesions in these areas. Ulcers occur less commonly in the descending, transverse, and ascending colon; rectal lesions occur infrequently. Aphthous ulcers of the esophagus, stomach, and small bowel, although rarely described in people living along the Silk Route, are not so rare among American patients. The pathology of these ulcers is nonspecific. In addition to causing ulcers of the GI tract, Behçet's disease can cause arteritis that can result in rupture of an abdominal aneurysm or in bowel ischemia. Behçet's disease is one of the few forms of vasculitis that also can involve large veins, which explains why some patients with Behçet's disease develop hepatic vein thrombosis leading to the Budd-Chiari syndrome.

The most frequently noted symptoms of Behçet's disease of the bowel are abdominal pain, anorexia, rectal bleeding, vomiting, and diarrhea. Given the predilection for ileocecal involvement, it is not surprising that as many as 20 percent of patients with GI Behçet's disease initially are thought to have appendicitis. Constipation can signal inflammation or stricture formation in the ileocecal area. Vomiting is more frequent with small bowel involvement. Weight loss of 5 to 10 kg can occur, testifying both to the sometimes insidious nature of the disease and to the challenge of making the diagnosis. Behçet's disease of the esophagus usually presents with odynophagia, and stricture formation in the esophagus can result in severe dysphagia and regurgitation.

The physical examination and laboratory tests are nonspecific. Fever is common and usually low grade. The patient may or may not have active disease in other tissues, such as the skin, eye, or mouth. Abdominal tenderness usually is mild (especially in patients already on prednisone) and most often develops in the right lower quadrant. Peritoneal signs are absent unless perforation has occurred. Anemia, mild leukocytosis, and an elevated erythrocyte sedimentation rate typically are present. Patients with ileocecal disease show signs of localized edema and thickening of the bowel on computed tomography. Colonoscopy usually reveals aphthous ulcers in the ileocecal area. Other areas of involvement, such as the esophagus, also appear ulcerated on endoscopy.

Behçet's Disease versus Inflammatory Bowel Disease

Distinguishing Behçet's disease from inflammatory bowel disease, especially Crohn's disease, often is difficult and sometimes is impossible. Both disorders share many extra-intestinal features (Table 137–2), including inflammation of the mucous membranes, skin, eye, and joints. Only neurologic disease and pathergy phenomenon, which is uncommon in Americans with Behçet's disease, are unique to Behçet's disease. The GI pathology of Behçet's disease is not specific and can mimic Crohn's disease or ulcerative colitis. The presence of granulomatous inflammation excludes Behçet's disease, whereas other clinical and pathologic features can be indicative of the diagnosis of Behçet's disease. Pathologists studying both Asian patients with Behçet's syndrome and American patients with Crohn's disease believe that there are subtle pathologic differences between the two illnesses.

Treatment

From a therapeutic standpoint, distinguishing GI Behçet's disease from inflammatory bowel disease is not crucial, because the medical treatments are similar. The few controlled trials in Behçet's disease that have been published have concerned either non-GI manifestations of Behçet's disease, such as uveitis, or multisystem Behçet's disease. No known trial has specifically evaluated the treatment of GI Behçet's disease.

Corticosteroids

Prednisone is the cornerstone of therapy for any severe inflammation in Behçet's disease, including GI disease. Initially, prednisone, 0.8 mg/kg/d, or about 60 mg/d in the average adult, is prescribed. Since the efficacy of corticosteroids is a function of the frequency of their administration, 30 mg is given twice daily for the sickest patients for 1 to 2 weeks before converting to a single daily dose. For those with upper GI involvement in whom swallowing is difficult and absorption is suspect, the dose is administered intravenously as methylprednisolone, usually without adjustment for the 20 percent greater potency of methylprednisolone compared with prednisone.

Although Behçet's disease generally is a relapsing and remitting disease, the GI manifestations usually follow a chronic course and require chronic therapy. Therefore, short courses of prednisone are almost never sufficient to achieve remission, and rapid tapering of corticosteroids almost invariably results in a flare. Prednisone is continued at 60 mg/d for 1 month before attempting to reduce the dose by 5 to 10 mg/wk to reach 20 to 30 mg/d by the end of the second month and 10 to 20 mg/d by the end of the third month. The dose is decreased less frequently and by smaller decrements thereafter.

Immunomodulators

Since patients still are apt to flare with this corticosteroid taper, and since most patients cannot tolerate corticosteroids at higher doses for longer periods, the patient usually is switched to immunosuppressive therapy. Clinical trials have established that azathioprine (AZA) is effective in treating various features of severe, albeit extra-intestinal, Behçet's disease. It also has been used successfully in patients with GI disease, beginning with 50 mg/d and increasing the daily dose by 50 mg every 1 to 2 weeks, while checking complete blood counts weekly, until the dose of 1.5 to 2.0 mg/kg is attained. Azathioprine is considered a potential teratogen, so patients must use effective birth control. Catabolism of AZA is reduced by allopurinol so the dose of AZA must be reduced in any patient taking both drugs, and the complete blood count should be monitored even more closely. If the patient tolerates the medication and does well, AZA is continued for 6 to 12 months before trying to taper it by 50 mg every 3 to 4 months. For patients who have recurrent flares, it may be best to continue treating with low doses of AZA (50 mg/d)

TABLE 137–3. Systemic Drug Therapy for Behçet's Disease

Drugs	Comment[*]
Prednisone	Used as cornerstone for all forms of active Behçet's disease
Colchicine	Effective for oral ulcers, genital ulcers
Thalidomide	Effective for oral and genital ulcers
Dapsone	Used for oral ulcers, erythema nodosum
Pentoxifylline	Used for mucocutaneous disease
Azathioprine	Effective for retinal vasculitis and arthritis; used for multi-system Behçet's disease
Chlorambucil	Used for severe eye and CNS disease
Methotrexate	Used for retinal and CNS vasculitis
Cyclosporine	Effective for retinal vasculitis
Interferon-alfa	Used for retinal vasculitis, arthritis, and mucocutaneous disease

*Effective indicates that the use is supported by clinical trials. CNS = central nervous system.
Adapted from Sakane T, Tekeno M, Suzuki N, Inaba G. Behçet's disease. N Engl J Med 1999;341:1284–91.

and low doses of prednisone (10 mg/d) or on alternate days indefinitely.

Most authorities also recommend adding sulfasalazine (1.0 to 2.0 g twice daily) for Behçet's disease that mimics inflammatory bowel disease. The slow-release forms of mesalamine (Pentasa®, Ferring-Shire Pharmaceuticals Inc., Florence, Kentucky, 750 mg to 1 g 3 times a day) are effective and well-tolerated alternatives. Thus, a combination of prednisone, AZA, and sulfasalazine (or substitute) is used for most patients with GI Behçet's disease.

The role of antibiotics, such as metronidazole (250 mg orally twice a day), has not been defined. Patients with extensive disease or resection of the ileum may require bowel rest and total parental nutrition, and eventually will need vitamin B_{12} replacement. All patients treated with prednisone should also be started on measures to prevent or lessen osteoporosis (such as calcium 1,500 mg/d and vitamin D 800 IU/d).

Other therapeutic choices in Behçet's disease are listed in Table 137–3. Colchicine has been effective chiefly for treating mucocutaneous disease. Since it has GI toxicity, most rheumatologists do not use it in patients with GI involvement. Thalidomide also has substantial toxicity and is known to be effective only for mucocutaneous disease. Whereas cyclosporine has been shown to be of help in ulcerative colitis, its established efficacy in Behçet's disease is limited to eye disease. Anecdotal reports and small studies suggest that methotrexate and interferon may be effective in some patients with Behçet's disease. Tumor necrosis factor (TNF) levels are elevated in Behçet's disease, so inhibitors of TNF may soon undergo evaluation. Pentoxifylline (Trental 400 mg each day) has benefited a small group of patients with multisystem Behçet's disease.

Although this agent's efficacy for GI disease is unknown, it is so well tolerated that it can be added for patients with active Behçet's disease of any form.

When medical therapy fails and the patient's bowel perforates, surgical resection is required. Unfortunately, there is a high rate of breakdown at the anastomosis. In addition, ulcers often recur and stricturing may develop.

Editor's Note

As the author describes, differentiation between Behçet's disease and Crohn's disease can be difficult. These patients often are treated for Crohn's disease with variations based on experience with Behçet's disease. The recent review by Sakane and colleagues (1999) is helpful. (TMB)

Reference

Sakane T, Tekeno M, Suzuki N, Inaba G. Behçet's disease. N Engl J Med 1999;341:1284–91.

Supplemental Reading

Frassanito MA, Dammacco R, Cafforio P, Dammacco F. Th1 polarization of the immune response in Behçet's disease. A putative pathogenetic role of interleukin-12. Arthritis Rheum 1999;42:1967–74.

Griffen JW Jr, Harrison HB, Tedesco FJ, et al. Behçet's disease with multiple sites of gastrointestinal involvement. South Med J 1982;75:1405–8.

Hamuryudan V, Özyazgan Y, Hizli N, et al. Azathioprine in Behçet's syndrome: effects on long-term prognosis. Arthritis Rheum 1997;40:769–74.

Kaklamani VG, Variopoulos G, Kaklamanis PG. Behçet's disease. Semin Arthritis Rheum 1998;27:197–217.

Kasahara Y, Tanaka S, Nishino M, et al. Intestinal involvement in Behçet's disease: review of 136 surgical cases in the Japanese literature. Dis Col Rectum 1981;24:103–6.

Masuda K, Nakajima A, Urayama A, et al. Double-masked trial of cyclosporin versus colchicine and long-term open study of cyclosporin in Behçet's disease. Lancet 1989;1:1093–6.

Mizuki N, Ota M, Katsuyama Y, et al. Association analysis between the MIC-A and HLA-B alleles in Japanese patients with Behçet's disease. Arthritis Rheum 1999;42:1961–6.

Mori S, Yoshihira A, Kawamura H, et al. Esophageal involvement in Behçet's disease. Am J Gastroenterol 1983;78:548–53.

O'Duffy JD, Calamia K, Cohen S, et al. Interferon-alpha treatment of Behçet's disease. J Rheumatol 1998;25:1938–44.

Shimizu T, Ehrlich G, Inaba G, Hayashi K. Behçet disease. Semin Arthritis Rheum 1979;8:223–60.

Yasui K, Ohta K, Kobayashi M, et al. Successful treatment of Behçet disease with pentoxifylline. Ann Intern Med 1996;124:891–3.

Yim CW, White RH. Behçet's syndrome in a family with inflammatory bowel disease. Arch Intern Med 1985;145:1047–50.

CHAPTER 138

THERAPY OF ULCERATIVE JEJUNOILEITIS

KONRAD H. SOERGEL, MD

Ulcerative jejunoileitis is a descriptive term that includes several poorly understood entities. Similar or identical cases have been published under the diagnosis of **chronic nongranulomatous ulcerative jejunoileitis** or **enterocolitis, unclassified sprue,** and **resistant sprue.**

If the clinical presentation of the disease is acute or life-threatening, prompt supportive measures take precedence over prolonged diagnostic studies. It is critical to determine whether a treatable primary disease is present. Conditions for which ulcerative jejunoileitis represents a complication of advancing disease include **intestinal lymphoma, celiac sprue,** and **hypogammaglobulinemia.** No associated condition and no exogenous cause, such as acquired immunodeficiency syndrome or nonsteroidal anti-inflammatory drug (NSAID) enteropathy, are present in 50 percent of cases. This entity has been termed **nongranulomatous chronic idiopathic enterocolitis** (NCIEC). Compared to patients with an underlying disease, those with idiopathic disease have a lower incidence of deep ulcerations and stricture formation (31% vs 64%) and intestinal perforation (16% vs 33%). In addition, patients with NCIEC may show delayed appearance of intestinal ulcerations. The colorectum is grossly inflamed in one-half of these patients. Nongranulomatous chronic idiopathic enterocolitis manifests with large-volume secretory diarrhea (mean stool weight: 4,425 g/d), malabsorption, and intestinal protein wasting. Colicky abdominal pain and vomiting with a diffusely dilatated, fluid-filled small bowel may be present initially and mimic ileal obstruction. The diagnostic hallmark of NCIEC is intense acute and chronic inflammation of the lamina propria and mucosa with varying degrees of villous atrophy but normal cytologic features of the enterocytes. Antibodies to gliadin, endomysium, and reticulin are absent.

Supportive Management

Parenteral hydration is provided without delay and admission to an intensive care unit may be necessary, owing to rapid changes in daily fluid losses per rectum and by vomiting. Fasting results in a 50 to 60 percent decrease in stool output; however, the authors have noted that 7 of 11 patients with NCIEC still produce daily stool volumes in excess of 1.5 L while receiving nothing by mouth. Total parenteral nutrition is required by the majority of patients, particularly in view of excessive intestinal protein losses. Opiate-type antidiarrheals, such as loperamide and codeine, as well as octreotide, have little or no effect. Intestinal perforation and bleeding, although rare in NCIEC, are feared complications and account for most of the early mortality rate of 50 percent in patients with underlying diseases. Emergency laparotomy is unavoidable in case of perforation. Massive gastrointestinal bleeding can arise from anywhere in the intestinal tract. Emergency endoscopy may identify bleeding sites in the duodenum or colorectum that can be treated endoscopically.

Therapy

Treatment of the disease depends only partly on the presence and type of an underlying cause. Options are limited. In patients with celiac sprue, a gluten-free diet will already have been instituted at the time of diagnosis. The diet either was ineffective from the start or the initial response was not maintained. In any event, most patients are not eating, and a de novo diagnosis of celiac sprue is difficult to establish in patients presenting with diffuse intestinal inflammation. In patients with intestinal lymphoma, chemotherapy and radiation therapy may damage the intestinal mucosa further and aggravate the diarrhea.

The treatment of choice for NCIEC is corticosteroids, orally or parenterally, in a dose of 40 to 60 mg/d of prednisone or its equivalent. In the study the authors conducted, 10 of 11 patients with this disease responded dramatically within days. Without any controlled therapeutic studies, this is the recommended treatment for all patients with ulcerative jejunoileitis. According to the literature, the response rate is about 50 percent in patients with an underlying condition. Further, several conditions that may be difficult to differentiate, such as autoimmune enteropathy and cryptogenic multifocal ulcerous stenotic enteritis, also are steroid responsive. By contrast, 5-aminosalicylic acid, cyclosporin A, metronidazole, ciprofloxacin, and doxycycline had no effect when each was given to two or three patients.

Maintenance Therapy

Patients with the idiopathic form of disease, NCIEC, tend to relapse after corticosteroid therapy has been discontinued. The authors have noted that the time to relapse ranges from weeks to 28 years and that, to date, all relapses have responded promptly to reinstitution of steroid therapy. In patients with NCIEC, prednisone was tapered to 10 mg/d a few weeks after clinical response had occurred and discontinued 3 to 6 months later. When relapses occurred early, maintenance therapy at 5 to 15 mg/d of prednisone was used. Four of eight surviving patients with NCIEC currently are receiving maintenance therapy.

Editor's Notes

As described, ulcerative jejunoileitis may describe various disorders. The patients described in the study seemingly had celiac disease and then developed multiple ulcerations, or had an unresponsive atypical malabsorption syndrome with ulcerations. Some experienced perforation and died while being treated with steroids. Others went on to develop T-cell lymphoma. As mentioned in the chapter on Crohn's jejunoileitis, a number of patients with malabsorption and multiple small bowel ulcers are referred to us. Among these patients are those who (1) have Crohn's disease; (2) are taking NSAIDs; (3) have lymphoma, including angiocentric lymphoma that causes an ischemic lesion; or (4) have nongranulomatous ulcerative jejunoileitis, some of whom have celiac disease. (TMB)

Supplemental Reading

Baer AN, Bayless TM, Yardley JH. Intestinal ulceration and malabsorption syndromes. Gastroenterology 1980;79:754–65.

Bayless TM, Kapelowitz RF, Shelley WM, et al. Intestinal ulceration: a complication of celiac disease. N Engl J Med 1967;276:996–1002.

Case Records of Massachusetts General Hospital. N Engl J Med 1999;341:1536–7.

Ruan EA, Komorowski RA, Hogan WJ, Soergel KH. Nongranulomatous chronic idiopathic enterocolitis: clinicopathologic profile and response to corticosteroids. Gastroenterology 1996;111:629–37.

Soergel KH. Nongranulomatous chronic idiopathic enterocolitis: a primary histologically defined disease. Dig Dis Sci 2000; in press.

INDEX

Abdominal sepsis, 203
Abscesses, 50, 61, 504
ADA. *See* American Disabilities Act
Addiction, 596
Adenoma-like masses, 261
Adherence, 9–11
Adhesion molecules, 37–38
Adolescents
    consultations, 23
    Crohn's disease in, 411, 415–19
    family-doctor interactions, 5–7
    growth impairment and enteral nutrition, 411
    with inflammatory bowel disease, 545, 562
    lifestyle issues, 532
    managing concerns, 528
    ulcerative colitis in, 155
Adrenocorticoids, 632–33
Advancement rectal flap, 517
Age, 204, 334, 337, 555
Agreeableness, 579
Allergic reactions, 375
Alternative medicine, 163–64, 552, 603–6
Amebic colitis, 95
American Disabilities Act (ADA), 558
Aminosalicylates, 66–67, 69, 145
    for children, 416
    for collagenous and lymphocytic colitis, 632
    compared to other agents, 348–49
    in Crohn's disease, 347–51, 416, 467–68
    for fistulae, 396
    for jejunoileitis, 426
    pharmcokinetics of, 347
    in pouchitis, 220–21
    and pregnancy, 608
    side effects, 350
    to spare corticosteroid use, 365
    in ulcerative colitis, 123–25
Amyloidosis, 270
Analgesics
    for arthritis, 281
    narcotic medications for pain, 590
Anal mucosectomy, 199–200
Anal stricture, 204
Anastomotic leak, 192, 210
Anemia, 269, 325–26, 626, 642
Anorectal stricture, 506
Anterior uveitis, 275, 276
Antibiotics, 145, 149–51

for children, 416
for Crohn's disease, 355–56, 359–62, 416, 435–36
for pouchitis, 220
in pregnancy, 608, 616–17
to spare corticosteroid use, 365
See also specific types
Anticonvulsants, 596
Anticytokine therapy, 389–92
Anti-infectious agents, 149–51
Anti-inflammatory agents, 63–67
Anti-tumor necrosis factor-alpha, 366
Anxiety, 574–75, 588–89
Aphthous stomatitis, 273, 641
Arthritis, 267–68, 279–82
Avascular necrosis of bone. *See* Ischemic necrosis of bone
Axial arthritis, 268, 279, 281
Azathioprine
    for children, 416–17
    for Crohn's disease, 134–36, 353–55, 373–76, 416–17, 436
    for distal colitis, 85, 103, 105, 106
    for fistulae, 397, 402–3
    for ileitis and ileocolitis, 339–40
    metabolism in inflammatory bowel disease, 377–80
    in pregnancy, 376, 617
    for sclerosing cholangitis, 301
    to spare corticosteroid use, 365
    for ulcerative colitis, 134–36, 139–41, 145

Bacterial cholangitis, 300
Balloon dilation, 510–11, 512
Barium studies, 24, 39–40
Beclomethasone dipropionate, 74
Behavior
    healthy, 584
    perspective, 579–80
    therapy, 589–90
Behçet's disease, 655–57
Bicarbonate, 482
Bilary tract infection, 314
Bile acid, 472, 474
Bile duct, 299–302
Biliary tract disease, 330
Biofeedback, 580, 588–89
Biologics, 285–86, 432–33
Biopsy
    colorectal, 631
    core decompression, 296–97

dysplasia, 259, 261
pouch, 230–31
Bismuth carbomer, 108, 222
Bisphosphonates, 291–92
Bleeding
    gastrointestinal, 325–26, 650
    from ileostomy, 188
    rectal, 83
    See also Hemorrhage
Blood coagulation, 326–27
Body image, 561–63
Bone marrow pressure, 296
Bone(s)
    ishchemic necrosis of, 293–97
    metabolic disease, 300
    mineral density, 249, 418
    and peripheral arthritis, 267–68
Bowel
    excessive movements, 209–13
    excluded, 519–21
    laparoscopically-assisted resection, 453–55
    obstruction, 200
    strictures, 59, 61
Bowel rest
    in Crohn's disease, 344–45
    and fistulae, 402, 407
    importance of, 410–11
    for jejunoileitis, 426
    and parenteral nutrition, 402, 405–8
    physiologic effects of, 405–6
    in ulcerative colitis, 145
Brooke ileostomy, 173, 176, 185–89
Brush cytology, 312–13
Budesonide, 339, 367–70
    combination therapy, 369–70
    in inflammatory bowel disease, 364–65
    long-term safety, 370
    maintenance therapy, 356, 370
    for ulcerative colitis, 74, 75
    versus standard steroid regimens, 368–69

Caffeine, 93
Calcitonin, 291
Calcium, 290, 481–82, 548
Calcium oxalate stones, 321
Calories, 548
Campylobacter jejuni, 96, 129–30
Cancer
    colorectal, 358, 496, 552–53
    and Crohn's colitis, 496
    and Crohn's disease, 50–51, 447
    dysplasia surveillance, 251–64
    and ileal pouch-anal anastomosis, 206
    and ileorectal anastomosis, 238
    neoplasms, 375–76
    prevention, 257–61
    renal cell carcinoma, 323
    and ulcerative colitis, 121, 205–6
Candidiasis, 183
Cannon, Walter B., 583–84

Carbomers, 108
Cataracts, 275
Catheter, 483
CCFA. *See* Crohn's and Colitis Foundation of America
CD. *See* Crohn's disease
Cecal disease, 497
Celiac disease, 646
Chemoradiotherapy, 313
Children
    Crohn's disease in, 247–48, 412, 415–19
    enteral nutrition, 412
    ileoanal pouch surgery, 215–18
    with inflammatory bowel disease, 5–7, 245–49, 543–45, 562
    lifestyle issues, 532
    managing concerns, 528
    nutrition for, 246–48, 417–18
    preparing for tests and procedures, 6–7
    and surgery, 215–18, 419
    ulcerative colitis in, 153–55
    See also Adolescents
Cholangiocarcinoma, 300, 306–8, 311–15
Cholangitis. *See* Sclerosing cholangitis
Chronic infectious colitides, 95–96
Chronic pain syndrome, 587–88
Chronic ulcerative colitis, 41
Ciprofloxacin, 360, 361, 397, 416, 435–36
Clarithromycin, 360–61
Clergy, 565–67
Clinical guidelines, 15–16
Closed loop obstruction, 445–46
Clostridium difficile, 96–97, 119, 149, 150, 620
Closure of ileostomy, 203–4
CMV. *See* Cytomegalovirus
Coagulation, 326–27
COBRA. *See* Consolidated Omnibus Budget Reconciliation Act
Colchicine, 301
Colectomy, 175–78, 197, 199, 440, 633
Colectomy and ileorectostomy, 173
Colitis
    cure of, 171–72
    in elderly, 619–22
    extensive with rectal sparing, 497–98
    in immunocompromised patients, 639–43
    mucosal protective and repair agents, 107–9
    See also specific types, e.g., Crohn's colitis
Collagenous colitis, 622, 631–33
Colon, 520–21
Colonic mucosal barrier, 107–9
Colonoscopy
    in Crohn's disease, 263, 357–58
    dysplasia surveillance, 258, 263
Colorectal biopsy, 631
Colorectal cancer, 358, 496, 552–53
Common variable immunodeficiency, 639–43
Compassion, 565–66
Complementary therapies, 603–6
Computed tomography (CT), 47–52, 312
Computer database, 29–33
Confidence, 567
Conscientiousness, 579

Consolidated Omnibus Budget Reconciliation Act (COBRA), 556
Constipation, 83
Consultations, 23–24
Continent ileostomy. *See* Kock pouch
Control, 6
Core decompression biopsy, 296–97
Corticosteroids
  appropriate use in inflammatory bowel disease, 363–66
  for Behçet's disease, 657
  for Crohn's disease, 333–34
  for Crohn's disease in children, 415–16
  for fistulae, 396
  for jejunoileitis, 426
  newer oral preparations, 75–76
  and osteoporosis in inflammatory bowel disease, 289–90
  and pregnancy, 608, 617
  for sclerosing cholangitis, 301
  systemic in inflammatory bowel disease, 127–31
  topically active preparations, 73–76, 367–70
  for ulcerative colitis, 73–76, 120–21, 144–45
  See also Glucocorticosteroids
Costs, 13–14
COX-2. *See* Cyclo-oxygenase 2
Crohn's and Colitis Foundation of America (CCFA), 539–42, 551, 552
Crohn's colitis, 342
  medical therapy for, 429–33
  segmental, 499
  surgery for, 495–99
Crohn's disease (CD)
  adherence issues, 9–11
  5-aminosalicyclic acid for, 347–51, 467–68
  anal and perianal, 441
  antibiotics for, 355–56, 359–62
  anticytokine therapy in, 389–92
  azathioprine and 6-mercaptopurine in, 134–36, 353–55, 373–76
  bowel rest, 405–8
  budesonide versus mesalazine in, 369
  cancer risk in, 263
  childhood, 247–48, 412, 415–19
  clinical questions not answered by control trials, 353–58
  cutaneous, 268–69, 272
  cyclosporine in, 135, 387–88
  diagnosis, 229, 244
  dietary factors, 547
  difference from ulcerative colitis, 551–52
  duodenal, 330
  in elderly, 623
  endoscopic management of strictures in, 509–12
  enteral nutrition, 247, 409–12
  extra-intestinal complications, 51–52
  fistulizing and perforating, 401–4, 435–38, 444, 446, 450
  gastroduodenal, 421–22, 461–63
  imaging, 42–45, 47–52
  intestinal transplantation for, 487–88
  and irritable bowel syndrome, 89
  laparoscopically-assisted bowel resection, 453–55
  measures of activity, 26–27
  medical-surgical collaboration for, 19–20
  methotrexate for, 384
  in ostomy, 188
  pain in, 594
  and patient-doctor interactions, 1–3
  perianal involvement, 501–7
  postoperative recurrence, 437–38, 465–69
  pouches for, 244
  and pregnancy, 613–14
  small bowel, 343–45, 443–47
  surgery for, 439–41, 443–47, 453–69
  therapeutic expectations of medical mangagement, 337–42
  therapeutic implications of subtypes, 333–35
  and transabdominal bowel sonography, 56–61
Crohn's Disease Activity Index, 429, 535
Crohn's jejunoileitis, 425–27
CT. *See* Computed tomography
Cuffitis, 200, 211
Cutaneous Crohn's disease, 268–69, 272
Cyclo-oxygenase 2 (COX-2), 283, 284–85
Cyclosporine
  for children, 417
  for Crohn's colitis, 432
  for Crohn's disease, 135, 387–88, 417, 436
  for distal colitis, 85
  for fistulae, 397–98, 403
  for inflammatory bowel disease, 135
  in pregnancy, 617–18
  for sclerosing cholangitis, 301
  to spare corticosteroid use, 365
  for ulcerative colitis, 120, 141–42, 146
Cytokines, 389–92
Cytomegalovirus (CMV), 96, 97

Dehydration, 600
Delirium, 573
Depression, 570, 573–74
Dermatosis-arthritis syndrome, 273
Diaphragmatic breathing, 585
Diarrhea
  following small bowel resection, 471–74
  Giardia-related, 641
  mechanism of, 631
  miscellaneous etiologies for, 79
  nocturnal, 83
  postcholecystectomy, 93–94
  unrelated to pouches, 213
Diet, 161–64, 181, 480, 552
  for children, 248–49
  elemental as substitute for bowel rest, 407
  exclusion, 163, 411, 547–48
  following small bowel resection, 473–74
  See also Nutrition
Disability programs, 557–58
Disease modifying anti-rheumatoid drugs (DMARDs), 283–84
Distal colitis
  immunomodulators in, 103–6
  management of, 69–70
  refractory, 81–85
Diverticulitis, 621–22

DMARDs. *See* Disease modifying anti-rheumatoid drugs
Doctor(s)
    as care givers, 544
    and denied payments, 16–17
    and late payments, 17–18
    and managed care, 13–18
    medical-surgical collaboration, 19–21
    and pain management, 588
    patient interactions, 1–3
    role in adjustment to disease, 528–29
    as source of information, 543
    surgical referrals, 24
    unionization by, 16
Dominant biliary strictures, 300, 312
D-penicillamine, 301
Drugs. *See* Medication(s)
Duodenal Crohn's disease, 330
Duodenocolic fistula, 404
Duodenum, 519
Dysplasia
    and endoscopy, 226–27
    and ileal pouch-anal anastomosis, 206, 226–27
    and pouchitis, 231–32
    surveillance/prevention, 251–64

Education, 1–2, 7, 540, 543–44, 558
Elderly, 533, 619–22
Electrolytes, 471–72, 477
Emergency kit, 182
Emergency surgery, 445, 499
Emotional needs, 418–19
End-loop modification, 187
Endoscopic balloon dilatation, 422
Endoscopic retrograde cholangiopancreatography (ERCP),
    303, 312, 510
Endoscopic ultrasound, 312
Endoscopy
    for cholangiocarcinoma, 313
    in evaluating ileal pouches, 225–27
    managment of small bowel, anastomotic, and colonic
        strictures in Crohn's disease, 509–12
    for sclerosing cholangitis, 303–4
Entamoeba histolytica, 95, 97
Enteral nutrition, 450, 451, 480
    in Crohn's disease, 247, 409–12
    cyclic, 411
    formula composition, 410
    and growth impairment, 411–12
    supplementary, 411
    in ulcerative colitis, 162, 163
Enteritis, 639–43
Enterostomal therapist, 186
Enterostomal therapy nurse, 179–83, 233
Enterovesical fistula, 322, 404
Epidermolysis bullosa acquisita, 273
Episcleritis, 276
EPO. *See* Recombinant human erythropoietin
ERCP. *See* Endoscopic retrograde cholangiopancreatography
Erythema nodosum, 268, 272
Escherichia coli, 96, 620

Estrogens, 291
Ethics, 14
Evacuation disorders, 200
Excluded bowel, 519–21
Exclusion diet, 163, 411, 547–48
Extroversion-introversion dimension, 578
Eye, 269, 275–76

Faith, 566–67
Family and Medical Leave Act (FMLA), 557
Family therapy, 590
Fats, 473, 480–81
Fecal diversion, 507, 516
Fecal enzymes, 107
Fecal incontinence, 83
Femoral head necrosis, 295
Fertility, 323, 607, 613
Fiber, dietary, 162, 163, 548
Fibrostenotic disease, 341–42
Fight-flight response, 583–84
Finney strictureplasty, 460
Fish oils, 162, 163, 248, 548
Fissures, 395, 503–4
Fistulae
    and bowel rest, 402, 407
    in Crohn's disease, 401–4, 435–38, 444, 446, 450
    CT scanning for, 49–50
    duodenocolic, 404
    enterovesical, 322, 404
    gastrocolic, 404
    ileal pouch, 492–93
    managing enteral, 401–4
    perianal, 395–99, 504–5
    perineal, 323, 492
    peristomal, 188, 492
    postoperative, 491–93
    and pouches, 192, 227
    rectovaginal, 395, 403–4, 438, 505–6, 515–18
    transabdominal bowel sonography for, 57, 59
    trans-valvular, 192
    vulvar, 395
Fistulizing ileitis, 355
Fitness programs, 599–601
Flap repair, 517–18
Fluids
    excessive losses, 479–80, 600
    malabsorption, 471–72, 641
FMLA. *See* Family and Medical Leave Act
Focally enhanced gastritis, 422
Food. *See* Diet; Nutrition

Gallstones, 317–20
Gastrocolic fistulae, 404
Gastroduodenal Crohn's disease, 421–22, 461–63
Gastroenterologist, 3, 24
Gastrointestinal bleeding, 325–26, 650
Gastrointestinal complications, 649–54
Gastrointestinal fistulae, 450
Gastrointestinal tract disease, 643
Genetics, 23, 523–26, 552, 609

Genitourinary tract, 321–23
GETAID Index, 27
Giardia lamblia, 97, 641
Glucocorticoids, 65–66, 84–85, 293–94
Glucocorticosteroids, 344, 367–70
Graft-versus-host disease, 486, 650–54
Growth, 245–46, 248, 411–12
Hartmann closure of rectum, 176
Harvey-Bradshaw (Simple) Index, 26
Health Insurance Portability and Accountabililty Act (HIPAA), 556
Health maintenance organizations. *See* HMOs
Helicobacter pylori, 422, 620, 645
Hematology, 269–70, 325–27
Hemorrhage, 175, 446, 496
Hemorrhoids, 395, 506–7
Heparin, 85, 120, 166
Hepatobiliary disease, 270
Hepatobiliary tract, 51
Hereditary factors. *See* Genetics
Herpes simplex virus, 97
High-risk insurance pools, 556–57
HIPAA. *See* Health Insurance Portability and Accountabililty Act
Histologic ileitis, 230
Histrionic patients, 575–76
HMOs (health maintenance organizations), 13–16
Hydrochlorothiazide, 290
Hyperalimentation, 449
Hypercoagulable state, 269–70
Hyperoxaluria, 475–78
Hypertriglyceridemia, 330
Hypertrophic osteoarthropathy, 268
Hypoalbuminemia, 626–27
Hypochromic anemia, 326

IAPP. *See* Ileoanal pouch procedure
Iatrogenic ureteral injury, 323
IBD. *See* Inflammatory bowel disease
IBS. *See* Irritable bowel syndrome
Ileal pouch-anal canal anastomosis (IPAA)
    and Crohn's disease, 492–93
    endoscopy in evaluating, 226–27
    and excessive bowel movements, 209–13
    long-term results, 203–6
    Mayo Clinic experience, 203–5
    pouch problems, 212–13, 219–22
    and restorative proctocolectomy, 199–201
    for ulcerative colitis, 171–73
Ileal pouch fistula, 492–93
Ileal stenosis, 354–55
Ileitis, 339–40
Ileoanal anastomosis, 93, 177–78, 197–201
Ileoanal pouch procedure (IAPP), 215–18
Ileoanal reservoir surgery, 234
Ileocolitis, 339–40
Ileorectal anastomosis, 237–39, 244
Ileostomy, 176, 197, 199, 203–4, 440
    See also Brooke ileostomy; Kock pouch
Ileum, 519–20

Imaging, 24, 36
    for cholangiocarcinoma, 312
    for ischemic necrosis of bone, 295–96
    of mucosal inflammation, 39–45
    See also specific types, e.g. Computed tomography
Immunocompromised patients, 639–43
Immunomodulators
    for Behçet's disease, 657
    for children, 153, 416–17
    for Crohn's colitis, 432
    for Crohn's disease, 416–17, 436
    for distal colitis, 103–6
    for jejunoileitis, 426
    in pregnancy, 617
    in ulcerative colitis, 139–42, 153
    See also specific types, e.g.
Immunosuppressives, 145–46, 221, 486, 608–9, 646–47
Incontinence, 83, 204, 227, 506
Indeterminate colitis, 119, 157–59
    diagnosis, 229–30
    surgical approaches, 241–44
Individualized therapy, 11
Induction of remission, 1, 111, 125
    methotrexate for, 384
    in small bowel Crohn's disease, 343–44
Inductive agents, 124
Infections, 375, 649–50
    See also specific types
Infectious agents, 95–97
Infectious colitis, 620–21
Infertility. *See* Fertility
Inflammation
    of anal transitional zone, 200
    antibiotics for, 359
    biochemical markers of, 35
    immunologic markers of, 37
    mucosal, 39–45
    radiographic and ultrasonic markers of, 36–37
    role of T cells in, 642
    and tumor necrosis factor, 63–65
Inflammatory bowel disease (IBD)
    adherence issues, 9–11
    anticytokine therapy, 389–90, 392
    arthritis associated with, 279–82
    azathioprine metabolism in, 377–80
    and Behçet's disease, 656
    bone mineral density in, 249
    cancer prevention strategies in, 257–61
    childhood, 5–7, 245–49, 543–45, 562
    and cholangiocarcinoma, 311–15
    and common variable immunodeficiency, 642
    complementary therapy, 603–4
    computer database, 29–33
    consultations, 23–24
    cutaneous manifestations, 271–73
    in elderly, 622–24
    and fertility, 607, 613
    fistulae in, 401–4
    gallstone management in, 317–20
    genetics, 523–26

hematologic problems, 325–27
infectious agents as aggravating factors, 95–97
and irritable bowel syndrome, 79, 87–94
lifestyle issues, 531–33
lymphoma in, 645–48
and managed care, 13–18
managing patients' concerns, 527–29
measures of activity, 25, 27, 35–38
methotrexate in, 383–85
nonsteroidal anti-inflammatory drugs in, 627–29
ocular manifestations, 275–76
osteoporosis and osteopenia with, 289–92
pain in, 588–90, 594–95
pancreatitis in, 329–32
and patient-doctor interactions, 1–3
and pregnancy, 607–10, 613–18
pseudo-intractability of, 77–80
psychological factors, 569–86
and radiation enterocolitis, 635
residual, 211
steroid use in, 127–31, 133–37, 363–66
University of Chicago approach, 20–21
Inflammatory mediator pathways, 165–68
Infliximab
   for Crohn's disease, 136, 340, 357, 436–37
   for fistulae, 398
   in pregnancy, 618
Information
   about complementary therapies, 606
   from Crohn's and Colitis Foundation of America, 539–42
   doctors as source of, 543
   about inflammatory bowel disease, 23, 527
Insurance, 553–58
Integrity, 565
Interleukin-2, 37
Interleukin-6, 37
Interleukin-10, 167
Internet, 234–35, 539–40
Interventional radiology, 313–14
Intestinal inflammation, 359, 412
Intestinal obstruction, 443, 445
Intestinal permeability, 36
Intestinal protein loss, 35–36
Intestinal transplantation, 483, 485–89
Intra-abdominal abscess, 444, 446–47
Intraosseous venography, 296
Intraspinal opioids, 596
Ionizing radiation, 608
IPAA. See Ileal pouch-anal canal anastomosis
Iron deficiency, 269, 325, 482, 548, 626
Irritable bowel syndrome (IBS)
   and Crohn's disease, 337
   following small bowel resection, 472
   and inflammatory bowel disorders, 79, 87–94, 551
   prevalence of, 92
   and ulcerative colitis, 119–21
Ischemia, 192
Ischemic colitis, 621
Ischemic necrosis of bone, 293–97

ISIS 2302 molecule, 167
Itching. See Pruritus

Jejunoileitis, 339, 425–27, 659–60
Jejunum, 519–20
Joints, 267–68, 297

Keratitis, 276
Kidneys, 600
Kock pouch, 93, 176–77, 191–94
   early problems, 192–93
   endoscopy in evaluating, 225–26
   late problems, 193
   patient selection, 192
   postoperative period, 191–92
   technique, 191

Lactose intolerance, 94, 161, 162, 548, 552
Laparoscopy, 440, 453–55
Large intestine, 440
Leflunomide, 284
Legal precedents, 14–15
Legislation, 15
Leukopenia, 375
Life story, 581
Lifestyle, 2, 531–33
Lignocaine carbomer, 108
Liver, 299–310
Locus of control, 561
Lymphocytic colitis, 622, 631–33
Lymphoma, 645–48
Lymphoproliferative disease, 486–87

Macrophages, 422
Magnesium, 482
Magnetic resonance imaging
   cholangiopancreatography, 312
   for ischemic necrosis of bone, 295–96
   for sclerosing cholangitis, 303
Maintenance of remission, 1, 9, 125
   in Crohn's disease, 341, 433
   and diet, 248
   with enteral nutrition, 411
   and immunmodulators in ulcerative colitis, 140
   and medical management of ulcerative colitis, 111–12
   methotrexate for, 384–85
   in small bowel Crohn's disease, 345
Malabsorption, 471–72, 641
MALT lymphoma, 645
Managed care, 13–18, 556
Mayo Clinic, 203–5
Medicaid, 556
Medical necessity decisions, 14–15
Medicare, 556
Medication(s)
   antidiarrheal, 474
   complementary therapies, 604
   nonadherence, 9
   pancreatitis induced by, 329–30

in pregnancy, 615–18
See also specific drugs
Mediterranean lymphoma, 645
6-Mercaptopurine
  for children, 416–17
  for Crohn's disease, 353–55, 373–76, 416–17, 436
  for distal colitis, 85, 103, 105–6
  for fistulae, 397, 402–3
  for ileitis and ileocolitis, 339, 340
  for inflammatory bowel disease, 134
  pharmacology of, 377–79
  in pregnancy, 376, 617
  to spare corticosteroid use, 365
  for ulcerative colitis, 139–41, 145
Mesalamine, 69, 84, 115–17, 124–25, 616
Mesalazine, 369
Mesenteric adenopathy, 48–49
Metabolic bone disease, 300
Methotrexate, 136, 281
  for children, 417
  for Crohn's colitis, 432
  for Crohn's disease, 417, 436
  for distal colitis, 85
  for fistulae, 397, 403
  for inflammtory bowel disease, 383–85
  in pregnancy, 609, 617–18
  for rheumatoid arthritis, 284–6
  for sclerosing cholangitis, 301–2
  to spare corticosteroid use, 365
Metronidazole
  for children, 416
  for Crohn's disease, 360, 361, 402, 416, 435–36
  for distal colitis, 85
  for fistulae, 396, 402
  for pouchitis, 220
Mineral deficiencies, 418
Mucosa, retained, 199
Mucosal inflammation, 39–45
Mucous membrane disorders, 273
Mucus gel barrier, 108–9
Musculoskeletal system, 52
Mycophenolate mofetil, 136
Myocarditis, 270

Necrolytic migratory erythema, 273
Neoplasms, 375–76
Nephrolithiasis, 270, 475–78
Neurolytic blockers, 597
Neuroticism-stability dimension, 578, 579
Nicotine, 85, 99–101, 108
Nodular lymphoid hyperplasia, 640–41
Nongranulomatous ulcerative jejunoileitis, 425–27
Nonsteroidal anti-inflammatory drugs (NSAIDs)
  in elderly, 623–24
  enteropathy, 625–27
  induced colonic damage, 627
  in inflammatory bowel disease, 627–29
  for pain, 596
Nothing by mouth, 406–7

NSAIDs. *See* Nonsteroidal anti-inflammatory drugs
Nurse advocate, 535–37
Nutrition, 2, 480
  awareness, 599–600
  for children, 246–48, 417–18
  consultation and guidance, 547–48
  parenteral, 162, 163, 405–8
  perioperative support, 449–51
  to spare corticosteroid use, 364
  See also Diet; Enteral nutrition; *specific nutrients*

Obsessive patient, 576
Octreotide, 402
Openness, 578–79
Opioids, 595–96
Oral rehydration solution, 480
Orofacial granulomatosis, 273
Osteomalacia, 268
Osteonecrosis. *See* Ischemic necrosis of bone
Osteopenia, 289–92
Osteoporosis, 268, 289–92
Oxalate nephrolithiasis, 475–78
Oxalates, 481
Oxford Index, 27

Pain
  definitions and taxonomy of, 593–94
  in distal colitis, 83–84
  management, 587–91, 595
  medical therapies, 595–97
  pathways, 594
  perineal, 83–84
  produced by inflammatory bowel disease, 594–95
Pancreatitis, 329–32, 375
Parenteral nutrition, 162, 163
  and bowel rest, 405–8
  See also Total parenteral nutrition
Parents, 5–6, 23, 545
Pediatrics. *See* Children
Pelvic infection, 203
Pelvic sepsis, 227
Pentoxifylline, 302
Percutaneous transhepatic colangiography, 312
Perforation, 175
Perianal disease, 501–7
Perianal Disease Index, 27
Perianal fistula, 395–99, 504–5
Pericarditis, 270
Perineal fistula, 323, 492
Perineal pain, 83–84
Perineal wound healing, 503
Perinuclear antineutrophil cytoplasmic antibody, 219
Peripheral arthritis, 267–68, 280–82
Peristomal fistula, 188, 492
Pernicious anemia, 642
Personality, 337
Personality disorder, 575–76
Photodynamic therapy, 313
Physical dependence, 596

Physicians. *See* Doctor(s)
Polypoid mucosa, 264
Polyps, 253–54
Postcholecystectomy diarrhea, 93–94
Postileal resection, 354–55
Potassium, 548
Pouches
  biopsy, 230–32
  construction, 199
  design, 205
  endoscopy in evaluating, 225–27
  and irritable bowel syndrome, 93
  options, 180–81
  role of pathologist in evaluating complications, 229–32
  See also Kock pouch; Pouchitis
Pouchitis, 192–93, 200, 204, 227
  chronic, 219–22
  and dysplasia, 231–32
  syndromes, 230–32
Prednisone, 339, 356, 486
Pregnancy
  and ileal pouch-anal anastomosis, 206
  and inflammatory bowel disease, 607–10, 613–18
  labor and delivery, 610
  medications during, 376, 615–18
Primary immunodeficiency, 639
Primary intestinal lymphoma, 645
Primary sclerosing cholangitis. *See* Sclerosing cholangitis
Probiotics, 109, 165, 221–22
Proctectomy, 503, 516
Proctitis, 70, 264, 498–99, 503, 505
Proctocolectomy
  and excessive bowel movements, 209–13
  and ileostomy, 176, 440
  for ulcerative colitis, 171–73, 176, 199
Proctocolitis, 498
Proctoscopy, 23–24
Progressive muscle relaxation, 579
Protein loss, 35–36
Pruritus, 299–300
Pseudoaddiction, 596
Pseudomembranous colitis, 620
Pseudopolyps, 261
Psychological factors, 569–86
  behavioral perspective, 579–80
  dimensional perspective, 578–79
  disease perspective, 577–78
  effects of dysfunction on disease, 570–71
  emotional needs of children, 418–19
  and ileal pouch-anal anastomosis, 206
  life story perspective, 581
  managing patients' concerns, 527–29
  prevalance of psychiatric disorders, 569
  psychiatric complications, 573–76
Psychological profile, 337
Publications, 539
Puerperium, 610–11
Pyoderma gangrenosum, 183, 188, 268, 271–73
Pyostomatitis vegetans, 273

Quality of life, 27, 153, 188, 205, 239

Radiation enterocolitis, 635–37
Radiologic techniques, 36
Radionuclide scanning, 295
Recombinant human erythropoietin (EPO), 418
Rectal bleeding, 83
Rectal sleeve advancement, 517–18
Rectovaginal fistulae, 395, 403–4, 438, 505–6, 515–18
Refractory colitis, 81–85, 120
Relaxation, 585, 588–89
Religion, 565–67
Remicade, 340, 366, 390–91, 426, 432
Remission maintenance. *See* Maintenance of remission
Renal cell carcinoma, 323
Research, 541–42
Restorative proctocolectomy, 197–201
Retroperitoneal abscess, 444
Rheumatoid arthritis, 283–87
Right colon, 497

St. Mark's Index, 25
Salmonella, 96, 620
Scleritis, 275
Sclerosing cholangitis, 299–302
  liver transplantation for, 305–10
  stricture management in, 303–4
Segmental colitis, 622
Selenium, 482
Self-esteem, 567
Sepsis, 200
Sexuality
  adjustments and body image, 561–63
  dysfunction with perianal disease, 503
  after ileal pouch-anal anastomosis, 204
  after ostomy, 181–82
Shigella, 96
Short-bowel syndrome, 426–27, 479–83
Short-chain fatty acids, 109, 161–63, 481
Siblings, 524–25
Sigmoidoscopy, 23–24, 82
Skin
  diseases associated with inflammatory bowel disease, 268–69
  perineal changes, 395
  peristomal problems, 182–83
Slipping rib syndrome, 595
Small bowel Crohn's disease, 343–45, 443–47
Small bowel obstruction, 203, 227, 341–42
Small bowel rejection, 486
Small bowel resection, 453–55, 471–74
Small intestine
  Crohn's disease of, 439–40
  radiation injury to, 635–37
  transplantation, 483, 485–89
Smoking, 335, 467
Social Security, 557–58
Sphincter, 210
Spirituality, 565–67
Steatorrhea, 300, 472, 473
Stem cell transplantation, 649–54

Stenosis, 192
Steroids
    for arthritis, 281
    for distal colitis, 70
    in pregnancy, 617
    therapeutic alternatives to, 134–37
    unresponsiveness in inflammatory bowel disease, 133–37
    See also Corticosteroids; Glucocorticosteroids
Stoma, 179–83, 187, 192
Stones. *See* Gallstones; Urinary tract calculi
Stool frequency, 83, 204, 209–13
Stress, 528, 552, 583–86, 588–89
Strictureplasty, 426, 457–60, 462–63
Strictures
    anal, 204
    anorectal, 506
    bowel, 59, 61
    colonic, 264
    dominant biliary, 300, 312
    endoscopic management of, 509–12
    formation, 227
    and nonsteroidal anti-inflammatory drugs, 627
    in primary sclerolsing cholangitis, 303–4
Subtotal colectomy, 176, 197
Sucralfate, 109
Sulfasalazine, 123, 124, 281, 416, 608, 616, 632
    See also Aminosalicylates
Sulfide, 161–62, 163
Support systems, 2, 233–35, 540–41, 544, 545
Surgery
    in children, 154–55, 215–18, 419
    for Crohn's colitis, 495–99
    for Crohn's disease, 439–41, 443–47, 453–69, 501–2
    for diarrheal symptoms, 633
    for distal colitis, 85
    enterostomal therapy nurse, 179–83
    and fitness programs, 599
    for indeterminate colitis, 241–44
    medical collaboration, 19
    referrals, 24
    support for patients after, 233–35
    for ulcerative colitis, 154–55, 171–78
    See also specific procedures
Sweet's syndrome, 273

TABS. *See* Transabdominal bowel sonography
Tacrolimus, 302, 417, 486
T cells, 642
Teenagers. *See* Adolescents
Telecommunication, 537
Tenesmus, 83
Thalidomide, 391–92, 417
6-Thioguanine, 379
Thiopurine methyltransferase (TPMT) activity, 339–40, 379
Tixocortol pivalate, 74
T-lymphocytes, 165–66
Tobacco, 99–101
Tolerance, 596
Total colectomy, 197, 199
Total parenteral nutrition

    in Crohn's disease, 407–8
    effect on operability, 450
    and fistulae, 402
    hypertriglyceridemia from, 330
    as primary therapy, 406–7
    and short-bowel syndrome, 482–83
Toxic megacolon, 175–76, 496
TPMT. *See* Thiopurine methyltransferase (TPMT) activity
Tranasabdominal repair, 518
Transabdominal bowel sonography (TABS), 55–61
Transabdominal ultrasound, 312
Transperineal repair, 518
Transvaginal advancement flaps, 517
Trans-valvular fistula, 192
Transverse colon, 497
Trefoil peptides, 107–8
Tricyclic antidepressants, 596
Truelove/Witts Index, 25
Tumor necrosis factor, 417
Tumor necrosis factor-alpha, 37, 63–65, 166–67, 285, 366, 390, 398, 403
UC. *See* Ulcerative colitis
Ulcerative colitis (UC)
    active, 162–64
    adherence issues, 9–11
    aminosalicylates for, 123–25
    antibiotics for, 149–51
    in children, 153–55
    corticosteroids for, 73–76, 120–21, 128–29, 144–45
    cyclosporine A for, 135
    diagnosis, 229, 241–42
    dietary factors, 161–64, 547
    difference from Crohn's disease, 551–52
    as diverse disease, 119–21
    in elderly, 622–23
    imaging, 39–41
    immunomodulators in, 139–42
    inactive, 161–62
    and irritable bowel syndrome, 89
    management of severe, 143–46
    measures of activity, 25–26
    medical management of, 111–13
    medical-surgical collaboration for, 19
    methotrexate for, 385
    pain in, 594
    and patient-doctor interactions, 1–3
    and pregnancy, 613–14
    and primary sclerosing cholangitis, 309–10
    sequential and combination therapy, 115–17
    severe acute, 128–29
    surgery for, 171–78, 197–99
    and transabdominal bowel sonography, 57
    use of nicotine and tobacco in, 99–101
    See also Distal colitis

Ulcerative jejunoileitis, 659–60
Ultrasound, 36, 55–61, 312
United Ostomy Association, 233–34
University of Chicago, 20–21
University of Pittsburgh, 487

Ureteral obstruction, 322–23
Uric acid stones, 321
Urinary tract, 51–52
Urinary tract calculi, 321–22
Urologic complications, 321–23
Ursodeoxycholic acid, 301

Vagotomy, 462
Valve disruption, 192
Valve prolapse, 193–94
Van Hees (Dutch) Index, 26
Vasculitis, 272–73
Vitamin B12, 269
Vitamin D, 290–91

Vitamins
    deficiency, 300
    fat-soluble, 481
    water-soluble, 482
    See also specific vitamins
Volvulus, 187–88
Vulvar fistula, 395

Water, 600–601
Web sites. *See* Internet

Yersinia, 95
Young adults, 532, 562

Zinc, 418, 482